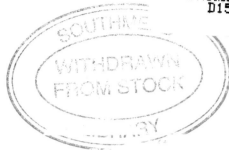

Bradley's Neurology
in Clinical Practice

Bradley's Neurology in Clinical Practice

Volume I: Principles of Diagnosis and Management

Sixth Edition

Robert B. Daroff, MD
Professor and Chair Emeritus of Neurology
School of Medicine
Case Western Reserve University
Cleveland, Ohio

Gerald M. Fenichel, MD
Professor of Neurology and Pediatrics
Department of Neurology/Pediatrics
Vanderbilt University School of Medicine
Neurologist-in-Chief
Monroe Carell Jr. Children's Hospital of Vanderbilt
Nashville, Tennessee

Joseph Jankovic, MD
Professor of Neurology
Distinguished Chair in Movement Disorders
Director, Parkinson Disease Center and Movement
Disorders Clinic
Department of Neurology
Baylor College of Medicine
Houston, Texas

John C. Mazziotta, MD, PhD
Chair, Department of Neurology
Pierson-Lovelace Investigator
Stark Chair in Neurology
Director, Brain Mapping Center
Associate Director, Semel Institute
David Geffen School of Medicine
University of California–Los Angeles
Los Angeles, California

ELSEVIER
SAUNDERS

1600 John F. Kennedy Blvd.
Ste 1800
Philadelphia, PA 19103-2899

Notices

Knowledge and best practice in this field are constantly changing. As new research and experience broaden our understanding, changes in research methods, professional practices, or medical treatment may become necessary.

Practitioners and researchers must always rely on their own experience and knowledge in evaluating and using any information, methods, compounds, or experiments described herein. In using such information or methods they should be mindful of their own safety and the safety of others, including parties for whom they have a professional responsibility.

With respect to any drug or pharmaceutical products identified, readers are advised to check the most current information provided (i) on procedures featured or (ii) by the manufacturer of each product to be administered, to verify the recommended dose or formula, the method and duration of administration, and contraindications. It is the responsibility of practitioners, relying on their own experience and knowledge of their patients, to make diagnoses, to determine dosages and the best treatment for each individual patient, and to take all appropriate safety precautions.

To the fullest extent of the law, neither the Publisher nor the authors, contributors, or editors assume any liability for any injury and/or damage to persons or property as a matter of products liability, negligence or otherwise, or from any use or operation of any methods, products, instructions, or ideas contained in the material herein.

Library of Congress Cataloging-in-Publication Data

Bradley's neurology in clinical practice.—6th ed. / [edited by] Robert B. Daroff ... [et al.].
       v. ; cm.
    Neurology in clinical practice
    Rev. ed. of: Neurology in clinical practice / edited by Walter G. Bradley ... [et al.]. 5th ed. c2008.
    Includes bibliographical references and index.
    Contents: v. 1. Principles of diagnosis and management—v. 2. Neurological disorders.
    ISBN 978-1-4377-0434-1 (set : hardcover : alk. paper)—ISBN 9996085309 (v. 1 : hardcover : alk. paper)—
ISBN 9996085368 (v. 2 : hardcover : alk. paper)
    I. Daroff, Robert B.   II. Bradley, W. G. (Walter George)   III. Neurology in clinical practice.   IV. Title: Neurology in clinical practice.
    [DNLM: 1. Nervous System Diseases.   2. Diagnostic Techniques, Neurological.   WL 140]
    616.8—dc23

                                                                    2011030671

Content Strategist: Charlotta Kryhl
Content Development Manager: Lucia Gunzel
Publishing Services Manager: Anne Altepeter
Project Manager: Cindy Thoms
Design Direction: Louis Forgione

Printed in China

Last digit is the print number: 9 8 7 6 5 4 3 2 1

Contributors

Bassel W. Abou-Khalil, MD
Professor of Neurology
Director, Epilepsy Division
Vanderbilt University
Nashville, Tennessee

Peter Adamczyk, MD
Vascular Neurology Fellow
Department of Neurology
University of California–Los Angeles Medical
Center
Los Angeles, California

Bela Ajtai, MD, PhD
Clinical Assistant Professor of Neurology
Neuroimager
Dent Neurologic Institute
Amherst, New York

Jeffrey C. Allen, MD
Professor of Pediatrics and Neurology
New York University
Langone Medical Center
New York, New York

Anthony A. Amato, MD
Vice-Chairman of Neurology
Brigham and Women's Hospital
Professor of Neurology
Harvard Medical School
Boston, Massachusetts

Michael J. Aminoff, MD, DSc
Professor, Department of Neurology
University of California–San Francisco
San Francisco, California

Liana G. Apostolova, MD, MSc
Assistant Professor of Neurology
Department of Neurology
David Geffen School of Medicine
University of California–Los Angeles
Los Angeles, California

Alon Y. Avidan, MD, MPH
Associate Professor of Neurology
Director, UCLA Sleep Disorders Center
Director, UCLA Neurology Clinic
UCLA, Department of Neurology
David Geffen School of Medicine at UCLA
Los Angeles, California

Joachim M. Baehring, MD, DSc
Associate Professor of Neurology, Medicine, and
Neurosurgery
Yale University School of Medicine
New Haven, Connecticut

Laura J. Balcer, MD, MSCE
Professor of Neurology, Ophthalmology, and
Epidemiology
Department of Neurology
University of Pennsylvania School of Medicine
Philadelphia, Pennsylvania

Robert W. Baloh, MD
Professor, Department of Neurology
Division of Head and Neck Surgery
University of California School of Medicine
Los Angeles, California

Garni Barkhoudarian, MD
Pituitary and Neuroendoscopy Fellow
Brigham and Women's Hospital
Boston, Massachusetts

J.D. Bartleson, MD
Consultant, Department of Neurology
Mayo Clinic
Associate Professor of Neurology
College of Medicine, Mayo Clinic
Rochester, Minnesota

Tracy T. Batchelor, MD
Professor of Neurology
Harvard Medical School
Chief of Neuro-Oncology
Massachusetts General Hospital
Boston, Massachusetts

J. David Beckham, MD
Assistant Professor
Division of Infectious Diseases
Department of Medicine, Neurology, and
Microbiology
University of Colorado
Anschultz Medical Campus
Aurora, Colorado

Leigh Beglinger, MD
Associate Professor, Neuropsychology
University of Iowa Hospitals and Clinics
Iowa City, Iowa

Joseph R. Berger, MD
Ruth L. Works Professor and Chairman
Neurology
University of Kentucky
Lexington, Kentucky

Marvin Bergsneider, MD
Professor
Department of Neurosurgery
Director, Adult Hydrocephalus Program
Co-Director, Benign Skullbase and Pituitary
Tumor Program
University of California–Los Angeles Medical
Center
Los Angeles, California

Francois Bethoux, MD
Director, Rehabiliation Services
The Mellen Center for Multiple Sclerosis
Treatment and Research
The Cleveland Clinic Foundation
Cleveland, Ohio

José Biller, MD, FACP, FAAN, FAHA
Professor and Chair
Department of Neurology
Loyola University Chicago
Stritch School of Medicine
Maywood, Illinois

David F. Black, MD
Assistant Professor of Neurology
Mayo Clinic
Rochester, Minnesota

Christopher J. Boes, MD
Associate Professor of Neurology
Consultant, Department of Neurology
Mayo Clinic
Rochester, Minnesota

Nicholas Boulis, MD
Assistant Professor, Department of Neurosurgery
Emory University
Atlanta, Georgia
Adjunct Assistant Professor of Neurology
University of Michigan School of Medicine
Ann Arbor, Michigan

Helen M. Bramlett, PhD
Associate Professor
University of Miami Miller School of Medicine
Miami, Florida

Michael H. Brooke, MD
Professor Emeritus, Departments of Medicine
and Neurology, University of Alberta
Edmonton, Alberta, Canada

Joseph Bruni, MD, FRCP(C)
Consultant Neurologist
Division of Neurology
St. Michael's Hospital
Associate Professor of Medicine
Division of Neurology
University of Toronto
Toronto, Ontario, Canada

W. Bryan Burnette, MD, MS
Assistant Professor of Neurology and Pediatrics
Vanderbilt University School of Medicine
Nashville, Tennessee

Edgar A. Buttner, MD, PhD
Instructor of Psychiatry
Harvard Medical School
Boston, Massachusetts
Director of the Pharmacogenomics Section
Molecular Pharmacology Laboratory
McLean Hospital
Belmont, Massachusetts

David J. Capobianco, MD
Associate Professor
Department of Neurology
Mayo Clinic College of Medicine
Jacksonville, Florida

Alan Carson, MBChB, MPhil, MD, FRCP
Consultant Neuropsychiatrist
Robert Fergusson Unit
Royal Edinburgh Hospital
Edinburgh, Scotland

Robert Cavaliere, MD
Assistant Professor of Neurology, Neurosurgery, and Oncology
Department of Neurosurgery
Ohio State University
Columbus, Ohio

David A. Chad, MD
Associate Professor of Neurology
Harvard Medical School
Neurologist
Massachusetts General Hospital
Boston, Massachusetts

Gisela Chelimsky, MD
Pediatric Gastroenterology
Rainbow Babies and Children's Hospital
Cleveland, Ohio

Thomas Chelimsky, MD
Professor of Neurology
Department of Neurology
Director, Autonomic Disorders, Neuromuscular Center, Neurologic Institute
University Hospitals Case Medical Center
Case School of Medicine
Cleveland, Ohio

William P. Cheshire, Jr., MD
Professor of Neurology
Mayo Clinic
Jacksonville, Florida

Tanuja Chitnis, MD
Assistant Professor in Neurology
Department of Neurology
Brigham and Women's Hospital
Boston, Massachusetts

Sudhansu Chokroverty, MD, FRCP
Professor of Neuroscience
Seton Hall University
South Orange, New Jersey
Professor and Co-Chair of Neurology
Program Director of Sleep Medicine and Clinical Neurophysiology
New Jersey Neuroscience Institute at JFK Medical Center
Edison, New Jersey
Clinical Professor of Neurology
Robert Wood Johnson Medical School
New Brunswick, New Jersey

Paul E. Cooper, MD, FRCPC
Professor of Neurology
Department of Clinical Neurological Sciences
Division of Neurology
Department of Medicine
Division of Endocrinology and Metabolism
University of Western Ontario
Interim Chair/Chief
London Health Sciences Centers and St. Joseph's Health Care
London, Ontario, Canada

Jeffrey L. Cummings, MD
Director
Cleveland Clinic Lou Ruvo Center
for Brain Health
Las Vegas, Nevada

F. Michael Cutrer, MD
Associate Professor
Mayo Medical School
Consultant in Neurology
Mayo Clinic
Rochester, Minnesota

Josep Dalmau, MD, PhD
Adjunct Professor of Neurology
University of Pennsylvania
Philadelphia, Pennsylvania
Research Professor at Institució Catalana de Recerca i Estudis Avançats (ICREA), IDIBAPS, Hospital Clínic
University of Barcelona
Barcelona, Spain

Robert B. Daroff, MD
Professor and Chair Emeritus of Neurology
School of Medicine
Case Western Reserve University
Cleveland, Ohio

Ranan DasGupta, MA, MD, MRCS, MBBChir
Consultant Urological Surgeon
St. Mary's Hospital
London, United Kingdom

Steven T. DeKosky, MD, FACP, FAAN
Vice President and Dean
James Carroll Flippin Professor of Medical Science
Professor of Neurology
University of Virginia School of Medicine
Physician in Chief
University of Virginia Medical Center
Charlottesville, Virginia

W. Dalton Dietrich, PhD
Scientific Director
The Miami Project to Cure Paralysis
Professor of Neurological Surgery, Neurology, and Cell Biology and Anatomy
University of Miami Miller School of Medicine
Miami, Florida

Bruce H. Dobkin, MD
Professor of Neurology
David Geffen School of Medicine
University of California–Los Angeles
Los Angeles, California

Richard L. Doty, BS, MA, PhD
Director
Smell and Taste Center
Professor, Department of Otorhinolaryngology: Head and Neck Surgery
University of Pennsylvania Medical Center
Philadelphia, Pennsylvania

Gary Duckwiler, MD
Professor of Radiology
Director of Clinical Affairs and Fellowship Director
Division of Interventional Neuroradiology
Fellowship Program
David Geffen School of Medicine
University of California–Los Angeles
Los Angeles, California

Joshua R. Dusick, MD
Research Associate
Department of Neurosurgery
University of California–Los Angeles
David Geffen School of Medicine
University of California—Los Angeles
Los Angeles, California

Ronald G. Emerson, MD
Attending Neurologist
Hospital for Special Surgery
New York, New York

Gerald M. Fenichel, MD
Professor of Neurology and Pediatrics
Department of Neurology/Pediatrics
Vanderbilt University School of Medicine
Neurologist-in-Chief
Monroe Carell Jr. Children's Hospital of Vanderbilt
Nashville, Tennessee

Richard G. Fessler, MD, PhD
Professor
Department of Neurosurgery
Northwestern University
Chicago, Illinois

Laura Flores-Sarnat, MD
Paediatric Neurologist
Division of Paediatric Neurology
Department of Paediatrics
Alberta Children's Hospital
Calgary, Alberta, Canada

Brent L. Fogel, MD, PhD
Assistant Professor
Neurology
University of California–Los Angeles
Los Angeles, California

Clare J. Fowler, MSc, FRCP, MBBS
Professor of Uro-Neurology
Institute of Neurology
University College London
Consultant
National Hospital for Neurology and
Neurosurgery
London, United Kingdom

Jennifer E. Fugate, DO
Department of Neurology
Mayo Clinic
Rochester, Minnesota

Martin J. Gallager, MD, PhD
Assistant Professor of Neurology
Vanderbilt University
Nashville, Tennessee

Sharon L. Gardner, MD
Associate Professor
Pediatrics
New York University
New York, New York

Ivan Garza, MD
Assistant Professor of Neurology
Mayo Clinic College of Medicine
Consultant, Department of Neurology
Mayo Clinic
Rochester, Minnesota

Carissa Gehl, PhD
Staff Neuropsychologist
Mental Health Service Line
Iowa City VA Health Care System
Iowa City, Iowa

David S. Geldmacher, MD, FACP
Patsy and Charles Collat Endowed
Scholar in Neuroscience
Professor of Neurology
University of Alabama at Birmingham
Birmingham, Alabama

Daniel H. Geschwind, MD
Gordon and Virginia MacDonald Distinguished
Chair
Professor of Neurology, Psychiatry, and Human
Genetics
University of California–Los Angeles
Los Angeles, California

Michael D. Geschwind, MD, PhD
Associate Professor
Neurology
Memory and Aging Center
University of California–San Francisco
San Francisco, California

Meredith R. Golomb, MD, MSc
Associate Professor
Department of Neurology, Division of Pediatric
Neurology
Indiana University School of Medicine
Indianapolis, Indiana

Nestor Gonzalez, MD
Assistant Professor of Neurosurgery and
Interventional Neuroradiology
Ruth and Raymond Stotter Chair in
Neurosurgery
Neurosurgery and Radiology
David Geffen School of Medicine
University of California–Los Angeles
Los Angeles, California

Mark Hallett, MD
Chief, Human Motor Control Section
National Institute of Neurological Disorders
and Stroke
National Institutes of Health
Bethesda, Maryland

Aline I. Hamati, MD
Clinical Assistant Professor of Pediatric
Neurology
Indiana University
James Whitcomb Riley Hospital for Children
Indianapolis, Indiana

Leif A. Havton, MD
Assistant Professor
Department of Neurology
University of California–Los Angeles
School of Medicine
Attending Neurologist, Neurologic Rehabilitation
and Research Unit
University of California–Los Angeles Medical
Center
Los Angeles, California

Reid R. Heffner, Jr., MD
Professor and Chair
Department of Pathology and Anatomical
Sciences
University of Buffalo School of Medicine
Buffalo, New York

Alan Hill, MD, PhD
Professor
Pediatric Division of Neurology
University of British Columbia
Vancouver, British Columbia, Canada

Fred H. Hochberg, MD
Neuro-Oncology
Attending Neuro-Oncologist
Massachusetts General Hospital
Boston, Massachusetts

Maria K. Houtchens, MD, M. Msci
Assistant Professor of Neurology
Harvard Medical School
Director, Women's Health Program
Partners Multiple Sclerosis Center
Brigham and Women's Hospital
Boston, Massachusetts

Monica P. Islam, MD
Assistant Professor
Clinical Pediatrics—Child Neurology
Ohio State University
Columbus, Ohio

Joseph Jankovic, MD
Professor of Neurology
Distinguished Chair in Movement Disorders
Director, Parkinson Disease Center and
Movement Disorders Clinic
Department of Neurology
Baylor College of Medicine
Houston, Texas

Michael Jansen, MBBCh (Witwatersrand),
DTM&H (Witwatersrand), FRCPath
Consultant Neuropathologist
Neuropathology
Beaumont Hospital
Dublin, Ireland

S. Andrew Josephson, MD
Associate Professor of Neurology
University of California–San Francisco
San Francisco, California

Matthias A. Karajannis, MD, MS
Assistant Professor of Pediatrics
New York University School of Medicine
New York, New York

Carlos S. Kase, MD
Professor of Neurology
Boston University School of Medicine
Neurologist-in-Chief
Boston Medical Center
Boston, Massachusetts

Bashar Katirji, MD
Director, Neuromuscular Center and EMG
Laboratory
Neurological Institute
University Hospitals Case Medical Center
Professor, Department of Neurology
Case Western Reserve University School
of Medicine
Cleveland, Ohio

Kevin A. Kerber, MD
Assistant Professor
University of Michigan Health System
Ann Arbor, Michigan

Geoffrey A. Kerchner, MD, PhD
Assistant Professor of Neurology and
Neurological Sciences
Stanford Center for Memory Disorders
Stanford University School of Medicine
Stanford, California

Samia J. Khoury, MD
Jack, Sadie and David Breakstone Professor
of Neurology
Brigham and Women's Hospital
Co-Director
Partners Multiple Sclerosis Center
Brigham and Women's Hospital
Boston, Massachusetts

Howard S. Kirshner, BA, MD
Professor and Vice Chair
Department of Neurology
Vanderbilt University Medical Center
Nashville, Tennessee

Daniel Koontz, MD
Neurological Institute
University Hospitals Case Medical Center
Assistant Professor
Case Western Reserve University
Cleveland, Ohio

Anita Koshy, MD
Instructor
Department of Medicine, Division of Infectious
Disease
Instructor
Department of Neurology and Neurological
Sciences
Stanford University School of Medicine
Stanford, California

Sarah A. Kremen, MD
Associate Physician
Department of Neurology
Mary S. Easton Center for Alzheimer's Disease
Research
David Geffen School of Medicine
University of California–Los Angeles
Los Angeles, California

Roger W. Kula, MD
Associate Professor of Neurology and
Neurosurgery
Hofstra North Shore–LIJ School of Medicine
Hempstead, New York
Medical Director, The Chiari Institute
Cushing Neuroscience Institutes
North Shore University Hospital
Great Neck, New York

Abhay Kumar, MD
Fellow, Department of Neurology
Barnes-Jewish Hospital
Washington University School of Medicine
St. Louis, Missouri

John F. Kurtzke, MD, FACP, FAAN
Professor Emeritus, Neurology
Georgetown University
Washington, DC
Distinguished Professor, Neurology
Uniformed Services University
Bethesda, Maryland
Consultant, Neurology Service
Veterans Affairs Medical Center
Washington, DC

Anthony E. Lang, MD, FRCPC
Professor
Department of Medicine, Neurology
University of Toronto
Director of Movement Disorders Center and the
Edmond J. Safra Program in Parkinson's Disease
Toronto Western Hospital
Toronto, Ontario, Canada

Patrick J.M. Lavin, MB, BCH, BAO, MRCPI
Professor of Neurology
Professor of Ophthalmology
Vanderbilt Eye Institute
Vanderbilt University Medical Center
Nashville, Tennessee

David S. Liebeskind, MD
Professor of Neurology
Neurology Director, Stroke Imaging
Co-Medical and Co-Technical Director, UCLA
Cerebral Blood Flow Laboratory
Program Director, Stroke and Vascular
Neurology Residency
Associate Neurology Director
UCLA Stroke Center
Los Angeles, California

Eric Lindzen, MD, PhD
Jacobs Neurological Institute
School of Medicine and Biomedical Sciences
State University of New York at Buffalo
Buffalo, New York

Alan H. Lockwood, MD
Emeritus Professor
Neurology and Nuclear Medicine
University at Buffalo
Buffalo, New York

David N. Louis, MD
Benjamin Castleman Professor of Pathology
Department of Pathology
Harvard Medical School
Pathologist-in-Chief, Pathology Service
Massachusetts General Hospital
Boston, Massachusetts

Betsy B. Love, MD
Adjunct Associate Professor
Department of Neurology
Loyola University Chicago
Stritch School of Medicine
Maywood, Illinois

Fred D. Lublin, MD
Saunders Family Professor of Neurology
Department of Neurology
Mount Sinai School of Medicine
Professor, Department of Neurology
Mount Sinai Hospital
Director, Department of Neurology
Corinne Goldsmith Dickinson Center for
Multiple Sclerosis
New York, New York

Robert L. Macdonald, PhD, MD
Professor and Chair of Neurology
Professor of Pharmacology
Professor of Molecular Physiology and
Biophysics
Vanderbilt University Medical Center
Nashville, Tennessee

William Mack, MD
Assistant Professor of Neurological Surgery
University of Southern California
Los Angeles, California

Neil Martin, MD
Professor and Chair of Neurosurgery
University of California–Los Angeles Stroke
Center
Director, Aneurysm and AVM Program
University of California–Los Angeles
Los Angeles, California

Joseph C. Masdeu, MD, PhD
Head, Molecular Neuroimaging Group
Section on Integrative Neuroimaging
National Institutes of Health
Bethesda, Maryland
Adjunct Professor of Neurology
New York Medical College
Valhalla, New York

John C. Mazziotta, MD, PhD
Chair, Department of Neurology
Pierson-Lovelace Investigator
Stark Chair in Neurology
Director, Brain Mapping Center
Associate Director, Semel Institute
David Geffen School of Medicine
University of California–Los Angeles
Los Angeles, California

Mario F. Mendez, MD, PhD
Director, Neurobehavior
Neurology
VA of Greater Los Angeles
Professor
Neurology, Psychiatry, and Biobehavioral
Sciences
David Geffen School of Medicine
University of California–Los Angeles
Los Angeles, California

Matthew N. Meriggioli, MD
Director
Division of Neuromuscular Medicine
Department of Neurology and Rehabilitation
University of Illinois
Chicago, Illinois

Philipp T. Meyer, MD, PhD
Department of Nuclear Medicine
University Hospital Freiburg
Freiburg, Germany

Dominique S. Michaud, ScD
Associate Professor of Epidemiology
Department of Epidemiology
Brown Public Health
Brown University
Providence, Rhode Island
Visiting Reader, School of Public Health
Imperial College
London, United Kingdom

Aaron E. Miller, MD
Professor, Department of Neurology
Maimonides Hospital
Brooklyn, New York
Professor, Department of Neurology
Mount Sinai School of Medicine
Mount Sinai Hospital
Medical Director, Department of Neurology
Corinne Goldsmith Dickinson Center for
Multiple Sclerosis
New York, New York

Karl E. Misulis, MD, PhD
Clinical Professor
Neurology
Vanderbilt University School of Medicine
Nashville, Tennessee
Neurologist
West Tennessee Neurosciences
West Tennessee Healthcare
Jackson, Tennessee

Hiroshi Mitsumoto, MD
Wesley J. Howe Professor of Neurology
Department of Neurology
Columbia University College of Physicians
and Surgeons
Director, The Eleanor and Lou Gehrig
MDA/ALS Research Center
Head, Neuromuscular Diseases Division
Columbia-Presbyterian Hospitals
New York, New York

Brian Murray, MB, BCh, BAO, MSc
Consultant Neurologist
Hermitage Medical Clinic
Blackrock Clinic
Dublin, Ireland

Evan D. Murray, MD
Instructor in Neurology
Harvard Medical School
Boston, Massachusetts
Consultant Neurologist
McLean Hospital
Belmont, Massachusetts
Assistant in Neurology
Massachusetts General Hospital
Boston, Massachusetts

Ruth Nass, MD
Professor of Child Neurology, Child and
Adolescent Psychiatry, and Pediatrics
New York University Langone Medical Center
New York, New York

John G. Nutt, MD
Professor of Neurology, Physiology, and
Pharmacology
Oregon Health and Science University
Portland VA Medical Center
Portland, Oregon

Marc R. Nuwer, MD, PhD
Professor, Department of Neurology
David Geffen School of Medicine
University of California–Los Angeles
Department of Clinical Neurophysiology
Ronald Reagan University of California–Los
Angeles Medical Center
Los Angeles, California

Michael S. Okun, MD
Associate Professor of Neurology
Departments of Neurology and Neurosurgery
University of Florida Center for Movement
Disorders and Neurorestoration
McKnight Brain Institute
Gainesville, Florida

Justin J.F. O'Rourke, MA
Departments of Psychiatry and
Counseling Psychology
University of Iowa
Iowa City, Iowa
Psychology Service
South Texas Veterans Health Care System
San Antonio, Texas

Ajay K. Pandey, MD
Neurology Resident
University of Florida College of Medicine
Gainesville, Florida

Jalesh N. Panicker, MD, DM, DNB,
MRCP(UK)
Consultant Neurologist
Department of Uro-Neurology
National Hospital for Neurology and
Neurosurgery
Honorary Senior Lecturer
UCL Institute of Neurology
London, United Kingdom

Gregory M. Pastores, MD
Associate Professor
Neurology and Pediatrics
New York University School of Medicine
New York, New York

Jane S. Paulsen, PhD
Professor
Psychiatry, Neurology, Neurosciences,
and Psychology
University of Iowa
Iowa City, Iowa

Timothy A. Pedley, MD
Professor of Neurology
Department of Neurology
Columbia University Medical Center
New York, New York

Arie Perry, MD
Associate Professor, Department of Pathology
Division of Neuropathology
Washington University School of Medicine
Associate Pathologist
Barnes-Jewish and St. Louis Children's Hospitals
Saint Louis, Missouri

Alan Pestronk, MD
Professor
Neurology, Immunology, and Pathology
Director
Neuromuscular Clinical Laboratory
Washington University School of Medicine
Saint Louis, Missouri

Ronald F. Pfeiffer, MD
Professor and Vice Chair
Neurology
University of Tennessee Health Science Center
Memphis, Tennessee

Sashank Prasad, MD
Instructor in Neurology and
Neuro-Ophthalmology
Brigham and Women's Hospital
Harvard Medical School
Boston, Massachusetts

David C. Preston, MD
Professor of Neurology
Program Director
Neurology Residency
University Hospitals Case Medical Center
Cleveland, Ohio

Bruce H. Price, MD
Associate Professor, Department of Neurology
Harvard Medical School
Boston, Massachusetts
Chief, Department of Neurology
McLean Hospital
Belmont, Massachusetts
Associate Neurologist
Massachusetts General Hospital
Boston, Massachusetts

Louis J. Ptáček, MD
John C. Coleman Distinguished Professorship
of Neurology
University of California–San Francisco
Investigator, Howard Hughes Medical Institute
San Francisco, California

Alejandro A. Rabinstein, MD
Professor of Neurology
Mayo Clinic College of Medicine
Consultant, St. Mary's Hospital–Mayo Clinic
Rochester, Minnesota

Tyler Reimschisel, MD
Assistant Professor of Pediatrics and Neurology
Director, Division of Developmental Medicine
Vanderbilt University School of Medicine
Nashville, Tennessee

Bernd F. Remler, MD
Professor of Neurology and Ophthalmology
Medical College of Wisconsin
Section of Neurology
Clement Zablocki VA Medical Center
Milwaukee, Wisconsin

Michel Rijntjes, MD
Department of Neurology
University Clinic Freiburg
Freiburg, Germany

E. Steve Roach, MD
Professor of Child Neurology
Ohio State University
College of Medicine
Columbus, Ohio

David Robertson, MD
Elton Yates Professor of Medicine,
Pharmacology, and Neurology
Director, Clinical Research Center
Vanderbilt University
Nashville, Tennessee

Lisa R. Rogers, DO
Director, Medical Neuro-Oncology
The Neurological Institute
University Hospitals Case Medical Center
Professor of Neurology
Case Western Reserve University School
of Medicine
Cleveland, Ohio

Michael Ronthal, MbBCh, FRCP, FRCPE
Neurology
Beth Israel Deaconess Medical Center
Professor of Neurology
Harvard Medical School
Boston, Massachusetts

Karen Roos, MD
John and Nancy Nelson Professor of Neurology
Indiana University School of Medicine
Indianapolis, Indiana

Richard B. Rosenbaum, MD
Neurology Division
The Oregon Clinic
Medical Director
Providence Center for Parkinson's Disease
Affiliate Professor of Neurology
Oregon Health and Science University
Portland, Oregon

Gary A. Rosenberg, MD
Professor of Neurology, Neurosciences, and Cell
Biology and Physiology
Chairman
Department of Neurology
University of New Mexico Health Sciences
Center
Albuquerque, New Mexico

Myrna R. Rosenfeld, MD, PhD
Professor of Neurology
Hospital Clinic/IDIBAPS, University of Barcelona
Barcelona, Spain
Adjunct Professor of Neurology
University of Pennsylvania
Philadelphia, Pennsylvania

Gail Ross, MD
Associate Professor of Psychology in Pediatrics
and Psychiatry
Weill Cornell Medical College
New York, New York

Janet C. Rucker, MD
Associate Professor of Neurology and
Ophthalmology
Mount Sinai Medical Center
New York, New York

Donald B. Sanders, MD
Professor, Medicine/Neurology
Duke University Medical Center
Durham, North Carolina

Harvey B. Sarnat, MD, FRCPC
Professor
Departments of Paediatrics, Pathology
(Neuropathology), and Clinical Neurosciences
University of Calgary Faculty of Medicine
Alberta Children's Hospital
Calgary, Alberta, Canada

Aman Savani, MD
Neurology Center for Sleep Disorders
Bethesda, Maryland

Anthony H.V. Schapira, MD, DSc, FRCP,
FMedSci
Professor
Department of Clinical Neurosciences
UCL Institute of Neurology
London, United Kingdom

David Schiff, MD
Harrison Distinguished Teaching Professor of
Neurology, Neurological Surgery, and Medicine
(Hematology-Oncology)
Co-Director, Neuro-Oncology Center
University of Virginia
Charlottesville, Virginia

James W. Schmidley, MD
Professor of Neurology
Virginia Tech Carilion School of Medicine
Roanoke, Virginia

Michael J. Schneck, MD
Professor of Neurology and Neurosurgery
Vice Chair, Department of Neurology
Loyola University Chicago
Stritch School of Medicine
Medical Director, Neurointensive Care Unit
Associate Director, Stroke Unit
Loyola University Medical Center
Maywood, Illinois

D. Malcolm Shaner, MD, FAAN
Consultant in Neurology
Southern California Permanente Medical Group
Associate Clinical Professor of Neurology
David Geffen School of Medicine
Los Angeles, California

Barbara E. Shapiro, MD, PhD
Associate Professor of Neurology
Department of Neurology
Case Western Reserve University
School of Medicine
Director, Neuromuscular Research
Department of Neurology
University Hospitals Case Medical Center
Cleveland, Ohio

Patrick Shih, MD
Clinical Instructor
Neurological Surgery
Northwestern University
Chicago, Illinois

Roger P. Simon, MD
Adjunct Professor
Departments of Neurology, Physiology, and
Pharmacology
Oregon Health and Sciences University
Director and Chair
Robert S. Dow Neurobiology Laboratories
Legacy Research
Portland, Oregon

Yuen T. So, MD, PhD
Professor
Neurology and Neurological Sciences
Stanford University
Stanford, California

Young H. Sohn, MD, PhD
Professor
Yonsei University College of Medicine
Seoul, Korea

Marylou V. Solbrig, MD, MS
Professor of Medicine (Neurology) and Medical
Microbiology
University of Manitoba
Winnipeg, Manitoba, Canada

Martina Stippler, MD
Assistant Professor
Director of Neurotrauma
Department of Neurosurgery
University of New Mexico
Albuquerque, New Mexico

**A. Jon Stoessl, CM, MD, FRCPC, FAAN,
FCAHS**
Professor and Head, Neurology
Canada Research Chair in Parkinson's Disease
Director, Pacific Parkinson's Research Center and
National Parkinson Foundation Center of
Excellence
University of British Columbia and Vancouver
Coastal Health
Vancouver, British Columbia, Canada

Jon Stone, MB, ChB, FRCP, PhD
Consultant Neurologist and Honorary Senior
Lecturer
Department of Clinical Neurosciences
University of Edinburgh
Western General Hospital
Edinburgh, United Kingdom

S.H. Subramony, MD
Professor of Neurology
McKnight Brain Institute at the University
of Florida
Gainesville, Florida

Jerry W. Swanson, MD, FACP
Professor of Neurology
College of Medicine, Mayo Clinic
Consultant, Neurology
Mayo Clinic
Rochester, Minnesota

Satoshi Tateshima, MD, DMSc
Associate Clinical Professor
Interventional Neuroradiology
Ronald Reagan University of California–Los
Angeles Medical Center
Los Angeles, California

Philip D. Thompson, MB, BS, PhD, FRACP
Department of Neurology
Royal Adelaide Hospital
Professor of Neurology
University Department of Medicine
University of Adelaide
Adelaide, South Australia

**Matthew J. Thurtell, BSc(Med), MBBS,
MSc(Med), FRACP**
Fellow
Neuro-Ophthalmology
Emory University Hospital
Atlanta, Georgia

Robert L. Tomsak, MD, PhD
Professor of Ophthalmology and Neurology
Wayne State University School of Medicine
Neuro-Ophthalmologist
Kresge Eye Institute
Detroit, Michigan

Po-Heng Tsai, MD
Department of Neurology
Cleveland Clinic Florida
Weston, Florida

Bryan Tsao, MD
Chair, Department of Neurology
Associate Professor of Neurology
Loma Linda University School of Medicine
Loma Linda, California

Chris Turner, BSc, MB, CHb, MRCP, PhD
Consultant Neurologist
MRC Center for Neuromuscular Disease
National Hospital for Neurology and
Neurosurgery
London, United Kingdom

Kenneth L. Tyler, MD
Reuler-Lewin Family Professor and Chair
of Neurology
Professor of Medicine and Microbiology
University of Colorado School of Medicine
Aurora, Colorado
Neurology Service
Denver Veterans Affairs Medical Center
Denver, Colorado

Bert B. Vargas, MD
Neurology Department
Mayo Clinic Arizona
Phoenix, Arizona

Ashok Verma, MD, DM, MBA
Professor of Neurology
Medical Director, Kessenich Family MDA ALS
Center
University of Miami Miller School of Medicine
Attending Neurologist
Jackson Memorial Hospital
Miami, Florida

Fernando Vinuela, MD
Professor of Radiology
Department of Radiological Sciences
Ronald Reagan University of California–Los
Angeles Medical Center
Los Angeles, California

Michael Wall, MD
Professor of Neurology and Ophthalmology
University of Iowa
Staff Physician
Department of Neurology
VA Health Care System
Iowa City, Iowa

Mitchell T. Wallin, MD, MPH
Associate Professor of Neurology
Georgetown University School of Medicine
Neurology Department
VA Medical Center
Washington, DC

Leo H. Wang, MD, PhD
Assistant Professor
Department of Neurology
University of Washington School of Medicine
Seattle, Washington

Cornelius Weiller, MD
Director, Neurological Clinic
University Medical Center
Freiburg, Germany

Patrick Wen, MD
Professor of Neurology
Harvard Medical School
Director, Center for Neuro-Oncology
Dana-Farber/Brigham and Women's Cancer
Institute
Director, Division of Cancer
Department of Neurology
Brigham and Women's Hospital
Boston, Massachusetts

Eelco F.M. Wijdicks, MD, PhD, FACP
Professor of Neurology
Mayo Clinic College of Medicine
Chair, Division of Critical Care Neurology
Mayo Clinic
Rochester, Minnesota

Guangbin Xia, MD
Assistant Professor
Department of Neurology
College of Medicine
University of Florida
Gainesville, Florida

Marco Zenteno, MD
Division of Surgical Neurology and
Neuroradiology
National Institute of Neurology and
Neurosurgery
Mexico City, Mexico

Jiachen Zhou, MD
PhD Candidate
Department of Epidemiology
Brown University
Providence, Rhode Island

YiLi Zhou, MD, PhD
Medical Director
Florida Pain and Rehabilitation Center
Courtesy Research Associate Professor
University of Florida
Gainesville, Florida

Foreword

The first ideas that led to *Neurology in Clinical Practice* (NICP) originated in Newcastle upon Tyne in the mid-1970s. Professor John Walton—now Lord Walton of Detchant, then professor of neurology and dean of the university's medical school—and several of us on the faculty believed we should write a Newcastle neurology textbook. We decided that the first section would describe how experienced neurologists approach common neurological conditions such as headache, walking difficulty, loss of vision, and so on. The second section would deal with neurological investigations such as neurophysiology and neuroimaging. The third section would provide an introduction to related neuroscience disciplines such as neurogenetics and neuroimmunology. The fourth section would outline the principles of management of neurological conditions, and the fifth would cover all the individual neurological diseases. The textbook would be divided into two volumes, with volume I containing the first four sections and volume II the neurological diseases.

The "Newcastle textbook" never got beyond the planning stage, and in 1977 I moved to Tufts New England Medical Center. There I started the journal, *Muscle and Nerve*, and was its founding editor for 10 years. However, the concept of an innovative practical textbook of neurology remained at the back of my mind. The opportunity to return to this project presented itself in 1987 when a small medical publisher approached me to write a book about neurology. A multi-author textbook of the magnitude that I conceived needed at least four editors who were not only clinicians and research workers with expertise in the major neurological subspecialties, but who were also established leaders across the breadth of neurology. I approached Bob Daroff, Gerry Fenichel, and David Marsden—all giants in the field—and they agreed to join me in this project.

We chose the title, *Neurology in Clinical Practice*, because we wanted the book to be used not only by neurologists in training and practice but also by others whose specialties border upon neurology, such as internists and neurosurgeons. Together, Bob, Gerry, David, and I selected the authors for the 84 chapters that made up the first edition and laid out guidelines for the chapter, its content, and format. We set tough time schedules, and Bob Daroff, in particular, ensured that our authors met the deadlines. All four editors reviewed the manuscript for every submitted chapter to ensure uniformity of style and content.

During this time, the small medical publishing company was bought by Houghton Mifflin, which was then acquired by Butterworth (later Butterworth-Heinemann), which eventually became part of the Elsevier group. Nancy Megley was the publishing editor with Butterworth for the first edition. The fact that NICP was published at the end of 1990 with a 1991 copyright is proof of the support we had from our contributors and Butterworth.

We devoted a great deal of attention to the technical aspects of textbook production. For instance, we wished to have the highest quality reproduction of halftone illustrations and chose top-quality china clay paper for the book. The first edition, divided into Volume I, Principles of Diagnosis and Management, and Volume II, The Neurological Disorders, encompassed 1941 pages plus 88 pages of index and weighed 16 pounds; we may have been responsible for a number of hernias among our readers. The first edition of NICP received the Most Outstanding Book award for 1991 from the Association of American Publishers and was greeted with very favorable reviews by all the neurological journals. It soon established itself as a leading international textbook of neurology.

Wishing to keep NICP up to date, we published the second edition in 1996. We were fortunate to be joined by Susan Pioli, then director of medical publishing for Butterworth-Heinemann and later neurology publisher for Elsevier. Susan continued to work with us through the fifth edition. For the second edition, we selected a number of new authors, and the text was completely rewritten. In editing it, we embraced the digital age and went electronic with an added CD version. The five sections were merged into three: Part 1, Approach to Common Neurological Problems; Part 2, Neurological Investigations and Related Clinical Neurosciences; and Part 3, Neurological Diseases. By slightly reducing the grade of paper, we were able to produce a lighter book and accommodate much new material in 2128 pages plus a 117-page index. We also produced the *Pocket Companion to Neurology in Clinical Practice, Second Edition,* which was almost entirely the work of Gerry Fenichel. It became very popular with residents, who came to refer to it as "the Baby Bradley."

For the third edition (published in 2000), besides recruiting new authors and adding new material, we persuaded Butterworth-Heinemann to publish NICP online, and it became the first major neurology textbook to be available in that format. Our initial discussions had revolved around how much material we could get onto a CD—at that time, 500 MB was the maximum capacity—but that was enough space to include only the text and not the illustrations. In the end, we leapfrogged straight into online publishing with www.expertconsult.com, thereby allowing us to add much more content, particularly videos of electroencephalograms, electromyograms, and eye movements. Tragically, we were in the final stages of production on the third edition when David Marsden died; that edition was dedicated to his memory.

For the fourth edition, published in 2004, we invited Joe Jankovic to join us in David's place. Joe brought his expertise in movement disorders and was responsible for adding videos of these fascinating conditions to www.expertconsult.com. This unparalleled teaching tool greatly expanded the educational role of NICP. Following the publication of our fourth edition, in collaboration with Karl Misulis, we launched the *Review Manual for Neurology in Clinical Practice,* a book of questions and answers intended as an introduction to board examinations.

Butterworth-Heinemann completely revamped the fifth edition of NICP, published in 2008. It was printed in color with completely redrawn figures to bring it into line with standard textbook format. Again, with rigorous editing we incorporated much new material and removed out-of-date work. Despite the major explosion of knowledge in the clinical and basic neurosciences in the previous 17 years, the NICP fifth edition had expanded to only 2488 pages.

In the 22 years since the first publication of NICP, it has become the major international textbook of neurology and been translated into Spanish, Italian, Polish, and Turkish. When making academic visits to medical centers in other countries, I have found myself lauded as an editor of "the bible, *Neurology in Clinical Practice*." I know that Bob Daroff, Gerry Fenichel, and Joe Jankovic have had the same experience.

When I stepped down as chair of the Neurology Department at the University of Miami in 2007, I decided it was time to move on to other interests and retire from the editorship of NICP. It had been an exciting and satisfying 20 years, and editing each new edition provided me personally with a complete neurological update course. For this, the sixth edition of NICP, my editorial colleagues and the publishers have been fortunate to persuade John Mazziotta to take my place. He brings a wealth of knowledge about the expanding field of functional imaging of the nervous system. The NICP sixth edition retains the structure of the textbook that was conceptualized nearly 40 years ago in Newcastle, but the clinical and scientific contents remain ever new. I have no doubt of the continuing success of our textbook and wish it well.

Walter G. Bradley DM, FRCP
Professor and Chairman Emeritus
Department of Neurology
Miller School of Medicine
University of Miami
Miami, Florida

Preface

Neurology in Clinical Practice is a practical textbook of neurology that covers all the clinical neurosciences and provides not only a description of neurological diseases and their pathophysiology but also a practical approach to their diagnosis and management. In the preface to the 1991 first edition of this book, we forecasted that major technological and research advances would soon reveal the underlying cause and potential treatment of an ever-increasing number of neurological diseases.

The 20 years that have passed since that prediction have been filled with the excitement of new discoveries resulting from the blossoming of neurosciences. Clinical neuroscience has taken on the important and challenging problems of neuroprotection in both neurodegenerative disorders and acute injuries to the nervous system, such as stroke, multiple sclerosis, and trauma. In line with this effort, basic science progress in areas of neuroplasticity and neural repair are yielding important results that should translate into clinical utility in the near future. Advances in the genetics of neurological diseases have not only facilitated genetic testing but also provided important insights into the pathogenesis of diseases and helped identify potential therapeutic targets. Significant advances have taken place in the management of patients with both ischemic and hemorrhagic stroke. When the first edition of this textbook was published, there was essentially no effective means of treating acute ischemic stroke. Today we have numerous opportunities to help such patients, and a campaign has begun to educate the general public about the urgency of seeking treatment when stroke symptoms occur.

The advent of teleneurology is also beginning to provide treatment for patients who lack access to neurological specialists or whose problems are too complicated for routine management in the community. Teleneurology consults are beginning to be provided nationwide across all subspecialties of our discipline, with a particular emphasis on patients who need intraoperative monitoring, critical care neurology, and stroke interventions.

To the benefit of patients, clinical neuroscience has partnered with engineering. Neuromodulation has become an important part of clinical therapy for patients with movement disorders and has applications in pain management and seizure control. Along these same lines, brain-controlled devices will soon help provide assistance to individuals whose mobility or communication skills are compromised. Recent advances in optogenetics have led to development of techniques that allow exploration and manipulation of neural circuitry, which may have therapeutic applications in a variety of neurologic disorders.

Finally, a search for biomarkers that reliably identify a preclinical state and track progression of disease is a promising goal in many neurodegenerative disorders.

Neurodegenerative disease, Alzheimer disease (AD) in particular, continues to be a worldwide crisis. The financial aspects associated with AD alone are staggering and have the capacity to bankrupt the modern world. For example, if no treatment or means to delay AD is found by 2050, the annual cost of care for such patients in the United States will exceed $1 trillion, and the 40-year interval aggregate cost will exceed $20 trillion. The costs in terms of suffering and hardship for patients and their families is too immense to quantify. As such, there is an urgent need for basic and clinical neuroscience to make progress in finding ways to delay the onset of neurodegenerative disorders and, ultimately, prevent them.

There is evidence of some startling new advances in neuroscience that are only just being considered today. The engineering of nanotechnologies into strategies to treat patients with neurological disorders is just beginning. One can envision a future that includes smart nanoimaging agents, nanopumps that can help regulate deranged circuitry on a local basis, and nanostimulators to participate in the growing field of neuromodulation. In addition, other partnerships with nanoengineers will produce sensors that can monitor not only the external condition of a patient by tracking movements, vital signs, and sleep behaviors but also internal states when such sensors are developed on a nano scale.

We still have a long way to go to reach the ultimate goal of being able to understand and treat all neurological diseases. Neurology remains an intellectually exciting discipline, both because of the complexity of the nervous system and because of the insight that the pathophysiology of neurological disease provides into the workings of the brain and mind. Accordingly, we offer the sixth edition of *Neurology in Clinical Practice* as the updated comprehensive and most authoritative presentation of both the art and the science of neurology.

For this edition, the text has been completely rewritten, and almost a fifth of the chapters have been prepared by authors new to the cadre of contributors. The layout of the pages has been completely redesigned to provide a user-friendly environment for accessing the material. The companion website, www.expertconsult.com, has been refined and expanded and includes video and audio material, additional illustrations and references, and chapters on key related material from other established neurology texts. It also is regularly updated with minireviews of important new publications in the neurological literature.

A work of this breadth would not have been possible without the contributions of many colleagues throughout the world. We are deeply grateful to them for their selfless devotion to neurological education. We are also grateful to our Elsevier counterparts, Lotta Kryhl, content strategist, and Lucia Gunzel, content development manager, who were key in drawing this project together. Additionally, we thank Cindy Thoms, project manager, without whose energy and efficiency the high quality of production and rapidity of publication of this work would not have been achieved. Finally, we gratefully acknowledge the contributions of our readers, whose feedback regarding *Neurology in Clinical Practice* and the website has been invaluable in enhancing our educational goals.

Robert B. Daroff, MD
Gerald M. Fenichel, MD
Joseph Jankovic, MD
John C. Mazziotta, MD, PhD

Contents

Volume II: Neurological Disorders

Part III
Neurological Diseases

Video Contents

Bradley's Neurology
in Clinical Practice

Part I

Approach to Common Neurological Problems

Chapter 1

Diagnosis of Neurological Disease

Robert B. Daroff, Gerald M. Fenichel, Joseph Jankovic, John C. Mazziotta

Neurological diagnosis is sometimes easy, sometimes quite challenging, and specialized skills are required. If a patient shuffles into the physician's office, demonstrating a pill-rolling tremor of the hands and loss of facial expression, Parkinson disease comes readily to mind. Although making such a "spot diagnosis" can be very satisfying, it is important to consider that this clinical presentation may have another cause entirely—such as neuroleptic-induced parkinsonism—or that the patient may be seeking help for a totally different neurological problem. Therefore, an evaluation of the whole problem is always necessary.

In all disciplines of medicine, the history of symptoms and clinical examination of the patient are key to achieving an accurate diagnosis. This is particularly true in neurology. Standard practice in neurology is to record the patient's chief complaint and the history of symptom development, followed by the history of illnesses and previous surgical procedures, the family history, personal and social history, and a review of any clinical features involving the main body systems. From these data, one formulates a hypothesis to explain the patient's illness. The neurologist then performs a neurological examination, which should support the hypothesis generated from the patient's history. Based on a combination of the history and physical findings, one proceeds with the differential diagnosis to generate a list of possible causes of the patient's clinical features.

What is unique to neurology is the emphasis on *localization* and *phenomenology*. When a patient presents to an internist or surgeon with abdominal or chest symptoms, the localization is practically established by the symptoms, and the etiology then becomes the primary concern. In clinical neurological practice, however, a patient with a weak hand may have a lesion localized to muscles, neuromuscular junctions, nerves in the upper limb, brachial plexus, spinal cord, or brain. The formal neurological examination allows localization of the offending lesion. Similarly, a neurologist skilled in recognizing phenomenology should be able to differentiate between tremor and stereotypy, both rhythmical movements; among tics, myoclonus, and chorea, all jerk-like movements; and among other rhythmical and jerk-like movement disorders, such as seen in dystonia. In general, the history provides the best clues to etiology, and the examination is essential for localization and appropriate disease categorization—all critical for proper diagnosis and treatment.

This diagnostic process consists of a series of steps, as depicted in **Fig. 1.1**. Although standard teaching is that the patient should be allowed to provide the history in his or her own words, the process also involves active questioning of the patient to elicit pertinent information. At each step, the neurologist should consider the possible anatomical localizations and particularly the etiology of the symptoms (see **Fig. 1.1**). From the patient's chief complaint and a detailed history, an astute neurologist can derive clues that lead first to a hypothesis about the location and then to a hypothesis about the etiology of the neurological lesion. From these hypotheses, the experienced neurologist can predict what neurological abnormalities *should be present* and what *should be absent*, thereby allowing confirmation of the site of the dysfunction. Alternatively, analysis of the history may suggest two or more possible anatomical locations and diseases, each with a different predicted constellation of neurological signs. The findings on neurological examination can be used to determine which of

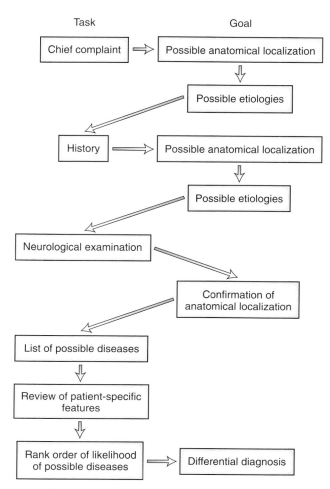

Task   Goal

Fig. 1.1 The diagnostic path is illustrated as a series of steps in which the neurologist collects data (Task) with the objective of providing information on the anatomical localization and nature of the disease process (Goal).

these various possibilities is the most likely. To achieve a diagnosis, the neurologist needs to have a good knowledge of not only the anatomy, physiology, and biochemistry of the nervous system but also of the clinical features and pathology of the neurological diseases.

Neurological Interview

The neurologist may be an intimidating figure for some patients. To add to the stress of the neurological interview and examination, the patient may already have a preconceived notion that the disease causing the symptoms may be progressively disabling and possibly life threatening. Because of this background, the neurologist should present an empathetic demeanor and do everything possible to put the patient at ease. It is important for the physician to introduce himself or herself to the patient and exchange social pleasantries before leaping into the interview. A few opening questions can break the ice: "Who is your doctor, and who would you like me to write to?" "What type of work have you done most of your life?" "How old are you?" "Are you right- or left-handed?" After this, it is easier to ask, "How can I be of service?" "What brings you to see me?" or "What is bothering you the most?" Such questions establish the physician's role in the relationship and

encourage the patient to volunteer an initial history. At a follow-up visit, it often is helpful to start with more personalized questions: "How have you been?" "Have there been any changes in your condition since your last visit?"

Another technique is to begin by asking, "How can I help you?" This establishes that the doctor is there to provide a service and allows patients to express their expectations for the consultation. It is important for the physician to get a sense of the patient's expectations from the visit. Usually the patient wants the doctor to find or confirm the diagnosis and cure the disease. Sometimes the patient comes hoping that something is *not* present ("Please tell me my headaches are *not* caused by a brain tumor!"). Sometimes the patient claims that other doctors "never told me anything" (which may sometimes be true, although in most cases the patient did not hear or did not like what was said).

Chief Complaint

The chief complaint (or the several main complaints) is the usual starting point of the diagnostic process. For example, the patient may present with the triad of complaints of headache, clumsiness, and double vision. The complaints serve to focus attention on the questions to be addressed in taking the history and provide the first clue to the anatomy and etiology of the underlying disease. In this case, the neurologist would be concerned that the patient may have a tumor in the posterior fossa affecting the cerebellum and brainstem.

The mode of onset is critically important in investigating the etiology. For example, a sudden onset usually indicates a stroke in the vertebrobasilar arterial system. A course characterized by exacerbations and remissions may suggest multiple sclerosis, whereas a slowly progressive course points to a neoplasm. Paroxysmal episodes suggest the possibility of seizures, migraines, or some form of paroxysmal dyskinesia, ataxia, or periodic paralysis.

History of Present Illness

A critical aspect of the information obtained from this portion of the interview has to do with establishing the temporal-severity profile of each symptom reported by the patient. Such information allows the neurologist to categorize the patient's problems based on the profile. For example, a patient who reports the gradual onset of headache and slowly progressive weakness of one side of the body over weeks to months could be describing the growth of a space-occupying lesion in a cerebral hemisphere. The same symptoms occurring rapidly, in minutes or seconds, with maximal severity from the onset, might be the result of a hemorrhage in a cerebral hemisphere. The symptoms and their severity may be equal at the time of the interview, but the temporal-severity profile leads to totally different hypotheses about the etiology.

Often the patient will give a very clear history of the temporal development of the complaints and will specify the location and severity of the symptoms and the current level of disability. In some instances, however, the patient, particularly if elderly, will provide a tangential account and insist on telling what other doctors did or said, rather than relating specific signs and symptoms. Direct questioning often is needed to clarify the symptoms, but it is important not to "lead" the patient. Patients frequently are all too ready to give a positive response to an authority figure, even if it is patently incorrect. It is important to consider whether the patient is reliable. Reliability depends on the patient's intelligence, memory, language function, and educational and social status and on the presence of secondary gain issues, such as a disability claim or pending lawsuit.

The clinician should suspect a *somatoform* or *psychogenic* disorder in any patient who claims to have symptoms that started suddenly, particularly after a traumatic event, manifested by clinical features that are incongruous with an organic disorder, or with involvement of multiple organ systems. The diagnosis of a psychogenic disorder is based not only on the exclusion of organic causes but also on positive criteria. Getting information from an observer other than the patient is important for characterizing many neurological conditions such as seizures and dementia. Taking a history from a child is complicated by shyness with strangers, a different sense of time, and a limited vocabulary. In children, the history is always the composite perceptions of the child and the parent.

Patients and physicians may use the same word to mean very different things. If the physician accepts a given word at face value without ensuring that the patient's use of the word matches the physician's, misinterpretation may lead to misdiagnosis. For instance, patients often describe a limb as being "numb" when it is actually paralyzed. Patients often use the term "dizziness" to refer to lightheadedness, confusion, or weakness, rather than vertigo as the physician would expect. Although a patient may describe vision as being "blurred," further questioning may reveal diplopia. "Blackouts" may indicate loss of consciousness, loss of vision, or simply confusion. "Pounding" or "throbbing" headaches are not necessarily pulsating.

The neurologist must understand fully the nature, onset, duration, and progression of each sign or symptom and the temporal relationship of one finding to another. Are the symptoms getting better, staying the same, or getting worse? What relieves them, what has no effect, and what makes them worse? In infants and young children, the temporal sequence also includes the timing of developmental milestones.

An example may clarify how the history leads to diagnosis: A 28-year-old woman presents with a 10-year history of recurrent headaches associated with her menses. The unilateral quality of pain in some attacks and the association of flashing lights, nausea, and vomiting together point to a diagnosis of migraine. On the other hand, in the same patient, a progressively worsening headache on wakening, new-onset seizures, and a developing hemiparesis suggest an intracranial space-occupying lesion. Both the absence of expected features and the presence of unexpected features may assist in the diagnosis. A patient with numbness of the feet may have a peripheral neuropathy, but the presence of backache combined with loss of sphincter control suggests that a spinal cord or cauda equina lesion is more likely. Patients may arrive for a neurological consultation with a folder of results of previous laboratory tests and neuroimaging studies. They often dwell on these test results and their interpretation by other physicians. The opinions of other doctors should never be accepted without question, however, because they may have been wrong! The careful neurologist takes a new history and makes a new assessment of the problem.

The history of how the patient or caregiver responded to the signs and symptoms may be important. A pattern of overreaction may be of help in evaluating the significance of the complaints. Nevertheless, a night visit to the emergency department for a new-onset headache should not be dismissed without investigation. Conversely, the child who was *not* brought to the hospital despite hours of seizures is likely to be the victim of child abuse, or at least of neglect.

Review of Patient-Specific Information

Information about the patient's background often greatly helps the neurologist make a diagnosis of the cause of the signs and symptoms. This information includes the history of medical and surgical illnesses; current medications and allergies; a review of symptoms in non-neurological systems of the body; the personal history in terms of occupation, marital status, and alcohol, tobacco, and illicit drug use; and the medical history of the parents, siblings, and children, looking for evidence of familial diseases. The order in which these items are considered is not important, but consistency avoids the possibility that something will be forgotten.

In the outpatient office, the patient can be asked to complete a form with a series of questions on all these matters before starting the consultation with the physician. This expedites the interview, although more details often are needed. What chemicals is the patient exposed to at home and at work? Did the patient *ever* use alcohol, tobacco, or prescription or illegal drugs? Is there excessive stress at home, in school, or in the workplace, such as divorce, death of a loved one, or loss of employment? Are there hints of abuse or neglect of children or spouse? Sexual preference is important information in this era of human immunodeficiency virus infection. The doctor should question children and adolescents away from their parents if obtaining more accurate information about sexual activity and substance abuse seems indicated.

Review of Systems

The review of systems should include the elements of nervous system function that did not surface in taking the history. The neurologist should have covered the following: cognition, personality, and mood change; hallucinations; seizures and other impairments of consciousness; orthostatic faintness; headaches; special senses; speech and language function; swallowing; limb coordination; slowness of movement; involuntary movements or vocalizations; strength and sensation; pain; gait and balance; and sphincter, bowel, and sexual function. A positive response may help clarify a diagnosis. For instance, if a patient complaining of ataxia and hemiparesis admits to unilateral deafness, an acoustic neuroma should be considered. Headaches in a patient with paraparesis suggest a parasagittal meningioma rather than a spinal cord lesion.

The developmental history must be assessed in children and also may be of value in adults whose illness started during childhood. The review must include all organ systems. Neurological function is adversely affected by dysfunction of many systems, including the liver, kidney, gastrointestinal tract, heart, and blood vessels. Multiorgan involvement characterizes several neurological disorders such as vasculitis, sarcoidosis, mitochondrial disorders, and storage diseases.

History of Previous Illnesses

Specific findings in the patient's medical and surgical history may help explain the present complaint. For instance, seizures and worsening headaches in a patient who previously had surgery for lung cancer suggest a brain metastasis. Chronic low back pain in a patient complaining of numbness and weakness in the legs on walking half a mile suggests neurogenic claudication from lumbar canal stenosis. The record of the history should include dates and details of all surgical procedures, significant injuries including head trauma and fractures, hospitalizations, and conditions requiring medical consultation and medications. For pediatric patients, record information on the pregnancy and state of the infant at birth.

Certain features in the patient's history should always alert the physician to the possibility that they may be responsible for the neurological complaints. Gastric surgery may lead to vitamin B_{12} deficiency. Sarcoidosis may cause Bell palsy, diabetes insipidus, ophthalmoplegia, and peripheral neuropathy. Disorders of the liver, kidney, and small bowel can be associated with a wide variety of neurological disorders. Systemic malignancy can cause direct and indirect (paraneoplastic) neurological problems. The physician should not be surprised if the patient fails to remember previous medical or surgical problems. It is common to observe abdominal scars in a patient who described no surgical procedures until questioned about the scars.

Medications often are the cause of neurological disturbances, particularly chemotherapy drugs. In addition, isoniazid may cause peripheral neuropathy. Lithium carbonate may produce tremor and ataxia. Neuroleptic agents can produce a parkinson-like syndrome or dyskinesias. Most patients do not think of vitamins, oral contraceptives, nonprescription analgesics, and herbal compounds as "medications," and specific questions about these agents are necessary.

Family History

Many neurological disorders are hereditary. Accordingly, a history of similar disease in family members or of consanguinity may be of diagnostic importance. The expression of a gene mutation, however, may be quite different from one family member to another with respect not only to the severity of neurological dysfunction but also to the organ systems involved. For instance, the mutations of the gene for Machado-Joseph disease (SCA3) can cause several phenotypes. A patient with Charcot-Marie-Tooth disease (hereditary motor-sensory neuropathy) may have a severe peripheral neuropathy, whereas relatives may demonstrate only pes cavus.

Reported diagnoses may be inaccurate. In families with dominant muscular dystrophy, affected individuals in earlier generations are often said to have had "arthritis" that put them into a wheelchair. Some conditions, such as epilepsy or Huntington disease, may be "family secrets." Therefore, the physician should be cautious in accepting a patient's assertion that a family history of a similar disorder is lacking. If the possibility exists that the disease is inherited, it is helpful to obtain information from parents and grandparents and to examine relatives at risk. Some patients wrongly attribute symptoms in family members to a normal consequence of aging or to other conditions such as alcoholism. This is particularly true in patients with essential tremor. At a minimum, historical data

for all first- and second-degree relatives should include age (current or at death), cause of death, and any significant neurological or systemic diseases.

Social History

It is important to discuss the social setting in which neurological disease is manifest. Marital status and changes in such can provide important information about interpersonal relationships and emotional stability. Employment history is often quite important. Has an elderly patient lost their job because of cognitive dysfunction? Does the patient's daily activities put them or others at risk if their vision, balance, or coordination is impaired or if they have alterations in consciousness? Does the patient's job expose them to potential injury or toxin exposure? Are they in a profession where the diagnosis of a neurological disorder would require reporting them to a regulatory agency (e.g., airline pilot, professional driver)? A travel history is important, particularly if infectious diseases are a consideration. Hobbies can be a source of toxin exposure (e.g., welding sculpture). Level and type of exercise provide useful clues to overall fitness and can also suggest potential exposures to toxins and infectious agents (e.g., hiking and Lyme disease).

Examination

Neurological Examination

Neurological examination starts during the interview. A patient's lack of facial expression (hypomimia) may suggest parkinsonism or depression, whereas a worried or astonished expression may suggest progressive supranuclear palsy. Unilateral ptosis may suggest myasthenia gravis or a brainstem lesion. The pattern of speech may suggest dysarthria, aphasia, or spasmodic dysphonia. The presence of abnormal involuntary movements may indicate an underlying movement disorder. Neurologist trainees must be able to perform and understand the complete neurological examination, in which every central nervous system region, peripheral nerve, muscle, sensory modality, and reflex is tested. However, the full neurological examination is too lengthy to perform in practice. Instead, the experienced neurologist uses the *focused neurological examination* to examine in detail the neurological functions relevant to the history and then performs a *screening neurological examination* to check the remaining parts of the nervous system. This approach should confirm, refute, or modify the initial hypotheses of disease location and causation derived from the history (see **Fig. 1.1**).

Both the presence and absence of abnormalities may be of diagnostic importance. If a patient's symptoms suggest a left hemiparesis, the neurologist should search carefully for a left homonymous hemianopia and for evidence that the blink or smile is slowed on the left side of the face. Relevant additional findings would be that rapid, repetitive movements are impaired in the left limbs, that the tendon reflexes are more brisk on the left than the right, that the left abdominal reflexes are absent, and that the left plantar response is extensor.

Along with testing the primary modalities of sensation on the left side, the neurologist may examine the higher integrative aspects of sensation, including graphesthesia, stereognosis, and sensory extinction with double simultaneous stimuli. The presence or absence of some of these features can separate

Table 1.1 Outline of the Screening Neurological Examination

Examination Component	Description/Observation/Maneuver
Mental status	Assessed while recording the history
Cranial nerves:	
CN I	Should be tested in all persons who experience spontaneous loss of smell, in patients suspected to have Parkinson disease, and in patients who have suffered head injury
CN II	*Each eye:* Gross visual acuity Visual fields by confrontation Funduscopy
CN III, IV, VI	Horizontal and vertical eye movements Pupillary response to light Presence of nystagmus or other ocular oscillations
CN V	Pinprick and touch sensation on face, corneal reflex
CN VII	Close eyes, show teeth
CN VIII	Perception of whispered voice in each ear or rubbing of fingers; if hearing is impaired, look in external auditory canals, and use tuning fork for lateralization and bone-versus-air sound conduction
CN IX, X	Palate lifts in midline, gag reflex present
CN XI	Shrug shoulders
CN XII	Protrude tongue
Limbs	*Separate testing of each limb:* Presence of involuntary movements Muscle mass (atrophy, hypertrophy) and look for fasciculations Muscle tone in response to passive flexion and extension Power of main muscle groups Coordination Finger-to-nose and heel-to-shin testing Performance of rapid alternating movements Tendon reflexes Plantar responses Pinprick and light touch on hands and feet Double simultaneous stimuli on hands and feet Joint position sense in hallux and index finger Vibration sense at ankle and index finger
Gait and balance	Spontaneous gait should be observed; stance, base, cadence, arm swing, tandem gait should be noted Postural stability should be assessed by the pull test
Romberg test	Stand with eyes open and then closed

a left hemiparesis arising from a lesion in the right cerebral cortex or from one in the left cervical spinal cord.

The screening neurological examination (**Table 1.1**) is designed for quick evaluation of the mental status, cranial nerves, motor system (strength, muscle tone, presence of involuntary movements, and postures), coordination, gait and balance, tendon reflexes, and sensation. More complex functions are tested first; if these are performed well, then it may not be necessary to test the component functions. The patient who can walk heel-to-toe (tandem gait) does not have a significant disturbance of the cerebellum or of joint position sensation. Similarly, the patient who can do a pushup, rise from the floor without using the hands, and walk on toes and heels will have normal limb strength when each muscle group is individually tested. Asking the patient to hold the arms extended in supination in front of the body with the eyes open allows evaluation of strength and posture. It also may reveal involuntary movements such as tremor, dystonia, myoclonus, or chorea. A weak arm is expected to show a downward or pronator drift. Repeating the maneuver with the eyes closed allows assessment of joint position sensation.

Of importance, the screening neurological examination may miss important neurological abnormalities. For instance, a bitemporal visual field defect may not be detected when the fields of both eyes are tested simultaneously; it will be found only when each eye is tested separately. Similarly, a parietal lobe syndrome may go undiscovered unless visuospatial function is assessed.

It is sometimes difficult to decide whether something observed in the neurological examination is normal or abnormal, and only experience prevents the neurologist from misinterpreting as a sign of disease something that is a normal variation. Every person has some degree of asymmetry. Moreover, what is abnormal in young adults may be normal in the elderly. Loss of the ankle reflex and loss of vibration sense at the big toe are common findings in patients older than 70 years. Conversely, children cannot detect the distal stimuli when the hand and face are simultaneously touched on the same side of the body until they are 7 years of age.

The experienced neurologist appreciates the normal range of neurological variation, whereas the beginner frequently records mild impairment of a number of different functions. Such impairments include isolated deviation of the tongue or uvula to one side and minor asymmetries of reflexes or sensation. Such *soft signs* may be incorporated into the overall synthesis of the disorder if they are consistent with other parts of the history and examination; otherwise, they should be disregarded. If an abnormality is identified, seek other features that usually are associated. For instance, ataxia of a limb may result from a corticospinal tract lesion, sensory defect, or cerebellar lesion. If the limb incoordination is due to a cerebellar lesion, findings will include ataxia on finger-to-nose and heel-to-shin testing, abnormal rapid alternating movements of the hands (dysdiadochokinesia), and often nystagmus and ocular dysmetria. If some of these signs of cerebellar dysfunction are missing, examination of joint position sense, limb strength, and reflexes may demonstrate that this incoordination is due to something other than a cerebellar lesion. At the end of the neurological examination, the abnormal physical signs should be classified as definitely abnormal (*hard signs*) or equivocally abnormal (*soft signs*). The hard signs, when combined with symptoms from the history, allow the neurologist to develop a hypothesis about the anatomical site of the lesion or at least about the neurological pathways involved. The soft signs can then be reviewed to determine whether they conflict with or support the initial conclusion. An important point is that the primary purpose of the neurological examination is to reveal functional disturbances that localize abnormalities. The standard neurological examination is less effective when used to monitor the course of a disease or its temporal response to treatment. Measuring changes in neurological function over time requires special quantitative functional tests and rating scales.

General Physical Examination

The nervous system is damaged in so many general medical diseases that a general physical examination is an integral part of the examination of patients with neurological disorders. Atrial fibrillation, valvular heart disease, or an atrial septal defect may cause embolic strokes in the central nervous system. Hypertension increases the risk for all types of stroke. Signs of malignancy raise the possibility of metastatic lesions of the nervous system or paraneoplastic neurological syndromes such as a subacute cerebellar degeneration or sensory peripheral neuropathy. In addition, some diseases such as vasculitis and sarcoidosis affect both the brain and other organs.

Assessment of the Cause of the Patient's Symptoms

Anatomical Localization

Hypotheses about lesion localization, neurological systems involved, and pathology of the disorder can be formed once the history is complete (see **Fig. 1.1**). The neurologist then uses the examination findings to confirm the localization of the lesion before trying to determine its cause. The initial question is whether the disease is in the brain, spinal cord, peripheral nerves, neuromuscular junctions, or muscles. Then it must be established whether the disorder is focal, multifocal, or systemic. A *system disorder* is a disease that causes degeneration of one part of the nervous system while sparing other parts of the nervous system. For instance, degeneration of the corticospinal tracts and spinal motor neurons with sparing of the sensory pathways of the central and peripheral nervous systems is the hallmark of the system degeneration termed *motor neuron disease*, or *amyotrophic lateral sclerosis*. Multiple system atrophy is another example of a system degeneration characterized by slowness of movement (parkinsonism), ataxia, and dysautonomia.

The first step in localization is to translate the patient's symptoms and signs into abnormalities of a nucleus, tract, or part of the nervous system. Loss of pain and temperature sensation on one half of the body, excluding the face, indicates a lesion of the contralateral spinothalamic tract in the high cervical spinal cord. A left sixth nerve palsy, with weakness of left face and right limbs, points to a left pontine lesion. A left homonymous hemianopia indicates a lesion in the right optic tract, optic radiations, or occipital cortex. The neurological examination plays a crucial role in localizing the lesion. A patient complaining of tingling and numbness in the feet initially may be thought to have a peripheral neuropathy. If examination shows hyperreflexia in the arms and legs and no vibration sensation below the clavicles, the lesion is likely to be in the spinal cord, and the many causes of peripheral neuropathy can be dropped from consideration. A patient with a history of weakness of the left arm and leg who is found on examination to have a left homonymous hemianopia has a right cerebral lesion, not a cervical cord problem.

The neurologist must decide whether the symptoms and signs could all arise from one focal lesion or whether several anatomical sites must be involved. The *principle of parsimony*, or *Occam's razor*, requires that the clinician strive to hypothesize only one lesion. The differential diagnosis for a single focal lesion is significantly different from that for multiple lesions. Thus, a patient complaining of left-sided vision loss and left-sided weakness is likely to have a lesion in the right cerebral hemisphere, possibly caused by stroke or tumor. On the other hand, if the visual difficulty is due to a central scotoma in the left eye, and if the upper motor neuron weakness affects the left limbs but spares the lower cranial nerves, two lesions must be present: one in the left optic nerve and one in the left corticospinal tract below the medulla—as seen, for example, in multiple sclerosis. If a patient with slowly progressive slurring of speech and difficulty walking is found to have ataxia of the arms and legs, bilateral extensor plantar responses, and optic atrophy, the lesion must be either multifocal (affecting brainstem and optic nerves, and therefore probably multiple sclerosis) or a system disorder, such as a spinocerebellar degeneration. The complex vascular anatomy of the brain can sometimes cause multifocal neurological deficits to result from one vascular abnormality. For instance, a patient with occlusion of one vertebral artery may suffer a stroke that produces a midbrain lesion, a hemianopia, and an amnestic syndrome.

Synthesis of symptoms and signs for anatomical localization of a lesion requires a good knowledge of neuroanatomy, including the location of all major pathways in the nervous system and their interrelationships at different levels. In making this synthesis, the neurologist trainee will find it helpful to refer to diagrams that show transverse sections of the spinal cord, medulla, pons, and midbrain; the brachial and lumbosacral plexuses; and the dermatomes and myotomes. Knowledge of the functional anatomy of the cerebral cortex and the blood supply of the brain and spinal cord also is essential.

Symptoms and signs may arise not only from disturbances caused at the focus of an abnormality—*focal localizing signs*—but also at a distance. One example is the damage that results from the shift of intracranial contents produced by an expanding supratentorial tumor. This may cause a palsy of the third or sixth cranial nerve, even though the tumor is located far from the cranial nerves. Clinical features caused by damage far from the primary site of abnormality sometimes are called *false localizing signs*. This term derives from the era before neuroimaging studies when clinical examination was the major means of lesion localization. In fact, these are not false signs but rather signs that the intracranial shifts are marked, alerting the clinician to the large size of the space-occupying lesion within the skull.

Differential Diagnosis

Once the likely site of the lesion is identified, the next step is to generate a list of diseases or conditions that may be responsible for the patient's symptoms and signs—the differential diagnosis (see **Fig. 1.1**). The experienced neurologist automatically first considers the most likely causes, followed by less common causes. The beginner is happy to generate a list of the main causes of the signs and symptoms in whatever order they come to mind. Experience indicates the most likely causes based on specific patient characteristics, the portions of the nervous system affected, and the relative frequency of each disease. An important point is that *rare presentations of common diseases are more common than common presentations of rare diseases*. Equally important, the neurologist must be vigilant to including in differential diagnosis less likely disorders that if overlooked can cause significant morbidity and/or mortality. A proper differential diagnosis list should include the most likely causes of the patient's signs and symptoms as well as the most ominous.

Sometimes only a single disease can be incriminated, but usually several candidate diseases can be identified. The list of possibilities should take into account both the temporal features of the patient's symptoms and the pathological processes known to affect the relevant area of the nervous system. For example, in a patient with signs indicating a lesion of the internal capsule, the cause is likely to be stroke if the hemiplegia was of sudden onset. With progression over weeks or months, a more likely cause is an expanding tumor. As another example, in a patient with signs of multifocal lesions whose symptoms have relapsed and remitted over several years, the diagnosis is likely to be multiple sclerosis or multiple strokes (depending on the patient's age, sex, and risk factors). If symptoms appeared only recently and have gradually progressed, multiple metastases should be considered.

Again, the principle of parsimony or Occam's razor should be applied in constructing the differential diagnostic list. An example is that of a patient with a 3-week history of a progressive spinal cord lesion who suddenly experiences aphasia. Perhaps the patient had a tumor compressing the spinal cord and has incidentally incurred a small stroke. The principle of parsimony, however, would suggest a single disease, probably cancer with multiple metastases. Another example is that of a patient with progressive atrophy of the small muscles of the hands for 6 months before the appearance of a pseudobulbar palsy. This patient could have bilateral ulnar nerve lesions and recent bilateral strokes, but amyotrophic lateral sclerosis is more likely. Nature does not always obey the rules of parsimony, however.

The differential diagnosis generally starts with pathological processes such as a stroke, a tumor, or an abscess. Each pathological process may result from any of several different diseases. Thus, a clinical diagnosis of an intracranial neoplasm generates a list of the different types of tumors likely to be responsible for the clinical manifestations in the affected patient. Similarly, in a patient with a stroke, the clinical history may help discriminate among hemorrhage, embolism, thrombosis, vascular spasm, and vasculitis. The skilled diagnostician is justly proud of placing the correct diagnosis at the top of the list, but it is more important to ensure that all possible diseases are considered. If a disease is not even considered, it is unlikely to be diagnosed. Treatable disorders should always be kept in mind, even if they have a very low probability. This is especially true if they may mimic more common incurable neurological disorders such as Alzheimer disease or amyotrophic lateral sclerosis.

Laboratory Investigations

Sometimes the neurological diagnosis can be made without any laboratory investigations. This is true for a clear-cut case of Parkinson disease, myasthenia gravis, or multiple sclerosis. Nevertheless, even in these situations, appropriate laboratory documentation is important for other physicians who will see the patient in the future. In other instances, the cause of the disease will be elucidated only by the use of laboratory tests. These tests may in individual cases include hematological and biochemical blood studies; neurophysiological testing (Chapters 32A-E); neuroimaging (Chapters 33A-E); organ biopsy; and bacteriological and virological studies. The use of laboratory tests in the diagnosis of neurological diseases is considered more fully in Chapter 31.

Management of Neurological Disorders

Not all diseases are curable. Even if a disease is incurable, however, the physician will be able to reduce the patient's discomfort and assist the patient and family in managing the disease. Understanding a neurological disease is a science. Diagnosing a neurological disease is a combination of science and experience. Managing a neurological disease is an art, an introduction to which is provided in Chapter 43.

Experienced Neurologist's Approach to the Diagnosis of Common Neurological Problems

The skills of a neurologist are learned. Seeing many cases of a disease teaches us which symptoms and signs *should* be present and—just as important—which *should not* be present in a given neurological disease. Although there is no substitute for experience and pattern recognition, the trainee can learn the clues used by the seasoned practitioner to reach a correct diagnosis. Part 1 of this book covers the main symptoms and signs of neurological disease. These chapters describe how an experienced neurologist approaches common presenting problems such as a movement disorder, a speech disturbance, or diplopia to arrive at the diagnosis. Part 2 of this book comprises the major fields of investigation and management of neurological disease. Part 3 provides a compendium of the neurological diseases themselves.

Chapter 2

Episodic Impairment of Consciousness

Joseph Bruni

Temporary loss of consciousness may be caused by impaired cerebral perfusion (syncope, fainting), cerebral ischemia, migraine, epileptic seizures, metabolic disturbances, sudden increases in intracranial pressure (ICP), or sleep disorders. Anxiety attacks, psychogenic seizures, panic disorder, and malingering may be difficult to distinguish from these conditions. Detailed laboratory examinations and prolonged periods of observation may not always clarify the diagnosis.

Syncope may result from cardiac causes and several noncardiac causes. Often, no cause is determined. Specific causes include decreased cardiac output secondary to cardiac arrhythmias, outflow obstruction, hypovolemia, orthostatic hypotension, or decreased venous return. Cerebrovascular disturbances from transient ischemic attacks of the posterior or anterior cerebral circulations, or cerebral vasospasm from migraine, subarachnoid hemorrhage, or hypertensive encephalopathy, may result in temporary loss of consciousness. Situational syncope may occur in association with cough, micturition, defecation, swallowing, Valsalva maneuver, or diving. Metabolic disturbances due to hypoxia, drugs, anemia, and hypoglycemia may result in frank syncope or, more frequently, the sensation of an impending faint (presyncope).

Absence seizures, generalized tonic-clonic seizures, and complex partial seizures are associated with alterations of consciousness and are usually easily distinguished from syncope. Epileptic seizures may be difficult to distinguish from pseudoseizures (psychogenic seizures), panic attacks, and malingering. In children, breath-holding spells, a form of syncope (discussed later under "Miscellaneous Causes of Altered Consciousness"), can cause a transitory alteration of consciousness that may mimic epileptic seizures. Although rapid increases in ICP (which may result from intermittent hydrocephalus, severe head trauma, brain tumors, intracerebral hemorrhage, or Reye syndrome) may produce sudden loss of consciousness, affected patients frequently have other neurological manifestations that lead to this diagnosis.

In patients with episodic impairment of consciousness, diagnosis relies heavily on the clinical history described by the patient and observers. Laboratory investigations, however, may provide useful information. In a small number of patients, a cause for the loss of consciousness may not be established, and these patients may require longer periods of observation. **Table 2.1** compares the clinical features of syncope and seizures.

Syncope

The pathophysiological basis of syncope is the gradual failure of cerebral perfusion, with a reduction in cerebral oxygen availability. *Syncope* refers to a symptom complex characterized by lightheadedness, generalized muscle weakness, giddiness, visual blurring, tinnitus, and gastrointestinal (GI) symptoms. The patient may appear pale and feel cold and "sweaty." The onset of loss of consciousness generally is gradual but may be rapid if related to certain conditions such as a cardiac arrhythmia. The gradual onset may allow patients to protect themselves from falling and injury. Factors precipitating a simple faint are emotional stress, unpleasant visual stimuli, prolonged standing, or pain. Although the duration of unconsciousness is brief, it may range from seconds to minutes. During the faint, the patient may be motionless or display myoclonic jerks, but never tonic-clonic movements. Urinary incontinence is uncommon. The pulse is weak and often slow. Breathing may be shallow and the blood pressure barely obtainable. As the fainting episode corrects itself by the patient becoming horizontal, normal color returns, breathing becomes more regular, and the pulse and blood pressure return to normal. After the faint, the patient experiences some residual weakness, but unlike the postictal state, confusion,

Table 2.1 Comparison of Clinical Features of Syncope and Seizures

Features	Syncope	Seizure
Relation to posture	Common	No
Time of day	Diurnal	Diurnal or nocturnal
Precipitating factors	Emotion, injury, pain, crowds, heat, exercise, fear, dehydration, coughing, micturition	Sleep loss, drug/alcohol withdrawal
Skin color	Pallor	Cyanosis or normal
Diaphoresis	Common	Rare
Aura or premonitory symptoms	Long	Brief
Convulsion	Rare	Common
Other abnormal movements	Minor twitching	Rhythmic jerks
Injury	Rare	Common (with convulsive seizures)
Urinary incontinence	Rare	Common
Tongue biting	No	Can occur with convulsive seizures
Postictal confusion	Rare	Common
Postictal headache	No	Common
Focal neurological signs	No	Occasional
Cardiovascular signs	Common (cardiac syncope)	No
Abnormal findings on EEG	Rare (generalized slowing may occur during the event)	Common

EEG, Electroencephalogram.

headaches, and drowsiness are uncommon. Nausea may be noted when the patient regains consciousness. The causes of syncope are classified by their pathophysiological mechanism (**Box 2.1**), but cerebral hypoperfusion is always the common final pathway. Wieling et al. (2009) reviewed the clinical features of the successive phases of syncope.

History and Physical Examination

The history and physical examination are the most important components of the initial evaluation of syncope. Significant age and sex differences exist in the frequency of the various types of syncope. Syncope occurring in children and young adults is most frequently due to hyperventilation or vasovagal (vasodepressor) attacks and less frequently due to congenital heart disease (Lewis and Dhala, 1999). Fainting associated with benign tachycardias without underlying organic heart disease also may occur in children. Syncope due to basilar migraine is more common in young females. When repeated syncope begins in later life, organic disease of the cerebral circulation or cardiovascular system usually is responsible.

A careful history is the most important step in establishing the cause of syncope. The patient's description usually establishes the diagnosis. The neurologist should always obtain as full a description as possible of the first faint. The clinical features should be established, with emphasis on precipitating factors, posture, type of onset of the faint (including whether it was abrupt or gradual), position of head and neck, the presence and duration of preceding and associated symptoms, duration of loss of consciousness, rate of recovery, and sequelae. If possible, question an observer about clonic movements, color changes, diaphoresis, pulse, respiration, urinary incontinence, and the nature of recovery.

Box 2.1 Classification and Etiology of Syncope

Cardiac:
    Arrhythmias:
        Bradyarrhythmias
        Tachyarrhythmias
        Reflex arrhythmias
    Decreased cardiac output:
        Outflow obstruction
        Inflow obstruction
        Cardiomyopathy
Hypovolemic
Hypotensive:
    Vasovagal attack
    Drugs
    Dysautonomia
Cerebrovascular:
    Carotid disease
    Vertebrobasilar disease
    Vasospasm
    Takayasu disease
Metabolic:
    Hypoglycemia
    Anemia
    Anoxia
Hyperventilation
Multifactorial:
    Vasovagal (vasodepressor) attack
    Cardiac syncope
    Situational: Cough, micturition, defecation, swallowing, diving
    Valsalva maneuver

Clues in the history that suggest cardiac syncope include a history of palpitations or a fluttering sensation in the chest before loss of consciousness. These symptoms are common in arrhythmias. In vasodepressor syncope and orthostatic hypotension, preceding symptoms of lightheadedness are common. Episodes of cardiac syncope generally are briefer than vasodepressor syncope, and the onset usually is rapid. Episodes due to cardiac arrhythmias occur independently of position, whereas in vasodepressor syncope and syncope due to orthostatic hypotension, the patient usually is standing.

Attacks of syncope precipitated by exertion suggest a cardiac etiology. Exercise may induce arrhythmic syncope or syncope due to decreased cardiac output secondary to blood flow obstruction, such as may occur with aortic or subaortic stenosis. Exercise syncope also may be due to cerebrovascular disease, aortic arch disease, congenital heart disease, pulseless disease (Takayasu disease), pulmonary hypertension, anemia, hypoxia, and hypoglycemia. A family history of sudden cardiac death, especially in females, suggests the long QT-interval syndrome. Postexercise syncope may be secondary to situational syncope or autonomic dysfunction. A careful and complete medical and medication history is mandatory to determine whether prescribed drugs have induced either orthostatic hypotension or cardiac arrhythmias. To avoid missing a significant cardiac disorder, consider a comprehensive cardiac evaluation in patients with exercise-related syncope.

The neurologist should inquire about the frequency of attacks of loss of consciousness and the presence of cerebrovascular or cardiovascular symptoms between episodes. Question the patient whether all episodes are similar, because some patients experience more than one type of attack. In the elderly, syncope may cause unexplained falls lacking prodromal symptoms. With an accurate description of the attacks and familiarity with clinical features of various types of syncope, the physician should correctly diagnose most patients (Brignole et al., 2006; Shen et al., 2004). Seizure types that must be distinguished from syncope include orbitofrontal complex partial seizures, which can be associated with autonomic changes, and complex partial seizures that are associated with sudden falls and altered awareness, followed by confusion and gradual recovery (temporal lobe syncope). Features that distinguish syncope from seizures and other alterations of consciousness are discussed later in the chapter.

After a complete history, the physical examination is of next importance. Examination during the episode is very informative but frequently impossible unless syncope is reproducible by a Valsalva maneuver or by recreating the circumstances of the attack, such as by position change. In the patient with suspected cardiac syncope, pay particular attention to the vital signs and determination of supine and erect blood pressure. Normally, with standing, the systolic blood pressure *rises* and the pulse rate may *increase*. An orthostatic drop in blood pressure greater than 15 mm Hg may suggest autonomic dysfunction. Assess blood pressure in both arms when suspecting cerebrovascular disease, subclavian steal, or Takayasu arteritis.

During syncope due to a cardiac arrhythmia, a heart rate faster than 140 beats per minute usually indicates an ectopic cardiac rhythm, whereas a bradycardia with heart rate of less than 40 beats per minute suggests complete atrioventricular (AV) block. Carotid sinus massage sometimes terminates a supraventricular tachycardia, but this maneuver is not advisable because of the risk of cerebral embolism from atheroma

in the carotid artery wall. In contrast, a ventricular tachycardia shows no response to carotid sinus massage. Stokes-Adams attacks may be of longer duration and may be associated with audible atrial contraction and a first heart sound of variable intensity. Heart disease as a cause of syncope is more common in the elderly patient (Brady and Shen, 1999). The patient should undergo cardiac auscultation for the presence of cardiac murmurs and abnormalities of the heart sounds. Possible murmurs include aortic stenosis, subaortic stenosis, or mitral valve origin. An intermittent posture-related murmur may be associated with an atrial myxoma. A systolic click in a young person suggests mitral valve prolapse. A pericardial rub suggests pericarditis.

All patients should undergo observation of the carotid pulse and auscultation of the neck. The degree of aortic stenosis may be reflected at times in a delayed carotid upstroke. Carotid, ophthalmic, and supraclavicular bruits suggest underlying cerebrovascular disease. Carotid sinus massage may be useful in older patients suspected of having carotid sinus syncope, but it is important to keep in mind that up to 25% of asymptomatic persons may have some degree of carotid sinus hypersensitivity. Carotid massage should be avoided in patients with suspected cerebrovascular disease, and when performed, it should be done in properly controlled conditions with electrocardiographic (ECG) and blood pressure monitoring. The response to carotid massage is either vasodepressor, cardioinhibitory, or mixed.

Causes of Syncope
Cardiac Arrhythmias

Both bradyarrhythmias and tachyarrhythmias may result in syncope, and abnormalities of cardiac rhythm due to dysfunction from the sinoatrial (SA) node to the Purkinje network may be involved. Always consider arrhythmias in all cases in which an obvious mechanism is not established. Syncope due to cardiac arrhythmias generally occurs more quickly than syncope from other causes. Cardiac syncope may occur in any position, is occasionally exercise induced, and may occur in both congenital and acquired forms of heart disease.

Although palpitations sometimes occur during arrhythmias, others are unaware of any cardiac symptoms. Syncopal episodes secondary to cardiac arrhythmias may be more prolonged than benign syncope. The most common arrhythmias causing syncope are AV block, SA block, and paroxysmal supraventricular and ventricular tachyarrhythmias. *AV block* describes disturbances of conduction occurring in the AV conducting system, which include the AV node to the bundle of His and the Purkinje network. *SA block* describes a failure of consistent pacemaker function of the SA node. *Paroxysmal tachycardia* refers to a rapid heart rate secondary to an ectopic focus outside the SA node; this may be either supra- or intraventricular.

Atrioventricular Block

Atrioventricular block is probably the most common cause of arrhythmic cardiac syncope. The term *Stokes-Adams attack* describes disturbances of consciousness occurring in association with a complete AV block. Complete AV block occurs primarily in elderly patients. The onset of a Stokes-Adams attack generally is sudden, although a number of visual, sensory, and perceptual premonitory symptoms may be experienced.

During the syncopal attack, the pulse disappears and no heart sounds are audible. The patient is pale and, if standing, falls down, often with resultant injury. If the attack is sufficiently prolonged, respiration may become labored, and urinary incontinence and clonic muscle jerks may occur. Prolonged confusion and neurological signs of cerebral ischemia may be present. Regaining of consciousness generally is rapid.

The clinical features of complete AV block include a slow-collapsing pulse and elevation of the jugular venous pressure, sometimes with cannon waves. The first heart sound is of variable intensity, and heart sounds related to atrial contractions may be audible. An ECG confirming the diagnosis demonstrates independence of atrial P waves and ventricular QRS complexes. During Stokes-Adams attacks, the ECG generally shows ventricular standstill, but ventricular fibrillation or tachycardia also may occur.

Sinoatrial Block

Sinoatrial block may result in dizziness, lightheadedness, and syncope. It is most frequent in the elderly. Palpitations are common, and the patient appears pale. Patients with SA node dysfunction frequently have other conduction disturbances, and certain drugs (e.g., verapamil, digoxin, beta-blockers) may further impair SA node function. On examination, the patient's pulse may be regular between attacks. During an attack, the pulse may be slow or irregular, and any of a number of rhythm disturbances may be present.

Paroxysmal Tachycardia

Supraventricular tachycardias include atrial fibrillation with a rapid ventricular response, atrial flutter, and the Wolff-Parkinson-White syndrome. These arrhythmias may suddenly reduce cardiac output enough to cause syncope. Ventricular tachycardia or ventricular fibrillation may result in syncope if the heart rate is sufficiently fast and if the arrhythmia lasts longer than a few seconds. Patients generally are elderly and usually have evidence of underlying cardiac disease. Ventricular fibrillation may be part of the long QT syndrome, which has a cardiac-only phenotype or may be associated with congenital sensorineural deafness in children. In most patients with this syndrome, episodes begin in the first decade of life, but onset may be much later. Exercise may precipitate an episode of cardiac syncope. Long QT syndrome may be congenital or acquired and manifests in adults as epilepsy. Acquired causes include cardiac ischemia, mitral valve prolapse, myocarditis, and electrolyte disturbances (Ackerman, 1998) as well as many drugs (Goldschlager et al., 2002). In the short QT syndrome, signs and symptoms are highly variable, ranging from complete absence of clinical manifestations to recurrent syncope to sudden death. The age at onset often is young, and affected persons frequently are otherwise healthy. A family history of sudden death indicates a familial short QT syndrome inherited as an autosomal dominant mutation. The ECG demonstrates a short QT interval and a tall and peaked T wave, and electrophysiological studies may induce ventricular fibrillation (Gaita et al., 2003). Brugada syndrome may produce syncope as a result of ventricular tachycardia or ventricular fibrillation (Brugada, 2000). The ECG demonstrates an incomplete right bundle-branch block in leads V_1 and V_2, with ST-segment elevation in the right precordial leads.

Reflex Cardiac Arrhythmias

A hypersensitive carotid sinus may be a cause of syncope in the elderly, most frequently men. Syncope may result from a reflex sinus bradycardia, sinus arrest, or AV block; peripheral vasodilatation with a fall in arterial pressure; or a combination of both. Although 10% of the population older than 60 years of age may have a hypersensitive carotid sinus, not all such patients experience syncope. Accordingly, consider this diagnosis only when the clinical history is compatible. Carotid sinus syncope may be initiated by wearing a tight collar or by carotid sinus massage on clinical examination. When syncope occurs, the patient usually is upright, and the duration of the loss of consciousness generally is a few minutes. On regaining consciousness, the patient is mentally clear. Unfortunately, no accepted diagnostic criteria exist for carotid sinus syncope, and the condition is overdiagnosed.

Syncope in certain patients can be induced by unilateral carotid massage or compression or by partial occlusion (usually atherosclerotic) of the contralateral carotid artery or a vertebral artery or by the release of atheromatous emboli. Because of these risks, carotid artery massage is contraindicated.

The rare syndrome of glossopharyngeal neuralgia is characterized by intense paroxysmal pain in the throat and neck accompanied by bradycardia or asystole, severe hypotension, and, if prolonged, seizures. Episodes of pain may be initiated by swallowing but also by chewing, speaking, laughing, coughing, shouting, sneezing, yawning, or talking. The episodes of pain always precede the loss of consciousness (see Chapter 18). Rarely, cardiac syncope may be due to bradyarrhythmias consequent to vagus nerve irritation caused by esophageal diverticula, tumors, and aneurysms in the region of the carotid sinus or by mediastinal masses or gallbladder disease.

Decreased Cardiac Output

Syncope may occur as a result of a sudden and marked decrease in cardiac output. Causes are both congenital and acquired. Tetralogy of Fallot, the most common congenital malformation causing syncope, does so by producing hypoxia due to right-to-left shunting. Other congenital conditions associated with cyanotic heart disease also may cause syncope. Ischemic heart disease and myocardial infarction (MI), aortic stenosis, idiopathic hypertrophic subaortic stenosis, pulmonary hypertension, and other causes of obstruction of pulmonary outflow, atrial myxoma, and cardiac tamponade may sufficiently impair cardiac output to cause syncope. Exercise-induced or effort syncope may occur in aortic or subaortic stenosis and other states in which there is reduced cardiac output and associated peripheral vasodilatation induced by the exercise. Exercise-induced cardiac syncope and exercise-induced cardiac arrhythmias may be related.

In patients with valvular heart disease, the cause of syncope may be arrhythmias. Syncope also may be due to reduced cardiac output secondary to myocardial failure, to mechanical prosthetic valve malfunction, or to thrombus formation. Mitral valve prolapse generally is a benign condition, but rarely, cardiac arrhythmias can occur. The most significant arrhythmias are ventricular. In atrial myxoma or with massive pulmonary embolism, a sudden drop in left ventricular output may occur. In atrial myxoma, syncope frequently is positional and occurs when the tumor falls into the AV valve opening during a change in position of the patient, thereby causing obstruction of the left ventricular inflow.

Decreased cardiac output also may be secondary to conditions causing in inflow obstruction or reduced venous return. Such conditions include superior and inferior vena cava obstruction, tension pneumothorax, constrictive cardiomyopathies, constrictive pericarditis, and cardiac tamponade. Syncope associated with aortic dissection may be due to cardiac tamponade but also may be secondary to hypotension, obstruction of cerebral circulation, or a cardiac arrhythmia.

Hypovolemia

Acute blood loss, usually due to GI tract bleeding, may cause weakness, faintness, and syncope if sufficient blood is lost. Blood volume depletion by dehydration may cause faintness and weakness, but true syncope is uncommon except when combining dehydration and exercise.

Hypotension

Several conditions cause syncope by producing a fall in arterial pressure. Cardiac causes were discussed earlier. The common faint (synonymous with *vasovagal* or *vasodepressor syncope*) is the most frequent cause of a transitory fall in blood pressure resulting in syncope. It often is recurrent, tends to occur in relation to emotional stimuli, and may affect 20% to 25% of young people. Less commonly, it occurs in older patients with cardiovascular disease (Fabian and Benditt, 1999; Fenton et al., 2000; Kosinski and Grubb, 2000).

The common faint may or may not be associated with bradycardia. The patient experiences impairment of consciousness, with loss of postural tone. Signs of autonomic hyperactivity are common, including pallor, diaphoresis, nausea, and dilated pupils. After recovery, patients may have persistent pallor, sweating, and nausea; if they get up too quickly, they may black out again. Presyncopal symptoms of lethargy and fatigue, nausea, weakness, a sensation of an impending faint, yawning, and blurred vision may occur. It is more likely to occur in certain circumstances such as in a hot crowded room, especially if the affected person is tired or hungry and upright or sitting. Venipuncture, the sight of blood, or a sudden painful or traumatic experience may precipitate syncope. When the patient regains consciousness, there usually is no confusion or headache, although weakness is frequent. As in other causes of syncope, if the period of cerebral hypoperfusion is prolonged, urinary incontinence and a few clonic movements may occur (convulsive syncope).

Orthostatic syncope occurs when autonomic factors that compensate for the upright posture are inadequate. This can result from a variety of clinical disorders. Blood volume depletion or venous pooling may cause syncope when the affected person assumes an upright posture. Orthostatic hypotension resulting in syncope also may occur with drugs that impair sympathetic nervous system function. Diuretics, antihypertensive medications, nitrates, arterial vasodilators, sildenafil, calcium channel blockers, phenothiazines, L-dopa, alcohol, and tricyclic antidepressants all may cause orthostatic hypotension. Patients with postural tachycardia syndrome (POTS) frequently experience orthostatic symptoms without orthostatic hypotension, but syncope can occur occasionally. Data suggest that there is sympathetic activation in this syndrome (Garland et al., 2007). Autonomic nervous system dysfunction resulting in syncope due to orthostatic hypotension may be a result of primary autonomic failure due to the Shy-Drager or the Riley-Day syndrome. Neuropathies that affect the autonomic nervous system include those of diabetes mellitus, amyloidosis, Guillain-Barré syndrome, acquired immunodeficiency syndrome (AIDS), chronic alcoholism, hepatic porphyria, beriberi, and autoimmune subacute autonomic neuropathy and small fiber neuropathies. Rarely, subacute combined degeneration, syringomyelia, and other spinal cord lesions may damage the descending sympathetic pathways, producing orthostatic hypotension. Accordingly, conditions that affect both the central and peripheral baroreceptor mechanisms may cause orthostatic hypotension (Benafroch, 2008).

Cerebrovascular Ischemia

Syncope occasionally may result from reduction of cerebral blood flow in either the carotid or vertebrobasilar system in patients with extensive occlusive disease. Most frequently, the underlying condition is atherosclerosis of the cerebral vessels, but reduction of cerebral blood flow due to cerebral embolism, mechanical factors in the neck (e.g., severe osteoarthritis), and arteritis (e.g., Takayasu disease or cranial arteritis) may be responsible. In the subclavian steal syndrome, a very rare impairment of consciousness is associated with upper extremity exercise and resultant diversion of cerebral blood flow to the peripheral circulation. In elderly patients with cervical skeletal deformities, certain head movements such as hyperextension or lateral rotation can result in syncope secondary to vertebrobasilar arterial ischemia. In these patients, associated vestibular symptoms are common. Occasionally, cerebral vasospasm secondary to basilar artery migraine or subarachnoid hemorrhage may be responsible. Insufficiency of the cerebral circulation frequently causes other neurological symptoms, depending on the circulation involved.

Reduction in blood flow in the carotid circulation may lead to loss of consciousness, lightheadedness, giddiness, and a sensation of an impending faint. Reduction in blood flow in the vertebrobasilar system also may lead to loss of consciousness, but dizziness, lightheadedness, drop attacks without loss of consciousness, and bilateral motor and sensory symptoms are more common. Dizziness and lightheadedness alone, however, are not symptoms of vertebrobasilar insufficiency. Syncope due to compression of the vertebral artery during certain head and neck movements may be associated with episodes of vertigo, disequilibrium, or drop attacks. Patients may describe blackouts on looking upward suddenly or on turning the head quickly to one side. Generally, symptoms persist for several seconds after the movement stops.

In Takayasu disease, major occlusion of blood flow in the carotid and vertebrobasilar systems may occur; in addition to fainting, other neurological manifestations are frequent. Pulsations in the neck and arm vessels usually are absent, and blood pressure in the arms is unobtainable. The syncopal episodes characteristically occur with mild or moderate exercise and with certain head movements. Cerebral vasospasm may result in syncope, particularly if the posterior circulation is involved. In basilar artery migraine, usually seen in young women and children, a variety of brainstem symptoms also may be experienced, and it is associated with a pulsating headache. The loss of consciousness usually is gradual, but a confusional state may last for hours (see Chapter 51A).

Metabolic Disorders

A number of metabolic disturbances including hypoglycemia, anoxia, and hyperventilation-induced alkalosis may predispose affected persons to syncope, but usually only lightheadedness and dizziness are experienced. The abruptness of onset of loss of consciousness depends on the acuteness and reversibility of the metabolic disturbances. Syncope due to hypoglycemia usually develops gradually. The patient has a sensation of hunger; there may be a relationship to fasting, a history of diabetes mellitus, and a prompt response to ingestion of food. Symptoms are unrelated to posture but may increase with exercise. During the syncopal attack, no significant change in blood pressure or pulse occurs. Hypoadrenalism may give rise to syncope by causing orthostatic hypotension. Disturbances of calcium, magnesium, and potassium metabolism are other rare causes of syncope. Anoxia may produce syncope because of the lack of oxygen or through the production of a vasodepressor type of syncope. A feeling of lightheadedness is common, but true syncope is less common. Patients with underlying cardiac or pulmonary disease are susceptible. In patients with chronic anemia or certain hemoglobinopathies that impair oxygen transport, similar symptoms may occur. Syncopal symptoms may be more prominent with exercise or physical activity.

Hyperventilation-induced syncope usually has a psychogenic origin. During hyperventilation, the patient may experience paresthesia of the face, hands, and feet, a buzzing sensation in the head, lightheadedness, giddiness, blurring of vision, mouth dryness, and occasionally tetany. Patients often complain of tightness in the chest and a sense of panic. Symptoms can occur in the supine or erect position and are gradual in onset. Rebreathing into a paper bag relieves the symptoms. During hyperventilation, a tachycardia may be present, but blood pressure generally remains normal.

Miscellaneous Causes of Syncope

More than one mechanism may be responsible in certain types of syncope. Both vasodepressor and cardioinhibitory factors may be operational in common syncope. In cardiac syncope, a reduction of cardiac output may be due to a single cause such as obstruction to inflow or outflow or a cardiac arrhythmia, but multiple factors are frequent.

Situational syncope, such as is associated with cough (tussive syncope) and micturition, are special cases of reflex syncope. In cough syncope, loss of consciousness occurs after a paroxysm of severe coughing. This is most likely to occur in obese men, usually smokers or patients with chronic bronchitis. The syncopal episodes occur suddenly, generally after repeated coughing but occasionally after a single cough. Before losing consciousness, the patient may feel lightheaded. The face often becomes flushed secondary to congestion, and then pale. Diaphoresis may be present, and loss of muscle tone may occur. Syncope generally is brief, lasting only seconds, and recovery is rapid. Several factors probably are operational in causing cough syncope. The most significant is blockage of venous return by raised intrathoracic pressure. In weightlifting syncope, a similar mechanism is operational.

Micturition syncope most commonly occurs in men during or after micturition, usually after arising from bed in the middle of the night to urinate in the erect position. There may be a history of drinking alcohol before going to bed. The syncope may result from sudden reflex peripheral vasodilatation caused by the release of intravesicular pressure and bradycardia. The relative peripheral vasodilatation from recent alcohol use and a supine sleeping position is contributory because blood pressure is lowest in the middle of the night. The syncopal propensity may increase with fever. Rarely, micturition syncope with headache may result from a pheochromocytoma in the bladder wall. Defecation syncope is uncommon, but it probably shares the underlying pathophysiological mechanisms responsible for micturition syncope. Convulsive syncope is an episode of syncope of any cause that is sufficiently prolonged to result in a few clonic jerks; the other features typically are syncopal and should not be confused with epileptic seizures. Other causes of situational syncope include diving and the postprandial state. Syncope during sexual activity may be due to neurocardiogenic syncope, coronary artery disease, or the use of erectile dysfunction medications.

Investigations of Patients with Syncope

In the investigation of the patient with episodic impairment of consciousness, the diagnostic tests performed depend on the initial differential diagnosis (Kapoor, 2000). Individualize investigations, but some measurements such as hematocrit, blood glucose, and ECG are always appropriate. A resting ECG may reveal an abnormality of cardiac rhythm or the presence of underlying ischemic or congenital heart disease. In the patient suspected of cardiac syncope, a chest radiograph may show evidence of cardiac hypertrophy, valvular heart disease, or pulmonary hypertension. Other noninvasive investigations include radionuclide cardiac scanning, echocardiography, and prolonged Holter monitoring for the detection of cardiac arrhythmias. Echocardiography is useful in the diagnosis of valvular heart disease, cardiomyopathy, atrial myxoma, prosthetic valve dysfunction, pericardial effusion, aortic dissection, and congenital heart disease. Holter monitoring detects twice as many ECG abnormalities as those discovered on a routine ECG and may disclose an arrhythmia at the time of a syncopal episode. Holter monitoring typically for a 24-hour period is usual, although longer periods of recording may be required. Implantable loop recordings can provide long-term rhythm monitoring in patients suspected of having a cardiac arrhythmia (Krahn et al., 2004).

Exercise testing and electrophysiological studies are useful in selected patients. Exercise testing may be useful in detecting coronary artery disease, and exercise-related syncopal recordings may help localize the site of conduction disturbances. Consider tilt-table testing in patients with unexplained syncope in high-risk settings or with recurrent faints in the absence of heart disease (Kapoor, 1999). False positives occur, and 10% of healthy persons may faint. Tilt testing frequently employs pharmacological agents such as nitroglycerin or isoproterenol. The specificity of tilt-table testing is approximately 90%. In patients suspected to have syncope due to cerebrovascular causes, noninvasive diagnostic studies including Doppler flow studies of the cerebral vessels and magnetic resonance imaging (MRI) or magnetic resonance angiography may provide useful information. Cerebral angiography is sometimes useful. Electroencephalography (EEG) is useful in differentiating syncope from epileptic seizure disorders. An EEG should be obtained only when a seizure disorder is suspected and generally has a low diagnostic yield (Poliquin-Lasnier and Moore, 2009). A systematic evaluation can establish a definitive diagnosis in 98% of patients (Brignole et al., 2006). Neurally mediated (vasovagal or vasodepressor) syncope was found in 66% of patients, orthostatic hypotension in 10%, primary arrhythmias in 11%, and structural cardiopulmonary disease in 5%. Initial history, physical examination, and a standard ECG established a diagnosis in 50% of patients. A risk score such as the San Francisco Syncope Rule (SFSR) can help identify patients who need urgent referral. The presence of cardiac failure, anemia, abnormal ECG, or systolic hypotension helps identify these patients (Parry and Tan, 2010).

Seizures

Epileptic seizures cause sudden, unexplained loss of consciousness in a child or an adult (see Chapter 67). Seizures and syncope are distinguishable clinically; pallor is not associated with seizures.

History and Physical Examination

The most definitive way to diagnose epilepsy and the type of seizure is clinical observation of the seizure, although this often is not possible, except when seizures are frequent. The history of an episode, as obtained from the patient and an observer, is of paramount importance. The neurologist should obtain a family history and should inquire about birth complications, central nervous system (CNS) infection, head trauma, and previous febrile seizures, because they all may have relevance.

The neurologist should obtain a complete description of the episode and inquire about any warning before the event, possible precipitating factors, and other neurological symptoms that may suggest an underlying structural cause. Important considerations are the age at onset, frequency, and diurnal variation of the events. Seizures generally are brief and have stereotypical patterns, as described previously. With complex partial seizures and tonic-clonic seizures, a period of postictal confusion is highly characteristic. Unlike some types of syncope, seizures are unrelated to posture and generally last longer. In a tonic-clonic seizure, cyanosis frequently is present, pallor is uncommon, and breathing may be stertorous.

Tonic-clonic and complex partial seizures may begin at any age from infancy to late adulthood, although young infants may not demonstrate the typical features because of incomplete development of the nervous system.

The neurological examination may reveal an underlying structural disturbance responsible for the seizure disorder. Birth-related trauma may result in asymmetries of physical development, cranial bruits may indicate an arteriovenous malformation, and space-occupying lesions may result in papilledema or in focal motor, sensory, or reflex signs. In the pediatric age group, mental retardation occurs in association with birth injury or metabolic defects. The skin should be examined for abnormal pigment changes and other dysmorphic features characteristic of some of the neurodegenerative disorders.

If examination is immediately after a suspected tonic-clonic seizure, the neurologist should search for abnormal signs such as focal motor weakness and reflex asymmetry and for pathological reflexes such as a Babinski sign. Such findings may help

confirm that the attack was a seizure and suggest a possible lateralization or location of the seizure focus.

Absence Seizures

The onset of absence seizures is usually between the ages of 5 and 15 years, and a family history of seizures is present in 20% to 40% of patients. The absence seizure is a well-defined clinical and EEG event. The essential feature is an abrupt, brief episode of decreased awareness without any warning, aura, or postictal symptoms. At the onset of the absence seizure, there is an interruption of activity. A simple absence seizure is characterized clinically only by an alteration of consciousness. Characteristic of a complex absence seizure is an alteration of consciousness and other signs such as minor motor automatisms. During a simple absence seizure, the patient remains immobile, breathing is normal, skin color remains unchanged, postural tone is not lost, and no motor manifestations occur. After the seizure, the patient immediately resumes the previous activities and may be unaware of the attack. An absence seizure generally lasts 10 to 15 seconds, but it may be shorter or as long as 40 seconds.

Complex absence seizures have additional manifestations such as diminution of postural tone that may cause the patient to fall, an increase in postural tone, minor clonic movements of the facial musculature or extremities, minor face or extremity automatisms, or autonomic phenomena such as pallor, flushing, tachycardia, piloerection, mydriasis, or urinary incontinence.

If absence seizures are suspected, office diagnosis is frequently possible by having the patient hyperventilate for 3 to 4 minutes, which often induces an absence seizure.

Tonic-Clonic Seizures

The tonic-clonic seizure is the most dramatic manifestation of epilepsy and characterized by motor activity and loss of consciousness. Tonic-clonic seizures may be the only manifestation of epilepsy or may be associated with other seizure types. In a primary generalized tonic-clonic seizure, the affected person generally experiences no warning or aura, although a few myoclonic jerks may occur in some patients. The seizure begins with a tonic phase, during which there is sustained muscle contraction lasting 10 to 20 seconds. Following this phase is a clonic phase that lasts approximately 30 seconds and is characterized by recurrent muscle contractions. During a tonic-clonic seizure, a number of autonomic changes may be present, including an increase in blood pressure and heart rate, apnea, mydriasis, urinary or fecal incontinence, piloerection, cyanosis, and diaphoresis. Injury may result from a fall or tongue biting. In the postictal period, consciousness returns slowly, and the patient may remain lethargic and confused for a variable period. Pathological reflexes may be elicitable.

Some generalized motor seizures with transitory alteration of consciousness may have only tonic or only clonic components. Tonic seizures consist of an increase in muscle tone, and the alteration of consciousness generally is brief. Clonic seizures have a brief impairment of consciousness and bilateral clonic movements. Recovery may be rapid, but if the seizure is more prolonged, a postictal period of confusion may be noted.

Complex Partial Seizures

In a complex partial seizure, the first seizure manifestation may be an alteration of consciousness, but the patient frequently experiences an aura or warning symptom. The seizure may have a simple partial onset that may include motor, sensory, visceral, or psychic symptoms. The patient initially may experience hallucinations or illusions, affective symptoms such as fear or depression, cognitive symptoms such as a sense of depersonalization or unreality, or aphasia.

The complex partial seizure generally lasts 1 to 3 minutes but may be shorter or longer. It may become generalized and evolve into a tonic-clonic convulsion. During a complex partial seizure, automatisms, generally more complex than those in absence seizures, may occur. The automatisms may involve continuation of the patient's activity before the onset of the seizure, or they may be new motor acts. Such new automatisms are variable but frequently consist of chewing or swallowing movements, lip smacking, grimacing, or automatisms of the extremities, including fumbling with objects, walking, or trying to stand up. Rarely, patients with complex partial seizures have drop attacks; in such cases, the term *temporal lobe syncope* often is used. The duration of the postictal period after a complex partial seizure is variable, with a gradual return to normal consciousness and normal response to external stimuli. **Table 2.2** provides a comparison of absence seizures and complex partial seizures.

Investigations of Seizures

In the initial investigations of the patient with tonic-clonic or complex partial seizures, perform a complete blood cell count, urinalysis, biochemical screening, and determinations of blood glucose level and serum calcium concentration. Laboratory investigations generally are not helpful in establishing a diagnosis of absence seizures. In infants and children, consider biochemical screening for amino acid disorders.

MRI is the imaging modality of choice for the investigation of patients with suspected seizures. It is superior to computed tomography and increases the yield of focal structural disturbances. Cerebrospinal fluid examination is not necessary in every patient with a seizure disorder and should be reserved for those in whom a recent seizure may relate to an acute CNS infection.

An EEG provides laboratory support for a clinical impression and helps classify the type of seizure. Epilepsy is a clinical diagnosis; therefore, an EEG study cannot confirm the diagnosis with certainty unless the patient has a clinical event during the recording. Normal findings on the EEG do not exclude epilepsy, and minor nonspecific abnormalities do not confirm epilepsy. Some patients with clinically documented seizures show no abnormality even after serial EEG recordings, sleep recordings, and special activation techniques. The EEG is most frequently helpful in the diagnosis of absence seizures. EEG supplemented with simultaneous video monitoring documents ictal events, allowing for a strict correlation between EEG changes and clinical manifestations. Simultaneous EEG and video monitoring also is useful in distinguishing epileptic seizures from nonepileptic phenomena.

In most patients, an accurate diagnosis requires only the clinical history and the foregoing investigations. Others present a diagnostic dilemma. A 24-hour ambulatory EEG recording differentiates an epileptic seizure from nonepileptic phenomena and also helps classify the specific type of seizure.

Psychogenic or Pseudoseizures (Nonepileptic Seizures)

Pseudoepileptic seizures are paroxysmal episodes of altered behavior that superficially resemble epileptic seizures but lack the expected EEG epileptic changes (Ettinger et al., 1999). However, as many as 40% of patients with pseudo- or nonepileptic seizures also experience true epileptic seizures.

A diagnosis often is difficult to establish based on the initial history alone. Establishing the correct diagnosis often requires observation of the patient's clinical episodes, but complex partial seizures of frontal lobe origin may be difficult to distinguish from nonepileptic seizures. Nonepileptic seizures occur in children and adults and are more common in females. Most frequently, they superficially resemble tonic-clonic seizures. They generally are abrupt in onset, occur in the presence of other people, and do not occur during sleep. Motor activity is uncoordinated, but urinary incontinence and physical injury are uncommon. Nonepileptic seizures tend to be more

---

Table 2.2 Comparison of Absence and Complex Partial Seizures

Feature	Absence Seizure	Complex Partial Seizure
Neurological status	Normal	May have positive history or examination
Age at onset	Childhood or adolescence	Any age
Aura or warning	No	Common
Onset	Abrupt	Gradual
Duration	Seconds	Up to minutes
Automatisms	Simple	More complex
Provocation by hyperventilation	Common	Uncommon
Termination	Abrupt	Gradual
Frequency	Possibly multiple seizures per day	Occasional
Postictal phase	No	Confusion, fatigue
Electroencephalogram	Generalized spike and wave	Focal epileptic discharges or nonspecific abnormalities
Neuroimaging	Usually normal findings	May demonstrate focal lesions

prolonged than true tonic-clonic seizures. Pelvic thrusting is common. Ictal eye closing is common in nonepileptic seizures, whereas the eyes tend to be open in true epileptic seizures (Chung et al., 2006). During and immediately after the seizure, the patient may not respond to verbal or painful stimuli. Cyanosis does not occur, and focal neurological signs and pathological reflexes are absent.

In the patient with known epilepsy, consider the diagnosis of nonepileptic seizures when previously controlled seizures become medically refractory. The patient should undergo psychological assessments because most affected persons are found to have specific psychiatric disturbances. In this patient group, a high frequency of hysteria, depression, anxiety, somatoform disorders, dissociative disorders, and personality disturbances is recognized. A history of physical or sexual abuse is also more prevalent in nonepileptic seizure patients. At times, a secondary gain is identifiable. In some patients with psychogenic seizures, the clinical episodes frequently precipitate by suggestion and by certain clinical tests such as hyperventilation, photic stimulation, intravenous saline infusion, tactile (vibration) stimulation, or pinching the nose to induce apnea. Hyperventilation and photic stimulation also may induce true epileptic seizures, but their clinical features usually are distinctive. Some physicians avoid the use of placebo procedures, because this could have an adverse effect on the doctor-patient relationship (Parra et al., 1998).

Findings on the interictal EEG in patients with pseudoseizures are normal and remain normal during the clinical episode, demonstrating no evidence of a cerebral dysrhythmia. With the introduction of long-term ambulatory EEG monitoring, correlating the episodic behavior of a patient with the EEG tracing is possible, and psychogenic seizures are distinguishable from true epileptic seizures. **Table 2.3** compares the features of psychogenic seizures with those of epileptic seizures.

As an auxiliary investigation of suspected psychogenic seizures, plasma prolactin concentrations may provide additional supportive data. Plasma prolactin concentrations frequently are elevated after tonic-clonic seizures, peaking in 15 to 20 minutes, and less frequently after complex partial seizures. Serum prolactin levels almost invariably are normal after psychogenic seizures, although such a finding does not exclude the diagnosis of true epileptic seizures (Chen et al., 2005). Elevated prolactin levels, however, also may be present after syncope and with the use of drugs such as antidepressants, estrogens, bromocriptine, ergots, phenothiazines, and antiepileptic drugs.

Although several procedures are employed to help distinguish epileptic from nonepileptic seizures, none of these procedures have both high sensitivity and high specificity. No procedure attains the reliability of EEG-video monitoring, which remains the standard diagnostic method for distinguishing between the two (Cuthill and Espie, 2005).

Table 2.3 Comparison of Psychogenic and Epileptic Seizures

Attack Feature	Psychogenic Seizure	Epileptic Seizure
Stereotypy of attack	May be variable	Usually stereotypical
Onset or progression	Gradual	More rapid
Duration	May be prolonged	Brief
Diurnal variation	Daytime	Nocturnal or daytime
Injury	Rare	Can occur with tonic-clonic seizures
Tongue biting	Rare (tip of tongue)	Can occur with tonic-clonic seizures (sides of tongue)
Ictal eye closure	Common	Rare (eyes generally open)
Urinary incontinence	Rare	Frequent
Vocalization	May occur	Uncommon
Motor activity	Prolonged, uncoordinated; pelvic thrusting	Automatisms or side-to-side head movements, flailing, coordinated tonic-clonic activity
Prolonged loss of muscle tone	Common	Rare
Postictal confusion	Rare	Common
Postictal headache	Rare	Common
Postictal crying	Common	Rare
Relation to medication changes	Unrelated	Usually related
Relation to menses in women	Uncommon	Occasionally increased
Triggers	Emotional disturbances	No
Frequency of attacks	More frequent, up to daily	Less frequent
Interictal EEG findings	Normal	Frequently abnormal
Reproduction of attack by suggestion	Sometimes	No
Ictal EEG findings	Normal	Abnormal
Presence of secondary gain	Common	Uncommon
Presence of others	Frequently	Variable
Psychiatric disturbances	Common	Uncommon

EEG, electroencephalogram.

Miscellaneous Causes of Altered Consciousness

In children, alteration of consciousness may accompany breath-holding spells and metabolic disturbances. Breath-holding spells and seizures are easily distinguished. Most spells start at 6 to 28 months of age, but they may occur as early as the first month of life; they usually disappear by 5 or 6 years of age. Breath-holding spells may occur several times per day and appear as either cyanosis or pallor.

The trigger for cyanotic breath-holding spells is usually a sudden injury or fright, anger, or frustration. The child initially is provoked, cries vigorously for a few breaths, and stops breathing in expiration, whereupon cyanosis rapidly develops. Consciousness is lost because of hypoxia. Although stiffening, a few clonic movements, and urinary incontinence occasionally are observed, these episodes can be clearly distinguished from epileptic seizures by the history of provocation and by noting that the apnea and cyanosis occur before any alteration of consciousness. In these children, findings on the neurological examination and the EEG are normal.

The provocation for pallid breath-holding is often a mild painful injury or a startle. The infant cries initially and then becomes pale and loses consciousness. As in the cyanotic type, stiffening, clonic movements, and urinary incontinence may rarely occur. In the pallid infant syndrome, loss of consciousness is secondary to excessive vagal tone, resulting in bradycardia and subsequent cerebral ischemia, as in a vasovagal attack.

Breath-holding spells do not require treatment, but when intervention is required, levetiracetam (Keppra) is effective for prophylaxis at ordinary anticonvulsant doses.

Several pediatric metabolic disorders may have clinical manifestations of alterations of consciousness, lethargy, or seizures (see Chapter 62).

References

The complete reference list is available online at www.expertconsult.com.

Chapter 3

Falls and Drop Attacks

Bernd F. Remler, Robert B. Daroff

Everyone occasionally loses balance and sometimes falls, but repeated and unprovoked falls signal a potentially serious neurological problem. Considering the large number of potential etiologies, it is helpful to determine whether a patient has suffered a drop attack or an accidental fall. The term *drop attack* describes a sudden fall occurring without warning that may or may not be associated with loss of consciousness. Falls, on the other hand, reflect an inability to remain upright during a postural challenge. This most commonly affects individuals with chronic neurological impairment. When associated with loss of consciousness, drop attacks are likely due to a syncopal or epileptic event. Patients with preserved consciousness during a drop attack may harbor midline tumors in the third ventricle or in the posterior fossa. Transient ischemic attacks (TIAs) involving the posterior circulation or the anterior cerebral artery distribution can manifest in the same monosymptomatic manner. Narcoleptics experience cataplexy, and patients with Meniere disease may fall abruptly as a result of otolith dysfunction. Patients with lower-extremity weakness, spasticity, rigidity, sensory loss, or ataxia frequently fall. Middle-aged women may fall with no discernible cause. Finally, the elderly, with their inevitable infirmities, fall frequently and with potentially disastrous consequences. These associations permit a classification of falls and drop attacks, presented in **Box 3.1**.

The medical history is essential in evaluating patients with falls and drop attacks. The situational and environmental circumstances of the event must be ascertained. To help establish a diagnosis from among the wide range of possible causes, a detailed interview of the patient or of a witness to the fall is required. Aside from the patient's gender and age, which affect fall risk, answers to the following basic questions should be elicited:

- Has the patient fallen before?
- Did the patient lose consciousness? If so, for how long?
- Did lightheadedness or palpitations precede the event?
- Is there a history of a seizure disorder, startle sensitivity, or of falls precipitated by strong emotions?
- Has the patient had excessive daytime sleepiness?
- Does the patient have headaches or migraine attacks associated with weakness?
- Does the patient have vascular risk factors, and were there previous symptoms suggestive of TIAs?
- Are there symptoms of sensory loss, limb weakness, or stiffness?
- Is there a history of visual impairment, hearing loss, vertigo, or tinnitus?

The neurological examination is equally important and can establish whether falls may be related to a disorder of the central or peripheral nervous system. Specific abnormalities include motor or sensory deficits in the lower limbs; the rigidity, tremor, and ocular motor abnormalities associated with Parkinson disease (PD) or progressive supranuclear palsy (PSP); ataxia, spasticity, cognitive impairment, and other signs suggestive of a neurodegenerative disorder or multiple sclerosis. Patients with normal findings on the neurological examination and no history of associated neurological or cardiac symptoms present a special challenge. In such patients, magnetic resonance imaging (MRI) and vascular imaging can be considered to rule out a clinically silent midline cerebral neoplasm, hindbrain malformation, or vascular occlusive disease. The workup is otherwise tailored to the clinical circumstance and may include cardiac and autonomic studies, nocturnal polysomnography, and in rare

---

Box 3.1 Causes and Types of Falls and Drops

Drop Attacks

With loss of consciousness:
  Syncope
  Seizures
Without loss of consciousness:
  Transient ischemic attacks:
    Vertebrobasilar insufficiency
    Anterior cerebral artery ischemia
  Third ventricular and posterior fossa tumors
  Chiari malformation
  Otolithic crisis

Falls

Basal ganglia disorders
Neuromuscular disorders (neuropathy, radiculopathy, and myopathy)
Other cerebral or cerebellar disorders
Cryptogenic falls in the middle-aged
Aged state

---

circumstances, genetic and metabolic testing if related conditions are suspected. Patients who frequently experience near-falls without injuries may have a psychogenic disorder of station and gait.

Loss of Consciousness

Syncope

The manifestations and causes of syncope are described in Chapter 2. Severe ventricular arrhythmias and hypotension lead to cephalic ischemia and falling. With sudden-onset third-degree heart block (Stokes-Adams attack), the patient loses consciousness and falls without warning. Less severe causes of decreased cardiac output, such as bradyarrhythmias or tachyarrhythmias, are associated with a prodromal sensation of faintness before the loss of consciousness. Elderly patients with cardioinhibitory sinus syndrome ("sick sinus syndrome"), however, often describe dizziness and falling rather than faintness, because of amnesia for the syncopal event. Thus, the history alone may not reveal the cardiovascular etiology of the fall. By contrast, cerebral hypoperfusion due to peripheral loss of vascular tone usually is associated with a presyncopal syndrome of progressive lightheadedness, faintness, dimming of vision, and "rubbery"-feeling legs. But even in the context of positive tilt table testing, up to 37% of patients report a clinically misleading symptom of true vertigo (Newman-Toker et al., 2008). So-called "cardiogenic vertigo" and downbeat nystagmus may also occur with asystole (Choi et al., 2010).

Orthostatic hypotension conveys a markedly increased risk of falling in the elderly and is particularly problematic in frail persons with additional risk factors for falling (Mussi et al., 2009) (see "Aged State" later in this chapter). Sudden drops in young persons, particularly when engaged in athletic activities, suggest a cardiac etiology. Exertional syncope requires a detailed cardiac evaluation to rule out valvular disease, right ventricular dysplasia, and other cardiomyopathies.

Seizures

Epileptic drop attacks are caused by several mechanisms, including asymmetrical tonic contractions of limb and axial muscles, loss of tone of postural muscles, and seizure-related cardiac arrhythmias. Arrhythmia-related drop attacks mimic cardiogenic syncope and, like temporal lobe drop attacks, typically are associated with a period of altered consciousness after the drop. Video-EEG monitoring of epileptic patients with a history of falls permits characterization of the various motor phenomena that cause loss of posture. For the clinician, however, the precise nature of these events is less important than establishing a diagnosis of seizures. This is straightforward in patients with long-standing epilepsy, but falls in patients with poststroke hemiparesis may be falsely attributed to motor weakness rather than to new-onset seizures. Destabilizing extensor spasms of spasticity can also be difficult to distinguish from focal seizures.

In children and adolescents with a history of drop attacks, a tilt-table test should be considered to avoid overdiagnosing epilepsy (Sabri et al., 2006). True epileptic drop attacks in young patients with severe childhood epilepsies may respond favorably to callosotomy (Sunaga, Shimizu, and Sugano, 2009). Falling as a consequence of the tonic axial component of startle-induced seizures may be controllable with lamotrigine. Paradoxically, some antiseizure drugs can precipitate drop attacks, such as carbamazepine in rolandic epilepsy.

Transient Ischemic Attacks

Drop attacks secondary to TIAs are sudden falls occurring without warning or obvious explanation such as tripping. Loss of consciousness either does not occur or is only momentary; the sensorium and lower limb strength are intact immediately or shortly after the patient hits the ground. The neurological examination should not reveal lower limb motor or sensory dysfunction between episodes. If such abnormalities are present, it can be impossible to distinguish drop attacks from the falls associated with sensorimotor impairment of the lower limbs. The vascular distributions for drop attacks from TIAs are the posterior circulation and the anterior cerebral arteries.

Vertebrobasilar Insufficiency

Drop attacks caused by posterior circulation insufficiency result from transient ischemia to the corticospinal tracts or the paramedian reticular formation. They are rarely an isolated manifestation of vertebrobasilar insufficiency, because most patients have a history of TIAs, including the more common signs and symptoms of vertigo, diplopia, ataxia, weakness, and hemisensory loss. Occasionally a drop attack may herald progressive thrombosis of the basilar artery hours before major and permanent neurological changes evolve.

Anterior Cerebral Artery Ischemia

Anterior cerebral artery ischemia causes drop attacks by impairing perfusion of the parasagittal premotor and motor cortex controlling the lower extremities. Origination of both anterior cerebral arteries from the same root occurs in approximately 20% of the population and predisposes to ischemic drop attacks from a single embolus. Paraparesis and even tetraparesis can result from simultaneous infarctions in bilateral ACA territories (Kang and Kim, 2008).

Third Ventricular and Posterior Fossa Tumors

Drop attacks can be a manifestation of colloid cysts of the third ventricle, Chiari malformation ("Chiari drop attack"), or mass lesions within the posterior fossa. With colloid cysts, unprovoked falling is the second most common symptom, after position-induced headaches. This history may be the only clinical clue to the diagnosis because the neurological examination can be entirely normal. Abrupt neck flexion may precipitate drop attacks in otherwise asymptomatic patients who are harboring posterior fossa tumors. Drop attacks occur in 2% to 3% of patients with Chiari malformation. These may be associated with loss of consciousness and often resolve after decompression surgery (Straus et al., 2009). Drops induced by rapid head turning were considered pathognomonic of cysticercosis of the fourth ventricle in the early 20th century (Brun sign). Other intracranial mass lesions such as parasagittal meningiomas, foramen magnum tumors, or subdural hematomas can also be associated with sudden drops. However, baseline abnormalities of gait and motor functions coexist, and falling may occur consequent to these impairments rather than to acute loss of muscle tone.

Otolithic Crisis

During attacks of vertigo, patients often lose balance and fall. Meniere disease (see Chapter 37) may be complicated by "vestibular drop attacks" unassociated with preceding or accompanying vertigo (Tumarkin otolithic crisis) in approximately 6% of patients. Presumably, stimulation of otolithic receptors in the saccule triggers inappropriate postural reflex adjustments via vestibulospinal pathways, leading to the falls. Affected patients report feeling as if, without warning, they are being thrown to the ground. They may fall straight down or be propelled in any direction. Indeed, one of the authors had a patient who reported suddenly seeing and feeling her legs moving forward in front of her as she did a spontaneous backflip secondary to an otolithic crisis. Vestibular drop attacks may also occur in elderly patients with unilateral vestibulopathies who do not satisfy diagnostic criteria for Meniere disease (Lee et al., 2005).

Disorders of the Basal Ganglia

Parkinson Disease

Patients with PD fall with a frequency of 81% over the long term and suffer twice as many fractures compared to age-matched controls. The forward-flexed posture, muscular rigidity, and bradykinesia of PD prevent compensatory weight shifts when balance is offset. Patients may also, without warning, drop directly to the ground. This phenomenon is most commonly related to dopamine-induced motor fluctuations, particularly peak-dose dyskinesias and off periods (see Chapter 71). Dopaminergic substitution and deep brain stimulation (DBS) improve step length and walking speed but have less effect on axial (vertical) locomotive components (Chastan et al., 2009). Vertical breaking speed, however, corresponds with an individual's ability to control falling and appears to depend on non-dopaminergic pathways. Positron emission tomography (PET) studies comparing PD patients with and without a history of falls indicate cortical and thalamic cholinergic hypofunction in those who fall, but no difference in nigrostriatal dopaminergic activity. Degeneration of the cholinergic pedunculopontine nucleus appears to be a key factor leading to impaired postural control in PD (Bohnen et al., 2009). These findings offer an explanation why DBS surgery does not appear to diminish fall risk (Hausdorff et al., 2009). Retropulsive tests are not fully predictable for falls in PD patients, but in combination with a self-reported fall history and risk factors such as dementia, disease duration, and benzodiazepine use, fallers can be reliably identified. Unfortunately, falling remains intractable in many PD patients, and prevention programs have demonstrated only limited benefit.

Progressive Supranuclear Palsy and other Parkinsonian Syndromes

Patients with PSP (see Chapter 71) have parkinsonian features, axial rigidity, nuchal dystonia, spasticity, and ophthalmoparesis. The fall frequency is 100%, and falling occurs early in the course of the illness (Williams, Watt, and Lees, 2006). Patients with PSP are more likely to fall backward than those with PD, even with equivalent functional impairment. Idiopathic rapid eye movement sleep behavior disorder (see Chapter 68) is a precursor of PSP and an underrecognized cause of nocturnal falls in the elderly. Clonazepam is commonly effective in the treatment of this parasomnia. Mechanisms similar to those described with PD and PSP contribute to falls in patients with other neurodegenerative disorders causing parkinsonism. Recurrent falls are a prominent feature of multiple system atrophy, the pure akinesia syndrome, corticobasal ganglionic degeneration, and especially of Lewy body disease (see Chapter 71), because of the additional cognitive dimension of neurological disability.

Neuromuscular Disorders and Myelopathy

Myopathies characteristically involve proximal muscles and increase the tendency to fall. The multiple causes of neuropathy and myopathy (genetically determined or acquired) are discussed in Chapters 76 and 79, respectively. Most lumbosacral radiculopathies and neuropathies are mixed (i.e., motor and sensory) in type. Regardless of cause, these conditions predispose patients to falling because of lower limb weakness and impaired afferent sensations from feet, joints, and muscles. Sensory neuropathies delay or reduce the relay of sensory signals from the lower limbs and promote falling when postural imbalance occurs. Falling may herald the onset of acute polyneuropathies such as Guillain-Barré syndrome. Aging polio survivors have a high annual frequency of falling that may exceed 60% (Silver and Aiello, 2002). Patients with spinal cord disease (see Chapter 24) are at particularly high risk of falling because all descending motor and ascending sensory tracts traverse the cord. Aside from weakness, spasticity, and impaired sensory input from the lower limbs, there is disruption of vestibulospinal and cerebellar pathways. A high rate of injurious falls is reported by MS patients aged 55 and older (Peterson et al., 2008).

Stroke

Motor, sensory, vestibular, and cerebellar dysfunction occur in isolation or in any combination in patients with stroke. Acute lesions of central otolithic pathways in the brainstem and basal ganglia produce contralateral tilting of variable intensity that can lead to falls. Weakness, truncal ataxia, extensive visual field defects and hemineglect due to right hemispheric stroke are obvious risk factors of falling. In the chronic state, depression and diminished arm function further enhance this risk, which is at least twice as high compared to age-matched controls. The poststroke risk of a hip fracture is increased by the same factor and is particularly high in women and within 3 months of the ischemic event (Pouwels et al., 2009).

In October of 2008, the CMS (Centers for Medicare and Medicaid in the United States) implemented payment changes to encourage avoidance of high-cost and high-volume complications in hospitalized patients, including falls and related injuries. The shift in associated financial burden to hospitals has resulted in increased efforts to reduce such events. But even well-implemented programs, on average, have prevention rates not exceeding 20%, and the absolute number of fractures may not be reduced (Oliver et al., 2007). Concerns about adverse financial consequences could lead to excessive restrictions of patient mobility in acute care and rehabilitation facilities (Inouye, Brown, and Tinetti, 2009), as falls typically occur when patients attempt to get out of bed, stand up, or walk.

Other Cerebral or Cerebellar Disorders

Metabolic encephalopathies may cause a characteristic transient loss of postural tone (asterixis). If this is extensive and involves the axial musculature, episodic loss of the upright posture can mimic drop attacks in patients with chronic uremia. Cerebellar disease causes truncal instability and represents a prime cause of falling. Patients with degenerative cerebellar ataxias (see Chapter 72) have a 50% frequency of falls in any 3-month period of observation. Episodic ataxia syndromes and familial hemiplegic migraine are also associated with recurrent falls (Black, 2006). Severe attacks of hyperekplexia, a familial disorder of startle sensitivity, are associated with generalized hypertonia that can lead to an uncontrollable fall. Effective prevention with clonazepam, valproate, or piracetam is available. Beneficial treatment can also be offered to properly diagnosed patients with normal-pressure hydrocephalus; ventriculoperitoneal shunting leads to dramatic improvement of gait and decreased risk of falls.

Cataplexy, the sudden loss of lower limb tone, is a part of the tetrad of narcolepsy that also includes excessive daytime sleepiness, hypnagogic hallucinations, and sleep paralysis (see Chapter 68). Consciousness is preserved during a cataplectic attack, which may vary in severity from slight lower limb weakness to generalized and complete flaccid paralysis with abrupt falling. Once on the ground, the patient is unable to move but continues to breathe. The attacks usually last less

than 1 minute, only rarely exceeding several minutes in duration. Cataplectic attacks are provoked by strong emotion and associated with laughter, anger, surprise, or startle. Occasionally they interrupt or follow sexual orgasm. During the attack, electromyographic silence in antigravity muscles is seen, and deep tendon reflexes and the H-reflex (see Chapter 32B) cannot be elicited. Cataplexy occurs in the absence of narcolepsy when associated with cerebral disease (symptomatic cataplexy), as in Niemann-Pick disease, Norrie disease, brainstem lesions, or as a paraneoplastic disorder (Farid et al., 2009). It may rarely occur as an isolated problem in normal persons in whom the predisposition may be familial. A liquid formulation of gamma-hydroxybutyrate (sodium oxybate), an agent infamous for its use in "date rape," is available for the treatment of cataplexy.

Cryptogenic Falls in the Middle-Aged

A diagnostic enigma is the occurrence of falls of unknown etiology among a subset of women older than 40 years of age. The fall usually is forward and occurs without warning during walking. The knees are often bruised (Thijs, Bloem, and van Dijk, 2009). Affected women report no loss of consciousness, dizziness, or even a sense of imbalance. They are convinced that they have not tripped but that their legs suddenly gave way. Gait is normal after the fall. This condition is estimated to affect 3% of women and develops after the age of 40 in the majority of affected patients. Familial occurrence has been reported. Originally described as a disorder of unknown causality, more recent inquiry into the frequency of falls in middle-aged and older women in the general population has elicited fall frequencies from 8% in women in their forties to 47% in their seventies. Age and number of comorbidities such as diabetes and neuropathies are most predictive of falling (Nitz and Choy, 2008).

Vestibular dysfunction of variable severity is also unexpectedly common in the adult population and can be seen in 35% of individuals over the age of 40. Symptomatic (dizzy) patients have a 12-fold increase in the odds of falling (Agrawal et al., 2009). Fibromyalgia is associated with vestibular symptoms and an increased fall frequency (Jones et al., 2009). These observations suggest that risk factors for falls are prevalent already in middle age and may correlate with falling later in life. Maintenance of good health is mandatory to contain the inevitable progression toward greater susceptibility to falls as age progresses.

Aged State

Most patients presenting to neurologists with a chief complaint of falling are elderly and chronically impaired. About one-third of persons older than 65 fall at least once every year (CDC, 2008). As the likelihood of falling increases with age, so does the severity of injury, as well as the number of chronic disabilities predisposing to falls. Next to fractures, falls are the single most disabling condition leading to admission to long-term care facilities. As would be expected, elderly in sheltered accommodations have the highest frequency of falls, affecting up to 50% every year. Many of these patients fall repeatedly, with women bearing a higher risk than men. Women also experience more fractures after falling, while men are more likely to suffer traumatic brain injury (TBI) (CDC, 2010). The high prevalence of anticoagulant and antiplatelet use in the elderly raises questions about the risk of intracranial bleeding in fall-related TBI. Paradoxically, low-dose aspirin may be protective in this regard (Gangavati et al., 2009) but can also cause delayed intracranial bleeding within 12 to 24 hours after head trauma (Tauber et al., 2009). The presence of an intracranial hemorrhage in conjunction with warfarin use indicates an increased risk of further clinical deterioration, even if the patient is awake upon admission (Howard et al., 2009). In the very old, falls constitute the leading cause of injury-related deaths, with TBI causing at least one-third of 15,000+ fall-related fatalities every year. Complications of hip fractures cause most of the other fatalities (Deprey, 2009). The direct and indirect cost of fall injuries is staggering and may rise from an estimated $19 billion in 2000 to over $50 billion by 2020 (CDC, 2010).

The normal aging process is associated with a decline in multiple physiological functions that alter body mechanics and diminish the ability to compensate for challenges to the upright posture. Decreased proprioception; loss of muscle bulk; arthritic joints; cardiovascular disturbances; deteriorating visual, ocular, motor, and vestibular functions (Serrardor et al., 2009); cognitive impairment; and failing postural reflexes (presbyastasis) summate to increase the risk of falling. Even the healthy elderly demonstrate significant alterations in quantitative gait characteristics (Chong et al., 2009). It is estimated that by the age of 65, only 1 in 10 persons show gait abnormalities , but by the age of 85, only 1 in 10 have a normal gait. The increased risk of injuries and fractures with falling is explained by a declining ability to absorb fall energy with the upper extremities (Sran et al., 2010), the diminishing size of soft-tissue pads around joints (in particular the hips), and osteoporosis.

Aside from age-related physical changes, the fall risk in elderly persons is further enhanced by numerous acquired neurological and medical conditions. Among more recently recognized disease states are chronic obstructive pulmonary disease (COPD) (Beauchamp et al., 2009), fatigue associated with fragmented sleep (Stone et al., 2008), and sleep apnea (Onen et al., 2009). The role of diffuse cerebral white matter disease as a contributing factor to gait abnormalities is reflected by strong correlations between bilateral frontal and periventricular changes with poorer gait (Srikanth et al., 2010). In turn, white matter disease and slower gait are associated with impaired cerebral vasoreactivity (Sorond et al., 2010). Other abnormal laboratory results evolving as markers of fall risk include asymptomatic hyponatremia, increased parathyroid levels, reduced testosterone levels in men, evidence for urinary tract infection, and vitamin D deficiency (LeBoff et al., 2008).

Walking requires attentional resources, which are stressed during dual tasks. The "stops walking when talking" sign as an indicator of fall risk is based on this physiological relationship (Beauchet et al., 2009). In the cognitively impaired, visuospatial dysfunction further enhances the fall risk. In part, this explains the much higher fall rates in elderly with Alzheimer disease and Lewy body disease.

The neurologist examining a patient after a fall needs to identify predisposing medical conditions and differentiate an accidental from an endogenous fall event. A detailed inventory of medications is essential, and a description of environmental factors contributing to the fall should be obtained from the patient or from a person familiar with the living circumstances. In elderly persons, the majority of falls are accidental, reflecting an interaction between an impaired individual and environmental or situational (attempting to get up and walk) hazards. In the absence of an overt explanation for falls, a syncopal event for which the patient may be amnestic becomes more likely. The immense burden of falling to patients and society necessitates recognition of an increased risk of future falls. Detailed practice parameters and guidelines have been published (Thurman et al., 2008; American Geriatric Society and British Geriatric Society Panel, 2011) and reiterate that a history of falls and the presence of motor, sensory, coordinative, and cognitive dysfunction are predictive. This risk is further enhanced by medications, in particular sedatives, hypnotics, antidepressants, and benzodiazepines (Woolcott et al., 2009).

Intervention for falling elders requires a multifaceted approach (Tinetti and Kumar, 2010; American Geriatric Society and British Geriatric Society Panel, 2011). Depending on the clinical situation, this may include provision of assistive devices (orthotics, canes, and walkers), treatment of orthostasis or cardiac dysrhythmias, and modification of environmental hazards identified during home visits. All unnecessary medications that increase the risk of falls should be discontinued. High-risk behavior such as the use of ladders and moving about at low levels of illumination is discouraged, and women are advised to wear sturdy low-heeled shoes. Balance training such as Tai Chi and exercises aimed at improving strength and endurance diminish fall rates. Behavioral intervention for the development of fear of falling after such events can be effective and is strongly encouraged (Dukyoo, Juhee, and Lee, 2009). Further useful interventions include vitamin D substitution (>800 International Units/day), improvement of vision with cataract surgery (Foss et al., 2006), and statin treatment for prevention of osteoporotic fractures. However, none of these measures abolish the risk of falling, and even well-intended interventions may be associated with an increased fall risk. Unexpectedly, this was shown in some patients who received new prescription eyeglass lenses (Campbell, Sanderson, and Robertson, 2010) and for the convenient annual dosing of 500,000 International Units of vitamin D, which not only enhanced the risk of falls but also fractures (Sanders et al., 2010). Use of walkers is associated with the highest fall risk, raising the question whether these ubiquitous devices have inherent design flaws that are contributory (Stevens et al., 2009).

Presently, falls in the elderly remain an intractable problem. Moderate benefit on fall rates and cost-effectiveness of interventional programs has been demonstrated (Tinetti and Kumar, 2010; Hektoen, Aas, and Luras, 2009). However, populations at high risk for falls and those with dementia may not benefit at all (deVries et al., 2010). The efficacy of interventional programs could potentially be improved by broader involvement of falling elderly, ongoing program participation, and regular home visits. Biomedical engineers are developing devices that aim to diminish adverse consequences of falls, including sensors that detect and announce falling, low-stiffness flooring, and soft, protective shells that are more acceptable than currently available hard shells worn on the hips. Advances like these, along with screening of elderly persons for fall risk and preventive program enrollment, may eventually diminish the burden of this epidemic.

Summary

A careful history and physical examination should in most cases uncover the cause of falls and drop attacks. Unfortunately, with middle-aged women and the elderly, the cause may be merely a function of gender or age. Patients with fixed motor or sensory impairments must be advised honestly about their almost unavoidable tendency to fall. Nevertheless, some specific treatments for falls and drop attacks exist. Environmental adjustments, participation in fall prevention programs, and use of protective devices can reduce the frequency of falls and related injuries.

References

The complete reference list is available online at www.expertconsult.com.

Delirium

Mario F. Mendez, Sarah A. Kremen

Delirium is an acute mental status change characterized by abnormal and fluctuating attention. There is a disturbance in level of awareness and reduced ability to direct, focus, sustain, and shift attention (American Psychiatric Association, DSM-V, Proposed Revision, 2013). These difficulties additionally impair other areas of cognition. The syndrome of delirium can be a physiological consequence of a medical condition or stem from a primary neurological cause.

Delirium is by far the most common behavioral disorder in a medical-surgical setting. In general hospitals, the prevalence ranges from 11% to 33% on admission. The incidence ranges between 6% and 56% of hospitalized patients, 15% to 53% postoperatively in elderly patients, and 80% or more of intensive care unit (ICU) patients (Fong, Tulebaev, and Inouye, 2009; Michaud et al., 2007). The consequences of delirium are serious: They include prolonged hospitalizations, increased mortality, high rates of discharges to other institutions, severe impact on caregivers and spouses, and between $38 billion and $152 billion annually in direct healthcare costs in the United States (Breitbart, Gibson, and Tremblay, 2002; Fong, Tulebaev, and Inouye, 2009; Inouye et al., 1999).

Physicians have known about this disorder since antiquity. Hippocrates referred to it as *phrenitis*, the origin of our word *frenzy*. In the 1st century AD, Celsus introduced the term *delirium*, from the Latin for "out of furrow," meaning derailment of the mind, and Galen observed that delirium was often due to physical diseases that affected the mind "sympathetically." In the 19th century, Gowers recognized that these patients could be either lethargic or hyperactive. Bonhoeffer, in his classification of organic behavioral disorders, established that delirium is associated with clouding of consciousness. Finally, Engel and Romano (1959) described alpha slowing with delta and theta intrusions on electroencephalograms (EEGs) and correlated these changes with clinical severity. They noted that treating the medical cause resulted in reversal of both the clinical and EEG changes of delirium.

Despite this long history, physicians, nurses, and other clinicians often fail to diagnose delirium (Cole, 2004; Inouye et al., 2001), and up to two-thirds of delirium cases go unidentified (Inouye, 2004). Healthcare providers often miss this syndrome more from lack of recognition than misdiagnosis. The elderly in particular may have a "quieter," more subtle presentation of delirium that may evade detection. Adding to the confusion about delirium are the many terms used to describe this disorder: acute confusional state, acute organic syndrome, acute brain failure, acute brain syndrome, acute cerebral insufficiency, exogenous psychosis, metabolic encephalopathy, organic psychosis, ICU psychosis, toxic encephalopathy, toxic psychosis, and others.

Clinicians must take care to distinguish delirium from dementia, the other common disorder of cognitive functioning. Delirium is acute in onset (usually hours to a few days) whereas dementia is chronic (usually insidious in onset and progressive). The definition of delirium must emphasize an acute behavioral decompensation with fluctuating attention, regardless of etiology or the presence of baseline cognitive deficits or dementia. Complicating this distinction is the fact that underlying dementia is a major risk factor for delirium.

Clinicians must also take care to define the terms used with delirium. *Attention* is the ability to focus on specific stimuli to the exclusion of others. *Awareness* is the ability to perceive or be conscious of events or experiences. *Arousal*, a basic prerequisite for attention, indicates responsiveness or excitability into action. *Coma*, *stupor*, *wakefulness*, and *alertness* are states of arousal. *Consciousness*, a product of arousal, means clarity of awareness of the environment. *Confusion* is the inability for clear and coherent thought and speech.

Clinical Characteristics

The essential elements of delirium are summarized in **Boxes 4.1 and 4.2**. Among the proposed American Psychiatric

Box 4.1 Clinical Characteristics of Delirium

Acute onset of mental status change with fluctuating course
Attentional deficits
Confusion or disorganized thinking
Altered level of consciousness
Perceptual disturbances
Disturbed sleep/wake cycle
Altered psychomotor activity
Disorientation and memory impairment
Other cognitive deficits
Behavioral and emotional abnormalities

Box 4.2 *Diagnostic and Statistical Manual of Mental Disorders*, Fifth edition, Proposed Revision, Criteria for Delirium due to a General Medical Condition

A. Disturbance in level of awareness and reduced ability to direct, focus, sustain, and shift attention
B. A change in cognition (such as deficits in orientation, executive ability, language, visuoperception, learning, and memory):
  ▪ Cannot be assessed in face of severely reduced level of awareness
  ▪ Should not be better accounted for by a preexisting neurocognitive disorder
C. There is evidence from the history, physical examination, or laboratory findings that the disturbance is caused by the direct physiological consequences of a general medical condition
D. The disturbance develops over a short period of time (usually hours to a few days) and tends to fluctuate in severity during the course of a day

NOTE: The following supportive features are commonly present in delirium but are not key diagnostic features: sleep/wake cycle disturbance, psychomotor disturbance, perceptual disturbances (e.g., hallucinations, illusions), emotional disturbances, delusions, labile affect, dysarthria, and EEG abnormalities (generalized slowing of background activity)

Modified from American Psychiatric Association. Diagnostic and Statistical Manual of Mental Disorders, fifth ed., proposed revision. American Psychiatric Association, Washington, DC.

Association's criteria (DSM-V Proposed Revision, 2013) for this disorder is a disturbance that develops over a short period of time; tends to fluctuate; and impairs awareness, attention, and other areas of cognition. In general, awareness, attention, and cognition fluctuate over the course of a day. Furthermore, delirious patients have disorganized thinking and an altered level of consciousness, perceptual disturbances, disturbance of the sleep/wake cycle, increased or decreased psychomotor activity, disorientation, and memory impairment. Other cognitive, behavioral, and emotional disturbances may also occur as part of the spectrum of delirium. Delirium can be summarized into the 10 clinical characteristics that follow.

Acute Onset with Fluctuating Course

Delirium develops rapidly over hours or days, but rarely over more than a week, and fluctuations in the course occur throughout the day. There are lucid intervals interspersed with the daily fluctuations. Gross swings in attention and awareness, arousal, or both occur unpredictably and irregularly and become worse at night. Because of potential lucid intervals, medical personnel may be misled by patients who exhibit improved attention and awareness unless these patients are evaluated over time.

Cognitive and Related Abnormalities
Attentional Deficits

A disturbance of attention and consequent altered awareness is the cardinal symptom of delirium. Patients are distractible, and stimuli may gain attention indiscriminately, trivial ones often getting more attention than important ones. All components of attention are disturbed, including selectivity, sustainability, processing capacity, ease of mobilization, monitoring of the environment, and the ability to shift attention when necessary. Although many of the same illnesses result in a spectrum of disturbances from mild inattention to coma, delirium is not the same as disturbance of arousal.

Confusion or Disorganized Thinking

Delirious patients are unable to maintain the stream of thought with accustomed clarity, coherence, and speed. There are multiple intrusions of competing thoughts and sensations, and patients are unable to order symbols, carry out sequenced activity, and organize goal-directed behavior.

The patient's speech reflects this jumbled thinking. Speech shifts from subject to subject and is rambling, tangential, and circumlocutory, with hesitations, repetitions, and perseverations. Decreased relevance of the speech content and decreased reading comprehension are characteristic of delirium. Confused speech is further characterized by an abnormal rate, frequent dysarthria, and nonaphasic misnaming, particularly of words related to stress or illness, such as those referable to hospitalization.

Altered Level of Consciousness

Consciousness, or clarity of awareness, may be disturbed. Most patients have lethargy and decreased arousal. Others, such as those with delirium tremens, are hyperalert and easily aroused. In hyperalert patients, the extreme arousal does not preclude attentional deficits because patients are indiscriminate in their alertness, are easily distracted by irrelevant stimuli, and cannot sustain attention. The two extremes of consciousness may overlap or alternate in the same patient or may occur from the same causative factor.

Perceptual Disturbances

The most common perceptual disturbance is decreased perceptions per unit of time; patients miss things that are going on around them. Illusions and other misperceptions result from abnormal sensory discrimination. Perceptions may be multiple, changing, or abnormal in size or location. Hallucinations also occur, particularly in younger patients and in those in the hyperactive subtype. They are most common in the visual sphere and are often vivid, three-dimensional, and in full color. Patients may see lilliputian animals or people that appear to move about. Hallucinations are generally unpleasant, and some patients attempt to fight them or run away with fear. Some hallucinatory experiences may be release phenomena, with intrusions of dreams or visual imagery into wakefulness. Psychotic auditory hallucinations with voices commenting on the patient's behavior are unusual.

Disturbed Sleep/Wake Cycle

Disruption of the day/night cycle causes excessive daytime drowsiness and reversal of the normal diurnal rhythm. "Sundowning"—with restlessness and confusion during the night—is common, and delirium may be manifest only at night. Nocturnal peregrinations can result in a serious problem when the delirious patient, partially clothed in a hospital gown, has to be retrieved from the hospital lobby or from the street in the middle of the night. This is one of the least specific symptoms and also occurs in dementia, depression, and other behavioral conditions. In delirium, however, disruption of circadian sleep cycles may result in rapid eye movement or dream-state overflow into waking.

Altered Psychomotor Activity

There are two subtypes of delirium, based on changes in psychomotor activity. The hypoactive-hypoalert subtype is characterized by psychomotor retardation. These are the patients with lethargy and decreased arousal. The hyperactive-hyperalert subtype is usually hyperalert and agitated and has prominent overactivity of the autonomic nervous system. Moreover, the hyperactive type is more likely to have delusions and perceptual disorders such as hallucinations. About half of patients with delirium manifest elements of both subtypes or fluctuate between the two. Only about 15% are strictly hyperactive. In addition to the patients being younger, the hyperactive subtype has more drug-related causes, a shorter hospital stay, and a better prognosis.

Disorientation and Memory Impairment

Disturbances in orientation and memory are related. Patients are disoriented first to time of day, followed by other aspects of time, and then to place. They may perceive abnormal juxtapositions of events or places. Disorientation to person—in the sense of loss of personal identity—is rare. Disorientation is one of the most common findings in delirium but is not specific for delirium; it occurs in dementia and amnesia as well. Among patients with delirium, recent memory is disrupted in large part by the decreased registration caused by attentional problems.

In delirium, reduplicative paramnesia, a specific memory-related disorder, results from decreased integration of recent observations with past memories. Persons or places are "replaced" in this condition. In general, delirious patients tend to mistake the unfamiliar for the familiar. For example, they tend to relocate the hospital closer to their homes. In a form of reduplicative paramnesia known as *Capgras syndrome*, however, a familiar person is mistakenly thought to be an unfamiliar impostor.

Other Cognitive Deficits

Disturbances occur in visuospatial abilities and in writing. Higher visual-processing deficits include difficulties in visual object recognition, environmental orientation, and organization of drawings and other constructions.

Writing disturbance may be the most sensitive language abnormality in delirium. The most salient characteristics are abnormalities in the mechanics of writing: The formation of letters and words is indistinct, and words and sentences sprawl in different directions (**Fig. 4.1**). There is a reluctance to write, and there are motor impairments (e.g., tremors, micrographia) and spatial disorders (e.g., misalignment, leaving insufficient space for the writing sample). Sometimes the writing shows perseverations of loops or aspects of the writing. Spelling and syntax are also disturbed, with spelling errors particularly involving consonants, small grammatical words (prepositions and conjunctions), and the last letters of words. Writing is easily disrupted in these disorders, possibly because it depends on multiple components and is the least used language function.

Behavioral and Emotional Abnormalities

Behavioral changes include poorly systematized delusions, often with persecutory and other paranoid ideation and personality alterations. Delusions, like hallucinations, are probably release phenomena and are generally fleeting, changing, and readily affected by sensory input. These delusions are most often persecutory. Some patients exhibit facetious humor and playful behavior, lack of concern about their illness, poor insight, impaired judgment, and confabulation.

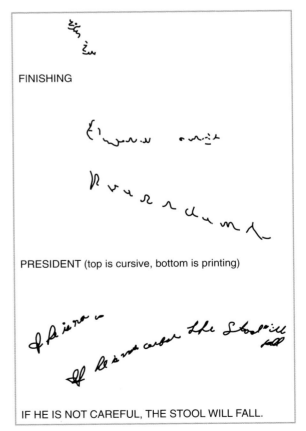

FINISHING

PRESIDENT (top is cursive, bottom is printing)

IF HE IS NOT CAREFUL, THE STOOL WILL FALL.

Fig. 4.1 Writing disturbances in delirium. Patients were asked to write indicated words to dictation. *(Reprinted with permission from Chédru, J., Geschwind, N., 1972. Writing disturbances in acute confusional states. Neuropsychologia 10, 343-353.)*

There can be marked emotional lability. Sometimes patients are agitated and fearful or depressed or quite apathetic. Dysphoric (unpleasant) emotional states are the more common, and emotions are not sustained. Up to half of elderly delirious patients display symptoms of depression with low mood, loss of interests, fatigue, decreased appetite and sleep, and other feelings related to depression. There may be mood-congruent delusions and hallucinations. The mood changes of delirium are probably due to direct effects of the confusional state on the limbic system and its regulation of emotions.

Finally, more elementary behavioral changes may be the principal symptoms of delirium. This is especially the case in the elderly, in whom decreased activities of daily living, urinary incontinence, and frequent falls are among the major manifestations of this disorder.

Pathophysiology

The pathophysiology of delirium is not entirely understood, but it depends on widely distributed neurological dysfunction. Delirium is the final common pathway of many pathophysiological disturbances that reduce or alter cerebral oxidative metabolism. These metabolic changes result in diffuse impairment in multiple neuronal pathways and systems.

Several brain areas involved in attention are particularly disturbed in delirium. Dysfunction of the anterior cingulate cortex is involved in disturbances of the management of attention (Reischies et al., 2005). Other areas include the bilateral or right prefrontal cortex in attentional maintenance and executive control, the temporoparietal junction region in disengaging and shifting attention, the thalamus in engaging attention, and the upper brainstem structures in moving the focus of attention. The thalamic nuclei are uniquely positioned to screen incoming sensory information, and small lesions in the thalamus may cause delirium. In addition, there is evidence that the right hemisphere is dominant for attention. Cortical blood flow studies suggest that right hemisphere cortical areas and their limbic connections are the "attentional gate" for sensory input through feedback to the reticular nucleus of the thalamus.

Another explanation for delirium is alterations in neurotransmitters, particularly a cholinergic-dopaminergic imbalance. There is extensive evidence for a cholinergic deficit in delirium (Inouye, 2006). Anticholinergic agents can induce the clinical and EEG changes of delirium, which are reversible with the administration of cholinergic medications such as physostigmine. The beneficial effects of donepezil, rivastigmine, and galantamine—acetylcholinesterase-inhibitor medications used for Alzheimer disease—may be partly due to an activating or attention-enhancing role. Moreover, cholinergic neurons project from the pons and the basal forebrain to the cortex and make cortical neurons more responsive to other inputs. A decrease in acetylcholine results in decreased perfusion in the frontal cortex. Hypoglycemia, hypoxia, and other metabolic changes may differentially affect acetylcholine-mediated functions. Other neurotransmitters may be involved in delirium, including dopamine, serotonin, norepinephrine, γ-aminobutyric acid, glutamine, opiates, and histamine. Dopamine has an inhibitory effect on the release of acetylcholine, hence the delirium-producing effects of L-dopa and other antiparkinsonism medications (Trzepacz and van der Mast, 2002). Opiates may induce the effects by increasing dopamine and glutamate activity. Recently, polymorphisms in genes coding for a dopamine transporter and two dopamine receptors have been associated with the development of delirium (van Munster et al., 2010).

Inflammatory cytokines such as interleukins, interferon, and tumor necrosis factor alpha (TNF-α), may contribute to delirium by altering blood-brain barrier permeability and further affecting neurotransmission (Cole, 2004; Fong et al., 2009; Inouye, 2006). The combination of inflammatory mediators and dysregulation of the limbic-hypothalamic-pituitary axis may lead to exacerbation or prolongation of delirium (Maclullich et al., 2008). Finally, secretion of melatonin, a hormone integral to circadian rhythm and the sleep/wake cycle, may be abnormal in delirious patients compared to those without delirium (van Munster, de Rooij, and Korevaar, 2009).

Diagnosis

Diagnosis is a two-step process. The first step is the recognition of delirium, which requires a thorough history, a bedside mental status examination focusing on attention, and a review of established diagnostic scales or criteria for delirium. The second step is to identify the cause from a large number of potential diagnoses. Because the clinical manifestations offer few clues to the cause, crucial to the differential diagnosis are the general history, physical examination, and laboratory assessments.

The general history assesses several elements. An abrupt decline in mentation, particularly in the hospital, should be presumed to be delirium. Although patients may state that they cannot think straight or concentrate, family members or other good historians should be available to describe the patient's behavior and medical history. The observer may have noted early symptoms of delirium such as inability to perform at a usual level, decreased awareness of complex details, insomnia, and frightening or vivid dreams. It is crucial to obtain accurate information about systemic illnesses, drug use, recent trauma, occupational and environmental exposures, malnutrition, allergies, and any preceding symptoms leading to delirium. Furthermore, the clinician should thoroughly review the patient's medication list.

Predisposing and Precipitating Factors

The greater the number of predisposing factors, the fewer or milder are the precipitating factors needed to result in delirium (Anderson, 2005) (**Box 4.3**). Four factors independently predispose to delirium: vision impairments (<20/70 binocular), severity of illness, cognitive impairment, and dehydration (high ratio of blood urea to creatinine) (Inouye, 2006). Among these, cognitive impairment or dementia is worth emphasizing. Elderly patients with dementia are five times more likely to develop delirium than those without dementia (Elie et al., 1998). Patients with dementia may develop delirium after minor medication changes or other relatively insignificant precipitating factors (Inouye, 2006). Moreover, premorbid impairment in executive functions may be independently associated with greater risk of developing delirium (Rudolph et al., 2006). Other important predisposing factors for delirium are advanced age, especially older than 80 years, and the presence of chronic medical illnesses (Johnson, 2001). Many of these elderly patients predisposed to delirium have cerebral atrophy or white matter and basal ganglia ischemic changes

---

Box 4.3 Predisposing and Precipitating Factors for Delirium

Elderly, especially 80 years or older

Dementia, cognitive impairment, or other brain disorder

Fluid and electrolyte disturbances and dehydration

Other metabolic disturbance, especially elevated BUN level or hepatic insufficiency

Number and severity of medical illnesses including cancer

Infections, especially urinary tract, pulmonary, and AIDS

Malnutrition, low serum albumin level

Cardiorespiratory failure or hypoxemia

Prior stroke or other nondementia brain disorder

Polypharmacy and use of analgesics, psychoactive drugs, or anticholinergics

Drug abuse, alcohol or sedative dependency

Sensory impairment, especially visual

Sensory overstimulation and "ICU psychosis"

Sensory deprivation

Sleep disturbance

Functional impairment

Fever, hypothermia

Physical trauma or severe burns

Fractures

Male gender

Depression

Specific surgeries:

    Cardiac, especially open heart surgery

    Orthopedic, especially femoral neck and hip fractures, bilateral knee replacements

    Ophthalmological, especially cataract surgery

    Noncardiac thoracic surgery and aortic aneurysmal repairs

    Transurethral resection of the prostate

AIDS, Acquired immunodeficiency syndrome; *BUN*, blood urea nitrogen; *ICU*, intensive care unit.

on neuroimaging. Additional predisposing factors are the degree of physical impairment, hip and other bone fractures, serum sodium changes, infections and fevers, and the use of multiple drugs, particularly those with narcotic, anticholinergic, or psychoactive properties. The predisposing factors for delirium are additive, each new factor increasing the risk considerably. Moreover, frail elderly patients often have multiple predisposing factors, the most common being functional dependency, multiple medical comorbidities, depression, and polypharmacy (Laurila et al., 2008).

In most cases, the cause of delirium is multifactorial, resulting from the interaction between patient-specific predisposing factors and multiple precipitating factors (Inouye and Charpentier, 1996; Laurila et al., 2008). Five specific factors that can independently precipitate delirium are use of physical restraints, malnutrition or weight loss (albumin levels less than 30 g/L), use of indwelling bladder catheters, adding more than three medications within a 24-hour period, and an iatrogenic medical complication (Inouye and Charpentier, 1996). Other precipitating factors for incident delirium after hospitalization include electrolyte disturbances (hyponatremia, hypercalcemia, etc.), major organ system disease, occult respiratory failure, occult infection, pain, specific medications such as sedative-hypnotics or histamine-2 blockers, sleep

disturbances, and alterations in the environment. Novel situations and unfamiliar surroundings contribute to sensory overstimulation in the elderly, and sensory overload may be a factor in producing "ICU psychosis." Ultimately, delirium occurs in patients from a synergistic interaction of predisposing factors with precipitating factors.

In addition to the risk factors already discussed, heritability of delirium is a new area of investigation. The presence of genes such as apolipoprotein E (APOE), dopamine receptor genes DRD2 and DRD3, and the dopamine transporter gene, SLC6A3, are possible pathophysiological vulnerabilities for delirium (van Munster et al., 2009; van Munster et al., 2010). Despite conflicting data, there is evidence for an association between APOE ε4 carriers and a longer duration of delirium (van Munster et al., 2009). Polymorphisms in SLC6A3 and DRD2 have occurred in association with delirium from alcohol and in elderly delirious patients with hip fractures (van Munster et al., 2009; van Munster et al., 2010).

Mental Status Examination

Initial general behavioral observations are an important part of the neurological mental status examination. The most important are observations of attentiveness and arousability. Attention may wander so much that it must constantly be brought back to the subject at hand. General behavior may range from falling asleep during the interview to agitation and combativeness. Slow and loosely connected thinking and speech may be present, with irrelevancies, perseverations, repetitions, and intrusions. Patients may propagate their errors in thinking and perception by elaboration or confabulation. Finally, the examiner should evaluate the patient's general appearance and grooming, motor activity and spontaneity, mood and affect, propriety and witticisms, and the presence of any special preoccupations or inaccurate perceptions.

Bedside tests of attention can be divided into serial recitation tasks, continuous performance tasks, and alternate response tasks. The digit span test is a serial recitation task in which a series of digits is presented, one digit per second, and the patient is asked to repeat the entire sequence immediately after presentation. Perceptual clumping is avoided by the use of random digits and a regular rhythm of presentation. Correct recitation of seven (plus or minus two) digits is considered normal. The serial reversal test is a form of recitation task in which the patient recites backward a digit span, the spelling of a word such as *world*, or the results of counting by ones, threes, or sevens from a predetermined number. Continuous performance tasks include the *A* vigilance test, in which the patient must indicate whenever the letter *A* is heard among random letters presented one per second. This can also be done visually by asking the patient to cross out every instance of a particular letter in a magazine or newspaper paragraph. Alternate response tasks are exemplified by the repetition of a three-step motor sequence (palm-side-fist), which is also a test of frontal functions. These attentional tests are not overly sensitive or specific, and they can be affected by the patient's educational background, degree of effort, or presence of other cognitive deficits. In sum, the best assessment of attention may be general behavioral observations and an appraisal of how "interviewable" the patient is.

Attentional or arousal deficits may preclude the opportunity to pursue the mental status examination much further, but the examiner should attempt to assess orientation and other areas of cognition. Patients who are off 3 days on the date, 2 days on the day of the week, or 4 hours on the time of day may be significantly disoriented to time. The examiner should inquire whether the patient knows where he or she is, what kind of place it is, and under what circumstances he or she is there. Disturbed recent memory is demonstrated by asking the patient to retain the examiner's name or three words for 5 minutes. A language examination should distinguish between the language of confusion and that of a primary aphasia (see Special Problems in Differential Diagnosis, later in this chapter). Attempts at simple constructions such as copying a cube may be unsuccessful. Hallucinations can sometimes be brought out by holding a white piece of paper or an imaginary string between the fingers and asking the patient to describe what he or she sees.

Diagnostic Scales and Criteria

The usual mental status scales and tests may not help in differentiating delirium from dementia and other cognitive disturbances. Specific criteria and scales are available for the diagnosis of delirium. Foremost among these are the *Diagnostic and Statistical Manual of Mental Disorders* (DSM-V, Proposed Revision, 2013) criteria for delirium (see **Box 4.2**). The Confusion Assessment Method (CAM) is a widely used instrument for screening for and diagnosing delirium (Ely et al., 2001) (**Box 4.4**). The Delirium Rating Scale-Revised-98 (DRS-R-98), a revision of the earlier Delirium Rating Scale (DRS), is a 16-item scale with 13 severity items and three diagnostic items that reliably distinguish delirium from dementia, depression, and schizophrenia (Trzepacz et al., 2001). Both the CAM and the DRS-R-98 are best used in combination with a cognitive test (Adamis et al., 2010). The Memorial Delirium Assessment Scale (MDAS) is a 10-item scale designed to quantify the severity of delirium in medically ill patients (Breitbart et al., 1997). While it may also be useful as a diagnostic tool, it is best used after the initial delirium diagnosis is made (Adamis et al., 2010). The Delirium Symptom Interview is also a valuable instrument but may not distinguish delirium from dementia. The Neelon and Champagne (NEECHAM) Confusion Scale (Neelon et al., 1996) is an easily administered screening tool widely used in the nursing community. It combines behavioral and physiological signs of delirium, but it has been suggested that the NEECHAM measures acute confusion rather than delirium (Adamis et al., 2010). The diagnosis of delirium is facilitated by the use of the CAM, DRS-R-98, MDAS, the Delirium Symptom Interview, the

---

Box 4.4 Confusion Assessment Method

1. Acute onset and fluctuating course (mental status changes from hours to days)
2. Difficulty in focusing (easily distracted, unable to follow interview)
3. Disorganized thinking (rambling, irrelevant conversation)
4. Altered level of consciousness (from hyperalert to decreased arousal)

A positive confusion assessment method (CAM) test for delirium requires items 1 and 2 plus either item 3 or item 4 (Inouye, 2006; supplementary material).

Delirium Index (McCusker et al., 2004), or the NEECHAM, along with the history from collateral sources such as family and nursing notes, a mental status examination focusing on attention, and specific tests such as a writing sample.

Physical Examination

The physical examination should elicit any signs of systemic illness, focal neurological abnormalities, meningismus, increased intracranial pressure (ICP), extracranial cerebrovascular disease, or head trauma. In delirium, less specific findings include an action or postural tremor of high frequency (8-10 Hz), asterixis or brief lapses in tonic posture (especially at the wrist), multifocal myoclonus or shock-like jerks from diverse sites, choreiform movements, dysarthria, and gait instability. Patients may manifest agitation or psychomotor retardation, apathy, waxy flexibility, catatonia, or carphologia ("lint-picking" behavior). The presence of hyperactivity of the autonomic nervous system may be life threatening because of possible dehydration, electrolyte disturbances, or tachyarrhythmias.

Laboratory Tests

Despite false-positive and false-negative rates on single tracings (Inouye, 2006), EEG changes virtually always accompany delirium when several EEGs are obtained over time (see Chapter 32A). Disorganization of the usual cerebral rhythms and generalized slowing are the most common changes, as illustrated in Romano and Engel's classic paper (1944). The mean EEG frequency or degree of slowing correlates with the degree of delirium. Both hypoactive and hyperactive subtypes of delirium have similar EEG slowing; however, predominant low-voltage fast activity is also present on withdrawal from sedative drugs or alcohol. Additional EEG patterns from intracranial causes of delirium include focal slowing, asymmetric delta activity, and paroxysmal discharges (spikes, sharp waves, and spike-wave complexes). Periodic complexes such as triphasic waves and periodic lateralizing epileptiform discharges may help in the differential diagnosis (see Chapter 32A). EEGs are of value in deciding whether confusional behavior may be due to an intracranial cause, in making the diagnosis of delirium in patients with unclear behavior, in evaluating demented patients who might have a superimposed delirium, in differentiating delirium from schizophrenia and other primary psychiatric states, and in following the course of delirium over time.

Other essential laboratory tests include a complete blood cell count; measurements of glucose, electrolytes, blood urea nitrogen, creatinine, transaminase, and ammonia levels; thyroid function tests; arterial blood gas studies; chest radiographs; electrocardiogram; urinalysis; and urine drug screening. Less routine tests, such as antibody tests against Hu or NMDA receptors, should be considered when routine labs are unrevealing and there is a suspicion for malignancy. Although they are nonspecific, evoked potential studies often show prolonged latencies.

Since most cases of delirium are due to medical conditions, lumbar puncture and neuroimaging are needed in only a minority of delirious patients (Inouye, 2006). The need for a lumbar puncture, however, deserves special comment. This valuable test, which is often neglected in the evaluation of delirious patients, should be performed as part of the workup when the cause is uncertain. The lumbar puncture should be preceded by a computed tomographic (CT) or magnetic resonance imaging (MRI) scan of the brain, especially if there are focal neurological findings or suspicions of increased ICP, a space-occupying lesion, or head trauma. The yield of functional imaging is variable, showing global increased metabolism in patients with delirium tremens and global decreased metabolism or focal frontal hypoactivity in many other delirious patients.

Differential Diagnosis

Common Causes of Delirium

The following discussion is a selective commentary that illustrates some basic principles and helps organize the approach to working through the large differential diagnosis. Almost any sufficiently severe medical or surgical illness can cause delirium, and the best advice is to follow all available diagnostic leads (**Table 4.1**). (For further discussion of individual entities, the reader should refer to corresponding chapters in this book.) The confusion-inducing effects of these disturbances are additive, and there may be more than one causal factor, the individual contribution of which cannot be elucidated. Nearly half of elderly patients with delirium have more than one cause of their disorder, and clinicians should not stop looking for causes when a single one is found. Of the causes for delirium, the most common among the elderly are metabolic disturbances, infection, stroke, and drugs, particularly anticholinergic and narcotic medications. The most common causes among the young are drug abuse and alcohol withdrawal.

Metabolic Disturbances

Metabolic disturbances are the most common causes of delirium (see Chapters 49 and 55-58). Fortunately, the examination and routine laboratory tests screen for most acquired metabolic disturbances that might be encountered. Because of the potential for life-threatening or permanent damage, some of these conditions—particularly hypoxia and hypoglycemia—must be considered immediately. Also consider dehydration, fluid and electrolyte disorders, and disturbances of calcium and magnesium. The rapidity of change in an electrolyte level may be as important a factor as its absolute value for the development of delirium. For example, some people tolerate chronic sodium levels of 115 mEq/L or less, but a rapid fall to this level can precipitate delirium, seizures, or even central pontine myelinolysis, particularly if the correction of hyponatremia is too rapid. Hypoxia from low cardiac output, respiratory insufficiency, or other causes is another common source of delirium. A cardiac encephalopathy may ensue from heart failure, increased venous pressure transmitted to the dural venous sinuses and veins, and increased ICP (Caplan, 2006). Also consider other major organ failures such as liver and kidney failure, including the possibility of unusual causes such as undetected portocaval shunting or acute pancreatitis with the release of lipases. Delirium due to endocrine dysfunction often has prominent affective symptoms such as hyperthyroidism and Cushing syndrome. Delirium occasionally results from toxins including industrial agents, pollutants, and heavy metals such as arsenic, bismuth, gold, lead, mercury, thallium, and zinc. Other considerations are inborn errors of metabolism such as acute intermittent porphyria. Finally, it is particularly important to consider thiamine deficiency. In alcoholics and others at risk, thiamine must be given immediately to avoid precipitating Wernicke encephalopathy with the administration of glucose.

Drugs

Drug intoxication and drug withdrawal are among the most common causes of delirium. Approximately 50% of patients over the age of 65 take five or more chronic medications daily,

---

Table 4.1 Major Causes of Delirium

Metabolic disorders	Cardiac encephalopathy, hepatic encephalopathy, uremia, hypoglycemia, hypoxia, hyponatremia, hypo-/hypercalcemia, hypo-/hypermagnesemia, other electrolyte disturbances, acidosis, hyperosmolar coma, endocrinopathies (thyroid, parathyroid, pituitary), porphyria, vitamin deficiencies (thiamine, vitamin B_{12}, nicotinic acid, folic acid), toxic and industrial exposures (carbon monoxide, organic solvent, lead, manganese, mercury, carbon disulfide, heavy metals)
Drug related	Withdrawal syndromes (alcohol, benzodiazepines, barbiturates, other), amphetamines, cocaine, coffee, phencyclidine, hallucinogens, inhalants, meperidine and other narcotics, antiparkinsonism drugs, sedative-hypnotics, corticosteroids, anticholinergic and antihistaminic drugs, cardiovascular agents (beta-blockers, clonidine, digoxin), psychotropics (phenothiazines, clozapine, lithium, tricyclic antidepressants, trazodone), 5-fluorouracil and cytotoxic antineoplastics, anticonvulsants (phenobarbital, phenytoin, valproate), cimetidine, disulfiram, ergot alkaloids, salicylates, methyldopa, and selected antiinfective agents (acyclovir, amphotericin B, cephalexin, chloroquine, isoniazid, rifampin)
Infections	Meningitis, encephalitis, brain abscess, neurosyphilis, Lyme neuroborreliosis, cerebritis, systemic infections with septicemia
Neurological	Strokes, epilepsy, head injury, hypertensive encephalopathy, brain tumors, migraine, other neurovascular disorders
Perioperative	Specific surgeries (cardiac, orthopedic, ophthalmological), anesthetic and drug effects, hypoxia and anemia, hyperventilation, fluid and electrolyte disturbances, hypotension, embolism, infection or sepsis, pain, fragmented sleep, sensory deprivation or overload
Miscellaneous	Cerebral vasculitides, paraneoplastic and limbic encephalitis, hyperviscosity syndromes, trauma, cardiovascular, dehydration, sensory deprivation

and medications contribute to delirium in up to 39% of these patients (Inouye and Charpentier, 1996). Drug effects are additive, and drugs that are especially likely to cause delirium are those with anticholinergic properties, including many over-the-counter cold preparations, antihistamines, antidepressants, and neuroleptics. Patients with anticholinergic intoxication present "hot as a hare, blind as a bat, dry as a bone, red as a beet, and mad as a hatter," reflecting fever, dilated pupils, dry mouth, flushing, and delirium. Other important groups of drugs associated with delirium, especially in the elderly, are sedative-hypnotics such as long-acting benzodiazepines, narcotic analgesics and meperidine, and histamine-2 receptor blockers. Antiparkinsonism drugs result in confusion with prominent hallucinations and delusions in patients with Parkinson disease who are particularly susceptible. Corticosteroid psychosis may develop in patients taking the equivalent of 40 mg/day or more of prednisone. The behavioral effects of corticosteroids often begin with euphoria and hypomania and proceed to a hyperactive delirium. Any drug administered intrathecally, such as metrizamide, is prone to induce confusional behavior. Drug withdrawal syndromes can be caused by many agents including barbiturates and other minor tranquilizers, sedative-hypnotics, amphetamines, cocaine or "crack," and alcohol. Delirium tremens begins 72 to 96 hours after alcohol withdrawal, with profound agitation, tremulousness, diaphoresis, tachycardia, fever, and frightening visual hallucinations.

Infections

Infections and fevers often produce delirium. The main offenders are urinary tract infections, pneumonia, and septicemia. In a sporadic encephalitis or meningoencephalitis, important causal considerations are herpes simplex virus, Lyme disease, and acquired immunodeficiency syndrome (AIDS) (see Chapter 53A). Patients with AIDS may be delirious because of the human immunodeficiency virus (HIV) itself or because of an opportunistic infection. Immunocompromised patients are at greater risk of infection, and any suspicion of infection should prompt culture of urine, sputum, blood, and cerebrospinal fluid.

Strokes

Delirium can be the nonspecific consequence of any acute stroke, but most postinfarct confusion usually resolves in 24 to 48 hours (see Chapter 51B). Sustained delirium can result from specific strokes, including right middle cerebral artery infarcts affecting prefrontal and posterior parietal areas, and posterior cerebral artery infarcts resulting in either bilateral or left-sided occipitotemporal lesions (fusiform gyrus). The latter lesions can lead to agitation, visual field changes, and even Anton syndrome (see Chapter 14). Delirium may also follow occlusion of the anterior cerebral artery or rupture of an anterior communicating artery aneurysm with involvement of the anterior cingulate gyrus and septal region. Thalamic or posterior parietal cortex strokes may present with severe delirium, even with small lesions.

Other cerebrovascular conditions that can produce delirium include high-grade bilateral carotid stenosis, hypertensive encephalopathy, subarachnoid hemorrhage, and central nervous system (CNS) vasculitides such as systemic lupus erythematosus, temporal arteritis, and Behçet syndrome. Migraine can present with delirium, particularly in children. It must be emphasized that the frequency of delirium in transient ischemic attacks, even in vertebrobasilar insufficiency, is low. Transient ischemic attacks should not be considered the cause of delirium unless there are other neurological signs and an appropriate time course.

Epilepsy

Abnormal brain electrical activity is associated with delirium in four conditions: (1) ictally, with absence status, complex partial status, tonic status without convulsions, or periodic lateralizing epileptiform discharges; (2) postictally, after complex partial or generalized tonic-clonic seizures; (3) interictally manifested as increasing irritability, agitation, and affective symptoms associated with the prodrome of impending seizures; and (4) from the cognitive effects of anticonvulsant medications.

Postoperative Causes

The cause of delirium in postoperative patients is often multifactorial (Robinson et al., 2009; Winawer, 2001). Predisposing factors to postoperative delirium include age older than 70 years, preexisting CNS disorders such as dementia and Parkinson disease, severe underlying medical conditions, a history of alcohol abuse, impaired functional status, and hypoalbuminemia. Precipitating factors include residual anesthetic and drug effects (especially after premedication with anticholinergic drugs), postoperative hypoxia, perioperative hypotension, electrolyte imbalances, infections, psychological stress, and multiple awakenings with fragmented sleep. There is no clear correlation of delirium with specific anesthetic route. Postoperative delirium may start at any time but often becomes evident about the third day and abates by the seventh, although it may last considerably longer.

A number of surgeries are associated with a high rate of postoperative delirium. Between 30% and 40% of patients experience delirium after open heart or coronary artery bypass surgery. Patients older than 60 years are at special risk for postoperative delirium after cardiac surgery. Additional factors are decreased postoperative cardiac output and length of time on cardiopulmonary bypass machine, with its added risk for microemboli. In addition to an already high rate of delirium following fractures (up to 35.6% after hip fracture), orthopedic surgeries, particularly femoral neck fractures and bilateral knee replacements, further increase the frequency of delirium by about 18%. Emergency hip fracture repair is associated with a higher risk of delirium than elective hip surgery (Bruce et al., 2007). Elective noncardiac thoracic surgery is also associated with a 9% to 14% frequency of delirium in the elderly. Cataract surgery is associated with a 7% frequency of delirium, possibly because of sensory deprivation. Patients who have undergone prostate surgery may develop delirium associated with water intoxication as a result of absorption of irrigation water from the bladder.

Other Neurological Causes

Other CNS disturbances predispose to delirium. In general, patients with dementia, Lewy body disease, Parkinson disease, and atrophy or subcortical ischemic changes on neuroimaging are particularly susceptible. Electroconvulsive therapy often produces a delirium of one week or more. Head trauma can result in delirium as a consequence of brain concussion, brain contusion, intracranial hematoma, or subarachnoid hemorrhage (see Chapters 51B and 51C). Moreover, subdural hematomas can occur in the elderly with little or no history of head injury. Rapidly growing tumors in the supratentorial region are especially likely to cause delirium with increased ICP. Paraneoplastic processes produce limbic encephalitis and multifocal leukoencephalitis. Delirium can result from acute demyelinating diseases and other diffuse multifocal lesions, and from communicating or noncommunicating hydrocephalus. Some patients with transient global amnesia have initial delirium before the pathognomonic and prominent anterograde amnesia. Transient global amnesia patients also have limited retrograde amnesia for the preceding hours and improve within 24 hours. In Wernicke encephalopathy, delirium accompanies oculomotor paresis, nystagmus, ataxia, and frequently residual amnesia (Korsakoff psychosis).

Miscellaneous Causes

Various other disturbances can produce delirium. Bone fractures are associated with delirium in the elderly, and about 50% of those admitted with a hip fracture have delirium. Time from admission to operation in these patients is an additional risk factor for development of preoperative delirium (Juliebo et al., 2009). In orthopedic cases, the possibility of fat emboli requires evaluation of urine, sputum, or cerebrospinal fluid for fat. ICU psychosis is associated with sleep deprivation, immobilization, unfamiliarity, fear, frightening sensory overstimulation or sensory deprivation, isolation, transfer from another hospital ward, mechanical ventilation, psychoactive medications, and use of drains, tubes, and catheters (Van Rompaey et al., 2009). Delirium results from blood dyscrasias including anemia, thrombocytopenia, and disseminated intravascular coagulopathy. Finally, physical factors such as heatstroke, electrocution, and hypothermia may be causal.

Special Problems in Differential Diagnosis

Delirium must be distinguished from dementia, Wernicke aphasia, and psychiatric conditions (see Chapters 6, 8, 9, and 12A). The main differentiating features of dementia are the longer time course and the absence of prominent fluctuating attentional and perceptual deficits. Chronic confusional states lasting 6 months or more are a form of dementia. Patients with delirium that becomes chronic tend to settle into a lethargic state without the prominent fluctuations throughout the day, and they have fewer perceptual problems and less disruption of the day/night cycle. In addition, delirium and dementia often overlap because demented patients have increased susceptibility for developing a superimposed delirium. Demented patients who suddenly get worse should always be evaluated for delirium. Moreover, distinguishing delirium from certain forms of dementia such as vascular dementia and dementia with Lewy bodies may be particularly difficult. Patients with vascular dementia may have an acute onset or sharp decline in cognition similar to delirium. Patients with dementia with Lewy bodies have fluctuations in attention and alertness and visual hallucinations that can look identical to delirium. Most of these patients, however, have parkinsonism, repeated falls, or other supportive features. Nevertheless, the differential diagnosis of delirium and dementia with Lewy bodies may not be possible until after a diagnostic workup is completed.

The language examination should distinguish Wernicke aphasia from the language of delirium. Aphasics have prominent paraphasias of all types, including neologisms, and they have relatively preserved response to axial or whole-body commands. Their agraphia is also empty of content and is paragraphic compared with the mechanical and other writing disturbances previously described in patients with delirium.

Psychiatric conditions that may be mistaken for delirium include schizophrenia, depression, mania, attention deficit disorder, autism, dissociative states, and Ganser syndrome, which is characterized by ludicrous or approximate responses (see Chapter 8). In general, patients with psychiatric conditions lack the fluctuating attentional and related deficits associated with delirium. Schizophrenic patients may have a very disturbed verbal output, but their speech often has an underlying bizarre theme. Schizophrenic hallucinations are more often consistent persecutory voices rather than fleeting visual images, and their delusions are more systematized and have personal reference. Conversely, delirious hallucinations are usually visual, and the delusions are more transitory and fragmented. Mood disorders may also be mistaken for delirium, particularly if there is an acute agitated depression or a predominantly irritable mania. A general rule is that psychiatric behaviors such as psychosis or mania may be due to delirium, especially if they occur in someone who is 40 years or older without a prior psychiatric history. They should be regarded as delirium until proven otherwise.

Table 4.2 outlines the special problems that must be considered in the differential diagnosis of delirium.

Prevention and Management

As many as 30% to 40% of cases of delirium may be prevented with provision of high-quality care (Inouye, 2006). Misdiagnosis of delirium results in inadequate management in up to 80% of patients (Michaud et al., 2007), and about half of elderly patients affected by delirium actually develop symptoms *after* admission to the hospital. Early identification of patients with predisposing risk factors is important, especially in a frail geriatric population (Laurila et al., 2008). In addition, early intervention by geriatricians and admission to geriatric-focused inpatient hospital wards have been shown to reduce delirium rates (Bo et al., 2009; Marcantonio et al., 2001). Multifactorial intervention programs can reduce the duration of delirium, length of hospital stay, and mortality (Bergmann et al., 2005; Inouye et al., 1999; Lundstrom et al., 2005). These programs focus on managing risk factors such as cognitive impairment, sleep deprivation, immobility, visual and hearing impairment, and dehydration, particularly in intermediate-risk patients (Inouye et al., 1999). They also focus on educational programs for physicians and nurses in the detection and management of delirium. Nurses in particular spend more time with patients than physicians do, and they may be in a better position to recognize delirium.

There are several steps in the management of delirium. First, attention is aimed at finding the cause and eliminating it. Second, the delirium is managed with symptomatic

Table 4.2 Special Problems in the Differential Diagnosis of Delirium*

Clinical Feature	Delirium	Dementias	Stroke with Wernicke Aphasia	Schizophrenia	Depression
Course	Acute onset; hours, days, or more	Insidious onset[†]; months or years; progressive	Sudden onset; chronic, stable deficit	Insidious onset, 6 months or more; acute psychotic phases	Insidious onset, at least 2 weeks, often months
Attention	Markedly impaired attention and arousal	Normal early; impairment later	Normal	Normal to mild impairment	Mild impairment
Fluctuation	Prominent in attention arousal; disturbed day/night cycle	Prominent fluctuations absent; lesser disturbances in day/night cycle	Absent	Absent	Absent
Perception	Misperceptions; hallucinations, usually visual, fleeting; paramnesia	Perceptual abnormalities much less prominent[‡]; paramnesia	Normal	Hallucinations, auditory with personal reference	May have mood-congruent hallucinations
Speech and language	Abnormal clarity, speed, and coherence; disjointed and dysarthric; misnaming; characteristic dysgraphia	Early anomia; empty speech; abnormal comprehension	Prominent paraphasias and neologisms; empty speech; abnormal comprehension	Disorganized, with a bizarre theme	Decreased amount of speech
Other cognition	Disorientation to time, place; recent memory and visuospatial abnormalities	Disorientation to time, place; multiple other higher cognitive deficits	No other necessary deficits	Disorientation to person; concrete interpretations	Mental slowing; indecisiveness; memory retrieval difficulty
Behavior	Lethargy or delirium; nonsystematized delusions; emotional lability	Disinterested; disengaged; disinhibited; delusions and other psychiatric symptoms	Paranoia possibly ensuing	Systematized delusions; paranoia; bizarre behavior	Depressed mood; anhedonia; lack of energy; sleep and appetite disturbances
Electroencephalogram	Diffuse slowing; low-voltage fast activity; specific patterns	Normal early; mild slowing later	Normal	Normal	Normal

*The characteristics listed are the relative and usual ones and are not exclusive.
[†]Patients with vascular dementia may have an abrupt decline in cognition.
[‡]Patients with dementia with diffuse cortical Lewy bodies often have a fluctuating mental status and hallucinations.

measures involving attention to fluid and electrolyte balance, nutritional status, and early treatment of infections. Third, management focuses on environmental interventions. Reduce unfamiliarity by providing a calendar, a clock, family pictures, and personal objects. Maintain a moderate sensory balance in the patient by avoiding sensory overstimulation or deprivation. Minimize staff changes, limit ambient noise and the number of visits from strangers, and provide a radio or a television set, a nightlight, and where necessary, eyeglasses and hearing aids. Other environmental measures include providing soft music and warm baths and allowing the patient to take walks when possible. Physical restraints should be avoided if possible and a sitter used instead. Fourth, proper

communication and support are critical with these patients. As much as possible, everything should be explained. Delusions and hallucinations should be neither endorsed nor challenged. Patients should receive emotional support including frequent family visits. They also benefit from frequent reorientation to place, time, and situation.

In general, it is best to avoid the use of drugs in confused patients, because they further cloud the picture and may worsen delirium. All the patient's medications should be reviewed, and any unnecessary drugs should be discontinued. When medication is needed, the goal is to make the patient manageable, not to decrease loud or annoying behavior or to sedate them (Inouye, 2006). These patients should receive the lowest possible dose and should not get drugs such as phenobarbital or long-acting benzodiazepines. In particular, use of benzodiazepines can have a paradoxical effect in the elderly, causing agitation and confusion. Medication may be necessary if the patient's behavior is potentially dangerous, interferes with medical care, or causes the patient profound distress. Clinicians most often use haloperidol (starting at 0.25 mg daily) for these symptoms. Haloperidol may be repeated every 30 minutes, PO or IM, up to a maximum of 5 mg/day. After the first 24 hours, 50% of the loading dose may be given in divided doses over the next 24 hours, then the dose should be tapered off over the next few days (Inouye, 2004). The atypical antipsychotics—risperidone, olanzapine, quetiapine, and aripiprazole—may be used at low doses (Attard, Ranjith, and Taylor, 2008). Safety and efficacy of the atypical and typical antipsychotics are similar (Fong, Tulebaev, and Inouye, 2009). Results in favor of acetylcholinesterase inhibitors for delirium management have not been borne out in controlled trials, though in some cases, such as in patients with Lewy body dementia, they can be helpful (Attard, Ranjith, and Taylor, 2008; Tabet and Howard, 2009). Other medications such as valproate, ondansetron, or melatonin may be effective and safe in selected cases. Finally, there is no evidence for the preventive use of haloperidol or related medications prior to the development of delirium, though it may reduce severity and duration postoperatively, as well as duration of hospital stay (Kalisvaart et al., 2005). Evidence for preventive use of acetylcholinesterase inhibitors after surgery is also not supportive, though this conclusion is based only on small pilot studies (Attard, Ranjith, and Taylor, 2008; Tabet and Howard, 2009).

Prognosis

The prognosis for recovery from delirium is variable. If the causative factor is rapidly corrected, recovery can be complete, with an average duration of delirium of about 8 days (2 days to 2 weeks). Delirium present at discharge is associated with a 2.6-fold increased risk of death or nursing home placement (McAvay et al., 2006), and delirium persisting after hospital discharge is associated with a 2.9-fold risk of death within the following year. This risk appears to be reversible with the resolution of delirium (Kiely et al., 2009). The link between delirium and subsequent long-term cognitive impairment is also firmly established (MacLullich et al., 2009).

In the elderly, delirium may not be a transient disorder. For them, the duration of delirium is often longer than that of their underlying medical problem. Moreover, after hospital discharge, older patients who are delirious may not recover back to baseline (Fong, Tulebaev, and Inouye, 2009; MacLullich et al., 2009; McCusker et al., 2002). In one study, 14.8% still met criteria for delirium 12 months after discharge (Rockwood et al., 1999). A partial delirium with some but not all criteria for delirium may persist in many elderly patients.

Delirium is an independent predictor of adverse outcomes in older hospitalized patients; particularly in the presence of baseline cognitive impairment or dementia, it is associated with an increased mortality rate and may accelerate cognitive decline (Adamis et al., 2006; MacLullich et al., 2009; McCusker et al., 2002). Delirium in the elderly predicts sustained poor cognitive and functional status and increased likelihood of nursing home placement after a medical admission. Hypoactive delirious patients appear to be at particular risk because of complications from aspiration and inadequate oral nutrition as well as falls and pressure sores. In general, however, clinicians can greatly improve prognosis with increased awareness of delirium, more rapid diagnosis of the causative factor(s), and better overall management.

References

The complete reference list is available online at www.expertconsult.com.

Stupor and Coma

Joseph R. Berger

Definitions

Consciousness may be defined as a state of awareness of self and surroundings. Alterations in consciousness are conceptualized into two types. The first type affects arousal and is the subject of this chapter. The second type involves cognitive and affective mental function, sometimes referred to as the "content" of mental function. Examples of the latter type of alteration in consciousness are dementia (see Chapter 6), delusions, confusion, and inattention (see Chapter 9). These altered states of consciousness, with the exception of advanced dementia, do not affect the level of arousal. Sleep, the only normal form of altered consciousness, is discussed in Chapter 68.

The term *delirium* describes a clouding of consciousness with reduced ability to sustain attention to environmental stimuli. Diagnostic criteria for delirium from the American Psychiatric Association's *Diagnostic and Statistical Manual of Mental Disorders* (DSM-IV-R) include at least two of the following: (1) perceptual disturbance (misinterpretations, illusions, or hallucinations), (2) incoherent speech at times, (3) disturbance of sleep/wake cycle, and (4) increased or decreased psychomotor activity. Delirium is a good example of a confusional state in which a mild decline in arousal may be clinically difficult to separate from a change in cognitive or affective mental function. In clinical practice, the exact boundary between different forms of altered consciousness may be vague. Alterations in arousal, though often referred to as "altered levels of consciousness," do not actually form discrete levels but rather are made up of a continuum of subtly changing behavioral states that range from alert to comatose. These states are dynamic and thus may change with time. Four

points on the continuum of arousal are often used in describing the clinical state of a patient: alert, lethargic, stuporous, and comatose. *Alert* refers to a perfectly normal state of arousal. *Lethargy* lies between alertness and stupor. *Stupor* is a state of baseline unresponsiveness that requires repeated application of vigorous stimuli to achieve arousal. *Coma* is a state of complete unresponsiveness to arousal in which the patient lies with the eyes closed. The terms *lethargy* and *stupor* cover a broad area on the continuum of behavioral states and thus are subject to misinterpretation by subsequent observers of a patient when used without further qualification. In clinical practice, in which relatively slight changes in arousal may be significant, only the terms *alert* and *comatose* (the endpoints of the continuum) have enough precision to be used without further qualification.

Conditions That May Mimic Coma

Several different states of impaired cognition or consciousness may appear similar to coma or be confused with it (**Table 5.1**). Moreover, patients who survive the initial coma may progress to certain of these syndromes after varying lengths of time. Once sleep/wake cycles become established, true coma is no longer present. Differentiation of these states from true coma is important to allow administration of appropriate therapy and help determine prognosis.

In the *locked-in syndrome* (de-efferented state), patients are alert and aware of their environment but are quadriplegic, with lower cranial nerve palsies resulting from bilateral ventral pontine lesions that involve the corticospinal, corticopontine,

Table 5.1 Behavioral States Confused with Coma

Behavioral State	Definition	Lesion	Comments
Locked-in syndrome	Alert and aware, quadriplegic with lower cranial nerve palsy	Bilateral ventral pontine	A similar state may be seen with severe polyneuropathies, myasthenia gravis, and neuromuscular blocking agents
Persistent vegetative state	Absent cognitive function but retained "vegetative" components	Extensive cortical gray or subcortical white matter with relative preservation of brain stem	Synonyms include apallic syndrome, coma vigil, cerebral cortical death
Abulia	Severe apathy, patient neither speaks nor moves spontaneously	Bilateral frontal medial	Severe cases resemble akinetic mutism, but patient is alert and aware
Catatonia	Mute, with marked decrease in motor activity	Usually psychiatric	May be mimicked by frontal lobe dysfunction or drugs
Pseudocoma	Feigned coma		

and corticobulbar tracts. These patients are awake and alert but are voluntarily able only to move their eyes vertically or blink. The locked-in syndrome most often is observed as a consequence of pontine infarction due to basilar artery thrombosis. Other causes include central pontine myelinolysis and brainstem mass lesions. A state similar to the locked-in syndrome also may be seen with severe polyneuropathy—in particular, acute inflammatory demyelinating polyradiculo-neuropathy, myasthenia gravis, and poisoning with neuro-muscular blocking agents.

In the *persistent vegetative state* (PVS), patients have lost cognitive neurological function but retain vegetative or non-cognitive neurological function such as cardiac action, respiration, and maintenance of blood pressure. This state follows coma and is characterized by absence of cognitive function or awareness of the environment despite a preserved sleep/wake cycle. Spontaneous movements may occur, and the eyes may open in response to external stimuli, but the patient does not speak or obey commands. Diagnostic criteria for PVS are provided in **Box 5.1**. Diagnosis of this condition should be made cautiously and only after extended periods of observation. A number of poorly defined syndromes have been used synonymously with PVS, including *apallic syndrome* or *state*, *akinetic mutism*, *coma vigil*, *alpha coma*, *neocortical death*, and *permanent unconsciousness*. These terms, used variously by different authors, probably are best avoided because of their lack of precision.

A condition that has been estimated to be 10 times more common than PVS is the *minimally conscious state*, in which severe disability accompanies minimal awareness. A set of diagnostic criteria for the minimally conscious state has been proposed (**Box 5.2**). *Abulia* is a severe apathy in which patients have blunting of feeling, drive, mentation, and behavior such that they neither speak nor move spontaneously.

Catatonia may result in a state of muteness with dramatically decreased motor activity. The maintenance of body posture, with preserved ability to sit or stand, distinguishes it from organic pathological stupor. It generally is a psychiatric manifestation but may be mimicked by frontal lobe dysfunction or drug effect.

Pseudocoma is the term for a condition in which the patient appears comatose (i.e., unresponsive, unarousable, or both) but has no structural, metabolic, or toxic disorder.

Box 5.1 Criteria for Diagnosis of Persistent Vegetative State

1. No evidence of awareness of themselves or their environment; they are incapable of interacting with others
2. No evidence of sustained, reproducible, purposeful, or voluntary behavioral responses to visual, auditory, tactile, or noxious stimuli
3. No evidence of language comprehension or expression
4. Intermittent wakefulness manifested by the presence of sleep/wake cycles
5. Sufficiently preserved hypothalamic and brainstem autonomic functions to survive if given medical and nursing care
6. Bowel and bladder incontinence
7. Variably preserved cranial nerve (pupillary, oculocephalic, corneal, vestibulo-ocular, and gag) and spinal reflexes

Data from The Multi-Society Task Force on PVS, 1994. Medical aspects of the persistent vegetative state. N Engl J Med 330, 1499-1508, 1572-1579.

Box 5.2 Criteria for the Minimally Conscious State

To diagnose a minimally conscious state, limited but clearly discernible evidence of self- or environmental awareness must be demonstrated on a reproducible or sustained basis by one or more of the following behaviors:

1. Follows simple commands
2. Gestural or verbal yes/no responses (regardless of accuracy)
3. Intelligible verbalization
4. Purposeful behavior, including movements or affective behaviors that occur in contingent relationship to relevant environmental stimuli and are not due to reflexive activity

Data from Giacino, J.T., Ashwal, S., Childs, N., et al., 2002. The minimally conscious state: definition and diagnostic criteria. Neurology 58, 349-353.

Approach to the Patient in Coma

The initial clinical approach to the patient in a state of stupor or coma is based on the principle that *all* alterations in arousal constitute acute life-threatening emergencies until vital functions such as blood pressure and oxygenation are stabilized, potentially reversible causes of coma are treated, and the underlying cause of the alteration in arousal is understood. Urgent steps may be necessary to avoid or minimize permanent brain damage from reversible causes. In view of the urgency of this situation, every physician should develop a diagnostic and therapeutic routine to use with a patient with an alteration in consciousness. A basic understanding of the mechanisms that lead to impairment in arousal is necessary to develop this routine. The anatomical and physiological bases for alterations in arousal are discussed in Chapter 68.

Although it is essential to keep in mind the concept of a spectrum of arousal, for the sake of simplicity and brevity only the term *coma* is used in the rest of this chapter. **Table 5.2** lists many of the common causes of coma. More than half of all cases of coma are due to diffuse and metabolic brain dysfunction. In Plum and Posner's landmark study (1980, see 2007 revision) of 500 patients initially diagnosed as having coma of unknown cause (in whom the diagnosis was ultimately established), 326 patients had diffuse and metabolic brain dysfunction. Almost half of these had drug poisonings. Of the remaining patients, 101 had supratentorial mass lesions, including 77 hemorrhagic lesions and 9 infarctions; 65 had subtentorial lesions, mainly brainstem infarctions; and 8 had psychiatric coma.

A logical decision tree often used in searching for the cause of coma divides the categories of diseases that cause coma into three groups: structural lesions, which may be above or below the tentorium; metabolic and toxic causes; and psychiatric causes. The history and physical examination usually provide sufficient evidence to determine the presence or absence of a structural lesion and quickly differentiate the general categories to either decide what further diagnostic tests are needed or allow for immediate intervention if necessary.

Serial examinations are needed, with precise description of the behavioral state at different points in time to determine whether the patient is improving or—a more ominous finding—worsening, and to decide whether a change in therapy or further diagnostic testing is necessary. Subtle declines in the intermediate states of arousal may herald precipitous changes in brainstem function, which may affect regulation of vital functions such as respiration or blood pressure. The dynamic quality of alterations of consciousness and the need for accurate documentation at different points in time cannot be overemphasized.

Rapid Initial Examination and Emergency Therapy

A relatively quick initial assessment is conducted to ensure that the comatose patient is medically and neurologically stable before a more detailed investigation is undertaken. This rapid initial examination is essential to rule out the need for immediate medical or surgical intervention. In addition, various supportive or preventive measures may be indicated.

Urgent and sometimes empirical therapy is given to prevent further brain damage. Potential immediate metabolic needs of the brain are supplied by empirical use of supplemental oxygen, intravenous (IV) thiamine (at least 100 mg), and IV 50% dextrose in water (25 g). A baseline serum glucose level should be obtained before glucose administration.

The use of IV glucose in patients with ischemic or anoxic brain damage is controversial. Extra glucose may augment local lactic acid production by anaerobic glycolysis and may worsen ischemic or anoxic damage. Clinically, however, we currently recommend empirical glucose administration when the cause of coma is unknown. There are two reasons for this approach: (1) the frequent occurrence of alterations in arousal due to hypoglycemia and the relatively good prognosis for coma due to hypoglycemia when it is treated expeditiously; and (2) the potentially permanent consequences if it is not treated. By comparison, the prognosis for anoxic or ischemic coma generally is poor and probably will remain poor regardless of glucose supplementation.

Thiamine must always be given in conjunction with glucose to prevent precipitation of Wernicke encephalopathy. Naloxone hydrochloride may be given parenterally, preferably IV, in doses of 0.4 to 2 mg if opiate overdose is the suspected cause of coma. An abrupt and complete reversal of narcotic effect may precipitate an acute abstinence syndrome in persons who are physically dependent on opiates.

Initial examination should include a check of general appearance, blood pressure, pulse, temperature, respiratory rate and breath sounds, best response to stimulation, pupil size and responsiveness, and posturing or adventitious movements. The neck should be stabilized in all instances of trauma until cervical spine fracture or subluxation can be ruled out. The airway should be protected in all comatose patients and an IV line placed.

In coma, however, the classic sign of an acute condition in the abdomen—namely, abdominal rigidity—may be subtle or absent. In addition, the diagnosis of blunt abdominal trauma is difficult in patients with a change in mental status. Therefore, in unconscious patients with a history of trauma, peritoneal lavage by an experienced surgeon may be warranted.

Hypotension, marked hypertension, bradycardia, arrhythmias causing depression of blood pressure, marked hyperthermia, and signs of cerebral herniation mandate immediate therapeutic intervention.

Hyperthermia or meningismus prompts consideration of urgent lumbar puncture (LP). Examination of the fundus of the eye for papilledema and a computed tomography (CT) scan of the brain should be performed before LP in any comatose patient. Although the only absolute contraindication to LP is the presence of an infection over the site of puncture, medicolegal considerations make a CT scan mandatory before LP. To avoid a delay in therapy required to perform a CT scan, some authorities recommend initiating antibiotics immediately when acute bacterial meningitis is strongly suspected, though this may prevent subsequent identification of the responsible organism.

The risk of herniation from an LP in patients with evidence of increased intracerebral pressure is difficult to ascertain from the literature; estimates range from 1% to 12%, depending on the series (Posner et al., 2007). It is important to recognize that both central and tonsillar herniation may increase neck tone.

Despite an elevated intracranial pressure (ICP), sufficient cerebrospinal fluid (CSF) should always be obtained to perform the necessary studies; bacterial culture and cell count, essential in cases of suspected bacterial meningitis, requires but a few milliliters of fluid. Intravenous access and IV mannitol should be ready in the event unexpected herniation begins after the LP. When the CSF pressure is greater than 500 mm H_2O, some authorities recommend leaving the needle

Table 5.2 Causes of Coma

I. SYMMETRICAL-NONSTRUCTURAL

Toxins

Lead
Thallium
Mushrooms
Cyanide
Methanol
Ethylene glycol
Carbon monoxide

Drugs

Sedatives
Barbiturates*
Other hypnotics
Tranquilizers
Bromides
Alcohol
Opiates
Paraldehyde
Salicylate
Psychotropics
Anticholinergics
Amphetamines
Lithium
Phencyclidine
Monoamine oxidase inhibitors

II. SYMMETRICAL-STRUCTURAL

Supratentorial

Bilateral internal carotid occlusion
Bilateral anterior cerebral artery occlusion

III. ASYMMETRICAL-STRUCTURAL

Supratentorial

Thrombotic thrombocytopenic purpura†
Disseminated intravascular coagulation
Nonbacterial thrombotic endocarditis marantic endocarditis
Subacute bacterial endocarditis
Fat emboli
Unilateral hemispheric mass (tumor, bleed) with herniation

Metabolic

Hypoxia
Hypercapnia
Hypernatremia
Hyponatremia*
Hypoglycemia*
Hyperglycemic nonketotic coma
Diabetic ketoacidosis
Lactic acidosis
Hypercalcemia
Hypocalcemia
Hypermagnesemia
Hyperthermia
Hypothermia
Reye syndrome encephalopathy

Aminoacidemia
Wernicke encephalopathy
Porphyria
Hepatic encephalopathy*
Uremia
Dialysis encephalopathy
Addisonian crisis

Subarachnoid Hemorrhage

Thalamic hemorrhage*
Trauma—contusion, concussion*
Hydrocephalus

Subdural Hemorrhage, Bilateral

Intracerebral bleed
Pituitary apoplexy†
Massive or bilateral supratentorial infarction
Multifocal leukoencephalopathy
Creutzfeldt-Jakob disease
Adrenal leukodystrophy
Cerebral vasculitis
Cerebral abscess

Infections

Bacterial meningitis
Viral encephalitis
Postinfectious encephalomyelitis
Syphilis
Sepsis
Typhoid fever
Malaria
Waterhouse-Friderichsen syndrome

Psychiatric

Catatonia

Other

Postictal
Diffuse ischemia (myocardial infarction, congestive heart failure, arrhythmia)
Hypotension
Fat embolism
Hypertensive encephalopathy
Hypothyroidism

Infratentorial

Basilar occlusion*
Midline brainstem tumor
Pontine hemorrhage*

Subdural Empyema

Thrombophlebitis†
Multiple sclerosis
Leukoencephalopathy associated with hemotherapy
Acute disseminated encephalomyelitis
Infratentorial
Brainstem infarction
Brainstem hemorrhage

Data from Plum, F., Posner, J.B., 1980. The Diagnosis of Stupor and Coma, third ed. F.A. Davis, Philadelphia; and from Fisher, C.M., 1969. The neurological examination of the comatose patient. Acta Neurol Scand 45, 1-56.
*Relatively common asymmetrical presentation.
†Relatively symmetrical.

in place to monitor the pressure and administering IV mannitol to lower the pressure. If focal signs develop during or after the LP, immediate intubation and hyperventilation also may be necessary to reduce intracerebral pressure urgently until more definitive therapy is available.

Ecchymosis, petechiae, or evidence of ready bleeding on general examination may indicate coagulation abnormality or thrombocytopenia. This increases the risk of epidural hematoma after an LP, which may cause devastating spinal cord compression. Measurements of prothrombin time, partial thromboplastin time, and platelet count should precede LP in these cases, and the coagulation abnormality or thrombocytopenia should be corrected before proceeding to LP.

Common Presentations

Coma usually manifests in one of three ways. Most commonly, it occurs as an expected or predictable progression of an underlying illness. Examples are focal brainstem infarction with extension; chronic obstructive pulmonary disease in a patient who is given too high a concentration of oxygen, thereby decreasing respiratory drive and resulting in carbon dioxide narcosis; and known barbiturate overdose when the ingested drug cannot be fully removed and begins to cause unresponsiveness. Second, coma occurs as an unpredictable event in a patient whose prior medical conditions are known to the physician. The coma may be a complication of an underlying medical illness, such as in a patient with arrhythmia who suffers anoxia after a cardiac arrest. Alternatively, an unrelated event may occur, such as sepsis from an IV line in a cardiac patient or stroke in a hypothyroid patient. Finally, coma can occur in a patient whose medical history is totally unknown to the physician. Sometimes this type of presentation is associated with a known probable cause such as head trauma incurred in a motor vehicle accident, but often the unknown comatose patient presents to the physician without an obvious associated cause. Although the patient without an obvious cause of coma may seem most challenging, thorough objective systematic assessment must be applied in every comatose patient. Special care must be taken not to be lulled or misled by an apparently predictable progression of an underlying illness or other obvious cause of coma.

History

Once the patient is relatively stable, clues to the cause of the coma should be sought by briefly interviewing relatives, friends, bystanders, or medical personnel who may have observed the patient before or during the decrease in consciousness. Telephone calls to family members may be helpful. The patient's wallet or purse should be examined for lists of medications, a physician's card, or other information.

Attempts should be made to ascertain the patient's social background and prior medical history and the circumstances in which the patient was found. The presence of drug paraphernalia or empty medicine bottles suggests a drug overdose. Newer recreational drugs, such as γ-hydroxybutyrate (GHB), must be considered in the differential diagnosis. An oral hypoglycemic agent or insulin in the medicine cabinet or refrigerator implies possible hypoglycemia. Antiarrhythmic agents such as procainamide or quinidine suggest existing coronary artery disease with possible myocardial infarction (MI) or warn that an unwitnessed arrhythmia may have caused cerebral hypoperfusion, with resulting anoxic encephalopathy. Warfarin, typically prescribed for patients with deep venous thrombosis or pulmonary embolism, those at risk for cerebral embolism, and those with a history of brainstem or cerebral ischemia, may be responsible for massive intracerebral bleeding. In patients found to be unresponsive at the scene of an accident such as a car crash, the unresponsive state may be due to trauma incurred in the accident, or sudden loss of consciousness may have precipitated the accident.

The neurologist often is called when patients do not awaken after surgery or when coma supervenes following a surgical procedure. Postoperative causes of coma include many of those listed in **Table 5.4**. In addition, the physician also must have a high index of suspicion for certain neurological conditions that occur in this setting, including fat embolism, addisonian crisis, hypothyroid coma (precipitated by acute illness or surgical stress), Wernicke encephalopathy from carbohydrate loading without adequate thiamine stores, and iatrogenic overdose of a narcotic analgesic.

Attempts should be made to ascertain whether the patient complained of symptoms before onset of coma. Common signs and symptoms include headache preceding subarachnoid hemorrhage, chest pain with aortic dissection or MI, shortness of breath from hypoxia, stiff neck in meningoencephalitis, and vertigo in brainstem stroke. Nausea and vomiting are common in poisonings. Coma also may be secondary to increased ICP. Observers may have noted head trauma, drug abuse, seizures, or hemiparesis. Descriptions of falling to one side, dysarthria or aphasia, ptosis, pupillary dilatation, or dysconjugate gaze may help localize structural lesions. The time course of the disease as noted by family or friends may help differentiate the often relatively slow, progressive course of toxic-metabolic or infectious causes from abrupt catastrophic changes seen most commonly with vascular events.

Finally, family members or friends may be invaluable in identifying psychiatric causes of unresponsiveness. The family may describe a long history of psychiatric disease, previous similar episodes from which the patient recovered, current social stresses on the patient, or the patient's unusual idiosyncratic response to stress. Special care must be taken with psychiatric patients because of the often biased approach to these patients, which may lead to incomplete evaluation. Psychiatric patients are subject to all the causes of coma listed in **Table 5.4**.

General Examination

A systematic, detailed general examination is especially helpful in the approach to the comatose patient who is unable to describe prior or current medical problems. This examination begins in the initial rapid examination with evaluation of blood pressure, pulse, respiratory rate, and temperature.

Blood Pressure Evaluation
HYPOTENSION

Cerebral hypoperfusion secondary to hypotension may result in coma if the mean arterial pressure falls below the value for which the brain is able to autoregulate (normally 60 mm Hg). This value is substantially higher in chronically hypertensive persons, in whom the cerebral blood flow–mean arterial pressure curve is shifted to the right. Among the causes of hypotension are hypovolemia, massive external or internal hemorrhage, MI, cardiac tamponade, dissecting aortic aneurysm, intoxication with alcohol or other drugs (especially barbiturates), toxins, Wernicke encephalopathy, Addison disease, and sepsis. Although most patients with hypotension are cold because of peripheral vasoconstriction, patients with Addison disease or sepsis may have warm shock due to peripheral vasodilation. Medullary damage also may result in hypotension due to damage to the pressor center.

HYPERTENSION

Hypertension is the cause of alterations in arousal in hypertensive crisis and is seen secondarily as a response to cerebral infarction, in subarachnoid hemorrhage, with certain brainstem infarctions, and with increased intracerebral pressure. The Kocher-Cushing (or Claude Bernard) reflex is the development of hypertension associated with bradycardia and respiratory irregularity due to increased ICP. This response occurs more commonly in the setting of a posterior fossa lesion and in children. It results from compression or ischemia of the pressor area lying beneath the floor of the fourth ventricle. Hypertension is a common condition and thus may be present but unrelated to the cause of coma.

Heart Rate

In addition to the Kocher-Cushing reflex, bradycardia can result from myocardial conduction blocks, with certain poisonings, and from effects of drugs such as the beta-blockers. Tachycardia is a result of hypovolemia, hyperthyroidism, fever, anemia, and certain toxins and drugs including cocaine, atropine, and other anticholinergic medications.

Respiration

The most common causes of decreased respiratory rate are metabolic or toxic, such as carbon dioxide narcosis or drug overdose with central nervous system (CNS) depressants. Increased respiratory rate can result from hypoxia, hypercapnia, acidosis, hyperthermia, hepatic disease, toxins or drugs (especially those that produce metabolic acidosis, such as methanol, ethylene glycol, paraldehyde, and salicylates), sepsis, pulmonary embolism (including fat embolism), and sometimes is seen in psychogenic unresponsiveness. Brainstem lesions causing hypopnea or hyperpnea are discussed later in the chapter. Changes in respiratory rate or rhythm in a comatose patient may be deceiving because a metabolic disorder may coexist with a CNS lesion.

Temperature

Core temperature must be measured with a rectal probe in a comatose patient, because oral or axillary temperatures are unreliable. Pyrexia most often is a sign of infection. Accordingly, any evidence of fever in a comatose patient warrants strong consideration of LP. Absence of an elevated temperature does not rule out infection. Immunosuppressed patients, elderly patients, and patients with metabolic or endocrine abnormalities such as uremia or hypothyroidism may not experience an increase in temperature in response to overwhelming infection. Pure neurogenic hyperthermia is rare and usually is due to subarachnoid hemorrhage or diencephalic (hypothalamus) lesions. A clue to brainstem origin is shivering without sweating. Shivering in the absence of sweating, particularly when unilateral in nature, also may be observed with a deep intracerebral hemorrhage. Other causes of increased temperature associated with coma are heatstroke, thyrotoxic crisis, and drug toxicity. (Atropine and other anticholinergics elevate core temperature but decrease diaphoresis, resulting in a warm, dry patient with dilated pupils and diminished bowel sounds.)

Except in heatstroke and malignant hyperthermia, fever does not result in stupor or coma by itself. Conversely, hypothermia—regardless of cause—is anticipated to lead to altered consciousness. Hypothermia causes diminished cerebral metabolism and, if the temperature is sufficiently low, may result in an isoelectric electroencephalogram. Hypothermia usually is metabolic or environmental in cause; however, it also is seen with hypotension accompanied by vasoconstriction and may occur with sepsis. Other causes of hypothermia associated with coma are hypothyroid coma, hypopituitarism, Wernicke encephalopathy, cold exposure, drugs (barbiturates), and other poisonings. Central lesions causing hypothermia are found in the posterior hypothalamus. Absence of shivering or vasoconstriction or presence of sweating are clues to the central origin of these lesions.

General Appearance

The general appearance of the patient may provide further clues to the diagnosis. Torn or disheveled clothing may indicate prior assault. Vomiting may be a sign of increased ICP, drug overdose, or metabolic or other toxic cause. Urinary or fecal incontinence indicates an epileptic seizure or may result from a generalized autonomic discharge resulting from the same cause as for the coma. Examination of body habitus may reveal cushingoid patients at risk for an acute addisonian crisis with abrupt withdrawal of their medications or additional stress from intercurrent illness. Cachexia suggests cancer, chronic inflammatory disorders, Addison disease, hypothyroid coma, or hyperthyroid crisis. The cachectic patient also is subject to Wernicke encephalopathy in association with carbohydrate loading. Gynecomastia, spider nevi, testicular atrophy, and decreased axillary and pubic hair are common in the alcoholic with cirrhosis.

Head and Neck Examination

The head and neck must be carefully examined for signs of trauma. Palpation for depressed skull fractures and edema should be attempted, although this means of evaluation is not very sensitive. Laceration or edema of the scalp is indicative of head trauma. The term *raccoon eyes* refers to orbital ecchymosis due to anterior basal skull fracture. The *Battle sign* is a hematoma overlying the mastoid, originating from basilar skull fracture extending into the mastoid portion of the temporal bone. The ecchymotic lesions typically are not apparent until 2 to 3 days after the traumatic event.

Meningismus neck stiffness may be a sign of infectious or carcinomatous meningitis, subarachnoid hemorrhage, or central or tonsillar herniation. Neck stiffness may be absent, however, in coma from any cause but is likely to be present in less severe alterations in arousal. Scars on the neck may be from endarterectomy, implying vascular disease, or from thyroidectomy or parathyroidectomy, suggesting concomitant hypothyroidism, hypoparathyroidism, or both. Goiter may be found with hypothyroidism or hyperthyroidism.

Eye Examination

Examination of the eyes includes observation of the cornea, conjunctiva, sclera, iris, lens, and eyelids. Edema of the conjunctiva and eyelids may occur in congestive heart failure and nephrotic syndrome. Congestion and inflammation of the conjunctiva from exposure may occur in the comatose patient. Enophthalmos indicates dehydration. Scleral icterus is seen with liver disease, and yellowish discoloration of the skin without scleral involvement may be due to drugs such as rifampin. Band keratopathy is caused by hypercalcemia, whereas hypocalcemia is associated with cataracts. Kayser-Fleischer rings are seen in progressive lenticular degeneration (Wilson disease). Arcus senilis is seen in normal aging but also in hyperlipidemia. Fat embolism may cause petechiae in conjunctiva and eye grounds.

Funduscopic examination demonstrates evidence of hypertension or diabetes. Grayish deposits surrounding the optic disc have been reported in lead poisoning. The retina is congested and edematous in methyl alcohol poisoning, and the disc margin may be blurred. Subhyaloid hemorrhage appears occasionally as a consequence of a rapid increase in ICP due to subarachnoid hemorrhage (Terson syndrome). Papilledema results from increased ICP and may be indicative of an intracranial mass lesion or hypertensive encephalopathy.

Otoscopic Examination

Otoscopic examination should rule out hemotympanum or CSF otorrhea from a basilar skull fracture involving the petrous ridge, as well as infection of the middle ear. Infections of the middle ear, mastoid, and paranasal sinuses constitute the most common source of underlying infection in brain abscess. CSF rhinorrhea, which appears as clear fluid from the nose, may depend on head position. Presence of glucose in the watery discharge is virtually diagnostic, although false-positive results are possible.

Oral Examination

Alcohol intoxication, diabetic ketoacidosis (acetone odor), uremia, and hepatic encephalopathy (musty odor of cholemia or *fetor hepaticus*) may be suspected from the odor of the breath. Arsenic poisoning produces the odor of garlic. Poor oral hygiene or oral abscesses may be a source of sepsis or severe pulmonary infection with associated hypoxemia. Pustules on the nose or upper lip may seed the cavernous sinus with bacteria by way of the angular vein. Lacerations on the tongue, whether old or new, suggest seizure disorder. Thin, blue-black pigmentation along the gingival margin may be seen in certain heavy metal poisonings (bismuth, mercury, and lead).

Integument Examination

Systematic examination of the integument includes inspection of the skin, nails, and mucous membranes. A great deal of information can be gained by a brief examination of the skin (**Table 5.3**). Hot, dry skin is a feature of heatstroke. Sweaty skin is seen with hypotension or hypoglycemia. Drugs may cause macular-papular, vesicular, or petechial-purpuric rashes or bullous skin lesions. Bullous skin lesions most often are a result of barbiturates but also may be caused by imipramine, meprobamate, glutethimide, phenothiazine, and carbon monoxide. Kaposi sarcoma, anogenital herpetic lesions, or oral candidiasis should suggest the acquired immunodeficiency syndrome (AIDS), with its plethora of CNS abnormalities.

Examination of Lymph Nodes

Generalized lymphadenopathy is nonspecific; it may be seen with neoplasm, infection (including AIDS), collagen vascular disease, sarcoid, hyperthyroidism, Addison disease, and drug reaction (especially that due to phenytoin). Local lymph node enlargement or inflammation, however, may provide clues to a primary tumor site or source of infection.

Cardiac Examination

Cardiac auscultation will confirm the presence of arrhythmias such as atrial fibrillation, with its inherent increased risk of emboli. Changing mitral murmurs are heard with atrial myxomas and papillary muscle ischemia, which is seen with current or impending MI. Constant murmurs indicate valvular heart disease and may be heard with the valvular vegetation of bacterial endocarditis.

Abdominal Examination

Possibly helpful findings on abdominal examination include abnormal bowel sounds, organomegaly, masses, and ascites. Bowel sounds are absent in an acute abdominal condition, as well as with anticholinergic poisoning. Hyperactive bowel sounds may be a consequence of increased gastrointestinal (GI) motility from exposure to an acetylcholinesterase inhibitor (a common pesticide ingredient). The liver may be enlarged as a result of right heart failure or tumor infiltration. Nodules or a rock-hard liver may be due to hepatoma or metastatic disease. The liver may be small and hard in cirrhosis.

Splenomegaly is caused by portal hypertension, hematological malignancies, infection, and collagen vascular diseases. Intraabdominal masses may indicate carcinoma. Ascites occurs with liver disease, right heart failure, neoplasms with metastasis to the liver, or ovarian cancer.

Miscellaneous Examinations

Examination of the breasts in the female and of the testicles in the male and rectal examination may reveal common primary tumors. A positive result on tests for blood in stool obtained at rectal examination is consistent with GI bleeding and, possibly, bowel carcinoma. Large amounts of blood in the GI tract may be sufficient to precipitate hepatic encephalopathy in the patient with cirrhosis.

Neurological Examination

Neurological signs may vary depending on the cause of the impaired consciousness and its severity, and they may be partial or incomplete. For example, the patient may have a partial third nerve palsy with pupillary dilation, rather than a complete absence of all third nerve function, or muscle tone may be decreased but not absent. This concept is especially important in the examination of the stuporous or comatose patient, because the level of arousal may also influence the expression of neurological signs. In the stuporous or comatose patient, even slight deviations from normal should not be dismissed as unimportant. Such findings should be carefully considered to discover their pattern or meaning.

Table 5.3 Skin Lesions and Rashes in Coma

Lesion or Rash	Possible Cause	Lesion or Rash	Possible Cause
Antecubital needle marks	Opiate drug abuse	Petechial-purpuric rash	Meningococcemia, other bacterial sepsis (rarely), gonococcemia, staphylococcemia, *pseudomonas*, subacute bacterial endocarditis, allergic vasculitis, purpura fulminans, Rocky Mountain spotted fever, typhus, fat emboli
Pale skin	Anemia or hemorrhage		
Sallow, puffy appearance	Hypopituitarism		
Hypermelanosis (increased pigment)	Porphyria, Addison disease, chronic nutritional deficiency, disseminated malignant melanoma, chemotherapy	Macular-papular rash	Typhus, *candida*, *cryptococcus*, toxoplasmosis, subacute bacterial endocarditis, staphylococcal toxic shock, typhoid, leptospirosis, *pseudomonas* sepsis, immunological disorders: Systemic lupus erythematosus Dermatomyositis Serum sickness
Generalized cyanosis	Hypoxemia or carbon dioxide poisoning		
Grayish-blue cyanosis	Methemoglobin (aniline or nitrobenzene) intoxication		
Localized cyanosis	Arterial emboli or vasculitis	Other skin lesions: Ecthyma gangrenosum	Necrotic eschar often seen in the anogenital or axillary area in *Pseudomonas* sepsis
Cherry-red skin	Carbon monoxide poisoning		
Icterus	Hepatic dysfunction or hemolytic anemia	Splinter hemorrhages	Linear hemorrhages under the nail, seen in subacute bacterial endocarditis, anemia, leukemia, and sepsis
Petechiae	Disseminated intravascular coagulation, thrombotic thrombocytopenic purpura, drugs		
Ecchymosis	Trauma, corticosteroid use, abnormal coagulation from liver disease or anticoagulants	Osler nodes	Purplish or erythematous painful, tender nodules on palms and soles, seen in subacute bacterial endocarditis
Telangiectasia	Chronic alcoholism, occasionally vascular malformations of the brain	Gangrene of digits, extremities	Emboli to larger peripheral veins or arteries
Vesicular rash	Herpes simplex, varicella, behçet disease, drugs		

Data on diseases associated with rashes from Corey, L., Kirby, P., 1987. Rash and fever. In: Braunwald, E., Isselbacher, K.J., Petersdorf, R.G. (Eds.), Harrison's Principles of Internal Medicine, eleventh ed. McGraw-Hill, New York, pp. 240-244.

The neurological examination of a comatose patient serves three purposes: (1) to aid in determining the cause of coma, (2) to provide a baseline, and (3) to help determine the prognosis. For prognosis and localization of a structural lesion, the following components of the examination have been found to be most helpful: state of consciousness, respiratory pattern, pupillary size and response to light, spontaneous and reflex eye movements, and skeletal muscle motor response.

State of Consciousness

The importance of a detailed description of the state of consciousness is worth reemphasizing. It is imperative that the exact stimulus and the patient's specific response be recorded. Several modes of stimulation should be used, including auditory, visual, and noxious. Stimuli of progressively increasing intensity should be applied, with the maximal state of arousal noted and the stimuli, the site of stimulation, and the patient's exact response described. The examiner should start with verbal stimuli, softly and then more loudly calling the patient's name or giving simple instructions to open the eyes. If there is no significant response, more threatening stimuli such as taking the patient's hand and advancing it toward the patient's face are applied. However, a blink response to visual threat need not indicate consciousness (Vanhaudenhuyse et al., 2008). Finally, painful stimuli may be needed to arouse the patient. All patients in apparent coma should be asked to open or close the eyes and to look up and down; these voluntary movements are preserved in the locked-in syndrome but cannot be elicited in coma—an important distinction.

Supraorbital pressure evokes a response even in patients who may have lost afferent pain pathways as a result of peripheral neuropathy or spinal cord or some brainstem lesions. Pinching the chest or extremities may help localize a lesion when it evokes asymmetrical withdrawal responses. Care must be taken to avoid soft-tissue damage. Purposeful movements indicate a milder alteration in consciousness. Vocalization to pain in the early hours of a coma, even if only a grunt, indicates relatively light alteration in consciousness. Later, primitive vocalization may be a feature of the vegetative state.

The Glasgow Coma Scale (GCS; **Table 5.4**) is used widely to assess the initial severity of traumatic brain injury. This battery assesses three separate aspects of a patient's behavior: the stimulus required to induce eye opening, the best motor response, and the best verbal response. Degrees of increasing dysfunction are scored. Its reproducibility and simplicity make the GCS an ideal method of assessment for nonneurologists involved in the care of comatose patients, such as neurological intensive care nurses. Its failure to assess other essential neurological parameters, however, limits its utility. Additionally, in patients who are intubated or who have suffered facial trauma, assessment of certain components of the GCS, such as eye opening and speech, may be difficult or impossible. Wijdicks and colleagues (1998) have suggested two new tools—the *continuous performance test* and the *hand position test*—that may serve as substitutes for the GCS in such patients, as well as in those with fluctuating levels of consciousness. The continuous performance test monitors level of alertness and requires the patient to raise a hand every time he or she hears a certain letter sound in a standardized sentence spoken by the examiner. The hand position test is a test of praxis in which the patient must mimic three different hand positions demonstrated by the examiner.

Table 5.4 **The Glasgow Coma Scale**

BEST MOTOR RESPONSE	M
Obeys	6
Localizes	5
Withdraws	4
Abnormal flexion	3
Extensor response	2
Nil	1
VERBAL RESPONSE	**V**
Oriented	5
Confused conversation	4
Inappropriate words	3
Incomprehensible sounds	2
Nil	1
EYE OPENING	**E**
Spontaneous	4
To speech	3
To pain	2
Nil	1

Respiration

Normal breathing is quiet and unlabored. The presence of any respiratory noise implies airway obstruction, which must be dealt with immediately to prevent hypoxia. Normal respiration depends on (1) a brainstem mechanism, located between the midpons and cervical medullary junction, that regulates metabolic needs; and (2) forebrain influences that subserve behavioral needs such as speech production. The organization and function of brainstem mechanisms responsible for respiratory rhythm generation, as well as forebrain influences, are complex and beyond the scope of this chapter. Neuropathological correlates of respiration are presented in **Fig. 5.1**.

Respiratory patterns that are helpful in localizing levels of involvement include Cheyne-Stokes respiration, central neurogenic hyperventilation, apneustic breathing, cluster breathing, and ataxic respiration. *Cheyne-Stokes respiration* is a respiratory pattern that slowly oscillates between hyperventilation and hypoventilation. In 1818, Cheyne described his patient as follows: "For several days his breathing was irregular; it would entirely cease for a quarter of a minute, then it would become perceptible, though very low, then by degrees it became heaving and quick and then it would gradually cease again. This revolution in the state of his breathing occupied about a minute during which there were about 30 acts of respiration."

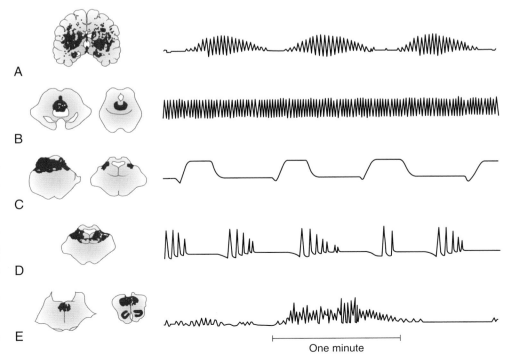

Fig. 5.1 Abnormal respiratory patterns associated with pathologic lesions (*shaded areas*) at various levels of the brain. The tracings were obtained by chest-abdomen pneumograph; inspiration reads up. **A,** Cheyne-Stokes respiration—diffuse forebrain damage. **B,** Central neurogenic hyperventilation—lesions of low midbrain ventral to aqueduct of Sylvius and of upper pons ventral to the fourth ventricle. **C,** Apneusis—dorsolateral tegmental lesion of middle and caudal pons. **D,** Cluster breathing—lower pontine tegmental lesion. **E,** Ataxic breathing—lesion of the reticular formation of the dorsomedial part of the medulla. *(Reprinted from Plum, F., Posner, J.B., 1995. The Diagnosis of Stupor and Coma, third ed. Oxford University Press, New York. Copyright 1966, 1972, 1980, 1996, Oxford University Press, Inc. Used by permission of Oxford University Press, Inc.)*

One minute

Cheyne-Stokes respiration is associated with bilateral hemispheric or diencephalic insults, but it may occur as a result of bilateral damage anywhere along the descending pathway between the forebrain and upper pons. It also is seen with cardiac disorders that prolong circulation time. Alertness, pupillary size, and heart rhythm may vary during Cheyne-Stokes respiration (Posner et al., 2007). Patients are more alert during the waxing portion of breathing.

A continuous pattern of Cheyne-Stokes respiration is a relatively good prognostic sign, usually implying that permanent brainstem damage has not occurred. However, the emergence of Cheyne-Stokes respiration in a patient with a unilateral mass lesion may be an early sign of herniation. A change in pattern from Cheyne-Stokes respiration to certain other respiratory patterns, described next, is ominous.

Two breathing patterns similar to Cheyne-Stokes respiration should not be confused with it. *Short-cycle periodic breathing* is a respiratory pattern with a shorter cycle (faster rhythm) than Cheyne-Stokes respiration, with one or two waxing breaths followed by two to four rapid breaths, then one or two waning breaths. It is seen with increased ICP, lower pontine lesions, or expanding lesions in the posterior fossa (Posner et al., 2007). A similar type of respiration, in which there are short bursts of seven to ten rapid breaths, then apnea without a waning and waxing prodrome, has been erroneously referred to as *Biot's breathing*. Biot, in fact, described an ataxic respiratory pattern, which is described later.

Central neurogenic hyperventilation refers to rapid breathing, from 40 to 70 breaths per minute, usually due to central tegmental pontine lesions just ventral to the aqueduct or fourth ventricle (Posner et al., 2007). This type of breathing is rare and must be differentiated from reactive hyperventilation due to metabolic abnormalities of hypoxemia secondary to pulmonary involvement. Large CNS lesions may cause neurogenic pulmonary edema with associated hypoxemia and increased respiratory rate. Increased intracerebral pressure causes spontaneous hyperpnea. Hyperpnea cannot be ascribed to a CNS lesion when arterial oxygen partial pressure is less than 70 to 80 mm Hg or carbon dioxide partial pressure is greater than 40 mm Hg.

Kussmaul breathing is a deep, regular respiration observed with metabolic acidosis. *Apneustic breathing* is a prolonged inspiratory gasp with a pause at full inspiration. It is caused by lesions of the dorsolateral lower half of the pons (Posner et al., 2007). *Cluster breathing*, which results from high medullary damage, involves periodic respirations that are irregular in frequency and amplitude, with variable pauses between clusters of breaths.

Ataxic breathing is irregular in rate and rhythm and usually is due to medullary lesions. The combination of ataxic respiration and bilateral sixth nerve palsy may be a warning sign of brainstem compression from an expanding lesion in the posterior fossa. This is an important sign because brainstem compression due to tonsillar herniation (or other causes) may result in abrupt loss of respiration or blood pressure. Ataxic and gasping respirations are signs of lower brainstem damage and often are preterminal respiratory patterns.

Pupil Size and Reactivity

Normal pupil size in the comatose patient depends on the level of illumination and the state of autonomic innervation.

The sympathetic efferent innervation consists of a three-neuron arc. The first-order neuron arises in the hypothalamus and travels ipsilaterally through the posterolateral tegmentum to the ciliospinal center of Budge at the T1 level of the spinal cord. The second-order neuron leaves this center and synapses in the superior cervical sympathetic ganglion. The third-order neuron travels along the internal carotid artery and then through the ciliary ganglion to the pupillodilator muscles. Parasympathetic efferent innervation of the pupil arises in the Edinger-Westphal nucleus and travels in the oculomotor nerve to the ciliary ganglion, from which it innervates the pupillosphincter muscle (see Figs. 16.1 and 16.2 in Chapter 16).

Afferent input to the papillary reflex depends on the integrity of the optic nerve, optic chiasm, optic tract, and projections into the midbrain tectum and efferent fibers through the Edinger-Westphal nucleus and oculomotor nerve. Abnormalities in pupil size and reactivity help delineate structural damage between the thalamus and pons (**Fig. 5.2**), act as a warning sign heralding brainstem herniation, and help differentiate structural causes of coma from metabolic causes.

Thalamic lesions cause small, reactive pupils, often referred to as *diencephalic pupils*. Similar pupillary findings are noted in many toxic-metabolic conditions resulting in coma. Hypothalamic lesions or lesions elsewhere along the sympathetic pathway result in *Horner syndrome*. Midbrain lesions produce three types of pupillary abnormality, depending on where the lesion occurs:

1. Dorsal tectal lesions interrupt the pupillary light reflex, resulting in *midposition pupils*, which are fixed to light but react to near vision; the latter is impossible to test in the comatose patient. Spontaneous fluctuations in size occur, and the ciliospinal reflex is preserved.
2. Nuclear midbrain lesions usually affect both sympathetic and parasympathetic pathways, resulting in *fixed, irregular midposition pupils*, which may be unequal.
3. Lesions of the third nerve fascicle in the brainstem, or after the nerve has exited the brainstem, cause *wide pupillary dilation* unresponsive to light. Pontine lesions interrupt sympathetic pathways and cause small, so-called pinpoint pupils which remain reactive, although magnification may be needed to observe this feature. Lesions above the thalamus and below the pons should leave pupillary function intact, except for Horner syndrome in medullary or cervical spinal cord lesions. The pathophysiology of pupillary response is discussed further in Chapters 16 and 36.

Asymmetry in pupillary size or reactivity, even of minor degree, is important. Asymmetry of pupil size may be due to dilation (mydriasis) of one pupil, such as with third nerve palsy, or contraction (miosis) of the other, as in Horner syndrome. This may be differentiated by the pupillary reactivity to light and associated neurological signs. A dilated pupil due to a partial third nerve palsy is less reactive and usually is associated with extraocular muscle involvement. The pupil in Horner syndrome is reactive; if the syndrome results from a lesion in the CNS, it may be associated with anhidrosis of the entire ipsilateral body. Cervical sympathetic chain lesions produce anhidrosis of only face, neck, and arm. A partial or complete third nerve palsy causing a dilated pupil may result

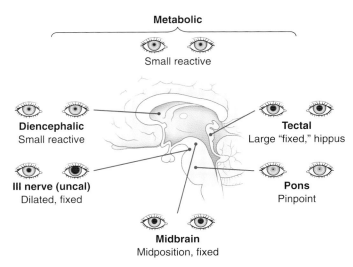

Metabolic

Small reactive

Diencephalic
Small reactive

Tectal
Large "fixed," hippus

III nerve (uncal)
Dilated, fixed

Pons
Pinpoint

Midbrain
Midposition, fixed

Fig. 5.2 Pupils in comatose patients. (*Reprinted from Plum, F., Posner, J.B., 1995. The Diagnosis of Stupor and Coma, third ed. Oxford University Press, New York. Copyright 1966, 1972, 1980, 1996, Oxford University Press, Inc. Used by permission of Oxford University Press, Inc.)*

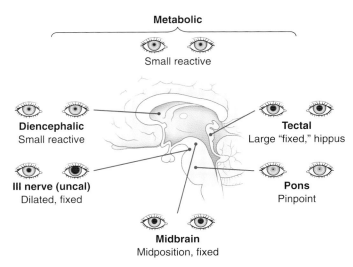

from an intramedullary lesion, most commonly in the midbrain (e.g., intramedullary glioma or infarction), uncal herniation compressing the third nerve, or a posterior communicating artery aneurysm. A sluggishly reactive pupil may be one of the first signs of uncal herniation, followed soon thereafter by dilation of that pupil, and later complete third nerve paralysis.

Several caveats are important in examining the pupil or assessing pupillary reflexes. A common mistake is using insufficient illumination. The otoscope may be useful in this regard, because it provides both adequate illumination and magnification. Rarely, preexisting ocular or neurological injury may fix the pupils or result in pupillary asymmetry. Seizures may cause transient anisocoria. Local and systemic medications may affect pupillary function. Topical ophthalmological preparations containing an acetylcholinesterase inhibitor, used in the treatment of glaucoma, produce miosis. The effect of a mydriatic agent placed by the patient or a prior observer may wear off unevenly, resulting in pupillary asymmetry. Some common misleading causes of a unilateral dilated pupil include prior mydriatic administration, old ocular trauma or ophthalmic surgery, and (more rarely) carotid artery insufficiency.

Ocular Motility

Normal ocular motility (see Chapters 16 and 35) depends on the integrity of a large portion of the cerebrum, cerebellum, and brainstem. Preservation of normal ocular motility implies that a large portion of the brainstem from the vestibular nuclei at the pontomedullary junction to the oculomotor nucleus in the midbrain is intact. Voluntary ocular motility cannot be judged in the comatose patient, so the examiner must rely on reflex eye movements that allow for assessment of the ocular motor system. The eye movements normally are conjugate, and eyes are in the midposition in the alert person. Sleep or obtundation alone may unmask a latent vertical or horizontal

strabismus, resulting in dysconjugacy; therefore, patients must be examined when maximally aroused. The eyes return to the midposition in brain-dead patients.

Evaluation of ocular motility consists of (1) observation of the resting position of the eyes, including eye deviation; (2) notation of spontaneous eye movements; and (3) testing of reflex ocular movements.

Abnormalities in Resting Position

Careful attention must be paid to the resting position of the eyes. Even a small discrepancy in eye position may represent a partial extraocular nerve palsy. Partial nerve palsies or combined nerve palsies predictably result in a more complex picture on examination. Unilateral third nerve palsy from either an intramedullary midbrain lesion or extramedullary compression causes the affected eye to be displaced downward and laterally. A sixth nerve palsy produces inward deviation. Isolated sixth nerve palsy, however, is a poor localizer because of the extensive course of the nerve and because this palsy may be caused by nonspecific increases in ICP, presumably from stretching of the extramedullary portion of the nerve. A fourth nerve palsy is difficult to assess in the comatose patient because of the subtle nature of the deficit in ocular motility. Extraocular nerve palsies often become more apparent with the "doll's eye maneuver" or cold caloric testing in the comatose patient.

Pontaneous eye deviation may be conjugate or dysconjugate. Conjugate lateral eye deviation usually is due to an ipsilateral lesion in the frontal eye fields but may be due to a lesion anywhere in the pathway from the ipsilateral eye fields to the contralateral parapontine reticular formation (see Chapter 35). Dysconjugate lateral eye movement may result from a sixth nerve palsy in the abducting eye, a third nerve palsy in the adducting eye, or an internuclear ophthalmoplegia. An internuclear ophthalmoplegia may be differentiated from a third nerve palsy by the preservation of vertical eye movements.

Downward deviation of the eyes below the horizontal meridian usually is due to brainstem lesions (most often from tectal compression); however, it also may be seen in metabolic disorders such as hepatic coma. Thalamic and subthalamic lesions produce downward and inward deviation of the eyes. Patients with these lesions appear to be looking at the tip of the nose. Sleep, seizure, syncope, apnea of Cheyne-Stokes respiration, hemorrhage into the vermis, and brainstem ischemia or encephalitis cause upward eye deviation, making this a poor localizing sign. *Skew deviation* is a maintained deviation of one eye above the other (hypertropia) that is not due to a peripheral neuromuscular lesion or a local extracranial problem in the orbit. It usually indicates a posterior fossa lesion (brainstem or cerebellar). Dysconjugate vertical eye position sometimes may occur in the absence of a brainstem lesion in the obtunded patient.

Spontaneous Eye Movements

Spontaneous eye movements (see Chapter 16) are of many types. Purposeful-appearing eye movements in a patient who otherwise seems unresponsive should lead to consideration of the locked-in syndrome, catatonia, pseudocoma, or PVS. *Roving eye movements* are slow, conjugate, lateral to-and-fro movements. For roving eye movements to be present, the ocular motor nuclei and their connections must be intact. Generally when roving eye movements are present, the brainstem is relatively intact and coma is due to a metabolic or toxic cause or bilateral lesions above the brainstem. Detection of roving eye movements may be complicated by ocular palsies or internuclear ophthalmoplegia. These superimposed lesions produce relatively predictable patterns but often obscure the essential roving nature of the movement for the inexperienced observer.

Nystagmus occurring in comatose patients suggests an irritative or epileptogenic supratentorial focus. An epileptogenic focus in one frontal eye field causes contralateral conjugate eye deviation. Nystagmus due to an irritative focus may rarely occur alone without other motor manifestations of seizures. In addition, inconspicuous movements of the eye, eyelid, face, jaw, or tongue may be associated with electroencephalographic status epilepticus. An electroencephalogram (EEG) is required to ascertain the presence of this condition.

Spontaneous conjugate vertical eye movements are separated into different types according to the relative velocities of their downward and upward phases. In *ocular bobbing*, rapid downward jerks of both eyes are observed, followed by a slow return to the midposition (Leigh and Zee, 2006). In the typical form, there is associated paralysis of both reflex and spontaneous horizontal eye movements. *Monocular* or *paretic bobbing* occurs when a coexisting ocular motor palsy alters the appearance of typical bobbing. The term *atypical bobbing* refers to all other variations of bobbing that cannot be explained by an ocular palsy superimposed on typical bobbing. Most commonly, this term is used to describe ocular bobbing when lateral eye movements are preserved. *Typical ocular bobbing* is specific but not pathognomonic for acute pontine lesions. Atypical ocular bobbing occurs with anoxia and is nonlocalizing. *Ocular dipping*, also known as *inverse ocular bobbing*, refers to spontaneous eye movements in which an initial slow downward phase is followed by a relatively rapid return. Reflex horizontal eye movements are preserved. It usually is associated with diffuse cerebral damage. In *reverse ocular bobbing*, there is a slow initial downward phase followed by a rapid return that carries the eyes past the midposition into full upward gaze. Then the eyes slowly return to the midposition. Reverse ocular bobbing is nonlocalizing.

Vertical nystagmus due to an abnormal pursuit or vestibular system is slow deviation of the eyes from the primary position, with a rapid (saccadic) immediate return to the primary position. It is differentiated from bobbing by the absence of latency between the corrective saccade and the next slow deviation. *Ocular-palatal myoclonus* (the palatal movement also is called *palatal tremor*) occurs after damage to the lower brainstem involving the Guillain-Mollaret triangle, which extends between the cerebellar dentate nucleus, red nucleus, and inferior olive. It consists of a pendular vertical nystagmus in synchrony with the palatal movements. *Ocular flutter* is back-to-back saccades in the horizontal plane and usually is a manifestation of cerebellar disease.

Reflex Ocular Movements

Examination of ocular movement is not complete in the comatose patient without assessment of reflex ocular movements, including the oculocephalic reflex ("doll's eye phenomenon") and, if necessary, caloric (thermal) testing. In practice, the terms *doll's eye phenomenon* and *doll's eye maneuver* are used synonymously to refer to the oculocephalic reflex, but these terms are often confusing to the neophyte neurologist. It is better to use the term *oculocephalic reflex* followed by a description of the response. To test for this reflex, the examiner briskly rotates the patient's head in both directions laterally, then flexes and extends the neck, continually observing the motion of the eyes. When supranuclear influences on the ocular motor nerves are removed, the eyes move in the orbit opposite to the direction of the head turn and maintain their position in space. *This maneuver should not be performed on any patient until the stability of the neck has been adequately assessed.* If there is any question of neck stability, a neck brace should be applied and caloric testing substituted. In the normal oculocephalic reflex (normal or positive doll's eye phenomenon), the eyes move conjugately in a direction opposite to the direction of movement of the head. Cranial nerve palsies predictably alter the response to this maneuver (**Table 5.5**).

Clinical caloric testing (as distinct from quantitative calorics, used to assess vestibular end-organ disorders; see Chapter 37) is commonly done by applying cold water to the tympanic membrane. With the patient supine, the head should be tilted forward 30 degrees to allow maximal stimulation of the lateral semicircular canal, which is most responsible for reflex lateral eye movements. After the ear canal is carefully checked to ensure that it is patent and the tympanic membrane is free of defect, 10 mL of ice-cold water is slowly instilled into one ear canal. For purposes of the neurological examination, irrigation of each ear with 10 mL of ice water generally is sufficient.

Cold water applied to the tympanic membrane causes currents to be set up in the endolymph of the semicircular canal. This results in a change in the baseline firing of the vestibular nerve and slow (tonic) conjugate deviation of the eyes toward the stimulated ear. In an awake person, the eye deviation is corrected with a resulting nystagmoid jerking of the eye toward the midline (fast phase). Warm-water irrigation produces reversal of flow of the endolymph, which causes conjugate eye deviation with a slow phase away from the stimulated ear and a normal corrective saccadic fast phase toward the ear. By tradition, the nystagmus is named by the direction of the fast phase. The mnemonic *COWS* (*c*old, *o*pposite; *w*arm, *s*ame) refers to the fast phases. Simultaneous bilateral cold water application results in slow downward deviation, whereas simultaneous bilateral warm water application causes upward deviation.

Oculocephalic or caloric testing may elicit subtle or unsuspected ocular palsies. Abnormal dysconjugate responses occur with cranial nerve palsies, intranuclear ophthalmoplegia, or restrictive eye disease. Movements may be sluggish or absent. Sometimes reinforcement of cold caloric testing with superimposed passive head turning after injection of cold water into the ear may reveal eye movement when either test alone shows none.

False-negative or misleading responses on caloric testing occur with preexisting inner ear disease, vestibulopathy such as that due to ototoxic drugs like streptomycin, vestibular paresis caused by illnesses such as Wernicke encephalopathy, and drug effects. Subtotal labyrinthine lesions decrease the response; there is no response when the labyrinth is destroyed. Lesions of the vestibular nerve cause a decreased or absent

Table 5.5 Oculocephalic Reflex*

Method	Response	Interpretation
Lateral head rotation	Eyes remain conjugate, move in direction opposite to head movement and maintain position in space	Normal
	No movement in either eye on rotating head to left or right	Bilateral pontine gaze palsy, bilateral labyrinthine dysfunction, drug intoxication, anesthesia
	Eyes move appropriately when head is rotated in one direction but do not move when head is rotated in opposite direction	Unilateral pontine gaze palsy
	One eye abducts, the other eye does not adduct	Third nerve palsy
		Internuclear ophthalmoplegia
Vertical head flexion and extension	Eyes remain conjugate, move in direction opposite to head movement and maintain position in space	Normal
	No movement in either eye	Bilateral midbrain lesions
	Only one eye moves	Third nerve palsy
	Bilateral symmetrical limitation of upgaze	Aging

*To be performed only after neck stability has been ascertained.

Table 5.6 Caloric Testing

Method	Response	Interpretation
Cold water instilled in right ear	Slow phase to right, fast (corrective) phase to the left	Normal
	No response (make sure canal is patent, apply warm-water stimulus to opposite ear)	Obstructed ear canal, "dead" labyrinth, eighth nerve or nuclear dysfunction, false-negative result (see text)
	Slow phase to right, no fast phase	Toxic-metabolic disorder, drugs, structural lesion above brainstem
	Downbeating nystagmus	Horizontal gaze palsy
Cold water instilled in left ear	Responses should be opposite those for right ear	Peripheral eighth nerve or labyrinth disorder on right (provided that right canal is patent)
Warm water instilled in left ear after no response from cold water in right ear	Slow phase to right, fast phase to left	

response. Drugs that suppress either vestibular or ocular motor function (or both) include sedatives, anticholinergics, anticonvulsants, tricyclic antidepressants, and neuromuscular blocking agents. If the response from one ear is indeterminate, both cold- and warm-water stimuli should be applied to the other ear. If the test remains equivocal, superimposition of the doll's eye maneuver is recommended. Interpretation of abnormal cold caloric responses is summarized in **Table 5.6**. An unusual ocular reflex that has been observed in the setting of PVS is reflex opening of both eyes triggered by flexion of an arm at the elbow. This reflex is distinct from reflex eye opening in the comatose patient induced by raising the head or turning it from side to side.

Motor System

Examination of the motor system of a stuporous or comatose patient begins with a description of the resting posture and adventitious movements. Purposeful and nonpurposeful movements are noted and the two sides of the body compared. Head and eye deviation to one side and contralateral hemiparesis suggests a supratentorial lesion, whereas ipsilateral paralysis indicates a probable brainstem lesion. External rotation of the lower limb is a sign of hemiplegia or hip fracture.

Decerebrate posturing is bilateral extensor posture with extension of the lower extremities and adduction and internal rotation of the shoulders and extension at the elbows and wrist. Bilateral midbrain or pontine lesions usually are responsible for decerebrate posturing. Less commonly, deep metabolic encephalopathies or bilateral supratentorial lesions involving the motor pathways may produce a similar pattern.

Decorticate posturing is bilateral flexion at the elbows and wrists, with shoulder adduction and extension of the lower extremities. It is a much poorer localizing posture, because it may result from lesions in many locations, although usually above the brainstem. Decorticate posture is not as ominous a sign as decerebrate posture, because the former occurs with many relatively reversible lesions.

Unilateral decerebrate or decorticate postures also are less ominous. Lesions causing unilateral posturing may be anywhere in the motor system from cortex to brainstem. Unilateral extensor posturing is common immediately after a cerebrovascular accident, followed in time by a flexor response.

Posturing may occur spontaneously or in response to external stimuli such as pain, or may even be set off by such minimal events as the patient's own breathing. These postures, though common, may also be variable in their expression because of other associated brainstem or more rostral brain damage.

Special attention should be given to posturing because it often signals a brainstem herniation syndrome. Emergency room personnel and inexperienced physicians may mistake these abnormal postures for convulsions (seizures) and institute anticonvulsant therapy, resulting in an unfortunate delay of appropriate therapy for the patient.

Adventitious movements in the comatose patient may be helpful in separating metabolic from structural lesions. Tonic-clonic or other stereotyped movements signal seizure as the probable cause of decreased alertness. *Myoclonic jerking*, consisting of nonrhythmical jerking movements in single or multiple muscle groups, is seen with anoxic encephalopathy or other metabolic comas such as hepatic encephalopathy. *Rhythmic myoclonus*, which must be differentiated from epileptic movements, usually is a sign of brainstem injury. Tetany occurs with hypocalcemia. *Cerebellar fits* result from intermittent tonsillar herniation and are characterized by deterioration of level of arousal, opisthotonos, respiratory rate slowing and irregularity, and pupillary dilatation.

The motor response to painful stimuli should be tested, but the pattern of response may vary depending on the site stimulated. Purposeful responses may be difficult to discriminate from more primitive reflexes. Flexion, extension, and adduction may be either voluntary or reflex in nature. In general, abduction is most reliably voluntary, with shoulder abduction stated to be the only definite nonreflex reaction. This is tested by pinching the medial aspect of the upper arm. Reflex flexor response to pain in the upper extremity consists of adduction of the shoulder, flexion of the elbow, and pronation of the arm. The *triple flexion response* in the lower extremities refers to reflex withdrawal, with flexion at the hip and knee and dorsiflexion at the ankle, in response to painful stimulation on the foot or lower extremity. Such reflexes seldom are helpful in localizing a lesion.

Spinal reflexes are reflexes mediated at the level of the spinal cord and do not depend on the functional integrity of the brain or brainstem. Most patients with absent cortical or brainstem function have some form of spinal reflex.

The *plantar reflex* may be extensor in coma from any cause, including drug overdoses and postictal states. It becomes flexor on recovery of consciousness if there is no underlying structural damage.

Muscle tone and asymmetry in muscle tone are helpful in localizing a focal structural lesion and may help differentiate metabolic from structural coma. Acute structural damage above the brainstem usually results in decreased or flaccid tone. In older lesions, tone usually is increased. Metabolic insults generally cause a symmetrical decrease in tone. Finally, generalized flaccidity is ultimately seen after brain death.

Coma and Brain Herniation

Herniation syndromes are explained in Chapter 50. Knowledge of some of the clinical signs of herniation is especially important in the clinical approach to coma. Traditional signs of herniation due to supratentorial masses usually are variations of either an uncal or a central pattern. Classically, the uncal pattern includes early signs of third nerve and midbrain compression. The pupil initially dilates as a result of third nerve compression but later returns to the midposition with midbrain compression that involves the sympathetic as well as the parasympathetic tracts. In the central pattern, the earliest signs are mild impairment of consciousness, with poor concentration, drowsiness, or unexpected agitation; small but reactive pupils; loss of the fast component of cold caloric testing; poor or absent reflex vertical gaze; and bilateral corticospinal tract signs, including increased tone of the body ipsilateral to the hemispheric mass lesion responsible for herniation (Posner et al., 2007).

Signs of herniation tend to progress generally in a rostrocaudal manner. An exception occurs when intraventricular bleeding extends to the fourth ventricle and produces a pressure wave, compressing the area around the fourth ventricle. Also, when an LP reduces CSF pressure suddenly in the face of a mass lesion that produced increased ICP, sudden herniation of the cerebellar tonsils through the foramen magnum may result (Posner et al., 2007). Both of these clinical scenarios may be associated with sudden unexpected failure of medullary functions that support respiration or blood pressure. In patients with herniation syndromes, the clinical picture may be confusing because of changing signs or the expression of scattered, isolated signs of dysfunction in separate parts of the brain. In addition, certain signs may be more prominent than others.

Increased ICP invariably accompanies brainstem herniation and may be associated with increased systolic blood pressure, bradycardia, and sixth nerve palsies. These signs, however, as well as many of the traditional signs of herniation described, actually occur relatively late. Earlier signs of potential herniation are decreasing level of arousal, slight change in depth or rate of respiration, and the appearance of a Babinski sign. Tonsillar herniation may be suggested by an altered level of consciousness, opisthotonic posturing, dilated pupils, and irregular breathing. It is important to suspect herniation early, because once advanced changes develop, structural injury is likely to have occurred; subsequently, there is less chance of reversal.

Differential Diagnosis

Differentiating Toxic-Metabolic Coma from Structural Coma

Many features of the history and physical examination help differentiate structural from metabolic and toxic causes of coma. Some features have already been mentioned. When the history is available, the patient's underlying illnesses and medications or the setting in which they are found often help guide the physician to the appropriate cause. The time course of the illness resulting in coma can be helpful. Generally, structural lesions have a more abrupt onset, whereas metabolic or toxic causes are more slowly progressive. Multifocal structural diseases such as vasculitis or leukoencephalopathy are an exception to this rule, as they may exhibit slow progression, usually in a stepwise manner. Supratentorial or infratentorial tumors characterized by slow growth and surrounding edema may also mimic metabolic processes.

The response to initial emergency therapy may help differentiate metabolic or toxic causes of coma. The hypoglycemic patient usually awakens after administration of glucose, the hypoxic patient responds to oxygen, and the patient experiencing an opiate drug overdose responds to naloxone.

In general, structural lesions have focal features or at least notable asymmetry on neurological examination. Toxic, metabolic, and psychiatric diseases are characterized by their symmetry. Bilateral and often multilevel involvement frequently is seen with metabolic causes. Asymmetries may be observed but generally are of small degree and tend to fluctuate over time.

Many features of the neurological examination differentiate metabolic or toxic causes from structural lesions:

- *State of consciousness.* Patients with metabolic problems often have milder alterations in arousal, typically with waxing and waning of the behavioral state. Patients with acute structural lesions tend to stay at the same level of arousal or progressively deteriorate. Toxins may also cause progressive decline in level of arousal.
- *Respiration.* Deep, frequent respiration most commonly is due to metabolic abnormalities, though rarely it is caused by pontine lesions or by neurogenic pulmonary edema secondary to acute structural lesions.
- *Funduscopic examination.* Subhyaloid hemorrhage or papilledema are almost pathognomonic of structural lesions. Papilledema due to increased ICP may be indicative of an intracranial mass lesion or hypertensive encephalopathy. Papilledema does not occur in metabolic diseases except hypoparathyroidism, lead intoxication, and malignant hypertension.
- *Pupil size.* The pupils usually are symmetrical in coma from toxic-metabolic causes. Patients with metabolic or toxic encephalopathies often have small pupils with preserved reactivity. Exceptions occur with methyl alcohol poisoning, which may produce dilated and unreactive pupils, or late in the course of toxic or metabolic coma if hypoxia or other permanent brain damage has occurred. In terminal asphyxia, the pupils dilate initially and then become fixed at midposition within 30 minutes. The initial dilation is attributed to massive sympathetic discharge.

- *Pupil reactivity.* Assessment of the pupillary reflex is one of the most useful means of differentiating metabolic from structural causes of coma. Pupillary reactivity is relatively resistant to metabolic insult and usually is spared in coma from drug intoxication or metabolic causes, even when other brainstem reflexes are absent. Hypothermia may fix pupils, as does severe barbiturate intoxication. Neuromuscular blocking agents produce midposition or small pupils, and glutethimide and atropine dilate them.
- *Ocular motility.* Asymmetry in oculomotor function typically is a feature of structural lesions.
- *Spontaneous eye movements.* Roving eye movements with full excursion are most often indicative of metabolic or toxic abnormalities.
- *Reflex eye movements.* Reflex eye movements normally are intact in toxic-metabolic coma, except rarely in phenobarbital or phenytoin intoxication or deep metabolic coma from other causes.
- *Adventitious movement.* Periods of motor restlessness, tremors, or spasm punctuating coma often are due to drugs or toxins such as chlorpromazine or lithium. Brainstem herniation or intermittent CNS ischemia also may produce unusual posturing movements. Myoclonic jerking generally is metabolic and often anoxic in origin.
- *Muscle tone.* Muscle tone usually is symmetrical and normal or decreased in metabolic coma. Structural lesions cause asymmetrical muscle tone. Tone may be increased, normal, or decreased by structural lesions.

The examiner should be aware of common structural lesions that mimic toxic-metabolic causes and, conversely, toxic or metabolic causes of coma that may be associated with focal abnormalities on examination. Structural lesions that may mimic toxic-metabolic causes include subarachnoid hemorrhage, sinus vein thrombosis, chronic or bilateral subdural hemorrhage, and other diffuse or multifocal disorders such as vasculitis, demyelinating diseases, or meningitis. Any toxic-metabolic cause of coma may be associated with focal features; however, such features most often are observed with barbiturate or lead poisoning, hypoglycemia, hepatic encephalopathy, and hyponatremia. Old structural lesions such as prior stroke may be the origin of residual abnormalities found on neurological examination in a patient who is comatose from toxic or metabolic causes. Moreover, metabolic abnormalities such as hypoglycemia may unmask relatively silent structural abnormalities. Detailed descriptions of the toxic and metabolic encephalopathies are provided in Chapter 56.

Differentiating Psychiatric Coma and Pseudocoma from Metabolic or Structural Coma

The patient who appears unarousable as a result of psychiatric disease and the patient who is feigning unconsciousness for other reasons may be difficult to differentiate from each other. In such instances, the history, when available, and findings on the physical examination may suggest to the physician that a nonphysiological mechanism is at work. Multiple inconsistencies are present on examination, and abnormalities that are found do not fit the pattern of usual neurological syndromes. Examinations of the eyelid, pupil, adventitious eye movements, and vestibulo-oculogyric reflex by cold caloric testing are especially useful to confirm the suspicion of pseudocoma.

Eyelid tone is difficult to alter voluntarily. In the patient with true stupor or coma, passive eyelid opening is easily performed and is followed by slow, gradual eyelid closure. The malingering or hysterical patient often gives active resistance to passive eye opening and may even hold the eyes tightly closed. It is nearly impossible for the psychiatric or malingering patient to mimic the slow, gradual eyelid closure. Blinking also increases in psychiatric and malingering patients but decreases in patients in true stupor.

The pupils normally constrict in sleep or (eyes-closed-type) coma but dilate with the eyes closed in the awake state. Passive eye opening in a sleeping person or a truly comatose patient (if pupillary reflexes are spared) results in pupillary dilation. Opening the eyes of an awake person produces constriction. This principle may help differentiate coma from pseudocoma.

Roving eye movements cannot be mimicked and thus also are a good sign of true coma. Finally, if during cold caloric testing, the eyes do not tonically deviate to the side of the caloric instillation, and the fast phases are preserved, stupor or true coma is essentially ruled out. Moreover, cold caloric testing with the resultant vertigo usually "awakens" psychiatric and malingering patients.

Helpful Laboratory Studies

Laboratory tests that are extremely helpful in evaluating the comatose patient are listed in **Table 5.7**. Arterial blood gas determinations rule out hypoxemia and carbon dioxide narcosis and help differentiate primary CNS problems from secondary respiratory problems. Liver disease, myopathy, and rhabdomyolysis all elevate alanine aminotransferase and aspartate aminotransferase levels. Liver function test results may be misleading in end-stage liver disease, as values may be normal or only mildly elevated with markedly abnormal liver function. Although the blood ammonia level does not correlate well with the level of hepatic encephalopathy, it often may

Table 5.7 Laboratory Tests Helpful in Differential Diagnosis for Coma

Laboratory Study	Result	Associated Disorders
Electrolytes (Na, K, Cl, CO_2)		See Chapters 49A and 56 for discussion of disorders associated with abnormalities of electrolytes, glucose, BUN, calcium, and magnesium
Glucose		
BUN		
Creatinine		
Calcium		
Magnesium		
Complete blood count with differential	Hematocrit: Increased	Volume depletion, underlying lung disorder, myeloproliferative disorder, cerebellar hemangioblastoma; may be associated with vascular sludging (hypoperfusion)
	Decreased	Anemia, hemorrhage
	White blood cell count: Increased	Infection, acute stress reaction, steroid therapy, after epileptic fit, myeloproliferative disorder
	Decreased	Chemotherapy, immunotherapy, viral infection, sepsis
	Lymphocyte count: Decreased	Viral infection, malnutrition, AIDS
Platelet count	Decreased	Sepsis, disseminated intravascular coagulation, thrombotic thrombo-cytopenic purpura, idiopathic thrombocytopenic purpura, drugs; may be associated with intracranial hemorrhage
PT	Increased	Coagulation factor deficiency, liver disease, anticoagulants, disseminated intravascular coagulation
PTT	Increased	Heparin therapy, lupus anticoagulant
Arterial blood gases		See text
Creatine phosphokinase		See text
Liver function studies		See text
Thyroid function studies		See text
Plasma cortisol level		See text
Drug and toxin screen		See text
Serum osmolality		See text

AIDS, Acquired immunodeficiency syndrome; *BUN*, blood urea nitrogen; *PT*, prothrombin time; *PTT*, partial thromboplastin time.

be markedly elevated and thus helpful in cases of suspected liver disease with relatively normal liver function studies. Hepatic encephalopathy may continue for up to 3 weeks after liver function values return to normal.

Thyroid function studies are necessary to document hypothyroidism or hyperthyroidism. When addisonian crisis is suspected, a serum cortisol level should be obtained. A low or normal level in the stressful state of coma or illness strongly suggests adrenal insufficiency. Further testing of adrenal function should be performed as appropriate.

When the cause of coma is not absolutely certain, or in possible medicolegal cases, a blood alcohol level and a drug and toxin screen are mandatory. The results of these tests usually are not available immediately but may be invaluable later. Serum osmolality can usually be measured rapidly by the laboratory and may be used to estimate alcohol level because alcohol is an osmotically active particle and increases the osmolar gap in proportion to its blood level. Serum osmolality can be calculated using the following:

$$\text{Serum osmolality} = 2\,Na + (mEq/L) + BUN\ (mg/dL)/2.8$$
$$+ \text{glucose}\ (mg/dL)/18$$

The osmolar gap, which is the difference between the measured serum osmolality and the calculated serum osmolality, represents unmeasured osmotically active particles.

Creatine kinase levels should routinely be measured in comatose patients initially and then at least daily for the first several days because of the great risk of rhabdomyolysis and subsequent preventable acute tubular necrosis in these patients. Measuring creatine kinase MB isoenzyme levels every 8 hours for the first 24 hours helps rule out an MI.

Other Useful Studies

Electrocardiography

The electrocardiogram is useful to show MI, arrhythmia, conduction blocks, bradycardia, or evidence of underlying hypertension or atherosclerotic coronary vascular disease. Hypocalcemia causes QT prolongation. Hypercalcemia shortens the QT interval. The heart rate is slow in hypothyroid patients with low-voltage QRS, flat or inverted T waves, and flattened ST segments. Hyperthyroid patients are generally tachycardic.

Neuroradiological Imaging

Once the patient is stabilized, necessary treatment is given, the initial examination is complete, and appropriate laboratory studies are ordered, the next test of choice is a CT scan of the brain, without contrast but with 5-mm cuts of the posterior fossa. Alternatively, magnetic resonance imaging (MRI) may be performed, depending on the clinical setting and the stability of the patient's condition. MRI provides superb visualization of the posterior fossa and its contents, an extremely useful feature when structural disease of the brainstem is suspected. MRI is not as specific as CT scanning for visualizing early intracranial hemorrhage, however, and it is limited at present by the length of time required to perform the imaging, image degradation by even a slight movement of the patient, and the relative inaccessibility of the patient during the imaging process. The CT scan, when performed as described, is currently the most expedient imaging technique, giving the physician the

most information about possible structural lesions with the least risk to the patient. Repeating the scan with IV dye may be necessary later to better define lesions seen on the initial scan.

The value of the CT scan in demonstrating mass lesions and hemorrhage is undeniable. Furthermore, it may demonstrate features of brain herniation. Uncal herniation is characterized on CT scan by (1) displacement of the brainstem toward the contralateral side, with increase in width of subarachnoid space between the mass and ipsilateral free edge, (2) medial stretching of the posterior cerebral and posterior communicating arteries, (3) obliteration of the interpeduncular cistern, (4) occipital lobe infarction, and (5) distortion and elongation of the U-shaped tentorial incisura. The clinician should be aware that the CT scan may miss early infarction, encephalitis, and isodense subdural hemorrhage. Special caution must be taken in evaluating CT scans in comatose patients, especially before LP, to rule out isodense subdural or bilateral subdural hemorrhage. Interpretation of CT scans is discussed in Chapter 33A.

In severe head injury, studies of cerebral metabolism employing single photon emission computed tomography (SPECT) may be of prognostic value (Della Corte et al., 1997). Although cerebral blood flow in the first 48 hours after trauma does not appear to correlate with severity or prognosis, the cerebral metabolic rate of oxygen ($CMRo_2$), like the GCS, may be useful in predicting prognosis.

Electroencephalography

The EEG is helpful in many situations and disorders: confirming underlying cortical structural damage in patients too unstable to travel to the CT scanner; postictal states in patients slow to wake after a presumed seizure; partial complex seizures; electroencephalographic or nonconvulsive status epilepticus, such as is seen in comatose patients after anoxic ischemic damage; and toxic-metabolic disturbances. With metabolic disorders, the earliest EEG changes typically are a decrease in the frequency of background rhythms and the appearance of diffuse theta activity that progresses to more advanced slowing in association with a decrease in the level of consciousness. In hepatic encephalopathy, bilaterally synchronous and symmetrical, medium- to high-amplitude, broad triphasic waves, often with a frontal predominance, may be observed. Herpes simplex encephalitis may be suggested by the presence of unilateral or bilateral periodic sharp waves with a temporal preponderance. The EEG also can help confirm a clinical impression of catatonia, pseudocoma, the locked-in syndrome, PVS, and brain death (Brenner, 2005). EEGs are discussed further in Chapter 32A.

Evoked Potentials

Evoked potentials may help in evaluating brainstem integrity and assessing prognosis for comatose patients. A study of 50 hemodynamically stable patients remaining in coma 4 hours after resuscitation from cardiopulmonary arrest with short-latency somatosensory evoked potentials within 8 hours after arrest found that none of the 30 patients without cortical potentials recovered cognition. Five of the 20 patients with cortical potentials recovered. Forty percent of the patients who did not recover had preserved brainstem reflexes, allowing some evaluation of prognosis in a group of patients in whom prognosis is difficult to assess by other means. Event-related potentials may prove particularly useful as an objective assessment of cognitive function in patients with the locked-in syndrome (Onofrj et al., 1997). The N100 component of the auditory evoked potential and cognitive evoked potentials (mismatch negativity obtained after novel stimuli) appear to have predictive value for awakening from coma, but the pupillary reflex remains the strongest prognostic variable (Fischer et al., 2004). Absence of evoked potentials in response to somatosensory stimuli also is highly predictive of nonawakening from coma (Robinson et al., 2003).

Intracranial Pressure Monitoring

ICP measurements provide an index of the degree of brain swelling and are particularly useful in the management of patients who have suffered severe head injury. Postmortem studies of fatal head injuries demonstrate a direct correlation between very elevated ICP and death due to tentorial herniation. In the absence of intracranial hematomas, however, comatose patients with normal findings on brain imaging studies have a low frequency of increased ICP and almost never develop uncontrolled intracranial hypertension.

Prognosis

In view of the current state of knowledge, outcome in any comatose patient cannot be predicted with 100% certainty unless that patient meets the criteria for brain death, as described later in the chapter. The available evidence is insufficient to permit a definitive statement that a particular non–brain-dead patient will *not* recover from coma, nor does it allow prognostication regarding how much recovery may occur in specific cases. However, based on serial examinations at various times after the onset of coma, general statistics on the outcome of coma have been compiled and give the examiner a general idea of how patients may do.

The natural history of coma can be considered in terms of three subcategories: drug-induced, nontraumatic, and traumatic coma. Drug-induced coma usually is reversible unless the patient has not had appropriate systemic support while comatose and has sustained secondary injury from hypoperfusion, hypoxia, or lack of other necessary metabolic substrates.

Nontraumatic Coma

Only about 15% of patients in nontraumatic coma make a satisfactory recovery. Functional recovery is related to the cause of coma. Diseases causing structural damage, such as cerebrovascular disease including subarachnoid hemorrhage, carry the worst prognosis; coma from hypoxia-ischemia due to such causes as cardiac arrest has an intermediate prognosis; coma due to hepatic encephalopathy and other metabolic causes has the best ultimate outcome. Age does not appear to be predictive of recovery. The longer a coma lasts, the less likely the patient is to regain independent functioning. Factors that adversely impact brain injury following cardiac arrest include cerebral edema, pyrexia, hyperglycemia, and seizures (Neumar et al., 2008).

In the early days after the onset of nontraumatic coma, it is not possible to predict with certainty which patients will ulti-

mately enter or remain in a vegetative state. Although rare cases have been reported of patients awakening after prolonged vegetative states, patients with nontraumatic coma who have not regained awareness by the end of 1 month are unlikely to do so. Even if they do regain consciousness, they have practically no chance of achieving an independent existence. A large multi-institutional study determined that within 3 days of cardiac arrest, evaluation in the intensive care unit is sufficiently predictive of neurological outcome to allow for informed decisions regarding life support. Absence of pupillary light or corneal reflexes, and motor response to noxious stimuli no greater than extension, suggest a poor prognosis for recovery. Other poor prognostic signs are myoclonic status epilepticus, bilateral absence of the N20 response from the somatosensory cortex, and several neuroimaging signs (Young, 2009).

Traumatic Coma

The prognosis for traumatic coma differs from that for nontraumatic coma in many ways. First, many patients with head trauma are young. Second, prolonged coma of up to several months does not preclude a satisfactory outcome in traumatic coma. Third, in relationship to their initial degree of neurological abnormality, traumatic coma patients do better than nontraumatic coma patients.

The prognosis for coma from head trauma may be considered in terms of survival. However, because many more patients survive traumatic coma than nontraumatic coma, it is equally important to consider the ultimate disabilities of the survivors; many who survive are left with profound disabilities. The GCS is a practical system for describing outcome in traumatic coma. As originally proposed, this scale includes five categories: (1) death, (2) PVS, (3) severe disability (conscious but disabled and dependent on others for activities of daily living), (4) moderate disability (disabled but independent), and (5) good recovery (resumption of normal life even though there may be minor neurological and psychiatric deficits).

In their landmark 1979 report, Jennett and colleagues studied 1000 patients in coma longer than 6 hours from severe head trauma: 49% of these patients died, 3% remained vegetative, 10% survived with severe disability, 17% survived with moderate disability, and 22% had good recovery. The most reliable predictors of outcome 6 months later were depth of coma as evaluated by the GCS; pupil reaction, eye movements, and motor response in the first week after injury; and patient age.

In summary, early predictors of the outcome of posttraumatic coma include patient's age, motor response, pupillary reactivity, eye movements, and depth and duration of coma. The prognosis worsens with increasing age. Cause of injury, skull fracture, lateralization of damage to one hemisphere, and extracranial injury appear to have little influence on the outcome.

Persistent Vegetative State

As a rule, PVS can be reliably diagnosed 12 months after a traumatic brain injury and 6 months after other cerebral insults. Recovery after 3 years for patients in PVS has not been reported (Wijdicks and Cranford, 2005). Those patients who have been reported to "improve" remain severely disabled, bed- or wheelchair-bound, and fully dependent on care. At 5 years, the mortality rate for PVS is in excess of 80%. Prolonged survival is rare and requires exquisite medical attention. Death typically results from untreated infection or overwhelming sepsis. "Miracle awakenings," such as with the sudden appearance of communicative speech, have been observed rarely in patients in the minimally conscious state but not in those in PVS (Wijdicks and Cranford, 2005).

Brain Death

Clinical Approach to Brain Death

A thorough knowledge of the criteria for brain death is essential for the physician whose responsibilities include evaluation of comatose patients. Despite differences in state laws, the criteria for the establishment of brain death are fairly standard within the medical community. These criteria include the following:

- *Coma.* The patient should exhibit an unarousable unresponsiveness. There should be no meaningful response to noxious, externally applied stimuli. The patient should not obey commands or demonstrate any verbal response, either reflexively or spontaneously. Spinal reflexes, however, may be retained.
- *No spontaneous respirations.* The patient should be removed from ventilatory assistance, and carbon dioxide should be allowed to build up because of the respiratory drive that hypercapnia produces. The diagnosis of absolute apnea requires the absence of spontaneous respiration at a carbon dioxide tension of at least 60 mm Hg. A safe means of obtaining this degree of carbon dioxide retention involves the technique of apneic oxygenation, in which 100% oxygen is delivered endotracheally through a thin sterile catheter for 10 minutes. Arterial blood gas levels should be obtained to confirm the arterial carbon dioxide pressure.
- *Absence of brainstem reflexes.* Pupillary, oculocephalic, corneal, and gag reflexes all must be absent, and there should not be any vestibulo-ocular responses to cold calorics.
- *Electrocerebral silence.* An isoelectric EEG should denote the absence of cerebrocortical function. Some authorities do not regard the performance of an EEG as mandatory in assessing brain death, and instances of preserved cortical function despite irreversible and complete brainstem disruption have been reported.
- *Absence of cerebral blood flow.* Cerebral contrast angiography or radionuclide angiography can substantiate the absence of cerebral blood flow, which is expected in brain death. These tests are considered confirmatory rather than mandatory. On rare occasions, in the presence of supratentorial lesions with preserved blood flow to the brainstem and cerebellum, findings on cerebral radionuclide angiography may be misleading.
- *Absence of any potentially reversible causes of marked CNS depression.* Such causes include hypothermia (temperature 32°C [89.6°F] or less), drug intoxication (particularly barbiturate overdose), and severe metabolic disturbance.

Brain Death Survival

Despite aggressive therapeutic measures, survival of "brain-dead" persons for more than 1 week has been considered unlikely. Shewmon (1998) reviewed a series of 175 cases surviving longer than 1 week after diagnosis of "brain death." Survival potential decreased exponentially, with an initial half-life of 2 to 3 months, followed at 1 year by a slow decline. One patient survived for more than 14 years. Survival was found to correlate inversely with age, and prolonged survival was more common with primary brain pathology. The tendency to cardiovascular collapse in brain death may be transient and is more likely to be attributable to systemic than to brain pathology.

References

The complete reference list is available online at www.expertconsult.com.

Chapter 6

Approaches to Intellectual and Memory Impairments

Howard S. Kirshner

The term *intellect* designates the totality of the mental or cognitive operations that comprise human thought—the higher cortical functions that make up the conscious mind. The intellect and its faculties, the subject matter of human psychology, are the qualities that most separate human beings from other animals. Memory is a specific cognitive function: the storage and retrieval of information. As such, it is the prerequisite for learning, the building block of all human knowledge. Other "higher" functions such as language, calculations, spatial topography and reasoning, executive function, music, and creativity all represent functions of specific brain systems. The relationship of the mind and brain has long been of philosophical interest. Recent advances in cognitive neuroscience have made mind-brain questions the subject of practical scientific and clinical study. It is now possible to study how the metabolic activation of brain regions and the firing patterns of neurons give rise to the phenomenon of consciousness, the sense of self, the ability to process information, and the development of decisions and attitudes. The pattern of an individual's habitual decisions and attitudes becomes one's personality.

Francis Crick (1994), who with James Watson won the Nobel Prize for the discovery of the structure of DNA, expressed the "astonishing hypothesis" that "you, your joys and your sorrows, your sense of personal identity and free will, are in fact no more than the behavior of a vast assembly of nerve cells and their associated molecules" (p. 3). This chapter considers our knowledge of intellect and memory, mind and brain, from the perspective of the clinical neurologist who must assess disorders of the higher functions.

Neural Basis of Cognition

Cerebral Cortex

The cognitive operations discussed in this chapter take place among a large network of cortical cells and connections, the neural switchboard that gives rise to conscious thinking. The cortical mantle of the human brain is very large compared with animal brains, containing more than 14 billion neurons. The information stored in the human cerebral cortex rivals that found in large libraries. Within the cortical mantle, the areas that have expanded the most from animal to human are the association cortices, cortical zones that do not carry out primary motor or sensory functions but rather interrelate the functions of the primary motor and sensory areas. According to Nauta and Feirtag's 1986 text, 70% of neurons in the human central nervous system reside in the cerebral cortex, and 75% of those are in the association cortex. Higher cortical functions, with few exceptions, take place in the association cortex.

The neuroanatomy of the cerebral cortex has been known in considerable detail since the 1800s. Primary cortical sensory areas include the visual cortex in the occipital lobe, the auditory cortex in the temporal lobe, the somatosensory cortex in the parietal lobe, and probably gustatory and olfactory cortices in the frontal and temporal lobes. Each of these primary cortices receives signals in only one modality (vision, hearing, or sensation) and has cortical-cortical connections only to adjacent portions of the association cortex also dedicated to this modality, called *unimodal association cortex*. Sensory information is sequentially processed in an increasingly complex fashion, leading from raw sensory data to a unified percept. Within each cortical area are columns of cells with similar function, called *modules*.

The organization of the primary sensory cortex and unimodal association cortex has been especially well worked out in the visual system through the Nobel Prize–winning research of Hubel and Wiesel and others. Retinal ganglion cells are activated by light within a bright center, with inhibition in the surround. These cells project through the optic nerve to the lateral geniculate body of the thalamus, then via the optic radiations to the primary visual cortex in the occipital lobes. In the primary visual cortex, a vertical band of neurons may be dedicated to the detection of a specific bright area, but in the cortex this is usually a bar or edge of light rather than a spot. These "simple" cells of the visual cortex respond to bright central bars with dark surrounds. Several such cells project to complex cells, which may detect an edge or line with a specific orientation or a specific direction of movement but with less specificity about the exact location within the visual field. Visual shapes are perceived by the operation of these cells. Complex cells in turn project to cells in the visual unimodal association cortex (the Brodmann areas 18 and 19), where cells may detect movement or patterns. Complex cells also respond to movement anywhere in the visual field, an important characteristic because of the organism's need to maintain visual attention for possible hazards in the environment. In the visual association cortex, columns may respond to specific shapes, colors, or qualities such as novelty. In this fashion, the functions of cell columns or modules become more sophisticated from the primary cortex to the association cortex. In Fodor's model, the modules of primary visual perception project to central systems. Cognitive science has made tremendous strides in the understanding of the neurobiology of specific functions such as vision, but it has yet to fathom the higher perceptual functions such as the concept of beauty in a starry sky or in a painting, or the cross-modality processes that underlie, for example, the adaptation of a ballet to a specific musical accompaniment.

Unimodal association cortices communicate with each other via still more complex connections to the heteromodal association cortex, of which there are two principal sites. The posterior heteromodal association cortex involves the posterior inferior parietal lobe, especially the angular gyrus. The posterior heteromodal cortex makes it possible to perceive an analogy between an association in one modality (e.g., a picture of a boat or the printed word *boat* in the visual modality) with a percept in a different modality (e.g., the sound of the spoken word *boat*). These intermodality associations are difficult for animals, even chimpanzees, but easy for human beings. Cross-sensory associations involve the functioning of *cortical networks* of multitudes of neurons; the analogy drawn by neuroscientists is to the vast arrays of circuits active in computer networks. The product of such associations is a concept.

The second heteromodal association cortex involves the lateral prefrontal region (Goldman-Rakic, 1996). This region is thought to be involved with attention or "working memory" and with sequential processes such as storage of temporally ordered stimuli and the planning of motor activities. This temporal sequencing of information and motor planning is referred to by neuropsychologists as the *executive function* of the brain—the decisions we make every instant regarding which of the myriad of sensory stimuli reaching the sensory cortices merit attention, which require a motor response, and in what sequence and timing these motor responses will occur.

Another frontal cortical area, the orbitofrontal portion of the prefrontal cortex, is thought to be involved in emotional states, appetites, and drives, or in the integration of internal bodily states with sensations from the external world. The orbitofrontal cortex is known as the *supramodal cortex* (Benson, 1996) because it relates the functions of the heteromodal cortex regarding attention and sequencing of responses with interoceptive inputs from the internal milieu of the body. The orbitofrontal area has close connections with the limbic system and autonomic, visceral, and emotional processes. In studying brain evolution from primitive reptiles to humans, the neurobiologist Paul MacLean hypothesized that the internal and emotional parts of the brain, the limbic system, must be tied into the newer neocortical areas responsible for intellectual function, and that the linking of these two systems must underlie the phenomenon of consciousness. In a review of neuronal mechanisms of consciousness, Ortinski and Meador (2004) defined *conscious awareness* as "the state in which external and internal stimuli are perceived and can be intentionally acted on" (p. 1017). Benson and Ardila (1996), in reviewing clinical data from individuals with frontal lobe damage, state that the supramodal cortex is the brain system that "anticipates, conjectures, ruminates, plans for the future, and fantasizes." In other words, this part of the brain brings specific cognitive processes to conscious awareness and may be responsible for the phenomena of consciousness and self-awareness themselves.

Consciousness

All human beings have a subjective understanding of what it means to be conscious and to have a concept of self, yet the neural basis for conscious awareness and the sense of self remain poorly understood. Until recently, many neuroscientists left the study of consciousness to the realm of religion and philosophy. Even Hippocrates knew that consciousness emanated from the brain, but "to consciousness the brain is messenger." Francis Crick devoted the last part of his career to the understanding of consciousness. For Crick, the best model for the study of consciousness is visual awareness because the anatomy and physiology of the visual system are well understood. Crick argued that neurons in the primary visual cortex likely do not have access to conscious awareness. Stated another way, we do not pay attention to much of what our eyes see and our visual cortex analyzes. A perceived object, however, excites neurons in several areas of the visual association cortex, each with associations that enter consciousness or are stored in short-term memory.

Crick and Koch (1995) hypothesized that activation of the frontal cortex is necessary for visual percepts to enter consciousness, although subconscious awareness in the form of blindsight may exist at the level of the occipital cortex. Conscious visual perception involves interactions between the visual parts of the brain and the prefrontal systems for attention and working memory (Ungerleider, Courtney, and Haxby, 1998). The orbitofrontal cortex contains neurons that integrate interoceptive stimuli related to changes in the internal milieu with exteroceptive sensory inputs such as vision. Ortinski and

Meader (2004) also point out the varying latencies of perception of specific sensory stimuli, such as color versus identification of a visual object. A synchronization of inputs through the thalamus to the cortex may be necessary before the perception becomes conscious. As stated earlier, the interaction between attention to external stimuli and internal stimuli underlies conscious awareness.

In the visual system, Goodale and Milner (1992; Milner and Goodale, 2008; see also McIntosh and Schenk, 2009) have divided the visual system, after processing in the occipital cortex, into a ventral and a dorsal stream. The ventral stream, involved in perception of objects, is usually subject to conscious awareness and involves an occipital-temporal pathway, whereas the dorsal stream, involved in spatial localization of perceived objects to plan action, is usually less conscious.

There are many clinical examples of "unconscious" mental processing, and a number of these involve vision. Patients with cortical blindness sometimes show knowledge of items they cannot see, a phenomenon called *blindsight*. Patients with right hemisphere lesions who extinguish objects in the left visual field when presented with bilateral stimuli nonetheless show activation of the right visual cortex by functional magnetic resonance imaging (MRI), indicating that the objects are perceived, although not with conscious awareness (Rees et al., 2000). Libet (1999) demonstrated experimentally that visual and other sensory stimuli have to persist at least 500 milliseconds to reach conscious awareness, yet stimuli of shorter duration can elicit reactions. An experimental example of unconscious visual processing comes from Gur and Snodderly (1997), who tested color vision in monkeys. When two colors were projected at a frequency of greater than 10 Hz, the monkey perceived a fused color, yet cellular recordings clearly demonstrated coding of information about the two separate colors in the monkey's visual cortex. Motor responses to sensory stimuli can occur before conscious awareness, as in the ability to pull one's hand away from a hot stove before feeling the heat. Racers begin running before they are aware of having heard the starting gun (Crick and Koch, 1998). A familiar example of unconscious visual processing is the drive home from work; most individuals can remember very little they see on the trip, yet they avoid oncoming vehicles and obstacles, stop for red lights, and drive without accidents. Crick and Koch (1998) refer to the unconscious visual processing as an "online" visual system. We shall discuss unconscious or "implicit" memories later in this chapter. In language syndromes, patients can match spoken to written words without knowledge of their meaning, suggesting that there are unconscious rules of language. Brust (2000) has called all of these unconscious mental processes the "non-Freudian unconscious."

Recent research has linked the right frontal cortex to the sense of self. Keenan and colleagues (2001) studied patients undergoing the Wada test, in which a barbiturate is injected into the carotid artery to determine cortical language dominance. They presented subjects with a self-photograph and a photograph of a famous person, followed by a "morphed" photograph of a famous person and the patient. When the left hemisphere was anesthetized, the subjects said that the morphed photograph represented the subject himself, whereas with right hemisphere anesthesia, the subject selected the famous face. Patients with frontotemporal dementia

also indicate a relationship between the right frontal lobe and self-concept. In the series by Miller and colleagues (2001), six of the seven patients who developed a major change in self-concept during their illness had predominant atrophy in the nondominant frontal lobe. A last example of the sense of self is the so-called Theory of Mind, which alludes to the understanding of another person as a conscious human being. Keenan and colleagues (2005) cite evidence that the right hemisphere frontotemporal cortex is dominant for both the sense of self and the recognition of other people.

The frontal lobes, as the executive center of the brain and the determining agent for attention and motor planning, are the origin of several critical networks for cognition and action. Cummings (1993) described five frontal networks for consciousness and behavior. The frontal cortex projects to the basal ganglia, then to thalamic nuclei, and back to the cortex.

Clinical neurology provides important information about how lesions in the brain impair consciousness. The functioning of the awake mind requires the ascending inputs referred to as the *reticular activating system*, with its way stations in the brainstem and thalamus, as well as an intact cerebral cortex. Bilateral lesions of the brainstem or thalamus produce coma. Very diffuse lesions of the hemispheres produce an "awake" patient who shows no responsiveness to the environment, a state sometimes called *coma vigil* or *persistent vegetative state*, as in the well-known Terri Schiavo case (Bernat, 2006; Perry, Churchill, and Kirshner, 2005). Patients with very slight responses to environmental stimuli are said to be in a *minimally conscious state* (Wijdicks and Cranford, 2005). Recently, functional brain imaging studies have suggested that at least in a few patients labeled as having persistent vegetative state or minimally conscious state after traumatic brain injury, patients can think of playing tennis or standing in their home and seeing the other rooms, and the brain areas activated are similar to those of normal subjects. These same subjects, a small minority of patients with chronically impaired consciousness secondary to traumatic brain injury, showed evidence of conscious modulation of brain activity to indicate "yes" or "no" responses (Monti et al., 2010). This report has engendered controversy over our ability to determine when a patient truly lacks consciousness. In an accompanying editorial, Ropper noted that activation on brain imaging studies does not equal conscious awareness, and the concept that "I have brain activation, therefore I am…would seriously put Descartes before the horse" (Ropper, 2010).

Still less severe diffuse abnormalities of the association cortex produce encephalopathy, delirium, or dementia. These topics involve very common syndromes of clinical neurology. Stupor and coma are discussed in Chapter 5, and encephalopathy, or delirium, is covered in Chapter 4.

Focal lesions of the cerebral cortex generally produce deficits in specific cognitive systems. A detailed listing of such disorders would include much of the subject matter of behavioral neurology. Examples include Broca aphasia from a left frontal lesion, Wernicke aphasia from a left temporal lesion, Gerstmann syndrome (acalculia, left-right confusion, finger agnosia, and agraphia) from a left parietal lesion, visual agnosia or failure to recognize visual objects (usually from bilateral posterior lesions), apraxia from a left parietal lesion, and constructional impairment from a right parietal lesion. Multiple focal lesions can affect cognitive function in a more global fashion, as in the dementias (Chapter 66). Some authorities separate "cortical" dementias such as Alzheimer disease, in which combinations of cortical deficits are common, from "subcortical" dementias, in which mental slowing is the most prominent feature.

The frontal lobes are heavily involved in integration of the functions provided by other areas of cortex, and lesions there may affect personality and behavior in the absence of easily discernible deficits of specific cognitive, language, or memory function. In severe form, extensive lesions of the orbitofrontal cortex may leave the individual awake but staring, unable to respond to the environment, a state called *akinetic mutism*. With lesser lesions, patients with frontal lobe lesions may lose their ability to form mature judgments, reacting impulsively to incoming stimuli in a manner reminiscent of animal behavior. Such patients may be inappropriately frank or disinhibited. A familiar example is the famous case of Phineas Gage, a worker who sustained a severe injury to the frontal lobes. Gage became irritable, impulsive, and so changed in personality that coworkers said he was "no longer Gage." Bedside neurological testing and even standard neuropsychological tests of patients with frontal lobe damage may reveal normal intelligence except for concrete or idiosyncratic interpretation of proverbs and similarities. Experimentally, subjects with frontal lobe lesions can be shown to have difficulty with sequential processes or shifting of cognitive sets, as tested by the Wisconsin Card Sorting Test or the Category Test of the Halstead-Reitan battery. Luria introduced a simple bedside test of sequential shapes (**Fig. 6.1**). In contrast to the subtlety of these deficits to the examiner, the patient's family may state that there is a dramatic change in the patient's personality.

Another clinical window into the phenomena of consciousness comes from surgery to separate the hemispheres by cutting the corpus callosum. In split-brain or commissurotomized patients, each hemisphere seems to have a separate consciousness. The left hemisphere, which has the capacity for speech and language, can express this consciousness in words. For example, a split-brain patient can report words or pictures that appear in the right visual field. The right hemisphere cannot produce verbal accounts of items seen in the left visual field, but the subject can choose the correct item by pointing with the left hand; at the same time, the subject claims to have no conscious knowledge of the item. In terms of the speaking left hemisphere, the right hemisphere has "unconscious" visual knowledge, or *blindsight*. At times, the left hand of the patient may seem to operate under a different agenda from the right hand. A split-brain patient may select a dress from a rack with the right hand while the left hand puts it back or selects a more daring fashion. This rivalry of the left hand with the right is called the *alien hand syndrome*, a striking example of the separate consciousnesses of the two divided

hemispheres (Gazzaniga, 1998). Callosal syndromes, including the alien hand syndrome, have also been described in patients with strokes involving the corpus callosum (Chan and Ross, 1997).

Memory

Memory Stages

Memory refers to the ability of the brain to store and retrieve information, the necessary prerequisite for all learning. Some memories are so vivid they seem like a reliving of a prior experience, as in Marcel Proust's sudden recollections of his youth on biting into a madeleine pastry. Other memories are more vague or bring up a series of facts rather than a perceptual experience. Memory has been divided into several types and stages, leading to a confusing set of terms and concepts. Clinical neurologists have historically divided memory into three temporal stages. The first stage, called *immediate memory span*, corresponds to Baddeley's concept of *working memory* (Baddeley, 2010). *Immediate memory* refers to the amount of information a subject can keep in conscious awareness without active memorization. The normal human being can retain seven digits in active memory span. Perhaps by coincidence, seven digits comprise a local telephone number. Most normal people can hear a telephone number, walk across the room, and dial the number without active memorization. Numbers of more than seven digits, called *supraspan numbers*, do require active memory processing, as do unnatural tasks such as reverse digit span. Disorders of attention affect digit span and very focal lesions of the superior frontal neocortex affecting Brodmann areas 8 and 9 may have profound effects on immediate memory (Goldman-Rakic, 1996). Many patients with aphasia secondary to left frontal lesions have impaired immediate memory. The items in immediate memory are normally forgotten as soon as the subject's attention switches to another topic (telephone numbers we look up and call once tend to be completely forgotten quickly unless we actively try to "memorize" them).

The second stage of memory, referred to by clinicians as *short-term* or *recent memory*, involves the ability to register and recall specific items such as words or events after a delay of minutes or hours. Synonyms for this type of memory include *declarative* and *episodic memory* (Squire and Zola, 1996; Dickerson and Eichenbaum, 2010). Some memory investigators and cognitive neuroscientists refer to immediate memory span as *short-term* and recent memory as *long-term*. This differs from clinical usage and causes confusion; for this reason, it is better to use the less ambiguous term, *episodic memory*. This second stage of memory requires the function of the hippocampus and parahippocampal areas of the medial temporal lobe for both storage and retrieval. The amygdala, a structure adjacent to the medial temporal cortex, is not essential for episodic memory but seems crucial for recall of emotional contexts of specific events and the reactions of fear or pleasure associated with those events. The familiar bedside test of recalling three unrelated memory items at 5 minutes demonstrates episodic (short-term) memory, as do questions about this morning's breakfast.

Long-term memory, also called *remote memory*, refers to long-known information such as where one grew up, who was one's first grade teacher, or the names of grandparents. In

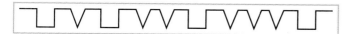

Fig. 6.1 Luria's test of alternating sequences. *(Adapted from Luria, A.R., 1969. Frontal lobe syndromes, In: Vynken P., Bruyn, G.W. (Eds.), Handbook of Clinical Neurology, vol. 2, Elsevier, New York. Reprinted with permission from Kirshner, H.S., 2002. Behavioral Neurology: Practical Science of Mind and Brain, second ed. Butterworth Heinemann, Boston.)*

Table 6.1 Memory Stages

Traditional Term	Cognitive Neuroscience Term	Awareness Level	Anatomy
Immediate memory	Working memory	Explicit	Prefrontal cortex
Short-term memory	Episodic memory	Explicit	Medial temporal lobe
Long-term memory	Semantic memory	Explicit	Lateral temporal and other cortices
Motor memory	Procedural memory	Implicit	Basal ganglia, cerebellum

Box 6.1 Amnestic Syndrome Features

Impaired recent memory (anterograde, retrograde)
Global amnesia
Spared procedural memory
Preserved immediate memory
Preserved remote memory
Intact general cognitive function
Disorientation to time or place
Confabulation

current parlance, the factual knowledge we recall consciously is called *semantic memory* (Budson and Price, 2005). Recall of famous figures or events, such as presidents or wars, and knowledge of semantic information, such as the definitions of words and the differences between words, are used to test semantic memory. Semantic memory differs from personal long-term memory in that the subject can continuously replenish such knowledge by reading and conversation.

Semantic memory is thought to reside in multiple cortical regions such as the visual association cortex for visual memories, the temporal cortex for auditory memories, and so on. This concept of multiple localizations of semantic memory is supported by functional brain imaging research (Cappa, 2008). Specific semantic knowledge of word meanings is thought to reside in the left lateral temporal cortex. Remote memory, as we shall see later, resists the effects of medial temporal damage; once memory is well stored in the neocortex, it can be retrieved without use of the hippocampal system.

Other categories of memory exist that do not fit into this temporal classification, such as motor and procedural memories. These will be discussed later in this chapter. **Table 6.1** is a classification of memory stages.

Amnestic Syndrome

The amnestic syndrome (**Box 6.1**) refers to profound loss of the second stage of memory, episodic, recent, or short-term memory. These patients, most of whom have bilateral hippocampal damage, have normal immediate memory span and largely normal ability to recall remote memories such as their childhood upbringing and education. Other cognitive or higher cortical functions may be completely intact, which distinguishes these patients from those with dementias such as Alzheimer disease. Motor memories (see Other Types of Memory) tend to be preserved in patients with amnestic syndrome, who may be taught to perform a new motor skill such

as mirror writing. When asked to perform it again, the patient will typically not recall knowing how to do it, but once he or she gets started, the action comes back (the memory is in the hands). Other more variable features of the amnestic syndrome include disorientation to time and sometimes place and *confabulation*, or making up information the memory system does not supply. Amnestic patients live in an eternal present in which they can interact, speak intelligently, and reason appropriately, but they do not remember anything about the interaction a few minutes after it ends. An amnestic patient may complete an IQ test with high scores but not recall taking the examination minutes later. These patients are condemned to repeat the same experiences without learning from them.

The registration of short-term or episodic memory involves a consolidation period during which a blow to the head, as in a football injury, can prevent memories from being stored or recalled. The recognition or recall of items appears to require the hippocampus. The site of storage of memories, as noted earlier, likely involves large areas of the neocortex specialized for specific cognitive functions such as auditory or visual analysis. Once processed in the neocortex and stored for a long period of time, items can be recalled even in the presence of hippocampal damage, as in the case of remote or semantic memories. After an injury producing hippocampal damage, a retrograde period of memory loss may extend back from minutes to years, and the subject cannot form new anterograde memories. As the ability to form new memories returns, the period of retrograde amnesia shortens or "shrinks" ("shrinking retrograde amnesia"). After a minor head injury, the permanent amnestic period may involve a few minutes of retrograde amnesia and a few hours or days of anterograde amnesia. In experimental studies in which amnestic subjects are shown famous people from past decades, a temporal gradient has been found in which subjects have excellent memory for remote personages but recall progressively less from periods dating up to the recent past.

The neuroanatomy of the amnestic syndrome is one of the best-studied areas of cognitive neuropsychology. In animal models, bilateral lesions of the hippocampus, parahippocampal gyrus, and entorhinal cortex produce profound amnesia (Squire and Zola, 1996). Human patients undergoing temporal lobectomy for epilepsy have shown very similar syndromes. In the early period of this surgery, a few patients were deliberately subjected to bilateral medial temporal ablations, with disastrous results for memory, as seen in the famous patient, H.M. (Corkin, 2002; Squire, 2009). In other cases, unilateral temporal lobectomy caused severe amnesia. In one such case, an autopsy many years later showed preexisting damage to the contralateral hippocampus. Patients currently

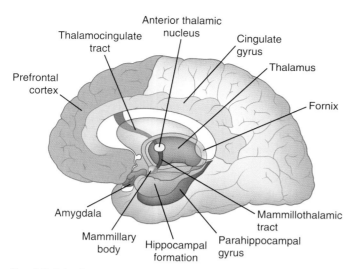

Fig. 6.2 Episodic memory. The medial temporal lobes, including the hippocampus and parahippocampus, form the core of the episodic memory system. Other brain regions are also necessary for episodic memory to function correctly. *(Adapted from Budson, A.E., Price, B.H., 2005. Memory dysfunction, N Engl J Med 352, 692-699.)*

receive extensive evaluation such as the Wada test (intracarotid barbiturate infusion) to ensure that ablation of one hippocampus will not result in the amnestic syndrome, although partial memory deficits still occur. Other common causes of the amnestic syndrome involving bilateral medial temporal lesions include bilateral strokes in the posterior cerebral artery territory, involving the hippocampus, and herpes simplex encephalitis, which has a predilection for the orbitofrontal and medial temporal cortices. Gold and Zola (2006) described three new cases of the amnestic syndrome with detailed neurobehavioral testing in life and neuropathology at autopsy. One had bilateral hippocampal damage, one had Wernicke-Korsakoff syndrome with damage in the mammillary bodies and dorsomedial thalamus, and one had bilateral thalamic infarctions; we will return to these other anatomic substrates of memory later.

Although the anatomy of memory storage and retrieval has been known for many years, numerous recent refinements have been made. **Fig. 6.2** shows a simplified diagram of the memory system in the human brain. The hippocampus on each side projects via the fornix to the septal areas, then to the mammillary bodies, which in turn project to the anterior nucleus of the thalamus and on to the cingulate gyrus of the frontal lobe, which projects back to the hippocampus. This circuit (Papez circuit) is critical for short-term memory registration and retrieval. Disease processes that affect extrahippocampal parts of this circuit also cause amnesia. One well-studied example is the Wernicke-Korsakoff syndrome induced by thiamine deficiency, usually in the setting of alcoholism, with damage to the mammillary bodies and dorsomedial thalamic nuclei (Gold and Squire, 2006). A second clinical example is that of patients with ruptured aneurysms of the anterior communicating artery, which are associated with damage to the deep medial frontal areas such as the septal nuclei. These two amnestic syndromes are commonly associated with confabulation. The anterior communicating artery aneurysm syndrome also involves frontal executive dysfunction (Diamond, DeLuca, and Kelley, 1997). Traumatic brain

injuries commonly produce memory loss, probably because the most common sites of damage are in the frontal and temporal lobes, but other deficits besides memory frequently occur. Of course, memory loss can be seen in several other neurological conditions, including brain tumors of the thalamus or temporal lobes, white matter diseases such as multiple sclerosis, and dementing diseases such as Alzheimer disease, which has a predilection for the hippocampus, basal frontal nuclei, and neocortex. In these other disorders, memory loss is usually not as isolated a deficit as in the amnestic syndrome.

Recently, use of functional brain imaging in awake patients has contributed to knowledge of the anatomy of memory function. According to an early positron emission tomography (PET) study, several brain regions show consistent activation in normal subjects during memory testing. These brain regions include (1) the prefrontal cortex, especially on the right; (2) the hippocampal and adjacent medial temporal regions; (3) the anterior cingulate cortex; (4) the posterior midline regions of the cingulate, precuneate, and cuneate gyri; (5) the inferior parietal cortex, especially on the right; and (6) the cerebellum, particularly on the left (Cabeza et al., 1997). A model for the functions of these areas in memory are as follows: the prefrontal cortex appears to relate to retrieval activation and attention, the hippocampi to conscious recollection, the cingulate cortex to the activation of memory and selection of a specific response, the posterior midline regions to visual imagery, the parietal cortex to spatial awareness, and the cerebellum to voluntary self-initiated retrieval (Cabeza et al., 1997; Wagner et al., 1998; Dickerson and Eichenbaum, 2010). In subjects asked to recognize previously presented pairs of associated words, the right prefrontal cortex, anterior cingulate cortex, and inferior parietal region were the most activated. When the subject had to recall the words, the basal ganglia and left cerebellum also became active. In similar studies using functional MRI, Wagner and colleagues (1998) found that the left prefrontal region was predominantly involved when words were semantically encoded in memory; the right frontal activations seen in the previous study reflected nonverbal memory stimuli. Even in the hippocampus, words elicited activation of the left hippocampus, objects evoked activation in both hippocampi, and faces mainly activated the right hippocampus (Fliessbach et al., 2010; Rosazza et al., 2009). In studies of the recognition of visual designs, Petersson and colleagues (1997) found that the medial temporal cortex activates more during new learning tasks than during previously trained and practiced memory tasks. Other areas activated during the new learning task included the prefrontal and anterior cingulate areas, more on the right side, and the parieto-occipital lobes bilaterally. Trained tasks activated the hippocampi much less but did activate the right inferooccipitotemporal region. This finding correlates with human studies indicating that overlearned memories gradually become less dependent on the hippocampus. Rugg and colleagues (1997) also found greater activation of the left medial temporal cortex in tasks in which the subject remembered words by "deep encoding" of their meaning compared to simpler "shallow" encoding of the specific word. Other studies have shown that the deeper the encoding of a word's meaning, the better the subject remembers it (Schacter, 1996). Finally, the amygdala appears necessary for affective aspects of memory items, such as recall of fear associated with a specific stimulus (Knight, Waters, and Bandettini, 2009).

Budson and Price (2005) provide a simple analogy for remembering the anatomical organization of episodic memory. By this analogy, the frontal lobes are the "filing clerk" of the memory system, deciding what memories to file or retrieve. The medial temporal lobes are the "recent memory filing cabinet," where recent memories are consolidated. More remote memories are stored in the "remote memory filing cabinet," thought to be located more diffusely in other cortical regions.

Basic research on animals has begun to unravel the fundamental biochemical processes involved in memory. Bailey and colleagues (1996) have studied memory formation in the giant snail, *Aplysia*. Development of long-term facilitation, a primitive form of memory, requires activation of a gene called CREB (cyclic adenosine monophosphate response element-binding protein) in sensory neurons. In this system and also in similar studies on the fruit fly, *Drosophila*, gene activation and protein synthesis are necessary for memory formation. Injection of protein-synthesis inhibitors into the hippocampus can prevent consolidation of memories (McGaugh, 2000). Although similar studies have not been performed in humans, it is likely that similar gene activation and protein synthesis, perhaps beginning in the hippocampi but proceeding through its neocortical connections, is necessary for the transition from immediate working memory to longer-term storage of memory (Bear, 1997). This field of research may hold promise for the development of drugs to enhance memory storage.

Syndromes of Partial Memory Loss

In contrast to the global amnesia seen in amnestic syndrome, patients have been described who have memory loss for selected classes of items. For example, patients who undergo left temporal lobectomy for intractable epilepsy usually have detectable impairment of short-term verbal memory, whereas those undergoing right temporal resection have impairment only of nonverbal memory. Isolated sensory-specific memory loss syndromes have also been described, such as pure visual or tactile memory loss. Ross described two patients with bilateral occipital lesions that disconnected the visual cortex from the memory structures. These patients could draw a diagram of their homes but could not learn new spatial layouts. Ross postulated that diagnosis of a selective visual recent memory deficit requires documentation of normal visual perception, absence of aphasia sufficient to impair testing, intact immediate visual memory, intact remote visual memory, and normal recent memory in other modalities. A similar syndrome of isolated tactile memory loss has also been described.

Transient Amnesia

Transient amnesia is a temporary version of amnestic syndrome. The most striking example of transient amnesia is the syndrome of transient global amnesia, lasting from several to 24 hours. In this syndrome, an otherwise cognitively intact individual suddenly loses memory for recent events, asks repetitive questions about his or her environment, and sometimes confabulates. During the episode, the patient has both anterograde and retrograde amnesia, as in the permanent amnestic syndrome. As recovery occurs, however, the retrograde portion "shrinks" to a short period, leaving a permanent gap in memory of the brief retrograde amnesia before the episode and the period of no learning during the episode. The syndrome is of unknown cause but can be closely imitated by disorders of known etiology such as partial complex seizures, migraine, and possibly transient ischemia of the hippocampus on one or both sides. Strupp and colleagues (1998) reported that 7 of 10 patients imaged during episodes of transient global amnesia showed abnormal diffusion MRI signal in the left hippocampus; 3 of these had bilateral hippocampal abnormalities. Permanent infarctions were not found. Yang and colleagues (2008) reported similar hippocampal lesions in the lateral or CA1 region in 17 of 20 cases of TGA. Other investigators have found frontal lobe abnormalities by diffusion-weighted MRI or PET. Gonzalez-Martinez and colleagues (2010) recently reported a case in which a small left thalamic infarction found by diffusion-weighted MRI was associated with hypometabolism in the left thalamic region, seen on FDG-PET. These studies do not prove an ischemic etiology for transient global amnesia; rather, they indicate transient dysfunction in the hippocampus or its connections. The last several patients with transient global amnesia observed at our hospital have had normal diffusion-weighted MRI studies, except for two patients who had incomplete recovery; these patients both had left medial temporal infarctions. Confusional migraine, partial epilepsy (Bilo et al., 2009), drug intoxication, alcoholic "blackouts," and minor head injuries can also produce transient amnesia.

Other Types of Memory (Nondeclarative or Implicit Memory)

A confusing array of memory classifications and terminology has arisen, as shown in **Table 6.2**. Several aspects of memory do not involve the conscious recall involved in the three temporal memory stages. A simple example is motor memory, such as the ability to ride a bicycle, which is remarkably resistant to hippocampal damage. Such motor memories probably reside in the basal ganglia and cerebellum. In Squire and Zola's (1996) classification, motor memories of this type are called *procedural* or *implicit nondeclarative memories*; note that all three of the temporal stages of memory—working (immediate) memory, episodic (short-term) memory, and semantic (long-term) memory—are *declarative, explicit*.

Table 6.2 Types of Memory and Their Localization

Types of Recent Memory	Localization
DECLARATIVE (EXPLICIT)	
Facts, events	Medial temporal lobe
NONDECLARATIVE (IMPLICIT)	
Procedural skills	Basal ganglia, frontal lobes
Classical conditioning	Cerebellum (+ amygdala)
Probabilistic classification learning	Basal ganglia
Priming	Neocortex

Another term for the class of memories for which subjects have no conscious awareness is *implicit* or *nondeclarative memory* (in contrast to the explicit declarative memory of episodic events). Implicit memories have in common storage and retrieval mechanisms that do not involve the hippocampal system; perhaps for this reason, the subject has no conscious knowledge of them. These procedural memories involve "knowing how" rather than "knowing that." Amnestic patients can learn new motor memories such as mirror drawing, which they can perform once started, although they have no recollection of knowing the task. Motor learning likely involves the supplementary motor cortex, basal ganglia, and cerebellum. Strokes in the territory of the recurrent artery of Heubner (affecting the caudate nucleus) can affect procedural memory (Mizuta and Motomura, 2006). Another type of memory localized to the cerebellum is *classical conditioning*, in which an unconditioned stimulus becomes associated with a reward or punishment given when the conditioned stimulus is presented (Thompson and Kim, 1996; Clark, Manns, and Squire, 2002). The conditioning itself clearly involves the cerebellum, but the emotional aspect of the reward or punishment stimulus may reside in the amygdala. Classical conditioning can continue to function after bilateral hippocampal damage. Squire and Zola (1996) outlined other types of nondeclarative memory that take place independent of the hippocampal system. Probabilistic classification learning (e.g., predicting the weather from a combination of cues that are regularly associated with sunny or rainy weather) is unaffected by hippocampal damage but impaired in diseases of the basal ganglia such as Huntington and Parkinson diseases (Thompson and Kim, 1996; Gluck, Myers, and Shohamy, 2002). Learning artificial grammar can also take place in the presence of amnestic syndrome, with functional imaging showing activation in the left parietal and occipital lobes (Skosnik et al., 2002). In all these memory experiments, the subject has no awareness of how he or she is able to answer the questions. The last form of nondeclarative memory is called *priming*, the presentation of a stimulus associated with the word or idea to be remembered, which then aids in retrieval of the item (e.g., recalling the word *doctor* when *nurse* appears on a priming list). Priming appears to involve the neocortex (Thompson and Kim, 1996; Levy et al., 2004). Schacter and Buckner (1998) have shown that deliberate use of priming can help amnestic patients compensate for their memory loss in everyday life.

Bedside Tests of Memory and Cognitive Function

The most important point to be made about bedside evaluations of cognition and memory is that they are an integral part of the neurological examination and a tool by which the neurologist localizes lesions affecting the higher cortical functions, just as the motor or cerebellar examinations localize neurological deficits. The most common error made by neurologists is to omit a systematic evaluation of mental function in patients who seem "alert and oriented." Deficits of memory, deficits in fund of knowledge, or focal deficits such as apraxia, agnosia, acalculia, or constructional impairment can be missed. Some patients have a "cocktail party" conversational pattern that belies such deficits; others become expert at deferring questions to a spouse or family member. Every neurologist

has the task of deciding which patients need formal cognitive testing and whether to make up an individual test routine or to rely on one of the standard tests. Again, it is more important to make the assessment than to follow a specific format.

Several versions of bedside mental status testing have been published. Perhaps the most widely used is Folstein's Mini-Mental State Examination (MMSE). The MMSE consists of 30 points: 5 for orientation to time (year, season, month, date, and day), 5 for orientation to place (state, county, town, hospital, and floor), 5 for attention (either serial 7s with 1 point for each of the first five subtractions or "spell *world* backward"), 3 for registration of three items, 3 for recall of three items after 5 minutes, 2 for naming a pencil and a watch, 1 for repeating "no ifs, ands, or buts," 3 for following a three-stage command, 1 for following a printed command ("close your eyes"), 1 for writing a sentence, 1 for copying a diagram of two intersecting pentagons.

The advantages of the MMSE are short time of administration and quantitation, useful in documentation for insurance benefits, such as rehabilitative therapies or drug therapy, and for disability assessment. Several disadvantages of the MMSE have been identified. First, the normal range of scores depends on education. The low-normal cutoff is estimated by Crum and colleagues (1993) to be 19 for uneducated people, 23 for graduates of elementary or junior high school, 27 for high school graduates, and 29 for college graduates. Age is also a factor. In addition, the test is weighted toward orientation and language, and results can be normal in patients with right hemisphere or frontal lobe damage. Finally, even an abnormal score does not distinguish a focal lesion from a more diffuse disorder such as an encephalopathy or dementia.

One answer to the dilemma of mental status testing is to use the MMSE as a screening test and then supplement it with more focused tests. **Box 6.2** lists the key elements of a mental status examination, whether the examiner chooses to adopt the MMSE, one of the other bedside cognitive instruments, or to create an individual test battery. Several texts provide further detail on such a battery. Although the mental status examination is the most neglected area of the neurological examination, it generally requires only a few minutes, and its cost-effectiveness compares well with brain imaging studies such as MRI or PET.

An experienced examiner can learn much about the subject's mental status by careful observation during the history. Considerable insight can be gained into the subject's recent memory, orientation, language function, affect or mood, insight, and judgment. Affect and mood are best assessed in this fashion; if there is doubt, the examiner should consider how the patient makes the examiner feel: a depressed patient

---

Box 6.2 **Bedside Mental Status Examination**

Orientation (time, place, person, situation)
Memory (immediate, short-term, long-term)
Fund of information
Speech and language
Praxis
Calculations
Visual-constructional abilities
Abstract reasoning, sequential processes

often makes the examiner feel depressed, whereas a manic patient makes the examiner feel happy and amused.

The formal mental status examination should always include explicit testing of orientation including the date, place, and situation. Memory testing should include an immediate attention test, of which the most popular are forward digit span, serial-7 subtractions from 100, or the MMSE test "spell *world* backward." Short-term memory should include recall of three unrelated words at 5 minutes. The subject should always be asked to say them back after presentation to make sure the three items have registered. At times, nonverbal short-term memory, such as recalling the locations of three hidden coins or reproducing drawings, can be useful to test. Remote memory can be tested by having the subject name children or siblings. Fund of information can be tested with recent presidents or other political figures. For patients who do not pay attention to politics, use of athletic stars or television celebrities may be more appropriate. Language testing should include spontaneous speech, naming, repetition, auditory comprehension, reading, and writing (the bedside language test is described in more detail in Chapter 12). In our practice, we like to show subjects more difficult naming items such as the drawings from the NIH Stroke Scale or body parts such as the thumb or the palm of the hand. Praxis testing should include the use of both imaginary and real (e.g., saw, hammer, pencil) objects. Both hands should be tested separately. Calculation tasks include the serial-7 subtraction test and simple change-making problems. Visual-spatial-constructional tasks can include line bisection, copying a cube or other design, and drawing a clock or a house (**Fig. 6.3**). The MMSE contains only one constructional task, the copying of intersecting pentagons. Many neurologists supplement this with the clock-drawing test. Insight and judgment are probably best tested by assessing the patient's understanding of his own illness. Artificial tests include interpretation of proverbs (e.g., "Those who live in glass houses should not throw stones") or stating why an apple and an orange are similar. An artificial test sometimes used to test frontal lobe processing is the copying and continuation of Luria's test of alternating sequences (sequential squares and triangles; see **Fig. 6.1**). With these tests, preliminary localization can be made in the deep memory structures of the medial temporal lobes, the frontal lobes (insight and judgment, proverbs, similarities, Luria's sequence test), the left hemisphere language cortex in the frontal and temporal lobes, the left parietal region (calculations), and the right parietal lobe (visual-constructional tasks).

In conclusion, this chapter considers the areas of neurology that most physicians find the most abstruse—namely, the higher cortical functions, intellect, and memory. As stated at the outset, this area of neurology can be treated as a series of specific functions to be analyzed at the bedside and localized,

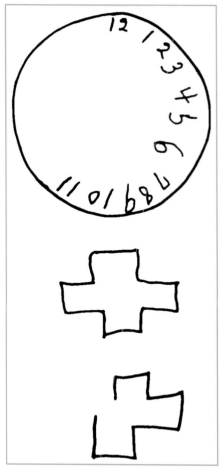

Fig. 6.3 Spontaneous clock drawing and copying of a cross by a patient with a right parietal infarction. The patient had only mild hemiparesis but dense left hemianopia and neglect of the left side of the body. The neglect of the left side of space is evident in both drawings. *(Reprinted with permission from Kirshner, H.S., 2002. Behavioral Neurology: Practical Science of Mind and Brain, second ed. Butterworth Heinemann, Boston.)*

just like other functions of the nervous system. In fact, the rapidly increasing knowledge of cognitive neuroscience and our vastly improved ability to image the brain both at rest and during functional activities promises a new era of practical diagnosis of higher cognitive disorders.

References

The complete reference list is available online at www.expertconsult.com.

Global Developmental Delay and Regression

Tyler Reimschisel

Developmental delay occurs in approximately 1% to 3% of children. Since developmental delay is common, monitoring a child's development is an essential component of well-child care. Ongoing assessment of the child's development at each well-child visit creates a pattern of development that is more useful than measuring the discrete milestone achievements at a single visit; therefore, developmental screening should be completed at each well-child visit (Council on Children with Disabilities, 2006). Identification of a child with developmental delays should be accomplished as early as possible, because the earlier a child is identified, the sooner the child can receive a thorough evaluation and begin therapeutic interventions that can improve the child's outcome. Developmental delay is common and one of the most frequent presenting complaints to a pediatric neurology clinic; neurologists should have a systematic approach to the child with developmental delay.

This chapter begins with a brief discussion of child development concepts related to typical and atypical development. Next, the clinical evaluation and management of developmental delay is reviewed. The chapter closes with a discussion of neurological regression.

Typical and Atypical Development

Child Development Concepts

Child development is a continuous process of acquiring new and advanced skills. This development depends on maturation of the nervous system. Although typical child development follows a relatively consistent sequence, it is not linear. Instead, there are spurts and lags. For example, motor development in the first year of life proceeds relatively rapidly. Babies typically mature from being completely immobile to walking in just over 12 months, but then motor development progresses less dramatically during the second year of life. Conversely, language development in the first year of life occurs slowly, but there is an explosion of language acquisition between a child's first and second birthdays.

On average, most children achieve each developmental milestone within a defined and narrow age range (**Table 7.1**). Usually physicians learn the average age for acquiring specific skills. However, since each developmental skill can be acquired within an age range, it is much more useful clinically to know when a child's development falls outside this range. These so-called red flags are important because they can be used to identify when a child has developmental delay for specific skills. For example, although the average age of walking is approximately 13 months, a child may walk as late as 17 months and still be within the typical developmental range. In this example, the red flag for independent walking is 18 months, and a child who is not walking by 18 months of age is delayed.

Global Developmental Delay
Developmental History

Child development is classically divided into five interdependent domains or streams: gross motor, fine motor and problem-solving, receptive language, expressive language, and socialization/adaptive. The approach to a child with possible developmental delays is based on a working knowledge of these domains and the typical age ranges for acquiring specific milestones within each domain. Therefore, the clinician should begin the evaluation of a child with developmental concerns by obtaining a developmental history, and emphasis should be placed on the pattern of milestone acquisition as well as the child's current developmental skills. Clinicians

Table 7.1 Normal Developmental Milestones by Age (50th-75th Percentile)

Age	Language	Socialization	Motor
2 mo	Coos (ooh, ah)	Smiles with social contact	Holds head up 45 degrees
4 mo	Laughs and squeals	Sustains social contact	Grasps objects, stands with support
6 mo	Imitates speech sounds	Prefers mother, enjoys mirror	Transfers objects between hands, uses a raking grasp, sits with support
8 mo	Jabbers (dadada)	Plays interactively	Sits alone, creeps or crawls
1 yr	Says "dada/mama" with meaning	Plays simple ball games, adjusts body to dressing	Stands alone, uses a thumb-finger pincer grasp
14 mo	Says 2-3 words	Indicates desires by pointing, hugs parents	Walks alone, stoops and recovers
18 mo	Says 6-10 words	Feeds self	Walks up steps with a hand held, imitates scribbling
2 yr	Combines words with a 250-word vocabulary	Helps to undress, listens to stories with pictures	Runs well, makes circular scribbles, copies a horizontal line
30 mo	Refers to self as "I," knows full name	Pretends in play, helps put things away	Climbs stairs with alternate feet, copies a vertical line
3 yr	Counts 3 objects, knows age and sex	Helps in dressing	Rides a tricycle, stands on one foot briefly, copies a circle
48 mo	Counts 4 objects, tells a story	Plays with other children, uses toilet alone	Hops on one foot, uses scissors to cut out pictures, copies a square and a cross
5 yr	Counts 10 objects, names 4 colors	Asks about word meanings, imitates domestic chores	Skips, copies a triangle

working in a busy clinical setting may need to base this history primarily on the caregiver's report of the child's developmental abilities. Clinicians may also use standardized tools to aid in this portion of the history, including the Ireton Child Development Inventory (CDI), the Ages and Stages Questionnaire (ASQ), and the Parents' Evaluation of Developmental Status (PEDS). However, if the clinician's history confirms a developmental disability, standardized testing by a developmental specialist or clinical psychologist should be strongly considered; this formal evaluation will provide a much better assessment of the child's developmental abilities.

When there is concern about developmental delay in a child, a developmental quotient should be calculated. The *developmental quotient* is the ratio of the child's developmental age over the chronological age. The developmental quotient should be calculated for each developmental stream. Typical development is a developmental quotient greater than 70%, and atypical development it is a developmental quotient less than 70%. Toddlers and young children with atypical development are at risk for lifelong developmental problems. The term *global development delay* is used if a child younger than 5 to 6 years of age has a developmental quotient less than 70% in two or more domains. Children with global developmental delay should receive a thorough medical evaluation to try to determine the cause of the delay and begin management for their developmental disabilities.

neurological history. Pertinent aspects of the history include the presence of any other neurological condition such as epilepsy, vision or hearing impairments, ataxia or a movement disorder, sleep impairment, and behavioral problems. The clinician should also inquire about prenatal, perinatal, and postnatal factors that can impact a child's development (**Tables 7.2 and 7.3**). The social history should probe for environmental factors that can affect development, including physical or other forms of abuse, neglect, psychosocial deprivation, family illness, impaired personalities in family members, sociocultural stressors, and the economic status of the family.

Though families now typically have fewer children, and the caregivers' knowledge of family history is frequently quite limited, the clinician should still make an effort to obtain a three-generation pedigree. The pertinent aspects of the family history include developmental disabilities, special education services or failure to graduate from school, neurodegenerative disorders, multiple miscarriages or early postnatal death, ethnicity, and consanguinity. If a specific genetic syndrome is suspected, the clinician should inquire about the presence in other family members of medical problems associated with that syndrome. For example, if the child has the features of fragile X syndrome, the family history should include questions about maternal premature ovarian failure, parkinsonism or ataxia of unknown etiology in the maternal grandfather, and intellectual disability or learning problems in an X-linked pattern.

Neurological and Other Medical History

For children with global developmental delay, the clinician should obtain a thorough medical history, including a detailed

Physical Examination

The growth parameters of the child should be measured, and the growth charts should be reviewed to determine the child's

Table 7.2 Etiology of Developmental Delay by Time of Onset

Prenatal/Perinatal	Examples
Congenital malformations of the CNS	Lissencephaly, holoprosencephaly
Chromosomal abnormalities	Down syndrome, Turner syndrome
Endogenous toxins	Maternal hepatic or renal failure
Exogenous toxins from maternal use	Anticonvulsants, anticoagulants, alcohol, drugs of abuse
Fetal infection	Congenital infections
Prematurity and/or fetal malnutrition	Periventricular leukomalacia
Perinatal trauma	Intracranial hemorrhage, spinal cord injury
Perinatal asphyxia	Hypoxic-ischemic encephalopathy
Postnatal	**Examples**
Inborn errors of metabolism	Aminoacidopathies, mitochondrial diseases
Abnormal storage of metabolites	Lysosomal storage diseases, glycogen storage diseases
Abnormal postnatal nutrition	Vitamin or calorie deficiency
Endogenous toxins	Hepatic failure, kernicterus
Exogenous toxins	Prescription drugs, illicit substances, heavy metals
Endocrine organ failure	Hypothyroidism, Addison disease
CNS infection	Meningitis, encephalitis
CNS trauma	Diffuse axonal injury, intracranial hemorrhage
Neoplasia	Tumor infiltration, radiation necrosis
Neurocutaneous syndromes	Neurofibromatosis, tuberous sclerosis complex
Neuromuscular disorders	Muscular dystrophy, myotonic dystrophy
Vascular conditions	Vasculitis, ischemic stroke, sinovenous thrombosis
Other	Epilepsy, mood disorders, schizophrenia

From Sherr, E.H., Shevell, M.I., 2006. Mental retardation and global developmental delay, in: Swaiman, K.F., Ashwal, S., Ferriero, D.I. (Eds.), Pediatric Neurology, Principles and Practice, fifth ed. Mosby, Philadelphia.
CNS, Central nervous system.

restricted or repetitive behaviors, and communication impairment may indicate that the child has an autism spectrum disorder, and the child should be referred to a psychologist for assessment or confirmation of this condition. Other abnormal behaviors such as hyperactivity, impulsivity, and inattention, as well as suboptimal parenting skills, may also be noted during these observations. However, the clinician should use caution when raising concerns about a behavior problem based solely on the child's behavior in clinic, since this stressful situation may lead the child to manifest uncharacteristic behaviors.

A complete general physical and neurological examination should be performed to the extent the child will allow. The general examination should include but not be limited to an evaluation for dysmorphic features; abnormalities of the eyes (**Table 7.4**), skin, and hair; and organomegaly (**Table 7.5**). The neurological examination should include signs of impairment in extraocular movements; hypertonia or hypotonia; focal or generalized weakness; abnormal posture or movements; abnormal or asymmetrical tendon reflexes; ataxia, incoordination or other signs of cerebellar dysfunction; and gait abnormalities (see **Table 7.5**).

Diagnostic Testing

Diagnostic testing in an individual with global developmental delay should be offered to the family, because the testing may provide an etiology for the developmental delays, could alert the physician and family to comorbid conditions the child is at risk for developing, can help provide recurrence information to the family, and may rarely lead to specific medical treatments or therapeutic interventions.

Genetic Testing

Based on the developmental history obtained, a diagnosis of global developmental delay can be made. In addition, the clinician should attempt to identify an underlying etiology for the delay. Occasionally, the history and examination suggest a specific recognizable genetic condition or other cause. In these situations, confirmatory testing should be performed if possible. For example, a girl with a history of global developmental delay who has acquired microcephaly, epilepsy, and midline hand wringing should be tested for Rett syndrome.

Frequently, however, the underlying cause is unknown despite the acquisition of a comprehensive history and physical examination. In these situations, a chromosomal microarray analysis (CMA) should be offered to the family, since it has the highest diagnostic yield of any single assay for children with global developmental delay: approximately 8% to 12%. A clinical CMA tests for submicroscopic deletions or duplications that can be associated with a variety of neurodevelopmental delays, including global developmental delay. This is also the first-line test for individuals with nonspecific intellectual disability, an autism spectrum disorder, and multiple congenital anomalies (Miller et al., 2010). Though this test has a relatively high diagnostic yield, it will typically not detect inversions and other balanced rearrangements. Consequently, if the microarray is within normal limits, a follow-up high-resolution karyotype should be considered.

The CMA is also unable to detect trinucleotide repeat expansions, point mutations, and imprinting abnormalities.

rate of growth. This is pertinent because many chromosomal anomalies and other genetic disorders that cause global developmental delay and intellectual disability are associated with failure to thrive or short stature, large stature, microcephaly, and macrocephaly.

In the mental status portion of the examination, the clinician should note the interactions the child has with his or her caregivers and the clinician. Abnormal behaviors such as impaired eye contact, limited or absent social reciprocity,

Table 7.3 Perinatal Risk Factors for Neurologic Injury

Maternal/Prenatal	Natal	Postnatal
Age <16 years or >40 years	Intrauterine hypoxia: prolapsed umbilical cord, abruptio placenta, circumvallate placenta	Abnormal feeding: poor sucking, weight gain, malnutrition, vomiting
Cervical or pelvic abnormalities	Midforceps delivery or breech presentation	Abnormal crying
Maternal illnesses: infection, shock, diabetes, nephritis, phlebitis, proteinuria, renal hypertension, thyroid disease, drug addiction, malnutrition	Poor Apgar scores: cyanosis, poor respiratory effort, bradycardia, poor reflexes, hypotonia	Abnormal exam: asymmetrical face, asymmetrical extremities, dysmorphic features, hypotonia, birth injuries, seizures
Maternal features: unmarried, uneducated, nonwhite, low-income, thin, short	Need for resuscitation: respiratory distress, bradycardia, hypotension	Abnormal findings: hyperbilirubinemia, fever, hypothermia, hypoxia
Consanguinity	Gestational age <30 weeks	
Prior abnormal pregnancy, miscarriages, stillbirths, abortions, neonatal deaths, infants less than 1500 g, abnormal placenta	Vaginal bleeding in the second or third trimester	
	Hypoxic-ischemic encephalopathy	
	Polyhydramnios or oligohydramnios	

From Sherr, E.H., Shevell, M.I., 2006. Mental retardation and global developmental delay, in: Swaiman, K.F., Ashwal, S., Ferriero, D.I. (Eds.), Pediatric Neurology, Principles and Practice, fifth ed. Mosby, Philadelphia.

Table 7.4 Ocular Findings Associated with Selected Syndromic Developmental Disorders

Finding	Examples
Cataracts	Cerebrotendinous xanthomatosis, galactosemia, Lowe syndrome, LSD, Wilson disease
Chorioretinitis	Congenital infections
Corneal opacity	Cockayne syndrome, Lowe syndrome, LSD, xeroderma pigmentosa, Zellweger syndrome
Glaucoma	Lowe syndrome, mucopolysaccharidoses, Sturge-Weber syndrome, Zellweger syndrome
Lens dislocation	Homocystinuria, sulfite oxidase deficiency
Macular cherry-red spot	LSD, multiple sulfatase deficiency
Nystagmus	Aminoacidopathies, AT, CDG, Chédiak-Higashi syndrome, Friedreich ataxia, Leigh syndrome, Marinesco-Sjögren syndrome, metachromatic leukodystrophy, neuroaxonal dystrophy, Pelizaeus-Merzbacher disease, SCD
Ophthalmoplegia	AT, Bassen-Kornzweig syndrome, LSDs, mitochondrial diseases
Optic atrophy	Alpers disease, Leber optic atrophy, leukodystrophies, LSDs, neuroaxonal dystrophy, SCD
Photophobia	Cockayne syndrome, Hartnup disease, homocystinuria
Retinitis pigmentosa or macular degeneration	AT, Bassen-Kornzweig syndrome, Cockayne syndrome, CDG, Hallervorden-Spatz syndrome, Laurence-Moon-Biedl syndrome, LSD, mitochondrial diseases, Refsum disease, Sjögren-Larsson syndrome, SCD

From Sherr, E.H., Shevell, M.I., 2006. Mental retardation and global developmental delay, in: Swaiman, K.F., Ashwal, S., Ferriero, D.I. (Eds.), Pediatric Neurology, Principles and Practice, fifth ed. Mosby, Philadelphia.
AT, Ataxia-telangiectasia; CDG, congenital disorders of glycosylation; LSD, lysosomal storage diseases; SCD, spinocerebellar degeneration.

Therefore, every child with nonspecific global developmental delay regardless of gender should also have fragile-X testing performed. Based on the phenotype, the clinician should also consider performing methylation testing for Angelman and Prader-Willi syndrome, since the microarray analysis will miss the uniparental disomy or imprinting center abnormalities associated with these syndromes. Based on the patient's constellation of clinical features, molecular testing for UBE3A (Angelman syndrome), MeCP2 (Rett syndrome), and other genetic disorders may be considered if the microarray analysis is within normal limits.

In children with global developmental delay, it is important to confirm that the universal newborn screening test was normal at birth. Nonetheless, the diagnostic yield of biochemical testing in a child with nonspecific global developmental delay is quite low (<1%) (Moeschler and Shevell, 2006). The

Table 7.5 Other Findings Associated with Selected Syndromic Developmental Disorders

Finding	Examples
Cerebellar dysfunction	Aminoacidopathies, AT, Bassen-Kornzweig syndrome, CDG, cerebrotendinous xanthomatosis, Chédiak-Higashi syndrome, Cockayne syndrome, Friedreich ataxia, Lafora disease, LSD, Marinesco-Sjögren syndrome, mitochondrial disease, neuroaxonal dystrophy, Pelizaeus-Merzbacher disease, Ramsay Hunt syndrome, SCD, Wilson disease
Hair abnormalities:	
Synophrys	Cornelia de Lange syndrome
Fine hair	Homocystinuria, hypothyroidism
Kinky hair	Argininosuccinic aciduria, Menkes disease
Hirsutism	LSD
Balding	Leigh syndrome, progeria
Gray hair	AT, Chédiak-Higashi syndrome, Cockayne syndrome, progeria
Hearing abnormalities:	
Hyperacusis	LSD, SSPE, sulfite oxidase deficiency
Conductive loss	Mucopolysaccharidoses
Sensorineural loss	Adrenoleukodystrophy, CHARGE, Cockayne syndrome, mitochondrial diseases, SCD, Refsum disease
Infantile hypotonia	Canavan disease, myopathies, LSD, Leigh syndrome, Menkes disease, neuroaxonal dystrophy, spinal muscular atrophy, Zellweger disease
Limb abnormalities:	
Micromelia	Cornelia de Lange syndrome
Broad thumbs	Rubinstein-Taybi syndrome
Macrocephaly	Alexander disease, Canavan histiocytosis X, LSD
Microcephaly	Alpers disease, CDG, Cockayne syndrome, incontinentia, pigmenti, neuronal ceroid lipofuscinoses, Crabbe disease, neuroaxonal dystrophy, Rett syndrome
Movement disorders	AT, LSD, dystonia musculorum deformans, Hallervorden-Spatz, juvenile Huntington disease, juvenile Parkinson disease, Lesch-Nyhan disease, phenylketonuria, Wilson disease, xeroderma pigmentosa
Odors:	
Cat urine	β-Methyl-crotonyl-CoA carboxylase deficiency
Maple	Maple syrup urine disease
Musty	Phenylketonuria
Rancid butter	Methionine malabsorption syndrome
Sweaty feet	Isovaleric acidemia
Organomegaly	Aminoacidopathies, CDG, galactosemia, glycogen storage diseases, LSD, Zellweger syndrome
Peripheral neuropathy	AT, Bassen-Kornzweig syndrome, cerebrotendinous xanthomatosis, Cockayne syndrome, LSD, Refsum disease
Short stature	Cockayne syndrome, Cornelia de Lange syndrome, hypothyroidism, leprechaunism, LSD, Prader-Willi syndrome, Rubinstein-Taybi syndrome, Seckel bird-headed dwarfism
Seizures	Aminoacidopathies, CDG, glycogen synthetase deficiency, HIE, LSD, Menkes disease, mitochondrial diseases, neuroaxonal dystrophy
Skin abnormalities:	
Hyperpigmentation	Adrenoleukodystrophy, AT, Farber disease, neurofibromatosis, Niemann-Pick disease, tuberous sclerosis complex, xeroderma pigmentosa
Hypopigmentation	
Nodules	Chédiak-Higashi syndrome, incontinentia pigmenti, Menkes disease, tuberous sclerosis complex
Thick skin	Cerebrotendinous xanthomatosis, Farber disease, neurofibromatosis, LSD, Refsum disease,
Thin skin	Sjögren-Larsson syndrome, AT, Cockayne syndrome, progeria, xeroderma pigmentosa

From Sherr, E.H., Shevell, M.I., 2006. Mental retardation and global developmental delay, in: Swaiman, K.F., Ashwal, S., Ferriero, D.I. (Eds.), Pediatric Neurology, Principles and Practice, fifth ed. Mosby, Philadelphia.

AT, Ataxia-telangiectasia; CDG, congenital disorders of glycosylation; CHARGE, coloboma, heart disease, choanal atresia, retardation, genital anomalies, ear anomalies; HIE, hypoxic-ischemic encephalopathy; LSD, lysosomal storage diseases; SCD, spinocerebellar degeneration; SSPE, subacute sclerosing panencephalitis.

yield may be slightly higher if there is a history of: (1) metabolic decompensation, hyperammonemia, hypoglycemia, protein aversion, acidosis or other evidence of an inborn metabolic disease; (2) neonatal seizures, stroke, movement disorder, or other neurological diagnosis; (3) a family history of unex-plained death or neurological disease in a first-degree relative; (4) parental consanguinity; or (5) prenatal history of acute fatty liver of pregnancy (AFLP) or toxemia with hemolysis, elevated liver enzymes, and low platelets (HELLP). Physical examina-tion findings that should increase the suspicion of a metabolic disease include microcephaly, macrocephaly, growth failure, unusual odor, coarse facial features, unusual birthmarks, abnormal hair, hypotonia, dystonia, and focal weakness.

Biochemical tests from the blood to consider in the evaluation of a child with global developmental delay include complete blood count, comprehensive metabolic panel, serum lactate (and possibly serum pyruvate if the result is reliable at the clinician's institution), plasma amino acids, serum creatinine kinase level, uric acid level, and creatine metabolites (in girls). Urine studies to consider include organic acid analysis, purine and pyrimidine metabolites, and creatine metabolites (in boys). Selective metabolic testing may be warranted in specific clinical cases, such as serum 7-dehydrocholesterol level for Smith-Lemli-Opitz syndrome, screening for congenital disorders of glycosylation, biotinidase activity in the blood, cerebrospinal fluid (CSF) neurotransmitter metabolites for neurotransmitter deficiencies, and white blood cell enzyme analysis and urine glycosaminoglycans and oligosaccharides for lysosomal storage diseases.

Neuroimaging

Magnetic resonance imaging (MRI) of the brain has a yield of 65% in children with developmental delay (Shevell et al., 2003). The abnormalities most frequently identified include cerebral malformations, cerebral atrophy, delayed myelination, other white matter changes, postischemic changes, widened Virchow-Robin spaces, and phakomatoses. However, many of these changes are nonspecific and do not lead to the diagnosis of a specific etiology for the developmental delay. The yield of a brain MRI is higher if the child has neurological abnormalities on physical examination such as microcephaly, macrocephaly, focal neurological deficits, epilepsy, strokes, or a movement disorder. Given the nonnegligible risk of sedation in a child with global developmental delay, neuroimaging with an MRI should be recommended as a first-line study in children with focal neurological findings and may be offered as a second-line study if genetic testing is nondiagnostic.

Because the diagnostic yield of head computed tomography (CT) is much lower than brain MRI, head CT is primarily indicated in children with global developmental delay who are suspected of having calcifications.

Other Tests

Electroencephalography (EEG) should be performed in children with global developmental delay who are suspected of having seizures. An EEG should also be obtained in children with regression, even in the absence of spells, to rule out treatable causes of regression including Landau-Kleffner syndrome, severe absence epilepsy, and electrical status epilepticus during slow-wave sleep. If the child has no history of spells or regression, an EEG is not indicated for routine evaluation of all children with global developmental delay.

Additional diagnostic tests are not typically warranted in children with nonspecific global developmental delay. However, depending on the presentation, the clinician may consider more invasive tests such as CSF analysis, electromyography (EMG) and nerve conduction studies, muscle and/or nerve biopsies, and cell culture for enzyme analysis or other biochemical testing. However, these studies are rarely indicated until the mentioned routine studies have been completed.

Management

Medical management of global developmental delay begins with a disclosure to the family of the clinician's concern for the diagnosis. As with any situation in which the physician discloses difficult news, this must be done gently but clearly. The clinician should be prepared to respond to a full range of emotions including doubt, denial, sorrow, and anger. Furthermore, the family will usually need time to process the information that their child has or is at risk for having lifelong developmental problems. Therefore, a follow up appointment should be scheduled to review the diagnosis and address additional questions or concerns the family may have.

In addition, any comorbid conditions should be treated, or the clinician should refer the patient to the appropriate subspecialist who can provide treatment for the comorbid condition. The clinician can also help facilitate social, community, or educational supports for the family. These may include family support groups, national parent organizations, and other resources in the community for families of children with developmental disabilities.

One of the most important aspects of the management of a child with global developmental delay is ensuring that the child receives early and appropriate therapeutic and educational interventions. Children younger than 3 years of age with developmental delays can be enrolled in early intervention programs. Each state's program includes a multidisciplinary team of therapists who complete a comprehensive assessment and provide appropriate interventions. Their assessment is summarized in a report called the *Individualized Family Service Plan*; this plan serves as the basis for provision of therapeutic services.

Children who are older than 3 years of age receive services through the special education program within the local school district. These services are usually provided by a multidisciplinary team of therapists as well as a psychologist. They also complete an assessment and summarize their findings in a report called the *Individualized Education Plan* (IEP). The IEP serves as the basis for the services that will be provided to the child within the school system. Federal law mandates that children receive the special services they need in the least restrictive environment possible. Therefore, many children with developmental disabilities are now educated in the regular ("mainstream") classroom with an aide instead of being placed in a separate classroom. However, some children with more significant intellectual or behavioral problems may require placement in a special education classroom for part or all of the day.

Prognosis

Once a child is diagnosed with global developmental delay, the family will inquire about the child's ultimate developmental outcome, including cognitive and motor abilities, future level of independence, and life expectancy. In young children with mild developmental delay, it is not prudent to predict a developmental outcome with certainty. Instead, the potential range of outcomes should be discussed. Depending on the severity of the delays and associated medical problems, this range may include typical development once the child is school-aged. In an otherwise healthy individual with developmental delay, the life expectancy is normal. Children with significantly impaired mobility or other neurological impairments may have a shortened life expectancy.

Though some toddlers and young children with developmental delay may "catch up" and ultimately have typical development, global developmental delay is associated with an increased risk for having a *developmental disability*—a lifelong and chronic condition due to impairments in mental and/or physical impairments that impacts major life activities such as language function, learning, mobility, self-help, and independent living. Several types of developmental disabilities exist, including cerebral palsy, learning disabilities like dyslexia, intellectual disability, autism spectrum disorders, attention deficit-hyperactivity disorder, hearing impairment, and vision impairment.

These developmental disabilities are predominantly impairments in a specific subset of the developmental domains. For example, cerebral palsy is primarily an impairment of gross and fine motor skills; intellectual disability is primarily an impairment of language, problem-solving, and social-adaptive abilities; and autism spectrum disorders are primarily disorders of social-adaptive behaviors with or without language and communication impairments.

Developmental disabilities are common. Approximately 16% to 18% of children have a developmental disability that includes behavior problems, and 1% to 3% of the population has an intellectual disability. Approximately 1 in 150 children have an autism spectrum disorder.

Toddlers or preschool children who are diagnosed with global developmental delay are at highest risk for being diagnosed with intellectual disability at an older age, especially as the developmental quotient worsens. *Intellectual disability* is defined as significantly subaverage general intellectual functioning (IQ less than 70) with limitations in adaptive functioning in at least two of the following skill areas: communication, self-help, social skills, academic skills, work, leisure, and health and/or safety. The incidence of intellectual disability is 1% to 3% in the general population. Males are more likely to be affected than females; occurrence rates are 1:4000 males and only 1:6000 females.

In general, the diagnosis of intellectual disability is not made in a toddler or preschool child unless they have been diagnosed with a specific genetic condition associated with intellectual disability. In the absence of a specific genetic diagnosis, the diagnosis of intellectual disability in most children is made once they are able to complete formal psychology testing at approximately 5 years of age.

In our practice, when the developmental delays of a child younger than 4 are very severe, we will occasionally tell the family that the child will likely have intellectual disability. In these situations, we may share this concern even if the child does not have a formal diagnosis of a genetic syndrome or before the child is old enough to complete formal psychology testing. Children with severe developmental delays may in fact be too impaired to perform formal psychology testing.

Recurrence Risk

Many couples are interested in knowing what their risk is for having another child with similar developmental concerns. A recurrence risk can only be provided with certainty if a specific etiology has been confirmed. Despite extensive genetic testing and other evaluations, the majority of children with develop-

mental delays will not be diagnosed with a specific named genetic condition or other etiology for the delays. Consequently, the clinician can only provide an empirical recurrence risk based on population data and family history information. Though each case is unique, the most prudent approach is to remind the family that 1% to 3% of the population has intellectual disability, and their risk for having another child with global developmental delay and subsequent intellectual disability is greater than the population risk. It is helpful to double frame the risk by also stating that it is more likely that they would have an *unaffected* child than an *affected* child.

Regression

A regressive or neurodegenerative disease should be suspected when a child has ongoing and relentless loss of developmental skills. In addition, a regressive disease may begin to manifest itself as the development of a new neurological problem, such as a new-onset seizure disorder or movement disorder, development of a different type of seizure in a child with epilepsy, vision impairment, behavior problems, and dementia or cognitive decline.

In a child with neurological regression, a thorough neurological history and examination is warranted. The history should focus on any modifiable factors that could contribute to neurological decline, including worsening of another medical problem, recent modification to an existing medication regimen or initiation of a new medication, recovery from a prolonged acute illness or surgery, or a psychosocial stressor. All children with neurological decline should receive an extensive physical examination, with attention to those aspects of the examination that could provide clues to an underlying neurodegenerative disease (see **Table 7.5**). A pediatric ophthalmologist should also examine the patient for ocular stigmata of a neurodegenerative disease (see **Table 7.4**). A brain MRI should be performed to assess for changes that can be seen in many regressive diseases—atrophy, ventriculomegaly, white matter changes, and infarcts. Additional studies should be considered based on the patient's clinical presentation: comprehensive metabolic panel, lipid panel, creatine kinase, EEG, EMG and nerve conduction studies, echocardiogram, and hearing test.

The need for genetic testing is based on the patient's presentation and results of the recommended studies. Categories of genetic diseases that should be considered include aminoacidopathies, organic acidurias, fatty acid oxidation defects, glycogen storage diseases, mitochondrial cytopathies, lysosomal storage diseases, neuronal ceroid lipofuscinoses, peroxisomal disorders, neurotransmitter synthesis disorders, spinal muscular atrophy syndromes, creatine synthesis disorders, congenital disorders of glycosylation, metal metabolism disorders (Menkes, Wilson, pantothenate kinase-associated neurodegeneration), and purine and pyrimidines disorders. Testing for most conditions can now be done on blood, urine, and/or CSF samples. Rarely, more invasive procedures may be warranted, including biopsies of the skin, muscle, liver, nerve, bone marrow, or conjunctiva.

Many reasons exist to aggressively pursue a diagnosis of an underlying neurodegenerative disease. Most regressive disorders are irreversible, and the treatment is symptomatic. However, early diagnosis can reverse the neurological impairment or prevent future morbidity is some conditions such as

Wilson disease, homocystinuria, and glutaric aciduria type I. Occasionally, pharmaceutical trials may be available to patients. Furthermore, a correct diagnosis can help the clinician provide better information about prognosis and life expectancy. Recurrence risk information and prenatal diagnosis may also be offered to families. For those conditions that are progressive and life limiting, the clinician should collaborate with a pediatric palliative care team to discuss end-of-life goals of care with the family.

References

The complete reference list is available online at www. expertconsult.com.

Behavior and Personality Disturbances

Carissa Gehl, Jane S. Paulsen

Behavioral and personality disturbances commonly occur in individuals with neurological disease or injury (**Table 8.1**). Identification and treatment of behavioral disturbances are critical because they are frequently associated with reduced functional capacity, decreased quality of life, and greater economic cost, caregiver burden, and morbidity. Dysfunction of various brain circuits, most notably the frontosubcortical and amygdaloid circuits, as well as psychological factors may contribute to increased rates of disturbances.

Historically, clear divisions between the fields of psychiatry and neurology have existed. Psychiatry focused on disruptions of behavior and personality resulting from "nonorganic" or psychological causes, whereas neurology focused on disease and injury with "organic" causes. The division between psychiatry and neurology has become blurred over the past few decades, however, because research shows neuroanatomic and biochemical correlates of behavior and personality disturbances. As a response, increased collaboration and partnership between these two fields has emerged. An example of this collaboration is the creation of the American Neuropsychiatric Association (ANPA), established in 1988.

The aim of this chapter is threefold. First, theoretical information linking brain circuitry to behavioral and personality disturbances is described. Second, methods of assessment of behavior and personality in cerebral dysfunction are detailed. Finally, information regarding the prevalence, phenomenology, and treatment of behavior and personality disturbances in dementia, movement disorders, epilepsy, stroke, and traumatic brain injury (TBI) is presented.

Frontosubcortical Circuitry

The frontosubcortical circuits provide a unifying framework for understanding the behavioral changes that accompany cortical and subcortical brain dysfunction. In the past 3 decades, a number of significant advances have been made in our understanding of the neuroanatomy, neurophysiology, and chemoarchitecture of the frontosubcortical circuits. An increasingly broad spectrum of neuropsychiatric phenomenology is now being interpreted in the context of dysfunction in this region. A brief overview of the frontosubcortical circuits and their signature behavioral syndromes is offered as a strategy to better understand the behavior and personality changes that accompany neurological conditions. Alexander and colleagues described five discrete parallel circuits linking regions of the frontal cortex to the striatum, the globus pallidus and substantia nigra, and the thalamus. These circuits consist of "direct" and "indirect" pathways. In general, the direct pathway facilitates the flow of information, and the indirect pathway inhibits it. The overall model for the frontosubcortical circuits can be observed in **Fig. 8.1**.

Five frontosubcortical circuits were initially described as motor, oculomotor, dorsolateral prefrontal, lateral orbitofrontal, and anterior cingulate gyrus. **Table 8.2** gives descriptions of specific neuroanatomic pathways for these circuits. Efforts to link functional domains to this brain circuitry have been developed and revised over the past few decades. Disruption of dorsolateral prefrontal, lateral orbitofrontal, and anterior cingulate gyrus circuits is associated with behavioral and

DOI: 10.1016/B978-1-4377-0434-1.00008-6

Table 8.1 Prevalence of Behavioral and Psychiatric Disturbances in Neurological Disorders

	Depression	Apathy	Anxiety	Psychosis	Aggression	PLC
AD	0%-86%	Up to 92%	—	10%-73%	33%-67%	—
ALS	40%-50%	—	—	—	—	10%-49%
FTD	—	95%	—	20% del., 7% hall.	—	—
VaD	32%	—	19%-70%	33% del., 13%-25% hall.	—	—
PD	40%–50%	16.5%-40.0%	—	16% del., 30% hall.	—	4%-6%
HD	Up to 63%	59%	—	3%-12%	19%-59%	—
TS	73%	—	—	—	—	—
MS	37%-54%	—	9.2%-25.0%	—	—	10%
Epilepsy	8%-63%	—	19%-50%	0.6%-7.0%	4.8%-50.0%	—
Stroke	30%-40%	—	Up to 27%	—	Up to 32%	11%-34%
TBI	6%-77%	10%-60%	11%-70%	2%-20%	11%-98%	5%-11%

AD, Alzheimer disease; *ALS,* amyotrophic lateral sclerosis; *del.,* delusions; *FTD,* frontotemporal dementia; *hall.,* hallucinations; *HD,* Huntington disease; *HIV,* human immunodeficiency virus and HIV dementia; *MS,* multiple sclerosis; *PD,* Parkinson disease; *PLC,* pathological laughing & crying; *TS,* Tourette syndrome; *TBI,* traumatic brain injury; *VaD,* vascular dementia.

Table 8.2 Frontal-Subcortical Circuitry

Circuit	Frontal lobe	Striatum	GPi and SNr	Thalamus
Dorsolateral	Dorsolateral PFC	Dorsolateral CN	Lateral Mediodorsal GPi Rostrolateral SNr	VA nucleus
Orbitofrontal	Orbitofrontal PFC	Ventromedial CN	Mediodorsal GPi Rostromedial SNr	VA nucleus
Anterior cingulate	Supracallosal anterior cingulate	Ventral striatum	Rostromedial GPi Ventral pallidum Rostrodorsal SNr	Mediodorsal nucleus

CN, Caudate nucleus; *GPi,* internal segment of the globus pallidus; *PFC,* prefrontal cortex; *SNr,* substantia nigra pars reticulata; *VA,* ventral anterior; *ventral striatum,* ventromedial caudate nucleus, ventral putamen, nucleus accumbens, and olfactory tubercle.

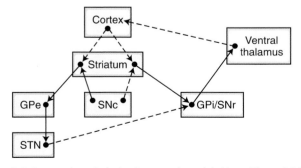

Fig. 8.1 Frontosubcortical circuit general model. NOTE: The solid line represents inhibitory neurons and dotted lines represent excitatory neurons. *GPe,* External segment of the globus pallidus; *GPi,* internal segment of the globus pallidus; *SNc,* substantia nigra pars compacta; *SNr,* substantia nigra pars reticulata; *STN,* subthalamic nucleus.

personality disruptions. Specific behavioral syndromes have been attributed to dysfunction in these circuits (**Box 8.1**) (Mega and Cummings, 2001). Disruptions at any point in the circuit (e.g., the frontal cortex, corpus striatum, globus pallidus) may result in alterations of behavior.

Disruption of the dorsolateral circuit (**Fig. 8.2**) is associated with executive dysfunction, including poor planning and organization skills, memory retrieval deficits, and poor set shifting. **Table 8.3** lists neurological disorders associated with disruption of this circuit. The orbitofrontal circuit (see **Fig. 8.2**) is associated with increased irritability, impulsivity, mood lability, tactlessness, and socially inappropriate behavior, whereas disruptions of the latter part of the orbitofrontal circuit may also result in mood disorder or obsessive-compulsive disorder (OCD) or both. See **Table 8.3** for disorders associated with disruption of this circuit. Finally, the anterior cingulate gyrus circuit is associated with decreased motivation, apathy, decreased speech, and akinesia. See **Table 8.3** for disorders associated with disruption of this circuit. Although these models may be heuristic in developing

Box 8.1 Behavioral Syndromes Associated with Dysfunction of the Motor Circuits

Symptoms Associated with Disruption of the Dorsolateral Circuit

Poor organizational strategies
Poor memory search strategies
Stimulus-bound behavior
Environmental dependency
Impaired set-shifting and maintenance

Symptoms Associated with Disruption of the Orbitofrontal Circuit

Emotional incontinence
Tactlessness
Irritability
Undue familiarity
Antisocial behavior
Environmental dependency
Mood disorders (depression, lability, mania)
Obsessive-compulsive disorder

Symptoms Associated with Disruption of the Anterior Cingulate Circuit

Impaired motivation
Akinetic mutism
Apathy
Poverty of speech
Psychic emptiness
Poor response inhibition

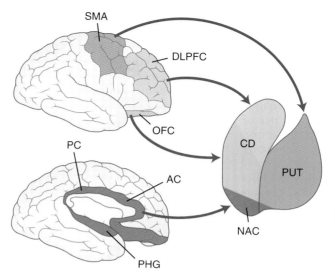

Fig. 8.2 Frontostriatal projections. *AC,* Anterior cingulate gyrus; *CD,* caudate nucleus; *DLPFC,* dorsal lateral prefrontal cortex; *NAC,* nucleus accumbens; *OFC,* orbital frontal cortex; *PC,* posterior cingulate gyrus; *PHG,* parahippocampal gyrus; *PUT,* putamen; *SMA,* supplementary motor area. *(Reprinted with permission from Brody, A.L., Saxena, S., 1996. Brain imaging in obsessive-compulsive disorder: evidence for the involvement of frontal-subcortical circuitry in the mediation of symptomatology. CNS. Spectr. 1, 27–41. Copyright 1996 by MBL Communications. Reproduced with permission.)*

Table 8.3 Disorders Associated with Disruptions of Frontal-Subcortical Circuitry

Syndrome	Disruption of Dorsolateral Frontal-Subcortical Circuit	Disruption of Orbitofrontal Frontal-Subcortical Circuit	Disruption of Anterior Cingulate Frontal-Subcortical Circuit
Alzheimer disease			X
Corticobasal degeneration	X		
Frontotemporal dementia	X	X	X
HIV dementia	X		
Huntington disease	X	X	X
Multiple sclerosis		X	X
Multiple symptom atrophy	X		
Obsessive-compulsive disorder		X	
Parkinson disease	X		X
Progressive supranuclear palsy	X		
Schizophrenia	X		X
Tourette syndrome		X	
Vascular dementia	X		

Modified with permission from Chow, T.W., Cummings, J.L., 1999. Frontal-subcortical circuits, in: Miller, B.L., Cummings, J.L. (Eds.), The Human Frontal Lobes: Functions and Disorders. New York, Guilford. Reproduced with permission of Guilford Publications, Inc.

function-structure hypotheses, it is unlikely that any current model is sufficient to explain the complex interface between behavior and brain circuitry.

Additionally, the role of the amygdala in behavior and personality disturbances is an area of increased interest and research. The amygdala exhibits a number of interconnections with the previously described frontosubcortical circuitry via the frontal cortex, thalamus, and ventromedial striatum (for a review, see Price and Drevets, 2010). Classic studies linking the amygdala and behavior include Kluver and Bucy's early work with monkeys with bitemporal lesions. Following selective lesions to the amygdala, monkeys exhibited less caution and fear when exposed to unfamiliar stimuli. Human case studies of individuals with amygdala lesions have also been described and have revealed similar findings. One individual with bilateral amygdala damage exhibited difficulty in recognition of fear and exhibited increased social interactions with features of disinhibition (Adolphs, 2010). Researchers have long implemented the amygdala in anxiety and fear. For example, changes in amygdala volume and functioning have been observed in posttraumatic stress disorder (PTSD) (Shin, Rauch, and Pitman, 2006). More recently, research has implemented the amygdala in a wider range of emotional and behavioral responses and syndromes. Although findings have been somewhat mixed, the amygdala has been implicated in mood disorders including depression and bipolar disorder (Hamidi, Drevets, and Price, 2004).

The current chapter focuses on behavioral and psychiatric changes in neurological disease and injury. Please see Chapter 34 for detailed information on assessment and description of common cognitive changes observed in neurological disease and injury.

Assessing Behavior and Personality Disturbances in Patients with Cerebral Dysfunction

Research on the incidence of behavioral and personality disturbances in patients with neurological disease and injury is encumbered by limitations within and across studies. Some limitations of the available research are that (1) treatment of symptoms such as a movement disorder may mask psychiatric and behavioral symptoms, and (2) most available neuropsychiatric assessment tools use conventional psychiatric terminology based on idiopathic psychiatric illness, which fails to distinctly reflect the symptoms associated with cerebral dysfunction secondary to acquired disease and/or trauma.

Several factors present challenges in the identification and diagnosis of behavior and personality disturbances in neurological samples. First, there is significant overlap between other symptoms of cerebral dysfunction and symptoms of behavior and personality disturbances. For example, psychomotor retardation or reduced energy, libido, or appetite might reflect the underlying illness or injury (i.e., TBI, Parkinson disease [PD]) or they may reflect a depressive disorder. Second, cognitive symptoms may confound the detection of behavioral changes. For example, language and cognitive deficits occurring in individuals with cerebral dysfunction can affect the ability to fully assess for changes in mood or insight. In these situations, observed behavior and collateral report must be heavily considered when assessing for behavioral or personality disturbances. Third, the validity of the behavioral dysfunction assessed can vary depending upon the source. Ample research shows that clinical ratings acquired from the patient, a collateral or spouse, and a healthcare worker can vary widely (see, for example, Hoth et al., 2007). Patients with cerebral dysfunction may have impaired insight; thus, they may underreport behavioral difficulties. Similarly, caregivers may also provide biased information, as their current mood or degree of caregiver burden may influence their reporting of behavioral symptoms.

Assessment of Depression

Symptoms of neurological illness or injury may manifest as depression. In fact, depression is frequently a very early symptom or precedes onset of illness in Huntington disease (HD) (Berrios et al., 2001), PD (Ishihara and Brayne, 2006), and Alzheimer disease (AD) (Green et al., 2003). There are several scales available for the assessment of mood disorders that might be useful in patients with acquired cerebral dysfunction. Although clinicians may not have enough time to thoroughly assess altered mood, self-report scales can be helpful in determining which symptoms are present and how bothersome or severe each symptom is. **Table 8.4** offers additional information regarding these scales. Individuals scoring highly on these self-report measures may benefit from referral for additional evaluation and possible intervention by mental health professionals.

Domains assessed by the different measures vary such that certain scales may not detect some symptoms of depression. Two of the most commonly used measures are the Beck Depression Inventory (BDI) and the Hamilton Depression Rating Scale (HDRS). Research suggests that the BDI may be a useful screening tool in PD and Tourette syndrome, and the HDRS may be an appropriate screening tool in PD. However, these measures assess several symptoms such as psychomotor retardation and reduced energy that are common in neurological illness and injury. Thus, care must be taken to be certain that these measures do not suggest the person is depressed based on symptoms of neurological syndrome or injury. The Geriatric Depression Scale (GDS) was developed to be used in elderly populations and may be a useful screening tool for patients with early dementia and PD. The Patient Health Questionnaire (PHQ-9) is a self-report measure designed to be used in primary care settings and may be appropriate in neurological settings. See Chapter 9 for more detailed information on depression in neurological settings.

Assessment of Other Behavioral and Personality Disturbances

In addition to depression, other behavioral and personality disturbances occur in patients with cerebral dysfunction, and several measures have been created to assess them (**Table 8.5**). These measures were specifically designed to assess behavioral symptoms in AD: Alzheimer's Disease Assessment Scale (ADAS); Behavioral Pathology in Alzheimer's Disease Rating Scale (BEHAVE-AD); CERAD Behavior Rating Scale for Dementia (C-BRSD); general dementia: Neuropsychiatric Inventory (NPI); frontal lobe dementia: Frontal Behavior Inventory (FBI); TBI: Neurobehavioral Rating Scale-Revised (NRS-R); and damage to frontal regions: Frontal Systems Behavior Scale (FrSBe). Some measures such as the NPI and the FrSBe have been implemented in diverse conditions including AD, PD, HD, and multiple sclerosis (MS). In addition, the NPI, which is available in an interview and a questionnaire format, has been frequently used as an outcome measure in clinical trials. These measures might be useful ways to screen for a wide variety of potential behavioral disruptions among patients with neurological illness or injury.

Table 8.4 Common Measures of Depression Symptom Severity

Scale	Method	Items	Domains Assessed
BDI-II	Self-administered	21	Cognitive symptoms Performance impairments Somatic symptoms
CES-D	Self-administered	20	Somatic symptoms Depressed affect Positive affect Interpersonal problems
GDS	Self-administered	30	Sad mood Lack of energy Positive mood Agitation/anxiety Social withdrawal
HADS	Self-administered	14	General depression Anxiety
HDRS	Interview	21	Anxiety General depression Insomnia Somatic symptoms
PHQ-9	Self-administered	9	Cognitive symptoms Somatic symptoms Level of functional impairment
ZDS	Self-administered	20	Positive affect Negative symptoms Somatic symptoms

BDI-II, Beck Depression Inventory, second ed.; CES-D, Center for Epidemiologic Studies Depression Scale; GDS, Geriatric Depression Scale; HADS, Hospital Anxiety and Depression Scale; HDRS, Hamilton Depression Rating Scale; PHQ-9, Patient Health Questionnaire; ZDS, Zung Depression Scale.

References
BDI-II: Beck, A.T., Steer, R.A., Brown, G.K., 1996. Beck Depression Inventory, second ed. The Psychological Corporation, San Antonio, TX.
CES-D: Radloff, L.S., 1997. A self-report depression scale for research in the general population. Appl Psychol Meas 1, 385-401.
GDS: Brink, T.L., Yesavage, J.A., Lum, O., et al., 1982. Screening tests for geriatric depression. Clin Gerontol 1, 37-44.
HADS: Zigmond, A.S., Snaith, R.P., 1983. The hospital anxiety and depression scale. Acta Psychiatr Scand 67, 361-370.
HDRS: Hamilton, M., 1960. A rating scale for depression. J Neurol Neurosurg Psychiatry 23, 56-61.
PHQ-9: Kroenke, K., Spitzer, R.L., Williams, J.B., 2001. The PHQ-9: validity of a brief depression severity measure. J Gen Intern Med 16, 606-613.
ZDS: Zung W.W.K., 1965. A self-rating depression scale. Arch Gen Psychiatry 12, 63-70.

Table 8.5 Common Measures to Assess Behavior and Personality in Patients with Cerebral Dysfunction

Scale	Administration		Behaviors Assessed				
	Source	Time (Minutes)	Depression	Apathy	Anxiety	Psychosis	Aggression
ADAS	Patient and caregiver Trained examiner	45	Yes	No	No	Yes	No
BEHAVE-AD	Caregiver interview	20	Yes	No	Yes	Yes	Yes
C-BRSD	Caregiver interview	20-30	Yes	Yes	No	Yes	Yes
FBI	Caregiver interview	10-15	No	Yes	No	No	Yes
FrSBe	Patient questionnaire Caregiver questionnaire	10	No	Yes	No	No	No
NPI	Caregiver interview	10	Yes	Yes	Yes	Yes	Yes
NPI-Q	Caregiver	5	Yes	Yes	Yes	Yes	Yes
NRS-R	Patient/caregiver interview	15-20	Yes	No	Yes	No	Yes

ADAS, Alzheimer Disease Assessment Scale; BEHAVE-AD, Behavioral Pathology in Alzheimer's Disease Rating Scale; C-BRSD, CERAD (Consortium to Establish a Registry for Alzheimer's Disease) Behavior Rating Scale for Dementia; FBI, Frontal Behavior Inventory; FrSBe, Frontal Systems Behavior Scale; NPI, Neuropsychiatric Inventory; NPI-Q, Neuropsychiatric Inventory-Questionnaire; NRS-R, Neurobehavioral Rating Scale-Revised.

Behavior and Personality Disturbances Associated with Cerebral Dysfunction

Alzheimer Disease

Based on 2000 census data, it is estimated that AD affects 5.1 million individuals in the United States (Hebert et al., 2003). Patients with AD experience a wide range of behavioral disturbances, including affective symptoms, agitation, aggression, and psychosis. Behavioral disturbances in AD are associated with increased caregiver burden, patient and caregiver abuse, greater use of psychotropic medications, more rapid cognitive decline, and earlier institutionalization. The relationship between behavioral changes in AD and neuropathological markers is equivocal. Some researchers report a correlation between behavioral changes in AD and increased white matter hyperintensities (WMH) (Berlow et al., 2009), while others have not observed this relationship (Staekenborg et al., 2008). Many studies do not document a correlation between the presence or absence of behavioral symptoms and whole brain or hippocampal volume (Berlow et al., 2009; Staekenborg et al., 2008). In contrast to frontotemporal dementia (FTD), social comportment is relatively spared in AD.

Use of atypical antipsychotic medications have historically been the preferred method of treatment for behavioral disturbances in AD including irritability, aggression, and psychosis. However, use of atypical antipsychotic medications in elderly adults may be associated with a nearly twofold increase in risk for mortality (Kuehn, 2005). Additionally, a multisite study of atypical antipsychotics (olanzapine, quetiapine, and risperidone) showed no significant difference in Clinical Global Impression Scale scores for any antipsychotic medication over a placebo group (Schneider et al., 2006). Moreover, significantly more participants found the side effects of the atypical antipsychotic medications to be intolerable compared to the placebo group (Schneider et al., 2006). In a retrospective observational study, behavioral symptoms were reduced in one-fifth to one-fourth of patients following treatment with antipsychotics, while a full half of participants exhibited worsening of symptoms (Kleijer et al., 2009). However, other retrospective observational studies have reported improvements in 33% to 43% of individuals with AD and behavioral disturbances treated with atypical antipsychotics (Rocca et al., 2007). The U.S. Food and Drug Administration (FDA) has issued a black-box warning on the use of antipsychotics in elderly persons with dementia. Antipsychotics may be beneficial in a small subgroup of individuals, but care must be taken in prescribing such medications, owing to the potential side effects in the context of questionable effectiveness. A review of the clinical trial literature for cholinesterase inhibitors and memantine suggests that individuals treated with these pharmaceuticals typically do experience a reduction in behavioral symptoms, including improved mood and abatement of apathy (Cummings, Mackell, and Kaufer, 2008).

Although the neurodegenerative process itself can be the cause of behavioral disturbances in AD, other causes must be explored: premorbid psychiatric diagnoses, medication side effects, or medical comorbidities to name a few. In many situations, behavioral disturbances may reflect an individual with impaired cognitive and language abilities attempting to communicate information to their providers (Sutor, Nykamp, and Smith, 2006). Given the nature of these behavioral disturbances and the limited availability of pharmacological interventions, behavioral interventions and environmental modifications may be among the most helpful strategies in managing undesired behaviors. Detailed discussion of such behavioral interventions is beyond the scope of this chapter, but for more detailed information, readers may wish to review Sutor and colleagues (2006).

Clinicians may wish to refer patients to geriatric psychiatry and/or neuropsychology providers for identification and implementation of behavioral and environmental interventions. Common environmental interventions include use of familiar and personal belongings readily viewable in the environment to reduce confusion and agitation. Similarly, minimizing background distracters and establishing a standard predictable routine may also be helpful in reducing confusion and agitation. It is not uncommon for undesired behaviors (e.g., aggression) to receive significant attention while preferred behaviors (e.g., working on quiet activity) receive no reinforcement. To successfully reduce undesired activities, individuals need to increase desired activities through reinforcing preferred behavior, offering desired activities, and reducing reinforcement of undesired behavior. Finally, redirection is frequently attempted in individuals with cognitive impairment who are engaging in undesired activities. Redirection is likely to be most successful if done in a multistep process involving validation of emotion, joining of behavior, distraction, and only then followed by redirection (Sutor, Nykamp, and Smith, 2006). **Table 8.6** lists more detailed information.

Depression

The true prevalence of depression in AD is controversial, with estimates up to 86%. One reason for the mixed findings lies in the different methods employed to assess depression in AD, such as family interviews and patient self-report. Some

Table 8.6 **Multistep Approach for Redirecting Patients with Dementia**	
Step	**Description and Example**
Validate	Validation of the individual's emotional state to establish rapport *Example:* "You look worried."
Join	Join the patient's behavior. *Example:* "You're looking for your children? Well, I'm trying to find something too. Let's look together."
Distract	Distraction is easier after establishing a common goal. This works best when individuals have significant cognitive impairment. *Example:* "Let's look over there where they are having coffee."
Redirect	At this stage, redirection may be possible. *Example:* "That coffee smells good; do you want a cup?"

Reprinted with permission from Sutor, B., Nykamp, L.J., Smith, G.E., 2006. Get creative to manage dementia-related behaviors. Curr Psychiatry 5, 81-96.

Table 8.7 Clinical Aspects Differentiating Dementia from Depression

Major Depression	Dementia
Acute, nonprogressive	Insidious and progressive
Affective before cognitive	Cognitive before affective
Attention impaired	Memory impaired
Orientation intact	Orientation impaired
Complains of memory	Minimizes/normalizes memory
Gives up on testing	Obvious effort on testing
Language intact	Aphasic errors
Better at night	Sundowning
Self-referred	Referred by others

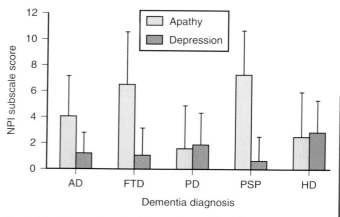

Fig. 8.3 Incidence of psychosis in patients with Alzheimer disease. *AD*, Alzheimer disease; *FTD*, frontotemporal dementia; *HD*, Huntington disease; *NPI*, Neuropsychiatric Inventory; *PD*, Parkinson disease; *PSP*, progressive supranuclear palsy. *(Reprinted with permission from Paulsen, J.S., Salmon, D.P., Thal, L.J., et al., 2000. Incidence of and risk factors for hallucinations and delusions in patients with probable AD. Neurology 54, 1965-1971.)*

symptoms of depression are confounded with components of AD (e.g., concentration, energy, interest). The probability of depression in AD appears to be greater if there is a history of depression either in the patient or in the family. **Table 8.7** suggests differences between the signs of depression and possibly confounding signs of dementia. Interestingly, there does not appear to be a clear relationship between depressive symptoms and severity of AD (Verkaik et al., 2007). Depression is associated with greater social and functional impairments in patients with AD (Starkstein et al., 2005), although others have not observed a correlation between depression and functional impairment (Landes, Sperry, and Strauss, 2005).

Selective serotonin reuptake inhibitors (SSRIs) are the preferred mode of treatment for depression in AD. Although clinical trials are relatively few, sertraline and citalopram have been shown to be effective (Lyketsos et al., 2000).

Apathy

Apathy, defined as diminished motivation not attributable to decreased level of consciousness, cognitive impairment, or emotional distress, is among the most common behavioral changes noted in AD. Assessment of apathy in AD may be difficult because it may be unclear whether decreased activity is due to apathy or inability to perform activities. Consistent with expectations based on frontal-subcortical circuitry, apathy in AD has been shown to be associated with bilateral reductions in gray matter volume in the anterior cingulate cortex, orbitofrontal cortex, dorsolateral prefrontal cortex, and putamen (Bruen et al., 2008). Apathy in AD is associated with greater functional and cognitive impairment (Landes et al., 2005) as well as lower quality of life (Hurt et al., 2008).

Aggression

Aggressive verbalizations and acts are common in AD. Reported prevalence rates range from 25% to 67%, and studies have indicated that verbal aggression is more common in men and in individuals with delusions or agitation (Eustace et al., 2001) and is associated with increased placement in skilled nursing facilities. Sertraline has been associated with a 38% response rate for the treatment of aggression and irritability in AD (Lanctot et al., 2002).

Psychosis

Prevalence rates of psychotic symptoms in AD range from 10% to 73%, with rates in clinical populations exceeding community-based samples. Interestingly, hallucinations and delusions are significantly less common among individuals with early-onset AD (Toyota et al., 2007). Once present, delusions recur or persist for several years in most patients with AD (**Fig. 8.3**). The presence of hallucinations is associated with increased placement in skilled nursing centers.

Previously it was believed that individuals with AD experienced delusions secondary to significant cognitive difficulties. However, more recent research has identified additional correlates and biological markers of psychosis. Evidence from neuropsychological investigations suggests more executive and frontal dysfunction in AD with psychotic symptoms than AD without these symptoms. For example, delusions have been associated with reduced gray matter volume in the inferior right frontal gyrus and the inferior parietal lobule (Bruen et al., 2008). The presence of delusions in AD is associated with poorer performance on the Frontal Assessment Battery (FAB) but was not related to global measures of cognitive impairment (i.e., MMSE) (Nagata et al., 2009). Persons with AD and hallucinations are at significantly increased risk for mortality; however, delusions alone are not associated with increased mortality (Wilson et al., 2005)

The most common psychotic symptoms reported in patients with AD are delusions and hallucinations. The delusions are typically paranoid-type, non-bizarre, and simple. Complex or bizarre delusions seen in patients with schizophrenia are conspicuously absent in patients with AD. Misidentification phenomena, however, are common in AD. Whereas hallucinations in AD are more often visual than auditory, the reverse is true for schizophrenia (**Table 8.8**).

Frontotemporal Dementia

Frontotemporal lobar degeneration (FTLD) is a heterogeneous group of syndromes including semantic dementia (SD), progressive nonfluent aphasia (PNFA), and behavioral variant frontotemporal dementia (bvFTD). Consensus criteria for

Table 8.8 Psychotic Symptoms in Alzheimer Disease versus Schizophrenia in Elderly Patients

	Psychosis in Alzheimer Disease	Schizophrenia in the Elderly
Incidence	30%-50%	<1%
Bizarre or complex delusions	Rare	Common
Misidentification of caregivers	Common	Rare
Common form of hallucinations	Visual	Auditory
Schneiderian first-rank symptoms	Rare	Common
Active suicidal ideation	Rare	Common
History of psychosis	Rare	Very common
Eventual remission of psychosis	Common	Uncommon
Need for many years of maintenance on antipsychotics	Uncommon	Very common
Average optimal daily dose of an antipsychotic	15%-25% of that in young adult with schizophrenia	40%-60% of that in a young adult with schizophrenia

Reprinted with permission from Jeste, D.V., Finkel, S.I., 2000. Psychosis of Alzheimer's disease and related dementias. Am J Geriatr Psychiatry 8, 29-34.

diagnosis of FTD have been described, with presence of behavioral change an important feature. While changes in personality and behavior are most commonly described in bvFTD, behavioral change has been reported across all FTLD syndromes to varying degrees. Caregiver distress is greater among individuals with FTLD and behavioral changes, particularly apathy and disinhibition, versus those with primarily aphasic difficulties (Massimo et al., 2009).

Behavioral Disruption

Atrophy within the frontal lobes leads to disruption of the frontosubcortical circuits and the characteristic behavioral syndromes in FTLD. Two classic behavioral syndromes have been described among individuals with FTD: an apathetic and a disinhibited subtype. Apathy is a very common symptom in individuals with FTD. Individuals may show little concern for personal hygiene and may appear unkempt. Moreover, symptoms of orbitofrontal syndrome, such as disinhibition, poor impulse control, tactlessness, and poor judgment are common. Loss of empathy, mental inflexibility, and stereotyped behaviors are also common. Symptoms similar to those observed in Klüver-Bucy syndrome, such as hyperorality and hypersexuality, may occur in late stages. Frequently the family members and caregivers are the ones who report these behavioral

disturbances, as many patients with FTD experience reduced insight into their current difficulties. Behavioral change to varying degrees has been described in all FTLD syndromes, including SD and PNFA (Kertesz et al., 2010), although they frequently are less severe and/or occur later in the progression of the illness.

No curative treatments exist for FTLD. However, there has been some success with pharmacological intervention for behavioral dyscontrol. Although few large-scale studies have been completed, evidence suggests that behavioral disturbances such as disinhibition, overeating, and compulsions may show some response to treatment with SSRIs (Huey, Putnam, and Grafman, 2006).

Anosognosia

As noted in the consensus criteria, individuals with FTD frequently exhibit anosognosia. This loss of insight may reflect psychological denial of illness, inability to perceive symptoms, or lack of concern for their current difficulties. Among individuals with FTLD, individuals with bvFTD exhibit greater anosognosia than individuals with the aphasic subtypes of FTLD (Zamboni et al., 2010). Patients with FTD frequently describe significantly fewer problems with cognition and behavior than what their caregivers describe. Moreover, this observed discrepancy between patient and caregiver report is greater among individuals with FTD than in individuals with AD, particularly for language, behavior, and functioning difficulties (Salmon et al., 2008). Severity of anosognosia is not typically associated with severity of dementia (Zamboni et al., 2010). The relationship between impaired awareness and specific neuropathology is somewhat unclear. Some studies have shown an association between impaired awareness and right frontal disruptions (Mendez and Shapira, 2005) while others have shown a link between anosognosia and involvement of the right temporoparietal cortex (Zamboni et al., 2010).

Relationship to Primary Pathology

From a pathological perspective, individuals with FTLD vary with regard to the degree to which the frontal versus temporal lobes and right versus left hemispheres are affected. Significant research has looked at the relationship between patterns of behavioral syndromes and underlying neuropathology (see Josephs, 2007 for a review). Individuals with bvFTD typically exhibit greater frontal versus temporal atrophy, which is typically symmetrical. There is emerging evidence to suggest that individuals with bvFTD and primarily apathetic behavioral changes show greater frontal involvement, particularly right dorsolateral prefrontal cortex (Zamboni et al., 2008; Massimo et al., 2009). Individuals with primarily disinhibited behavioral change show greater involvement of the right mediotemporal limbic and temporal lobe (Zamboni et al., 2008), although others have described increased atrophy within the left dorsolateral prefrontal cortex (Massimo et al., 2009). Individuals with SD most typically exhibit atrophy and dysfunction within the left anterior temporal lobe, while individuals with SD and behavioral changes are more likely to also exhibit changes in the ventromedial and superior frontal lobes. Individuals with PNFA are most likely to show changes in left frontal and perisylvian areas.

Vascular Dementia

Dementia secondary to vascular changes is among the most common causes of dementia in older adults. NINDS-AIREN diagnostic criteria for vascular dementia include the presence of dementia and cerebrovascular disease, including evidence of such disease on imaging with a documented relationship between these two criteria. Pathologically, vascular dementia (VaD) frequently involves small-vessel disease involving white matter hyperintensities and/or lacunar strokes, most commonly affecting subcortical regions; therefore, frontosubcortical circuits are frequently disrupted, and behavioral disturbances are common. Apathy, depression, and behavioral changes are common in VaD. The presence of significant cerebrovascular changes are observed among individuals with AD, suggesting that both pathologies may be present among a large subgroup of individuals with dementia.

Depression

The mean reported prevalence of depression in VaD is 32%, although rates vary widely between studies (Ballard and O'Brien, 2002). Sample source likely influences the reported prevalence rates, with community samples endorsing lower rates of depression than clinic samples. Individuals with VaD and depression are less likely to have had a stroke and are more likely to have a prior history of depression and impairments in memory or attention than patients with VaD without depression. The relationship between age and depression in VaD is unclear, with increased rates of depression being reported in both younger and older samples.

Additional Behavioral and Psychiatric Disorders

Apathy in VaD is associated with increased impairment in both basic and instrumental activities of daily living (Zawacki

et al., 2002). This relationship is particularly apparent in patients with VaD who have also experienced a stroke. Rates of psychotic symptoms are similar in AD and VaD. Delusions (33%) and visual hallucinations (13% to 25%) are reported in VaD and are associated with impaired cognitive functioning (Ballard and O'Brien, 2002). Care must be taken in the assessment of delusions in VaD and in dementia in general. It is important to differentiate delusions from confabulation or thought processes based on impaired cognitive functioning.

Parkinson Disease

Behavioral changes are common in PD, and while research has adequately characterized these difficulties, little controlled research has assessed the effectiveness of various interventions. **Table 8.9** offers more detailed information regarding characteristics of behavioral change observed in PD.

Depression

Depression is the most common psychiatric disturbance in persons with PD. Depending on threshold for diagnosis and sample assessed, reported rates vary depending on the threshold for diagnosis of depression that is used. Depression may predate the onset of motor symptoms in PD (Ishihara and Brayne, 2006). Risk factors for depression in PD include greater cognitive impairment, earlier disease onset, and family history of depression. Depression is *not* associated with increased motor symptom severity (Holroyd et al., 2005). The correlation between depression and disability is equivocal. Although the precise etiology is unknown, it is believed that depression in PD results from disruptions in dopamine (D2), noradrenaline, and serotonin pathways (Veazey et al., 2005).

Very few well-controlled studies have assessed antidepressant therapy in PD. Available research suggests that SSRIs are well tolerated and likely effective in the treatment of

Table 8.9 Neuropsychiatric Features and Treatment in Parkinson Disease

Syndrome	Subtype	Key Feature	Treatment
Depression	Major depression	Low mood or loss of interest/pleasure	No large controlled trials published to date. Nonpharmacological (counseling), dopamine agonists (pramipexole, ropinirole), antidepressants (tricyclics, trazodone, SSRIs, SSNRI, SNRI, mirtazapine)
	Minor depression	Low mood and/or loss of interest/pleasure	No available evidence
	Dysthymia	Low mood ≥ 2 years	No available evidence
Anxiety	Panic attacks	Episodic panic attacks	Poor evidence for benzodiazepines, clomipramine, nonpharmacological
	GAD	Excessive, often irrational anxiety or worry	Same as above
Psychosis	Hallucinations	Seeing imaginary people or animals	Clozapine: two randomized trials showing improvement
	Delusions	False, fixed idiosyncratic beliefs, maintained despite contrary evidence	Same as above
Apathy		Lack of initiative, motivation	Limited evidence: dopamine agonists, stimulants, modafinil

Modified with permission from Aarsland, D., Marsh, L., Schrag, A., 2009. Neuropsychiatric symptoms in Parkinson's disease. Mov Disord 24, 2175-2186.

depression in PD (see McDonald et al., 2003 for a review). SSRIs are frequently implemented as a first-line therapy for depression in patients with PD, although SSRIs may worsen motor symptoms. In such cases, tricyclic antidepressants may be an effective alternative. Successful treatment of depressive symptoms with an SSRI may also result in reductions in anxiety and decreased disability.

Psychosis

Hallucinations, typically visual, occur in up to 40% of patients with PD, with 16% reporting delusions (Fenelon et al., 2000). Psychotic symptoms are very uncommon early in the course of PD. Other diagnoses such as dementia with Lewy bodies (DLB) should be considered in patients exhibiting hallucinations early in the course of the disease. **Table 8.10** summarizes important distinctions between psychosis in PD and DLB. Psychotic symptoms are more common in PD patients with greater cognitive impairment, longer duration of illness, greater daytime somnolence, and older age and in those who

are institutionalized. Psychotic symptoms are strong predictors of nursing home placement and mortality in PD (Fenelon et al., 2000).

Historical accounts of PD rarely described psychotic symptoms, and it has been postulated that psychosis occurred secondary to dopamine agonist use. While dopamine agonists may contribute to the development of psychosis, additional factors are also important. For example, individuals with psychosis are more likely to exhibit cholinergic deficits and have Lewy bodies in the temporal lobe observed at autopsy (Aarsland et al., 2009).

Intervention for remediation of psychotic symptoms in PD can involve several processes. Discontinuation of anticholinergics, selegiline, and amantadine before reducing L-dopa is recommended. Following these discontinuations, reduction and simplification of dopamine agonists may be beneficial. Atypical antipsychotics are added only when a reduction of other medications has not resulted in improvement, as even atypical antipsychotics have been associated with worsening of PD motor symptoms (Goetz et al., 2000).

Apathy

Individuals with PD often experience increased rates of apathy. Estimates of apathy in PD have ranged from 16.5% to 40.0%. Individuals with apathy exhibit greater cognitive impairment (Dujardin et al., 2007). Controlled clinical trials for apathy in PD are very limited. Environmental and other behavioral interventions including establishment of a routine, structured schedule, and cuing from others can be helpful in some settings. Dopamine agonists, psychostimulants, modafinil, dopamine agonists, and testosterone have been reported to be helpful in decreasing apathy (see Aarsland et al., 2009 for more detailed information).

Dementia with Lewy Bodies

Dementia with lewy bodies is increasingly being recognized as a common cause of dementia in older adults. DLB is associated with fluctuating cognitive difficulties, parkinsonism, and hallucinations. Clinical presentation overlap occurs between the presentation of DLB with AD and PD. Research has observed greater overall behavioral symptoms among individuals with DLB compared to individuals with AD, particularly with regard to hallucinations and apathy (Ricci et al., 2009).

Psychosis

Psychotic symptoms, particularly hallucinations, are a hallmark feature of DLB. Insight is typically poor. Unlike patients with AD or PD, patients with DLB exhibit hallucinations early in the course of the illness. Delusions are also common in DLB. The neuropathological correlates of hallucinations in DLB are somewhat unclear. It has been suggested that hallucinations are likely due to decreased acetylcholine as well as changes in the basal forebrain and the ventral temporal lobe (Ferman and Boeve, 2007).

Hallucinations are correlated with poorer functioning with regard to instrumental activities of daily living (Ricci et al., 2009). Typical neuroleptics are avoided in DLB, because patients exhibit high sensitivity to these drugs and may experience severe parkinsonian symptoms and other side effects. In

Table 8.10 Differentiating Psychosis in Parkinson Disease and Dementia with Lewy Bodies

Psychosis in Parkinson Disease	Psychosis in Dementia with Lewy Bodies
• Psychosis occurs in many but not all patients.	• Psychosis is a core feature for diagnosis.
• Visual hallucinations are more common than delusions.	• Visual hallucinations and delusions occur at similar frequencies.
• Psychosis is generally medication induced.	• Psychosis occurs in the absence of antiparkinsonian medications.
• Hallucinations are usually fleeting and nocturnal.	• Hallucinations are generally persistent/recurrent.
• Fluctuating level of consciousness represents onset of delirium.	• Fluctuating level of consciousness can be a core feature.
• Dementia may or may not accompany psychosis.	• Presence of dementia is required for a diagnosis of DLB.
• Motor impairment virtually always precedes psychosis.	• Motor impairment may occur after psychosis.
• Neuroleptics worsen motor function, but "neuroleptic sensitivity" associated with DLB is not a feature of PD.	• Neuroleptic sensitivity characterized by dramatic motor and cognitive worsening and associated with increased morbidity and mortality has been reported.
• Disordered dopaminergic (and possibly serotonergic) transmission are the most frequently hypothesized underlying mechanisms.	• Disordered cholinergic transmission may be the most important underlying mechanism.

Table 8.11 Percentage of Patients with Huntington Disease Endorsing Psychiatric Symptoms by TFC Stage

Symptom	Stage 1 (n = 432)	Stage 2 (n = 660)	Stage 3 (n = 520)	Stage 4 (n = 221)	Stage 5 (n = 84)
Depression	57.5%	62.9%	59.3%	52.1%	42.2%
Suicide	6.0%	9.7%	10.3%	9.9%	5.5%
Aggression	39.5%	47.7%	51.8%	54.1%	54.4%
Obsessions	13.3%	16.9%	25.5%	28.9%	13.3%
Delusions	2.4%	3.5%	6.1%	9.9%	2.2%
Hallucinations	2.3%	4.2%	6.3%	11.2%	3.3%

Data provided by the Huntington Study Group.

Table 8.12 Ratings by Nursing Home Staff of Problematic Behaviors in Patients with Huntington Disease

Behavior Problem	Percentage	Rank
Agitation	76	2.0
Irritability	72	2.9
Disinhibition	59	3.3
Depression	51	4.2
Anxiety	50	4.4
Appetite	54	5.1
Delusions	43	5.5
Sleep disorders	50	5.5
Apathy	32	6.8
Euphoria	40	6.9

From Paulsen and Hamilton, unpublished data.

contrast, atypical neuroleptics such as clozapine and quetiapine, as well as cholinesterase inhibitors, are associated with improved cognition and decreased psychotic symptoms (McKeith, 2002).

Huntington Disease

Up to 79% of individuals with HD report psychiatric and behavioral symptoms as the presenting manifestation of the disease. Symptom presentation varies across stage of illness in HD (**Table 8.11**). Behavioral symptoms are commonly observed among institutionalized patients with HD (**Table 8.12**). The behavioral difficulties can lead to placement difficulties in these patients.

Depression

Depression is one of the most common concerns for individuals and families with HD, occurring in up to 63% of patients. Depression may precede the onset of neurological symptoms in HD by 2 to 20 years, although large-scale empirical research has been minimal. Depression is common immediately before diagnosis, when neurological soft signs and other subtle abnormalities become evident. Following a definite diagnosis of HD, however, depression is most prevalent in the middle stages of the disease (i.e., Shoulson-Fahn stages 2 and 3) and may diminish in the later stages (Paulsen et al., 2005b). Positron emission tomography (PET) studies indicate that patients with HD with depression have hypermetabolism in the inferior frontal cortex and thalamus relative to nondepressed patients with HD or normal age-matched controls.

Suicide

Suicide is more common in HD than in other neurological disorders with high rates of depression such as stroke and PD. Most studies have found a four- to sixfold increase of suicide in HD, with reports as high as 8 to 20 times greater than the general population. Two "critical periods" during which suicidal ideation in HD increased dramatically have been identified. First, frequency of suicidal ideation doubles from 10.4% in at-risk persons with a normal neurological examination to 20.5% in at-risk persons with soft neurological signs. Second, in persons with a diagnosis of HD, 16% had suicidal ideation in stage 1, whereas nearly 21% had suicidal ideation in stage 2. Although the underlying mechanisms for suicidal risk in HD are poorly understood, it may be beneficial for healthcare providers to be aware of periods during which patients may be at an increased risk of suicide (Paulsen et al., 2005a).

Psychosis

Psychosis occurs with increased frequency in HD, with estimates ranging from 3% to 12%. Psychosis is more common among early adulthood-onset cases than among those whose disease begins in middle or late adulthood. Psychosis in HD is more resistant to treatment than psychosis in schizophrenia. Huntington Study Group data suggest that psychosis may increase as the disease progresses (see **Table 8.11**), although psychosis can become difficult to measure in the later stages of disease.

Obsessive-Compulsive Traits

Although true OCD is rare in HD, obsessive and compulsive behaviors are prevalent (13% to 30%). Obsessional thinking often increases with proximity to disease onset and then remains stable throughout the illness. Obsessional thinking associated with HD is reminiscent of perseveration, such that individuals get "stuck" on a previous occurrence or need and are unable to shift.

Aggression

Aggressive behaviors ranging from irritability to intermittent explosive disorders occur in 19% to 59% of patients with HD. Although aggressive outbursts are often the principal reason for admission to a psychiatric facility, research on the prevalence and incidence of irritability and aggressive outbursts in HD is sparse. The primary limitation in summarizing these symptoms in HD is the varied terminology used to describe this continuum of behaviors. Clinicians and HD family members suggested that difficulty with placement attributable to the patient's aggression was among the principal obstacles to providing an effective continuum of care.

Apathy

Early signs of HD may include withdrawal from activities and friends, decline in personal appearance, lack of behavioral initiation, decreased spontaneous speech, and constriction of emotional expression. Frequently these symptoms are considered reflective of depression. Though difficult to distinguish, apathy is defined as diminished motivation not attributable to cognitive impairment, emotional distress, or decreased level of consciousness. Depression involves considerable emotional distress evidenced by tearfulness, sadness, anxiety, agitation, insomnia, anorexia, feelings of worthlessness and hopelessness, and recurrent thoughts of death. Both apathy (59%) and depression (70%) are common in HD. However, 53% of individuals experienced only one of these symptoms rather than the two combined. Furthermore, depression and apathy were not correlated.

Tourette Syndrome

Tourette syndrome (TS) is associated with disinhibition of frontosubcortical circuitry; as a result, it is not surprising that increased rates of psychiatric and behavioral symptoms are observed. These behavioral difficulties are more strongly associated with problems with psychosocial functioning than the presence of tics (Zinner and Coffey, 2009). Rates of psychiatric disorders vary widely; significantly higher rates of psychiatric disorders are reported when samples are drawn from psychiatric clinics than from movement disorder clinics. Given the correlation between psychiatric symptoms and changes in psychosocial functioning, treatments in TS that consider psychiatric and behavioral symptoms are encouraged.

Approximately 20% to 40% of individuals with TS meet criteria for OCD, while up to 90% of individuals in a clinic referred sample may exhibit subthreshold levels of obsessive-compulsive symptoms (Zinner and Coffey, 2009). The frequency and severity of tics often decrease as individuals enter adulthood, but the comorbid obsessive-compulsive symptoms are more likely to continue into adulthood and are associated with difficulties with psychosocial functioning (Cheung, Shahed, and Jankovic, 2007). Mood and anxiety symptoms are common in TS. The relationship between severity of depression and tics is unclear. The comorbid presence of obsessive-compulsive symptoms is associated with increased risk for depressive symptoms (Zinner and Coffey, 2009).

Multiple Sclerosis

The assessment of behavioral symptoms in MS is complicated because one of the hallmark symptoms of MS is variability of symptoms across time. Additionally, there is significant heterogeneity within patients with MS. Finally, a disconnection between the experience of emotion and the expression of emotion has historically been observed in individuals with MS.

Depression

Depression is the most common behavioral symptom in MS, occurring at rates of 37% to 54%. Patients with MS may report symptoms of depression even with outward signs of euphoria. While depression is frequently associated with reduced quality of life, the correlation between depressive symptoms and disability in MS is debated with equivocal research. Depression in MS is *not* consistently associated with increased rates of stressful events, disease duration, sex, age, or socioeconomic status. Among the subtypes of MS, depression may be most common in those with relapsing-remitting MS (Beiske et al., 2008). Fatigue is a strong predictor of depression among individuals with MS (Beiske et al., 2008).

Increased rates of suicidal ideation, suicide attempts, and completed suicides have been observed in individuals with MS. Suicide rates in MS are between two and seven times higher than in the general population (Bronnum-Hansen et al., 2005). Risk factors for suicidal ideation in MS include social isolation, current depression, and lifetime diagnosis of alcohol abuse disorder. Although suicide attempts occur throughout the progression of the disease, some have suggested that increased risk may be particularly high in the year following diagnosis (Bronnum-Hansen et al., 2005).

Biological factors likely contribute to depressive symptoms in MS. It has been hypothesized that the inflammatory process associated with MS may directly lead to depressive symptoms. Similarly, demyelination lesions in MS may directly contribute to the etiology of depression. Imaging studies in MS, however, have failed to show clear neuropathological correlates of depression. Disruptions have been observed in right parietal, right temporal, and right frontal areas (Zorzon et al., 2001) as well as the limbic cortex, implying disruption of frontosubcortical circuitry. It is likely that depression in MS results from a combination of psychosocial and biological factors.

Although controversial, depression may be a side effect for some individuals treated with interferon beta-1b (IFN-β-1b) (Feinstein, 2000). Patients with severe depression should be closely monitored while receiving IFN-β-1b. The relationship between depression and IFN-β-1a and interferon alfa (IFN-α) is equivocal, as conflicting results have been reported. In contrast, glatiramer acetate has not been associated with increased depressive symptoms (Feinstein, 2000). Because of the potential relationship between depression and treatment for MS, as well as the high rates of depression in MS, it is critical that physicians take care to thoroughly assess a patient's current and past history of depression. This may be particularly important prior to beginning IFN interventions, as patients with histories of depression may be more likely to experience symptoms of depression following IFN treatment.

Box 8.2 Strategies to Minimize Anxiety in Patients with Multiple Sclerosis

- Respect adaptive denial as a useful coping mechanism.
- Provide referrals to the National Multiple Sclerosis Society (1-800-Fight-MS) early in disease.
- Help patients to live "one day at a time," and restrict predictions regarding the future.
- Help patients manage stress with relaxation techniques.
- Involve occupational therapists for energy conservation techniques.
- Focus on the patient's abilities, not disabilities.
- Consider patient's educational and financial background when giving explanations and referrals.
- Realize that patients have access to the Internet, self-help groups, and medical journals, and may ask "difficult" questions.
- Expect grief reactions to losses.
- Deal with losses one at a time.
- Attend to the mental health needs of patients' families and caregivers.
- Respect the patient's symptoms as real.
- Avoid overmedicating.
- Focus supportive psychotherapy on concrete, reality-based cognitive and educational issues related to multiple sclerosis.
- Provide targeted pharmacotherapy.
- Refer appropriate patients for cognitive remediation training.
- Ask about sexual problems, as well as bowel and bladder dysfunction.
- Keep an open dialogue with the patient about suicidal thoughts.

Modified with permission from Riether, A.M., 1999. Anxiety in patients with multiple sclerosis. Semin Neuropsychiatry 4, 103-113.

Table 8.13 Neuroanatomical Structures and Pathological Laughing and Crying

Structure	Neuroanatomical Significance
Prefrontal cortex and anterior cingulate	A major component of the limbic lobe, with motor efferents to the brainstem structures involved in emotional expression
Internal capsule	A white matter structure consisting of pathways descending from the brain to the brainstem and spinal cord. Some of these pathways are related to the brainstem nuclei, some to the cerebellum (via basis pontis), and some reach the spinal cord.
Thalamus	A node in the pathways to the cortex originated from the brainstem, cerebellum, and basal ganglia
Subthalamic nucleus	A crucial node in the indirect pathways that carry signals from the striatum to the frontal lobe via the thalamus
Basis pontis	Relay center for pathways entering the cerebellum
Cerebellar white and gray matter	Receives inputs from many parts of the nervous system and sends its signals to the spinal cord, brainstem, and cerebral cortex (mostly frontal lobe and some to somatomotor parietal cortical areas) through the thalamus

Modified with permission from Parvizi, J., Coburn, K.L., Shillcutt, S.D., et al., 2009. Neuroanatomy of pathological laughing and crying: a report of the American Neuropsychiatric Association Committee on Research. J Neuropsychiatry. Clin Neurosci 21, 75-87. Copyright 2009, American Psychiatric Association.

Few randomly assigned clinical trials have been conducted for the treatment of depression in MS. Several open-label trials of SSRIs have been conducted, which suggest that SSRIs may be effective in the treatment of depression in MS (Siegert and Abernethy, 2005). In addition, psychotherapy, particularly that focusing on coping skills, is efficacious in the reduction of depressive symptoms.

Anxiety

Although common, anxiety is often overlooked because anxiety symptoms may be viewed as a result of poor coping skills. Some strategies to minimize anxiety in individuals with MS are described in **Box 8.2.** Comorbid anxiety and depression are associated with greater somatic complaints, social difficulties, and suicidal ideation than either anxiety or depression alone. Predictors of anxiety in individuals with MS include fatigue, pain, and younger age of onset (Beiske et al., 2008).

Euphoria

Increased rates of cheerfulness, optimism, and denial of disability may occur in MS. Early studies suggested that over 70% of individuals with MS experienced periods of euphoria. However, more recent studies suggest that prevalence rates of euphoria are between 10% and 25%. Euphoria frequently co-occurs with disinhibition, impulsivity, and emotional liability. Individuals with euphoria are more likely to have cerebral involvement, enlarged ventricles, poorer cognitive and neurological function, and increased social disability.

Pathological Laughing and Crying

Pathological laughing and crying (PLC) occurs when there is disparity between an individual's emotional *experience* and his or her emotional *expression*; affected individuals are unable to control laughter or crying. Approximately 10% of individuals with MS exhibit periods of PLC. (Parvizi et al., 2009). PLC is more common in MS patients who have entered the chronic-progressive disease course, have high levels of disability, and cognitive dysfunction. The neuropathological substrate for PLC is believed to involve several aspects of the frontosubcortical circuits as well as the cerebellum (Parvizi et al., 2009). **Table 8.13** gives more detailed information. Dextromethorphan/quinidine may be effective in treating such symptoms (Panitch et al., 2006). Additionally, tricyclic and SSRI antidepressant medications may be helpful in reducing PLC symptoms (Parvizi et al., 2009).

Amyotrophic Lateral Sclerosis

Historically, amyotrophic lateral sclerosis (ALS) was largely viewed as a pure motor neuron disease. More recently, however,

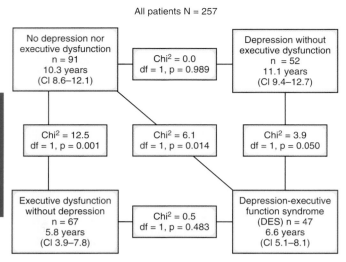

All patients N = 257

No depression nor executive dysfunction n = 91 10.3 years (CI 8.6–12.1)	Chi² = 0.0 df = 1, p = 0.989	Depression without executive dysfunction n = 52 11.1 years (CI 9.4–12.7)
Chi² = 12.5 df = 1, p = 0.001	Chi² = 6.1 df = 1, p = 0.014	Chi² = 3.9 df = 1, p = 0.050
Executive dysfunction without depression n = 67 5.8 years (CI 3.9–7.8)	Chi² = 0.5 df = 1, p = 0.483	Depression-executive function syndrome (DES) n = 47 6.6 years (CI 5.1–8.1)

Fig. 8.4 Poststroke survival by presence or absence of depression and executive dysfunction (endpoint, all causes of death). NOTE: determined by Kaplan Meier Logistic-Rank Analysis. *(Reprinted with permission from Melkas, S., Vataja R., Oksala N.K., et al., 2010. Depression-executive dysfunction syndrome relates to poor poststroke survival. Am J Geriatr Psychiatry 18, 1007-1016. Available at: http://dx.doi.org/10.1097/JGP.0b013e3181d695d7.)*

researchers have recognized that cognitive abilities in individuals with ALS can vary widely from normal cognition to dementia. In particular, a relationship between ALS and FTD has been described (Lomen-Hoerth, Anderson, and Miller, 2002).

Depression

Depressive symptoms occur in 40% to 50% of individuals with ALS (Kubler et al., 2005), although most individuals exhibit subsyndromal depression. Depression in ALS is associated with increased physical impairment, although these results are not always replicated. Individuals with low psychological well-being were at increased risk of mortality (**Fig. 8.4**). Mortality risk was more strongly associated with psychological distress than age and was similar to the association of risk associated with severity of illness. Depression is correlated with duration of illness; however, depression is not associated with ventilator use or tube feeding (Kubler et al., 2005).

Pathological Laughing and Crying

Up to 50% of individuals with ALS, most often those with pseudobulbar syndrome, report PLC (Parvizi et al., 2009). Individuals with PLC may be more likely to exhibit behavioral changes similar to those observed among individuals with FTD (Gibbons et al., 2008). Little research has assessed treatment of pseudobulbar affect. Potential pharmacological interventions include use of tricyclic and SSRI antidepressant medications (Parvizi et al., 2009). Dextromethorphan/quinidine may also be an effective treatment for PLC (Parvizi et al., 2009). Reduction in PLC symptoms was associated with improved quality of life and quality of relationships.

Personality Change

With recognition of the correlation between ALS and FTD, increased interest has been placed on assessing for potential behavioral changes in ALS. Minimal research has fully explored this question. Gibbons and colleagues (2008) assessed behavioral changes among a small group of individuals with ALS by using a structured interview of close family members of those with ALS. In this small study, 14/16 individuals with ALS exhibited behavioral changes. Of those with behavioral changes, 69% exhibited reduced concern for others, 63% exhibited increased irritability, and 38% exhibited increased apathy.

Epilepsy

Behavioral and personality disturbances occur in up to 50% of individuals with epilepsy. Identification and treatment of these behavioral disturbances remains inadequate, with less than half of individuals with epilepsy and major depressive disorder (MDD) being treated for depression. Presence of a psychiatric disorder is an independent predictor of quality of life in individuals with epilepsy (Kanner et al., 2010). In epilepsy, psychiatric disturbances are classified based on their chronological relationship to seizures. Ictal disturbances occur during the seizure. Peri-ictal disturbances occur immediately before (preictal) or after (postictal) a seizure. Finally, interictal disturbances are those that occur independent of seizure states (**Table 8.14**). To facilitate the patient's understanding and for accurate treatment of symptoms, it is important to recognize that behavioral and personality disturbances can occur during the ictal state. Individuals in the ictal period may experience episodes of anxiety, depression, psychosis, and aggression. However, because much of the research regarding psychiatric disturbances in epilepsy has focused on interictal behavioral and personality disturbances, these disturbances will be the focus of this section.

Depression

Depression is the most common psychiatric disorder in epilepsy. Rates of depression vary as a function of the sample assessed (clinical samples report higher rates of depression than population samples) and the measures used to diagnosis depression. Depression often goes undiagnosed in patients with epilepsy, because symptoms of depression may be viewed as a normal reaction to illness. However, accurate diagnosis of depression is critical because depression is associated with poorer quality of life, employment, and family functioning (Ettinger et al., 2004). Interestingly, presurgical depression is associated with poorer postsurgical seizure outcomes (Metternich et al., 2009).

Attempted and completed suicides are common in epilepsy. The suicide rate in epilepsy is two or more times greater than in the general population (Stefanello et al., 2010). Rates of suicide are even higher in temporal lobe epilepsy. Risk factors include history of self-harm, family history of suicide, stressful life situations, poor morale, stigma, and psychiatric disorders. Individuals with difficulties with comorbid anxiety and depression are at greater risk for suicidal ideation than individuals with only one syndrome (Stefanello et al., 2010).

The cause of depression in epilepsy is unclear. Psychosocial stressors, genetic disposition, and neuropathology may play contributing roles. Although psychosocial stressors have been suggested as important in the cause of depression in epilepsy, observed rates of depression in epilepsy are higher than those

Table 8.14 Psychiatric Disturbances in Ictal, Postictal, and Interictal States

Ictal	Postictal	Interictal
Anxiety	Agitation	Panic disorder
Intense feelings of horror		Generalized anxiety disorder
Panic attacks		Phobias
Depressed mood	Depression	Major depressive disorder
Tearfulness		Dysthymic disorder
		Atypical depressive syndromes
		Medication-induced mood changes
		Adjustment disorder
Paranoia	Paranoia	Psychotic syndromes
Hallucinations	Hallucinations	
Illusions		
Forced thoughts resembling obsessions		Obsessive-compulsive disorder
Obsessions		
Aggression/violence	Aggression/violence	Aggression/violence
Confusion	Confusion	
Sexual Excitement		
Laughter	Mania	
Déjà vu and other memory experiences		
		Conversion disorder
		Medication-induced conditions

Reprinted with permission from Marsh, L., Rao, V., 2002. Psychiatric complications in patients with epilepsy: a review. Epilepsy Res 49, 11-33.

in other chronically ill patient populations, lending support to theories of biological causes. Perception of seizure control is an important psychosocial variable to consider, as a lower perception of seizure control is associated with increased depressive symptoms. Though results are somewhat mixed, there appears to be no relationship between age of onset or duration of epilepsy and depression. Depression appears to be more common in individuals with focal epilepsy than in those with primarily generalized epilepsy. Lateralization of seizure foci may be related to depression, with left-sided foci being more commonly associated with depression.

Pharmacological treatment of epilepsy may contribute to depression and psychiatric symptoms in general. **Table 8.15** notes commonly used antiepileptic drugs and their psychotropic effects. Medications associated with sedation (e.g., barbiturates, benzodiazepines) may lead to depression, fatigue, and mental slowing.

Although the phenomenology of depression in epilepsy may prove dissimilar from that in patients with general depression, similar treatments are efficacious in the treatment of depression. Supportive psychotherapy may prove beneficial, particularly after initial diagnosis as patients begin to adapt to their illness. Few clinical trials have assessed the efficacy of antidepressant medications in patients with epilepsy. Older antidepressants and the antidepressant, bupropion, have been associated with increased seizures and thus should be avoided. Prueter and Norra (2005) suggest that citalopram and sertraline be considered first-line antidepressant medications in epilepsy because of their limited interactions with antiepileptic medication.

Anxiety

Increased rates of anxiety disorders occur in patients with epilepsy. Between 19% and 50% of individuals with epilepsy meet criteria for one or more DSM-IV anxiety disorder (Beyenburg et al., 2005). Individuals with comorbid anxiety and depressive disorders report lower quality of life than individuals with either disorder alone (Kanner et al., 2010). Common anxiety disorders include agoraphobia, generalized anxiety disorder, and social phobia. Fear of having a seizure and anticipatory anxiety are quite common. Care must be taken to distinguish between panic attacks and fear occurring in the context of a seizure ("ictal fear"). Fear is the most common psychiatric symptom to manifest during a seizure.

The relationship between antiepileptic drugs (AEDs) and anxiety is complex. Some AEDs appear to exacerbate anxiety symptoms, and others are associated with reduction in anxiety symptoms. Antidepressant medication, particularly the SSRIs, is the most common pharmacological treatment for anxiety in epilepsy. See the review by Beyenburg and colleagues (2005) for a more detailed discussion of treatment of anxiety in epilepsy.

Psychosis

The association between epilepsy and psychosis has been debated throughout the past century. Individuals with epilepsy onset before age 20 years, duration of illness greater than 10 years, history of complex partial seizures, and temporal lobe epilepsy are at increased risk of psychotic disturbances. Postictal and interictal psychosis are most commonly reported. Postictal psychosis most commonly develops after many years of epilepsy (Devinsky, 2003). Episodes of postictal psychosis are short in duration, lasting from a few hours to a few months. Postictal psychosis is more common with limbic lesions (Devinsky, 2003). In interictal psychosis, episodes of psychosis are not temporally tied to seizure onset and typically last for more than 6 months.

Aggression

The relationship between epilepsy and aggression remains controversial. Early research suggested that the prevalence of aggression in epilepsy ranged from 4.8% to 50.0%. Aggression occurring in the context of a seizure is quite rare (Devinsky, 2003). Rates of aggression are believed to be higher in individuals with temporal lobe epilepsy. Results vary owing to the definition of aggression used and the method of group selection. Interictal aggression may be described as episodic dyscontrol or, as in the DSM-IV nosology, intermittent explosive disorder (IED), which is characterized by periods of largely

Table 8.15 **Psychotropic Effects of Antiepileptic Drugs**

Drug	Positive Effects	Negative Effects	Complications
Barbiturates	—	Aggression, depression, withdrawal syndromes	ADHD in children
Benzodiazepines	Anxiolytic, sedative	Withdrawal syndromes	Disinhibition
Ethosuximide	—	Insomnia	Alternative psychoses
Phenytoin	—	—	Toxic schizophreniform psychoses, encephalopathy
Carbamazepine	Mood stabilizing/impulse control	Rarely, mania and depression	—
Valproate	Mood stabilizing, antimanic	—	Acute and chronic encephalopathy
Vigabatrin	—	Aggression, depression, psychosis, withdrawal syndromes	ADHD, encephalopathy, alternative psychoses
Lamotrigine	Mood stabilizing, antidepressive	Insomnia	Rarely psychoses
Felbamate	Stimulating?	Agitation	Psychoses possible
Gabapentin	Anxiolytic, antidepressive?	Rarely aggression in children	—
Tiagabine	—	Depression	Nonconvulsive status epilepticus
Topiramate	Mood stabilizing?	Depression	Psychoses
Levetiracetam	—	—	—

Reprinted with permission from Schmitz, B., 2002. Effects of antiepileptic drugs on behavior, in: Trimble, M., Schmitz, B., (Eds.), The Neuropsychiatry of Epilepsy. Cambridge University Press, Cambridge, UK.
?, Minimal data; —, not applicable; ADHD, attention-deficit/hyperactivity disorder.

unprovoked anger, rage, severe aggression, and violent behavior. Hippocampal sclerosis is less common in individuals with epilepsy and aggression (Tebartz van Elst et al., 2000). A subgroup of individuals with epilepsy and aggression have significant amygdala atrophy (Tebartz van Elst, 2002).

Stroke

Depression

Within the first year following a stroke, 30% to 40% of patients experience depression, with most developing depression within the first month (Ballard and O'Brien, 2002). Interestingly, rates appear to be similar for individuals in early, middle, and late stages following stroke. Depression after a stroke is associated with age, time since stroke, cognitive impairment, and social support. Significantly higher rates (5 to 6 times more likely) of poststroke depression have been reported among individuals with a premorbid diagnosis of depression (Ried et al., 2010).

Depression is associated with longer hospital stays, suggesting that it affects rehabilitation efforts. Depression is associated with poorer recovery of activities of daily living and increased morbidity. Depression and executive dysfunction commonly co-occur following a stroke. The presence of executive dysfunction with or without co-occurring depressive symptoms may be the strongest predictor of morbidity following stroke (Melkas et al., 2010) (see **Fig. 8.4**). Studies assessing the relationship between disability and depression in stroke patients have been equivocal. Depression is associated with poorer

quality of life in individuals who have had a stroke, even when neurological symptoms and disability are held constant.

The relationship between depression and lesion location has been the focus of significant research and controversy. Early research by Robinson and Price showed that left anterior lesions were associated with increased rates and severity of depression. Lesions nearer the left frontal pole or left caudate nucleus were associated with increased rates of depression. Some researchers have replicated these findings, but others have failed to do so. More recent review articles have not supported a relationship between lesion location and depression in poststroke patients (Bhogal et al., 2004). Of note, there is significant heterogeneity in previous studies, particularly between different sample sources.

If more homogeneous groups of patients are considered, some relationships emerge. Depression is associated with left-sided lesions in studies using hospital samples, whereas depression is associated with right-sided lesions in community samples (Bhogal et al., 2004). Time since stroke is an additional important variable to consider. Poststroke depression is associated with left-sided lesions in individuals in the first month following stroke (Bhogal et al., 2004). However, poststroke depression is associated with right-sided lesions in individuals more than 6 months after the stroke (Bhogal et al., 2004). Other differences in previous research, such as method of depression diagnosis, may contribute to the mixed results.

Few studies have assessed the effectiveness of various treatments for depression in these patients. A recent review suggests that there is no clear evidence that standard antidepressant medications are effective in the treatment of poststroke depression (Hackett et al., 2005). Although such interventions may not lead to effective cessation of depressive disorders, they may result in overall reductions in depressive severity. One study suggests that nortriptyline was more effective in the treatment of depression than either placebo or fluoxetine (Robinson et al., 2000). In this study, response to treatment with nortriptyline was associated with improvement in cognitive and functional abilities. This improvement in cognition and functional abilities following reduction in depressive symptoms has not always been replicated (Hackett et al., 2005).

Pathological Laughing and Crying

A portion of individuals experience PLC after a stroke. Between 11% and 35% of individuals experience emotional incontinence after stroke (Parvizi et al., 2009). Emotional incontinence is associated with lesions of the brainstem and cerebellar lesions (see Parvizi et al., 2009 for a review). Research assessing treatment for PLC has been largely limited to case studies. Preliminary evidence suggests that tricyclic and SSRI antidepressants may be helpful in alleviating symptoms of PLC (Parvizi et al., 2009).

Aggression

Reports have suggested that individuals have difficulty controlling aggression and anger following a stroke. Inability to control anger or aggression was associated with increased motor dysfunction and dysarthria. Aggression following stroke is associated with increased rates of MDD and generalized anxiety disorder. There is some evidence that lesions in the area supplied by the subcortical middle cerebral artery are associated with inability to control anger or aggression. Poststroke irritability and aggression are associated with lesions nearer to the frontal pole. Fluoxetine has been shown to successfully reduce levels of poststroke anger (Choi-Kwon et al., 2006). Similarly, reductions in irritability and aggression have been associated with reductions in depression following pharmacological intervention (Chan et al., 2006).

Traumatic Brain Injury

Traumatic brain injury is a significant public health concern, affecting approximately 1.4 million individuals, with 235,000 individuals hospitalized each year in the United States. Significant behavioral and psychiatric disturbances can be observed in individuals following TBI (**Table 8.16**). Kim and colleagues (2007) provide a comprehensive summary of recent literature regarding psychiatric symptoms following brain injury. Behavioral and psychiatric changes are common after TBI and can remain for decades following injury. Behavioral or mood disturbances are associated with decreased quality of life, increased caregiver burden, more challenges to the treating physician, and can significantly affect daily functioning including management of close relationships and employment. Psychiatric diagnoses following TBI are more common in individuals with a history of psychiatric illness, poor social functioning, alcoholism, arteriosclerosis, lower MMSE score, and fewer years of education. Many behavioral changes such as increased disinhibition are associated with dysfunction within the frontal cortex.

Table 8.16 Lifetime Prevalence of Major Psychiatric Disorders by Head Injury Status from the New Haven Epidemiologic Catchment Area Study (N = 5034)

	Head Injury (%)	No Head Injury (%)
Major depression (n = 242)	11.1	5.2
Dysthymia (n = 172)	5.5	2.9
Bipolar disorder (n = 45)	1.6	1.1
Panic disorder (n = 60)	3.2	1.3
Obsessive-compulsive disorder (n = 102)	4.7	2.3
Phobic disorder (n = 361)	11.2	7.4
Alcohol abuse/dependence (n = 412)	24.5	10.1
Drug abuse/dependence (n = 175)	10.9	5.2
Schizophrenia (n = 73)	3.4	1.9

Note: Adjusted for age, sex, marital status, socioeconomic status, alcohol abuse, and quality of life.

Reprinted with permission from Silver, J.M., Kramer, R., Greenwald, S., et al., 2001. The association between head injuries and psychiatric disorders: findings from the New Haven NIMH epidemiologic catchment area study. Brain Inj 15, 935-945.

Anosognosia

Although TBI is often associated with changes in motor, cognitive, and behavioral functioning, individuals with TBI frequently do not accurately assess these changes. Impairments in awareness have been associated with functional outcomes. Although it is most commonly reported that individuals with TBI underreport their difficulties, a subgroup of individuals appear to overreport their difficulties. It has been reported that individuals with mild to moderate TBI report greater impairments than their family members do of them, whereas those with more severe TBI report less impairments than their family member. Overreporting may be associated with depressive symptoms or litigation. Discussion of behavioral change following mild TBI is beyond the scope of the current discussion. Although symptoms of TBI frequently lead to difficulties in independent living and in the workplace, accurate assessment of these difficulties serves to mitigate this relationship. Thus, it is possible that improved levels of awareness may lead to reductions in disability.

Depression

Depression following TBI is common. Diagnosis of depression in TBI is complicated, because symptoms of depression (e.g., fatigue, concentration difficulties, sleep disturbances) are common following TBI. For further discussion regarding the diagnosis of depression in TBI, see Seel and colleagues (2010). MDD occurs in up to 60% of individuals who have suffered TBI (Kim et al., 2007). Rates of depression in TBI vary as a function of severity of TBI assessed, method of depression diagnosis, and sample source. The best predictor of depression after TBI is the presence of premorbid depression; however, some have failed to replicate this finding. Other factors associated with post-TBI depression include poor coping

Table 8.17 Core Features of Behavioral Symptoms in Traumatic Brain Injury

Core Features	Depression	Apathy	Anxiety	Dysregulation
Mood (Intensity, scope)	Sad, irritable, frustrated (Constant, global)	Flat, unexcited (Constant, global)	Worried, distressed (Frequent, situational)	Angry, Tense (Frequent, global)
Activity level	Low activity	Lack of initiative, behavior	Restless, "keyed up"	Impulsive, physically aggressive, argumentative
Attitude	Loss of interest, pleasure	Lack of concern	Overconcern	Argumentative
Awareness	Overestimates problems	Does not notice problems	Overestimates problems	Underestimates problems
Cognitions	Rumination on loss, failures	Unresponsive to events	Rumination on harm, danger	Rumination on tension, arousal
Physiological	Under- or hyperaroused	Underaroused	Hyperaroused	Underaroused or agitated
Coping style	Avoidance, social withdrawal	Compliant, dependent	Avoidance, checking behaviors	Uncontrolled outbursts

Modified from Seel, R.T., Macciocchi, S., Kreutzer, J.S., 2010. Clinical considerations for the diagnosis of major depression after moderate to severe TBI. J Head Trauma Rehabil 25, 99-112.

styles, social isolation, and increased stress (Kim et al., 2007). Depression in TBI is associated with increased suicidality, increased cognitive problems, greater disability, and aggression. See **Table 8.17** for additional information regarding differentiating features associated with depression in TBI.

Suicidal ideation (65%) and attempts (8.1%) are common following TBI (Silver et al., 2001). In contrast to sex differences reported in the general population, women with TBI are more likely to commit suicide than men with TBI. Furthermore, suicide was more common in individuals with more severe injury and those younger than 21 years or older than 60 years at the time of injury.

No large class I studies of use of antidepressant medications, particularly SSRIs, in TBI have been completed, but small studies provide preliminary support for their use to treat depressive symptoms following TBI. Care must be taken in certain situations, because some antidepressants (i.e., bupropion) are associated with increased risk of seizures. Close monitoring following the beginning of a trial of antidepressant medication is encouraged; in some settings, such medications can increase agitation or anxiety in individuals with TBI. Please see Alderfer and colleagues (2005) for more details regarding recommendations for treatment of depression following TBI.

Anxiety

Less research has assessed the prevalence of anxiety disorders in TBI; however, studies suggest that 11% to 70% of individuals meet criteria for anxiety. A meta-analysis suggested that the mean prevalence of anxiety disorders following TBI is 29%. Panic disorder occurs in 3.2% to 9.0% of individuals with a TBI (Silver et al., 2001).

Apathy

Symptoms of apathy are reported in 10% to 60% of individuals with a TBI. Among individuals with TBI referred to a

behavioral management program, lack of initiation was among the most common reported problems, occurring in approximately 60% of the sample (Kelly et al., 2008). Apathy in TBI is associated with depressive symptoms, although a significant number of individuals (28%) report experiencing apathy but not depression. Lesions affecting the right hemisphere and subcortical regions are more strongly associated with apathy than lesions affecting the left hemisphere.

Personality Change

Personality changes following TBI is common secondary to frequent injury to the frontal lobe and disruption of the frontosubcortical circuitry. Common changes include increased irritability, aggression, disinhibition, and inappropriate behavior. Although these difficulties can be among the most disabling for individuals with TBI, research in these areas is limited, and no uniform, agreed-upon diagnostic criteria for these behavioral changes exist.

Aggression within 6 months of TBI has been reported in up to 60% of individuals with TBI (Baguley et al., 2006). Among individuals referred to a TBI behavior management service, verbal aggression along with inappropriate social behavior were among the most commonly reported behavioral difficulties and occurred in more than 80% of individuals (Kelly et al., 2008). Aggression following TBI is associated with onset of depression following TBI, poorer psychosocial functioning, and greater disability (Rao et al., 2009).

A number of pharmacological interventions have been used to reduce and remediate behavioral changes following brain injury. See Nicholl and LaFrance (2009) for a review. One class of medication used in these settings is AEDs, now routinely used to treat aggression, disinhibition, and mania following TBI. Again, few large-scale studies have assessed the effectiveness of AEDs in the treatment of behavioral change following TBI. Historically, neuroleptic drugs were used in high doses to treat behavioral dyscontrol in individuals with cognitive impairment. More recently, there has been increased interest in the use of atypical neuroleptics to treat both psychosis and behavioral changes following TBI.

In addition to pharmacological interventions, behavioral and environmental interventions have been shown to be effective at remediating behavioral dyscontrol following TBI. The discussion of behavioral and environmental techniques aimed at decreasing behavioral dyscontrol, including aggression and irritability, is beyond the scope of this chapter (see Sohlberg and Mateer, 2001 for more information). Providers may find referrals for such interventions within rehabilitation programs. Briefly, interventions may seek to reduce stimulation in the environment, increase structure and predictability, reinforce good behavior with limited response to undesired behavior, and use of structured problem-solving strategies.

References

The complete reference list is available online at www.expertconsult.com.

Chapter 9

Depression and Psychosis in Neurological Practice

Evan D. Murray, Edgar A. Buttner, Bruce H. Price

The most widely recognized nomenclature used for discussion of mental disorders derives from the classification system developed for the *Diagnostic and Statistical Manual of Mental Disorders* (DSM). The American Psychiatric Association introduced the DSM in 1952 to facilitate psychiatric diagnosis through improved standardization of nomenclature. There have been consecutive revisions of this highly useful and relied-upon document since its inception, with the last revision being the DSM IV-TR in 2000 and a planned revision, the DSM V, scheduled for publication in 2013. Discussion about the potential secondary causes of depression and psychosis requires a familiarity with the most salient features of the primary psychiatric conditions. A brief outline of selected conditions derived from the DSM IV-TR is included in **Boxes 9.1** and **9.2**, which can be found at www.expertconsult.com, along with other content in this chapter marked "online only."

Principles of Differential Diagnosis

Emotional and cognitive processes are based on brain structure and physiology. Abnormal behavior can be attributable to the complex interplay of social influences, physical environment, and neural physiology. Psychosis, mania, depression, disinhibition, obsessive compulsive disorder (OCD), and anxiety all can occur as a result of neurological disease and can be indistinguishable from the idiopathic forms (Robinson and Travella, 1996). Neurological conditions must be considered in the differential diagnosis of any disorder with psychiatric symptoms.

Neuropsychiatric dysfunction can be correlated with altered functioning in anatomical regions. Any disease, toxin, drug, or process that affects a particular region can be expected to show changes in behavior mediated by the circuits within that region. The limbic system and the frontosubcortical circuits are most commonly involved in neuropsychiatric dysfunction. This neuroanatomical conceptual framework can provide useful information for localization and thus differential diagnosis. Klüver-Bucy syndrome, which consists of placidity, apathy, visual and auditory agnosia, hyperorality, and hypersexuality, occurs in processes that cause injury to the bilateral medial temporoamygdalar regions. A few of the most common causes of this syndrome include herpes encephalitis, traumatic brain injury (TBI), frontotemporal dementias (FTDs), and late-onset or severe Alzheimer disease (AD). Brain trauma, ischemic disease, demyelination, abscesses, or tumors, as well as degenerative dementias can also result in disinhibition. Damage to any portion of the circuit between the orbitofrontal cortex, ventral caudate nucleus, anterior globus pallidus, or mediodorsal thalamus can result in disinhibition (Tekin and Cummings, 2002).

Mood disorders, paranoia, disinhibition, and apathy derive from dysfunction in the limbic system and basal ganglia, which are phylogenetically more primitive (Mesulam, 2000). In some cases, the behavioral changes represent a response to

Table 9.1 Neuropsychiatric Symptoms and Corresponding Neuroanatomy

Symptom	Neuroanatomical Region
Depression	Frontal lobes, left anterior frontal cortex, anterior cingulate gyrus, subgenu of the corpus callosum, basal ganglia, left caudate
Mania	Inferomedial and ventromedial frontal cortex, right inferomedial frontal cortex, anterior cingulate, caudate nucleus, thalamus, and temporothalamic projections
Apathy	Anterior cingulate gyrus, nucleus accumbens, globus pallidus, thalamus
OCD	Orbital or medial frontal cortex, caudate nucleus, globus pallidus
Disinhibition	Orbitofrontal cortex, hypothalamus, septum
Paraphilia	Mediotemporal cortex, hypothalamus, septum, rostral brainstem
Hallucinations	Unimodal association cortex, orbitofrontal cortex, paralimbic cortex, limbic cortex, striatum, thalamus, midbrain
Delusions	Orbitofrontal cortex, amygdala, striatum, thalamus
Psychosis	Frontal lobes, left temporal cortex

OCD, Obsessive-compulsive disorder.

Table 9.2 Neurological Disorders and Associated Prominent Behavioral Features

Neurological Disorder	Associated Behavioral Disturbances
Alzheimer disease	Depression, irritability, anxiety, apathy, delusions, paranoia, psychosis
Lewy body dementia	Fluctuating confusion, hallucinations, delusions, depression, RBD
Vascular dementia	Depression, apathy, psychosis
Parkinson disease	Depression, anxiety drug-associated hallucinations and psychosis, RBD
FTD	Early impaired judgment, disinhibition, apathy, depression, delusions, psychosis
PSP	Disinhibition, apathy
TBI	Depression, disinhibition, apathy, irritability, psychosis uncommon
HD	Depression, irritability, delusions, mania, apathy, obsessive-compulsive disorder, psychosis
Corticobasal degeneration	Depression, irritability, RBD, alien hand syndrome
Epilepsy	Depression, psychosis
HIV infection	Apathy, depression, mania, psychosis
MS	Depression, irritability, anxiety, euphoria, psychosis
ALS	Depression, disinhibition, apathy, impaired judgment

ALS, Amyotrophic lateral selerosis; *FTD*, frontotemporal dementia; *HD*, Huntington disease; *HIV*, human immunodeficiency virus; *MS*, multiple sclerosis; *OCD*, obsessive-compulsive disorder; *PSP*, progressive supranuclear palsy; *RBD*, rapid eye movement behavior disorder; *TBI*, traumatic brain injury.

the underlying disability; in others, behavioral abnormalities are part of the disease. For example, studies have shown that apathy in Parkinson disease (PD) is probably related to the underlying disease process, rather than being a psychological reaction to disability or to depression, and is closely associated with cognitive impairment (Kirsch-Darrow et al., 2006). Positron emission tomographic (PET) and single-photon emission computed tomographic (SPECT) studies suggest similar regions of abnormality in acquired forms of depression, mania, OCD, and psychosis, compared with their primary psychiatric presentations (Hirono et al., 1998; Rubinsztein et al., 2001; Saxena et al., 1998). **Table 9.1** summarizes neuropsychiatric symptoms and their anatomical correlates. Additionally, the developmental phase during which a neurological illness occurs influences the frequency with which some neuropsychiatric syndromes are manifested. Adults with post-TBI sequelae tend to exhibit a higher rate of depression and anxiety. In contrast, post-TBI sequelae in children often involve attention deficits, hyperactivity, irritability, aggressiveness, and oppositional behavior (Geraldina et al., 2003). When temporal lobe epilepsy or Huntington disease (HD) begins in adolescence, a higher incidence of psychosis is noted than when their onset occurs later in life. Earlier onset of multiple sclerosis (MS) and stroke are associated with a higher incidence of depression (Rickards, 2005).

Patients with AD, PD, HD, and FTDs can develop multiple coexisting symptoms such as irritability, agitation, impulse-control disorders, apathy, depression, delusions, and psychosis that may be exacerbated by medications used to treat the underlying disorder (**Table 9.2**). For example, in patients with PD dopamine agonists such as pramipexole and ropinirole have been found to increase the risk of pathological gambling, compulsive shopping, hypersexuality, and other impulse-control disorders, sometimes referred to as *dopamine dysregulation* (Voon et al., 2006; Weintraub et al., 2006). Management outcome can be influenced by multiple factors. For instance, the complex relationship between behavioral changes and the caregiver's ability to cope play a role in illness management and nursing home placement (de Vugt et al., 2005; Smith et al., 2001). Behavioral disturbances in patients with neurological illness have been related to the severity of caregiver distress (Kaufer et al., 1998).

Principles of Neuropsychiatric Evaluation

A number of important principles must be taken into account when evaluating and treating a patient for behavioral disturbances.

1. A normal neurological examination does not exclude neurological conditions. Lesions in the limbic, para-limbic, and prefrontal regions may manifest with cognitive-behavioral changes in the absence of elemental neurological abnormalities.
2. Normal routine laboratory testing, brain imaging, electroencephalography, and cerebral spinal fluid analysis do not necessarily exclude diseases of neurological origin.
3. New neurological complaints or behavioral changes should not be dismissed as being of psychiatric origin in a person with a preexisting psychiatric history.
4. The possibility of iatrogenically induced conditions such as lethargy with benzodiazepines, parkinsonism with neuroleptics, or hallucinations with dopaminergic medications must be taken into account. Medication side effects can significantly complicate the clinical history and physical examination in both the acute and long-term setting. Medication side effects can also potentially be harbingers of underlying pathology or progression of illness. Marked parkinsonism occurring after neuroleptic exposure can be a feature of PD and dementia with Lewy bodies (Aarsland et al., 2005) before the underlying neurodegenerative condition becomes clinically apparent. PD patients may develop hallucinations as a side effect of dopaminergic medications (Papapetropoulos and Mash, 2005).
5. Treatment of primary psychiatric and neurological behavioral disturbances share common principles. A response to therapy does not constitute evidence for a primary psychiatric condition.

The medical evaluation of affective illness and psychotic disorders must be individualized based on the patient's family history, social environment, habits, risk factors, age, gender, clinical history, and examination findings. A careful review of the patient's medical history and a general physical examination as well as a neurological examination (Murray and Price, 2008; Ovsiew et al., 2008) should be performed to assess for possible neurological and medical causes. The most basic evaluation should include vital signs (blood pressure, pulse, respirations, and temperature) and a laboratory evaluation that minimally includes a complete blood cell count (CBC); electrolyte panel; determination of serum levels for glucose, blood urea nitrogen (BUN), creatinine, calcium, total protein, and albumin; liver function assessment; thyroid function assessment; and additional laboratory testing as clinically indicated. Consideration should be given to checking the patient's oxygen saturation on room air (especially in the elderly). Neurological abnormalities suggested by the clinical history or identified on examination, especially those attributable to the central nervous system (CNS), should prompt further evaluation for neurological and medical causes of psychiatric illness. A clear consensus has not been reached about when neuroimaging is indicated as part of the evaluation of new-onset depression in patients without focal neurological complaints and a normal neurological examination. This must be individualized based on clinical judgment. Treatment-resistant depression should prompt reassessment of the diagnosis and evaluation to rule out secondary causes of depressive illness. A careful history to rule out a primary sleep disorder such as sleep apnea should

be considered in the evaluation of refractory depressive symptoms (Haba-Rubio, 2005) or cognitive complaints. When new-onset psychosis presents in the absence of identifiable infectious/inflammatory, metabolic, toxic, or other causes, we recommend that magnetic resonance imaging (MRI) of the brain be incorporated into the evaluation. In our experience, 5% to 10% of such patients have MRI abnormalities that identify potential neurological contributions (particularly in those 65 years of age and older). The MRI will help exclude lesions (e.g., demyelination, ischemic disease, neoplasm, congenital structural abnormalities, evidence of metabolic storage diseases) in limbic, paralimbic, and frontal regions, which may not be associated with neurological abnormalities on elemental examination (Walterfang et al., 2005). An electroencephalogram (EEG) should be considered to evaluate for complex partial seizures if there is a history of intermittent, discrete, or abrupt episodes of psychiatric dysfunction (e.g., confusion, spells of lost time, psychotic symptoms), stereotypy of hallucinations, automatisms (e.g., lip smacking, repetitive movements) associated with episodes of psychiatric dysfunction (or confusion), or a suspicion of encephalopathy (or delirium). Sensitivity of the EEG for detecting seizure activity is highest when the patient has experienced the specific symptoms while undergoing the study. Selected cases may require 24-hour or longer EEG monitoring to capture a clinical event to clarify whether a seizure disorder is present.

Cognitive-Behavioral Neuroanatomy

We begin with a brief overview of cortical functional anatomy and perceptual, cognitive, and behavioral processing, after which will follow a synopsis of frontal lobe functional anatomy describing the distinct frontosubcortical circuits subserving important cognitive-behavioral domains.

The cerebral cortex can be subdivided into five major functional subtypes: primary sensory-motor, unimodal association, heteromodal association, paralimbic, and limbic. The primary sensory areas are the point of entry for sensory information into the cortical circuitry. The primary motor cortex conveys complex motor programs to motor neurons in the brainstem and spinal cord. Processing of sensory information occurs as information moves from primary sensory areas to adjacent unimodal association areas. The unimodal and heteromodal cortices are involved in perceptual processing and motor planning. The complexity of processing increases as information is then transmitted to heteromodal association areas which receive input from more than one sensory modality. Examples of heteromodal association cortex include prefrontal cortex, posterior parietal cortex, parts of the lateral temporal cortex, and portions of the parahippocampal gyrus. These cortical regions have a six-layered architecture. Further cortical processing occurs in areas designated as *paralimbic*. These regions demonstrate a gradual transition of cortical architecture from the six-layered to the more primitive and simplified allocortex of limbic structures. The paralimbic regions consist of orbito-frontal cortex, insula, temporal pole, parahippocampal cortex, and cingulate cortex. Cognitive, emotional, and visceral inputs merge in these regions. The limbic subdivision is composed

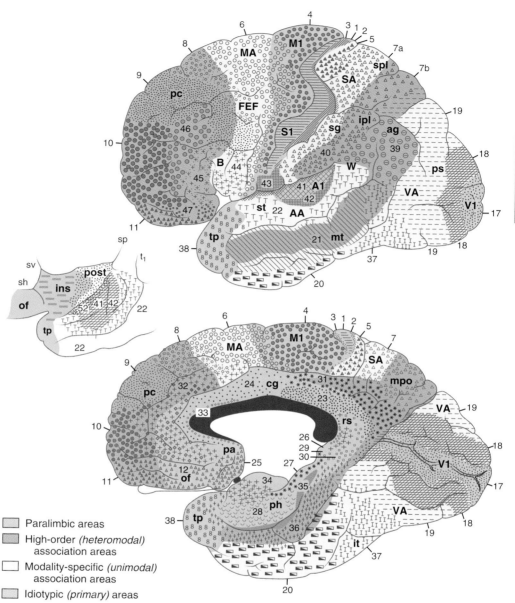

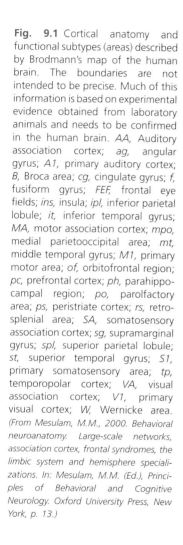

Fig. 9.1 Cortical anatomy and functional subtypes (areas) described by Brodmann's map of the human brain. The boundaries are not intended to be precise. Much of this information is based on experimental evidence obtained from laboratory animals and needs to be confirmed in the human brain. *AA*, Auditory association cortex; *ag*, angular gyrus; *A1*, primary auditory cortex; *B*, Broca area; *cg*, cingulate gyrus; *f*, fusiform gyrus; *FEF*, frontal eye fields; *ins*, insula; *ipl*, inferior parietal lobule; *it*, inferior temporal gyrus; *MA*, motor association cortex; *mpo*, medial parietooccipital area; *mt*, middle temporal gyrus; *M1*, primary motor area; *of*, orbitofrontal region; *pc*, prefrontal cortex; *ph*, parahippocampal region; *po*, parolfactory area; *ps*, peristriate cortex; *rs*, retrosplenial area; *SA*, somatosensory association cortex; *sg*, supramarginal gyrus; *spl*, superior parietal lobule; *st*, superior temporal gyrus; *S1*, primary somatosensory area; *tp*, temporopolar cortex; *VA*, visual association cortex; *V1*, primary visual cortex; *W*, Wernicke area. (From Mesulam, M.M., 2000. Behavioral neuroanatomy. Large-scale networks, association cortex, frontal syndromes, the limbic system and hemisphere specializations. In: Mesulam, M.M. (Ed.), Principles of Behavioral and Cognitive Neurology. Oxford University Press, New York, p. 13.)

■ Paralimbic areas

■ High-order (*heteromodal*) association areas

□ Modality-specific (*unimodal*) association areas

■ Idiotypic (*primary*) areas

of the hippocampus, amygdala, substantia innominata, prepiriform olfactory cortex, and septal area (**Figs. 9.1** and **9.2**). These structures are to a great extent reciprocally interconnected with the hypothalamus. The limbic region is intimately involved with regulation of emotion, memory, motivation, autonomic, and endocrine function. The highest level of cognitive processing occurs in regions referred to as *transmodal areas*. These areas are composed of heteromodal, paralimbic, and limbic regions, which are collectively linked, in parallel, to other transmodal regions. Interconnections among transmodal areas (e.g., Wernicke area, posterior parietal cortex, hippocampal-enterorhinal complex) allow integration of distributed perceptual processing systems, resulting in perceptual recognition such as scenes and events becoming experiences and words taking on meaning (Mesulam, 2000).

Cortical Networks

Five distinct cortical network regions govern various aspects of cognitive functioning: (1) the language network, which includes transmodal regions or "epicenters" in Broca and Wernicke areas; (2) spatial awareness, based in transmodal regions in the frontal eye fields and posterior parietal area; (3) the memory and emotional network, located in the hippocampal-enterorhinal region and amygdala; (4) the executive function–working memory network, based in transmodal regions in the lateral prefrontal cortex and possibly the inferior parietal cortices; and (5) the face-object recognition network, based in the temporopolar and midtemporal cortices (Mesulam, 1998).

Lesions of transmodal cortical areas result in global impairments such as hemineglect, anosognosia, amnesia, and multimodal anomia. Disconnection of transmodal regions from a

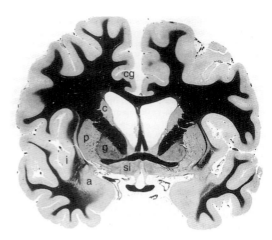

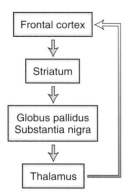

Fig. 9.3 General structure of frontal subcortical circuits.

Fig. 9.2 Coronal section through the basal forebrain of a 25-year-old human brain stained for myelin. The substantia innominata (si) and the amygdaloid complex (a) are located on the undersurface of the brain. c, Head of caudate nucleus; cg, cingulate gyrus; g, globus pallidus; I, insula. *(From Mesulam, M.M., 2000. Behavioral neuroanatomy. Large-scale networks, association cortex, frontal syndromes, the limbic system and hemisphere specializations. In: Mesulam, M.M. (Ed.), Principles of Behavioral and Cognitive Neurology. Oxford University Press, New York, p. 4.)*

specific unimodal input will result in selective perceptual impairments such as category-specific anomias, prosopagnosia, pure word deafness, or pure word blindness.

The ability to empathize with another person's psychological and physical circumstances is a foundation for social and moral behavior. The human mirror neuron system is now postulated to be involved in understanding the actions of others and the intentions behind the actions. It also may provide the basis for observational learning. The parietofrontal mirror system, which includes the parietal lobe and the premotor cortex plus the caudal part of the inferior frontal gyrus, is involved in recognition of voluntary behavior in other people, while the limbic mirror system, formed by the insula and the anterior mesial frontal cortex, is devoted to the recognition of affective behavior. Dysfunction of this system is postulated to underlie deficits in theory of mind and has been proposed as an explanation for the social deficits seen in autistic disorders (Cattaneo and Rizzolatti, 2009).

Frontosubcortical Networks

Five frontosubcortical circuits subserve cognition, behavior, and movement. Disruption of these networks at the cortical or subcortical level can be associated with similar neuropsychiatric symptoms. Each of these circuits shares the same components: (1) frontal cortex, (2) striatum (caudate, putamen, ventral striatum), (3) globus pallidus and substantia nigra, and (4) thalamus (which then projects back to frontal cortex) (Tekin and Cummings, 2002) (**Fig. 9.3**). Integrative connections also occur to and from other subcortical and distant cortical regions related to each circuit. Neurotransmitters such as dopamine (DA), glutamate, γ-aminobutyric acid (GABA), acetylcholine, norepinephrine, and serotonin are involved in various aspects of neural transmission and modulation in these circuits. The frontosubcortical networks are named according to their site of origin or function. Somatic motor function is subserved by the motor circuit originating in the supplementary motor area. Oculomotor function is governed by the oculomotor circuit originating in the frontal eye fields. Three of the five circuits are intimately involved in cognitive and behavioral changes: the dorsolateral prefrontal, the orbitofrontal, and the anterior cingulate circuits. Each circuit has both efferent and afferent connections with adjacent and distant cortical regions. The dorsolateral prefrontal circuit governs executive functions, including the ability to plan and maintain attention, problem solve, learn, retrieve remote memories, sequence the temporal order of events, shift cognitive and behavioral sets, and generate motor programs. Executive dysfunction is a principal component of subcortical dementias. Deficits identified in subcortical dementias include slowed information processing, memory retrieval deficits, mood and behavioral changes, gait disturbance, dysarthria, and other motor impairments. Vascular dementias, PD, and HD are a few examples of conditions that affect this circuit.

The orbitofrontal circuit connects frontal monitoring functions to the limbic system. This circuit governs appropriate responses to social cues, empathy, social judgment, and interpersonal sensitivity. It pairs thoughts, memories, and experiences with corresponding visceral and emotional states. This circuit is heavily involved in the process of decision making and evaluating the costs and benefits of specific behavioral responses to the environment. The medial orbitofrontal cortex (OFC) evaluates reward, whereas the lateral OFC monitors and decodes punishment as it pertains to motivating behavioral change. There is also an anterior-posterior gradient in which the reward value for more abstract and complex secondary reinforcing factors such as money are encoded in the anterior regions, and more concrete factors such as touch and taste are encoded in the posterior OFC areas. The posterior OFC is thought to have an important role in evaluating the emotional significance of stimuli (Barbas and Zikopoulos, 2007). Dysfunction in this circuit can lead to disinhibition, irritability, aggressive outbursts, inappropriate social responses, and impulsive decision making. Patients with OFC lesions show deficits in both the production and recognition of emotional expression from the face, voice, or gestures. Persons with bilateral OFC lesions may manifest "theory of mind" deficits. *Theory of mind* is a model of how a person understands and infers other people's intentions, desires, mental states, and emotions (Bodden et al., 2010). Conditions that exhibit impairment in this circuit include schizophrenia

(Bora et al., 2009), FTD (Adenzato et al., 2010), and HD. Other conditions that may affect this circuit include closed head trauma, rupture of anterior communicating aneurysms, and subfrontal meningiomas.

The anterior cingulate circuit includes the nucleus accumbens and has both afferent and efferent connections to the dorsolateral prefrontal cortex (DLPFC) and amygdala. It is involved in motivated behavior. Lesions in this circuit result in apathy, abulia, and akinetic mutism. There also is a reported decrease in the ability to understand new thoughts and participate in the creative thought process (Chow and Cummings, 1999; Mesulam, 2000). The medial prefrontal cortex is thought to play a significant role in generating emotions related to empathy, cognitive functions related to theory of mind, and the ability to recognize a moral dilemma (Robertson et al., 2007). The ventromedial frontal lobe evaluates the current relative value of stimuli helping to guide decision making by determining the goals toward which behavior is directed and through judging outcomes (Fellows, 2007). Some conditions that may affect this circuit include AD, FTD, PD, HD, head trauma, brain tumors, cerebral infarcts, and obstructive hydrocephalus.

Cerebrocerebellar Networks

The cerebellum is engaged in the regulation of cognition and emotion through a feed-forward and feedback loop. The cortex projects to pontine nuclei, which in turn project to the cerebellum. The cerebellum projects to the thalamus, which then projects back to the cortex. Cognitive processing tasks such as language, working memory, and spatial and executive tasks appear to activate the posterior cerebellar lobe. The posterior cerebellar vermis may function as a putative limbic cerebellum, modulating emotional processing (Stoodley and Schmahmann, 2010). Distractibility, executive and working memory problems, impaired judgment, reduced verbal fluency, disinhibition, irritability, anxiety, emotional lability or blunting, obsessive compulsive behaviors, depression, and psychosis have been reported in association with cerebellar pathology.

Biology of Psychosis

Among several etiological hypotheses for schizophrenia, the neurodevelopmental model is one of the most prominent. This model generally posits that schizophrenia results from processes that begin long before the onset of clinical symptoms and is caused by a combination of environmental and genetic factors (Murray and Lewis, 1987; Weinberger, 1987). Several postmortem and neuroimaging studies support this hypothesis with findings of brain developmental alterations such as agenesis of the corpus callosum, arachnoid cysts, and other abnormalities in a significant number of schizophrenic patients (Hallak et al., 2007; Kuloglu et al., 2008). Environmental factors are associated with an increased risk for schizophrenia. These factors include being a first-generation immigrant or the child of a first-generation immigrant, urban living, drug use, head injury, prenatal infection, maternal malnutrition, obstetrical complications during delivery, and winter birth (Tandon et al., 2008). Genetic risks are clearly present but not well understood. The majority of patients with schizophrenia lack a family history of the disorder. The

population lifetime risk for schizophrenia is 1%, 10% for first-degree relatives, and 4% for second-degree relatives. There is an approximately 50% concordance rate for monozygotic twins, compared to approximately 15% for dizygotic twins. Advancing paternal age increases risk in a linear fashion, which is consistent with the hypothesis that de novo mutations contribute to the genetic risk for schizophrenia. It is most likely that many different genes make small but important contributions to susceptibility. The disease only manifests when these genes are combined or certain environmental factors are present. A number of susceptibility genes show association with schizophrenia: catechol-O-methyl-transferase, neuroregulin 1, dysbindin, disrupted in schizophrenia 1 (DISC1), metabotropic glutamate receptor type 3 gene and G27/G30 gene complex (Nöthen et al., 2010; Tandon et al., 2008). Research in twins and first-degree relatives of patients has shown that genes predisposing to schizophrenia and related disorders affect heritable traits related to the illness. Such traits include neurocognitive functioning, structural MRI brain volume measures, neurophysiological informational processing traits, and sensitivity to stress (van Os and Kapur, 2009). A small proportion of schizophrenia incidence may be explained by genomic structural variations known as *copy number variants* (CNVs). CNVs consist of inherited or de novo small duplications, deletions, or inversions in genes or regulatory regions. CNV deletions generally show higher penetrance (more severe phenotype) than duplications, and larger CNVs often have higher penetrance and/or more clinical features than smaller CNVs. These genomic structural variations contribute to normal variability, disease risk, and developmental anomalies, as well as act as a major mutational mechanism in evolution. The most common CNV disorder, 22q11.2 deletion syndrome (velocardiofacial syndrome), has an established association with schizophrenia. Individuals with 22q11.2 deletions have a 20-fold increased risk for schizophrenia and constitute about 0.9% to 1% of schizophrenia patients. When this syndrome is present, genetic counseling is helpful (Bassett and Chow, 2008).

A wide variety of neurological conditions, medications, and toxins are associated with psychosis. No consensus is available in the literature regarding the precise anatomical localization of various psychotic syndromes. Evidence from neurochemistry, cellular neuropathology, and neuroimaging studies support that schizophrenia is a brain disease, but there is no universally accepted theory regarding the specific nature of the brain dysfunction. The two best-known neurotransmitter models offered to explain the various manifestations of schizophrenia include the "dopamine hypothesis," now in its third revision (Howes and Kapur, 2009), and the "glutamate hypothesis." Schizophrenia has been associated with frontal lobe dysfunction and abnormal regulation of subcortical DA (Goldman-Rakic et al., 2004) and glutamate systems (Weinberger, 2005).

Functional imaging studies in persons with schizophrenia show decreased cerebral blood flow (CBF) in the DLPFC during specific cognitive tasks (Andreasen, 1996; Lehrer et al., 2005). Schizophrenic patients with prominent negative symptoms display reduced glucose utilization in the frontal lobes. Functional imaging studies suggest that disruption in distributed functional circuits is important in the development of schizophrenia. These functional circuit locations include the DLPFC, orbitofrontal cortex, mediofrontal cortex, anterior cingulate gyrus, thalamus, temporal lobe subregions, and the cerebellum (Schultz and Andreasen, 1999). Several conditions that may manifest psychosis (e.g., HD, PD, frontotemporal degenerations, stroke) are commonly associated with frontal and subcortical dysfunction. Dorsolateral and mediofrontal hypoperfusion on functional imaging has been demonstrated in a subset of AD patients with delusions (Hirono et al., 1998).

Biology of Depression

The connection between psychiatry and neurology is nowhere more evident than the remarkable comorbidity of psychiatric illness, especially depression, in many neurological disorders, with a 20% to 60% prevalence rate of depression in patients with stroke, neurodegenerative diseases, MS, headache, human immunodeficiency virus (HIV), TBI, epilepsy, chronic pain, obstructive sleep apnea, intracranial neoplasms, and motor neuron disease. Depression amplifies the physiological response to pain, while pain-related symptoms and limitations frequently lead to the emergence of depressive symptoms. In a community-based study, almost 50% of adolescents with chronic daily headaches had at least one psychiatric disorder, most commonly major depression and panic. Women with migraine who have major depression are twice as likely as those with migraine alone to report being sexually abused as a child. If the abuse continued past age 12, women with migraine were five times more likely to report depression (Tietjen et al., 2007). Despite the proliferation of antidepressant therapeutics, major depression is often a chronic and/or recurrent condition that remains difficult to treat. Up to 70% of patients taking antidepressants in a primary care setting may be poorly compliant, most often due to adverse side effects during both short and long-term therapy.

Efforts to link single genes to major depressive disorder (MDD) have been unsuccessful despite exhaustive mapping attempts. Consequently, behavioral geneticists have turned to the study of genetic polymorphisms in establishing a predisposition to depression and in shaping the response to environmental stressors. Perlis and coworkers (2007) found a strong association between variation at the CREB1 locus and anger expression in MDD. The most extensive studies in this field have focused on polymorphisms in the serotonin transporter (5-HTT) gene. Recent work has demonstrated that patients with a single nucleotide polymorphism on the long allele that entails an A-to-G transposition (LG) have low expression of 5-HT. The risk for major depression among hurricane survivors with either short or LG alleles was four to five times that of low-risk survivors. Although conflicting results have been reported with regard to these polymorphisms, a recent meta-analysis found that the 44bp Ins/Del short/long polymorphism was associated with MDD, whereas the VNTR intron 2 polymorphism was not. This study also reported significant associations for polymorphisms in the apolipoprotein E, guanine nucleotide binding protein, methylenetetrahydrofolate reductase, and dopamine transporter genes (López-León et al., 2008).

Behavioral genetics research based on diathesis-stress models of depression demonstrate that the risk of depression after a stressful event is enhanced in populations carrying genetic risk factors and is diminished in populations lacking such risk factors. A gene's contribution to depression may be missed in studies that do not account for environmental interactions and may only be revealed when studied within the context of environmental stressors specifically mediated by that gene (Uher, 2008). Genotype-environment interactions are ubiquitous because genes not only impact the risk for depression by creating susceptibility to specific environmental stressors but also cause individuals to persistently place themselves in highly stressful environments.

The potential clinical relevance of neurogenesis in the adult mammalian brain represents the most recent major breakthrough in depression studies at the cellular neurobiological level. Imaging studies have demonstrated a 10% to 20% decrease in the hippocampal volume of human patients with chronic depression. Cell proliferation studies using 5-bromo-2′-deoxyuridine injection to label dividing cells show that antidepressants also lead to increased cell number in the mammalian hippocampus. This effect is seen with chronic but not acute treatment; the time course of the effect mirrors the known time course of the therapeutic action of antidepressants in humans (Czéh et al., 2001). Although a role for neurogenesis in the pathophysiology of depression appears to be a promising avenue of research, the relevance of animal studies described here remains controversial in the human (Reif et al., 2006).

Analysis at the systems level suggests that anterotemporal paralimbic and orbitofrontal regions are involved in mediating primary and acquired depression. Functional imaging studies of unmedicated patients with familial depression reveal increased CBF and glucose metabolism in the amygdala, orbital cortex, and medial thalamus and decreased CBF and glucose metabolism in the dorsomedial/dorsal anterolateral prefrontal cortex and anterior cingulate cortex (Charney and Manji, 2004). Damage to the prefrontal cortex from stroke or tumor, or to the striatum from degenerative diseases such as PD and HD, is associated with depression (Charney and Manji, 2004; Drevets, 2001). Functional imaging studies of subcortical disorders such as these reveal hypometabolism in paralimbic regions, including the anterotemporal cortex and anterior cingulate, which are correlated with depression seen in these patients (Ketter et al., 1996; Mayberg, 2003). Depression in PD, HD, and epilepsy has been correlated with reduced metabolic activity in the orbitofrontal cortex and caudatenucleus.

Mayberg (2003) proposed that primary depression is due to dysfunction in a network that includes two known pathways: the orbitofrontal–basal ganglia–thalamic circuit and the basotemporal limbic circuit that links the orbitofrontal cortex and the anterior temporal cortex by the uncinate fasciculus. Portions of this model are illustrated in **Fig. 9.4**. This has been expanded into a unifying depression circuit model that consists of four interconnected functional compartments. Each functional compartment consists of strongly interconnected anatomical structures upon which that compartment is dependent. Functional compartments are as follows: mood regulation (medial frontal, medial orbital-frontal and pregenu anterior cingulate cortex), mood monitoring (ventral striatum-caudate, amygdale, dorsomedial thalamus, midbrain-ventral tegmental area), interoception (subcallosal cingulated, ventral-anterior hippocampus, anterior insula, brain stem, hypothalamus) and exteroception (prefrontal, premotor, parietal, mid-cingulate and posterior cingulate cortices with dorsal-posterior hippocampus) (Mayberg, 2009).

Functional imaging studies of untreated depression have been extended to evaluate responses to pharmacological, cognitive-behavioral, and surgical treatments of depression.

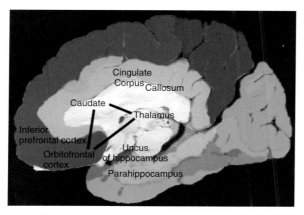

Fig. 9.4 Midline sagittal human brain. Frontal lobe, red; parietal lobe, dark blue; occipital lobe, green; temporal lobe, light blue; limbic cortex, orange. Thick black lines approximate a cortical-basal ganglia-thalamic-cortical loop (circuit) to the orbital frontal cortex.

Clinical improvement after treatment with serotonin-specific reuptake inhibitors such as fluoxetine correlates with increased activity on PET in brainstem and dorsal cortical regions including the prefrontal, parietal, anterior, and posterior cingulate areas, and with decreased activity in limbic and striatal regions including the subgenual cingulate, hippocampus, insula, and pallidum (Mathew et al., 2003). These findings are consistent with the prevailing model for involvement of a limbic-cortical-striatal-pallidal-thalamic circuit in major depression. The same group has shown that imaging can be used to identify patterns of metabolic activity predictive of treatment response. Hypometabolism of the rostral anterior cingulate characterized patients who failed to respond to antidepressants, whereas hypermetabolism characterized responders. Dougherty and coworkers (2003) used PET to search for neuroimaging profiles that might predict clinical response to anterior cingulotomy in patients with treatment-refractory depression. Responders displayed elevated preoperative metabolism in the left prefrontal cortex and the left thalamus. A combination of functional imaging and pharmacogenomic technologies might allow subsets of treatment responders to be classified and predicted more precisely than with either technology alone. Goldapple and coinvestigators (2004) used PET to study the clinical response of cognitive-behavioral therapy in patients with unipolar depression and found increases in hippocampus and dorsal cingulate and decreases in dorsal, ventral, and medial frontal cortex. The authors speculate that the same limbic-cortical-striatal-pallidal-thalamic circuit is involved but that differences in the direction of metabolic changes may reflect different underlying mechanisms of action of cognitive-behavioral therapy (CBT) and selective serotonin reuptake inhibitors (SSRIs).

Clinical Symptoms and Signs Suggesting Neurological Disease

Many neurological conditions have associated psychiatric symptoms. Psychiatrists and neurologists need to be intimately acquainted with features of the clinical history and examination that indicate the need for further investigation. **Box 9.3** outlines some key features that have historically suggested an underlying neurological condition. **Box 9.4** (online only at

www.expertconsult.com) reviews some key areas of the review of systems that can be helpful when assessing for neurological and medical causes of psychiatric symptoms. **Table 9.3** (online only at www.expertconsult.com) reviews abnormalities in the elemental neurological examination associated with diseases that can exhibit significant neuropsychiatric features.

Psychiatric Manifestations of Neurological Disease

Virtually any process that affects the neuroanatomical circuits described earlier can result in behavioral changes and psychiatric symptoms at some point. Psychiatric symptoms may be striking and precede any neurological manifestation by years. **Table 9.4** (online only at www.expertconsult.com) lists conditions that can be associated with psychosis or depression. **Box 9.5** summarizes some key points from the preceding discussion. A general overview and discussion of a number of

---

Box 9.5 Key Points

1. Affective and psychotic disorders may occur as a result of neurological disease and be indistinguishable from the idiopathic forms.
2. Neuropsychiatric and cognitive dysfunction can be correlated with altered functioning in anatomical regions.
3. Cortical processing of sensory information proceeds from its point of entry through association areas with progressively more complex interconnections with other regions having sensory, memory, cognitive, emotional, and autonomic information, resulting ultimately in perceptual recognition and emotional meaning for experiences.
4. Frontosubcortical circuits are heavily involved in cognitive and behavioral functioning. Disruption of frontal circuits at the cortical or subcortical level by various processes can be associated with similar neuropsychiatric symptoms.
5. Features of the patient's clinical history and examination can be suggestive of a medical or neurological cause of psychiatric symptoms.
6. Many medical and neurological conditions are associated with neuropsychiatric symptoms. Each condition may carry unique implications for prognosis, treatment, and long-term management.

---

major categories of neurological and systemic conditions with prominent neuropsychiatric features follows. More detailed information regarding the evaluation, natural history, pathology, and specific treatment recommendations for these conditions is beyond the scope of this chapter.

Stroke and Cerebral Vascular Disease

Stroke is the leading cause of neurological disability in the United States and one of the most common causes of acquired behavioral changes in adults. The neuropsychiatric consequences of stroke depend on the location and size of the stroke, preexisting brain pathology, baseline intellectual capacity and functioning, age, and premorbid psychiatric history. Neuropsychiatric symptoms may occur in the setting of first strokes and multiinfarct dementia. In general, interruption of bilateral frontotemporal lobe function is associated with an increased risk of depressive and psychotic symptoms. Specific stroke-related syndromes such as aphasia and visuospatial dysfunction are beyond the scope of this chapter, so only the abnormalities in mood and emotion after stroke will be discussed. A common misconception is that depressive symptoms can be explained as a response to the associated neurological deficits and impairment in function. Evidence supports a higher incidence of depression in stroke survivors than occurs in persons with other equally debilitating diseases. Minor depression is more closely related to the patient's elemental deficits. Emotional and cognitive disorders may occur independently of or in association with sensorimotor dysfunction in stroke. Poststroke depression (PSD) is the most common neuropsychiatric syndrome, occurring in 30% to 50% of survivors at 1 year, with irritability, agitation, and apathy often present as well. About half of patients with depressive symptoms will meet criteria for a major depressive episode. Onset of depression within the first few weeks after a stroke is most commonly associated with lesions affecting the frontal lobes, especially the prefrontal cortex and head of the caudate. The frequency and severity of depression increase with closer proximity to the frontal poles. Left prefrontal lesions are more apt to be associated with acute depression and may be complicated by aphasia, resulting in the patient's inability to express the symptoms. Mania is much less common but occurs usually in relation to lesions of the right hemisphere. Single manic events as well as recurrent manic and depressive episodes have been reported. Nondominant hemispheric strokes may also result in aprosody without associated depression. Currently, the standard treatment of PSD remains supportive psychotherapy and pharmacotherapy.

Psychosis or psychotic features may present as a rare complication of a single stroke, but the prevalence of these features is not well established. Manifestations may include paranoia, delusions, ideas of reference, hallucinations, or psychosis. Paranoia and psychosis have been reported in association with left temporal strokes that result in Wernicke aphasia. Other regions producing similar neuropsychiatric symptoms include the right temporoparietal region and the caudate nuclei. Right hemispheric lesions may also be more associated with visual hallucinations and delusions. Reduplicative paramnesia and misidentifications syndromes such as Capgras syndrome and Fregoli syndrome have also been reported. Reduplicative paramnesia is a syndrome in which patients claim that they are simultaneously in two or more locations. It has been observed to occur in patients with combined lesions of frontal and right temporal lobe but has also been described as due to temporal-limbic-frontal dysfunction (Moser et al., 1998). Capgras syndrome is the false belief that someone familiar, usually a family member or close friend, has been replaced by an identical-appearing imposter. It has been proposed that this results from right temporal-limbic-frontal disconnection resulting in a disturbance in recognizing familiar people and places (Feinberg et al., 1999). In Fregoli syndrome, the patient believes a persecutor is able to take on a variety of faces, like an actor. Psychotic episodes can also be a manifestation of complex partial seizures secondary to stroke. Patients with poststroke psychosis are more prone to have comorbid epilepsy than poststroke patients without associated psychosis. Lesions or infarcts of the ventral midbrain can result in a syndrome characterized by well-formed and complex visual hallucinations referred to as *peduncular hallucinosis*. Obsessive-compulsive features have also been reported with strokes. These symptoms have been postulated to be due to dysfunction in the orbitofrontal-subcortical circuitry (Saxena et al., 1998).

Consensus criteria for accurately diagnosing vascular cognitive impairments and dementia are lacking (Bowler and Gorelick, 2009; Wiederkehr et al., 2008). The vascular cognitive impairments can be conceptualized as being made up of three groups: vascular dementia, mixed vascular dementia and AD pathology, and vascular cognitive impairment not meeting criteria for dementia. These conditions may have variable contributions from mixed forms of small-vessel disease, large-vessel disease, and cardioembolic disease, which accounts for the clinical phenotypic heterogeneity. AD pathology is commonly found in association with cerebrovascular disease pathology, leading to uncertainty with respect to the relative contributions of each in some cases. A temporal relationship between a stroke and the onset of dementia or a stepwise progression of cognitive decline with evidence of cerebrovascular disease on examination and neuroimaging are considered most helpful. No specific neuroimaging profile exists that is diagnostic for pure cerebrovascular disease-related dementia. Vascular dementia may present with prominent cortical, subcortical, or mixed features. Cortical vascular dementia may manifest as unilateral sensorimotor dysfunction, abrupt onset of cognitive dysfunction and aphasia, and difficulties with planning, goal formation, organization, and abstraction. Subcortical vascular dementia often affects frontosubcortical circuitry, resulting in executive dysfunction, cognitive slowing, difficulties with abstraction, apathy, memory problems (recognition and cue recognition relatively intact), working memory impairment, and decreased ability to perform activities of daily living. Memory difficulties tend to be less severe than in AD. Limited data suggest that cholinesterase inhibitors are beneficial for treatment of vascular dementia, as demonstrated by improvements in cognition, global functioning, and performance of activities of daily living.

Infectious

An expansive list of infections could be generated that result in behavioral changes during early, middle, or late phases of illness or as a result of treatments or subsequent opportunistic infections. This portion will only focus on a few salient examples with contemporary relevance and illustrative complexity.

Human Immunodeficiency Virus

Individuals infected with HIV can be affected by a variety of neuropsychiatric and neurological problems independent of opportunistic infections and neoplasms. These include cognitive impairment, behavioral changes, and sensorimotor disturbances. Psychiatrists and neurologists must anticipate a spectrum of psychiatric phenomena that can include depression, paranoia, delusions, hallucinations, psychosis, mania, irritability, and apathy. *HIV-associated dementia* (HAD) is the term given to the syndrome that presents with bradyphrenia, memory decline, executive dysfunction, impaired concentration, and apathy. These features are compatible with a subcortical dementia with prominent dysfunction in the frontal-basal ganglia circuitry (Woods et al., 2004). *Minor cognitive motor disorder* (MCMD) refers to a milder form of this syndrome that has become more common since the advent of highly active antiretroviral therapy (HAART). HAD may be the acquired immunodeficiency virus syndrome (AIDS)-defining illness in up to 10% of patients. It has been estimated to occur in 20% to 30% of untreated adults. HAART has reduced its frequency by approximately 50%, but the frequency of pathologically proven HIV encephalitis remains high.

Lifetime prevalence of depression in HIV-positive individuals is 22% to 45%, with depressed individuals demonstrating reduced compliance with antiretroviral therapy and increased HIV-related morbidity. Antidepressants have been efficacious in treating HAD (Himelhoch and Medoff, 2005). Psychostimulants may also be a helpful adjunct in treating HAD. Evidence suggests that HIV-infected patients with new-onset psychosis usually respond well to typical neuroleptic medications, but they are more sensitive to the side effects of these medications, particularly extrapyramidal symptoms and tardive dyskinesias. This sensitivity is thought to be due to HIV's effect on the basal ganglia, resulting in a loss of dopaminergic neurons. When prescribing typical neuroleptics, caution is warranted owing to this sensitivity and the additional possible pharmacological interactions with antiretroviral medications. Atypical neuroleptics are favored.

HAART and other medications used in HIV patients can have neuropsychiatric side effects. For example, the nucleoside reverse transcriptase inhibitor, zidovudine (AZT), may lead to mania, delirium, or depression. Moreover, many medications used in the treatment of HIV inhibit or induce the cytochrome P450 system, thereby altering psychotropic drug levels. Therefore, drug interactions in HIV patients with psychiatric disorders are common and require close monitoring.

Creutzfeldt-Jakob Disease

Prion diseases are a group of fatal degenerative disorders of the nervous system caused by a conformational change in the prion protein, a normal constituent of cell membranes. They are characterized by long incubation periods followed by relatively rapid neurological decline and death (Johnson, 2005). Creutzfeldt-Jakob disease (CJD) is the most common human prion disease but is rare, with an incidence of between 0.5 and 1.5 cases per million people per year. The sporadic form of the disease accounts for about 85% of cases, typically occurs later in life (mean age, 60 years), and manifests with a rapidly progressive course characterized by cerebellar ataxia, dementia, myoclonus, seizures, and psychiatric symptoms progressing to akinetic mutism and complete disability within months after disease onset. Psychiatric symptoms such as personality changes, anxiety, depression, paranoia, obsessive-compulsive features, and psychosis occur in about 80% of patients during the first 100 days of illness (Wall et al., 2005). About 60% present with symptoms compatible with a rapidly progressive dementia. The mean duration of the illness is 6 to 7 months.

The autosomal dominant familial form of CJD accounts for 10% to 15% of cases, and iatrogenically caused cases account for about 1%. New-variant CJD is a new form of acquired spongiform encephalopathy that emerged in 1994 in the United Kingdom. This form has been linked with consumption of infected animal products. Patients with the new variant have a different course characterized by younger age at onset (mean age, 29 years), prominent psychiatric and sensory symptoms, and a longer disease course. (Spencer and colleagues, 2002) reported that 63% demonstrated purely psychiatric symptoms at onset (dysphoria, anxiety, anhedonia), 15% had purely neurological symptoms, and 22% had features of both. Median duration of illness was 13 months, and by the time of death, prominent neurological and psychiatric manifestations were universal.

Neurosyphilis

A resurgence of neurosyphilis has accompanied the AIDS epidemic in the industrialized world. Neurosyphilis may occur in any stage of syphilis. Early neurosyphilis, seen in the first weeks to years of infection, is primarily a meningitic process in which the parenchyma is not typically involved. It can coexist with primary or secondary syphilis and be asymptomatic. Inadequate treatment of early syphilis and coinfection with HIV predispose to early neurosyphilis. Epidemiological studies in HIV-positive patients have documented increased HIV shedding associated with genital ulcers, suggesting that syphilis increases the susceptibility of infected persons to HIV acquisition and transmission (Golden et al., 2003). Symptomatic early neurosyphilis may present with meningitis, with or without cranial nerve involvement or ocular changes, meningovascular disease, or stroke. Late neurosyphilis affects the meninges, brain, or spinal cord parenchyma and usually occurs years to decades after primary infection. Manifestations of late neurosyphilis include tabes dorsalis, a rapidly progressive dementia with psychotic features, or general paresis, or both. Dementia as a symptom of neurosyphilis is unlikely to improve significantly with treatment, yet the course of the illness can be arrested. Presenting psychiatric symptoms of neurosyphilis can include personality changes, hostility, confusion, hallucinations, expansiveness, delusions, and dysphoria. Symptoms also reported in association with neurosyphilis include explosive temper, emotional lability, anhedonia, social withdrawal, decreased attention to personal affairs, unusual giddiness, histrionicity, hypersexuality, and mania. A significant incidence of depression has been associated with general paresis.

There is no uniform consensus for the best approach to diagnosing neurosyphilis. Diagnosis usually depends on various combinations of reactive serological tests, cerebral spinal fluid (CSF) cell count or protein, CSF Venereal Disease Research Laboratories (VDRL) testing, and clinical manifestations. Some authorities argue that all patients with syphilis should have CSF examination, since asymptomatic neurosyphilis can only be identified by changes in the CSF. The CSF VDRL is the standard serological test for CSF and is highly specific but insensitive. When reactive in the absence of substantial contamination of CSF with blood, it is usually considered diagnostic. Its titer may be used to assess the activity of the disease and response to treatment. Two tests of CSF may be used to confirm a diagnosis of neurosyphilis: *Treponema pallidum* hemagglutination assay (TPHA) and fluorescent treponemal antibody absorption (FTA-ABS) assay. No single serology screen is perfect for diagnosing neurosyphilis. Other indicators of disease activity include CSF abnormalities such as elevated white blood cell count, elevated protein, and increased gamma globulin (IgG) levels. Treatment of neuro-

syphilis consists of a regimen of aqueous penicillin G, 18 to 24 million units/day, administered as 3 to 4 million units intravenously (IV) every 4 hours, or continuous infusion for 10 to 14 days. An alternative treatment is procaine penicillin G, 2 to 4 million units intramuscularly (IM) daily, with probenecid, 500 mg orally (PO), both daily for 10 to 14 days. A common recommendation to ensure an adequate response and cure is to repeat CSF studies 6 months after treatment.

Metabolic and Toxic

Essentially any metabolic derangement, if severe enough or combined with other conditions, can adversely affect behavior and cognition (**Table 9.5**). Metabolic disorders should remain within the differential diagnosis when evaluating patients with psychiatric symptoms.

Thyroid Disease

Hypothyroidism results from a deficiency in circulating thyroxine (T_4). It can result from impaired function at the level of the hypothalamus (tertiary hypothyroidism), the anterior pituitary (secondary hypothyroidism), or the thyroid gland (primary hypothyroidism, the most common cause of hypothyroidism). Neurological symptoms and signs can include headache, fatigue, apathy, inattention, slowness of speech and thought, sensorineural hearing loss, sleep apnea, and seizures. Some of these symptoms may be mistaken for depression. Hypothyroidism can worsen or complicate the course of depression, resulting in a seemingly refractory depression. More rare findings include polyneuropathy, cranial neuropathy, muscle weakness, psychosis (referred to as *myxedema madness*), dementia, coma, and death. Psychosis typically presents with paranoid delusions and auditory hallucinations.

Hyperthyroidism may be due to a number of causes that produce increased serum T_4. With mild hyperthyroidism, patients are typically anxious, irritable, emotionally labile, tachycardic, and tremulous. Other symptoms can include apathy, depression, panic attacks, feelings of exhaustion, inability to concentrate, and memory problems. When apathy and depression are present, the term *apathetic hyperthyroidism*

Table 9.5 Metabolic Disorders That May Cause Psychiatric and Neurological Symptoms

Abnormality	Mood Disorder	Mania	Delirium	Dementia	Psychotic Disorder	Anxiety Disorder	Personality Changes
Hyperthyroidism	+	+	++	+	++	+++	+
Hypothyroidism	+++		++	+	++		+
Hypercortisolism	+++	++	++	+	+++	+	+
Hypocortisolism	++		+	+	+		+
Hypercalcemia	++		++	++	++		
Hypoglycemia	++	+	+++	++	++	+++	+
Hyponatremia (SIADH)	++		++	++	+		

Adapted from Breitbart, W.B., 1989. Endocrine-related psychiatric disorders. In: Holland, J.C., Rowland, J.H. (Eds.), Handbook of Psycho-oncology: Psychological Care of the Patient with Cancer. Oxford University Press, New York, pp. 356-366; and from Breitbart W., Holland, J.C., 1993. Psychiatric Aspects of Symptom Management in Cancer Patients. APA Press, Washington, D.C., p. 29.

+++, Frequent; ++, common; +, rare; SIADH, syndrome of inappropriate antidiuretic hormone secretion.

is often used. Thyroid storm results from an abrupt elevation in T_4, often provoked by a significant stress such as surgery. It can be associated with fever, tachycardia, seizures, and coma; if untreated, it is often fatal. Psychosis and paranoia frequently occur during thyroid storm but are rare with milder hyperthyroidism, as is mania. Many patients usually will experience complete remission of symptoms 1 to 2 months after a euthyroid state is obtained, with a marked reduction in anxiety, sense of exhaustion, irritability, and depression. Some authors, however, report an increased rate of anxiety in patients, as well as persistence of affective and cognitive symptoms for several months to up to 10 years after a euthyroid state is established.

Hashimoto encephalopathy is a rare disorder involving thyroid autoimmunity. Antibodies associated with this condition include antithyroid peroxidase antibodies (previously known as *antithyroid microsomal antibodies*) and antithyroglobulin antibodies. The clinical syndrome may manifest with a progressive or relapsing and remitting course consisting of tremor, myoclonus, transient aphasia, stroke-like episodes, psychosis, seizures, encephalopathy, hypersomnolence, stupor, or coma. Encephalopathy usually develops over 1 to 7 days. The underlying mechanism of Hashimoto encephalopathy is unknown, and importantly, thyroid-stimulating hormone levels can be normal in this disorder. CSF most often shows an elevated protein level with almost no nucleated cells, whereas oligoclonal bands are often present. The EEG is abnormal in almost all cases, showing generalized slowing or frontal intermittent rhythmic delta activity. Triphasic waves, focal slowing, and epileptiform abnormalities may also be seen. MRI of the brain is often normal but may reveal hyperintensities on T2-weighted or fluid-attenuated inversion recovery (FLAIR) imaging in the subcortical white matter or at the gray/white matter junction. SPECT may show regions of hypoperfusion. The neurological and psychiatric symptoms respond well to treatment, which generally involves high-dose steroids. The associated abnormal findings on EEG, and often the MRI abnormalities, resolve with effective treatment.

Wilson Disease

Wilson disease (WD), also known as *hepatolenticular degeneration*, is an autosomal recessive disorder produced by a mutation on chromosome 13. The gene encodes a transport protein, the mutation of which causes abnormal deposition of copper in the liver, brain (especially the basal ganglia), and the cornea of the eyes. WD typically begins in childhood but in some cases has its onset as late as the fifth or sixth decade. About one-third of patients present with psychiatric symptoms, one-third present with neurological features, and one-third present with hepatic disease. Neurological manifestations are largely extrapyramidal, including chorea, tremor, and dystonia. Other symptoms include dysphagia, dysarthria, ataxia, gait disturbance, and a fixed (sardonic) smile. Seizures may also occur in a minority of patients. Potential neuropsychiatric symptoms are numerous, with at least half of patients manifesting symptoms early in the disease course. Personality and mood changes are the most common neuropsychiatric features, with depression occurring in approximately 30% of patients. Bipolar disorder occurs in about 20% of patients. Suicidal ideation is recognized in about 5% to 15%. WD patients can present with increased sensitivity to neuroleptics.

Other symptoms include irritability, aggression, and psychosis. Cognitively, the profile is consistent with disturbance of frontosubcortical systems. Even long-term-treated WD patients develop psychiatric symptoms in about 70% of cases (Srinivas et al., 2008; Svetel et al., 2009).

Diagnosis is suggested by identification of Kayser-Fleischer (KF) rings in patients with the appropriate clinical picture. The KF ring is a yellow-brown discoloration of the Descemet membrane in the limbic area of the cornea, best visualized with slit-lamp examination. A KF ring is present in 98% of patients with neurological disease and in 80% of all cases of WD. Reduced serum ceruloplasmin levels and elevated 24-hour urine copper excretion are consistent with this disorder. A liver biopsy is sometimes necessary to make the diagnosis. MRI studies may show abnormal T2 signal in the putamen, midbrain, pons, thalamus, cerebellum, and other structures. Atrophy is commonly present. The initial treatment for symptomatic patients is chelation therapy with either penicillamine or trientine. An estimated 20% to 50% of patients with neurological manifestations treated with penicillamine experience an acute worsening of their symptoms. A portion of these patients do not recover to their pretreatment neurological baseline. Alternatives that may have a lower incidence of neurological worsening include trientine or tetrathiomolybdate. Both may be used in combination with zinc therapy. Treatment of presymptomatic patients or maintenance therapy of successfully treated symptomatic patients can be accomplished with a chelating agent or zinc. Early treatment may result in partial improvement of the MRI changes as well as well as most of the neurological and psychiatric symptoms.

Vitamin B₁₂ and Folic Acid Deficiency

The true prevalence of vitamin B_{12} deficiency in the general population is unknown. The Framingham study demonstrated a prevalence of 12% among elderly persons living in the community. Other studies have suggested that the incidence may be as high as 30% to 40% among the sick and institutionalized elderly. The most common sign of vitamin B_{12} deficiency is macrocytic anemia. However, signs and symptoms attributed to the nervous system are diverse and can occur in the absence of anemia or macrocytosis. Furthermore, a normal serum cobalamin level does not exclude the possibility of a clinical deficiency. Serum homocysteine levels, which are elevated in more than 90% of deficiency states, and serum methylmalonic acid levels can be used to verify deficiency states in the appropriate settings.

Subacute combined degeneration (SCD) refers to the combination of spinal cord and peripheral nerve pathology associated with vitamin B_{12} deficiency. Patients often complain of unsteady gait and distal paresthesias. The examination may demonstrate evidence of posterior column, pyramidal tract, and peripheral nerve involvement. Cognitive, behavioral, and psychiatric manifestations can occur in isolation or together with the elemental signs and symptoms. Personality change, cognitive dysfunction, mania, depression, and psychosis have been reported. Prominent psychotic features include paranoid or religious delusions and auditory and visual hallucinations. Dementia is often comorbid with cobalamin deficiency; however, the causative association is unclear. There is little research data to support the existence of reversible dementia due to B_{12} deficiency. Cobalamin deficiency–associated cognitive impairment is more likely to improve when impairment is mild and of short duration. Folate deficiency can produce a clinical picture similar to cobalamin deficiency, although some investigators report that folate deficiency tends to produce more depression, whereas vitamin B_{12} deficiency tends to produce more psychosis. Elevated serum homocysteine is also seen with a functional folate deficiency state wherein folate utilization is impaired. Repletion of folate if comorbid vitamin B_{12} deficiency is not first corrected can result in an acute exacerbation of the neuropsychiatric symptoms.

Porphyrias

The porphyrias are caused by enzymatic defects in the heme biosynthetic pathway. Porphyrias with neuropsychiatric symptoms include acute intermittent porphyria (AIP), variegated porphyria (VP), hereditary mixed coproporphyria (HMP), and plumboporphyria (extremely rare and autosomal recessive), which may give rise to acute episodes of potentially fatal symptoms such as neurovisceral crisis, abdominal pain, delirium, psychosis, neuropathy, and autonomic instability. AIP, the most common type reported in the United States, follows an autosomal dominant pattern of inheritance and is due to a mutation in the gene for porphobilinogen deaminase. The disease is characterized by attacks that may last days to weeks, with relatively normal function between attacks. Infrequently, the clinical course may exhibit persisting clinical abnormalities with superimposed episodes of exacerbation. The episodic nature, clinical variability, and unusual features may cause symptoms to be attributed to somatization, conversion, or other psychiatric conditions. Attacks may be spontaneous but are typically precipitated by a variety of factors such as infection, alcohol use, pregnancy, anesthesia, and numerous medications that include antidepressants, anticonvulsants, and oral contraceptives.

Porphyric attacks usually manifest with a triad consisting of abdominal pain, peripheral neuropathy, and neuropsychiatric symptoms. Seizures may also occur. Abdominal pain is the most common symptom, which can result in surgical exploration if the diagnosis is unknown. A variety of cognitive and behavioral changes can occur, including anxiety, restlessness, insomnia, depression, mania, hallucinations, delusions, confusion, catatonia, and psychosis. The diagnosis can be confirmed during an acute attack of AIP, HMP, or VP by measuring urine porphobilinogens. Acute attacks are treated with avoidance of precipitating factors (e.g., medications), IV hemin, IV glucose, and pain control.

Drug Abuse

Common neurological manifestations are broad and include the direct effects of intoxication, side effects, and withdrawal syndromes, as well as indirect effects. Direct effects can range from somnolence with sedatives to psychosis from hallucinogens. Side effects may be as severe as stroke or vasculitis from stimulant abuse. Withdrawal may be lethal as in the case of alcohol withdrawal and delirium tremens. Indirect effects can occur as a result of trauma, such as head injury, suffered while under the influence. Substance abuse has a high comorbidity with a variety of psychiatric conditions. Neuropsychiatric manifestations occur with abuse of all classes of drugs and are summarized in **Box 9.6** (online only at www.expertconsult.com). The behavioral and cognitive manifestations of substance abuse may be transient but in a vulnerable subset of individuals may be chronic. Growing evidence suggests that drug use (e.g., 3,4-methylenedioxymethamphetamine [MDMA, "Ecstasy"]) may promote the development of chronic neuropsychiatric states such as depression and impaired cognition due to changes in structural and functional neuroanatomy (Montoya et al., 2002a). Although *Cannabis* use seems to be neither a sufficient nor a necessary cause of psychosis, it does confer an increased relative risk for developing schizophrenia later in life (Arseneault et al., 2004).

Autoimmune
Systemic Lupus Erythematosus

Systemic lupus erythematosus (SLE, lupus) is a multisystem inflammatory disorder that affects all ages, although young females are at a significantly elevated risk. CNS involvement is common, with clinical manifestations seen at some point during their disease course in up to 90% of patients. Primary neurological and psychiatric manifestations of SLE are likely due to a mixture of pathogenic mechanisms that include vascular abnormalities, autoantibodies, and the local production of inflammatory mediators. Secondary neurological and psychiatric manifestations occur as a result of various therapies (e.g., immunosuppression with steroids) or complications of the disease.

Neuropsychiatric symptoms are common, often episodic, and may occur in association with steroid treatment, which creates significant dilemmas in management. Depression and anxiety each occur in approximately 25% of SLE patients. Reports of the prevalence of overall mood disturbances range between 16% and 75%, and reports of anxiety disorders occur in 7% to 70%. Psychosis is more rare and tends to occur in the context of confusional states. Its overall prevalence has been reported to range from 5% to 8%. The incidence of psychotic symptoms in patients receiving prednisone doses between 60 mg and 100 mg/day is approximately 30%. These symptoms are reported to respond favorably to reduction in steroid dose and psychotropic management. Focal or generalized seizures may occur in the setting of active generalized SLE or as an isolated event. The prevalence of seizures ranges from 3% to 51%. Cognitive manifestations of SLE including temporary, fluctuating, or relatively stable characteristics eventually occur in up to 75% of patients; these manifestations range from mild attentional difficulties to dementia. In some patients, cognitive performance improves with resolution of any concurrent psychiatric disturbances. Cerebrovascular disease may underlie nonreversible cognitive dysfunction and when progressive may cause atrophy and multiinfarct dementia. Many patients with cognitive impairment have no demonstrable vascular lesions on neuroimaging. Cognitive impairment may manifest as subcortical features with deficits in processing speed, attention, learning and memory, conceptual reasoning, and cognitive flexibility. Reports of the prevalence of subclinical cognitive impairment range from 11% to 54% of patients. A number of brain-specific antibodies have been studied as potential diagnostic markers of psychosis associated with neuropsychiatric SLE (NPSLE), but none appear to be specific (Kimura et al., 2010). SLE patients identified as having a persistently positive immunoglobulin (Ig)G anticardiolipin antibody over a 5-year period have been demonstrated to have a greater reduction in psychomotor speed than antibody-negative SLE patients. Patients with a persistently elevated IgA anticardiolipin antibody level have been demonstrated to have poorer performance on tests of conceptual reasoning and executive function than antibody-negative SLE patients. Elevated IgG and IgA anticardiolipin antibody levels may be causative or a marker of long-term subtle deterioration in cognitive function in SLE patients. However, their role in routine evaluation and management remains controversial. Cerebrovascular disease is a well-known cause of neuropsychiatric dysfunction and is reported to occur in 5% to 18% of SLE patients.

The criteria set most widely used for diagnosing SLE is that developed by the American College of Rheumatology (ACR). An antinuclear antibody (ANA) titer to 1:40 or higher is the most sensitive of the ACR criteria and is present in up to 99% of persons with SLE at some point in their illness. The ANA, however, is not specific. It can be positive in several other rheumatological conditions as well as in relation to some medication exposures. There is also a significant incidence of false-positive tests. Anti–double-stranded DNA and anti–Smith antibodies, particularly in high titers, have high specificity for SLE, although their sensitivity is low. The rapid plasma reagin (RPR) test, a syphilis serology, may be falsely positive.

Treatment of NPSLE includes corticosteroids and immunosuppressive therapy, including pulse IV cyclophosphamide or plasmapheresis when NPSLE is thought to occur secondary to an inflammatory process. Anticoagulation is used in patients with thrombotic disease in the setting of antiphospholipid antibody syndrome.

Multiple Sclerosis

Multiple sclerosis is an inflammatory demyelinating disease that manifests the pathological hallmark findings of multifocal demyelinated plaques in the brain and spinal cord. MS lesions are typically disseminated throughout the CNS, with a predilection for the optic nerves, brainstem, spinal cord, cerebellum, and periventricular white matter. Its cause remains unknown but is thought to be an immune-mediated disorder affecting individuals with a genetic predisposition. The heterogeneity of clinical, pathological, and MRI findings suggest involvement of more than one pathological mechanism. It is the leading cause of nontraumatic disability among young adults. Socioepidemiological studies indicate that MS leads to unemployment within a 10-year disease course in as many as 50% to 80% of patients. Females are more affected than males at a 2:1 ratio. It is characterized either by attacks of neurological deficits with variable remittance or by a steady progressive course of neurological decline. Neuropsychiatric manifestations of MS are common, occurring in up to 60% of patients at some point in their disease. The lifetime prevalence of major depression in MS is approximately 50%. The lifetime prevalence of bipolar disorder is twice the prevalence in the general population. Euphoria may be present in more advanced MS, usually in association with cognitive deficits. *Pseudobulbar affect*—defined as outbursts of involuntary, uncontrollable, stereotypical episodes of

laughing or crying—occurs in varying degrees of severity in approximately 10% of patients. Other symptoms include anxiety, sleep disorder, emotional lability/irritability, apathy, mania, suicidality, and rarely psychosis. Occasionally, psychiatric symptoms may present as the major manifestation of an episode of demyelination. The presence of psychiatric symptomatology does not preclude the use of steroids to abbreviate clinical attacks of MS. There is presently ongoing debate about whether interferon therapy is associated with a higher incidence of depression in MS patients. Pharmacological and behavioral treatment mirrors the management of depression and psychosis in patients without MS.

Cognitive impairment is found in approximately 40% of patients. Deficits have been described in working, semantic, and episodic memory as well as in the person's ability to accurately assess his or her own memory function. Patients may also suffer from impaired attention, cognitive slowing, reduced verbal fluency, and difficulties with abstract reasoning and concept formation. Correlations between cognitive impairment and MRI location of lesions and indices of total lesion area have been noted. There is little data on the treatment of cognitive dysfunction in MS. The disease-modifying agent interferon beta-1a was noted to be associated with improvements in information-processing and problem-solving abilities over a 2-year longitudinal study. A small trial demonstrated an improvement in complex attention, concentration, and visual memory in a group of patients treated for 1 year with interferon beta-1b compared with controls (Barak and Achiron, 2002). Donepezil, 10 mg daily, has been reported to improve verbal learning and memory in some MS patients.

Neoplastic

A variety of neoplasms cause cognitive and behavioral disorders. Of particular relevance are mass lesions and paraneoplastic syndromes. Mass lesions can be single or multiple and can be primary to the CNS or metastatic. The most common intracranial primary tumors are astrocytomas (e.g., glioblastoma multiforme), meningiomas, pituitary tumors, vestibular schwannomas, and oligodendrogliomas. Common metastatic tumors include primary lung and breast tumors, melanoma, and renal and colon cancers. The number of patients presenting with a primary psychiatric diagnosis secondary to an unidentified brain tumor is likely to be less than 5%. However, 15% to 20% of patients with intracranial tumors may present with neuropsychiatric manifestations before the development of primary neurological problems such as motor or sensory deficits. The behavioral manifestations of mass lesions are diverse and related to a number of factors including direct disruption of local structures or circuits, rate of growth, seizures, and increased intracranial pressure. A relationship between tumor location and specific psychiatric symptoms has not been established. Meningiomas, given their slow growth over years, are classic examples of tumors that can present solely with behavioral manifestations. Common locations include the olfactory groove and sphenoid wings, which can disrupt adjacent limbic structures such as the orbital frontal gyri and medial temporal lobes.

Paraneoplastic syndromes represent remote nonmetastatic manifestations of malignancy. Neurological paraneoplastic syndromes are primarily immune-mediated disorders that may develop as a result of antigens shared between the nervous system and tumor cells. The most common primary malignancies that promote neurological paraneoplastic syndromes are ovarian and small-cell lung cancer (SCLC). These syndromes generally develop subacutely, often before the primary malignancy is identified, and may preferentially involve selected regions of the CNS. Typical sites of involvement include muscle, neuromuscular junction, peripheral nerve, cerebellum, and limbic structures. Limbic encephalitis, associated with SCLC and testicular cancer, produces a significant amnestic syndrome and neuropsychiatric symptoms including agitation, depression, personality changes, apathy, delusions, hallucinations, and psychosis. Complex partial and generalized seizures may also occur. Relevant markers include: (1) intracellular paraneoplastic antigens such as Hu, associated with SCLC, and Ta and Ma-2, associated with testicular cancer and (2) cell membrane antigens such as the N-methyl-D-aspartate receptor and voltage-gated potassium channels (Graus et al., 2010; Hoffmann et al., 2008). Paraneoplastic disorders are often progressive and refractory to therapy, although in some cases significant improvement follows tumor resection and immunotherapy. Significant neuropsychiatric sequelae can arise from the various chemotherapeutic and radiation therapies used for cancer treatment.

Degenerative

Neuropsychiatric symptoms are common in most degenerative disorders that produce significant dementia. The individual presentations of such symptoms are related to a number of factors specific to the disease: location of lesion burden, rate of progression of disease, and factors specific to the individual (e.g., premorbid personality, education level, psychiatric history, social support system, and coping skills).

Neurodegenerative diseases are increasingly recognized as involving abnormalities of protein metabolism. About 70% of dementias in the elderly and more than 90% of neurodegenerative dementias can be linked to abnormalities of three proteins: β-amyloid, α-synuclein, and τ. Disorders of protein metabolism have associated neuroanatomical regions of vulnerable cell populations that are related to the clinical manifestations. AD, for example, has associated disorders of β-amyloid, τ, and α-synuclein metabolism that involve specific anatomical regions. PD, dementia with Lewy bodies (DLB), and multisystem atrophies are synucleinopathies. α-Synuclein is the main component of Lewy bodies, which are a major histological marker seen in PD and DLB. In these disorders, Lewy bodies may be found in the substantia nigra, locus ceruleus, nucleus basalis, limbic system, and transitional and neocortex. Frontotemporal dementia, progressive supranuclear palsy (PSP), and corticobasal ganglionic degeneration implicate abnormal τ metabolism in their pathogenesis. Tauopathies are associated with selective involvement of the frontal and temporal cortex and frontosubcortical circuitry. **Table 9.6** lists associated regions of vulnerability and neuropsychiatric symptoms.

Alzheimer Disease and Mild Cognitive Impairment

Neuropsychiatric symptoms of AD may include paranoia, agitation, aggression, delusions, hallucinations, anxiety, apathy, social withdrawal, reduced speech output, reduction or alteration of long-standing family relationships, and loss of sense of humor. A review of 100 cases of autopsy-proven AD demonstrated that 74% of patients had behavioral symptoms detected at the time of the initial evaluation. Symptoms

Table 9.6 Correlations of Neuropsychiatric Symptoms to Regions of Vulnerability in Neurodegenerative Disorders

Neuropsychiatric Symptoms	Dementia Type	Protein Abnormality	Regional Vulnerability
Hallucinations	PD	α-Synuclein	Brainstem>limbic cortex>neocortex
	DLB		
Delusions	PD with dementia	α-Synuclein	Brainstem>limbic cortex>neocortex
	DLB AD with parkinsonism		
REM sleep behavior disorder	PD with dementia	α-Synuclein	Brainstem>limbic cortex>neocortex
	DLB		
Disinhibition	FTD	τ	Frontal cortex, frontal-subcortical systems, anterior temporal systems
	PSP AD (frontal variant)		
OCD	FTD PSP	τ	Frontal cortex or basal ganglia
Apathy	FTD PSP AD	τ	Frontal cortex or basal ganglia

Adapted from Cummings, J.L., 2003. Toward a molecular neuropsychiatry of neurodegenerative diseases. Ann. Neurol 54, 147-154.

AD, Alzheimer disease; *DLB,* dementia with lewy bodies; *FTD,* frontotemporal dementia; *OCD,* obsessive-compulsive disorder; *PD,* Parkinson disease; *PSP,* progressive supranuclear palsy; *REM,* rapid eye movement.

included apathy (51%), hallucinations (25%), delusions (20%), depressed mood (6.6%), verbal aggression (36.8%), and physical aggression (17%). The presence of behavioral symptoms at the initial evaluation was associated with greater functional impairment not directly related to their cognitive impairments. Depressive symptoms, dysphoria, or major depression eventually occur in approximately half of patients. Psychosis has been reported to occur in 30% to 50% of patients at some time during the course of the illness, more commonly in the later stages. Mania occurs in less than 5%. Behavioral changes have been shown to be problematic and to precipitate earlier nursing home placement. Social comportment has been viewed as being relatively spared in AD, but subtle personality changes occur in nearly every individual over time. Significant impairment in the ability to recognize facial expressions of emotion and an inability to repeat, comprehend, and discriminate affective elements of language have been reported. It has been hypothesized that 15% of AD patients may have a frontal variant wherein they present with difficulties attributable to frontal lobe circuitry rather than an amnestic syndrome. Impairments in driving ability (Dawson et al., 2009) and decision-making abilities such as medical decision making (Okonkwo et al., 2008) and financial management (Marson et al., 2009) may be present even in early AD.

Atypical antipsychotic drugs are widely used to treat psychosis, aggression, and agitation in patients with AD. Their benefits are uncertain, and concerns about safety have emerged. Adverse effects may offset advantages in the efficacy of atypical antipsychotic drugs for the treatment of psychosis, aggression, or agitation in AD patients. Limited evidence suggests that electroconvulsive therapy (ECT) may be effective for management of agitation (Sutor and Rasmussen, 2008).

The concept of mild cognitive impairment (MCI) was developed to characterize a population of individuals exhibiting symptoms that are between normal age-related cognitive decline and dementia. These patients have a very slight degree of functional impairment and minimal decline from their prior level of functioning and therefore do not meet criteria for dementia. MCI was initially defined as a condition of memory impairment beyond what was expected for age, in the absence of impairments in other domains of cognitive functioning such as working memory, executive function, language, and visual-spatial ability. This concept has since evolved and now includes a total of four subtypes of impairment that are not of sufficient severity to warrant the diagnosis of dementia. The second type of MCI, called *amnestic multiple domain*, is associated with memory impairment plus impairment in one or more other cognitive domains. The third subtype is called *nonamnestic single domain*, and the fourth is known as *nonamnestic multiple domain* MCI. In many cases, the natural history of these subtypes leads to different end-point conditions. Combining the clinical syndrome with the presumed cause may allow for reliable prediction of outcome of the MCI syndrome. When associated with only memory impairment, MCI may represent normal aging or depression or progress to AD. Amnestic MCI–multiple domains has a higher association with depression or progression to AD or vascular dementia. Nonamnestic single-domain MCI may have a higher likelihood of progression to frontal temporal dementia. Nonamnestic multiple-domain MCI may have a higher likelihood of progression to Lewy body dementia or vascular dementia (Petersen and Negash, 2008).

In 2008, it was estimated that more than 5 million people in the United States older than age 71 had MCI. The prevalence of MCI among persons younger than age 75 has been estimated to be 19% and for those older than 85 years, 29%. Almost a third of these individuals have amnestic MCI which may to progress to AD at a rate of 10% to 15% per year. The conversion rate of amnestic MCI to dementia over a 6-year period may be as high as 80%. Neuropsychiatric symptoms are common in persons with MCI. Depression occurs in 20%, apathy in 15%, and irritability in 15%. Increased levels of agitation and aggression are also present. Almost half of MCI patients demonstrate one of these neuropsychiatric symptoms coincident with the onset of cognitive impairment. Impaired awareness of memory dysfunction may also be present to a degree comparable to that found in persons with early AD. Evidence suggests that persons with MCI have an increased risk of motor vehicle accidents when risk factors such as a having a history of driving citations, crashes, reduced driving mileage, situational avoidance, or aggression or impulsivity are present. Difficulties with medical decision making have also been identified in some individuals with MCI (Okonkwo et al., 2008).

Frontotemporal Dementia

Frontotemporal dementia (FTD), the most common progressive focal cortical syndrome, is characterized by atrophy of the frontal and anterotemporal lobes. Age at presentation is usually between 45 and 65 years (almost invariably before age 65), and reports of its incidence range from being equal in males and females to (more recently) predominating in males by a ratio of 14:3. The prevalence of FTD is equal to that of AD for early-onset (age < 65) dementia. Behavioral features include apathy, social withdrawal, disinhibition, impulsivity, poor insight, anosognosia, obsessive tendencies, inappropriate sexual behavior, agitation, delusions, hallucinations, and psychosis. Elements of the Klüver-Bucy syndrome may be present. Memory and language are usually spared during the early disease course. Depressive symptoms occur in 30% to 40% of patients. SSRIs are somewhat effective in treating behavioral symptoms but are less effective in treating cognitive symptoms. About 30% of patients with FTD have a positive family history, and first-degree relatives of patients have a 3.5 times higher risk of developing dementia. Genes known to be mutated in this disorder include those encoding microtubule-associated protein τ and progranulin.

Idiopathic Parkinson Disease

Neuropsychiatric manifestations of PD are common. Depression is the most common psychiatric symptom, with a reported prevalence of 25% to 50%. Establishing the diagnosis of depression is complicated by the presence of comorbid confounding symptoms including dementia, facial masking, bradykinesia, apathy, and hypophonia. Menza et al. (2009) conducted a placebo-controlled trial in PD patients with depression and found that nortriptyline was efficacious, but paroxetine was not. Psychosis is also particularly prevalent and generally related to dopaminergic agents. The onset of motor impairment almost always precedes that of psychosis. Hallucinations, usually fleeting and nocturnal, are typically visual and occur in 30% of treated patients. Auditory and olfactory hallucinations, however, are rare. Visual hallucinations are associated with impaired cognition, use of anticholinergic medications, and impaired vision. In contrast to the hallucinations associated with DLB, patients with PD generally have at least partial insight into the nature of their hallucinations. Delusions occur less commonly and are often persecutory in nature. Management is complicated by neuroleptic sensitivity to both typical and atypical agents. Typical neuroleptics should be avoided. Novel atypical neuroleptics with potentially more favorable pharmacological properties, such as quetiapine and clozapine, may have theoretical advantages over other agents for treating PD. Evidence suggests that clozapine is effective, quetiapine may be effective, and olanzepine is not effective. Impulse-control disorders including pathological gambling, binge-eating, compulsive sexual behavior and buying are associated with dopamine agonist treatment in PD (Weintraub et al., 2010).

Many PD patients will develop dementia 10 years or more after the onset of motor symptoms. Up to 80% of PD patients will eventually develop frank dementia, a majority of whom will show comorbid AD pathology. Initial deficits may include cognitive slowing, memory retrieval deficits, attentional difficulties, visual-spatial deficits, and mild executive impairments. In advanced disease, memory encoding and storage can become impaired. Primary language difficulties are not involved until the disease has significantly progressed. Some evidence suggests that patients with an akinetic-dominant form of PD with hallucinations are at higher risk of developing dementia than patients with a tremor-dominant form who have no hallucinations. Dementia is a major prognostic factor for progressive disability and nursing home placement. In a placebo-controlled trial, rivastigmine (a cholinesterase inhibitor) has been shown to produce moderate but significant improvements in global ratings of dementia, cognition, and behavioral symptoms in patients with mild to moderate PD. Open-label drug data suggest that all three cholinesterase inhibitors may be effective.

Dementia with Lewy Bodies

By some accounts, DLB is the second most common cause of dementia. The revised consensus criteria for the clinical diagnosis of DLB reiterate dementia as an essential feature for the diagnosis of DLB occurring before or concurrently with parkinsonism. Criteria developed for research purposes to distinguish DLB from PD with dementia use an arbitrary period of 1 year within which the occurrence of dementia and extrapyramidal symptoms suggests the diagnosis of possible DLB. If the clinical history of parkinsonism is longer than 1 year before dementia occurs, a diagnosis of PD with dementia is more accurate. Deficits of attention, executive function, and visuospatial ability may be prominent. These deficits may be worse in DLB than in patients with AD. Prominent or persistent memory impairment may not necessarily occur in the early stages but is usually evident with progression. Memory impairment is a less prominent feature than in AD. According to the revised consensus criteria, two core features are sufficient for the diagnosis of probable DLB and one feature for the diagnosis of possible DLB. Core features include fluctuating cognition, recurrent visual hallucinations, and spontaneous features of parkinsonism. Other suggestive and supportive features associated with DLB include delusions, hallucinations

in other modalities, rapid eye movement (REM) sleep behavior disorder, depression, severe neuroleptic sensitivity, autonomic dysfunction, repeated falls/syncope, and episodes of unexplained transient loss of consciousness.

Hallucinations are characteristically seen early in the disease course and are persistent and recurrent. Visual hallucinations tend to occur early in the illness, are typically well formed and complex, and occur in 50% to 80% of patients. Auditory hallucinations occur in approximately 30% of patients and olfactory hallucinations in 5% to 10% of patients. Delusions may be systematized and are present in 50% of patients over the course of the disease. Psychotic symptoms are common and occur in the absence of medications. Depression is estimated to be nearly as common as that in AD. Treatment is complicated by hypersensitivity to the adverse effects of antidopaminergic neuroleptic agents (both typical and atypical). Typical agents should be avoided. Novel atypical neuroleptics with potentially more favorable pharmacological properties (e.g., quetiapine and clozapine) may have theoretical advantages over other agents in treating DLB as with PD. Cholinesterase inhibitors are helpful for managing neuropsychiatric symptoms and may be beneficial for treating fluctuating cognitive impairment and improving global functioning and activities of daily living.

Huntington Disease

Huntington Disease is a degenerative disorder of autosomal dominant inheritance resulting from an expanded trinucleotide (cytosine-adenine-guanine [CAG]) repeat on chromosome 4. Symptoms typically develop during the fourth or fifth decade, initially manifesting with neurological features, psychiatric features, or both. Neurologically, patients often demonstrate generalized chorea, motor impersistence, and oculomotor dysfunction. In the juvenile form, the Westphal variant, early parkinsonian features are prominent, as are seizures, ataxia, and myoclonus. Significant cognitive impairment is inevitable and is often present early in the disease. Features of a subcortical dementia are present with involvement of frontosubcortical circuits. Common features include cognitive slowing, memory retrieval deficits, attentional difficulties, and executive dysfunction. Patients often lack awareness of their chorea and their cognitive and emotional deficits. Psychiatric features such as personality changes, apathy, irritability, and depression are common. Depression may be exacerbated by tetrabenazine used for the treatment of chorea, since this drug is a dopamine-depleting agent. Psychosis may occur in up to 25% of patients with HD. Anxiety and obsessive tendencies also occur (Phillips et al., 2008).

Epilepsy

Behavioral and cognitive dysfunction is frequently observed in patients with epilepsy and represents an important challenge in treating these patients. A complex array of factors influence the neuropsychiatric effect of epilepsy: cause, location of epileptogenic focus, age at onset, duration of epilepsy, nature of the epilepsy syndrome, seizure type, frequency, medications used for treatment, and psychosocial factors. Epilepsies that develop subsequent to brain trauma and stroke may be associated with cognitive and behavioral changes due to brain injury quite apart from those associated with the secondary seizures. The localization of an epileptogenic focus is also an important determinant of cognitive deficits. For example, temporal lobe epilepsy may be associated with memory defects, and frontal lobe epilepsy may be associated with performance deficits in executive functioning. Behavioral disturbances are most common with complex partial seizures and seizures involving foci in the temporolimbic structures. The age of onset can affect cognitive and behavioral functioning; onset of epilepsy before 5 years of age appears to be a risk factor for a lower intelligence quotient (IQ). Attention-deficit hyperactivity disorder, inattentive type, has been observed to be 2.5 times more common in children younger than 16 years with newly diagnosed unprovoked seizures than in controls. Behavioral symptoms may be more prominent in later-onset seizures. Duration of epilepsy and seizure type and frequency are other factors that affect cognition and behavior. Individuals with generalized tonic-clonic seizures may have greater associated cognitive impairment than that observed in persons with partial seizures, and compared with patients experiencing fewer seizures, those who experience repeated generalized tonic-clonic seizures generally have increased cognitive impairment. A single seizure can be associated with postictal attentional deficits lasting 24 hours or longer. Antiepileptic medications add another level of complexity to management by introducing their associated side effects, which may include impairment of working memory, slowed cognitive processing, language disturbances, and behavioral changes. Anticonvulsants have been reported to be associated with a host of effects on sleep such as insomnia, alterations of sleep architecture, and in some cases, worsening of sleep disordered breathing (barbiturates and benzodiazepines). These may all adversely affect cognition. On the other hand, anticonvulsants may reduce seizure activity, interictal activity, and arousals from sleep, thereby contributing to improved cognitive function.

Cognitive adverse side effects are more prominent in patients receiving polytherapy and have been noted to improve with a switch to monotherapy. It is estimated that more than 60% of patients with epilepsy meet diagnostic criteria for at least one psychiatric disorder during their lifetime. Depression is the most common symptom, occurring with an estimated prevalence of 11% to 44%. Precise information regarding the prevalence and incidence of depression in patients with epilepsy is unavailable owing to the heterogeneity of patient populations studied and studies not distinguishing between depressive symptoms and depressive disorder. The prevalence of psychosis is estimated at between 2% and 8%. Other prominent psychiatric symptoms associated with epilepsy include anxiety, aggression, personality disorders, and panic disorders. Mania is considered rare. When evaluating mood disorder symptoms or psychosis in a patient with epilepsy, it is important to take into account the chronological relationship of the seizures with the symptoms. Conceptually, these symptoms can be classified into peri-ictal or preictal, ictal, postictal, and interictal. Paradoxically, depression or psychosis can follow remission of epilepsy, either after epilepsy surgery or the initiation of effective antiepileptic drug therapy, as part of the phenomenon of forced normalization. Peri-ictal or preictal dysphoric or depressive syndromes frequently precede a seizure. They may last hours to days and resolve with the occurrence of the seizure or persist for hours to days afterward. Peri-ictal depressive symptoms are more common in

focal seizures than in generalized seizures. Ictal depressive symptoms occur in approximately 10% of temporal lobe epilepsy patients. Ictal depression is most often characterized by a sudden onset of symptoms independent of outside stimuli. No associated hemispheric lateralization of the epileptic focus has been clearly demonstrated. Anxiety is the most common ictal psychiatric symptom. Treatment of preictal and ictal depressive symptoms does not usually require antidepressant therapy. Treatment should be directed at reducing the frequency of seizures.

The prevalence of postictal depression has not been established. Patients with poorly controlled simple focal seizures have been reported to have postictal depressive symptoms averaging approximately 37 hours. After a seizure, depressive symptoms have been known to last up to 2 weeks with some reports, suggesting increased suicide risk. Investigation of patients with postictal depression has revealed unilateral frontal or temporal foci without hemispheric predominance. Interictal depression is considered the most common type of depression in epileptic patients. Its estimated prevalence ranges from 20% to 70%, depending on the patient group characteristics. Episodic major depression and dysthymia are common, whereas bipolar affective symptoms are rare. Interictal depressive symptoms are often chronic and less prominent than those of MDD, resulting in patients not reporting their symptoms and healthcare providers not recognizing them. Treatment may be required for postictal depressive symptoms and usually is required for interictal depressive symptoms. Treatment should consist of an antidepressant medication and optimized seizure control. SSRIs have a lower risk of associated seizures and should be considered as first-line pharmacotherapy. Electroconvulsive therapy is not contraindicated in patients with epilepsy and should be considered for severe or treatment-refractory depression. The incidence of seizures in epilepsy patients after ECT is not increased compared to that in patients without epilepsy.

Psychosis is a rare primary manifestation of a seizure focus. When present, it is best treated by controlling the ictus and thus by antiepileptic medications. Psychosis may commonly manifest as a postictal phenomenon (representing approximately 25% of all psychosis associated with epilepsy). Diagnostic criteria for postictal psychosis (PIP) include (1) an episode of psychosis emerging within 1 week after the return of normal mental function following a seizure; (2) an episode length between 24 hours and 3 months; and (3) no evidence of EEG-supported nonconvulsive status epilepticus, anticonvulsant toxicity, previous history of interictal psychosis, recent head injury, or alcohol or drug intoxication. PIP may manifest affect-laden symptomatology. Commonly, there is a prompt response to low-dose antipsychotics or benzodiazepines. The annual incidence of PIP among patients who undergo inpatient video EEG monitoring was estimated to be approximately 6%. The prevalence of having experienced PIP among treatment-resistant partial epilepsy outpatients has been reported to be 7%. PIP is most commonly associated with temporal lobe epilepsy. Psychotic symptoms may include auditory, visual, or olfactory hallucinations. Abnormalities of thought content or form may include ideas of reference, paranoia, delusions, grandiosity, religious delusions, thought blocking, tangentiality, or loose associations. Manic symptoms may briefly occur in a minority of patients but are usually not of sufficient duration to meet criteria for a manic episode. In patients with temporal lobe epilepsy and PIP, studies have shown a higher incidence of bilateral cerebral injury or dysfunction, bilateral independent temporal region EEG discharges, and bifrontal and bitemporal hyperperfusion patterns on SPECT. These data suggest that bilateral cerebral abnormalities may be an important feature of PIP.

There has been speculation that PIP may sometimes be caused by complex partial (limbic) status (Elliott et al., 2009). When this is thought to be the case, acute therapy with antiepileptic medications would be advised, possibly in conjunction with antipsychotic medication. Risk factors for PIP include a cluster of seizures, insomnia within 1 week of onset of PIP (particularly within 1-3 days), epilepsy of more than 10 years' duration, generalized tonic-clonic seizures or secondarily generalized complex partial seizures, prior episodes of PIP, prior psychiatric hospitalizations or a history of psychosis, bilateral independent seizure foci (particularly temporal), history of TBI or encephalitis, and low intellectual function. PIP is usually short-lived, lasting several days to weeks, but chronic psychosis may develop after recurrent episodes or even after a single episode. Research data are lacking for treatment of PIP, and recommendations are based on expert opinion. Recommendations include vigilant monitoring of patients with risk factors for PIP after a cluster of seizures, ensuring that there is not ongoing seizure activity, early implementation of antipsychotic medications (preferably atypical agents) after the emergence of symptoms, consideration of treatment after a cluster of seizures in patients with a history of PIP, and consideration of treatment with the emergence of sleeplessness, which can be a harbinger of PIP. PIP can respond to ECT, but it is rarely necessary to utilize this resource.

Interictal psychosis manifesting the positive psychopathological phenomena of schizophrenia has been felt to be more common in patients with temporolimbic foci. This idea has been recently challenged by a population-based study using a cohort comprising 2.27 million people derived from the Danish longitudinal registers. These data support the premise that all types of epilepsy increase the risk of developing schizophrenia or a schizophrenia-like psychosis. Furthermore, compared with the general population, persons with epilepsy have nearly 2.5 times the risk of developing schizophrenia and almost 3 times the risk of developing a schizophrenia-like psychosis. The risk for psychosis also increases with an increasing number of hospital admissions for epilepsy and with people first admitted for epilepsy at later ages. Some experts have suggested that interictal psychosis differs from primary psychosis insofar as the former tends to be associated with preserved affect, fewer negative symptoms, and arguably greater insight. The greatest similarities can be seen in the presence of positive symptoms such as thought disorder, delusions, and hallucinations. The underlying causal mechanism for the association of epilepsy with schizophrenia or schizophrenia-like psychosis is unknown, but it may have features in common with PIP and likely involves bilateral cerebral dysfunction within frontal subcortical circuits and probably temporal subcortical circuits as well. Treatment for PIP is based primarily on use of antipsychotic medications once status epilepticus has been diagnostically eliminated from consideration.

Treatment of epilepsy-related psychosis is complicated by the propensity of antipsychotics to cause paroxysmal EEG abnormalities (Centorrino et al., 2002) and induce seizures. EEG changes occur in the nonepileptic population treated with antipsychotics but in most circumstances are of little consequence. Studies defining the effects of neuroleptics on the EEG of persons with epilepsy are lacking. The potential for increasing seizures has led to some anxiety about the use of antipsychotics in individuals with epilepsy. In most circumstances, the risk of increasing seizures is considered low, but formal studies investigating the efficacy of antipsychotic medications for treating epilepsy-related psychosis and the risks for precipitating seizures are lacking. The specific causes and characteristics of a given epilepsy have to be considered carefully, as these may increase risk. Seizure potential is generally dose related, so high-dose therapy should be avoided. Careful monitoring of anticonvulsants is advised. The lowest possible effective dose should be used, medications selected carefully, and psychiatric polypharmacy avoided if possible, since this may increase the risk of seizures. Seizure risk is particularly increased with use of clozapine and chlorpromazine. Potential problems with antipsychotic treatment in persons with epilepsy include pharmacokinetic interactions due to common metabolism with P450 isoenzymes, as well as side effects (sedation, weight gain, hyperlipidemia, decreased glycemic control, hematotoxicity, and hepatotoxicity).

Traumatic Brain Injury

Each year approximately 1.7 million people in the United States sustain a TBI. It is estimated that 80% of these are of mild severity, and the remaining 20% are about evenly split between moderate and severe injuries. The leading causes of TBI in the United States are motor vehicle accidents, falls, assaults, and recreational accidents. The wars in Iraq and Afghanistan have increased the numbers of injuries suffered by U.S. military personnel; 15% to 20% of military and civilian personnel serving in these theaters have experienced mild TBI during their deployments.

The pathological correlates of moderate to severe TBI are numerous and particular to the types and mechanisms of injuries suffered. Various types of pathology, which are often found in combinations, include penetrating wounds, depressed skull fractures, diffuse axonal injury (DAI), petechial hemorrhages, contusions, lacerations, hematomas (epidural, subdural, and intraparenchymal), subarachnoid hemorrhage, edema, herniation, and focal or diffuse hypoxic ischemic injury. Many of these specific types of injuries have their own prognosis and time course of recovery. Concussion or mild TBI occurs most frequently in young adults. There is no consensus about what clinical findings constitute mild TBI, with many practitioners advocating that loss of consciousness is not an absolute requirement. Others differ on the required duration of loss of consciousness, with ranges from 20 minutes to any event lasting less than 1 hour. Any traumatic process associated with a generalized alteration in cerebral function, including amnesia (retrograde or anterograde) or alteration in consciousness at the time of the accident, may be associated with brain injury. Persons who sustain a mild TBI often complain of a number of emotional/behavioral, cognitive, and physical symptoms, which can persist for months to years after the injury, and rarely may be permanent. Such symptoms can include anxiety, depression, irritability, mood lability, cognitive slowing, judgment problems, difficulty concentrating, memory problems, fatigue, sensitivity to noise, dizziness, and headaches. Postconcussive symptoms occur after moderate and severe TBI as well. It is estimated that 80% to 90% of persons sustaining a mild TBI make a favorable recovery. When symptoms persist, the patient is said to suffer from a *postconcussive syndrome*. The overall prevalence for postconcussive symptoms, self-limited and persistent at 3 months after injury, ranges from approximately 25% to 85%. Well-controlled research data are not available on optimal pharmacological management or rehabilitation strategies for post-TBI neuropsychiatric and cognitive difficulties. Limited evidence supports the effectiveness of methylphenidate for enhancing attention, processing speed, and memory function. Other medications such as D-amphetamine, amantadine, donepezil, levodopa, and bromocriptine may also have some benefit for treating symptoms that include attentional difficulties, cognitive slowing, poor initiation, aspects of poor memory, fatigue, or motor deficits. Cognitive rehabilitation may be helpful for management of attention and executive difficulties, as well as improving communication skills (Cicerone et al., 2009). Evidence-based reviews generally support holistic rehabilitation programs that support community reintegration, awareness of deficits, regulation of behavior and affect, improved physical and social function, and effective communication (Cernich et al., 2010). Psychiatric disorders occur at high rates in TBI patients, with criteria for axis I disorders (as defined by the DSM-IV-TR) being met in 50% to 80% of patients in a community sample of patients with a mixed level of severity. Axis II disorders were identified in 25% to 65% of patients (Price, 2004; Warriner and Velikonja, 2006). Axis I disorders include major mood and anxiety disorders, schizophrenia, and other psychoses; axis II disorders include major personality disorders and other maladaptive personality features. Psychiatric symptoms have been observed to occur immediately after injury up to decades later. It is likely that a complex interplay of factors results in the particular cognitive and psychiatric manifestations in a given individual. These factors include the nature and severity of the neurological injury, premorbid personality and cognition, preexisting psychiatric illness, substance abuse history, family psychiatric history, educational level, occupational status, coping strategies, age at injury, stressors, support systems, and the possibility of psychological or financial gains.

Post-TBI depression occurs in up to 60% of patients, with comorbid anxiety and aggressive behavior being common. Both right and left hemispheric lesions have been implicated. SSRIs are most commonly prescribed and may be helpful for management of depression, irritability, agitation, and aggression. CBT may decrease depression, anxiety, and anger and improve problem-solving skills (Silver et al., 2009). TBI-associated hypomania and mania have also been observed, although at much lower frequencies. Psychosis in association with TBI has a reported incidence ranging from 0.7% to 20%. Reliable incidence and prevalence information is unavailable. An increased risk of developing chronic psychosis has been observed in individuals suffering severe diffuse brain injury involving the temporal and frontal lobes. Patients undergoing evaluation for potential TBI-related psychosis need to be carefully distinguished from those with preexisting psychotic symptoms and schizophrenia. The mean delay to the onset of psychotic symptoms after injury has been reported to be about 4 years (Guerreiro et al., 2009). The latency of the injury to the onset of symptoms has been reported to range from 2 days

to 48 years. Delusions occur in more than 75%, and hallucinations occur in almost 50% of patients. Approximately 70% of affected individuals were noted to have abnormal findings on EEG. Neuropsychological testing demonstrated abnormalities in almost 90%. Psychosis in the majority of patients eventually improves with antipsychotics.

Depression-Related Cognitive Impairment

Depression-related cognitive impairment (DRCI) refers to the complex pattern of cognitive impairment seen in association with affective disorders such as major depression. Several factors are thought to be helpful in distinguishing DRCI from dementia. Patients with DRCI tend to complain of memory and concentration problems, whereas demented patients often deny that problems exist despite impairment that is obvious to their family members. The distinction between dementia and DRCI is often difficult to achieve because of the increased comorbidity of affective disorders in MCI and dementias. More recent research has added considerable complexity to the considerations involved in evaluating persons with DRCI. It is widely accepted that during an episode of MDD, patients can show deficits on neuropsychological testing in several domains including selective and sustained attention, alertness as assessed by reaction time tasks, memory, verbal and nonverbal learning, problem solving, planning, and monitoring. Recent data suggest that some deficits, particularly attentional and executive dysfunctions, do not remit in a subset of patients and may increase with recurrent episodes of depression or as the MDD proceeds. It has been postulated that persistent impaired performance in MDD patients experiencing remission could have a trait character.

The neuropsychology of late-life depression is poorly understood and may have some different considerations than its counterpart earlier in life. Impairments on measures of word generation, visuoconstruction, short-term memory, visual memory, executive functioning, and psychomotor and information-processing speed have been reported. Successful treatment of depression results in improvement of cognitive performance yet not necessarily to premorbid levels, particularly in memory and executive domains. A growing body of evidence suggests that late-life depression associated with cognitive dysfunction is due to deficits in frontosubcortical circuitry. Neuroimaging findings suggest a relationship among late-onset depression, executive dysfunction, and white-matter hyperintensities, particularly in the frontal lobe deep white matter and caudate nucleus. Neuropsychological impairments in patients with major depressive symptoms predict a less favorable outcome with antidepressant therapy and cognitive behavior therapy.

Converging evidence suggests that late-onset depressive symptoms may be both a prodrome of and an independent risk factor for cognitive decline as seen in AD and vascular dementia (Saczynski et al., 2010). Late-onset depression is also a risk factor for MCI (Dotson et al., 2010). Four possible mechanisms may underlie the association between depression and dementia/MCI. First, depression may cause cognitive impairment. For example, depression produces excessive release of glucocorticoids which may lead to hippocampal damage. Second, depression may be an emotional reaction on the part of the patient to the onset of dementia. Third, an underlying neurodegenerative process may cause both the depression and the dementia. Fourth, there may be a synergistic interaction between depression and a neurodegenerative process that produces dementia. Although a causal relationship between depression and dementia is speculative at this time, future studies may distinguish between these four possible mechanisms (Geda, 2010).

Delirium

Delirium or acute confusional state is considered to be a subacute- to acute-onset disorder of attentional mechanisms that subsequently affect all other aspects of cognition. Three primary features include disturbance of vigilance, inability to maintain a coherent stream of thought, and difficulty or inability to carry out goal-directed movements. Disturbances in vigilance and behavior may manifest as hyperalertness, agitation, lethargy, or fluctuations in arousal. An impaired sleep/wake cycle is often seen and may be a presenting symptom. Other manifestations may include mild anomia, slurred speech, dysgraphia, dyscalculia, constructional deficits, perceptual distortions leading to illusions and hallucinations (which may be florid and frequently visual), tremor, myoclonus, asterixis, or gait imbalance. Delirium represents one of the most common causes of acute neuropsychiatric disturbances in the hospital setting and is often multifactorial in nature. Advanced age is an independent risk factor for its development, as are metabolic derangements, infections, medications, withdrawal syndromes, toxic exposures, major surgeries, head trauma, other CNS disease, and sensory deprivation (especially impaired eyesight). Focal damage to the following regions may also be associated with a confusional state: unilateral or bilateral fusiform gyri and lingual gyri, nondominant posteroparietal regions, and inferoprefrontal regions. A common comorbidity of delirium is underlying dementia that may or may not have been diagnosed previously. In these patients, return to their predelirium cognitive state may be prolonged or incomplete despite elimination of the offending factor(s). The EEG findings are almost always abnormal, with changes paralleling the degree of behavioral impairment. Early EEG changes show slowing of alpha rhythms, which may be succeeded by further slowing described as medium- to high-voltage generalized activity in the theta-delta range. Triphasic waves may be seen in a number of conditions that commonly include hepatic and renal encephalopathy. Fast rhythms superimposed on slow activity is characteristic of sedative-hypnotic drug ingestion. The EEG is an indispensable tool for diagnosing nonconvulsive status epilepticus causing acute confusional states. Resolution of delirium is reflected by a reversal of these changes, although resolution may lag behind recovery, particularly in the elderly.

Catatonia

Catatonia, once felt to be rare, has been reported to occur among psychiatric inpatients with a prevalence ranging from 7% to 30%. Up to 20% of catatonia in psychiatric inpatients is associated with mania, and 5% to 15% is associated with schizophrenia. In general, catatonia is characterized by motor abnormalities that occur in association with changes in thought, mood, and vigilance. The specific manifestations vary and commonly include mutism, stupor, stereotypies, mannerisms, diminished motor function (including waxy

flexibility or rigidity), staring, negativism, automatic obedience, echopraxia, and echolalia. *Stereotypies* are purposeless repetitions of sounds, words, phrases, or movements. Unexplained foreign accents, whispered or robotic speech, and tiptoe walking have also been observed. There are two principal forms of catatonia: a hypokinetic retarded-stuporous variety and a hyperkinetic excited-delirious variety. Patients with the excited form can present with impulsive or combative behavior that may be difficult to distinguish from mania. If untreated, catatonia may progress to a malignant state marked by fever, hyperexcitability, and autonomic instability, which after several days can be followed by exhaustion, dehydration, coma, cardiac arrest, and death. Although the majority of catatonic patients have an underlying affective (most often mania) or psychotic disorder, some 10% to 20% have significant medical or neurological conditions that contribute to their catatonic state. Stroke, demyelinating disease, encephalitis, head trauma, medications, and CNS malignancy are individually associated with catatonia. Medical disorders that can result in catatonia include heat stroke, autoimmune disease, uremia, hyperthyroidism, diabetic ketoacidosis, porphyria, and Cushing disease. Catatonia has been reported in association with use of illicit recreational drugs, antipsychotics, and opiates, as well as withdrawal from benzodiazepines and dopaminergic drugs. Important considerations in the differential diagnosis include neuroleptic malignant syndrome, serotonin syndrome, and nonconvulsive status epilepticus. Treatment with IV benzodiazepines, IV sodium amobarbital, or ECT can result in dramatic improvement. Bilateral ECT is more effective than unilateral in patients who are febrile, delirious, or do not respond to benzodiazepines (Fink and Taylor, 2009).

Treatment Modalities

Persons with mild to moderate major depression may benefit equally from psychotherapy or medication. Patient preference remains the primary factor in choosing initial therapy. Severely depressed patients benefit more from antidepressant medication, alone or in combination with psychotherapy, than from psychotherapy alone. Three types of psychotherapeutic options have proven to be effective for treatment of depression: CBT, interpersonal therapy (IPT), and problem-solving therapy (PST). The aim of CBT is to modify thoughts and behaviors to yield positive emotions. It may help prevent relapse in patients with a history of recurrent depression. IPT requires the capacity for insight and targets conflicts and role transitions contributing to depression. In PST, patients learn to cope better with specific everyday problems.

Clinicians face a wide array of antidepressant drug options (**Table 9.7**). The most commonly prescribed drugs are the second-generation antidepressants: SSRIs, serotonin and norepinephrine reuptake inhibitors (SNRIs), and bupropion. First-generation antidepressants (tricyclic antidepressants [TCAs] and monoamine oxidase inhibitors [MAOIs]) offer similar effectiveness, but with more toxicity. Generally, TCAs are avoided because of considerable dry mouth, constipation, and dizziness. TCAs are relatively contraindicated in patients with coronary artery disease, congestive heart failure, and arrhythmias. They are also potentially fatal in overdose. MAOIs are also used infrequently, even by psychiatrists, because of the many dietary restrictions and the potential for hypertensive crisis. The selegiline patch (20-mg formulation)

Table 9.7 Medication Treatment for Depression

Agent, Daily Dose*	Benefits/Selected Side Effects
First-Generation Antidepressants:	As a class: dry mouth, dizziness, nausea, sedation, anticholinergic effects, orthostatic hypotension. Contraindicated with MAOIs. Do not use with prolonged QT interval. Use with caution in patients with cardiovascular disease or predisposition to urinary retention or narrow-angle glaucoma. Follow ECGs and orthostatic blood pressure changes.
Amitriptyline, 25-300 mg	May aid with sleep and treat neuropathic pain and migraines. Highly sedating and anticholinergic.
Clomipramine, 25-250 mg	Possibly useful in comorbid anxiety, panic disorders, and OCD.
Desipramine, 25-300 mg	
Imipramine, 25-300 mg	
Protriptyline, 15-60 mg	
MAOIs:	As a class: hypertensive crisis, orthostatic hypotension, insomnia, agitation, sedation, weight change, dry mouth, urinary hesitancy, and sexual dysfunction. Special dietary restrictions except for selegiline patch. Potential severe drug-drug interactions.
Phenelzine, 45-60 mg	
Tranylcypromine, 30-50 mg	
Selegiline transdermal patch, 6-12 mg/day	
Second-Generation Antidepressants:	Nausea, diarrhea, decreased appetite, nervousness, insomnia, somnolence, sweating, impaired sexual function; hyponatremia in the elderly.[†] Contraindicated with MAOIs. Potential for drug interactions with drugs metabolized in liver. Risk/benefit analysis needed in pregnancy.
Bupropion, 200-300 mg	NE/DA reuptake inhibitor. Less weight gain and fewer sexual side effects than other agents.
(75-225mg)	Lowers seizure threshold. Relatively contraindicated in patients with history of seizures, family history of seizures, or head trauma.
Citalopram, 20-40 mg (10-40 mg)	SSRI
Escitalopram, 5-20 mg (5-10 mg)	SSRI; similar to citalopram.
Duloxetine, 30-120 mg	SNRI; may be effective in comorbid pain and depression[‡]
Fluoxetine, 20-40 mg (5-40 mg)	SSRI; long half-life mitigates effects of missed doses. Withdrawal symptoms rare.
Mirtazapine, 15-45 mg (7.5-30 mg)	ARA; increased appetite and somnolence. Use caution with renal impairment. Avoid concomitant benzodiazepines and alcohol.
Paroxetine, 20-40 mg (5-40 mg)	SSRI; more weight gain and sexual adverse events. Withdrawal syndrome not uncommon.
Sertraline, 50-150 mg (25-150 mg)	SSRI
Trazodone, 50-400 mg (50-225 mg)	SRA/A; less effective in doses <300 mg. Somnolence, rare priapism in young men. Useful in low doses (50-100 mg) as a sleeping aid.
Venlafaxine, 75-300 mg (50-225 mg)	SNRI; higher incidence of nausea, vomiting, dry mouth, sexual side effects, and hypertension. Occasional hypertensive urgencies.

ARA, α₂-Receptor antagonist; *ECG*, electrocardiogram; *MAOI*, monoamine oxidase inhibitor; *NDRI*, norepinephrine and dopamine reuptake inhibitor; *OCD*, obsessive compulsive disorder; *SNRI*, serotonin and norepinephrine reuptake inhibitor; *SRA/A*, serotonin receptor antagonists/agonists; *SSRI*, selective serotonin reuptake inhibitor.

*Dose range for geriatric patients is in parentheses.

[†]Wright, S.K., Schroeter, S., 2008. Hyponatremia as a complication of selective serotonin reuptake inhibitors. J Am Acad Nurse Pract 20, 47–51.

[‡]Kroenke, K., Krebs, E.E., Bair, M.J., 2009. Pharmacotherapy of chronic pain: a synthesis of recommendations from systematic reviews. Gen Hosp Psychiatry 31, 206–19.

is a U.S. Food and Drug Administration (FDA)-approved MAOI that does not require dietary tyramine restrictions. Antidepressant selection is based on tolerability, safety, evidence of effectiveness in the patient or a first-degree relative, and cost. The goal of treatment is complete remission of symptoms and return to normal functioning. About 50% of patients achieve full remission with antidepressant therapy, while the other half achieves partial remission or are nonresponders. For the first episode, antidepressant treatment may take 1 to several months until remission is achieved, and medication should be continued for another 4 to 9 months. Some clinicians advocate treatment for at least 1 year to maintain remission for a full annual cycle of holidays and anniversaries. For patients older than 70 years who respond to an SSRI, consider treating for 2 years to prevent recurrence. Increasing the dose of the current medication or changing medications

is often necessary. For a partial response, the dose of the initial agent should be maximized as tolerated before switching to another medication or adding a second drug. When a partial response continues, the clinician can refer for psychotherapy, change antidepressants, or augment treatment with bupropion, mirtazapine, or a nontraditional agent. Compared with withdrawing one drug and initiating another, combination therapy offers faster effects and avoidance of withdrawal symptoms when stopping the first agent. Combinations of MAOIs and either SSRIs or TCAs are not recommended because of an increased risk for serotonin syndrome (with confusion, nausea, autonomic instability, and hyperreflexia). Adding adjunctive atypical antipsychotics, psychostimulants, and thyroid hormone remains controversial. Antipsychotics added to SSRIs for treatment-resistant depression show some benefit but also carry significant risks, so their use should be

Table 9.8 Antipsychotic Side Effects

	EPS	TD	Prolactin Elevation	Anticholinergic SE	Sedation	Weight Gain	Glucose Dysregulation	Dyslipidemia
Chlorpromazine	++	+++	+++	++++	++++	+++	+++	++
Perphenazine	+++	+++	+++	++	++	++	—	+
Haloperidol	++++	+++	+++	—	+	+	—	—
Clozapine	—	—	—	++++	++++	++++	++++	++++
Risperidone	++	+	++++	—	++	++	++	+
Olanzapine	+	+	+	+	+++	++++	++++	++++
Quetiapine	—	?	—	++*	+++	++	+++	+++

Adapted from Goff, D.C., Freudenreich, O., Henderson, D.C., 2008. Antipsychotic drugs. In: Stern, T.A., Rosenbaum, J.F., Fava, M., Rauch, S.L., et al. (Eds.), *Comprehensive Clinical Psychiatry*, first ed. Mosby, Philadelphia, pp. 577-594.

EPS, Extrapyramidal symptoms; *SE*, side effects; *TD*, tardive dyskinesia.

*Possibly not mediated via muscarinic acetylcholine receptors.

Key: — = negligible or absent association; + = low; ++ = moderate; +++ = high; ++++ = very high.

limited to psychiatrists (Shelton and Papakostas, 2008). A Cochrane review of monotherapy treatment with psychostimulants (dexamphetamine, methylphenidate, methyl amphetamine, and pemoline) for moderate to severe depression found short-term improvement in depression symptoms and fatigue (Candy et al., 2008). A second review of 19 controlled trials on adults older than 65 years supported this recommendation for methylphenidate (Hardy, 2009).

Studies are conflicting about the effectiveness of adding thyroid hormone (triiodothyronine [T_3] and levothyroxine [T_4]) to antidepressants. More research is needed before these therapies can be recommended. Augmentation with other nontraditional agents has also shown mixed results: omega-3 fatty acids added to sertraline in patients with coronary heart disease did not improve depressive outcomes (Carney et al., 2009). For seasonal depression, light therapy, 6000 to 10,000 lux for 30 to 90 minutes each morning may be helpful (Golden et al., 2005). Yoga, exercise (Mead et al., 2009), self-help books, and relaxation therapy (Morgan and Jorm, 2008) may also be useful. Specific types of side effects are more common with particular drugs and should guide choice of medications (see **Table 9.7**). Sexual side effects of SSRIs include decreased libido or interest (men and women), anorgasmia (women), and delayed ejaculation (men). To address these side effects, consider pretreatment counseling, switching to a drug with a different mechanism of action (e.g., bupropion, mirtazapine), or using sildenafil for SSRI-associated erectile dysfunction if there are no contraindications. Switching to bupropion can reduce undesired weight gain. Agitation or excessive activation may occur with fluoxetine and warrants a switch to a different SSRI.

Treatment for schizophrenia is most successful when antipsychotic medications are combined with psychological and social supports. These supports may include CBT, vocational interventions, and the use of multidisciplinary mental health professional teams who work with the patient and caregivers inside and outside the hospital to insure health and social care (van Os and Kapur, 2009). CBT may improve coping and reduce distress and affective symptoms associated with psychotic symptoms. Despite these interventions, about one-third may remain symptomatic. All antipsychotics share varying degrees of striatal D_2 receptor blockade. The first-generation antipsychotics (e.g., haloperidol, perphenazine, chlorpromazine) possess equivalent efficacy but differ in potency and side effects. All potentially produce extrapyramidal symptoms (EPS), tardive dyskinesia, and hyperprolactinemia. The second-generation antipsychotics (e.g., clozapine, risperidone, olanzapine, quetiapine), also known as *atypical antipsychotics*, generally produce fewer EPS, less risk of tardive dyskinesia, and less hyperprolactinemia. **Table 9.8** lists selected antipsychotic side effects. Some atypical antipsychotics such as clozapine and olanzapine have been associated with weight gain, impairment of glucose metabolism, and dyslipidemia. Clozapine has greater efficacy than first-generation drugs but requires regular blood test monitoring throughout the course of treatment owing to an increased risk for agranulocytosis (1%-4%). Risperidone is known for its association with hyperprolactinemia. The primary symptom targets for antipsychotics are psychotic symptoms, agitation, and negative symptoms (e.g., apathy, social withdrawal, diminished affect). Response times for psychotic symptoms may range from responding within hours of administration to several weeks of administration. Maximal response may require months. Some patients are nonresponders. Agitation responds well to most antipsychotics, but negative symptoms generally respond only modestly.

Electroconvulsive Therapy

MDD is the most common indication for ECT. The mechanisms by which this procedure alleviates depressive symptoms are not fully understood. Remission rates of 70% to 90% have been reported in clinical trials of ECT for MDD (Popeo, 2009). It is also an effective treatment for bipolar disorder but may uncommonly precipitate hypomania or mania. Suicidal thoughts respond favorably to ECT and are an indication for early transition from drug therapy. ECT is not routinely used for treatment of schizophrenia, but when combined with antipsychotic medications, it may result in improvement in 80% of drug-resistant chronic schizophrenia patients. Patients with mania also respond favorably to ECT. There are few absolute contraindications to ECT, but cardiac conditions may worsen and should be addressed. Conditions such as vascular aneurysms and aortic stenosis should preferably be repaired prior to ECT, but persons with such conditions have been reported to tolerate the procedure. Those with properly functioning cardiac pacemakers generally tolerate ECT well. Case reports of ECT performed on individuals with a recent cerebral infarction suggest a low complication rate and a favorable response to treatment. ECT has been successfully used in persons with mental retardation, MS, HD, arteriovenous malformations, and hydrocephalus. Patients with depression and PD may experience improvement of mood and motor symptoms with ECT. Some research supports the effectiveness of ECT for treatment of the core motor symptoms of PD (Popeo and Kellner, 2009). There is no evidence of structural brain damage due to ECT. Posttreatment memory difficulty (anterograde amnesia) is usually experienced during the course of ECT treatments but normally resolves within one month after the last treatment. Retrograde amnesia is more prominent for the events closer to the time of ECT treatment. Posttreatment confusion is variable and may be associated with bilateral electrode placement, high stimulus intensity, prolonged seizure activity, and inadequate oxygenation. There is controversy about whether unilateral electrode placement for ECT is as effective as bilateral placement. Several studies have shown equal efficacy so long as unilateral ECT is performed with a stimulus intensity well above seizure threshold (Lisanby, 2007). Studies also indicate a lower incidence of cognitive side effects with right unilateral electrode placement and electrical brief pulse waveform stimulus. There is uncertainty about the efficacy of ultra-brief pulse stimulus, but preliminary evidence suggests it is associated with a significant reduction in memory-related side effects (Peterchev et al., 2010).

Vagus Nerve Stimulation

The FDA approved vagus nerve stimulation (VNS) for treatment-refractory depression (TRD) in July 2005. Consensus criteria are unavailable for what constitutes TRD. Interest in VNS as a treatment for depression arose when it was noticed that persons being treated with VNS for treatment-resistant epilepsy (which is associated with an increased prevalence of depression) experienced improvements in their mood. Long-term studies of VNS for use as an adjunct to medications and therapy showed that it was well tolerated and resulted in a successful response in one-half of patients and complete remission in one-third (Andrade et al., 2010). The mechanism of VNS's effects are not completely understood. It is believed that input information from the vagus nerve projects to the solitary tract nucleus and follows an ascending pathway to modulate various structures such as the amygdala, dorsal raphe, locus coeruleus, and the ventromedial prefrontal cortex that produce its effects on mood. The solitary tract nucleus also communicates with the parabrachial nucleus (PBN), cerebellum, and periaquaductal gray matter. The PBN communicates with other regions implicated in the pathophysiology of depression such as the hypothalamus, thalamus, amygdala, and nucleus of the stria terminalis. Only the left vagus nerve is used for VNS, because the right vagus nerve has parasympathetic branches to the heart. Aside from standard surgical risks, the most common side effects are voice alteration (54%-60% of patients), cough, neck pain, paresthesia, and dyspnea. These side effects typically decrease over time. It is recommended that VNS be used as an adjunctive treatment to medications and psychotherapy. Right unilateral ECT has been well tolerated in persons with VNS (Sharma et al., 2009).

Repetitive Transcranial Magnetic Stimulation

Repetitive transcranial magnetic stimulation (rTMS) is an emerging and recently FDA-approved noninvasive, well-tolerated treatment modality for MDD in adults. It is being studied for potential therapeutic applications in OCD, post-traumatic stress disorder, and auditory hallucinations in schizophrenia. The rTMS procedure uses a pulsed magnetic field introduced on the scalp surface to generate focal electrical stimulation of the cortical surface; it does not require anesthesia, does not produce a seizure, and can be administered in the office setting. The mechanism of action for treatment of depression is not well understood. The rTMS field can be pulsed at different frequencies to produce excitatory or inhibitory effects on cortical neurons. Frequencies of less than or equal to 1 Hz (slow rTMS) are believed to have mostly inhibitory neuronal effects by means of preferentially activating GABA-ergic interneurons in the cortex; this may result in transsynaptic depression. Use of rTMS frequencies greater than 1 Hz (fast rTMS) are believed to have mostly glutamatergic or excitatory neuronal effects (Kim et al., 2009). In depression, the target area is the left DLPFC. Left DLPFC high-frequency rTMS has shown effectiveness in almost one-third of pharmacotherapy-resistant MDD patients (Andrade et al., 2010). Headaches and site application pain are the most common side effects; the risk for seizure is estimated at less than 1 per 10,000 rTMS sessions. Monotherapy with rTMS is associated with few adverse effects but significant antidepressant effects for unipolar depressed patients who do not respond to medications or who cannot tolerate them (George et al., 2010).

Psychiatric Neurosurgery or Psychosurgery

Neurosurgical procedures are not commonly used for treatment of neuropsychiatric symptoms but should be considered for selected conditions when patients have failed combined pharmacotherapy and psychotherapy. Psychosurgery, both ablative and by deep brain stimulation, is still experimental and should be performed at institutions supporting psychosurgery research, having multidisciplinary involvement, and appropriate follow-up. In the middle of the 20th century, procedures such as frontal lobotomy were performed without defined indications or an understanding of the limbic system. This resulted in severe adverse events, even death. During the latter half of the 20th century, smaller stereotactically targeted lesions were used, resulting in benefits for patients, useful research data, and a precipitous decline in adverse events. Currently used ablative procedures include anterior cingulotomy, subcaudate tractotomy, limbic leucotomy (combined anterior cingulotomy and subcaudate tractotomy), and anterior capsulotomy. Carefully selected patients with intractable mood and anxiety disorders have experienced response rates ranging from 30% to 70%. Postoperative side effects are mostly transient and include headache, nausea, and edema. More serious adverse events include infection, urinary dysfunction, seizures, cognitive deficits, and cerebral infarct or hemorrhage (Andrade, 2010).

Deep brain stimulation involves the placement of electrodes into targeted deep brain regions so electrical stimulation can be delivered. Its advantages over ablative procedures are its adjustability (by manipulation of stimulation parameters) and reversibility. Published brain targets include the subcallosal cingulate gyrus (Hamani et al., 2009), nucleus accumbens, ventral internal capsule/ventral striatum, inferior thalamic peduncle, and lateral habenula. Response rates for MDD range from 35% to 50% (Blomstedt et al., 2010). Targets for OCD include the anterior limb of the internal capsule, ventral striatum, nucleus accumbens, or subthalamic nucleus (Denys et al., 2010). Transient hypomania may occur with deep brain stimulation for OCD. Response rates for OCD range from 20% to 75% (Haynes and Mallet, 2010). Nine brain regions have been targeted for treatment of Gilles de la Tourette syndrome, with in most cases some diminution of tics (Hariz and Robertson, 2010; Porta et al., 2009). The effects on other neuropsychiatric comorbidities are uncertain.

Treatment Principles

The unique features of each condition discussed should be carefully taken into account when developing a treatment plan. Transient, progressive, or static impairments in abilities such as driving, medical decision making, and management of finances may be present. Increased vigilance when monitoring patients for these impairments may improve care and allow for earlier interventions to protect the welfare of the patient, their family, and society. Patients with underlying neurological conditions tend to be more susceptible to the adverse reactions of psychotropic medications, particularly to extrapyramidal and cognitive side effects. These adverse reactions tend to be minimized with initiation of medications at low doses and use of gentle titration. When clinically indicated, atypical antipsychotics are often preferred over typical agents because of their fewer adverse side effects, but longitudinal studies are needed to better confirm this impression (Lieberman et al., 2005; Tarsy and Baldessarini, 2006). Further options to consider for treatment of refractory primary depression and other carefully selected psychiatric conditions include ECT, VNS (Elger et al., 2000; Groves and Brown, 2005; Marangell et al., 2002; Rush et al., 2000), transcranial magnetic stimulation (Rosa et al., 2006), deep brain stimulation (Skidmore et al., 2006), or stereotactic ablative surgery (Dougherty et al., 2002, 2003; Montoya et al., 2002b; Price et al., 2001). There is currently little evidence to guide the optimal treatment approach for patients with neurological disease and comorbid psychiatric symptoms.

In conclusion, advances in neuroscience have improved our understanding of the neural substrates of cognition and emotional behavior. The traditional boundaries between neurology and psychiatry have become obsolete. The future of psychiatric and neurological care, training, and research will inevitably require effective collaboration between both disciplines (Cunningham et al., 2006; Price et al., 2000).

References

The complete reference list is available online at www.expertconsult.com.

Chapter 10

Limb Apraxias and Related Disorders

Mario F. Mendez, Po-Heng Tsai

Apraxia is an inability to correctly perform learned skilled movements. In the limb apraxias, there is an inability to correctly execute these movements in an arm or hand owing to neurological dysfunction. Apraxia is a cognitive deficit in motor programming and results in errors of either the spatiotemporal processing of the movements or in the content of the actions. In the context of an apraxia examination, these errors can help distinguish the major types of limb apraxias.

A first step in recognizing the limb apraxias is distinguishing them from other causes of impaired movement. First of all, it is not apraxia if the impaired movements result from elementary motor deficits such as weakness, hemipareses, spasticity, ataxia, or extrapyramidal disturbances. Second, apraxia is distinguishable from impaired movements due to primary sensory deficits, hemispatial neglect, spatial or object agnosia, or other complex visual disorder. Third, apraxia is distinct from abnormal movements or postures such as tremor, myoclonus, choreoathetosis, or dystonic posturing. Finally, it is not apraxia if the impaired movements result from other cognitive disorders involving attention, memory, language comprehension, or executive functions (Leiguarda and Marsden, 2000). Although these sensorimotor and cognitive disorders may coexist with limb apraxia, the clinician must first ascertain whether they account for the patient's inability to perform learned skilled movements.

Limb apraxia is not rare or insignificant. Apraxia occurs in about 50% to 80% of patients with left hemisphere lesions and can persist as a chronic deficit in 40% to 50% of these. Limb apraxia often results in major functional impairment, even when subtle, as it affects critical movements of the arms, hands, and fingers. Limb apraxia correlates with the level of caregiver dependence and greater need for help with activities of daily living (ADLs). It can also interfere with rehabilitation and therapy, including occupational therapy, physical therapy, and the use of gestural communication in aphasia rehabilitation.

Despite its importance, clinicians often fail to recognize limb apraxia. In many left hemisphere strokes, right hemiparesis masks the presence of right limb apraxia, and the assumption of normal non-dominant hand clumsiness masks the presence of left limb apraxia. Even when there are no masking factors, the presence of limb apraxia may still go undetected. Many examiners do not evaluate patients for limb apraxia, do not know how to test for apraxia, or cannot recognize the spatiotemporal or content errors produced by this condition. Yet apraxia is part of the diagnostic criteria of Alzheimer disease and corticobasal syndrome, as well as a manifestation of many other disorders.

This chapter is about the limb apraxias. The term *apraxia* occurs broadly in neurology and is usually interchangeable with *dyspraxia*. Apraxia describes non-learned motor dysfunctions including oculomotor movements, gait initiation (magnetic apraxia), and eyelid opening. It also describes skilled motor tasks that are dependent on visuospatial processing, including optic, constructional, and dressing apraxia. *Apraxia* is used as well for conditions that are more clearly consistent with the definition of disturbances in learned skilled movements but involve body parts other than the limbs, including orobucchal-facial and speech apraxias. These clinical entities are not included in this chapter, because they

DOI: 10.1016/B978-1-4377-0434-1.00010-4

are either not limb apraxias or not disorders of "praxis" in the sense of disturbances in learned skilled movements (Zadikoff and Lang, 2005). This chapter focuses on the seven major limb apraxias of the upper extremities, where apraxia is most evident. They include ideomotor apraxia, parietal variant; ideomotor apraxia, disconnection variant; dissociation apraxia; ideational apraxia; and conceptual apraxia. Also included is limb-kinetic apraxia, a disorder that some argue is not a true apraxia, but instead a more basic disturbance in fine motor movements. Callosal apraxias comprise a separate category because of their unique unilateral and varied manifestations.

Historical Perspective

Many clinicians and investigators helped develop the current concept of limb apraxia. In 1866, John Hughlings Jackson probably recognized the clinical phenomenon of apraxia in a patient (Pearce, 2009). Jackson observed that the patient had "power in his muscles and in the centres for coordination of muscular groups, but he – the whole man, or the 'will' – cannot set them agoing." In 1870, Carl Maria Finkelnburg used "asymbolia" to describe the clumsy and incomprehensible communicative gestures in aphasics, and in 1890, Meynert distinguished motor asymbolia from decreased motor "images" for movement. In 1899, D. De Buck used "parakinesia" to describe a patient who "though retaining the concepts for her actions, did not succeed in awakening the corresponding kinetic image." By this time, the stage was set for Hugo Karl Liepmann's seminal model of the limb apraxias.

In the early 1900s, Liepmann published a series of papers that led to the contemporary concept of limb apraxias. He proposed that the execution of purposeful movements could be divided into three steps (Goldenberg, 2003). First is the retrieval of the spatial and temporal representation or "movement formulas" of the intended action from the left hemisphere. Second is the transfer and association of these movement formulas via cortical connections with the "innervatory patterns" or motor programs located in the left "sensomotorium" (which includes premotor and supplementary motor areas). Third is the transmission of the information to the left primary motor cortex for performance of the intended actions in the right limb. Finally, in order for the left limb to perform the movements, the information traverses the corpus callosum to the right sensomotorium to activate the right primary motor cortex. Using Heymann Steinthal's term of "apraxia," Liepmann classified disturbances in these connections as "ideational, ideo-kinetic (melokinetic), and limb-kinetic apraxia." Over the years, this classification nomenclature has evolved and the application of these terms has shifted, but Liepmann's basic formulation of apraxia has persisted to the present day.

A Model for Praxis

The left parietal region retains its central role of converting mental images of intended action into motor execution (Heilman and Rothi, 2003) (**Fig. 10.1**). The inferior parietal lobule contains the spatial and temporal movement programs (praxicons, visuokinesthetic motor engrams, or movement formulas) needed to carry out learned skilled movements.

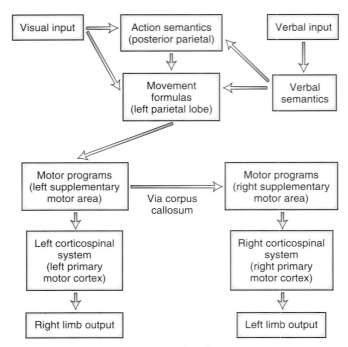

Fig. 10.1 A model of praxis.

Multiple input modalities including visual, verbal-auditory, and tactile can activate these movement formulas. Cells in the inferior parietal lobule fire selectively in response to hand movements, visually presented information about object size and shape, or the actual manipulation of objects (Rizzolatti et al., 1998), and functional neuroimaging studies show activity of this region in response to recognition of actions associated with object or tool use (transitive actions) (Damasio et al., 2001). The right parietal lobe participates in the integration of visual information and upper-extremity movement. In addition to movement formulas, the left parietal region appears to contain action semantics and conceptual systems such as tool action, tool-object association information, and general principles of tool use (Goldenberg and Spatt, 2009; Ochipa et al., 1992). If a movement involves the use of a tool or object, action semantics specify knowledge of tool action (turning, pounding, etc.) and the knowledge of which tool or object to use to choose for a task (Leiguarda and Marsden, 2000).

In the premotor region, the supplementary motor area (SMA) translates the movement formulas into motor programs before sending them on to primary motor cortex (Roy and Square, 1985). The SMA, which is involved in complex movements of the upper extremities, receives projections from parietal neurons and in turn projects axons to motor neurons in the primary motor cortex. The SMA programs a specific order of movements and is involved in bimanual coordination. It translates these time-space movement formulas to specific motor programs that activate the motor neurons such that the contralateral extremity moves in the proscribed spatial trajectory and timing. For movements in the opposite extremity, the brain further conveys these programs across the corpus callosum to the opposite premotor cortex and activates the motor neurons for the desired contralateral extremity movements.

Beyond this traditional model for praxis, apraxia may result from damage in other regions including the prefrontal cortex, right hemisphere, basal ganglia (putamen and globus pallidus), thalamus, and their white-matter connections. The prefrontal region participates in sequencing multiple arm, hand, and finger movements. The right parietal region participates in performing nonpurposeful movements. Although the left inferior parietal lobule is more active than the right during action imagery and actual discrimination of nonpurposeful gestures, the right parietal region is more active during imitation and when these gestures consist of finger postures (Buccino et al., 2001; Hermsdorfer et al., 2001). The role of basal ganglia and thalamus is less clear, but they function as part of cortical-subcortical motor loops. Apraxia could, theoretically, result from damage to any of these areas outside the traditional model of praxis.

Classification of Limb Apraxias

Beginning with Liepmann, there have been multiple attempts to classify and define the limb apraxias (Hanna-Pladdy and Rothi, 2001). The classification presented here is based on the seminal work of Heilman and associates, who have significantly contributed to the understanding of the limb apraxias (Heilman and Rothi, 2003). Depending on the location of the lesion, the patient has different patterns of ability to imitate and recognize gestures, perform sequential movements, and do fine motor activities (**Fig. 10.2**). The presence of production and content errors further characterize the subtypes of limb apraxia.

Ideomotor Apraxia, Parietal Variant

The parietal variant of ideomotor apraxia may be the most common and prototypical limb apraxia. Disruption of the movement formulas in the inferior parietal lobule impairs

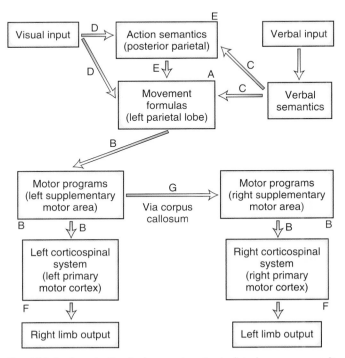

Fig. 10.2 Lesions in the limb apraxias. Praxis disturbances can result from various brain localizations as illustrated below. **A,** Ideomotor apraxia – parietal variant. **B,** Ideomotor apraxia – disconnection variant. **C,** Verbal dissociation apraxia. **D,** Visual dissociation apraxia. **E,** Conceptual apraxia. **F,** Limb-kinetic apraxia. **G,** Callosal apraxia.

skilled movements on command and to imitation, as well as the recognition of gestures (see **Fig. 10.2, A**). Patients make spatial and temporal errors while producing movements. There is a failure to adopt the correct posture or orientation of the arm and hand or to move the limb correctly in space and at the correct speeds. Spatial errors involve the configuration of the hand and fingers, the proper orientation of the limb to the tool or object, and the spatial trajectory of the motion. A major distinguishing feature of the parietal variant of ideomotor apraxia is difficulty recognizing or identifying gestures, implicating damage to the praxicons, visuokinesthetic motor engrams, or movement formulas themselves.

Ideomotor Apraxia, Disconnection Variant

The disconnection variant of ideomotor apraxia results from disruptions of motor programs in the SMA or in their intra- and interhemispheric connections (Heilman and Watson, 2008). This form of ideomotor apraxia is a disconnection of an intact parietal region from the pathways to primary motor cortices. These lesions result in impaired pantomime to verbal commands, impaired imitation of gestures, and the presence of spatiotemporal production errors. The movement formulas themselves are preserved, but in contrast to the parietal variant of ideomotor apraxia, these patients can recognize and identify gestures. The lesions lie along the route from the left inferior parietal cortex to primary motor cortices (see **Fig. 10.2, B**). Although SMA lesions tend to affect both upper extremities, if the SMA lesion is limited to the right, apraxia may be limited to the left upper extremity.

Dissociation Apraxia

Patients with dissociation apraxia only exhibit errors when the movement is evoked by stimuli in one specific modality, usually verbal. Dissociation apraxia is a special type of disconnection apraxia where the disconnection is between language areas and movement formulas in the inferior parietal lobule. Information, however, can reach the inferior parietal lobe via other input modalities than language. Patients with dissociation apraxia may be impaired when attempting to perform skilled movements in response to verbal commands, but they are able to imitate gestures and to indicate or use actual objects correctly. Their errors are often unrecognizable movements rather than spatiotemporal or content errors. In addition to verbal dissociation apraxia (see **Fig. 10.2, C**), there can be visual (see **Fig. 10.2, D**) and tactile dissociation apraxias as well.

Ideational Apraxia

Ideational apraxia is the inability to correctly order or sequence a series of movements to achieve a goal. It is a disturbance in an overall ideational action plan. When these patients are given components necessary to complete a multistep task, they have trouble carrying out the steps in the proper order, such as preparing, addressing, and then mailing a letter. The lesion responsible for ideational apraxias is not clear; the deficits usually occur in patients with diffuse cerebral processes such as dementia, delirium, or extensive lesions in the left hemisphere that involve the frontal lobe and SMA. Unfortunately, use of the term *ideational apraxia* has been confusing, with the term erroneously applied to conceptual apraxia and other disorders. Ideational apraxia is not a conceptual problem in the proper application or use of tools or objects, but rather a problem in sequencing of actions in multistep behaviors.

Conceptual Apraxia

Conceptual apraxia results in errors in content of the action, such as in tool-selection errors or in tool-object knowledge. Whereas dysfunction of praxis production results in ideomotor apraxia, defects in the conceptual knowledge needed to successfully select tools and objects results in conceptual apraxia. Although conceptual apraxia often co-occurs with ideomotor apraxia, it can occur by itself, indicating that praxis production and praxis conceptual systems are independent. Patients with conceptual apraxia are unable to name or point to a tool when its function is discussed, or recall the type of actions associated with specific tools, utensils, or objects. They make content errors in which they substitute the action associated with the wrong tool for the requested tool. For example, when asked to demonstrate the use of a hammer or a saw either by pantomiming or using the tool, the patient with the loss of tool-object action knowledge may pantomime a screwing twisting movement as if using a screwdriver. Other terms used to describe these errors include *disturbances in mechanical knowledge* or *in action semantics* (see **Fig. 10.2, *E***). Conceptual apraxia is most common in Alzheimer disease, other dementias (Ochipa et al., 1992), and in patients with diffuse posterior cerebral lesions, particularly involving the left hemisphere.

Limb-Kinetic Apraxia

Limb-kinetic apraxia is the inability to make finely graded, precise, coordinated individual finger movements. Limb-kinetic apraxia may not be a real apraxia in the traditional definition, but it is prominently considered in the differential diagnosis of the limb apraxias. Patients with limb-kinetic apraxia complain of a loss of dexterity or deftness that makes fine motor movements such as buttoning or tying shoes difficult. Weakness or changes in muscle tone do not account for this "clumsiness," and limb-kinetic apraxia may be intermediate between paresis and other limb apraxias. Limb-kinetic apraxia is usually confined to the limb contralateral to a hemispheric lesion; however, when limb-kinetic apraxia occurs in the preferred hand, it may also be present in the non-preferred hand (Hanna-Pladdy et al., 2002). Clinicians need to distinguish limb-kinetic apraxia from right parietal functions such as nonsymbolic gestures (e.g., copying meaningless fine finger movements) and from optic ataxia, or decreased coordination of the hands under visual guidance. Limb-kinetic apraxia results from lesions in the primary motor cortex or corticospinal system (see **Fig. 10.2, *F***). Liepmann (1920) also thought that limb-kinetic apraxia could result from lesions in the sensory motor cortex, and Kleist (1931) attributed it to damage in the premotor areas.

Callosal Apraxia

Several limb apraxia syndromes can result from callosal lesions (see **Fig. 10.2, *G***). What distinguishes these patients is that their apraxia is confined to the non-dominant limb, usually the left arm or hand in right-handed individuals. The right limb may be affected in left-handed individuals, or they may have a similar lateralization as right-handers. Liepmann and others described left-sided disconnection-variant ideomotor apraxia due to callosal lesions and strokes (Heilman and Watson, 2008). These patients cannot pantomime with their left hand to verbal command or imitate but can recognize and identify gestures. Others described left-sided dissociative apraxia due to callosal lesions (Gazzaniga et al., 1967; Geschwind and Kaplan, 1962). Patients who have had surgical disconnection of the corpus callosum could not gesture normally to command with their left arm and hand but performed well with imitation and actual tools. Some patients have had a combination of both ideomotor and dissociative apraxia of their left arm and hand manifested by unrecognizable movements on verbal command and spatiotemporal errors on imitation. Other patients have a callosal "alien limb" with independent movements of the non-dominant limb, sometimes with "diagonistic apraxia" or the intermanual conflict of the hands acting in opposition to each other. The classic example of this is the split-brain patient who has undergone a corpus callosotomy who finds that his or her left hand is unbuttoning his shirt or blouse while the right one is trying to button it. Finally, there is a rare description of callosal lesions resulting in conceptual apraxia, indicating that conceptual knowledge as well as movement formulas have lateralized representations, and that such representations are contralateral to the preferred hand (Heilman et al., 1997).

Testing for Limb Apraxias

Apraxia testing involves a systematic approach (**Box 10.1**). Prior to testing of praxis, a neurological examination excludes the presence of significant motor, sensory, or cognitive disorders that could explain the inability to perform learned skilled movements. First, the testing of praxis itself begins with asking the patient to pantomime to command. The movements are transitive (associated with tool or instrument use) and intransitive (associated with communicative gestures such as waving goodbye). For transitive movements, the examiner asks the patient to demonstrate how to comb their hair, brush their teeth, or use a pair of scissors. For intransitive movements, the examiner asks the patient to demonstrate how to wave goodbye, beckon somebody to come, or hitchhike. The testing involves the right and left limb independently. The examiner observes the patient for the presence of temporal-spatial or content errors. Second, if the patient has difficulty pantomiming movements, the examiner tests their ability to imitate gestures. For gesture imitation, the examiner performs both transitive and intransitive movements and asks the patient to copy the movements. Third, for gesture knowledge, the examiner performs the same transitive and intransitive gestures and asks the patient to identify the gesture. The patient must identify the gesture and discriminate between those that are well and poorly performed. Fourth, the patient must perform tasks that require several motor acts in sequence, such as making a sandwich or preparing a letter for mailing. Fifth, the examiner shows the patient pictures of tools or objects or the actual tools or objects themselves. The examiner then requests that the patient pantomime the action associated with the tool or object. Finally, the examiner checks for fine finger movements by asking the patient to do repetitive tapping, picking up a coin with a pincer grasp, and twirling

Box 10.1 The Examination for Limb Apraxias

I. DOMINANT UPPER EXTREMITY
  1. PANTOMIME TO VERBAL COMMAND
    a. Transitive actions:
       Comb hair
       Brush teeth
       Flip a coin
       Use scissors
       Use a hammer
       Use a screwdriver
    b. Intransitive actions:
       Wave goodbye
       Beckon someone to come
       Indicate someone to stop
       Salute
       Show how to hitchhike
       Give the victory sign
  2. IMITATION OF GESTURES
    The examiner demonstrates the same actions without naming them and asks the patient to copy them.
  3. GESTURE KNOWLEDGE
    The examiner demonstrates different actions and asks the patient to identify their function/purpose and how well they were performed.
  4. SEQUENTIAL ACTIONS
    The examiner asks the patient to show how to prepare a letter for mailing, a sandwich for lunch, a pipe for smoking. The examiner instructs the patient that the imaginary elements needed for the task are laid out in front of them.
  5. CONCEPTUAL KNOWLEDGE
    The examiner show the patient either pictures or the actual tools or objects and asks the patient to pantomime or demonstrate their use or function. The examiner may also show a task, such as holding a nail, and ask the patient to pantomime the correct tool use and action.
  6. LIMB-KINETIC MOVEMENTS
    Finger tapping
    Alternate touching each finger tip with thumb
    Pick up a coin without sliding
    Twirl coin between thumb, index, and middle fingers
  7. REAL OBJECT USE
    If limb apraxia is present, test with real object use. Most limb apraxias improve when using real objects for transitive actions and when gesturing spontaneously with intransitive actions.
II. NON-DOMINANT UPPER EXTREMITY
  The examiner repeats the same procedures as for the dominant upper extremity.

the coin. Additional impairment in the patient's ability to use real objects indicates marked severity of the limb apraxia. The pattern of deficits will determine the types of apraxia (**Table 10.1**). Specialists in occupational therapy, physical therapy, speech pathology, and neuropsychology can further assess and quantify the deficits in limb apraxia using instruments like the Apraxia Battery for Adults-2 and the Florida Apraxia Battery (Power et al., 2010).

Testing for Ideomotor Apraxia, Parietal and Disconnection Variants

Patients with the ideomotor apraxias cannot pantomime to command or imitate the examiner's gestures. These patients improve only partially with intransitive acts, imitation, and real object use. Ideomotor apraxia results in spatiotemporal errors in the positioning and orientation of the arm, hand, and fingers to the target and in the timing of the movements, but the goal of the action is still recognizable. In addition to poor positioning of the limb in relation to an imagined object, patients with ideomotor apraxia have an incorrect trajectory of their limb through space owing to poor coordination of multiple joint movements. Patients with ideomotor apraxia also have hesitant, stuttered movements rather than smooth, effortless ones. Unlike patients with the parietal variant of ideomotor apraxia, patients with the disconnection variant can both comprehend gestures and pantomimes and discriminate between correctly and incorrectly performed pantomimes.

On attempting to pantomime, patients with ideomotor apraxia may substitute a body part for the tool or object (Raymer et al., 1997). For example, when attempting to pantomime combing their hair or brushing their teeth, they substitute their fingers for the comb or toothbrush. Normal subjects may make the same errors, so the examiner should ask patients not to substitute their fingers or other body parts but to pantomime using a "pretend tool." Patients with ideomotor apraxia may not improve with these instructions and continue to make body-part substitution errors. The substitution of a body part for a tool or object activates the right inferior parietal lobe, hence patients with ideomotor apraxia with left parietal injury appear to be using their normal right parietal lobe in order to pantomime gestures (Ohgami et al., 2004).

Testing for Dissociation Apraxia

The testing for dissociation apraxia is the same as for ideomotor apraxia. An important feature of dissociation apraxia when attempting to pantomime is the absence of recognizable movements. When asked to pantomime to verbal command, some patients may look at their hands but fail to perform any pertinent actions. Unlike patients with ideomotor apraxia, however, these patients can imitate the use of objects. Given the language-motor disconnection, it is important to evaluate the patient for language disorders and to exclude aphasia. Similar defects in other modalities are possible as well. For example, some patients who are asked to pantomime in response to visual or tactile stimuli may be unable to do so but can correctly pantomime to verbal command.

Testing for Ideational Apraxia

The test for ideational apraxia involves pantomiming multi-step sequential tasks to verbal command. Examples are asking the patient to demonstrate how to prepare a letter for mailing or a sandwich for lunch. The examiner instructs the patient that the imaginary elements needed for the task are laid out in front of them; the patient is then observed to see whether the correct sequence of events is performed. Ideational apraxia manifests as a failure to perform each step in the correct order. If disturbed, the examiner repeats this testing with a real object, such as providing the patient with a letter and stamp.

Table 10.1 Testing in Limb Apraxias

	Ideomotor-Parietal	Ideomotor-Disconnection1	Dissociation1	Ideational	Conceptual1	Limb-Kinetic
Pantomime to verbal command	Abnormal2	Abnormal2	Abnormal3	Normal4	Abnormal5	Normal
Imitation of gestures	Abnormal2	Abnormal2	Normal	Normal4	Normal	Normal6
Gesture knowledge	Abnormal	Normal	Normal	Normal	Normal	Normal
Sequential actions	Normal2	Normal	Abnormal	Abnormal	Abnormal	Normal
Conceptual knowledge of tool use	Normal	Normal	Normal	Abnormal Normal4	Abnormal	Normal
Limb-kinetic movement	Normal	Normal	Normal	Normal	Normal	Abnormal
Real object use	Normal/Abnormal7	Normal/Abnormal7	Normal	Normal/Abnormal7	Abnormal5	Normal/Abnormal7

1 Callosal apraxia, which is limited to the non-dominant limb, can present as disconnection-variant ideomotor apraxia, a dissociative apraxia, or (rarely) a conceptual apraxia.
2 Spatiotemporal production errors on single, individual ideomotor tasks.
3 Unrecognizable movements or attempts.
4 Errors on performing sequential actions only (i.e., individual actions and their conceptual knowledge are normal).
5 Content and tool use errors on individual ideomotor tasks.
6 Decreased dexterity in fine finger movements.
7 Errors depend on severity. In general, errors are worse with verbal commands>imitation>real spontaneous object use and worse for transitive than intransitive actions.

Testing for Conceptual Apraxia

Patients with conceptual apraxia make content errors and demonstrate the actions of tools or objects other than the one they were asked to pantomime. For example, the examiner shows the patient either pictures or the actual tools or objects and asks the patient to pantomime or demonstrate their use or function. Patients with conceptual apraxia pantomime the wrong use or function, but they are able to imitate gestures without spatiotemporal errors (see **Table 10.2**).

Testing for Limb-Kinetic Apraxia

For limb-kinetic apraxia testing, the examiner asks the patient to perform fine finger movements and looks for evidence of incoordination. For example, the examiner asks the patient to pick up a small coin such as a dime from the table with the thumb and the index finger only. Normally, people use the pincer grasp to pick up a dime by putting a forefinger on one edge of the coin and the thumb on the opposite edge. Patients with limb-kinetic apraxia will have trouble doing this without sliding the coin to the edge of the table or using multiple fingers. Another test involves the patient rotating a nickel between the thumb, index, and middle fingers 10 times as rapidly as they can. Patients with limb-kinetic apraxia are slow and clumsy at these tasks (Hanna-Pladdy et al., 2002).

Testing for Callosal Apraxia

The examination for callosal apraxias is the same as for the other limb apraxias except that the abnormalities are limited to the non-dominant hand in most cases. The testing for cal-losal apraxia may reveal a disconnection-variant ideomotor apraxia, a dissociative apraxia, or even a conceptual apraxia in the non-dominant limb (Heilman et al., 1997).

Pathophysiology of Limb Apraxias

Ideomotor apraxia is associated with lesions in a variety of structures including the inferior parietal lobe, the frontal lobe, and the premotor areas, particularly the SMA. There are reports of ideomotor apraxia due to subcortical lesions in the basal ganglia (caudate-putamen), thalamus (pulvinar), and associated white-matter tracts including the corpus callosum. Limb apraxias can be caused by a variety of central nervous system disorders that affect these regions. The different forms of limb apraxia result from cerebrovascular lesions, especially right middle cerebral artery strokes with right hemiparesis. There may be left-sided limb apraxia in these patients. Right anterior cerebral artery strokes and paramedian lesions could produce ideomotor apraxia, disconnection variant. Ideomotor apraxia and limb-kinetic apraxia can be the initial or presenting manifestation of disorders such as corticobasal syndrome, primary progressive aphasia, or parietal-variant Alzheimer disease (Rohrer et al., 2010). Tumors, traumatic brain injury, infections, and other pathologies can also lead to limb apraxias.

There are effects of hemispheric specialization and handedness on praxis. Early investigators proposed that handedness was related to the hemispheric laterality of the movement formulas. The greatest evidence is for the left hemisphere localization of the movement formulas. Studies using functional imaging have provided converging evidence that in people who are right-handed, it is the left inferior parietallobe that appears to store the movement representation needed for learned skilled movements (Muhlau et al., 2005). Left-handed people, however, may demonstrate an ideomotor apraxia from a right hemisphere lesion, because their movement formulas are stored in their right hemisphere. It is not unusual to see right-handed patients with large left hemisphere lesions who are not apraxic, and there are rare reports of right-handed patients with right hemisphere lesions and limb apraxia. These findings suggest that hand preference is not entirely determined by the laterality of the movement formulas, and praxis and handedness can be dissociated.

Rehabilitation for Limb Apraxias

Because many instrumental and routine ADLs depend on learned skilled movements, patients with limb apraxia usually have impaired functional abilities. The presence of limb apraxia, more than any other neuropsychological disorder, correlates with the level of caregiver assistance required 6 months after a stroke, whereas the absence of apraxia is a significant predictor of return to work after a stroke (Saeki et al., 1995). The treatment of limb apraxia is therefore important for improving the quality of life of the patient.

Even though many treatments have been studied, none has emerged as the standard. There are no effective pharmacotherapies for limb apraxia, and treatments primarily involve rehabilitation strategies. Buxbaum and associates (2008) surveyed the literature on the rehabilitation of limb apraxia and identified 10 studies with 10 treatment strategies: multiple cues, error type reduction, 6-stage task hierarchy, conductive education, strategy training, transitive/intransitive gesture training, rehabilitative treatment, error completion, exploration training, and combined error completion and exploration training. Most of these approaches emphasize cueing with multiple modalities, with verbal, visual, and tactile inputs, repetitive learning, and feedback and correction of errors. Patients with post-stroke apraxia have had generalization of cognitive strategy training to other activities of daily living (Geusgens et al., 2006), but others have not (Bickerton et al., 2006). Although most studies have shown positive treatment effects, fewer studies have demonstrated the effects to be generalizable compared to those that have not. It is also unclear whether the benefits can be sustained long term. In sum, patients can learn and produce new gestures, but the newly learned gestures may not generalize well to contexts outside the rehabilitation setting. Nevertheless, some patients with ideomotor apraxia have improved with gesture-production exercises (Smania et al., 2000), and patients with apraxia would benefit from referral to a rehabilitation specialist with experience in treating apraxias.

Additional important interventions for the management of limb apraxias involve making environmental changes. This includes removing unsafe tools or implements, providing a limited number of tools to select from, replacing complex tasks with simpler ones that require few or no tools and fewer steps, as well as similar modifications.

Related Disorders

Other movement disturbances may be related to or confused with the limb apraxias. The *alien limb phenomenon*, mentioned previously as a potential result of callosal lesions, is the experience that a limb feels foreign and has involuntary semipurposeful movements, such as spontaneous limb levitation. This disorder can occur from neurodegenerative conditions, most notably corticobasal syndrome. *Akinesia* is the inability to initiate a movement in the absence of motor deficits, and *hypokinesia* is a delay in initiating a response. Akinesia and hypokinesia can be directional, with decreased initiation of movement in a specific spatial direction or hemifield. Akinesia and hypokinesia result from a failure to activate the corticospinal system due to Parkinson disease and diseases that affect the frontal lobe cortex, basal ganglia, and thalamus.

Several other movement disturbances are associated with frontal lobe dysfunction. *Motor impersistence* is the inability to sustain a movement or posture and occurs with dorsolateral frontal lesions. *Magnetic grasp and grope reflexes* with automatic reaching for environmental stimuli are primitive release signs. In *echopraxia*, some patients automatically imitate observed movements. Along with utilization behavior, echopraxia may be part of the environmental dependency syndrome of some patients with frontal lesions. *Catalepsy* is the maintenance of a body position into which patients are placed (waxy flexibility). Two related terms are *mitgehen* ("going with"), where patients allow a body part to move in response to light pressure, and *mitmachen* ("doing with"), where patients allow a body part to be put into any position in response to slight pressure, then return the body part to the original resting position after the examiner releases it. *Motor perseveration* is the inability to stop a movement or a series of movements after the task is complete. In recurrent motor perseveration, the patient keeps returning to a prior completed motor program, and in afferent or continuous motor perseveration, the patient cannot end a motor program that has just been completed.

Summary

Limb apraxia, or the disturbance of learned skilled movements, is an important but often missed or unrecognized impairment. Clinicians may misattribute limb apraxia to weakness, hemiparesis, clumsiness, or other motor or cognitive disturbance. Apraxia may only be evident in natural or real situations, with actual tool or object use, or on fine, sequential, or specific movements of the upper extremities (Zadikoff and Lang, 2005). Apraxia is an important cognitive disturbance and a salient sign in patients with strokes, Alzheimer disease, corticobasal syndrome, and other conditions. The model of left parietal movement formulas and disconnection syndromes introduced by Liepmann over 100 years ago continues to be compelling today. This model, in the context of a dedicated apraxia examination and analysis for spatiotemporal or content errors, clarifies and classifies the limb apraxias. Although more effective treatments need to be developed, rehabilitation strategies can be helpful interventions for these disturbances. Fortunately, recent advances in technology and rehabilitation promise to enhance our understanding and management of the limb apraxias.

References

The complete reference list is available online at www.expertconsult.com.

Agnosias

Howard S. Kirshner

Agnosias are disorders of recognition. The general public is familiar with agnosia from Oliver Sacks's patient, who not only failed to recognize his wife's face but also mistook it for a hat. Sigmund Freud originally introduced the term *agnosia* in 1891 to denote disturbances in the ability to recognize and name objects, usually in one sensory modality in the presence of intact primary sensation. Another definition, that of Milner and Teuber in 1968, referred to agnosia as a "normal percept stripped of its meaning." The agnosic patient can perceive and describe sensory features of an object yet cannot recognize or identify the object.

Criteria for the diagnosis of agnosia include: (1) failure to recognize an object; (2) normal perception of the object, excluding an elementary sensory disorder; (3) ability to name the object once it is recognized, excluding anomia as the principal deficit; and (4) absence of a generalized dementia. In addition, agnosias usually affect only one sensory modality, and the patient can identify the same object when presented in a different sensory modality. For example, a patient with visual agnosia may fail to identify a bell by sight but readily identifies it by touch or by the sound of its ring.

Agnosias are defined in terms of the specific sensory modality affected—usually visual, auditory, or tactile—or they may be selective for one class of items within a sensory modality, such as color agnosia or prosopagnosia (agnosia for faces). To diagnose agnosia, the examiner must establish that the deficit is not a primary sensory disorder, as documented by tests of visual acuity, visual fields, auditory function, and somatosensory functions, and not part of a more general cognitive disorder such as aphasia or dementia, as established by the bedside mental status examination. Naming deficits in aphasia or dementia are, with rare exceptions, not restricted to a single sensory modality.

Clinically, agnosias seem complex and arcane, yet they are important in understanding the behavior of neurological patients, and they provide fascinating insights into brain mechanisms related to perception and recognition. Part of their complexity derives from the underlying neuropathology; agnosias frequently result from bilateral or diffuse lesions such as hypoxic encephalopathy, multiple strokes, major head injuries, and neurodegenerative disorders and dementias.

Agnosias have aroused controversies since their earliest descriptions. Some authorities have attributed agnosic deficits to primary perceptual loss in the setting of general cognitive dysfunction or dementia. Abundant case studies, however, argue in favor of true agnosic deficits. In each sensory modality, a spectrum of disorders can be traced from primary sensory dysfunction to agnosia. We approach agnosias by sensory modality, with progression from primary sensory deficits to disorders of recognition.

Visual Agnosias

Cortical Visual Disturbances

Patients with bilateral occipital lobe damage may have complete "cortical" blindness. Some patients with cortical blindness are unaware that they cannot see, and some even confabulate visual descriptions or blame their poor vision on dim lighting or not having their glasses (Anton syndrome, originally described in 1899). Patients with Anton syndrome may describe objects they "see" in the room around them but walk immediately into the wall. The phenomena of this syndrome suggest that the thinking and speaking areas of the brain are not consciously aware of the lack of input from visual centers. Anton syndrome can still be thought of as a perceptual deficit rather than a visual agnosia, but one in which there is unawareness or neglect of the sensory deficit. Such visual unawareness is also frequently seen with hemianopic visual field defects (e.g., in patients with R hemisphere strokes), and it even has a correlate in normal people; we are not conscious of a visual field defect behind our heads, yet we know to turn when we hear a noise from behind. In contrast to Anton syndrome, some cortically blind patients actually have preserved ability to react to visual stimuli, despite the lack of any conscious visual perception, a phenomenon termed *blindsight* or *inverse Anton syndrome* (Ro and Rafal, 2006). Blindsight may be considered an agnosic deficit, because the patient fails to recognize what he or she sees. Residual vision is usually absent in blindness caused by disorders of the eyes, optic nerves, or optic tracts. Patients with cortical vision loss may react to more elementary visual stimuli such as brightness, size, and movement, whereas they cannot perceive finer attributes such as shape, color, and depth. Subjects sometimes look toward objects they cannot consciously see. One study reported a woman with postanoxic cortical blindness who could catch a ball without awareness of seeing it. Blindsight may be mediated by subcortical connections such as those from the optic tracts to the midbrain.

Lesions causing cortical blindness may also be accompanied by visual hallucinations. Irritative lesions of the visual cortex produce unformed hallucinations of lines or spots, whereas those of the temporal lobes produce formed visual images. Visual hallucinations in blindness are referred to as *Bonnet syndrome* (Teunisse et al., 1996). Although Bonnet originally described this phenomenon in his grandfather, who had ocular blindness, complex visual hallucinations occur more typically with cortical visual loss (Manford and Andermann, 1998). Visual hallucinations can occur during recovery from cortical blindness; positron emission tomography (PET) has shown metabolic activation in the parieto-occipital cortex associated with hallucinations, suggesting hyperexcitability of the recovering visual cortex (Wunderlich et al., 2000).

In practice, we diagnose cortical blindness by the absence of ocular pathology, the preservation of the pupillary light reflexes, and the presence of associated neurological symptoms and signs. In addition to blindness, patients with bilateral posterior hemisphere lesions are often confused, agitated, and have short-term memory loss. Amnesia is especially common in patients with bilateral strokes within the posterior cerebral artery territory, which involves not only the occipital lobe but also the hippocampi and related structures of the medial temporal region. Cortical blindness occurs as a transient phenomenon after traumatic brain injury, in migraine, in epileptic seizures, and as a complication of iodinated contrast procedures such as arteriography. Cortical blindness can develop in the setting of hypoxic-ischemic encephalopathy (Wunderlich et al., 2000), meningitis, systemic lupus erythematosus, dementing conditions such as the Heidenhain variant of Creutzfeldt-Jakob disease, or the posterior cortical atrophy syndrome described in Alzheimer disease and other dementias (Kirshner and Lavin, 2006).

Cortical Visual Distortions

Positive visual phenomena frequently develop in patients with visual field defects and even in migraine: distortions of shape called *metamorphopsia*, scintillating scotomas, irregular shapes (teichopsia, or fortification spectra), macropsia and micropsia, peculiar changes of shape and size known as the *Alice in Wonderland syndrome* (described by Golden in 1979), achromatopsia (loss of color vision), akinetopsia (loss of perception of motion), palinopsia (perseveration of visual images), visual allesthesia (spread of a visual image from a normal to a

hemianopic field), and even polyopia (duplication of objects). All these phenomena are disturbances of higher visual perception rather than agnosias.

Two types of color vision deficit are associated with occipital lesions. First, a complete loss of color vision, or achromatopsia, may occur either bilaterally or in one visual hemifield with lesions that involve portions of the visual association cortex (Brodmann areas 18 and 19). Second, patients with pure alexia and lesions of the left occipital lobe fail to name colors, although their color matching and other aspects of color perception are normal. Patients often confabulate an incorrect color name when asked what color an object is. This deficit can be called *color agnosia*, in the sense that a normally perceived color cannot be properly recognized. Although this deficit has been termed *color anomia*, these patients can usually name the colors of familiar objects such as a school bus or the inside of a watermelon.

Balint Syndrome and Simultanagnosia

In 1909, Balint described a syndrome in which patients act blind, yet can describe small details of objects in central vision (Rizzo and Vecera, 2002). The disorder is usually associated with bilateral hemisphere lesions, often involving the parietal and frontal lobes. Balint syndrome involves a triad of deficits: (1) psychic paralysis of gaze, also called *ocular motor apraxia*, or difficulty directing the eyes away from central fixation; (2) optic ataxia, or incoordination of extremity movement under visual control (with normal coordination under proprioceptive control; and (3) impaired visual attention. These deficits result in the perception of only small details of a visual scene, with loss of the ability to scan and perceive the "big picture." Patients with Balint syndrome literally cannot see the forest for the trees. Some but not all patients have bilateral visual field deficits. In bedside neurological examination, helpful tests include asking the patient to interpret a complex drawing or photograph, such as the "Cookie Theft" picture from the Boston Diagnostic Aphasia Examination and the National Institutes of Health Stroke Scale.

Partial deficits related to Balint syndrome have also been described, including isolated optic ataxia, or impaired visually guided reaching toward an object. Optic ataxia likely results from disruption of the transmission of visual information for visual direction of motor acts from the occipital cortex to the premotor areas. This function involves portions of the dorsal occipital and parietal areas as part of the "dorsal visual stream" (Himmelbach et al., 2009). A second partial Balint syndrome deficit is simultanagnosia, or loss of ability to perceive more than one item at a time, first described by Wolpert in 1924. The patient sees details of pictures, but not the whole. Many such patients have left occipital lesions and associated pure alexia without agraphia; these patients can often read "letter-by-letter," or one letter at a time, but they cannot recognize a word at a glance (see Chapter 12). Robertson and colleagues (1997) emphasized deficient spatial organization as a contributing factor to the perceptual difficulties of a patient with Balint syndrome secondary to bilateral parieto-occipital strokes. Balint syndrome has also been reported in patients with posterior cortical atrophy and related neurodegenerative conditions involving the posterior parts of both hemispheres (Kirshner and Lavin, 2006; McMonagle et al., 2006).

Visual Object Agnosia

Visual object agnosia is the quintessential visual agnosia: the patient fails to recognize objects by sight, with preserved ability to recognize them through touch or hearing in the absence of impaired primary visual perception or dementia (Biran and Coslett, 2003). In 1890, Lissauer distinguished two subtypes of visual object agnosia: *apperceptive visual object agnosia*, referring to the synthesis of elementary perceptual elements into a unified image, and *associative visual object agnosia*, in which the meaning of a perceived stimulus is appreciated by recall of previous visual experiences.

Apperceptive Visual Agnosia

The first type, apperceptive visual agnosia, is difficult to separate from impaired perception or partial cortical blindness. Patients with apperceptive visual agnosia can pick out features of an object correctly (e.g., lines, angles, colors, movement), but they fail to appreciate the whole object (Grossman et al., 1997).Warrington and Rudge (1995) pointed to the right parietal cortex for its importance in visual processing of objects, and they found this area critical to apperceptive visual agnosia. A patient described by Luria misnamed eyeglasses as a bicycle, pointing to the two circles and a crossbar. Another study considered apperceptive visual agnosia related to bilateral occipital lesions a "pseudoagnosic syndrome" associated with visual processing defects, as compared to true visual agnosias, in which the right parietal cortex is deficient in identifying and recognizing visual objects. Recent evidence of the functions of specific cortical areas has included the specialization of the medial occipital cortex for appreciation of color and texture, whereas the lateral occipital cortex is more involved with shape perception. Deficits in these specific visual functions can be seen in patients with visual object agnosia (Cavina-Pratesi et al., 2010). On the other hand, a patient reported by Karnath et al. (2009) had visual form agnosia with bilateral medial occipitotemporal lesions.

Another way of analyzing apperceptive visual agnosia is by the focusing of visual attention. Theiss and DeBleser in 1992 distinguished two features of visual attention: a wide-angle attentional lens that sees the figure generally but perceives only gross features (the forest), and a narrow-angle spotlight that focuses on the fine visual details (the trees). They described a patient with a faulty wide-angle attentional beam; she could identify small objects within a drawing but missed what the drawing represented. Fink and colleagues (1996), in PET studies of visual perception in normal subjects, found that right hemisphere sites, particularly the lingual gyrus, activated during global processing of figures, whereas left hemisphere sites, particularly the left inferior occipital cortex, activated during more local processing. The ability of patients with apperceptive visual agnosia to perceive fine details but not the whole picture (missing the forest for the trees) is closely related to Balint syndrome and simultanagnosia.

As with most cortical visual syndromes, apperceptive visual agnosia usually occurs in patients with bilateral occipital lesions. It may represent a stage in recovery from complete cortical blindness. Deficits in recognition of visual objects may be especially apparent with recognition of degraded images, such as drawings rather than actual objects. Apperceptive visual agnosia can also be part of dementing

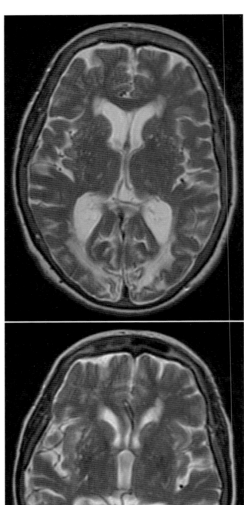
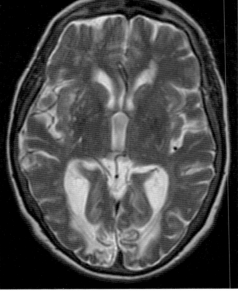

Fig. 11.1 T2-weighted magnetic resonance images from a patient with progressive loss of vision, misidentification of objects, and inability to describe the whole of a picture, mentioning only small details. The clinical diagnosis was posterior cortical atrophy, a neurodegenerative condition.

syndromes (Kirshner and Lavin, 2006; McMonagle et al., 2006) (**Fig. 11.1**).

Associative Visual Agnosia

Associative visual agnosia, Lissauer's second type, has to do with recognition of appropriately perceived objects. Some patients can copy or match drawings of objects they cannot name, thus excluding a primary defect of visual perception. Aphasia is excluded because the patient can identify the same object presented in the tactile or auditory modality. Patients with associative visual agnosia often have other related recognition deficits such as color agnosia, prosopagnosia, and alexia. Associative visual agnosia is usually associated with bilateral posterior hemisphere lesions, often involving the fusiform or occipitotemporal gyri, sometimes the lingual gyri and adjacent white matter. Jankowiak and colleagues described a patient with bilateral parieto-occipital damage from gunshot injuries. Visual acuity was nearly normal except for bilateral upper "altitudinal" visual field defects. He had difficulty recognizing and naming colors, faces, objects, and pictures. He could copy drawings he could not recognize, and he could draw images from memory or after tachistoscopic presentation. The crux of this patient's deficit was an inability to match an internal visual percept with representations of visual objects; in other words, he could perceive visual stimuli normally but failed to assign meaning or identity to them.

Geschwind postulated in 1965 that visual agnosia results from a disconnection syndrome in which bilateral lesions prevent visual information from the occipital lobes from reaching the left hemisphere language areas. Most but not all cases of associative visual agnosia have involved the fusiform or occipitotemporal gyri bilaterally, presumably interrupting connections between the visual cortex and the language areas for naming, or the medial temporal region for identification from memory. The disconnection hypothesis of visual agnosia is likely an oversimplification of the complexities of visual perception and recognition, but it provides a simple way to remember the syndrome.

Optic Aphasia

The syndrome of optic aphasia, or optic anomia, is intermediate between agnosias and aphasias. The patient with optic aphasia cannot name objects presented visually but can demonstrate recognition of the objects by pantomiming or describing their use. The preserved recognition of the objects distinguishes optic aphasia from associative visual agnosia. Like visual agnosics, patients with optic aphasia can name objects presented in the auditory or tactile modalities, distinguishing them from anomic aphasics. In optic aphasia, information about the object must reach parts of the cortex involved in recognition, perhaps in the right hemisphere, but the information is not available to the language cortex for naming. This explanation also fits Geschwind's disconnection hypothesis. Patients with optic aphasia may confabulate incorrect names when asked to name an object they clearly recognize, just as the patient with color agnosia confabulates incorrect color names. The language cortex appears to supply a name from the class of items when specific information is not forthcoming, without the conscious awareness that the information is not correct. Patients with optic aphasia frequently manifest associated deficits of alexia without agraphia and color agnosia, suggesting a left occipital lesion. Optic aphasia bears great similarity to pure alexia without agraphia; just as optic aphasics may recognize objects they cannot name, pure alexics sometimes recognize words they cannot read.

Prosopagnosia

Prosopagnosia refers to the inability to recognize faces. Patients fail to recognize close friends and relatives or pictures of famous people, except by memorizing details of shape or hairstyle, but they learn to compensate by identifying a person by voice, mannerisms, gait patterns, and apparel. Prosopagnosia is restricted not only to the visual modality but also to the class of faces.

Facial recognition is a complex function. First, patients who cannot match pictures of faces must have defective face processing, or apperceptive prosopagnosia, whereas those who can match faces but simply fail to recognize familiar examples (either friends and relatives or famous personages) have associative prosopagnosia (Barton et al., 2004). There has been some opinion that faces are not a unique perceptual entity but just representative of complex stimuli, but a recent study by Busigny and colleagues (2010) found that their patient performed normally in perceptual tasks involving cars, objects, and geometric shapes, while deficient with faces. Another aspect of facial recognition is the perception of emotion in facial expressions, a function that appears localized to the right hemisphere. A recent study suggested that white matter lesions disconnecting the occipital cortex from "emotion-related regions" might be responsible for agnosia for emotional facial expression (Philippi et al., 2009).

In clinical studies, prosopagnosia may occur either as an isolated deficit or as part of a more general visual agnosia for objects and colors. Faces are likely the most complex and individualized visual displays to recognize, but some patients with visual object agnosia can recognize faces, suggesting that there may be a specific brain area devoted to facial recognition. Humphreys (1996) reviewed evidence that living things may be recognized in a different part of the occipital cortex from nonliving things.

The anatomical localization of prosopagnosia parallels that of the other visual agnosias. Most studies have reported bilateral temporo-occipital lesions, often involving the fusiform or occipitotemporal gyri, but cases with unilateral posterior right hemisphere lesions have also been described. Facial perception seems localized to the fusiform gyri, but recognition of familiar faces may require anterior temporal memory stores (Barton, 2003). A recent study involving both functional magnetic resonance imaging (fMRI) and neuropsychological testing found the inferior occipital ("occipital face area") lobe critical for the identification of specific individual faces, whereas the "fusiform face area" in the middle fusiform gyrus was involved in other aspects of face perception (Steeves et al., 2009). The disconnection hypothesis has been invoked in prosopagnosia, reflecting interruption of fibers passing from the occipital cortices to the centers where memories of faces are stored. Prosopagnosia also occurs in dementing illnesses such as frontotemporal dementia (Joubert et al., 2004) and posterior cortical atrophy (Kirshner and Lavin, 2006).

Klüver-Bucy Syndrome

Another form of visual agnosia is the psychic blindness syndrome described by Klüver and Bucy in 1939. They reported the syndrome originally in monkeys with bilateral temporal lobectomies, but similar symptoms develop in humans with bilateral temporal lesions (Trimble et al., 1997). An animal may inappropriately try to eat or mate with objects or fail to show customary fear when confronted with a natural enemy. Human Klüver-Bucy patients manifest visual agnosia and prosopagnosia as well as memory loss, language deficits, and changes in behavior such as placidity, altered sexual orientation, and excessive eating. Cases of the human Klüver-Bucy syndrome have been reported with bitemporal damage from surgical ablation, herpes simplex encephalitis, and dementing conditions such as Pick disease. Patients with Klüver-Bucy syndrome appear to have no major deficits of primary visual perception, but connections appear to be disrupted between vision and memory and limbic structures, so visual percepts do not arouse their ordinary associations.

Auditory Agnosias

Like cortical visual syndromes, cortical auditory disorders range from primary auditory syndromes of cortical deafness to partial deficits of recognition of specific types of sound. As with the visual agnosias, most cortical auditory deficits require bilateral cerebral lesions, usually involving the temporal lobes, especially the primary auditory cortices in the Heschl gyri.

Cortical Deafness

Profound hearing deficits are seen in patients with acquired bilateral lesions of the primary auditory cortex (Heschl gyrus, Brodmann areas 41 and 42) or of the auditory radiations projecting to the Heschl gyri. In general, unilateral lesions of the auditory cortex have little effect on hearing. Only rarely are patients with bilateral auditory cortex lesions completely deaf, even to loud noises; most retain some pure tone hearing but have deficits in higher-level acoustic processing such as identification of meaningful sounds, temporal sequencing, and sound localization. As in visual agnosia, the cortical hearing deficits blend imperceptibly into the auditory agnosias.

A patient with auditory agnosia can hear noises but not appreciate their meanings, as in identifying animal cries or sounds associated with specific objects, such as the ringing of a bell. Most such patients also cannot understand speech or appreciate music. Auditory agnosias can be divided into (1) pure word deafness, (2) pure auditory nonverbal agnosia, (3) phonagnosia, or inability to identify persons by their voices (Polster and Rose, 1998; Hailstone et al., 2010), and (4) pure amusia. Patients may have one or a mixture of these deficits.

Pure Word Deafness

The syndrome of pure word deafness involves an inability to comprehend spoken words, with preserved ability to hear and recognize nonverbal sounds. Pure word deafness often evolves out of an initial deficit of cortical deafness or severe cortical auditory disorder. Pure word deafness has traditionally been explained as a disconnection of both primary auditory cortices from the left hemisphere Wernicke area. Engelien and colleagues (2000) showed activation on PET scanning during auditory stimulation in a patient with extensive bilateral temporal lesions, a phenomenon they referred to as *deaf hearing* (analogous to blindsight). Unilateral left hemisphere lesions have also been associated with pure word deafness; by Geschwind's disconnection theory, such a lesion might be strategically placed so as to disconnect both primary auditory cortices from the Wernicke area. Occasionally patients with Wernicke aphasia have more severe involvement of auditory comprehension than reading comprehension, also resembling pure word deafness. In fact, most cases of pure word deafness also have paraphasic speech, further linking the syndrome to Wernicke aphasia (**Fig. 11.2**).

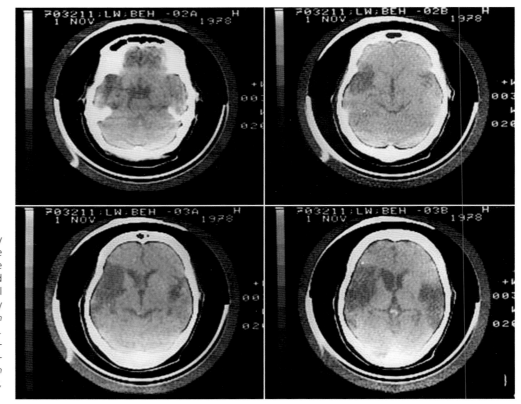

Fig. 11.2 A computed tomography scan from a patient with extensive bilateral infarctions involving the temporal lobes. The patient could hear pure tones and nonverbal sounds, but she was completely unable to comprehend speech. *(From Kirshner, H.S., Webb, W.G., 1981. Selective involvement of the auditory-verbal modality in an acquired communication disorder: benefit from sign language therapy, Brain Lang 13, 161–170.)*

Auditory Nonverbal Agnosia

Auditory nonverbal agnosia refers to patients who have lost the ability to identify meaningful nonverbal sounds but have preserved pure tone hearing and language comprehension. These cases also tend to have bilateral temporal lobe lesions. A recently reported case had a unilateral left temporal lesion with evidence of reorganization of auditory word perception involving adjacent left and contralateral right temporal cortex (Saygin et al., 2010).

Phonagnosia

Phonagnosia is analogous to prosopagnosia in the visual modality; it is a failure to recognize familiar people by their voices. Again, apperceptive deficits can occur in the matching of unfamiliar voices, usually reflecting unilateral or bilateral temporal damage, but failure to recognize a familiar voice may involve a right parietal locus corresponding to the specific area for recognition of faces. A related deficit is auditory affective agnosia, or failure to recognize the emotional intonation of speech, usually associated with right hemisphere lesions (Polster and Rose, 1998). Two cases of progressive phonagnosia have been reported in frontotemporal dementia (Hailstone et al., 2010).

Amusia

The loss of musical abilities after focal brain lesions is another complex topic, reflecting the complexity of musical appreciation and analysis (Alossa and Castelli, 2009). Traditional lesion-deficit analysis has suggested that recognition of melodies and musical tones is a right temporal function, whereas analysis of pitch, rhythm, and tempo involves the left temporal lobe. In a recent study of patients with temporal lobe lesions and epilepsy, those with left hemisphere lesions were more impaired in temporal sequencing of music as well as speech (Samson et al., 2001). The left hemisphere is likely more activated when a trained musician listens to music, as compared to an untrained listener. In a study of PET brain imaging during musical performance in 10 professional pianists, sight-reading of music activated both visual association cortices and the superior parietal lobes, areas distinct from those utilized in reading words. Listening to music activated both secondary auditory cortices, and playing music activated frontal and cerebellar areas. The authors commented that widespread as these areas were, the study did not examine the whole of musical experience, let alone the pleasure afforded by music.

The composer Maurice Ravel, whose case was originally described in 1948 by Alajouanine, suffered a progressive fluent aphasia that gradually took his ability to read or write music but spared his capacity to listen to and appreciate it. Another study also reported progressive musical dysfunction in two professional musicians with dementing illness.

Tactile Agnosias

As we have seen with the syndromes of cortical loss of visual and auditory perception, a range of somatosensory deficits is seen with cortical lesions. Patients with lesions of the parietal cortex may have preserved ability to feel pinprick, temperature, vibration, and proprioception, yet they fail to identify objects palpated by the contralateral hand or to recognize numbers or letters written on the opposite side of the body. These deficits, called *astereognosis* and *agraphesthesia*, represent deficits of cortical sensory loss rather than agnosias. Alternatively, they could be considered as apperceptive tactile agnosias. Rarely patients have been reported who can describe the shape and features of a palpated object, yet cannot identify the object. The patient can readily identify the object by sound or sight, thereby fulfilling the criteria for associative tactile agnosia (Bottini et al., 1995).

Caselli investigated 84 patients with unilateral hemisphere lesions for deficits in tactile perception. Seven patients had tactile agnosia for objects palpated by the contralateral hand. These deficits occurred in the absence of primary somatosensory loss. Some patients had severe hemiparesis or hemianopia yet performed well in tactile object recognition, but patients with neglect secondary to right hemisphere lesions tended to have more severe deficits. A second study reported that only patients with neglect had bilateral tactile object recognition deficits, whereas patients with left parietal lesions had tactile agnosia only for items in the right hand. The study did not include patients with bilateral lesions, however, and agnosia in the visual and auditory modalities is clearly more profound when bilateral lesions are present.

The mechanisms of tactile agnosia may vary. First, appreciation of shape may be a property of the sensory cortex. In the studies of Bottini and colleagues (1995), matching of shapes (an apperceptive task) was more sensitive to right hemisphere damage, whereas matching of meaningful shapes (the associative task) was more sensitive to left hemisphere lesions. Second, the right parietal cortex is also involved in spatial and topographical functions, and spatial disorders may account for some of the tactile recognition deficits of patients with right parietal lesions. Third, attentional deficits and neglect seen with right hemisphere lesions may increase the lack of tactile recognition. Fourth, disconnection syndromes may be involved in tactile agnosia. The famous 1962 patient of Geschwind and Kaplan with a lesion of the corpus callosum could not identify objects with the left hand but could point to the correct object in a group. Patients with surgical section of the corpus callosum have similar deficits; these patients can feel the object with the left hand but cannot name it, presumably because the callosal lesion disconnects the right parietal cortex from left hemisphere language centers.

Tactile Aphasia

Tactile aphasia is an inability to name a palpated object despite intact recognition of the object and intact naming when the object is presented in another sensory modality. This syndrome is closely analogous to optic aphasia and has been recognized only rarely.

Summary

Agnosias are disorders of sensory perception and recognition. The cortical mechanisms of the agnosias span a spectrum from primary sensory cortical deficits to disorders of the association cortex, or disconnection syndromes between cortical areas. Recognition of objects requires not only primary sensation but also association of the perceived item with previous sensory experiences and associative memories. The agnosias open a window into the brain's ability to perceive and recognize aspects of the world around us.

Acknowledgment

Portions of this chapter appeared in Kirshner, H.S., 2002. Agnosias, In: Behavioral Neurology: Practical Science of Mind and Brain. Butterworth Heinemann, Boston, pp. 137-158.

References

The complete reference list is available online at www.expertconsult.com.

Language and Speech Disorders
Aphasia and Aphasic Syndromes

Howard S. Kirshner

Language Disorders: Overview

The study of language disorders involves analysis of that most human of attributes, the ability to communicate through common symbols. Language has provided the foundation of human civilization and learning, and its study has been the province of philosophers as well as physicians. When language is disturbed by neurological disorders, analysis of the patterns of abnormality has practical usefulness in neurological diagnosis. Historically, language was the first higher cortical function to be correlated with specific sites of brain damage. It continues to serve as a model for the practical use of a cognitive function in localizing brain lesions and for understanding human cortical processes in general.

Definitions

Aphasia is defined as a disorder of language acquired secondary to brain damage. This definition, adapted from Alexander and Benson (1997), separates aphasia from several related disorders. First, aphasia is distinguished from congenital or developmental language disorders, called *dysphasias*. (In contrast with British usage, in the United States the term *dysphasia* applies to developmental language disorders rather than partial or incomplete aphasia.)

Second, aphasia is a disorder of language rather than speech. *Speech* is the articulation and phonation of language sounds; *language* is a complex system of communication symbols and rules for their use. Aphasia is distinguished from motor speech disorders (the subject of Part B of this chapter), which include dysarthria, dysphonia (voice disorders), stuttering, and speech apraxia. *Dysarthrias* are disorders of articulation of single sounds; causes of these disorders may include mechanical disturbance of the tongue or larynx and neurological disorders such as dysfunction of the muscles, neuromuscular junction, cranial nerves, bulbar anterior horn cells, corticobulbar tracts, cerebellar connections, or basal ganglia. *Apraxia of speech* is a syndrome of misarticulation of phonemes, especially consonant sounds. Unlike dysarthria, in which certain phonemes are consistently distorted, apraxia of speech is characterized by inconsistent distortions and substitutions of phonemes. The disorder is called an *apraxia* because there is no primary motor deficit in articulation of individual phonemes. Clinically, speech-apraxic patients produce inconsistent articulatory errors, usually worse on the initial phonemes of a word and with polysyllabic utterances. Apraxia of speech, so defined, is commonly involved in speech production difficulty in the aphasias.

Third, aphasia is distinguished from disorders of thought. Thought involves the mental processing of images, memories, and perceptions, usually but not necessarily involving language symbols. Psychiatric disorders derange thought and alter the content of speech without affecting its linguistic structure. Schizophrenic patients, for example, may manifest bizarre and individualistic word choices, with loose associations and a loss of organization in discourse together with

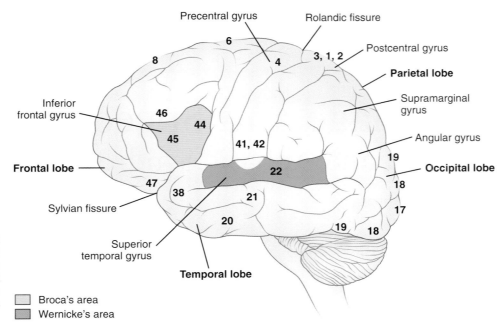

Fig. 12A.1 Lateral surface of the left hemisphere, showing a simplified gyral anatomy and the relationships between the Wernicke area and Broca area. Not shown is the arcuate fasciculus, which connects the two cortical speech centers via the deep subcortical white matter.

☐ Broca's area
■ Wernicke's area

vague or unclear references and communication failures (Docherty et al., 1996). Elementary language and articulation, however, are intact. Abnormal language content in psychiatric disorders is therefore not considered to represent aphasia, because the disorder is more one of thought than of language. Language disorders associated with diffuse brain diseases such as encephalopathies and dementias do qualify as aphasias, but the involvement of other cognitive functions distinguishes them from aphasia secondary to focal brain lesions.

An understanding of language disorders requires an elementary review of linguistic components. *Phonemes* are the smallest meaning-carrying sounds; *morphology* is the use of appropriate word endings and connector words for tenses, possessives, and singular versus plural; *semantics* refers to word meanings; the *lexicon* is the internal dictionary; and *syntax* is the grammatical construction of phrases and sentences. *Discourse* refers to the use of these elements to create organized and logical expression of thoughts. *Pragmatics* refers to the proper use of speech and language in a conversational setting, including pausing while others are speaking, taking turns properly, and responding to questions. Specific language disorders affect one or more of these elements.

Relevant Neuroanatomy

Language processes have a clear neuroanatomical basis. In simplest terms, the reception and processing of spoken language take place in the auditory system, beginning with the cochlea and proceeding through a series of way stations to the auditory cortex, the Heschl gyrus, in each superior temporal gyrus. Decoding sounds into linguistic information involves the posterior part of the left superior temporal gyrus, the Wernicke area or Brodmann area 22, which gives access to a network of cortical associations to assign word meanings. For both repetition and spontaneous speech, auditory information is transmitted to the Broca area in the posterior inferior frontal gyrus. This area of cortex "programs" the neurons in

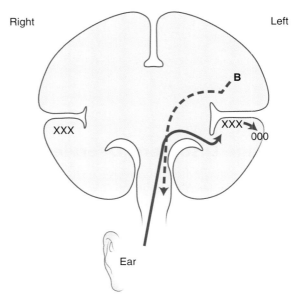

Fig. 12A.2 Coronal plane diagram of the brain, indicating the inflow of auditory information from the ears to the primary auditory cortex in both superior temporal regions (xxx), and then to the Wernicke area (ooo) in the left superior temporal gyrus. The motor outflow of speech descends from the Broca area (B) to the cranial nerve nuclei of the brainstem via the corticobulbar tract *(dashed arrow)*. In actuality, the Broca area is anterior to the Wernicke area, and the two areas would not appear in the same coronal section.

the adjacent motor cortex subserving the mouth and larynx, from which descending axons travel to the brainstem cranial nerve nuclei. The inferior parietal lobule, especially the supramarginal gyrus, also may be involved in phoneme processing in language comprehension and in phoneme production for repetition and speech (Hickok and Poeppel, 2000). These anatomical relationships are shown in **Figs. 12A.1** and **12A.2**. Reading requires perception of visual language stimuli by the occipital cortex, followed by processing into auditory language information via the heteromodal association cortex of the angular gyrus. Writing involves activation of motor neurons projecting to the arm and hand. A French study that used aphasia testing and magnetic resonance imaging (MRI) scans to evaluate 107 stroke patients confirmed the general themes of nearly 150 years of clinical aphasia research: that frontal lesions caused nonfluent aphasia, whereas posterior temporal lesions affected comprehension (Kreisler et al., 2000).

These pathways, and doubtless others, constitute the cortical circuitry for language comprehension and expression. In addition, other cortical centers involved in cognitive processes project into the primary language cortex, influencing the content of language. Finally, subcortical structures play increasingly recognized roles in language functions. The thalamus, a relay for the reticular activating system, appears to alert the language cortex, and lesions of the dominant thalamus frequently produce fluent aphasia. Nuclei of the basal ganglia involved in motor functions, especially the caudate nucleus and putamen, participate in expressive speech. No wonder, then, that language disorders are seen with a wide variety of brain lesions and are important in practical neurological diagnosis and localization.

In right-handed people, and in a majority of left-handers as well, clinical syndromes of aphasia result from left hemisphere lesions. Rarely, aphasia may result from a right hemisphere lesion in a right-handed patient, a phenomenon called *crossed aphasia* (Bakar et al., 1996). In left-handed persons, language disorders are usually similar to those of right-handed persons with similar lesions, but occasional cases manifest with atypical syndromes that suggest a right hemisphere capability for at least some language functions. For example, a patient with a large left frontotemporoparietal lesion may have preserved comprehension, suggesting right hemisphere language comprehension. For the same reason, recovery from aphasia may be better in some left-handed than in right-handed patients with left hemisphere strokes.

Diagnostic Features

Muteness, a total loss of speech, may represent severe aphasia (see Aphemia later in the chapter). Muteness also can be a sign of dysarthria, frontal lobe dysfunction with akinetic mutism, severe extrapyramidal system dysfunction (as in Parkinson disease), non-neurological disorders of the larynx and pharynx, or even psychiatric syndromes such as catatonia. Caution must therefore be taken in diagnosing the mute patient as aphasic. A good rule of thumb is that if the patient can write or type and the language form and content appear normal, the disorder is probably not aphasic in origin. If the patient cannot speak or write but makes apparent effort to vocalize, and if there is also evidence of deficient comprehension, aphasic muteness is likely. Associated signs of a left hemisphere injury, such as right hemiparesis, also aid in diagnosis. Finally, if the patient gradually begins to make sounds containing paraphasic errors, aphasia can be identified with confidence.

Hesitant speech is a feature of aphasia but also of motor speech disorders such as dysarthria or stuttering, and it may be a manifestation of a psychogenic disorder. A second rule of thumb is that if the utterances of a hesitant speaker can be transcribed into normal language, the patient is not aphasic.

Hesitancy occurs in many aphasia syndromes for various reasons, including difficulty in speech initiation, imprecise articulation of phonemes, deficient syntax, and word-finding difficulty.

Anomia, or inability to produce a specific name, is generally a reliable indicator of language disorder, although it also may reflect memory loss. Anomia is manifested in aphasic speech by word-finding pauses and circumlocutions, or use of a phrase when a single word would suffice (e.g., "the thing you tell time with" for watch).

Paraphasic speech refers to the presence of errors in the patient's speech output. Paraphasic errors are divided into literal or phonemic errors involving substitution of an incorrect sound (e.g., "shoon" for "spoon") and verbal or semantic errors involving substitution of an incorrect word (e.g., "fork" for "spoon"). A related language symptom is *perseveration*, the inappropriate repetition of a previous response. Occasionally, aphasic utterances involve nonexistent word forms called *neologisms*. A pattern of paraphasic errors and neologisms that so contaminate speech that the meaning cannot be discerned is called *jargon speech*.

Another cardinal symptom of aphasia is failure to comprehend the speech of others. Most aphasic patients also have difficulty with comprehension and production of written language (reading and writing). Fluent paraphasic speech usually makes an aphasic disorder obvious. The chief considerations in the differential diagnosis here include aphasia, psychosis, acute encephalopathy or delirium, and dementia. Aphasic patients usually do not appear confused and do not exhibit inappropriate behavior; they are not agitated and do not misuse objects, with occasional exceptions in acute syndromes of Wernicke or global aphasia. In contrast, most psychotic patients speak in an easily understood, grammatically appropriate manner, but their behavior and speech content are abnormal. Only rarely do schizophrenics speak in "clang association" or "word salad" speech. Sudden onset of fluent paraphasic speech in a middle-aged or elderly patient should always be suspected of representing a left hemisphere lesion with aphasia.

Patients with acute encephalopathy or delirium may manifest paraphasic speech and "higher" language deficits, such as the inability to write, but the grammatical expression of language is less disturbed than its content. These language symptoms, moreover, are less prominent than accompanying behavioral disturbances such as agitation, hallucinations, drowsiness, or excitement, and cognitive difficulties such as disorientation, memory loss, or delusional thinking.

Chronic encephalopathies, or dementias, pose a more difficult diagnostic problem because involvement of the language cortex produces readily detectable language deficits, especially involving naming, reading, and writing. These language disorders (see Language in Dementing Diseases later in this chapter) differ from aphasia secondary to focal lesions mainly by the involvement of other cognitive functions such as memory and visuospatial processes.

Bedside Language Examination

The first part of any bedside examination of language is observing the patient's speech and comprehension during the clinical interview. A wealth of information about language function can be obtained if the examiner pays deliberate

---

Box 12A.1 Bedside Language Examination

1. Spontaneous speech
   a. Informal interview
   b. Structured task
   c. Automatic sequences
2. Naming
3. Auditory comprehension
4. Repetition
5. Reading
   a. Reading aloud
   b. Reading comprehension
6. Writing
   a. Spontaneous sentences
   b. Writing to dictation
   c. Copying

---

attention to the patient's speech patterns and responses to questions. In particular, minor word-finding difficulty, occasional paraphasic errors, and higher-level deficits in discourse planning and in the pragmatics of communication—turn-taking in conversation and the use of humor and irony, for example—can be detected principally during the informal interview.

D. Frank Benson and Norman Geschwind popularized a bedside language examination of six parts, updated by Alexander and Benson (1997) (**Box 12A.1**). This examination provides useful localizing information about brain dysfunction and is well worth the few minutes it takes.

The first part of the examination is assessment of spontaneous speech. A speech sample may be elicited by asking the patient to describe the weather or the reason for coming to the doctor. If speech is sparse or absent, recitation of lists (e.g., counting or listing days of the week) may be helpful. The most important variable in spontaneous speech is fluency. Fluent speech flows rapidly and effortlessly; nonfluent speech is uttered in single words or short phrases, with frequent pauses and hesitations. Attention should first be paid to such elementary characteristics as initiation difficulty, articulation, phonation or voice volume, rate of speech, prosody or melodic intonation of speech, and phrase length. Second, the content of speech utterances should be analyzed in terms of the presence of word-finding pauses, circumlocutions, and errors such as literal and verbal paraphasias and neologisms.

Naming, the second part of the bedside examination, is tested by asking the patient to name objects, object parts, pictures, colors, or body parts to confrontation. A few items from each category should be tested because anomia can be specific to word classes. Proper names of persons are often affected severely. The examiner should ask questions to be sure the patient recognizes the items or people he or she cannot name.

Auditory comprehension is tested first by asking the patient to follow a series of commands of one, two, and three steps. An example of a one-step command is "Stick out your tongue"; a two-step command is "Hold up your left thumb and close your eyes." Successful following of commands ensures adequate comprehension, at least at this simple level, but failure to follow commands does not automatically establish a loss of comprehension. The patient must hear the command, understand the language the examiner speaks, and possess the motor ability to execute it, including the absence of apraxia. *Apraxia* (see Chapter 10 for full discussion) is defined operationally as the inability to carry out a motor command despite normal comprehension and normal ability to carry out the motor act in another context, such as for imitation or with use of a real object. Because apraxia is difficult to exclude with confidence, it is advisable to test comprehension by tasks that do not require a motor act, such as yes/no questions, or by commands that require only a pointing response. The responses to nonsense questions (e.g., "Do you vomit every day?") quickly establish whether the patient comprehends. Nonsense questions often produce surprising results because of the tendency of some aphasics to cover up comprehension difficulty with social chatter.

Repetition of words and phrases should be deliberately tested. Dysarthric patients and those with apraxia of speech (see Chapter 12B) have difficulty with rapid sequences of consonants, such as in "Methodist Episcopal," whereas aphasic persons have special difficulty with grammatically complex sentences. The phrase "no ifs, ands, or buts" is especially challenging for aphasics. Often, aphasics can repeat familiar or "high-probability" phrases much better than unfamiliar ones.

Reading should be tested both aloud and for comprehension. The examiner should carry a few printed commands to facilitate a rapid comparison of auditory and reading comprehension. Of course, the examiner must have some idea of the patient's premorbid reading ability.

Writing, the element of the bedside examination most often omitted, not only provides a further sample of expressive language but also allows an analysis of spelling, which is not possible with spoken language. A writing specimen may be the most sensitive indicator of mild aphasia, and it provides a permanent record for future comparison. Spontaneous writing, such as a sentence describing why the patient has come for examination, is especially sensitive for the detection of language difficulty. When spontaneous writing fails, writing to dictation and copying should be tested as well.

Finally, the neurologist combines the results of the bedside language examination with those of the rest of the mental status examination and of the neurological examination in general. These "associated signs" help classify the type of aphasia and localize the responsible brain lesion.

Aphasic Syndromes

Broca Aphasia

In 1861, the French physician Paul Broca described two patients, establishing the aphasia syndrome that now bears his name. The speech pattern is nonfluent; on bedside examination, the patient speaks hesitantly, often producing the principal meaning-containing nouns and verbs but omitting small grammatical words and morphemes. This pattern is called *agrammatism* or "telegraphic speech." An example is "wife come hospital." Patients with acute Broca aphasia may be mute or may produce only single words, often with dysarthria and apraxia of speech. They make many phonemic errors, inconsistent from utterance to utterance, with substitution of phonemes usually differing only slightly from the correct target (e.g., /p/ for /b/). Naming is deficient, but the patient often manifests a "tip-of-the-tongue" phenomenon, getting out the first letter or phoneme of the correct name. Paraphasic errors in naming more frequently are of literal than of verbal type. Auditory comprehension seems intact, but detailed testing usually reveals some deficiency, particularly in the comprehension of complex syntax. For example, for persons with Broca aphasia, sentences with embedded clauses involving prepositional relationships cause difficulty in comprehension as well as in expression ("The rug that Bill gave to Betty tripped the visitor"). A positron emission tomography (PET) study in normal persons (Caplan et al., 1998) showed activation of the Broca area in the frontal cortex during tests of syntactic comprehension; the Broca area thus appears to be involved in syntactical operations, both expressively and receptively. Repetition is hesitant in these patients, resembling their spontaneous speech. Reading often is impaired despite relatively preserved auditory comprehension. Benson termed this reading difficulty of Broca aphasics the "third alexia," in contradistinction to the two classical types of alexia (see Aphasic Alexia later in the chapter). Patients with Broca aphasia may have difficulty with syntax in reading, just as in auditory comprehension and speech. Writing is virtually always deficient in Broca aphasics. Most patients have a right hemiparesis necessitating use of the nondominant left hand for writing, but this left-handed writing is far more abnormal than the awkward renditions of a normal right-handed person attempting to write left-handed. Many patients can scrawl only a few letters.

Associated neurological deficits of Broca aphasia include right hemiparesis, hemisensory loss, and apraxia of the oral apparatus and the nonparalyzed left limbs. Apraxia in response to motor commands is important to recognize because it may be mistaken for comprehension disturbance. As mentioned earlier, comprehension should also be tested by responses to yes/no questions or commands to point to an object. The common features of Broca aphasia are listed in **Table 12A.1**.

An important clinical feature of Broca aphasia is its frequent association with depression (Robinson, 1997). Patients with Broca aphasia typically are aware of and frustrated by their deficits. At times they become withdrawn and refuse help or therapy. Usually the depression lifts with recovery from the deficit, but it may be a limiting factor in rehabilitation.

The lesions responsible for Broca aphasia usually include the traditional Broca area in the posterior part of the inferior frontal gyrus, along with damage to adjacent cortex and subcortical white matter. Most patients with lasting Broca aphasia, including Broca's original cases, have much larger left frontoparietal lesions, including most of the territory of the upper division of the left middle cerebral artery. In such patients, the deficit typically evolves from global to Broca aphasia over weeks to months. Patients who manifest Broca aphasia immediately after their strokes, by contrast, have smaller lesions of the inferior frontal region, and their deficits generally resolve quickly. In computed tomography (CT) scan analyses at the Boston Veterans Administration Medical Center, lesions restricted to the lower precentral gyrus produced only dysarthria and mild expressive disturbance. Lesions involving the traditional Broca area (Brodmann areas 44 and 45) resulted in difficulty initiating speech, and lesions combining the Broca area, the lower precentral gyrus, and subcortical white matter yielded the full syndrome of Broca aphasia. In other studies at the center, damage to two subcortical white matter sites—the rostral subcallosal fasciculus deep to the Broca area and the periventricular white matter adjacent to the body of the left lateral ventricle—was required to cause permanent nonfluency. These concepts concerning the Broca area and its mainly temporary role in Broca aphasia have been confirmed by a recent MRI study, indicating that MRI lesions in the Broca area correlate with Broca or global aphasia in acute stroke, but not in the chronic period (Ochfeld et al., 2010). **Fig. 12A.3** shows an MRI scan of the brain from a patient with Broca aphasia.

Aphemia

A rare variant of Broca aphasia is *aphemia*, a nonfluent syndrome in which the patient initially is mute and then becomes able to speak with phoneme substitutions and pauses. All other language functions are intact, including writing. This rare and usually transitory syndrome results from small lesions of the Broca area or its subcortical white matter or of the inferior precentral gyrus. Because written expression and auditory comprehension are normal, aphemia is not a true language disorder; aphemia may be equivalent to pure apraxia of speech.

Wernicke Aphasia

Wernicke aphasia may be considered the opposite of Broca aphasia in that expressive speech is fluent, but comprehension is impaired. The speech pattern is effortless and sometimes even excessively fluent ("logorrhea"). A speaker of a foreign language would notice nothing amiss, but a listener who shares the patient's language detects speech empty of meaning, containing verbal paraphasias, neologisms, and jargon productions. Neurolinguists refer to this pattern as *paragrammatism*. In milder cases, the intended meaning of an utterance may be discerned, but the sentence goes awry with paraphasic substitutions. Naming in Wernicke aphasia is deficient, often with bizarre, paraphasic substitutions for the correct name. Auditory comprehension is impaired, sometimes even for simple nonsense questions. Deficient semantics is the major cause of the comprehension disturbance in Wernicke aphasia, along with disturbed access to the internal lexicon. Repetition is impaired; whispering a phrase in the patient's ear, as in a hearing test, may help cue the patient to attempt repetition.

Table 12A.1 Bedside Features of Broca Aphasia

Feature	Syndrome
Spontaneous speech	Nonfluent, mute or telegraphic, usually dysarthric
Naming	Impaired
Comprehension	Intact (mild difficulty with complex grammatical phrases)
Repetition	Impaired
Reading	Often impaired ("third alexia")
Writing	Impaired (dysmorphic, dysgrammatical)
Associated signs	Right hemiparesis
	Right hemisensory loss ± Apraxia of left limbs

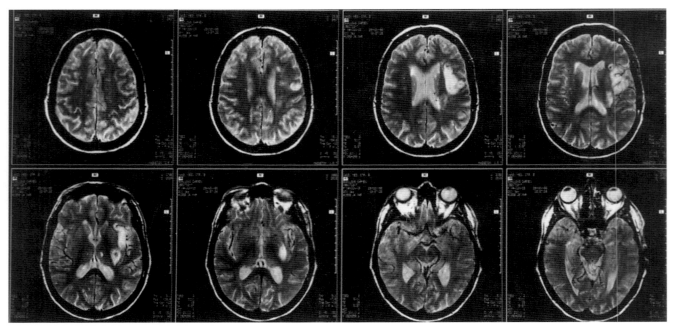

Fig. 12A.3 Magnetic resonance imaging study of the brain of a patient with Broca aphasia. In this patient, the cortical Broca area, subcortical white matter, and the insula all were involved in the infarction. The patient made a good recovery.

Reading comprehension is usually affected in a fashion similar to that observed for auditory comprehension, but occasionally patients show greater deficit in one modality than in the other. The discovery of spared reading ability in Wernicke aphasics is important in allowing these patients to communicate. In addition, neurolinguistic theories of reading must account for the access of visual language images to semantic interpretation, even in the absence of auditory comprehension. Writing also is impaired, but in a manner quite different from that of Broca aphasia. The patient usually has no hemiparesis and can grasp the pen and write easily. Written productions are even more abnormal than oral ones, however, in that spelling errors are also evident. Writing samples are especially useful in the detection of mild Wernicke aphasia.

Associated signs are limited in Wernicke aphasia; most patients have no elementary motor or sensory deficits, although a partial or complete right homonymous hemianopia may be present. The characteristic bedside examination findings in Wernicke aphasia are summarized in **Table 12A.2**.

The psychiatric manifestations of Wernicke aphasia are quite different from those of Broca aphasia. Depression is less common; many Wernicke aphasics seem unaware of or unconcerned about their communicative deficits. With time, some patients become angry or paranoid about the inability of family members and medical staff to understand them. This behavior, like depression, may hinder rehabilitative efforts.

The lesions of patients with Wernicke aphasia usually involve the posterior portion of the superior temporal gyrus, sometimes extending into the inferior parietal lobule. **Fig. 12A.4** shows a typical example. The exact confines of the Wernicke area have been much debated. Damage to this area (Brodmann area 22) has been reported to correlate most closely with persistent loss of comprehension of single words, although only larger temporoparietal lesions have been found in patients with lasting Wernicke aphasia. In the acute phase,

Table 12A.2 Bedside Features of Wernicke Aphasia

Feature	Syndrome
Spontaneous speech	Fluent with paraphasic errors; usually not dysarthric, sometimes logorrheic
Naming	Impaired (often bizarre paraphasic misnaming)
Comprehension	Impaired
Repetition	Impaired
Reading	Impaired for comprehension, reading aloud
Writing	Well formed, paragraphic
Associated signs	± Right hemianopia
	Motor, sensory signs usually absent

the ability to match a spoken word to a picture is quantitatively related to decreased perfusion of the Wernicke area on perfusion-weighted MRI, indicating less variability during the acute phase than after recovery has taken place (Hillis et al., 2001). Electrical stimulation of the Wernicke area produces consistent interruption of auditory comprehension, supporting the importance of this region for decoding auditory language. A receptive speech area in the left inferior temporal gyrus has also been suggested by electrical stimulation studies and by a few descriptions of patients with seizures involving this area (Kirshner et al., 1995), but aphasia has not been recognized with destructive lesions of this area. Extension of the lesion of Wernicke aphasia into the inferior parietal region may predict greater involvement of reading comprehension.

In terms of vascular anatomy, the Wernicke area lies within the territory of the inferior division of the left middle cerebral artery.

Pure Word Deafness

Pure word deafness is a rare but striking syndrome of isolated loss of auditory comprehension and repetition, without any abnormality of speech, naming, reading, or writing. Hearing for pure tones and nonverbal noises (e.g., animal cries) is intact. Most cases have mild aphasic deficits, especially paraphasic speech. Classically, the anatomical substrate is a bilateral lesion isolating the Wernicke area from input from both

the Heschl gyri. Pure word deafness is thus an example of a "disconnection syndrome" in which the deficit results from loss of white matter connections rather than of gray matter language centers. In some cases of pure word deafness, however, the underlying cause is a unilateral left temporal lesion. These cases closely resemble Wernicke aphasia, with greater impairment of auditory comprehension than of reading.

Global Aphasia

Global aphasia may be thought of as a summation of the deficits of Broca aphasia and Wernicke aphasia. Speech is

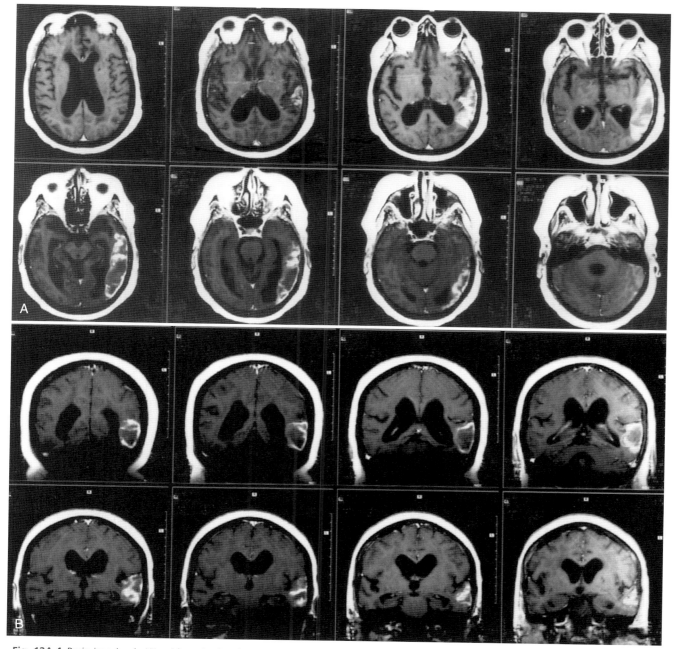

Fig. 12A.4 Brain imaging in Wernicke aphasia. The patient was an elderly woman. **A** and **B,** Axial and coronal magnetic resonance images.

Continued

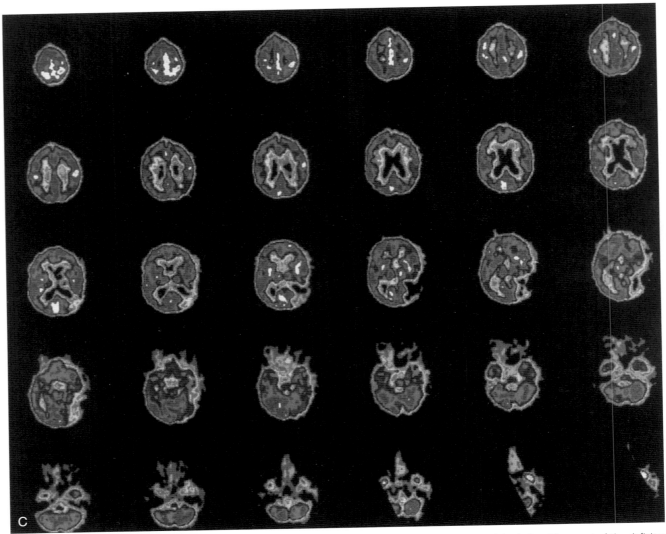

Fig. 12A.4, cont'd C, Axial positron emission tomography (PET) scan. There is a large left superior temporal lobe lesion. The onset of the deficit was not clear, and the PET scan was useful in showing that the lesion had reduced metabolism, favoring a stroke over a tumor.

nonfluent or mute, but comprehension also is poor, as are naming, repetition, reading, and writing. Most patients have dense right hemiparesis, hemisensory loss, and often hemianopia, although occasional patients have mild or no hemiparesis. Milder aphasic syndromes in which all modalities of language are affected often are called *mixed aphasias*. The lesions of patients with global aphasia are usually large, involving both the inferior frontal and superior temporal regions, and often much of the parietal lobe in between. This lesion represents most of the territory of the left middle cerebral artery. Patients in whom the superior temporal gyrus is spared tend to recover their auditory comprehension, with evolution of the deficit toward the syndrome of Broca aphasia. Recovery in global aphasia may be prolonged; in patients with global aphasia, more clinical improvement may occur during the second 6 months than in the first 6 months after a stroke. Characteristics of global aphasia are presented in **Table 12A.3**.

Table 12A.3 Bedside Features of Global Aphasia

Feature	Syndrome
Spontaneous speech	Mute or nonfluent
Naming	Impaired
Comprehension	Impaired
Repetition	Impaired
Reading	Impaired
Writing	Impaired
Associated signs	Right hemiparesis
Right hemisensory loss
Right hemianopia

Conduction Aphasia

Conduction aphasia is an uncommon but theoretically important syndrome that can be recognized by its striking deficit of repetition. Most patients have relatively normal spontaneous speech, although some make literal paraphasic errors and hesitate frequently for self-correction. Naming is impaired to varying degrees, but auditory comprehension is preserved. Repetition may be disturbed to seemingly ridiculous extremes such that a patient who is capable of self-expression at a sentence level and can comprehend conversation may be unable to repeat even single words. One such patient could not repeat the word "boy" but said "I like girls better." Reading and writing are somewhat variable, but reading aloud may share some of the same difficulty as repeating. Associated deficits include hemianopia in some patients; right-sided sensory loss may be present, but right hemiparesis usually is mild or absent. Some patients have limb apraxia, creating a misimpression that comprehension is impaired. Bedside examination findings in conduction aphasia are summarized in **Table 12A.4**.

The lesions of conduction aphasia usually involve either the superior temporal or inferior parietal region. Benson and associates suggested that patients with limb apraxia have parietal lesions, whereas those without apraxia have temporal lesions. Conduction aphasia may represent a stage of recovery in patients with Wernicke aphasia in whom the damage to the superior temporal gyrus is not complete.

Conduction aphasia has been advanced as a classical disconnection syndrome. Wernicke originally postulated that a lesion disconnecting the Wernicke and Broca areas would produce this syndrome; Geschwind later pointed to the arcuate fasciculus, a white-matter tract traveling from the deep temporal lobe, around the sylvian fissure, to the frontal lobe, as the site of disconnection. Anatomical involvement of the arcuate fasciculus is present in most if not all cases of conduction aphasia, but doubt has arisen as to the importance of the arcuate fasciculus to this syndrome. Bernal and Ardila (2009) cite evidence that the arcuate fasciculus terminates in the premotor/motor areas, and not in the Broca area. In addition, there is usually also cortical involvement of the supramarginal

gyrus or temporal lobe. The supramarginal gyrus appears to be involved in auditory immediate memory and in phoneme perception related to word meaning as well as phoneme generation (Hickok and Poeppel, 2000). Lesions in this area are associated with conduction aphasia and phonemic paraphasic errors. Other investigators have pointed out that lesions of the arcuate fasciculus do not always produce conduction aphasia. Another theory of conduction aphasia suggests a defect in auditory verbal short-term memory.

Anomic Aphasia

Anomic aphasia refers to aphasic syndromes in which naming, or access to the internal lexicon, is the principal deficit. Spontaneous speech is normal except for the pauses and circumlocutions produced by the inability to name. Comprehension, repetition, reading, and writing are intact except for the same word-finding difficulty in written productions. Anomic aphasia is common but less specific in localization than the other aphasic syndromes. Isolated severe anomia may indicate focal left hemisphere pathology. Alexander and Benson (1997) refer to the angular gyrus as the site of lesions producing anomic aphasia, but lesions there usually produce other deficits as well, including alexia and the four elements of the Gerstmann syndrome: agraphia, right-left disorientation, acalculia, and finger agnosia, or inability to identify fingers. Isolated lesions of the temporal lobe can produce pure anomia, and PET studies of naming in normal persons also have shown consistent activation of the superior temporal lobe. Inability to produce nouns is characteristic of temporal lobe lesions, whereas inability to produce verbs occurs more often with frontal lesions. Even specific classes of nouns may be selectively affected in some cases of anomic aphasia. Anomia also is seen with mass lesions elsewhere in the brain, and in neurodegenerative disorders such as Alzheimer disease. Anomic aphasia also is a common stage in the recovery of many aphasic syndromes. Anomic aphasia thus serves as an indicator of left hemisphere or diffuse brain disease, but it has only limited localizing value. The typical features of anomic aphasia are presented in **Table 12A.5**.

Transcortical Aphasias

The transcortical aphasias are syndromes in which repetition is normal, presumably because the causative lesions do not

Table 12A.4 Bedside Features of Conduction Aphasia

Feature	Syndrome
Spontaneous speech	Fluent, some hesitancy, literal paraphasic errors
Naming	May be moderately impaired
Comprehension	Intact
Repetition	Severely impaired
Reading	± Inability to read aloud; some reading comprehension
Writing	Variable deficits
Associated signs	± Apraxia of left limbs ± Right hemiparesis, usually mild ± Right hemisensory loss ± Right hemianopia

Table 12A.5 Bedside Features of Anomic Aphasia

Feature	Syndrome
Spontaneous speech	Fluent, some word-finding pauses, circumlocution
Naming	Impaired
Comprehension	Intact
Repetition	Intact
Reading	Intact
Writing	Intact except for anomia
Associated signs	Variable or none

Table 12A.6 Bedside Features of Transcortical Aphasias

Feature	Isolation Syndrome	Transcortical Motor	Transcortical Sensory
Speech	Nonfluent, echolalic	Nonfluent	Fluent, echolalic
Naming	Impaired	Impaired	Impaired
Comprehension	Impaired	Intact	Impaired
Repetition	Intact	Intact	Intact
Reading	Impaired	± Intact	Impaired
Writing	Impaired	± Intact	Impaired

disrupt the perisylvian language circuit from the Wernicke area through the arcuate fasciculus to the Broca area. Instead, these lesions disrupt connections from other cortical centers into the language circuit—hence the name *transcortical*. The transcortical syndromes are easiest to think of as analogs of the syndromes of global, Broca, and Wernicke aphasias, with intact repetition.

Mixed transcortical aphasia, or the "syndrome of the isolation of the speech area," is a global aphasia in which the patient repeats, often echolalically, but has no propositional speech or comprehension. This syndrome is rare, occurring predominantly with large watershed infarctions of the left hemisphere or both hemispheres that spare the perisylvian cortex, or in advanced dementias.

Transcortical motor aphasia is an analog of Broca aphasia in which speech is hesitant or telegraphic, comprehension is relatively spared, but repetition is fluent. This syndrome occurs with lesions in the frontal lobe anterior to the Broca area, in the deep frontal white matter, or in the medial frontal region in the vicinity of the supplementary motor area. All of these lesion sites are within the territory of the anterior cerebral artery, separating this syndrome from the aphasia syndromes of the middle cerebral artery (Broca, Wernicke, global, and conduction aphasias). This syndrome has also been reported with watershed infarctions, reflecting carotid artery stenosis.

The third transcortical syndrome, transcortical sensory aphasia, is an analog of Wernicke aphasia in which fluent paraphasic speech, paraphasic naming, impaired auditory and reading comprehension, and abnormal writing coexist with normal repetition. This syndrome is relatively uncommon, occurring with strokes of the left temporo-occipital area and in dementias. "Watershed" infarctions between the left middle and posterior cerebral artery territories may produce this syndrome. Bedside examination findings in the transcortical aphasias are summarized in **Table 12A.6**.

Subcortical Aphasias

A current area of interest in aphasia research involves the "subcortical" aphasias. Although all the syndromes discussed so far are defined by behavioral characteristics that can be diagnosed at bedside examination, the subcortical aphasias are defined by lesion localization in the basal ganglia or deep cerebral white matter; in other words, diagnosis of this aphasia syndrome is based on brain imaging. As knowledge about subcortical aphasia has accumulated, two major groups of aphasic symptomatology have been described: aphasia with

thalamic lesions and aphasia with lesions of the subcortical white matter and basal ganglia.

Left thalamic hemorrhages frequently produce a Wernicke-like fluent aphasia with better comprehension than in cortical Wernicke aphasia. A fluctuating or "dichotomous" state has been described, alternating between an alert state with nearly normal language and a drowsy state in which the patient mumbles paraphasically and comprehends poorly. Luria has referred to this state as a "quasi-aphasic abnormality of vigilance." One way of thinking of thalamic aphasia is that the thalamus plays a role in alerting the language cortex such that the language cortex, in effect, goes to sleep. Thalamic aphasia can occur even with a right thalamic lesion in a left-handed patient, indicating that hemispheric language dominance extends to the thalamic level. Although some skeptics have attributed thalamic aphasia to pressure on adjacent structures and secondary effects on the cortex, cases of thalamic aphasia have been described with small ischemic lesions, especially those involving the paramedian or anterior nuclei of the thalamus in the territory of the tuberothalamic artery. Because these lesions produce little or no mass effect, such cases indicate that the thalamus and its connections play a definite role in language function (Carrerra and Bogousslavsky, 2006).

Lesions of the left basal ganglia and deep white matter also cause aphasia. As in thalamic aphasia, the first syndromes described were in basal ganglia hemorrhages, especially those involving the putamen, the most common site of hypertensive intracerebral hemorrhage. Here the aphasic syndromes are more variable, but most commonly involve global or Broca-like aphasia. As in thalamic lesions, ischemic strokes have provided better localizing information than hemorrhage cases. The most common lesion is an infarct involving the anterior putamen, caudate nucleus, and anterior limb of the internal capsule. Patients with this lesion have an "anterior subcortical aphasia syndrome" involving dysarthria, decreased fluency, mildly impaired repetition, and mild comprehension disturbance. This syndrome most closely resembles Broca aphasia, but with greater dysarthria and less language dysfunction. **Fig. 12A.5** shows imaging findings in an example of this syndrome. More restricted lesions of the anterior putamen, head of caudate, and periventricular white matter produce hesitancy or slow initiation of speech but little true language disturbance. More posterior lesions involving the putamen and deep temporal white matter, referred to as the *temporal isthmus*, are associated with fluent paraphasic speech and impaired comprehension, resembling the features of Wernicke aphasia. Small lesions in the posterior limb of the internal capsule and adjacent putamen cause mainly dysarthria, but mild aphasic

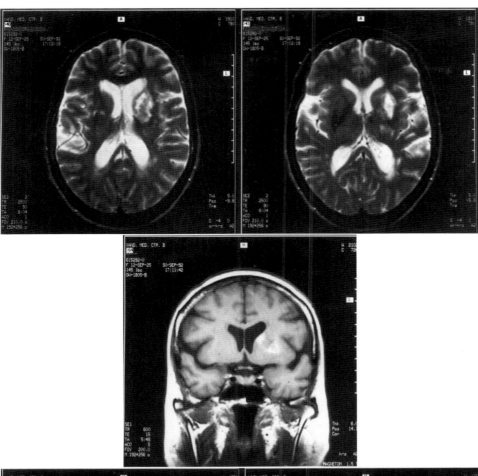

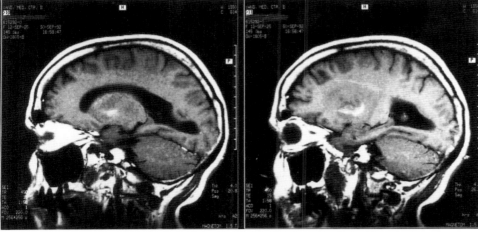

Fig. 12A.5 Magnetic resonance imaging (MRI) study of the brain with slices in the axial, coronal, and sagittal planes in subcortical aphasia. The lesion is an infarction involving the anterior caudate, putamen, and anterior limb of the left internal capsule. The patient presented with dysarthria and mild, nonfluent aphasia with anomia, with good comprehension. The advantage of MRI in permitting visualization of the lesion in all three planes is apparent.

deficits may occasionally occur. Finally, larger subcortical lesions involving both the anterior and posterior lesion sites produce global aphasia. A wide variety of aphasia syndromes can thus be seen with subcortical lesion sites. Nadeau and Crosson (1997) presented an anatomical model of basal ganglia involvement in speech and language, based on the known motor functions and fiber connections of these structures. Evidence from PET indicates that basal ganglia lesions affect language, both directly and indirectly, via decreased activation of cortical language areas.

The insula, a cortical structure that shares a deep location with the subcortical structures, may also be important to speech and language function. Dronkers (1996) reported that involvement of this area is closely associated with the presence of apraxia of speech in aphasic patients. Hillis and colleagues (2004), however, in MRI studies of brain in acute stroke patients, found that the left frontal cortex correlates more with speech apraxia than does the insula.

In clinical terms, subcortical lesions do produce aphasia, although less commonly than cortical lesions do, and the language characteristics of subcortical aphasias often are atypical. The presentation of a difficult-to-classify aphasic syndrome, in the presence of dysarthria and right hemiparesis, should lead to suspicion of a subcortical lesion.

Pure Alexia without Agraphia

Alexia, or acquired inability to read, is a form of aphasia, according to the definition given at the beginning of this chapter. The classic syndrome of alexia, pure alexia without agraphia, was described by the French neurologist Dejerine in 1892. This syndrome may be thought of as a linguistic blind-folding (or "pure word blindness") in that patients can write but cannot read their own writing. On bedside examination, speech, auditory comprehension, and repetition are normal. Naming may be deficient, especially for colors. Patients initially cannot read at all; as they recover, they learn to read letter by letter, spelling out words laboriously. They cannot read words at a glance as normal readers do. By contrast, they quickly understand words spelled orally to them, and they can spell normally, both orally and in writing. Some patients can match words to pictures, indicating that some subconscious awareness of the word is present, perhaps in the right hemisphere. Associated deficits include a right hemianopia or right upper quadrant defect in nearly all patients and frequently a deficit of short-term memory. There usually is no hemiparesis or sensory loss.

The causative lesion in pure alexia is nearly always a stroke in the territory of the left posterior cerebral artery, with infarction of the medial occipital lobe, often the splenium of the corpus callosum, and often the medial temporal lobe. Dejerine postulated a disconnection between the intact right visual cortex and left hemisphere language centers, particularly the angular gyrus. **Fig. 12A.6** is an adaptation of Dejerine's original diagram; **Fig. 12A.7** shows an MRI of a patient with alexia without agraphia. Geschwind later rediscovered this "disconnection" hypothesis. Although Damasio and Damasio found splenial involvement in only 2 of 16 cases, they postulated a disconnection within the deep white matter of the left occipital lobe. As in the disconnection hypothesis for conduction aphasia, the theory fails to explain all the behavioral phenomena, such as the sparing of single-letter reading. A deficit in immediate memory span for visual language elements or an inability to perceive multiple letters at once (simultanagnosia) also can explain many features of the syndrome. Typical features of pure alexia without agraphia are presented in **Table 12A.7**.

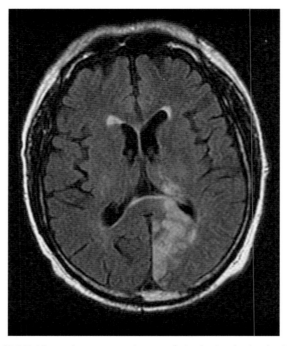

Fig. 12A.7 Magnetic resonance image of the brain obtained using a fluid-attenuated inversion recovery (FLAIR) sequence. The patient was an 82-year-old man with alexia without agraphia. The infarction involves the medial occipital lobe and the splenium of the corpus callosum, within the territory of the left posterior cerebral artery.

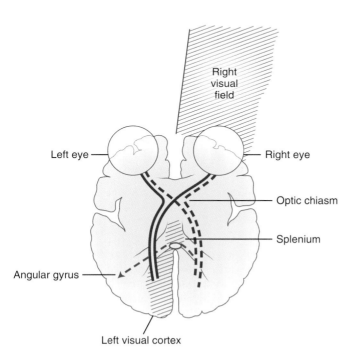

Fig. 12A.6 Horizontal brain diagram of pure alexia without agraphia, adapted from that of Dejerine, 1892. Visual information from the left visual field reaches the right occipital cortex but is "disconnected" from the left hemisphere language centers by the lesion in the splenium of the corpus callosum.

Table 12A.7 **Bedside Features of Pure Alexia without Agraphia**	
Feature	**Syndrome**
Spontaneous speech	Intact
Naming	± Impaired, especially colors
Comprehension	Intact
Repetition	Intact
Reading	Impaired (some sparing of single letters)
Writing	Intact
Associated signs	Right hemianopia or superior quadrantanopia Short-term memory loss Motor, sensory signs usually absent

Alexia with Agraphia

The second classic alexia syndrome, alexia with agraphia, described by Dejerine in 1891, may be thought of as an acquired illiteracy in which a previously literate patient is rendered unable to read or write. The oral language modalities of speech, naming, auditory comprehension, and repetition are largely intact, but in many cases the patient demonstrates a fluent paraphasic speech pattern with impaired naming. This syndrome thus overlaps Wernicke aphasia, especially in cases in which reading is more impaired than auditory comprehension. Associated deficits include right hemianopia and elements of the Gerstmann syndrome: agraphia, acalculia, right-left disorientation, and finger agnosia. The lesions typically involve the inferior parietal lobule, especially the angular gyrus. Etiologic disorders include strokes in the territory of the angular branch of the left middle cerebral artery and mass lesions in the same region. Characteristic features of the syndrome of alexia with agraphia are summarized in **Table 12A.8**.

Aphasic Alexia

In addition to the two classic alexia syndromes, many patients with aphasia have associated reading disturbance. Examples already cited are the "third alexia" of Broca aphasia and the reading deficit of Wernicke aphasia. Neurolinguists and cognitive psychologists have divided alexias according to breakdown in specific stages of the reading process. The linguistic concepts of surface structure versus the deep meanings of words have been instrumental in these new classifications. Four patterns of alexia (or "dyslexia" in British usage) have been recognized: letter-by-letter, deep, phonological, and surface dyslexia. **Fig. 12A.8** diagrams the steps in the reading process and the points of breakdown in the four syndromes. Letter-by-letter dyslexia is equivalent to pure alexia without agraphia. Deep dyslexia is a severe reading disorder in which patients recognize and read aloud only familiar words, especially concrete, imageable nouns and verbs. They make semantic or visual errors in reading and fail completely in reading nonsense syllables or nonwords. Word reading is not affected by word length or regularity of spelling; one patient, for example, could read "ambulance" but not "am." Most cases are characterized by severe aphasia, with extensive left frontoparietal damage.

Phonological dyslexia is similar to deep dyslexia, with poor reading of nonwords, but single nouns and verbs are read in a nearly normal fashion, and semantic errors are rare. Patients appear to read words without understanding. The fourth type, surface dyslexia, involves spared ability to read laboriously by grapheme-phoneme conversion but inability to recognize words at a glance. These patients can read nonsense syllables but not words of irregular spelling, such as "colonel" or "yacht." Their errors tend to be phonological rather than semantic or visual (e.g., pronouncing "rough" and "though" alike).

Agraphia

Like reading, writing may be affected either in isolation (pure agraphia) or in association with aphasia (aphasic agraphia). In addition, writing can be impaired by motor disorders, apraxia, and visuospatial deficits. Isolated agraphia has been described with left frontal or parietal lesions.

Agraphias can be analyzed in the same way as alexias (**Fig. 12A.9**). Thus, phonological agraphia involves the inability to convert phonemes into graphemes or to write pronounceable nonsense syllables in the presence of ability to write familiar words. Deep dysgraphia is similar to phonological agraphia, but the patient can read nouns and verbs better than articles, prepositions, adjectives, and adverbs. In lexical or surface dysgraphia, patients can write regularly spelled words and pronounceable nonsense words but not irregularly spelled words. These patients have intact phoneme-grapheme conversion but cannot write by a whole-word or "lexical" strategy.

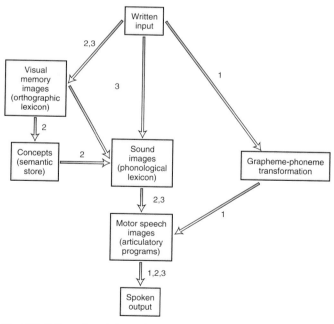

Fig. 12A.8 Neurolinguistic model of the reading process. Evidence from studies of the alexias points to three separate routes to reading: 1, the phonological (or grapheme-phoneme conversion) route; 2, the semantic (or lexical-semantic-phonological) route; and 3, the nonlexical phonological route. In deep dyslexia, only route 2 can operate; in phonological dyslexia, 3 is the principal pathway; in surface dyslexia, only 1 is functional. *(Adapted with permission from Margolin, D.I., 1991. Cognitive neuropsychology. Resolving enigmas about Wernicke's aphasia and other higher cortical disorders. Arch Neurol 48, 751-765.)*

Table 12A.8 Bedside Features of Alexia with Agraphia

Feature	Syndrome
Spontaneous speech	Fluent, often some paraphasia
Naming	± Impaired
Comprehension	Intact or less impaired than reading
Repetition	Intact
Reading	Severely impaired
Writing	Severely impaired
Associated signs	Right hemianopia Motor, sensory signs usually absent

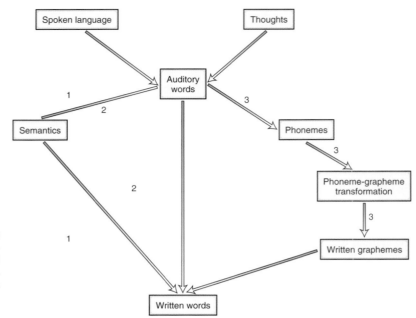

Fig. 12A.9 Neurolinguistic model of writing and the agraphias. In deep agraphia, only the semantic (phonological-semantic-lexical) route (1) is operative. In phonological agraphia, route 2, the nonlexical phonological route, produces written words directly from spoken words. In surface agraphia, only route 3, the phoneme-grapheme pathway, can be used to generate writing.

Language in Right Hemisphere Disorders

Language and communication disorders are important even in patients with right hemisphere disease. First, left-handed patients may have right hemisphere language dominance and may acquire aphasic syndromes due to right hemisphere lesions. Second, right-handed patients occasionally become aphasic after right hemisphere strokes, a phenomenon called *crossed aphasia* (Bakar et al., 1996). These patients presumably have crossed or mixed dominance. Third, even right-handed persons with typical left hemisphere dominance for language have subtly altered language function after right hemisphere damage. Such patients are not aphasic in that the fundamental mechanisms of speech production, repetition, and comprehension are undisturbed. Affective aspects of language are impaired, however, such that the speech sounds flat and unemotional; the normal prosody or emotional intonation of speech is lost. Syndromes of loss of emotional aspects of speech are termed *aprosodias*. Motor aprosodia involves loss of expressive emotion with preservation of emotional comprehension; sensory aprosodia involves loss of comprehension of affective language, also called *affective agnosia*. In addition to emotional tone, stress and emphasis within a sentence are affected by right hemisphere dysfunction. Of greater importance, such vital aspects of human communication as metaphor, humor, sarcasm, irony, and related constituents of language that transcend the literal meaning of words are especially sensitive to right hemisphere dysfunction. These deficits significantly impair patients in the pragmatics of communication. In other words, right hemisphere–damaged patients understand what is said, but not how it is said. They may have difficulty following a complex story. Such higher-level language deficits are related to the right hemisphere disorders of inattention and neglect, discussed in Chapters 4 and 36.

Language in Dementing Diseases

Language impairment is commonly seen in patients with dementia. Despite considerable variability from patient to patient, two patterns of language dissolution can be described. The first, the common presentation of Alzheimer disease (AD), involves early loss of memory and general cognitive deterioration. In these patients, mental status examinations are most remarkable for deficits in short-term memory, insight, and judgment, but language impairments can be found in naming and in discourse, with impoverished language content and loss of abstraction and metaphor. The mechanics of language, grammatical construction of sentences, receptive vocabulary, auditory comprehension, repetition, and oral reading tend to remain preserved until later stages. By aphasia testing, patients with early AD have anomic aphasia. In later stages, language functions become more obviously impaired. In terms of the components of language mentioned earlier in this chapter, the semantic aspects of language tend to deteriorate first, then syntax, and finally phonology. Reading and writing, the last-learned language functions, are among the first to decline. Auditory comprehension later becomes deficient, whereas repetition and articulation remain normal. The language profile may then resemble that of transcortical sensory or Wernicke aphasia. In terminal stages, speech is reduced to the expression of simple biological wants; eventually, even muteness can develop. By this time, most patients are institutionalized or bedridden.

The second pattern of language dissolution in dementia, considerably less common than the first, involves the gradual onset of a progressive aphasia, often without other cognitive deterioration. Auditory comprehension may be involved early in the illness, and specific aphasic symptoms are evident, such as paraphasic or nonfluent speech, misnaming, and errors of repetition. These deficits worsen gradually, mimicking the course of a brain tumor or mass lesion rather than that of a typical dementia (Grossman et al., 1996; Mesulam, 2001, 2003). The syndrome generally is referred to as *primary progressive aphasia*. CT scans may show focal atrophy in the left perisylvian region, whereas electroencephalographic studies may show focal slowing. PET has shown prominent areas of decreased metabolism in the left temporal region and adjacent cortical areas.

Primary progressive aphasia (PPA) is now considered a variant of a more general category of dementing illnesses called *frontotemporal dementia* (FTD) (Neary and Snowden, 1996; Neary et al., 1998; Josephs, 2008). There are several variants. Mesulam's patients with PPA had largely nonfluent, Broca-like patterns of aphasia (2001, 2003). A progressive fluent aphasia with impaired naming and loss of understanding of words has been termed *semantic dementia*, often associated with surface alexia (Hodges and Patterson, 2007). A third type of progressive aphasia, the logopenic phonological type (Gorno-Tempini et al., 2008), is associated with AD. In general, patients with fluent aphasia who come to autopsy may have either AD or FTD, whereas those with nonfluent aphasia generally have non-Alzheimer disorders. The two most common subtypes in progressive nonfluent aphasia are those with tau staining and those with ubiquitin staining. Many familial cases of FTD have had genetic mutations in the tau gene on chromosome 17 (Heutink et al., 1997), whereas those with ubiquitin pathology may have mutations in the progranulin gene, related to the TAR-DNA binding protein (TDP-43) (Baker et al., 2006; Cruts et al., 2006; Hodges et al., 2004). Other variants include corticobasal degeneration and mixed FTD with motor neuron disease. In one study of 10 patients with PPA followed prospectively until they became nonfluent or mute, Kertesz and Munoz (2003) found that at autopsy, all had evidence of FTD: corticobasal degeneration in four, Pick body dementia in three, and tau and synuclein negative ubiquinated inclusions of the motor neuron disease in three. Kertesz and colleagues (2000) have proposed that Pick disease, FTD, corticobasal degeneration, and PPA should be linked together under the term *Pick complex*. Imaging studies have shown that primary progressive aphasia often is associated with atrophy in the left frontotemporal region, and other areas such as the fusiform and precentral gyri and intraparietal sulcus are activated, possibly as a compensatory neuronal strategy (Sonty et al., 2003). Whitwell and colleagues (2006) have used voxel-based MRI morphometry to delineate different patterns of atrophy in FTD associated with motor neuron disease versus ubiquitin pathology. Cases of isolated aphasia secondary to Creutzfeldt-Jakob disease have been reported, but these usually progress to dementia over a period of months.

Clinical Investigations in the Aphasic Patient

Preliminary Evaluation

The bedside language examination is useful in forming a preliminary impression of the type of aphasia and the localization of the causative lesion. Follow-up examinations also are helpful; as in all neurological diagnosis, the evolution of a neurological deficit over time is the most important clue to the specific disease process. For example, an embolic stroke and a brain tumor both may produce Wernicke aphasia, but strokes occur suddenly, with improvement thereafter, whereas tumors produce gradually worsening aphasia.

Other Useful Tests

In addition to the bedside examination, a large number of standardized aphasia test batteries have been published. The physician should think of these tests as more detailed extensions of the bedside examination. They have the advantage of quantitation and standardization, permitting comparison over time and, in some cases, even a diagnosis of the specific aphasia syndrome. Research on aphasia depends on these standardized tests.

For neurologists, the most helpful battery is the Boston Diagnostic Aphasia Examination or its Canadian adaptation, the Western Aphasia Battery. Both tests provide subtest information analogous to that obtained with the bedside examination, and therefore meaningful to neurologists, as well as aphasia syndrome classification. The Porch Index of Communicative Ability quantitates performance in many specific functions, allowing comparison over time. Other aphasia tests are designed to evaluate specific language areas. For example, the Boston Naming Test evaluates a wide variety of naming stimuli, whereas the Token Test evaluates higher-level comprehension deficits. Further information on neuropsychological tests can be found in Chapter 34.

More specific diagnosis in the aphasic patient rests on the confirmation of a brain lesion by neuroimaging (**Fig. 12A.10**). The CT brain scan (discussed in Chapter 33A) revolutionized the localization of aphasia by permitting "real-time" delineation of a focal lesion in a living patient; previously, the physician had to outlive the patient to obtain a clinical-pathological correlation at autopsy. MRI provides better resolution of areas difficult to see on CT images, such as the temporal cortex adjacent to the petrous bones, and more sensitive detection of tissue pathology, such as early changes of infarction. The anatomical distinction of cortical from subcortical aphasia is best made by MRI. Acute strokes are visualized early on diffusion-weighted MRI.

The electroencephalogram (EEG) is helpful in aphasia in localizing seizure discharges, interictal spikes, and slowing seen after destructive lesions such as traumatic contusions and infarctions. The EEG can provide evidence that aphasia is an ictal or a postictal phenomenon and can furnish early clues in aphasia secondary to mass lesions or herpes simplex encephalitis. In research applications, electrophysiological testing via subdural grid and depth electrodes or stimulation mapping of epileptic foci in preparation for epilepsy surgery have aided in the identification of cortical areas involved in language.

Cerebral arteriography is useful in the diagnosis of aneurysms, arteriovenous malformations (AVMs), arterial occlusions, vasculitis, and venous outflow obstructions. In preparation for epilepsy surgery, the Wada test, or infusion of amobarbital through an arterial catheter, is useful in the determination of language dominance. Other related studies using language activation with functional MRI (fMRI) or PET are beginning to rival the Wada test for the study of language dominance (Abou-Khalil and Schlaggar, 2002).

Single photon emission CT (SPECT), PET, and functional MRI (fMRI; see Chapter 33C) are contributing greatly to the

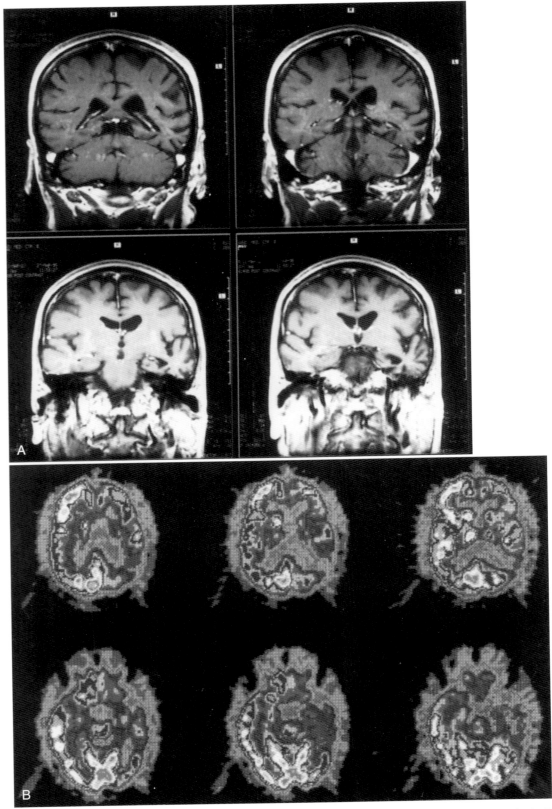

Fig. 12A.10 A, Coronal T1-weighted magnetic resonance imaging study of the brain of a patient with primary progressive aphasia. Note the marked atrophy of the left temporal lobe. **B,** Axial fluorine-2 deoxyglucose positron emission tomography (PET) scans showing extensive hypometabolism in the left cerebral hemisphere, especially marked in the left temporal lobe.

study of language. Patterns of brain activation in response to language stimuli have been recorded, mainly in normal persons, and these studies have largely confirmed the localizations based on clinicopathological findings in disorders such as stroke over the past 140 years. In addition, these techniques can be used to map areas of the brain that activate during language functions after insults such as strokes, and the pattern of recovery can be studied. Some such studies have indicated right hemisphere activation in patients recovering from aphasia (Cappa et al., 1997), whereas others have found that only left hemisphere activation is associated with full recovery (Heiss et al., 1999). A recent fMRI study (Saur et al., 2006) has suggested hypometabolism in the language cortex shortly after an ischemic insult, followed by increased activation of homologous areas in the contralateral hemisphere, and then a shift back to the more normal pattern of left hemisphere activation. Subcortical contributions to aphasia and language in degenerative conditions have been studied with PET. These techniques provide the best correlation between brain structure and function currently available and should help advance our understanding of language disorders and their recovery.

Differential Diagnosis

Vascular lesions, especially ischemic strokes, constitute the most common cause of aphasia. Historically, most research studies in aphasia have used stroke patients because stroke is an "experiment" of nature in which one area of the brain is damaged while the rest remains theoretically intact. Strokes are characterized by the abrupt onset of a neurological deficit in a patient with vascular risk factors. The precise temporal profile is important: most embolic strokes are sudden and maximal at onset, whereas thrombotic strokes typically wax and wane or increase in steps. The bedside aphasia examination is helpful in delineating the vascular territory affected. For example, the sudden onset of Wernicke aphasia nearly always indicates an embolus to the inferior division of the left middle cerebral artery. Global aphasia may be caused by an embolus to the middle cerebral artery stem, thrombosis of the internal carotid artery, or even a hemorrhage into the deep basal ganglia. Whereas most aphasic syndromes involve the territory of the left middle cerebral artery, transcortical motor aphasia is specific to the anterior cerebral territory, and pure alexia without agraphia is specific to the posterior cerebral artery territory. The clinical features of the aphasia are thus of crucial importance to the vascular diagnosis.

Hemorrhagic strokes also are an important cause of aphasia, most commonly the basal ganglionic hemorrhages associated with hypertension. The deficits tend to worsen gradually over minutes to hours, in contrast with the sudden or stepwise onset of ischemic strokes. Headache, vomiting, and obtundation are more common with hemorrhages. Because hemorrhages compress cerebral tissue without necessarily destroying it, the ultimate recovery from aphasia often is better in hemorrhages than in ischemic strokes, although hemorrhages more often are fatal. Other potential causes of intracerebral hemorrhage include anticoagulants, head injury, blood dyscrasias, thrombocytopenia, and bleeding into structural lesions, such as infarctions, tumors, AVMs, and aneurysms. Hemorrhages from AVMs mimic strokes, with abrupt onset of focal neurological deficit. Ruptured aneurysms, on the other hand, manifest with severe headache and stiff neck or with coma; most

patients have no focal deficits, but delayed deficits (e.g., aphasia) may develop secondary to vasospasm. Lobar hemorrhages may occur in elderly patients without hypertension. These hemorrhages occur near the cortical surface, sometimes extending into the subarachnoid space, and they may be recurrent. Histopathological studies have shown amyloid deposition in small arterioles, or amyloid angiopathy. A final vascular cause of aphasia is cerebral vasculitis (see Chapter 51E).

Traumatic brain injury is a common cause of aphasia. Cerebral contusions, depressed skull fractures, and hematomas of the intracerebral, subdural, and epidural spaces all cause aphasia when they disrupt or compress left hemisphere language structures. Trauma tends to be less localized than ischemic stroke; accordingly, aphasia often is admixed with the general effects of the head injury, such as depressed consciousness, encephalopathy or delirium, amnesia, and other deficits. Head injuries in young people may be associated with severe deficits but excellent long-term recovery. Language deficits, especially those that involve discourse organization, can be found in most cases of significant closed head injury. Gunshot wounds produce focal aphasic syndromes, which rival stroke as a source of clinical-anatomical correlation. Subdural hematomas are infamous for mimicking other neurological syndromes. Aphasia occasionally is associated with subdural hematomas overlying the left hemisphere, but it may be mild and may be overlooked because of the patient's more severe complaints of headache, memory loss, and drowsiness.

Tumors of the left hemisphere frequently manifest with aphasia. The onset of the aphasia is gradual, and edema and mass effect may result in other cognitive deficits. Aphasia secondary to an enlarging tumor may thus be difficult to distinguish from a diffuse encephalopathy or early dementia. Any syndrome of abnormal language function should therefore be investigated for a focal, dominant hemisphere lesion.

Infections of the nervous system may cause aphasia. Brain abscesses can mimic tumors in every respect, and those in the left hemisphere can manifest with progressive aphasia. Chronic infections such as tuberculosis or syphilis can result in focal abnormalities that run the entire gamut of central nervous system symptoms and signs. Herpes simplex encephalitis has a predilection for the temporal lobe and orbital frontal cortex, and aphasia can be an early manifestation, along with headache, confusion, fever, and seizures. Aphasia often is a permanent sequela in survivors of herpes encephalitis. Acquired immunodeficiency syndrome (AIDS) is rapidly becoming a common cause of language disorders. Opportunistic infections can cause focal lesions anywhere in the brain, and the neurotropic human immunodeficiency virus (HIV) agent itself produces a dementia (AIDS dementia complex) in which language deficits play a part.

Aphasia frequently is caused by the degenerative central nervous system diseases. Reference has already been made to the focal progressive aphasia in patients with FTD, versus the more diffuse cognitive deterioration characteristic of AD. Language dysfunction in AD may be more common in familial cases and may predict poor prognosis. Cognitive deterioration in patients with Parkinson disease (PD) also may include language deterioration similar to that of AD, although PD tends to involve more fluctuation in orientation and greater tendency to active hallucinations and delusions. A striking abnormality of speech—that is, initial stuttering followed by true aphasia and dementia—has been described in the dialysis dementia syndrome, which has all but disappeared in recent years after removal of aluminum from dialysis fluids. This disorder may be associated with spongiform degeneration of the frontotemporal cortex similar to that in Creutzfeldt-Jakob disease. Paraphasic substitutions and nonsense speech also are occasionally encountered in acute encephalopathies such as hyponatremia or lithium toxicity.

A final cause of aphasia is seizures. Seizures can be associated with aphasia in children as part of the Landau-Kleffner syndrome or in adults as either an ictal or postictal Todd phenomenon. Epileptic aphasia is important to recognize because anticonvulsant drug therapy can prevent the episodes, and unnecessary investigation or treatment for a suspected new lesion, such as a stroke, can be avoided. As mentioned earlier, localization of language areas in epileptic patients has contributed greatly to the knowledge of language organization in the brain. Greater than 15% of young epileptic patients have no Broca or Wernicke area. In addition, a new language area, the basal temporal language area (BTLA) has been discovered through epilepsy stimulation studies and only later confirmed in patients with spontaneous seizures (Kirshner et al., 1995).

Recovery and Rehabilitation of the Patient with Aphasia

Patients with aphasia from acute disorders such as stroke generally show spontaneous improvement over days, weeks, and months. In general, the greatest recovery occurs during the first 3 months, but improvement may continue over a prolonged period, especially in young patients and in persons with global aphasia. The aphasia type often changes during recovery: global aphasia evolves into Broca aphasia, and Wernicke aphasia into conduction or anomic aphasia. Language recovery may be mediated by shifting of functions to the right hemisphere or to adjacent left hemisphere regions. As mentioned earlier, studies of language activation PET and SPECT scanning techniques are advancing our understanding of the neuroanatomy of language recovery (Heiss et al., 1999). In addition, study of patients in the very acute phase of aphasia with techniques of diffusion and perfusion-weighted MRI has suggested less variability in the correlation of comprehension impairment with left temporal ischemia than has been suggested from testing of patients with chronic aphasia, after recovery and compensation have commenced (Hillis et al., 2001).

Speech therapy provided by speech/language pathologists attempts to facilitate language recovery by a variety of techniques and to help the patient compensate for lost functions (see Chapter 48). Repeated practice in articulation and comprehension tasks traditionally has been used to stimulate improvement. Other techniques include melodic intonation therapy, which uses melody to involve the right hemisphere in speech production; visual action therapy, which uses gestural expression; and treatment of aphasic perseveration, which aims to reduce repetitive utterances. Two other therapeutic techniques are functional communication therapy, which takes advantage of extralinguistic communication, and cVIC or Lingraphica, a computer program originally developed for primate communication. Patients who cannot speak can learn to produce simple sentences via computer. Augmentative devices make language expression possible through use of printers or voice simulators.

Speech therapy has remained controversial. Some studies have suggested that briefly trained volunteers can induce as much improvement as that achieved by speech/language pathologists, but large randomized trials have clearly indicated that patients who undergo formal speech therapy recover better than untreated patients (Robey, 1998). A recent Cochrane review also supports the efficacy of intensive speech/language therapy over conventional therapy (Kelly, Brady, and Enderby, 2010).

A new approach to language rehabilitation is the use of pharmacological agents to improve speech. In 1998, Albert and colleagues first reported that the dopaminergic drug, bromocriptine, promotes spontaneous speech output in transcortical motor aphasia. Several other studies have supported use of this drug in nonfluent aphasias, although a recent controlled study showed no benefit (Ashtary et al., 2006). Stimulant drugs also are being tested in aphasia rehabilitation. As new information accumulates on the neurochemistry of cognitive functions, other pharmacological therapies may be forthcoming.

Other new approaches to aphasia therapy include both transcranial magnetic stimulation (Martin, Naeser, and Ho, 2009) and transcranial direct-current stimulation (Baker et al., 2010). These are preliminary exploratory studies, and it remains to be seen from larger studies how effective these stimulation techniques will be.

References

The complete reference list is available online at www.expertconsult.com.

Language and Speech Disorders
Motor Speech Disorders: Dysarthria and Apraxia of Speech

Howard S. Kirshner

Motor Speech Disorders: Overview

Motor speech disorders are syndromes of abnormal articulation, the motor production of speech, without abnormalities of language. A patient with a motor speech disorder can produce normal expressive language in writing and can comprehend both spoken and written language. If a listener transcribes the speech of a patient with a motor speech disorder into print or type and then reads it, the text should sound normal. Motor speech disorders include *dysarthrias*, disorders of speech articulation, and *apraxia of speech*, a motor programming disorder for speech, as well as four rarer syndromes: *aphemia, the foreign accent syndrome, acquired stuttering,* and *the opercular syndrome.* Duffy (1995), in an analysis of speech and language disorders at the Mayo Clinic, reported that 46.3% of the patients had dysarthria, 27.1% aphasia, 4.6% apraxia of speech, 9% other speech disorders (such as stuttering), and 13% other cognitive or linguistic disorders.

Dysarthrias

Dysarthrias involve the abnormal articulation of sounds or phonemes. The pathogenic mechanism in dysarthria is abnormal neuromuscular activation of the speech muscles, affecting the speed, strength, timing, range, or accuracy of movements involving speech (Duffy, 1995). The most consistent finding in dysarthria is the distortion of consonant sounds. Speech disorders can be mechanical, as in patients with physical disorders of the pharynx and larynx, but dysarthrias are neurogenic, related to dysfunction of the central nervous system, nerves, neuromuscular junction, or muscle, with a contribution of sensory deficits in some cases. Dysarthria can affect not only articulation but also phonation, breathing, and prosody (emotional tone) of speech. Total loss of ability to articulate is called *anarthria.*

Like the aphasias, dysarthrias can be analyzed in terms of the brain lesion sites associated with specific patterns of speech impairment. Analysis of dysarthria at the bedside is useful for the localization of neurological lesions and the diagnosis of neurological disorders. An experienced examiner should be able to recognize the major types of dysarthria, rather than referring to "dysarthria" as a single disorder.

The examination of speech at the bedside should include having the patient repeat syllables, words, and sentences. Repeating consonant sounds (such as /p/, /p/, /p/) or shifting consonant sounds (/p/, /t/, /k/) can help identify which consonants consistently cause trouble. Repetition of polysyllabic words such as "impossibility" or "catastrophe" 4 or 5 times can elicit both the consistent errors of dysarthria and the inconsistent errors of apraxia of speech (see later discussion).

The Mayo Clinic classification of dysarthria (Duffy, 1995), widely used in the United States, includes six categories: (1) flaccid, (2) spastic and "unilateral upper motor neuron," (3) ataxic, (4) hypokinetic, (5) hyperkinetic, and (6) mixed dysarthria. These types of dysarthria are summarized in **Table 12B.1.**

DOI: 10.1016/B978-1-4377-0434-1.00043-8

Table 12B.1 Classification of the Dysarthrias

Type	Localization	Auditory Signs	Characteristic Disease(s)
Flaccid	Lower motor neuron	Breathy, nasal voice, imprecise consonants	Stroke, myasthenia gravis
Spastic	Bilateral motor neuron	Strain-strangle, harsh voice; slow rate; imprecise consonants	Bilateral strokes, tumors, primary lateral sclerosis
	Unilateral upper motor neuron	Consonant imprecision, slow rate, harsh voice quality	Stroke, tumor
Ataxic	Cerebellum	Irregular articulatory breakdowns, excessive and equal stress	Stroke, degenerative disease
Hypokinetic	Extrapyramidal	Rapid rate, reduced loudness, monopitch and monoloudness	PD
Hyperkinetic	Extrapyramidal	Prolonged phonemes, variable rate, inappropriate silences, voice stoppages	Dystonia, HD
Spastic and flaccid	Upper and lower motor neuron	Hypernasality, strain-strangle, harsh voice, slow rate, imprecise consonants	ALS, multiple strokes

Adapted from Duffy, J.R., 1995. Motor Speech Disorders: Substrates, Differential Diagnosis, and Management. Mosby, St. Louis; and from Kirshner, H.S., 2002. Behavioral Neurology: Practical Science of Mind and Brain. Butterworth Heinemann, Boston.
ALS, Amyotrophic lateral sclerosis; HD, Huntington disease; PD, Parkinson disease.

Flaccid dysarthria is associated with disorders involving lower motor neuron weakness of the bulbar muscles, such as polymyositis, myasthenia gravis, and bulbar poliomyelitis. The speech pattern is breathy and nasal, with indistinctly pronounced consonants. In the case of myasthenia gravis, the patient may begin reading a paragraph with normal enunciation, but by the end of the paragraph the articulation is soft, breathy, and frequently interrupted by labored respirations.

Spastic dysarthria occurs in patients with bilateral lesions of the motor cortex or corticobulbar tracts, such as bilateral strokes. The speech is harsh or "strain-strangle" in vocal quality, with reduced rate, low pitch, and consonant errors. Patients often have associated features of pseudobulbar palsy, including dysphagia, exaggerated jaw jerk and gag reflexes, and easy laughter and crying (synonyms: emotional incontinence, pseudobulbar affect, or pathological laughter and crying). Another variant is the opercular syndrome, described later in this chapter.

A milder variant of spastic dysarthria, unilateral upper motor neuron (UUMN) dysarthria, is associated with unilateral upper motor neuron lesions, such as strokes (Duffy, 1995). This type of dysarthria has similar features to spastic dysarthria, but UUMN dysarthria is less severe. Unilateral upper motor neuron dysarthria is one of the most common types of dysarthria, since it occurs in patients with unilateral strokes. In a study by Urban and colleagues (2006), left hemisphere strokes were more likely than right hemisphere strokes to be associated with dysarthria.

Ataxic dysarthria, associated with cerebellar disorders, is characterized by one of two patterns: irregular breakdowns of speech with explosions of syllables interrupted by pauses, or a slow cadence of speech with excessively equal stress on every syllable. The second pattern of ataxic dysarthria is referred to as *scanning speech*. A patient with ataxic dysarthria, attempting to repeat the phoneme /p/ as rapidly as possible, for example, produces either an irregular rhythm, resembling popcorn popping, or a very slow rhythm. Causes of ataxic dysarthria include cerebellar strokes, tumors, multiple sclerosis, and cerebellar and spinocerebellar degenerations. A recent report localized ataxic dysarthria to the upper cerebellar loci of the quadrangularis and simplex lobules by magnetic resonance imaging (MRI) (Ogawa et al., 2010).

Hypokinetic dysarthria, the typical speech pattern in Parkinson disease (PD), is notable for decreased and monotonous loudness and pitch, rapid rate, and occasional consonant errors. In a study of brain activation by positron emission tomography (PET) methodology, Liotti and colleagues (2003) described premotor and supplementary motor area activation in patients with PD and untreated hypokinetic dysarthria, but not in normal subjects. After completion of a voice treatment protocol, these premotor and motor activations diminished, whereas right-sided basal ganglia activations increased.

Hyperkinetic dysarthria, a pattern in some ways the opposite of hypokinetic dysarthria, is characterized by marked variation in rate, loudness, and timing, with distortion of vowels, harsh voice quality, and occasional sudden stoppages of speech. This speech pattern is seen in hyperkinetic movement disorders such as Huntington disease (HD) and dystonia musculorum deformans.

The final category, *mixed dysarthria*, involves combinations of the other five types. One common mixed dysarthria is a spastic-flaccid dysarthria, seen in amyotrophic lateral sclerosis (ALS). The ALS patient has the harsh, strain-strangle voice quality of spastic dysarthria, combined with the breathy and hypernasal quality of flaccid dysarthria. Multiple sclerosis may feature a spastic-flaccid-ataxic or spastic-ataxic mixed dysarthria, in which slow rate or irregular breakdowns are added to the other characteristics seen in spastic and flaccid dysarthria. Wilson disease can involve hypokinetic, spastic, and ataxic features.

The management of dysarthria includes speech therapy techniques to strengthen muscles, train more precise articulations, slow the rate of speech to increase intelligibility, or teach the patient to stress specific phonemes. Devices such as pacing boards to slow articulation, palatal lifts to reduce hypernasality, amplifiers to increase voice volume, communication boards for subjects to point to pictures, and augmentative communication devices and computer techniques can be used when the patient is unable to communicate in speech. Visual cues may help dysarthric speakers become more intelligible

(Hustad and Garcia, 2005). Surgical procedures such as a pharyngeal flap to reduce hypernasality or vocal fold Teflon injection or transposition surgery to increase loudness may help the patient speak more intelligibly. Treatment of PD can improve dysarthria in terms of both speech therapy and pharmacological treatments (DeLetter et al., 2005; Pinto et al., 2004; Trail et al., 2005), but surgical or deep brain stimulation procedures occasionally result in worsened intelligibility (Farrell et al., 2005; Guehl et al., 2006). In general, few randomized trials have examined the efficacy of speech therapy techniques for dysarthria (Sellars et al., 2005). A more detailed discussion of dysarthria can be found in Kirshner (2002).

Apraxia of Speech

Apraxia of speech is a disorder of the programming of articulation of sequences of phonemes, especially consonants. The motor speech system makes errors in selection of consonant phonemes in the absence of any weakness, slowness, or incoordination of the muscles of speech articulation. The term *apraxia of speech* implies that the disorder is one of a skilled, sequential motor activity (as in other apraxias) rather than a primary motor disorder. Consonants frequently are substituted rather than distorted, as in dysarthria. Patients have special difficulty with polysyllabic words and consonant shifts as well as in initiating articulation of a word. Errors are inconsistent from one attempt to the next, in contrast with the consistent distortion of phonemes in dysarthria (Ogar et al., 2005).

The four cardinal features of apraxia of speech are (1) effortful, groping, or trial-and-error attempts at speech with efforts at self-correction, (2) dysprosody, (3) inconsistencies in articulation errors, and (4) difficulty with initiating utterances. Usually the patient has the most difficulty with the first phoneme of a polysyllabic utterance. The patient may make an error in attempting to produce a word on one trial, a different error the next time, and a normal utterance the third time. Apraxia of speech involves primarily consonant transitions; vowels are relatively unaffected (Jacks et al., 2010). A study of the diagnosis of apraxia of speech by speech pathologists viewing videoclips of patients showed very good reliability and consistency of diagnosis (Mumby et al., 2007).

Apraxia of speech is rare in isolated form, but it frequently contributes to the speech and language deficit of Broca aphasia. A patient with apraxia of speech in addition to aphasia often can write better than he or she can speak, and comprehension is relatively preserved. Dronkers (1996) presented evidence from CT and MRI scans indicating that although the anatomical lesions vary, patients with apraxia of speech virtually always have damage in the left hemisphere insula, whereas patients without apraxia of speech do not. More recent MRI correlations of apraxia of speech in acute stroke patients by Hillis and colleagues (2004), however, have pointed to the traditional Broca area in the left frontal cortex as the site of damage in apraxia of speech.

Apraxia of speech also occurs in neurodegenerative disorders. In a recent review of 17 cases of progressive aphasia or apraxia of speech, Josephs and colleagues (2006) found apraxia of speech in 11 cases, all with conditions associated with tau pathology, such as progressive supranuclear palsy, corticobasal degeneration, and frontotemporal dementia or Pick disease.

Voxel-based morphometric studies of the MRIs from these patients showed predominant atrophy in the precentral and supplementary cortices with apraxia of speech and in the perisylvian cortex in primary progressive aphasia.

Other Motor Speech Disorders

Oral or Buccolingual Apraxia

Apraxia of speech is not the same as oral-buccal-lingual apraxia, or ideomotor apraxia for learned movements of the tongue, lips, and larynx. Oral apraxia can be elicited by asking the affected person to lick the upper lip, smile, or stick out the tongue. Both oral apraxia and apraxia of speech can coexist with Broca aphasia.

Aphemia

Another consideration in the differential diagnosis with both apraxia of speech and dysarthria is the syndrome of *aphemia*. Broca first used this term *(aphemie* in French) to designate the syndrome later called *Broca aphasia*, but in recent years, *aphemia* has been reserved for a syndrome of near-muteness, with normal comprehension, reading, and writing. Aphemia clearly is a motor speech disorder rather than an aphasia if written language and comprehension are indeed intact. Patients often are anarthric with no speech whatever, and then effortful, nonfluent speech emerges. Some patients have persisting dysarthria with dysphonia and sometimes distortions of articulation that sound similar to foreign accents (as described next). Pure anarthria may be associated with lesions of the face area of the motor cortex. Functional imaging studies also suggest that articulation is mediated at the level of the primary motor face area (Riecker et al., 2000), and disruption of speech articulation can be produced by transcranial magnetic stimulation over the motor face area (Epstein et al., 1999). Controversy remains as to whether aphemia is equivalent to apraxia of speech. In general, aphemia is likely to involve lesions in the vicinity of the primary motor cortex and perhaps the Broca area, whereas apraxia of speech may be localized to the insula (although, see Hillis et al., 2004).

Foreign Accent Syndrome

The *foreign accent syndrome* is an acquired form of motor speech disorder related to the dysarthrias, in which the patient acquires a dysfluency resembling a foreign accent, usually after a unilateral stroke (Kurowski et al., 1996). The syndrome has also been reported in multiple sclerosis (Chanson et al., 2009), traumatic brain injury (Lippert-Gruener et al., 2005), and in the degenerative disorder known as *primary progressive aphasia* or *frontotemporal dementia* (Luzzi et al., 2008). Lesions may involve the motor cortex of the left hemisphere. The dysfluency also can be mixed with aphasia.

Acquired Stuttering

Another uncommon motor speech disorder associated with acquired brain lesions is a pattern resembling developmental stuttering, referred to as *acquired stuttering* or *cortical stuttering*. Both developmental and acquired stuttering are associated with hesitancy in producing initial phonemes, pauses in speech, contortions of the face, and sometimes repetition of phonemes and associated dysrhythmia of speech. Acquired stuttering clearly overlaps with apraxia of speech but may lack the other features of apraxia of speech. Acquired stuttering has been described most often in patients with left hemisphere cortical strokes (Franco et al., 2000; Sahin et al., 2005; Turgut et al., 2002), but the syndrome also has been reported with subcortical lesions including infarctions of the pons, basal ganglia, and subcortical white matter (Ciabarra et al., 2000). Acquired stuttering also follows traumatic brain injury (Yeoh et al., 2006) and seizures, especially involving the supplementary motor area (Chung et al., 2004).

The neurobiology of developmental stuttering, a much more common disorder than acquired stuttering, is poorly understood. Stuttering appears to be a genetic disorder involving mutations in genes governing lysosomal metabolism (Kang et al., 2010). A functional MRI study suggested that patterns of cerebral activation during articulation in persons who stutter are different from those in normal persons, with greater right hemisphere activation in stutterers (Van Borsel et al., 2003). PET imaging studies have revealed either reduced left perisylvian hypometabolism (Wu et al., 1998), or increased right hemisphere activation (Fox et al., 2000). Abnormalities in the basal ganglia and in dopamine metabolism have also been suggested (Wu et al., 1997). MRI studies with diffusion anisotropy have suggested delayed or impaired myelination (Cykowski et al., 2010).

The treatment of stuttering involves behavioral techniques (reviewed in Prins and Ingram, 2009); altered auditory feedback techniques (Antipova et al., 2008; Lincoln et al., 2010); and pharmacological therapies with dopamine-blocking drugs such as risperidone, olanzapine (Maguire et al., 2004), or pimozide (Stager et al., 2005), or selective serotonin reuptake inhibitors such as paroxetine (Busan et al., 2009). A new antagonist at the γ-aminobutyric acid (GABA)-A receptor, pagoclone, currently under testing for anxiety disorders, has shown positive results in stuttering (Maguire et al., 2010). Overall, however, pharmacological therapies for stuttering have had limited success (Prasse and Kikano, 2008). In very refractory cases, deep brain stimulation in the vicinity of the centromedial thalamus may be of help (Bhatnagar and Andy, 1989, Bhatnagar and Mandybur, 2005).

Opercular Syndrome

The opercular syndrome, also called *Foix-Chavany-Marie syndrome* or *cheiro-oral syndrome* (Bakar et al., 1998), is a severe form of pseudobulbar palsy in which patients with bilateral lesions of the perisylvian cortex or subcortical connections become completely mute. These patients can follow commands involving the extremities but not those mediated by the cranial nerves. For example, they may be unable to open or close the eyes or mouth or to smile voluntarily, yet they smile when amused, yawn spontaneously, and even utter cries in response to emotional stimuli. The ability to follow limb commands shows that the disorder is not an aphasic disorder of comprehension. The discrepancy between automatic activation of the cranial musculature and inability to perform the same actions voluntarily has been called an *automatic-voluntary dissociation.*

References

The complete reference list is available online at www.expertconsult.com.

Neurogenic Dysphagia

Ronald F. Pfeiffer

Swallowing is like a wristwatch. It appears at first glance to be a simple, even mundane, mechanism, but under its unassuming face is a process that is both tremendously complex and fascinating. Swallowing occurs once every minute on average; when operating properly, it functions unobtrusively and is afforded scant attention. Malfunction can go completely unnoticed for a time, but when it finally becomes manifest, serious—sometimes catastrophic—consequences can ensue.

Impaired swallowing, or *dysphagia*, can originate from disturbances in the mouth, pharynx, or esophagus and can involve mechanical, musculoskeletal, or neurogenic mechanisms. Although mechanical dysphagia is an important topic, this chapter primarily focuses on neuromuscular and neurogenic causes of dysphagia because processes in these categories are most likely to be encountered by the neurologist.

Dysphagia is surprisingly common and has been reported to be present in 5% to 8% of persons over age 50. Dysphagia occurs quite frequently in neurological patients and can occur in a broad array of neurological or neuromuscular conditions. It has been estimated that neurogenic dysphagia develops in approximately 400,000 to 800,000 people per year, and that dysphagia is present in roughly 50% of inhabitants of long-term care units. Moreover, dysphagia can lead to superimposed problems such as inadequate nutrition, dehydration, recurrent upper respiratory infections, and frank aspiration with consequent pneumonia and even asphyxia. It thus constitutes a formidable and frequent problem confronting the neurologist in everyday practice.

Normal Swallowing

Swallowing is a surprisingly complicated and intricate phenomenon. It comprises a mixture of voluntary and reflex, or automatic, actions engineered and carried out by a combination of the 55 muscles of the oropharyngeal, laryngeal, and esophageal regions, along with five cranial nerves and two cervical nerve roots that in turn receive directions from centers within the central nervous system (Schaller et al., 2006). Reflex swallowing is coordinated and carried out at a brainstem level, where centers act directly on information received from sensory structures within the oropharynx and esophagus. Volitional swallowing is, not surprisingly, accompanied by additional activity that originates not only in motor and sensory cortices, but also in other cerebral structures (Hamdy et al., 1999; Zald and Pardo, 1999).

The process of swallowing can conveniently be broken down into three distinct stages or phases: oral, pharyngeal, and esophageal. These components have also been distilled into what have been termed the *horizontal and vertical subsystems*, reflecting the direction of bolus flow in each component (when the individual is upright when swallowing). The *oral phase* of swallowing comprises the horizontal subsystem and is largely volitional in character; the *pharyngeal and esophageal phases* comprise the vertical subsystem and are primarily under reflex control.

In the oral, or swallow-preparatory phase, food is taken into the mouth and, if needed, chewed. Saliva is secreted to provide both lubrication and the initial "dose" of digestive enzymes, and the food bolus is formed and shaped by the tongue. The tongue then propels the bolus backward to the pharyngeal inlet where, in a piston-like action, it delivers the bolus into the pharynx. This initiates the pharyngeal phase, in which a cascade of intricate, extremely rapid, and exquisitely coordinated movements seal off the nasal passages and protect the trachea while the cricopharyngeal muscle, which functions as the upper esophageal sphincter (UES), relaxes and allows the bolus to

DOI: 10.1016/B978-1-4377-0434-1.00013-X

enter the pharynx. As an example of the intricacy of movements during this phase of swallowing, the UES, prompted in part by traction produced by elevation of the larynx, actually relaxes just prior to arrival of the food bolus, creating suction that assists in guiding the bolus into the pharynx. The bolus then enters the esophagus where peristaltic contractions usher it distally and, on relaxation of the lower-esophageal sphincter, into the stomach. Synchronization of swallowing with respiration such that expiration rather than inspiration immediately follows a swallow, thus reducing the risk of aspiration, is another example of the finely tuned coordination involved in the swallowing mechanism(Mehanna and Jankovic, 2010).

Neurophysiology of Swallowing

Central control of swallowing has traditionally been ascribed to brainstem structures, with cortical supervision and modulation emanating from the inferior precentral gyrus. However, recent positron emission tomography (PET) and transcranial magnetic stimulation (TMS) studies of volitional swallowing reveal a considerably more complex picture in which a broad network of brain regions are active in the control and execution of swallowing.

It is perhaps not surprising that the strongest activation in PET studies of volitional swallowing occurs in the lateral motor cortex within the inferior precentral gyrus, wherein lie the cortical representations of tongue and face. There is disagreement among investigators, however, in that some have noted bilaterally symmetrical activation of the lateral motor cortex (Zald and Pardo, 1999), whereas others have noted a distinctly asymmetrical activation, at least in a portion of subjects tested (Hamdy et al., 1999).

Some additional and perhaps somewhat surprising brain areas are also activated during volitional swallowing (Hamdy et al., 1999; Schaller et al., 2006; Zald and Pardo, 1999). The supplementary motor area may play a role in preparation for volitional swallowing, and the anterior cingulate cortex may be involved with monitoring autonomic and vegetative functions. Another area of activation during volitional swallowing is the anterior insula, particularly on the right. It has been suggested that this activation may provide the substrate that allows gustatory and other intraoral sensations to modulate swallowing. Lesions in the insula may also increase the swallowing threshold and delay the pharyngeal phase of swallowing (Schaller et al., 2006). PET studies also consistently demonstrate distinctly asymmetrical left-sided activation of the cerebellum during swallowing. This activation may reflect cerebellar input concerning coordination, timing, and sequencing of swallowing. Activation of putamen has also been noted during volitional swallowing, but it has not been possible to differentiate this activation from that seen with tongue movement alone.

Within the brainstem, swallowing appears to be regulated by central pattern generators that contain the programs directing the sequential movements of the various muscles involved. The *dorsomedial pattern generator* resides in the medial reticular formation of the rostral medulla and the reticulum adjacent to the nucleus tractus solitarius and is involved with the initiation and organization of the swallowing sequence (Schaller et al., 2006). A second central pattern generator, the *ventrolateral pattern generator*, lies near the nucleus ambiguus and its surrounding reticular formation (Prosiegel et al., 2005; Schaller et al., 2006). It serves primarily as a connecting pathway to motor nuclei such as the nucleus ambiguus and the dorsal motor nucleus of the vagus, which directly control motor output to the pharyngeal musculature and proximal esophagus.

It has become evident that a large network of structures participates in the act of swallowing, especially volitional swallowing. The presence of this network presumably accounts for the broad array of neurological disease processes that can produce dysphagia as a part of their clinical picture.

Mechanical Dysphagia

Structural abnormalities, both within and adjacent to the mouth, pharynx, and esophagus, can interfere with swallowing on a strictly mechanical basis, despite fully intact and functioning nervous and musculoskeletal systems (**Box 13.1**).

Box 13.1 Mechanical Dysphagia

Oral

Amyloidosis
Congenital abnormalities
Intraoral tumors
Lip injuries:
    Burns
    Trauma
Macroglossia
Scleroderma
Temporomandibular joint dysfunction
Xerostomia:
    Sjögren syndrome

Pharyngeal

Cervical anterior osteophytes
Infection:
    Diphtheria
Thyromegaly
Retropharyngeal abscess
Retropharyngeal tumor
Zenker diverticulum

Esophageal

Aberrant origin of right subclavian artery
Caustic injury
Esophageal carcinoma
Esophageal diverticulum
Esophageal infection:
    Candida albicans
    Herpes simplex virus
    Cytomegalovirus
    Varicella-zoster virus
Esophageal intramural pseudodiverticula
Esophageal stricture
Esophageal ulceration
Esophageal webs or rings
Gastroesophageal reflux disease
Hiatal hernia
Metastatic carcinoma
Posterior mediastinal mass
Thoracic aortic aneurysm

Within the mouth, macroglossia, temporomandibular joint dislocation, certain congenital anomalies, and intraoral tumors can impede effective swallowing and produce mechanical dysphagia. Pharyngeal function can be compromised by processes such as retropharyngeal tumor or abscess, cervical anterior osteophyte formation, Zenker diverticulum, or thyroid gland enlargement. An even broader array of structural lesions can interfere with esophageal function, including malignant or benign esophageal tumors, metastatic carcinoma, esophageal stricture from numerous causes, vascular abnormalities such as aortic aneurysm or aberrant origin of the subclavian artery, or even primary gastric abnormalities such as hiatal hernia or complications from gastric banding procedures. Gastroesophageal reflux can also produce dysphagia. Individuals with these problems, however, are more likely to be seen by the gastroenterologist rather than the neurologist.

Neuromuscular Dysphagia

A variety of neuromuscular disease processes of diverse etiology can involve the oropharyngeal and esophageal musculature and produce dysphagia as part of their broader neuromuscular clinical picture (**Box 13.2**). Certain muscular dystrophies, inflammatory myopathies, and mitochondrial myopathies all can display dysphagia, as can disease processes affecting the myoneural junction, such as myasthenia gravis.

Box 13.2 Neuromuscular Dysphagia

Oropharyngeal

Inflammatory myopathies:
    Dermatomyositis
    Inclusion-body myositis
    Polymyositis
Mitochondrial myopathies:
    Kearns-Sayre syndrome
    MNGIE
Muscular dystrophies:
    Duchenne
    Facio-scapulohumeral
    Limb girdle
    Myotonic
    Oculopharyngeal
Neuromuscular junction disorders:
    Botulism
    Lambert-Eaton syndrome
    Myasthenia gravis
    Tetanus
Scleroderma
Stiff man syndrome

Esophageal

Amyloidosis
Inflammatory myopathies:
    Dermatomyositis
    Polymyositis
Scleroderma

MNGIE, Mitochondrial neurogastro-intestinal encephalomyopathy.

Oculopharyngeal Muscular Dystrophy

Oculopharyngeal muscular dystrophy (OPMD) is a rare autosomal dominant disorder that has a worldwide distribution. It was initially described and is most frequently encountered in individuals with a French-Canadian ethnic background, although its highest reported prevalence is among the Bukhara Jews in Israel (Abu-Baker and Rouleau, 2007). It is the consequence of a GCG trinucleotide repeat expansion in the polyadenylate-binding protein, nuclear 1 gene (PABPN1; also known as *poly(A)-binding protein 2* [PABP2]) on chromosome 14. OPMD is unique among the muscular dystrophies because of its appearance in older individuals, with symptoms typically first appearing between ages 40 and 60. It is characterized by slowly progressive ptosis, dysphagia, and proximal limb weakness. Because of the ptosis, patients with OPMD may assume an unusual posture characterized by raised eyebrows and extended neck.

Dysphagia in OPMD is due to impaired function of the oropharyngeal musculature. Although it evolves slowly over many years, OPMD can eventually result not only in difficulty or discomfort with swallowing, but also in weight loss, malnutrition, and aspiration. No specific treatment for the muscular dystrophy itself is available, but cricopharyngeal myotomy affords dysphagia relief in over 80% of treated individuals (Fradet et al., 1997). More recently, botulinum toxin injections have been successfully used to treat dysphagia in OPMD.

Myotonic Dystrophy

Myotonic dystrophy is an autosomal dominant disorder whose phenotypic picture includes not only skeletal muscle but also cardiac, ophthalmological, and endocrinological involvement. Mutations at two distinct locations have now been associated with the clinical picture of myotonic dystrophy (Turner and Hilton-Jones, 2010). Type 1 myotonic dystrophy is due to a CTG expansion in the myotonic dystrophy protein kinase (DMPK) gene on chromosome 19; type 2 is the consequence of a CCTG repeat expansion in the zinc finger protein 9 (ZNF9) gene on chromosome 3.

Gastrointestinal (GI) symptoms develop in more than 50% of individuals with the clinical phenotype of myotonic dystrophy. These may be the most disabling component of the disorder in 25% of individuals with type 1 myotonic dystrophy, and GI symptoms may actually antedate the appearance of other neuromuscular features (Turner and Hilton-Jones, 2010). Subjective dysphagia is one of the most prevalent GI features and has been reported in 37% to 56% of patients (Ertekin et al., 2001b). Coughing when eating, suggestive of aspiration, may occur in 33%. Objective measures paint a picture of even more pervasive impairment, demonstrating disturbances in swallowing in 70% to 80% of persons with myotonic dystrophy (Ertekin et al., 2001b). In one study, 75% of patients asymptomatic for dysphagia were still noted to have abnormalities on objective testing (Marcon et al., 1998).

A variety of abnormalities in objective measures of swallowing have been documented in myotonic dystrophy. Abnormal cricopharyngeal muscle activity is present in 40% of patients during electromyographic (EMG) testing (Ertekin et al., 2001b). Impaired esophageal peristalsis has also been noted in affected individuals studied with esophageal manometry. On videofluoroscopic testing, incomplete relaxation of the UES and esophageal hypotonia are the most frequently noted abnormalities (Marcon et al., 1998). Both muscle weakness and myotonia are felt to play a role in the development of dysphagia in persons with myotonic dystrophy (Ertekin et al., 2001b), and in at least one study, a correlation was noted between the size of the CTG repeat expansion and the number of radiological abnormalities in myotonic patients (Marcon et al., 1998).

Other Muscular Dystrophies

Although less well characterized, dysphagia also occurs in other types of muscular dystrophy. Difficulty swallowing and choking while eating occur with increased frequency in children with Duchenne muscular dystrophy. Dysphagia has also been documented in patients with limb-girdle dystrophy and facioscapulohumeral dystrophy.

Inflammatory Myopathies

Dermatomyositis and polymyositis are the most frequently occurring of the inflammatory myopathic disorders. Both are characterized by progressive, usually symmetrical, weakness affecting proximal muscles more prominently than distal. Fatigue and myalgia may also occur. Malignant disease is associated with the disorder in 10% to 15% of patients with dermatomyositis and 5% to 10% of those with polymyositis. In individuals older than age 65 with these inflammatory myopathies, more than 50% are found to have cancer.

Although dysphagia can develop in both conditions, it more frequently is present in dermatomyositis and when present is more severe. Dysphagia is present in 20% to 55% of individuals with dermatomyositis but in only 18% with polymyositis (Parodi et al., 2002). It is the consequence of involvement of striated muscle in the pharynx and proximal esophagus. Involvement of pharyngeal and esophageal musculature in polymyositis and dermatomyositis is an indicator of poor prognosis and can be the source of significant morbidity. A 1-year mortality rate of 31% has been reported in individuals with inflammatory myopathy and dysphagia (Williams et al., 2003), although other investigators have reported a 1-year survival rate of 89% (Oh et al., 2007).

Dysphagia in persons with inflammatory myopathy may be due to restrictive pharyngo-esophageal abnormalities such as cricopharyngeal bar, Zenker diverticulum, and stenosis. In fact, in one study of 13 patients with inflammatory myopathy, radiographic constrictions were noted in 9 (69%) individuals, compared with 1 of 17 controls with dysphagia of neurogenic origin (Williams et al., 2003). Aspiration was also more common in the patients with myositis (61% versus 41%). The resulting dysphagia can be severe enough to require enteral feeding. Acute total obstruction by the cricopharyngeal muscle has been reported in dermatomyositis, necessitating cricopharyngeal myotomy. Other investigators have reported improvement in 50% of individuals 1 month following cricopharyngeal bar disruption; improvement was still present in 25% at 6 months (Williams et al., 2003). The reason for the formation of restrictive abnormalities in inflammatory myopathy is uncertain, but it may be that long-standing inflammation of the cricopharyngeus muscle impedes its compliance and ability to open fully (Williams et al., 2003).

Dysphagia may also develop in inclusion body myositis. It may even be the presenting symptom (Cox et al., 2009). In the late stages of the disorder, the frequency of dysphagia may actually exceed that seen in dermatomyositis and polymyositis. In a group of individuals in whom inclusion-body myositis mimicked and was confused with motor neuron disease, dysphagia was present in 44% (Dabby et al., 2001). In another study, dysphagia was documented in 37 of 57 (65%) patients with inclusion-body myositis (Cox et al., 2009). Abnormal function of the cricopharyngeal sphincter, probably due to inflammatory involvement of the cricopharyngeal muscle, with consequently reduced compliance, was documented in 37%. A focal inflammatory myopathy involving the pharyngeal muscles and producing isolated pharyngeal dysphagia has also been described in individuals older than age 69. It has been suggested that this is a distinct clinical entity characterized by cricopharyngeal hypertrophy, although polymyositis localized to the pharyngeal musculature has also been reported.

Dysphagia in both dermatomyositis and polymyositis may respond to corticosteroids and other immunosuppressive drugs, and these remain the mainstay of treatment. Intravenous immunoglobulin therapy has produced dramatic improvement in dysphagia in individuals who were unresponsive to steroids. However, inclusion-body myositis typically responds poorly to these agents, and myotomy is often necessary (Ebert, 2010; Oh et al., 2007).

Mitochondrial Disorders

The mitochondrial disorders are a family of diseases that develop as a consequence of dysfunction in the mitochondrial respiratory chain. Most are the result of mutations in mitochondrial deoxyribonucleic acid (DNA) genes, but nuclear DNA mutations may be responsible in some. Mitochondrial disorders are by nature multisystemic, but myopathic and neurological features often predominate, and symptoms may vary widely even between individuals within the same family.

In addition to the classic constellation of symptoms that includes progressive external ophthalmoplegia, retinitis pigmentosa, cardiac conduction defects, and ataxia, individuals with Kearns-Sayre syndrome may also develop dysphagia. Severe abnormalities of pharyngeal and upper-esophageal peristalsis have been documented in this disorder. Cricopharyngeal dysfunction is common, and impaired deglutitive coordination may also develop.

Dysphagia has also been described in other mitochondrial disorders, but descriptions are only anecdotal, and formal study has not been undertaken.

Myasthenia Gravis

Myasthenia gravis (MG) is an autoimmune disorder characterized by the production of autoantibodies directed against the α_1 subunit of the nicotinic postsynaptic acetylcholine receptors at the neuromuscular junction, with destruction of the receptors and reduction in their number. The clinical consequence of this process is the development of fatigable muscle weakness that progressively increases with repetitive muscle action and improves with rest. MG occurs more frequently in women than men; although symptoms can develop at any age, the reported mean age of onset in women is between 28 and 35, and in men, between age 42 and 49. Although myasthenic symptoms remain confined to the extraocular muscles in approximately 20% of patients, more widespread muscle weakness becomes evident in most individuals.

Involvement of bulbar musculature, with resultant dysphagia, is relatively common in MG. In approximately 6% to 30% of patients, bulbar involvement is evident from the beginning (Koopman et al., 2004); with disease progression, most eventually develop bulbar symptoms such as dysphagia and dysarthria. Dysphagia in MG can be due to dysfunction at oral, pharyngeal, or even esophageal levels, and many patients experience it at multiple levels. In a study of 20 myasthenic patients experiencing dysphagia, abnormalities in the oral preparatory phase were evident in 13 individuals (65%), oral phase dysphagia in 18 (90%), and pharyngeal phase involvement in all 20 (100%) (Koopman et al., 2004). Oral phase involvement can be due to fatigue and weakness of the tongue or masticatory muscles. In MG patients with bulbar symptoms, repetitive nerve stimulation studies of the hypoglossal nerve have demonstrated abnormalities, as have studies utilizing EMG of the masticatory muscles recorded while chewing. Pharyngeal dysfunction is also common in MG patients who have dysphagia, as demonstrated by videofluoroscopy. Aspiration, often silent, may be present in 35% or more of these individuals (Colton-Hudson et al., 2002); in elderly patients the frequency of aspiration may be considerably higher. Bedside speech pathology assessment is not a reliable predictor of aspiration (Koopman et al., 2004). Motor dysfunction involving the striated muscle of the proximal esophagus has also been documented in MG. In one study that used testing with esophageal manometry, 96% of patients with MG demonstrated abnormalities such as decreased amplitude and prolongation of the peristaltic wave in this region. Cricopharyngeal sphincter pressure was also noted to be reduced.

It is important to remember that dysphagia can also precipitate myasthenic crisis in individuals with MG. In fact, in one study, dysphagia was considered to be a major precipitant of myasthenic crisis in 56% of patients (Koopman et al., 2004).

Neurogenic Dysphagia

A variety of disease processes originating in the central and peripheral nervous systems can also disrupt swallowing mechanisms and produce dysphagia. Processes affecting cerebral cortex, subcortical white matter, subcortical grey matter, brainstem, spinal cord, and peripheral nerves all can elicit dysphagia as a component of their clinical picture (**Box 13.3**).

In individuals with neurogenic dysphagia, prolonged swallow response, delayed laryngeal closure, and weak bolus propulsion combine to increase the risk of aspiration and the likelihood of malnutrition (Clavé et al., 2006)

Stroke

Cerebrovascular disease is an extremely common neurological problem, and stroke is the third leading cause of death in the United States. It has been estimated that 500,000 to 750,000 strokes occur in the United States each year, and approximately 150,000 persons die annually following stroke. The mechanism of stroke is ischemic in 80% to 85% of cases; in the remaining 15% to 20% it is hemorrhagic. Approximately

---

Box 13.3 Neurogenic Dysphagia

Oropharyngeal

Arnold-Chiari malformation
Basal ganglia disease:
   Biotin-responsive
   Corticobasal degeneration
   DLB
   HD
   Multiple system atrophy
   Neuroacanthocytosis
   PD
   PSP
   WD
Central pontine myelinolysis
Cerebral palsy
Drug related:
   Cyclosporin
   Tardive dyskinesia
   Vincristine
Infectious:
   Brainstem encephalitis
   Listeria
   Epstein-Barr virus
   Diphtheria
   Poliomyelitis
   Progressive multifocal leukoencephalopathy
   Rabies
Mass lesions:
   Abscess
   Hemorrhage
   Metastatic tumor
   Primary tumor
Motor neuron diseases:
   ALS
MS
Peripheral neuropathic processes:
   Charcot-Marie-Tooth disease
   Guillain-Barré syndrome (Miller Fisher variant)
Spinocerebellar ataxias
Stroke
Syringobulbia

Esophageal

Achalasia
Autonomic neuropathies:
   Diabetes mellitus
   Familial dysautonomia
   Paraneoplastic syndromes
Basal ganglia disorders:
   PD
Chagas disease
Esophageal motility disorders
Scleroderma

ALS, Amyotrophic lateral sclerosis; *DLB*, dementia with lewy bodies; *HD*, Huntington disease; *MS*, multiple sclerosis; *PD*, Parkinson disease; *PSP*, progressive supranuclear palsy; *WD*, Wilson disease.

25% of ischemic strokes are due to small-vessel disease, 50% to large-vessel disease, and 25% to a cardioembolic source. Although stroke can occur at all ages, 75% of strokes occur in individuals older than 75.

Dysphagia develops in 45% to 57% of individuals following stroke, and its presence is associated with increased likelihood of severe disability or death (Runions et al., 2004; Schaller et al., 2006). Aspiration is the most widely recognized complication of dysphagia following stroke, but undernourishment and even malnutrition occur with surprising frequency (Finestone and Greene-Finestone, 2003). Reported frequencies of nutritional deficits in patients with dysphagia following stroke range from 48% to 65%. The presence of dysphagia following stroke results in a threefold prolongation of hospital stay and increases the complication rate during hospitalization (Runions et al., 2004). It is also an independent risk factor for severe disability and death.

Finestone and Greene-Finestone (2003) have delineated a number of warning signs that can alert physicians to the presence of post-stroke dysphagia. Some are obvious, others more subtle. They include drooling, excessive tongue movement or spitting food out of the mouth, poor tongue control, pocketing of food in the mouth, facial weakness, slurred speech, coughing or choking when eating, regurgitation of food through the nose, wet or "gurgly" voice after eating, hoarse or breathy voice, complaints of food sticking in the throat, absence or delay of laryngeal elevation, prolonged chewing, prolonged time to eat or reluctance to eat, and recurrent pneumonia.

Although it is commonly perceived that the presence of dysphagia following stroke indicates a brainstem localization for the stroke, this is not necessarily so. Impaired swallowing has been documented in a significant proportion of strokes involving cortical and subcortical structures. The pharyngeal phase of swallowing is primarily impaired in brainstem infarction; in hemispheric strokes, the most striking abnormality often is a delay in initiation of voluntary swallowing. Strokes involving the right hemisphere tend to produce more impairment of pharyngeal motility, whereas left hemisphere lesions have a greater effect on oral stage function (Ickenstein et al., 2005). Dysphagia has been reported as the sole manifestation of infarction in both medulla and cerebrum.

Approximately 50% to 55% of patients with lesions in the posterior inferior cerebellar artery distribution, with consequent lateral medullary infarction (Wallenberg syndrome), develop dysphagia (Teasell et al., 2002). The fact that unilateral medullary infarction can produce bilateral disruption of the brainstem swallowing centers suggests that they function as one integrated center. Infarction in the distribution of the anterior inferior cerebellar artery can also result in dysphagia.

Following stroke within the cerebral hemispheres, dysphagia can develop by virtue of damage to either cortical or subcortical structures involved with volitional swallowing. Bilateral hemispheric damage is more likely to produce dysphagia, but it can also occur in the setting of unilateral damage. Bilateral infarction of the frontoparietal operculum may result in the anterior operculum syndrome (Foix-Chavany-Marie syndrome), which is characterized by inability to perform voluntary movements of the face, jaw, tongue, and pharynx but fully preserved involuntary movements of the same muscles. Impairment of volitional swallowing may be a component of this syndrome. Individuals with subcortical strokes have a higher incidence of dysphagia and aspiration than those with cortical damage. In one study, more than 85% of individuals with unilateral subcortical strokes demonstrated videofluoroscopic evidence of delayed initiation of the pharyngeal stage of swallowing; in 75%, some radiographic aspiration was noted. Although tongue deviation is classically associated with medullary lesions damaging the hypoglossal nucleus, it has also been documented in almost 30% of persons with hemispheric infarctions. When present in hemispheric stroke, tongue deviation is always associated with facial weakness, and dysphagia is present in 43% of affected patients.

Aspiration is a potentially life-threatening complication of stroke. Studies have documented its occurrence in 30% to 55% of stroke patients. In one study, videofluoroscopic evidence of aspiration was observed in 36% of patients with unilateral cerebral stroke, 46% with bilateral cerebral stroke, 60% with unilateral brainstem stroke, and 50% with bilateral brainstem lesions. Other studies have suggested that the incidence of aspiration in brainstem strokes may be considerably higher—more than 80%—and that subcortical strokes may result in aspiration in 75% of cases. The risk of developing pneumonia is almost seven times greater in persons experiencing aspiration following stroke compared with those who do not. Individuals in whom aspiration occurs post stroke do not always experience clinical symptoms such as coughing or choking during food or liquid ingestion. Furthermore, an absent gag reflex does not help to differentiate those aspirating from those who are not (Finestone and Greene-Finestone, 2003). In a recent study, only 44% of patients with suspected oropharyngeal dysphagia following stroke had an impaired gag reflex, and only 47% coughed during oral feeding (Terre and Mearin, 2006). Therefore, the employment of objective testing measures to detect the presence and predict the risk of aspiration has been advocated. Modified barium swallow testing using videofluoroscopy is the standard method of diagnosis used, but simple bedside techniques such as a water swallowing test have also been advocated as practical, though somewhat less sensitive, alternatives.

Ickenstein and colleagues (2010) emphasize the value of a stepwise assessment of swallowing in patients admitted to the hospital with stroke, with the assessment beginning on the first day of admission. The first step is a modified swallowing assessment performed by the nursing staff on the day of admission; the second step is a clinical swallowing examination performed within 72 hours of admission by a swallowing therapist; the third step is performance of flexible transnasal swallowing endoscopy performed by a physician within 5 days of admission. Appropriate diet and treatment are then determined after each step. Employment of such a stepwise assessment of dysphagia resulted in a significant reduction in the rate of pneumonia and in antibiotic consumption in a stroke unit (Ickenstein et al., 2010).

Swallowing often improves spontaneously in the days and weeks after stroke. Improvement is more likely to occur after cortical strokes, compared with those of brainstem origin; the improvement is probably the result of compensatory reorganization of undamaged brain areas (Schaller et el., 2006). Nasogastric tube feeding can temporarily provide adequate nutrition and buy time until swallowing improves sufficiently to allow oral feeding, but it entails some risks itself, such as increasing the possibility of reflux with consequent aspiration. For individuals in whom significant dysphagia persists after stroke, percutaneous endoscopic gastrostomy (PEG) tube placement may become necessary. Ickenstein and colleagues (2005) documented this necessity in 77 of 664 (11.6%) stroke patients admitted to their rehabilitation hospital. Continued need for a PEG tube after discharge from the unit carried with it a somber prognosis. Various methods of behavioral swallowing therapy can be useful in managing persistent post-stroke dysphagia. Recent studies have provided some tantalizing hints that sensory pharyngeal stimulation and repetitive transcranial magnetic stimulation (rTMS) may improve some aspects of swallowing, but in a small percentage of individuals, placement of a PEG tube will be necessary.

Dysphagia can also develop in the setting of other cerebrovascular processes. Within the anterior circulation, dysphagia has been reported with carotid artery aneurysms. Within the posterior circulation, processes such as elongation and dilatation of the basilar artery, posterior inferior cerebellar artery aneurysm, intracranial vertebral artery dissections, giant dissecting vertebrobasilar aneurysms, and cavernous malformations within the medulla may produce dysphagia in addition to other symptoms.

Dysphagia is also a potential complication of carotid endarterectomy, not on the basis of stroke but due to laryngeal or cranial nerve injury. In one study, careful otolaryngologic examination demonstrated such deficits in almost 60% of patients postoperatively (Monini et al., 2005). Most deficits were mild and transient, but some persistent impairment was noted in 17.5% of those studied, and 9% required some rehabilitative procedures.

Multiple Sclerosis

Multiple sclerosis (MS) is an inflammatory demyelinating disease of the central nervous system that primarily, though not exclusively, affects young adults. The mean age of onset is approximately age 30. In its most common guise, MS is characterized by exacerbations and remissions, although some individuals may follow a chronic progressive course right from the start. The etiology of MS is uncertain, but an autoimmune process is presumed.

Dysphagia is a frequent but often overlooked problem in MS. Survey studies have indicated the presence of dysphagia in 24% to 34% of individuals with MS (Calcagno et al., 2002; Prosiegel et al., 2004). The prevalence of dysphagia in MS rises with increasing disability; about 15% of individuals with mild disability may develop neurogenic dysphagia (Prosiegel et al., 2004), with the percentage escalating to 65% in the most severely affected. Individuals with severe brainstem involvement as part of their MS are especially likely to experience dysphagia.

Objective studies demonstrate a somewhat higher frequency of dysphagia than their survey study counterparts. In one study, approximately 50% of individuals with objective abnormalities were not aware of any difficulty swallowing; in another that used videofluoroscopic analysis, some alteration of swallowing efficiency or safety was present in over 80% of 23 patients studied (Terre-Boliart et al., 2004). Abnormalities in oral, pharyngeal, and even esophageal phases of swallowing have been documented. Rare instances of the

anterior operculum syndrome with buccolinguofacial apraxia have been reported in MS. Abnormalities in the oral phase of swallowing are common in MS patients with mild disability, but additional pharyngeal phase abnormalities develop in those with more severe disability. Disturbances in both the sequencing of laryngeal events and function of the pharyngeal constrictor muscles are typically present in persons experiencing dysphagia. Pharyngeal sensory impairment may also play a role in the development of dysphagia in some patients.

Parkinson Disease

Parkinson disease (PD) is a neurodegenerative disorder in which symptoms typically emerge between ages 55 and 65. The most prominent neuropathology in PD involves the pigmented dopaminergic neurons in the substantia nigra, but neuronal loss in other areas of the nervous system, including within the enteric nervous system, has also been documented.

Dysphagia was first documented in PD by none other than James Parkinson himself in his original description of the illness in 1817. Recent survey studies have confirmed that dysphagia is indeed a frequent phenomenon in PD. Reported frequencies of dysphagia in these studies range from 30% to 82% (Pfeiffer, 2003), with the broad range probably reflecting differences in the detail within questionnaires. Objective testing indicates an even higher frequency of dysphagia in PD and has allowed its separation into two categories, oropharyngeal and esophageal.

Studies using modified barium swallow have demonstrated some abnormality in the oropharyngeal phase of swallowing in 75% to 97% of persons with PD (Pfeiffer, 2003). Even individuals asymptomatic for dysphagia frequently display abnormalities on modified barium swallow testing. Within the oral phase, difficulty with bolus formation, delayed initiation of swallowing, repeated tongue pumping, and other abnormalities have been described. Pharyngeal dysmotility and impaired relaxation of the cricopharyngeal muscle constitute examples of abnormalities noted in the pharyngeal phase. Individuals with PD are more likely to swallow during inspiration and also to inhale post swallow, both of which increase the risk of aspiration (Gross et al., 2008).

Esophageal dysfunction can also trigger dysphagia in PD. Esophageal manometry has demonstrated abnormalities in 61% to 73% of PD patients studied; videofluoroscopic studies show a broader range, with some abnormality reported in 5% to 86% of individuals (Pfeiffer, 2003). A wide variety of abnormalities of esophageal function has been described, including slowed esophageal transit, both segmental and diffuse esophageal spasm, ineffective or tertiary contractions, and even aperistalsis. Lower-esophageal sphincter dysfunction may also be present in PD and can produce not only symptoms of reflux but also dysphagia.

Aspiration has been noted to be present in 15% to 56% of patients with PD, and completely silent aspiration in 15% to 33% (Pfeiffer, 2003). Even more striking is a study in which vallecular residue, believed to indicate an increased risk of aspiration, was found to be present in 88% of PD patients without clinical dysphagia. Silent aspiration and laryngeal penetration of saliva have also been noted to occur in a significant percentage (10.7% and 28.6%, respectively) of individuals with PD who exhibit daily drooling (Rodrigues et al.,

2010). In another study by the same group of investigators, a 9.75-fold increased risk of respiratory infection was documented in PD patients with daily drooling and silent aspiration or silent laryngeal penetration of food who were followed for 1 year (Nóbrega et al., 2008). Hypesthesia of laryngeal structures has also been noted in PD patients, possibly contributing to the risk of aspiration (Rodrigues et al., 2010).

Dysphagia demonstrates an inconsistent response to levodopa or dopamine agonist therapy. Objective improvement in swallowing, documented by modified barium swallow testing, has been observed in 33% to 50% of patients in some but not all studies. A recent meta-analysis, however, concluded that levodopa intake was not associated with improvement in swallowing (Menezes and Melo, 2009). In patients with cricopharyngeal muscle dysfunction, both cricopharyngeal myotomy and botulinum toxin injections have been used successfully. Behavioral swallowing therapy approaches are of benefit to some individuals. On rare occasions, PEG tube placement may be necessary.

Other Basal Ganglia Disorders

In the parkinsonism-plus syndromes, such as progressive supranuclear palsy (PSP), multiple system atrophy, corticobasal degeneration, and dementia with Lewy bodies (DLB), dysphagia is a frequent problem and, in contrast to PD, often develops relatively early in the course of the illness. The median latency to the development of dysphagia in PD is more than 130 months, whereas it is 67 months in multiple system atrophy, 64 months in corticobasal degeneration, 43 months in DLB, and 42 months in PSP (Muller et al., 2001). In fact, the appearance of dysphagia within 1 year of symptom onset virtually eliminates PD as a diagnostic possibility, although it does not help distinguish between the various parkinsonism-plus syndromes (Muller et al., 2001). In persons with PSP, the presence and severity of dysphagia does not correlate well with the presence and severity of dysarthria, so the decision to evaluate swallowing function should not be based on the presence or absence of speech impairment (Warnecke et al., 2010).

Dysphagia can be a prominent problem in patients with Wilson disease and is frequently a component of the clinical picture in neuroacanthocytosis. A unique basal ganglia process characterized by the presence of subacute encephalopathy, dysarthria, dysphagia, rigidity, dystonia, and eventual quadriparesis has been shown to improve promptly and dramatically after biotin administration. Dysphagia may also develop in the setting of spinocerebellar ataxia.

Dysphagia is also a well-documented complication of botulinum toxin injections for cervical dystonia, presumably as a consequence of diffusion of the toxin (Comella and Thompson, 2006). It should be noted, however, that 11% of patients with cervical dystonia experience dysphagia as part of the disease process itself, and 22% may display abnormalities on objective testing. Whether the dysphagia in individuals with cervical dystonia is mechanical or neurogenic has been the topic of debate. In a study of 25 patients with cervical dystonia, clinical assessment suggested the presence of dysphagia in 36%; electrophysiological evaluation demonstrated abnormalities in 72% (Ertekin et al., 2002). The electrophysiological abnormalities strongly suggested a neurogenic basis for the dysfunction.

Amyotrophic Lateral Sclerosis

Amyotrophic lateral sclerosis (ALS) is the most common form of motor neuron disease. It is characterized by progressive loss of motor neurons in the cortex, brainstem, and spinal cord, which results in a clinical picture of progressive weakness that combines features of both upper motor neuron dysfunction with spasticity and hyperreflexia, and lower motor neuron dysfunction with atrophy, fasciculations, and hyporeflexia. The mean age of symptom onset is between ages 54 and 58.

Although dysphagia eventually develops in most individuals with ALS, bulbar symptoms can be the presenting feature in approximately 25% of patients. A sensation of solid food sticking in the esophagus may provide the initial clue to emerging dysphagia, but abnormalities in the oral phase of swallowing are most often evident in patients with early ALS. Impaired function of the lips and tongue (particularly the posterior portion of the tongue) due to evolving muscle weakness typically appears first, followed next by involvement of jaw and suprahyoid musculature, and finally by weakness of pharyngeal and laryngeal muscles. Lip weakness can result in spillage of food from the mouth; tongue weakness leads to impaired food bolus formation and transfer. Inadequate mastication due to the jaw muscle weakness adds to the difficulty with bolus formation, and the eventual development of pharyngeal and laryngeal weakness opens the door for aspiration. Neurophysiological testing in patients with ALS who have dysphagia demonstrates delay in, and eventual abolishment of, triggering of the swallowing reflex for voluntarily initiated swallows, with relative preservation of spontaneous reflexive swallows until the terminal stages of the disease (Ertekin et al., 2000). Although videofluoroscopy is the most precise means of evaluating dysphagia in individuals with ALS, scales such as the Norris ALS Scale provide an adequate venue to decide on the need for dysphagia treatment.

Spasm of the UES, with hyperreflexia and hypertonicity of the cricopharyngeal muscle, has been reported in ALS patients with bulbar dysfunction, presumably as a consequence of upper motor neuron involvement, and has been considered to be an important cause of aspiration (Ertekin et al., 2000; Ertekin et al., 2001a). This has prompted the employment of cricopharyngeal myotomy as a treatment measure in such patients, but this approach should be limited to those with objectively demonstrated UES spasm.

Control of oral secretions can be a difficult problem for patients with ALS. Peripherally acting anticholinergic drugs such as glycopyrrolate are the first line of treatment for this problem. Because β-adrenergic stimulation increases production of protein and mucus-rich secretions that may thicken saliva and make it especially difficult for patients to handle, administration of beta-blockers such as metoprolol has been proposed to reduce thickness of oral, nasal, and pulmonary secretions. Surgical procedures to reduce salivary production (e.g., tympanic neurectomy, submandibular gland resection) have also been employed but have not been extensively studied.

Behavioral therapy approaches can be useful in treating mild to moderate dysphagia in ALS. Alterations in food consistency (e.g., thickening liquids), swallowing compensation techniques, and voluntary airway protection maneuvers all provide benefit and can be taught by speech/swallowing therapists. Eventually, however, enteral feeding becomes necessary in many individuals with advanced ALS. Placement of a PEG tube can stabilize weight loss, relieve nutritional deficiency, and improve quality of life for individuals with advanced ALS and severe dysphagia.

Cranial Neuropathies

Pathological processes involving the lower cranial nerves can produce dysphagia, usually as a part of a broader clinical picture. Dysphagia can be prominent in the Miller Fisher variant of acute inflammatory demyelinating polyneuropathy (Guillain-Barré syndrome). Response to plasmapheresis is expected in this situation. Dysphagia may also be present in herpes zoster infection, where it has been attributed to cranial ganglionic involvement. Examples of other processes in which cranial nerve involvement can result in dysphagia include Charcot-Marie-Tooth disease and primary or metastatic tumors involving the skull base. Severe but reversible dysphagia with significantly prolonged esophageal transit time has been attributed to vincristine therapy.

Brainstem Processes

Any process damaging the brainstem swallowing centers or lower cranial nerve nuclei can lead to dysphagia. Therefore, in addition to stroke and MS, a number of other processes affecting brainstem function may display dysphagia as part of their clinical picture. Brainstem tumors, both primary and metastatic, may be responsible for dysphagia, as can central pontine myelinolysis, progressive multifocal leukoencephalopathy, and leukoencephalopathy due to cyclosporin toxicity. Brainstem encephalitis produced by organisms such as *Listeria* and Epstein-Barr virus, may also result in dysphagia.

Cervical Spinal Cord Injury

Dysphagia may develop in individuals with cervical spinal cord injury, especially if the injury is associated with respiratory insufficiency. In a study of 51 persons with cervical spinal cord injury and respiratory insufficiency, 21 (41%) suffered from severe dysphagia with aspiration and another 20 (39%) had mild dysphagia (Wolf and Meiners, 2003). Individuals with higher spinal cord injury were statistically more likely to experience more prominent dysphagia after undergoing therapy, although this difference was not evident on admission. With treatment and time, most patients demonstrate improvement in their dysphagia.

Dysphagia may also develop in the setting of nontraumatic cervical spinal column disease. For example, dysphagia is one of the most frequent symptoms experienced by individuals with diffuse idiopathic skeletal hyperostosis (DISH, Forestier disease).

Other Processes

Although rare in developed countries, rabies is encountered more frequently in developing nations. In endemic areas, approximately 10% of affected individuals do not report any prior exposure to animal bite (Kietdumrongwong and Hemachudha, 2005). Dysphagia, typically accompanying phobic spasms in the classic "furious" form of rabies, is a well-recognized feature of the human disease. A hyperactive gag reflex is usually also present in this situation. However, dysphagia may also develop in the "paralytic" form of rabies, which may be more difficult to diagnose because the classically recognized features are often absent.

Neurogenic oropharyngeal dysphagia has also been reported as a consequence of severe hypothyroid coma (Urquhart et al., 2001).

Evaluation of Dysphagia

Various diagnostic tests ranging from simple bedside analysis to sophisticated radiological and neurophysiological procedures have been developed to evaluate dysphagia (**Box 13.4**). Although most are actually performed by specialists other than neurologists, it is important for neurologists to have an awareness of them so that they can be employed when clinical circumstances are appropriate (**Box 13.5**).

Clinical examination is somewhat limited because of the inaccessibility of some structures involved with swallowing, but both history and examination can provide useful clues to localization and diagnosis (**Table 13.1**). In fact, it has been reported that a good history will accurately identify the location and cause of dysphagia in 80% of cases (Cook, 2008). Difficulty initiating swallowing, the need for repeated attempts to succeed at swallowing, the presence of nasal regurgitation during swallowing, and coughing or choking immediately after attempted swallowing all suggest an oropharyngeal source for the dysphagia. A sensation of food "hanging up" in a retrosternal location implicates esophageal dysfunction, whereas a perception of the bolus "sticking" in the neck may indicate either pharyngeal or esophageal localization (**Fig. 13.1**). Individuals who report dysphagia for solid food but not liquids are more likely to have a mechanical obstruction, whereas equal dysphagia for both solids and liquids is more typical for an esophageal motility disorder. Lip and tongue function can be easily assessed during routine neurological examination, and both palatal and gag reflexes can be evaluated.

Cervical auscultation is not widely used to evaluate swallowing, but it may be useful to assess coordination between respiration and swallowing. In the normal situation,

---

Box 13.4 Diagnostic Tests

Oropharyngeal

Clinical examination
Cervical auscultation
Timed swallowing tests
3-ounce water swallow test
Modified barium swallow test
Pharyngeal videoendoscopy
Pharyngeal manometry
Videomanofluorometry
Electromyographic recording
Dysphagia limit

Esophageal

Endoscopy
Esophageal manometry
Videofluoroscopy

Box 13.5 Dysphagia Testing

If Oral Phase Dysfunction Suspected:

Screening tests:
  Clinical examination
  Cervical auscultation
  3-oz water swallow
Primary test:
  Modified barium swallow

If Pharyngeal Phase Dysfunction Suspected:

Screening tests:
  Clinical examination
  3-oz water swallow
  Timed swallowing
Primary test:
  Modified barium swallow
Complementary tests:
  Pharyngeal videoendoscopy
  Pharyngeal manometry
  Electromyography
  Videomanofluorometry

If Esophageal Dysfunction Suspected:

Primary tests:
  Videofluoroscopy
  Endoscopy
Complementary test:
  Esophageal manometry

swallowing occurs during exhalation, which reduces the risk of aspiration. Conversely, discoordinated swallowing in the midst of inhalation increases the possibility that food might be drawn into the respiratory tract.

Timed swallowing tests that require repetitive swallowing of specific amounts of water have also been employed to evaluate dysphagia. Individuals with swallowing impairment may display a number of abnormalities including slower swallowing speed (<10 mL/sec) and coughing, which may indicate the presence of dysphagia or aspiration. Some concern has been voiced, however, that the relatively large amounts of fluid used

Table 13.1 Dysphagia Clues

Clue	Cause of Dysphagia
Difficulty initiating swallowing	Oropharyngeal dysfunction
Repetitive swallowing	Oropharyngeal dysfunction
Retrosternal "hanging-up" sensation	Esophageal dysfunction
Difficulty with solids but not liquids	Mechanical obstruction
Difficulty with both solids and liquids	Esophageal dysmotility
Regurgitation of undigested food	Zenker diverticulum
Halitosis	Zenker diverticulum

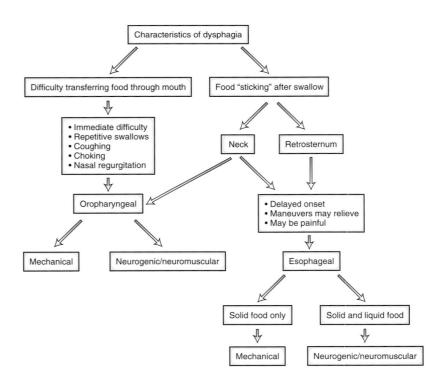

Fig. 13.1   Dysphagia assessment.

in these timed tests could present a significant risk for pulmonary complications due to of aspiration, even if it is water that is used.

A standardized 3-ounce water swallow test has been advocated as a simple bedside evaluation for oropharyngeal dysphagia. The presence of cough on swallowing during this test has been reported to provide a positive predictive value of 84% with regard to the presence of aspiration, and a negative predictive value of 78%. The test, however, does not provide any information regarding the specific mechanism of dysphagia in the patient.

The modified barium swallow test has become a standard method for assessing oropharyngeal dysphagia. Patients are observed via videofluoroscopy swallowing barium-impregnated food of differing consistencies (thin liquid, pudding, cookie). Both oral and pharyngeal function can be characterized and the presence of aspiration accurately documented; the response to corrective measures such as positioning techniques can also be evaluated. Increasing bolus viscosity typically improves swallowing function in individuals with neurogenic dysphagia (Clave et al., 2006).

Videoendoscopy of the pharynx via the nasal passageway allows direct visualization of the pharyngeal component of swallowing before and after passage of the food bolus. Its primary value is to demonstrate the presence of residual material in the pharynx after a swallow, indicative of increased risk of aspiration.

Pharyngeal manometry provides physiological information regarding function of both the pharynx and the UES; the information derived is complementary to that obtained by videofluoroscopy. A combined procedure termed *videomanofluorometry*, in which videofluoroscopy and manometry are performed simultaneously, can also be utilized. Although useful, this procedure is not always readily available.

Esophageal function can be assessed by endoscopy, esophageal manometry, and videofluoroscopy. Scintigraphic procedures can also be employed to evaluate oral, pharyngeal, and esophageal function but are not widely utilized. It has been suggested that scintigraphic examination with documentation of piecemeal deglutition and determination of the dysphagia limit may be particularly useful in centers where more sophisticated electrophysiological techniques are not available (Argon et al., 2004).

More sophisticated electrodiagnostic procedures have also been developed to study dysphagia. EMG recording of cricopharyngeal function and integrated submental activity has been useful in a research setting to characterize aspects of swallowing. Ertekin and colleagues (2002) have used EMG recordings to define an indicator of dysphagia they term the *dysphagia limit*. Normal subjects can swallow a 20-mL bolus of water in a single attempt, but persons with dysphagia must divide the bolus into two or more parts in order to complete the swallow. If individuals are administered stepwise increases in bolus volume, the volume of fluid at which the division of the bolus first occurs is labeled the dysphagia limit. The investigators consider a dysphagia limit of less than 20 mL as abnormal and indicative of dysphagia.

In conclusion, because of the broad network of structures involved with the control and execution of swallowing, dysphagia can be an important component of the clinical picture in patients with a wide variety of neurological diseases. Determining the specific mechanism responsible for dysphagia in individual patients can be of great value in both diagnosis and treatment of this disorder.

References

The complete reference list is available online at www.expertconsult.com.

I

Chapter **14**

Visual Loss

Matthew J. Thurtell, Robert L. Tomsak

Visual loss commonly accompanies neurological disease and is one of the most disturbing symptoms a patient may experience. While visual loss is often due to a benign or treatable process, it can be the first sign of a blinding or life-threatening disease. Common causes of visual loss include uncorrected refractive error, corneal disease, cataract, glaucoma, retinal and choroidal disease, and amblyopia. Ophthalmic causes of visual loss are often not apparent to the neurologist, whereas neurological causes of visual loss often confuse ophthalmologists. Thus, the approach to evaluating visual loss must be systematic, so that important causes are not missed and simple causes are not overinvestigated. In this chapter, we discuss the patterns and temporal profiles of visual loss; examination techniques are discussed in Chapter 36 and funduscopic abnormalities are discussed in Chapter 15.

Pattern of Visual Loss

Central Visual Loss

A defect in the visual field surrounded by normal vision is called a *scotoma*, from the Greek word meaning "darkness." Loss of central vision, resulting in a central or cecocentral scotoma, is usually quickly noticed and reported. Peripheral visual field defects, such as homonymous hemianopia, can be asymptomatic but when noticed are frequently referred to the eye with the greater extent of field loss (i.e., the eye with temporal field loss) (**Fig. 14.1**). Central and cecocentral scotomas are usually due to lesions of the central retina or optic nerve. When the lesion is at the junction of the optic nerve and chiasm, there will be an ipsilateral central scotoma due to optic nerve involvement, and a contralateral temporal defect due to chiasmal involvement; this highly-localizing visual field defect is known as a *junctional scotoma* (**Fig. 14.2**). Patients with junctional scotomas are often unaware of the contralateral temporal defect, emphasizing the importance of assessing each eye separately during history taking and visual field evaluation.

In general, scotomas caused by retinal disease are so-called positive scotomas, since they are perceived as a black or gray spot in the visual field. Patients with macular pathology can also have metamorphopsia, where there is distortion of images such that straight edges or geometrical figures appear warped. Metamorphopsia is almost always caused by retinal disease. In contrast, optic nerve lesions characteristically produce negative scotomas, areas of absent vision that are otherwise not perceivable, in conjunction with decreased color vision, contrast vision, and light brightness perception. On occasion, paradoxical photophobia, especially with fluorescent lighting, can occur with optic nerve lesions. Photopsias (light flashes) can occur with vitreoretinal traction (e.g., posterior vitreous detachment), retinal disease (e.g., cancer-associated retinopathy), toxicity from certain drugs (e.g., digitalis), or optic nerve disease (e.g., in the healing phase of optic neuritis, in which case they may be evoked by sound). Photopsias can also occur as part of migrainous visual aura. Aside from ocular diseases, bilateral central visual loss can result from lesions involving both optic nerves, the optic chiasm, or the part of the occipital cortex concerned with central vision. The possibility of nonorganic visual loss must also be considered, but it remains a diagnosis of exclusion (see Chapter 36).

Peripheral Visual Loss

For simplicity, visual field defects can be classified into one of three groups: prechiasmal, chiasmal, or retrochiasmal. Unilateral prechiasmal lesions affect the visual field of one eye only, chiasmal lesions affect the fields of both eyes in a non-homonymous bitemporal fashion, and retrochiasmal lesions cause homonymous field defects with variable degrees of congruity (i.e., similarity) depending on their location (**Fig. 14.3**). See Chapter 36 for further discussion of patterns of visual field loss.

Temporal Profile of Visual Loss

Sudden-Onset Visual Loss

Visual loss of sudden onset can be divided into three temporal patterns: transient (**Box 14.1**) (Thurtell and Rucker, 2009), nonprogressive, and progressive.

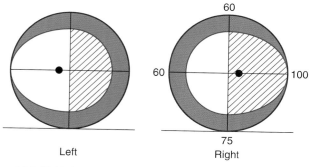

Fig. 14.1 Right homonymous hemianopia. The visual loss is often referred to the right eye, because the right temporal visual field is larger than the left nasal visual field. *Numbers* refer to the normal extent of the visual field in degrees.

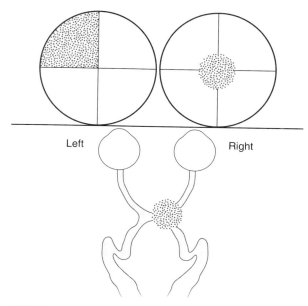

Fig. 14.2 Junctional scotoma from a lesion at the junction of the optic nerve and chiasm. The lesion affects both the right optic nerve, producing a cecocentral scotoma in the right eye, and crossing fibers in the optic chiasm, producing an upper temporal visual field defect in the left eye. The temporal field defect of a junctional scotoma often goes unnoticed by the patient and may only be detected with visual field testing (see Chapter 36).

Transient Monocular Visual Loss

AMAUROSIS FUGAX

The term *amaurosis fugax* is often used to describe the transient monocular visual loss (TMVL) caused by emboli from the carotids, aortic arch, or heart to the retinal circulation. Typically, these attacks are sudden in onset, last from several to 15 minutes, and are characterized by altitudinal visual field loss that is often described as being like a curtain descending over the eye (Donders, 2001). Patients may also describe having separate attacks with hemispheric symptoms, such as weakness and speech disturbance, rather than visual loss.

RETINAL ARTERY VASOSPASM

Transient monocular visual loss can be caused by retinal artery vasospasm and is called *retinal migraine* when accompanied by migraine headache (Hill et al., 2007). Vasospastic TMVL is

---

Box 14.1 Causes of Transient Monocular Visual Loss

Embolic cerebrovascular disease
Migraine/vasospasm
Hypoperfusion (hypotension, hyperviscosity, hypercoagulability)
Ocular (optic disc edema, intermittent angle-closure glaucoma, hyphema, impending central retinal vein occlusion)
Vasculitis (e.g., giant cell arteritis)
Other (Uhthoff phenomenon, idiopathic, nonorganic)

---

usually benign and often responds to calcium channel blockers (Winterkorn et al., 1993).

ANGLE-CLOSURE GLAUCOMA

Subacute attacks of angle-closure glaucoma should also be considered in the differential diagnosis of TMVL, especially if the patient reports seeing halos around lights or has associated eye pain, infection, or vomiting. Urgent ophthalmic consultation should be obtained to prevent irreversible visual loss.

VISUAL LOSS IN BRIGHT LIGHT

Some patients with reduced blood supply to the eye due to a high-grade stenosis or occlusion of the internal carotid artery report TMVL in bright light, which is likely due to impaired regeneration of photopigments secondary to ocular ischemia (Kaiboriboon et al., 2001). The TMVL can also occur following meals or with postural changes. A variety of ophthalmic abnormalities, including midperipheral retinal hemorrhages, can be present and collectively comprise the *ocular ischemic syndrome* (Chen and Miller, 2007). Other retinal diseases, such as cone dystrophies and age-related macular degeneration, can cause evanescent visual loss in bright light, also known as *hemeralopia* or *day blindness*. The visual loss in these diseases is usually bilateral, whereas it is unilateral in patients with unilateral carotid disease.

UHTHOFF PHENOMENON

Transient monocular visual loss with increases in body temperature is known as the Uhthoff phenomenon and most commonly occurs in patients with optic neuritis associated with demyelinating disease, but it can also occur in patients with other optic neuropathies. The phenomenon is thought to arise as a result of transient conduction block within the optic nerve. Vision returns to baseline when the body temperature returns to normal.

TRANSIENT VISUAL OBSCURATIONS

Transient visual obscurations are brief episodes of monocular or binocular visual loss in patients with optic disc edema. The visual loss is frequently precipitated by postural changes or Valsalva-like maneuvers (e.g., coughing, straining) and probably occurs secondary to transient hypoperfusion of the edematous optic nerve head. The visual loss lasts for only a few seconds, with vision rapidly returning to baseline thereafter. Similar episodes of visual loss can occur with systemic hypotension, giant cell arteritis, or retinal venous stasis. Gaze-evoked transient visual loss has been reported with orbital tumors but can occasionally occur with optic disc edema.

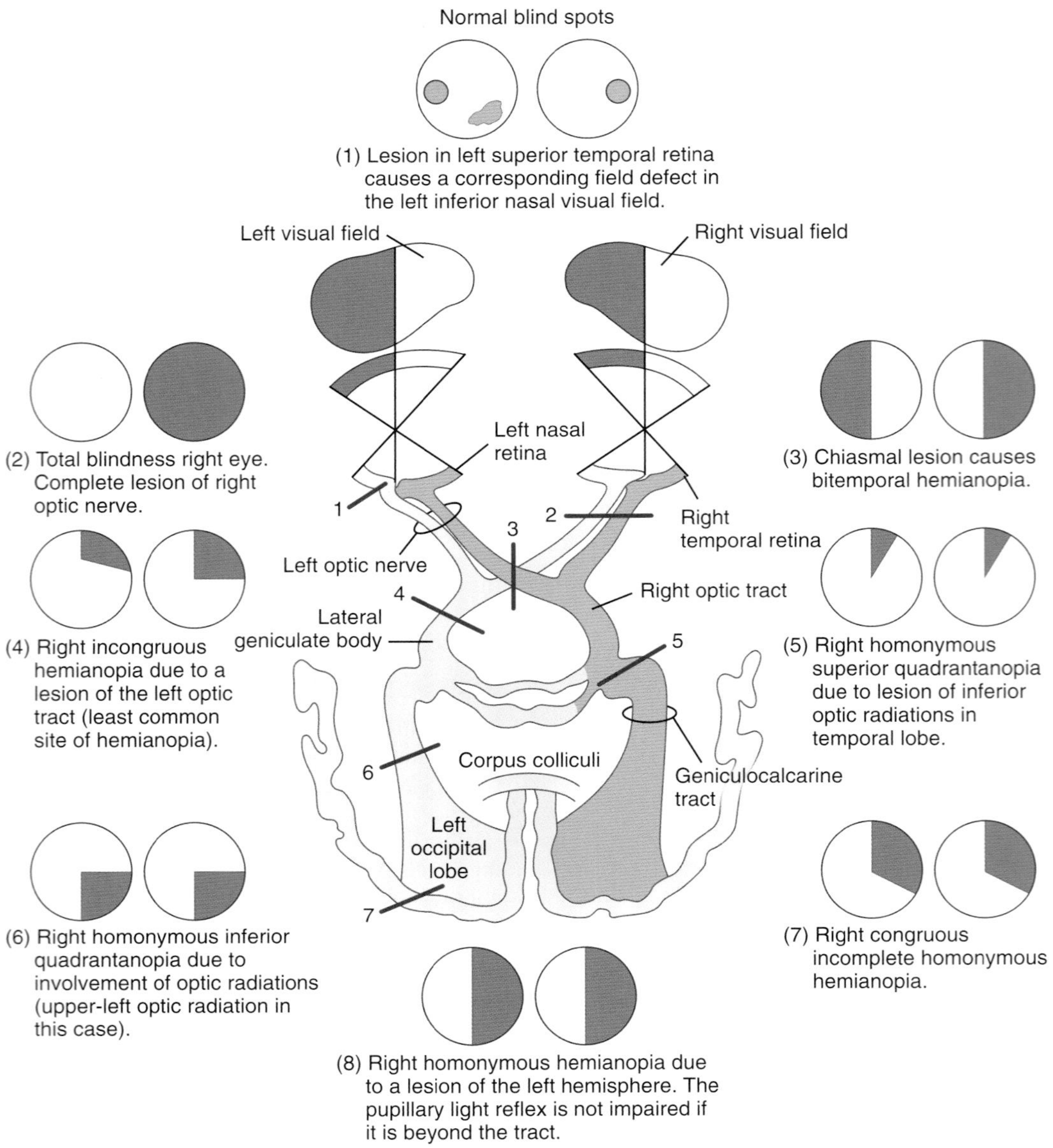

Fig. 14.3 Topographical diagnosis of visual field defects. *(Reprinted with permission from Vaughn, C., Asbury, T., Tabbara, K.F., 1989. General Ophthalmology, twelfth ed. Appleton & Lange, Norwalk, CT, p. 244.)*

OTHER CAUSES OF TRANSIENT VISUAL LOSS

Transient visual loss can also occur with cystic lesions such as sphenoid sinus mucoceles, craniopharyngiomas, and pituitary tumors. Other ophthalmic causes of TMVL include impending central retinal vein occlusion and recurrent hyphema, although it is important to note that some causes (e.g., corneal basement membrane dystrophy, tear film dysfunction) produce visual blurring or distortion rather than actual visual loss.

Transient Binocular Visual Loss

Other than transient visual obscurations occurring in patients with bilateral optic disc edema, simultaneous complete or incomplete transient binocular visual loss is almost always due to transient dysfunction of the visual cortex. Visual migraine aura is probably the most common cause of transient binocular visual loss, especially in patients younger than 40 years (see Chapter 69). Transient binocular visual loss can also result from cerebral hypoperfusion due to vasospasm, thromboembolism, systemic hypotension, hyperviscosity, or vascular compression (**Box 14.2**) (Thurtell and Rucker, 2009). Transient binocular visual loss can occur in association with seizures, although they more commonly cause visual hallucinations, which can be elementary or complex depending on the location of the seizure focus (Bien et al., 2000). Transient cortical blindness can occur in association with headache, altered mental status, and seizures in the posterior reversible encephalopathy syndrome (Hinchey et al., 1996). Transient cortical blindness can sometimes occur after head trauma, especially in children. Lastly, transient bilateral visual loss can occasionally be nonorganic in etiology, but this should remain a diagnosis of exclusion.

Box 14.2 Causes of Transient Binocular Visual Loss

Migraine
Cerebral hypoperfusion:
    Thromboembolism
    Systemic hypotension
    Hyperviscosity
Seizures
Posterior reversible encephalopathy syndrome
Head trauma
Optic disc edema (transient visual obscurations)

Sudden Monocular Visual Loss without Progression

Visual loss due to optic nerve or retinal ischemia is characteristically sudden in onset (**Box 14.3**) and is usually nonprogressive, although a stuttering decline in vision may occur over several weeks in approximately 10% of patients with anterior ischemic optic neuropathy. *Anterior ischemic optic neuropathy* is a common cause of optic neuropathy and occurs secondary to loss of blood supply to the optic nerve head, resulting in optic disc edema (Rucker et al., 2004). In affected patients younger than 60 years, it is usually nonarteritic in etiology, being caused by a combination of factors that impair blood supply to the optic nerve head. In patients older than 60 years, giant cell (temporal or cranial) arteritis must be considered; urgent investigations and empirical treatment with high-dose steroids may be required in these patients to prevent further devastating visual loss. Retrobulbar optic nerve infarction, also known as *posterior ischemic optic neuropathy*, is far less common but can result from perioperative hypotension (e.g., with spinal surgery or cardiac bypass surgery) and other causes of hemodynamic shock (Rucker et al., 2004). Giant cell arteritis should be specifically considered in elderly patients with posterior ischemic optic neuropathy.

Optic nerve ischemia very rarely results from embolism or migraine. In contrast, central or branch retinal artery occlusions are caused mostly by embolic or thrombotic events. Opacification of the retinal nerve fiber layer with a cherry-red spot at the macula is the classic funduscopic appearance of acute central retinal artery occlusion (see Chapter 15). Retinal arterial occlusions can produce altitudinal, quadrantic, or complete monocular visual loss. The triad of branch retinal artery occlusions, hearing loss, and encephalopathy results from a rare microangiopathy known as *Susac syndrome* (Susac et al., 2007). A distinctive pattern of white-matter lesions with involvement of the corpus callosum is seen on magnetic resonance imaging in this disease.

Occlusion of the central retinal vein results in sudden visual loss and an unmistakable hemorrhagic retinopathy. It usually occurs in adults with risk factors for atherosclerosis and results from venous thrombosis at the level of the lamina cribrosa of the sclera. It characteristically causes a dense central scotoma with sparing of peripheral vision.

Idiopathic central serous retinopathy can manifest as a positive scotoma of sudden onset, often with symptoms of metamorphopsia or micropsia and a positive light-stress test result (see Chapter 36). It results from leakage of fluid into the subretinal space and most often occurs in young adult men with

---

Box 14.3 Causes of Sudden Monocular Visual Loss without Progression

Central or branch retinal artery occlusion
Anterior ischemic optic neuropathy, arteritic or nonarteritic
Posterior ischemic optic neuropathy
Branch or central retinal vein occlusion
Traumatic optic neuropathy
Central serous retinopathy
Retinal detachment
Vitreous hemorrhage
Nonorganic (functional) visual loss

Box 14.4 Causes of Sudden Binocular Visual Loss without Progression

Occipital lobe stroke
Bilateral ischemic optic neuropathies
Pituitary apoplexy
Head trauma
Nonorganic (functional) visual loss

---

type-A personalities. The diagnosis can be difficult to make without the aid of fluorescein angiography or optical coherence tomography, as the retinal findings are subtle. Spontaneous recovery usually occurs within weeks to months, but occasionally laser photocoagulation is required to seal leaking vessels.

Traumatic optic neuropathy (TON) usually results in sudden permanent optic nerve dysfunction. The trauma can be severe or deceptively minor, causing a contusion or laceration of the optic nerve in its canal or a shearing of its nutrient vessels with subsequent ischemia. Treatments for TON, such as steroids, remain controversial and mostly ineffective (Levin et al., 1999).

Sudden Binocular Visual Loss without Progression

Sudden, permanent, binocular visual loss, if not caused by trauma, most commonly results from a stroke involving the retrochiasmal visual pathways and causes an homonymous visual field defect (**Box 14.4**) (Rizzo and Barton, 2005). In patients who have no other neurological symptoms or signs, the lesion usually involves the occipital lobe. Bilateral occipital lobe infarcts can result in tubular visual field defects, checkerboard visual field defects, or complete loss of vision in both eyes, a condition called *cortical blindness*. Cortical blindness, especially from infarction, can be accompanied by a denial of the visual loss and confabulation, a condition known as *Anton syndrome*.

Sudden binocular visual loss can result from simultaneous bilateral ischemic optic neuropathies and chiasmal compression due to *pituitary apoplexy*. Pituitary apoplexy can also cause headache, diplopia, altered mental status, and hemodynamic shock (Sibal et al., 2004), but the presentation can be subtle such that the diagnosis is missed.

Sudden Visual Loss with Progression

Sudden-onset, painful monocular visual loss that subsequently worsens is commonly due to optic nerve inflammation (optic neuritis). The visual loss typically progresses over hours to

Box 14.5 Causes of Progressive Visual Loss

Anterior visual pathway inflammation:
  Optic neuritis
  Sarcoidosis
  Meningitis
Anterior visual pathway compression:
  Tumors
  Aneurysms
  Thyroid-associated orbitopathy
Hereditary optic neuropathies:
  Leber hereditary optic neuropathy
  Dominant optic atrophy
Optic nerve head drusen
Glaucoma and low-tension glaucoma
Chronic papilledema
Toxic (e.g., ethambutol) and nutritional optic neuropathies
Radiation damage to anterior visual pathways
Paraneoplastic retinopathy or optic neuropathy

days before stabilizing and then improving. Optic neuritis is well known to be associated with multiple sclerosis and may be the first sign of the disease. The prognosis for visual recovery without treatment is excellent in most patients, although there is a poor recovery in some, such as those with optic neuritis occurring in association with neuromyelitis optica (Wingerchuk et al., 2007).

Leber hereditary optic neuropathy (LHON), a maternally transmitted disease resulting from mutations in the mitochondrial deoxyribonucleic acid (DNA) genes encoding subunits of respiratory chain complex I, can also cause sudden visual loss with subsequent progression. Primary mutations have been identified at positions 11778, 3460, 15257, and 14484 in the mitochondrial DNA. Many other mutations have been reported but occur less frequently (Yu-Wai-Man et al., 2009). LHON produces acute or subacute painless, often permanent, central visual loss, usually in young adult men. The visual loss is initially monocular, but the other eye usually becomes affected within 6 months. Visual recovery is variable and infrequent, and depends on the mitochondrial DNA mutation. The 11778 mutation carries the worst visual prognosis and the 14484 mutation the best. In the acute phase, the classic triad of ophthalmic findings includes telangiectatic vessels around the optic disc, nonedematous elevation of the optic disc, and absence of leakage from the disc on fluorescein angiography. Arteriolar narrowing can be marked, and vascular tortuosity is often a clue early in the disease. LHON can also cause loss of vision in women, but it tends to be less severe than in men.

Careful questioning of the patient with "sudden" visual loss may reveal a long-standing deficit that has suddenly been noticed (e.g., when covering the good eye) or that has worsened over time. In such cases, the clinician should evaluate for a slow-growing compressive lesion (**Box 14.5**).

Progressive Visual Loss

Progressive visual loss is the hallmark of a lesion compressing the afferent visual pathways. Common compressive lesions include pituitary tumors, aneurysms, craniopharyngiomas,

and meningiomas (see **Box 14.5**) (Gittinger, 2005; Glaser, 1999). Granulomatous disease of the optic nerve from sarcoidosis or tuberculosis can cause chronic progressive visual loss. Optic nerve compression at the orbital apex from thyroid-associated orbitopathy can occur with minimal orbital signs or ocular motility disturbance. In each of these cases, the visual loss can be so insidious as to go unnoticed until it is fortuitously discovered during a routine examination.

Hereditary or degenerative diseases of the optic nerves or retina must be included in the differential diagnosis of gradual-onset visual loss. The hereditary optic neuropathies are bilateral and are usually diagnosed during the first 2 decades of life (Yu-Wai-Man et al., 2009). The most common inherited optic neuropathy is the autosomal dominant variety, known as *dominant optic atrophy*. A number of mutations involving the OPA1 gene have been described in dominant optic atrophy (Yu-Wai-Man et al., 2009). The visual loss can range from mild to severe and can sometimes be asymmetrical. Characteristically, there are central or cecocentral scotomas with sparing of the peripheral fields, and temporal pallor and cupping of the optic discs. Color vision is usually abnormal. Other ophthalmic and neurological abnormalities may be present.

Drusen of the optic nerve head are extracellular deposits of plasma proteins and a variety of inorganic materials that can compress optic nerve axons near the surface of the nerve head as they enlarge (Auw-Haedrich et al., 2002). Drusen are a common cause of pseudopapilledema and can produce visual field defects including arcuate defects, sectorial scotomas, blind spot enlargement, and generalized visual field constriction (Lee and Zimmerman, 2005). Loss of visual acuity is atypical but can result from development of a secondary choroidal neovascular membrane, with subsequent hemorrhage into the macula, or anterior ischemic optic neuropathy. "Buried" drusen (i.e., those not visible with the ophthalmoscope) can also cause visual field loss; the diagnosis can be confirmed by identifying calcified deposits in the optic nerve head on ophthalmic ultrasound. Buried drusen can occasionally be seen with computed tomography if they are large enough, and appear as calcifications. If central visual loss occurs in patients with optic disc drusen and no obvious retinal lesion, a search for a retrobulbar lesion should be undertaken.

Normal-tension glaucoma (NTG) is a controversial entity that creates a diagnostic and therapeutic conundrum, since a number of conditions can give rise to a similar clinical picture (Tomsak, 1997). In true NTG, glaucomatous optic disc and visual field changes develop despite normal intraocular pressure. NTG is bilateral in 70% of patients, and the average age at diagnosis is 66 years. Women are affected approximately twice as frequently as men. NTG can be either progressive or static (Anderson et al., 2001).

Chronic papilledema from any cause of intracranial hypertension can produce progressive optic neuropathy (see Chapter 59). The optic discs often develop a milky gray color, and there is sheathing of peripapillary retinal vessels. The visual fields become constricted, with nasal defects occurring initially, followed by gradual constriction, with central vision being spared until late. Optociliary collateral vessels can develop, and sudden visual loss from ischemic optic neuropathy can rarely occur. On occasion, optic atrophy develops in the absence of papilledema or despite a decrease in intracranial pressure, possibly due to retrobulbar optic nerve compression (Thurtell et al., 2010).

Toxic and nutritional optic neuropathies are bilateral and usually progressive (Phillips, 2005; Tomsak, 1997). The nutritional variety is characterized by a history of inadequate diet, a gradual onset of painless visual loss over weeks to months, prominent dyschromatopsia, cecocentral scotomas, and development of optic atrophy late in the disease. Most cases of so-called tobacco-alcohol amblyopia are probably related to vitamin B deficiencies. Other conditions that lead to nutritional deficiency, such as bariatric surgery and keto-genic diet, can also cause bilateral optic neuropathies. Medications that are toxic to the optic nerves, including ethambutol, amiodarone, isoniazid, chloramphenicol, and iodoquinol (formerly diiodohydroxyquin), can cause a gradual onset of painless visual loss (Phillips, 2005). Retinal toxins such as vigabatrin, digitalis, chloroquine, hydroxychloroquine, and phenothiazines can also cause painless progressive binocular visual loss.

Slowly progressive visual loss from radiation damage to the anterior visual pathways, especially the retina, can result from direct radiation therapy to the eye for primary ocular tumors or metastases, or can occur after periocular irradiation for basal cell carcinomas, sinus carcinomas, and related malignancies. It can also occur after whole-brain irradiation for metastases or gliomas, or after parasellar radiation therapy for pituitary or other parasellar neoplasms (Lessell, 2004). Radiation retinopathy becomes clinically apparent after a variable latent period of several months to a few years following the radiation therapy and is usually irreversible. Its incidence relates to the fraction size, total radiation dose, and use of concomitant chemotherapy. Radiation-induced retinal capillary endothelial cell damage is the initial event that triggers the retinopathy, which is usually indistinguishable from diabetic retinopathy.

Rapidly progressive bilateral visual loss in patients with cancer can be caused by paraneoplastic processes that affect the retina or optic nerves (Ko et al., 2008). Small cell carcinoma of the lung is the most commonly associated tumor, but gynecological, endocrine, breast, and other tumors have been implicated. The visual loss is usually accompanied by photopsias, often precedes the diagnosis of cancer, and is associated with circulating antibodies to the tumor and retinal or optic nerve antigens (see Chapter 52G). Findings similar to those of retinitis pigmentosa are present, including night blindness, constricted visual fields, and an extinguished electroretinogram. No effective treatment is available.

References

The complete reference list is available online at www.expertconsult.com.

Chapter 15

Abnormalities of the Optic Nerve and Retina

Laura J. Balcer, Sashank Prasad

Disorders of the optic nerve and retina are common causes of afferent visual loss in clinical neurology. The diagnosis of optic neuropathy should be considered when visual loss (affecting visual acuity, color vision, or visual field) is accompanied by abnormal optic disc appearance or a relative afferent pupillary defect (RAPD; see Chapter 17). The specific cause for an optic neuropathy often can be established on the basis of clinical history (i.e., character, progression of vision loss) and examination (i.e., pattern of visual field loss and optic disc appearance). Furthermore, optic neuropathies are classifiable by appearance of the optic disc: normal, swollen, or pale. Chapter 14 describes the various patterns of visual field loss and clinical history typically elicited in patients with specific optic nerve disorders. This chapter presents the differential diagnosis for optic neuropathies based on the optic disc appearance and discusses retinal disorders of particular interest in neurology. Chapter 36 discusses many of the entities described in this chapter in more detail.

Optic Nerve Anatomy and Physiology

Light stimulates retinal photoreceptors whose signal reaches a ganglion cell after being modulated by bipolar, horizontal, and amacrine cells (**Fig. 15.1**). Two main types of retinal ganglion cells exist: *parasol cells* (which project to the magnocellular layer and are specialized for motion perception and coarse stereopsis) and *midget cells* (which project to the parvocellular layer and are specialized for high spatial resolution, color vision,

and fine stereopsis). Temporal retinal fibers form arcuate bundles around the fovea, respecting the midline horizontal raphe, and then enter the optic disc superiorly and inferiorly (**Fig. 15.2**). Optic nerve fibers exit the globe at the scleral canal, where they receive physical support from the lamina cribrosa and receive metabolic support from intertwining astrocytes. Once nerve fibers pass the lamina cribrosa, they are supported by oligodendrocytes and become myelinated. After exiting the orbit, the nerve enters the optic canal within the lesser sphenoid wing. In this space, the nerve is particularly vulnerable to trauma or compressive lesions (Balcer, 2001; Sarkies, 2004).

Effective axonal transport is essential for maintenance of the ganglion cell axon's structure and function. Orthograde transport (away from the ganglion cell body) occurs at two speeds: 400 mm per day for proteins and neurotransmitters packaged in vesicles, and 1 to 4 mm per day for structural elements of the cytoskeleton. Interference of axonal transport, for example from elevated intracranial pressure (ICP), ultimately damages axons of the optic nerve and causes atrophy (Hayreh, 1977).

The ophthalmic artery, arising from the internal carotid artery, provides blood supply to the eye via multiple short posterior ciliary arteries and the central retinal artery (Hayreh and Zimmerman, 2007) (**Fig. 15.3**). The short posterior ciliary arteries provide blood supply to the optic nerve head and the subretinal choroid. Each posterior ciliary artery supplies a variable segmental territory of the optic nerve head, and because anastomoses in this blood supply are scant, it can suffer watershed ischemia during hypoperfusion. Furthermore, the segmental blood supply underlies the sectoral disc

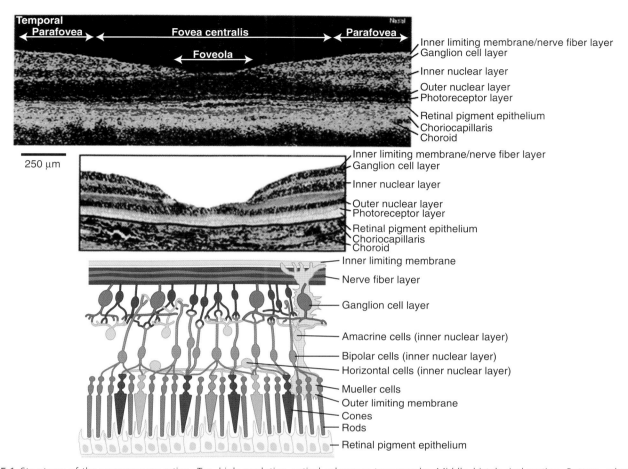

Fig. 15.1 Structures of the neurosensory retina. *Top*, high-resolution optical coherence tomography. *Middle*, histological section. *Bottom*, schematic depiction of retinal layers. *(Adapted and reprinted with permission from Jaffe and Caprioli [2004] and www.webvision.med.utah.edu.)*

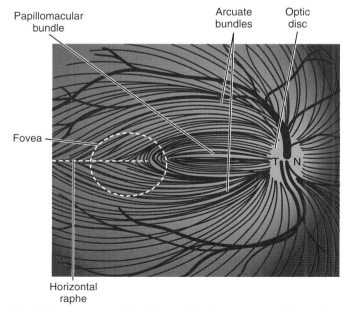

Fig. 15.2 Arrangement of retinal nerve fiber layer, composed of ganglion cell axons. The papillomacular bundle conveys axons from the fovea directly to the temporal margin (T) of the optic disc. The remainder of temporal ganglion cell axons are arranged in arcuate bundles above and below the fovea, arriving at the superior and inferior disc margins. Finally, axons originating nasal to the disc arrive at its nasal border (N).

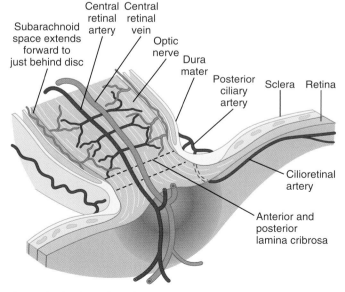

Fig. 15.3 Blood supply to the optic nerve. *(Reprinted with permission from Patten [2004].)*

swelling or atrophy that results from interrupted flow of a posterior ciliary artery and subsequent optic nerve infarction (Balcer, 2001; Fontal et al., 2007).

The Swollen Optic Disc

In assessing an elevated optic disc, the examiner must first make the important distinction between true disc swelling and pseudopapilledema. Disc swelling caused by elevated ICP is referred to as *papilledema* and may be accompanied by headache, transitory visual obscurations with change in posture, nausea, and vomiting. In addition, papilledema commonly is bilateral, in contrast with other optic neuropathies including optic neuritis or nonarteritic ischemic optic neuropathy. Causes of pseudopapilledema include congenital anomalies, myelinated nerve fibers, and optic nerve head drusen (discussed later).

Unilateral Optic Disc Swelling

The most common causes of unilateral optic disc edema are nonarteritic anterior ischemic optic neuropathy (NAION), optic neuritis, and orbital compressive lesions. Although characteristics of the optic disc appearance may overlap among NAION, optic neuritis, and compressive optic neuropathies, certain features may suggest a specific diagnosis. These are described and illustrated in the following sections. Briefly, in NAION the disc typically has a pale, edematous appearance which is often sectoral, and disc hemorrhages are likely to be present. On the other hand, only one-third of patients with optic neuritis will have optic disc swelling, and, when present, it is typically mild. Disc hemorrhages are uncommon in these patients, and this finding should suggest an alternative diagnosis. Finally, compressive lesions may lead to chronic disc edema, optociliary shunt vessels, and glistening white bodies on the disc surface (pseudodrusen from extruded axoplasm).

Despite suggestive patterns in the appearance of the optic nerve, it often is not possible to distinguish NAION, optic neuritis, and compressive optic neuropathies on this basis alone. Typically these diagnoses also rely on data from the clinical history and the pattern of the visual field deficit (**Fig. 15.4**). Vision loss generally is slowly progressive in patients with compressive lesions; it is rapidly progressive with subsequent improvement in those with optic neuritis; and it is maximal at onset with minimal improvement in patients with NAION. Both optic neuritis and compressive lesions generally produce central visual loss, whereas NAION typically produces a nerve fiber bundle–type field defect (originating from the physiological blind spot and respecting the horizontal meridian, owing to the arrangement of retinal ganglion cell axons traveling to the optic disc). However, considerable overlap exists in the patterns of visual field loss caused by the different forms of optic neuropathy.

Optic Neuritis

Typical *optic neuritis* is an inflammatory optic neuropathy caused by demyelinating disease (Balcer, 2006) (**Fig. 15.5**). Visual loss in the affected eye typically occurs rapidly over several hours to a few days. Decreased color vision and contrast sensitivity are highly characteristic (Baier et al., 2005; Trobe et al., 1996). In addition, pain with eye movements precedes the vision loss in approximately 90% of cases (Optic Neuritis Study Group, 1991). The pain typically lasts 3 to 5 days; if it persists for longer than 7 days, optic neuritis should be considered less likely, and further workup should be pursued. Visual field defects commonly are present; they can be either diffuse or discrete scotomas and are nonspecific. Fundus examination reveals mild disc swelling in approximately one-third of affected eyes, which is considerably less prominent than the disc swelling associated with papilledema

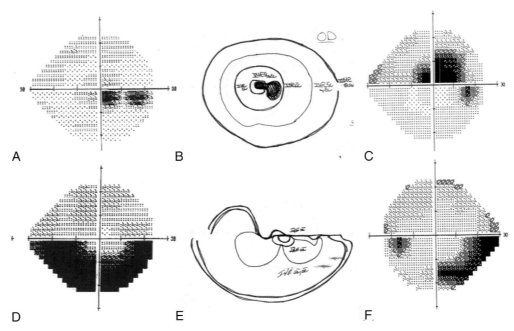

Fig. 15.4 Visual field defects in patients with optic neuropathies (grayscale output of Humphrey automated perimetry [**A, C, D,** and **F**] and kinetic Goldmann perimetry [**B** and **E**]). **A,** Central scotoma in a patient with right optic neuritis. **B,** Centrocecal scotoma (connecting to physiological blind spot) in a patient with optic neuropathy due to B$_{12}$ deficiency. **C,** Superior altitudinal central scotoma in a patient with inferior optic nerve compression due to a meningioma. **D,** Inferior arcuate altitudinal scotoma in a patient with nonarteritic ischemic optic neuropathy. **E,** Superior altitudinal scotoma in a patient with arteritic ischemic optic neuropathy. **F,** Inferonasal step in a patient with glaucomatous optic neuropathy. *(Reprinted with permission from Prasad, S., Volpe, N.J., Balcer, L.J., 2010. Approach to optic neuropathies: clinical update. Neurologist 16, 23-34.)*

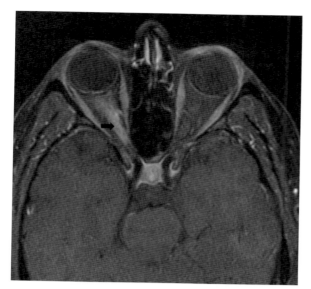

Fig. 15.5 Axial T1-weighted post-gadolinium MRI with fat saturation in a patient with right optic neuritis. Note swelling and enhancement of the right optic nerve *(black arrow)* consistent with inflammation. *(Reprinted with permission from Prasad et al., 2010.)*

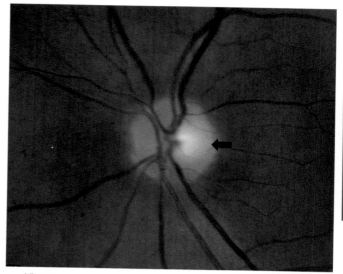

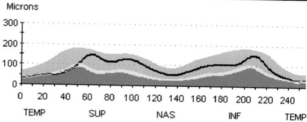

Fig. 15.7 *Top,* Fundus photographs of the left eye in a patient with prior left optic neuritis, demonstrating mild temporal pallor *(black arrow). Below,* Optical coherence tomography (OCT) measurement of retinal nerve fiber layer thickness confirms and quantifies temporal nerve fiber layer thinning (corresponding to the papillomacular bundle). Thickness measurement is shown in black line, with normal range depicted in green zone; measurements within the yellow zone are borderline, and within the red zone are abnormally low. *(Reprinted with permission from Prasad et al., 2010.)*

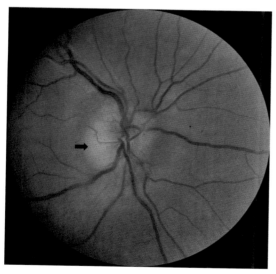

Fig. 15.6 Fundus photograph of the right eye in a patient with acute right optic neuritis. Note mild nerve fiber layer swelling, greatest at the temporal portion of the disc *(black arrow)*, without hemorrhages or cotton-wool spots. *(Reprinted with permission from Prasad et al., 2010.)*

(Balcer, 2006; Beck, 1998) (**Fig. 15.6**). In the majority of patients, the fundus appearance is normal.

The prognosis for recovery of vision generally is good but is in relation to the severity of the initial deficit. Recovery typically begins within 1 month. The likelihood of progression of optic neuritis to multiple sclerosis (MS) is best predicted by brain magnetic resonance imaging (MRI) at the time of diagnosis. In the Optic Neuritis Treatment Trial, the risk of developing MS within 15 years was 72% among patients with one or more characteristic brain lesions, whereas it was 25% if the MRI was normal (Optic Neuritis Study Group, 2008). With features that are atypical for optic neuritis, however (e.g.,

painless visual loss, severe disc edema, disc or peripapillary hemorrhages, macular exudate), the risk of developing MS is significantly lower (Beck et al., 2003).

Following an episode of optic neuritis, the optic nerve often demonstrates pallor, suggesting that axonal loss has accompanied the episode of demyelination (**Fig. 15.7**). Optical coherence tomography (OCT) is a noninvasive imaging method that quantifies the atrophy of the nerve fiber layer (Balcer, 2006). It provides a reliable structural marker that complements clinical assessments of visual function.

Neuromyelitis optica (NMO), or Devic disease, is characterized by necrotizing demyelinating lesions of bilateral optic nerves and the spinal cord (Wingerchuk, 2006). It is believed to be a humorally mediated disease distinct from MS. The spinal lesion characteristic of NMO often extends contiguously over three or more vertebral segments. A serum antibody, neuromyelitis optica immunoglobulin G (NMO-IgG), which targets the autoantigen aquaporin 4 (AQP4), may be a useful marker in diagnosing the condition, although the exact specificity remains unknown (Jarius et al., 2008). Treatment with rituximab, a chemotherapeutic monoclonal antibody, may be of particular benefit in this group of patients (Wingerchuk, 2006).

Treating optic neuritis with high-dose intravenous (IV) corticosteroids reduces the risk of developing MS over the following 2 years (Beck et al., 1992). In the long term, however, this acute treatment is unlikely to affect the likelihood of progression to MS. In addition, IV corticosteroid treatment may hasten visual recovery, particularly for visual fields and contrast sensitivity, but does not significantly affect long-term visual outcomes. Because low-dose oral corticosteroids may be associated with an increased risk of recurrence of optic neuritis, this therapy should be avoided (Beck et al., 1992). In addition to IV corticosteroids, recent studies support the early use of immunomodulating treatments for high-risk patients to reduce the likelihood of progression to MS within 2 to 5 years (Balcer, 2006).

Ischemic Optic Neuropathy

Arteritic anterior ischemic optic neuropathy (AAION) is usually related to giant cell arteritis (GCA), also referred to as *temporal arteritis*. Its incidence increases with age, with most patients being older than 70.

GCA typically affects the extracranial medium- to large-caliber arteries, because they possess elastic lamina, which is the initial site of inflammation in this disorder (Salvarani et al., 2008). The condition is associated with polymyalgia rheumatica, consisting of proximal muscle ache, arthralgia, and stiffness, as well as with jaw claudication, fever, malaise, and scalp tenderness. The diagnosis is suggested by an elevated erythrocyte sedimentation rate and C-reactive protein and is confirmed by evidence of giant cells and endovascular inflammation on temporal artery biopsy. Acute vision loss is the presenting symptom in 7% to 60% of cases and is generally more severe than in NAION. In approximately 25% of cases, vision is limited to hand motion perception or worse (Balcer et al., 2003). In suspected cases, treatment with corticosteroids should not be delayed until a biopsy is obtained. Intraveous corticosteroids may help delay the progression of visual loss and decrease the likelihood of fellow eye involvement. The prognosis for recovery in the affected eye, however, is poor despite treatment (Hall and Balcer, 2004).

The optic disc in AAION typically has a chalky-white edematous appearance, and disc hemorrhages are likely to be present (**Fig. 15.8**). Coexisting retinal ischemia with cotton-wool spots is very typical for AAION. Fluorescein angiography reveals choroidal hypoperfusion (**Fig. 15.9**). Occasionally, GCA can be limited to the retro-orbital nerve and present without disc swelling; this situation is termed *arteritic posterior ischemic optic neuropathy* (PION).

Nonarteritic AION is the most common cause of unilateral optic nerve swelling in adults older than 50 and is commonly associated with vascular risk factors such as diabetes or hypertension (Fontal et al., 2007). Other risk factors include a crowded optic nerve head and nocturnal hypotension, possibly precipitated by antihypertensive therapy (Arnold, 2003; Mathews, 2005). Swelling of a crowded optic nerve within the scleral canal may provoke a cycle of further vascular compression, ischemia, and swelling.

Although the clinical profile of NAION may occasionally overlap with the findings of optic neuritis (Rizzo et al., 1991), typical features of NAION include nerve fiber hemorrhages, altitudinal visual field loss, moderate to severe disc edema, and the absence of pain (**Figs. 15.10 and 15.11**). Because the optic

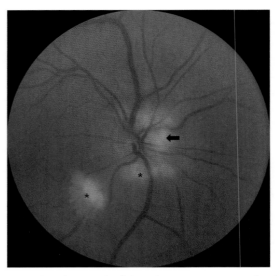

Fig. 15.8 Fundus photograph of the right eye in a patient with ischemic optic neuropathy from temporal arteritis. Note blurring of the nasal disc margin, with pallor and swelling of the nerve head *(black arrow)*. The patient also has inner retinal ischemia evidenced by large cotton-wool spots *(black asterisks)*. *(Reprinted with permission from Prasad et al., 2010.)*

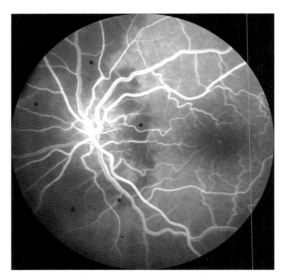

Fig. 15.9 Late-phase fluorescein angiography of the left eye in a patient with giant cell arteritis, revealing nonperfused choroid *(black asterisks)* consistent with occlusion of posterior ciliary vessels. *(Reprinted with permission from Prasad et al., 2010.)*

nerve head is supplied by an end-arterial system of short posterior ciliary arteries and the circle of Zinn-Haller, sectoral ischemic disc swelling is common. NAION may follow ocular surgery, because an associated increase in intraocular pressure may compromise optic nerve head perfusion (Fontal et al., 2007).

Many patients with NAION will have a stable deficit, although one minority may experience visual loss progressing over one month. Spontaneous improvement may occur in the first 6 months, although in many patients this reflects improved ability with eccentric fixation (Hayreh and Zimmerman, 2008). In 30% to 40% of patients, subsequent

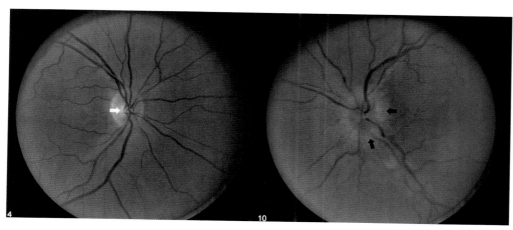

Fig. 15.10 Fundus photographs in a patient with acute nonarteritic ischemic optic neuropathy in the right eye, demonstrating peripapillary edema *(black arrows)* with a small cup-to-disc ratio in the left eye *(white arrow)*, suggesting a "disc at risk." *(Reprinted with permission from Prasad et al., 2010.)*

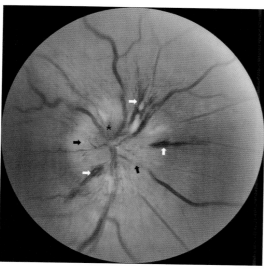

Fig. 15.11 Fundus photographs of the right eye in a patient with right nonarteritic anterior ischemic optic neuropathy. Note blurring of the disc margin and swelling of the optic nerve head *(black arrows)*, splinter hemorrhages *(white arrows)*, as well as dilated capillaries and luxury perfusion of the nerve head *(asterisk)*. *(Reprinted with permission from Prasad et al., 2010.)*

involvement of the fellow eye also occurs, and this rate is increased by the presence of vascular risk factors. When the second eye is affected in AION, optic atrophy has already developed in one eye, and acute disc edema occurs in the fellow eye; this clinical presentation is called the *pseudo–Foster Kennedy syndrome.* (A true Foster Kennedy syndrome is produced by optic atrophy due to compression, typically from an expanding tumor, and papilledema in the fellow eye secondary to increased ICP.) Occasionally, premonitory disc swelling in an asymptomatic eye will be noted, which may progress to frank visual loss or remit spontaneously (Hayreh and Zimmerman, 2007). Recurrence of NAION in an affected eye, however, is rare, possibly because optic nerve atrophy following the initial event decompresses the nerve. There does not appear to be a significantly higher rate of stroke in patients with nonarteritic ischemic optic neuropathy, suggesting that its pathophysiology may differ from simple vasoocclusion (Arnold and Levin, 2002).

Other Causes

Inflammatory conditions are an important cause of subacute optic neuropathy. Optic discs may appear swollen or normal, the latter indicating retrobulbar involvement. Optic nerve involvement is common in neurosarcoidosis, which can be accompanied by anterior uveitis or posterior segment vitritis (Prasad et al., 2008) (**Fig. 15.12**). Visual loss due to this condition is often steroid responsive. Optic neuropathy and retinal involvement may also occur with other inflammatory disorders, such as systemic lupus erythematosus and Sjögren disease (**Fig. 15.13**). Occasionally, optic nerve infiltration produces optic disc edema without affecting visual function, but more often there is a decrease in visual acuity and visual field loss.

Infectious conditions are another frequent cause of optic neuropathy (March and Lessell, 1996). Neuroretinitis, in which optic neuropathy coexists with characteristic peripapillary or macular exudates, should be distinguished from acute demyelinating optic neuritis (**Fig. 15.14**). The initial clinical presentation of these conditions may be similar, but the characteristic macular star of neuroretinitis will appear within 1 to 2 weeks, establishing the diagnosis. The distinction is critical because neuroretinitis has no association with an increased risk of MS and may be due to cat scratch disease (*Bartonella henselae*), syphilis (*Treponema pallidum*), or Lyme disease (*Borrelia burgdorferi*). In most cases, *Bartonella* infection is self-limited and does not require treatment, but in severe cases doxycycline may be effective (Balcer et al., 2003). Other infectious causes of optic neuropathy include human immunodeficiency virus (HIV) and opportunistic infections including toxoplasmosis, cytomegalovirus, and cryptococcosis. Paranasal sinusitis or mucocele may lead to either compressive or inflammatory optic neuropathy.

Paranasal sinus disease can cause a condition that mimics optic neuritis, with acute optic neuropathy and pain on eye movements, or can cause a progressive optic neuropathy resulting from compression (Rothstein et al., 1984). Consider optic neuropathy due to sinusitis and mucocele in patients who have clinical evidence of optic neuritis with seemingly atypical features, particularly elderly patients with severe sinus disease, a history of fevers, ophthalmoplegia, or progression of vision loss beyond 2 weeks.

Several compressive mass lesions cause a progressive optic neuropathy. The optic disc swells in cases of intraorbital compression, but in cases of retro-orbital compression, disc

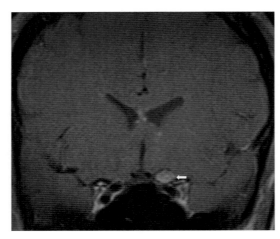

Fig. 15.12 Coronal T1-weighted post-gadolinium MRI in a patient with left optic neuropathy from neurosarcoidosis. Note swelling and enhancement of right optic nerve *(white arrow)*. *(Reprinted with permission from Prasad et al., 2010.)*

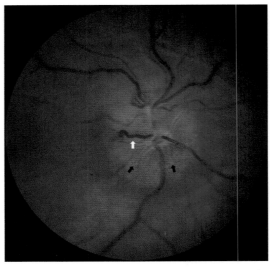

Fig. 15.15 Fundus photograph of the right eye in a patient with chronic disc swelling. Note blurred disc margins *(black arrows)* and an optociliary shunt vessel *(white arrow)*. *(Reprinted with permission from Prasad et al., 2010.)*

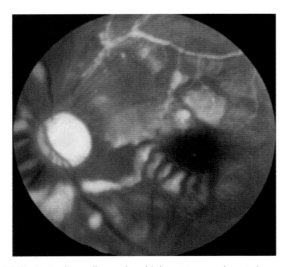

Fig. 15.13 Optic disc pallor and multiple cotton-wool spots in a patient with systemic lupus erythematosus.

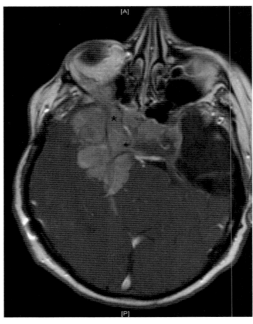

Fig. 15.16 Axial T1-weighted postcontrast MRI in a patient with an extensive sphenoid wing meningioma *(asterisk)* causing left optic nerve compression, ocular motor palsies, and proptosis. *(Reprinted with permission from Prasad et al., 2010.)*

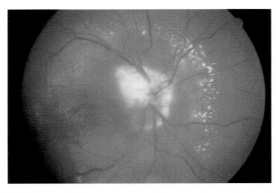

Fig. 15.14 Neuroretinitis in a 6-year-old boy. Such exudates, although usually not present in optic neuritis, indicate an inflammatory cause for the disc edema. *(Reprinted with permission from Beck, R.W., Smith, C.H., 1988. Neuro-Ophthalmology: A Problem-Oriented Approach. Little, Brown, Boston.)*

swelling only occurs if ICP is elevated. Chronic disc edema due to compressive lesions may be accompanied by optociliary shunt vessels and glistening white bodies on the disc surface (pseudodrusen from extruded axoplasm) (**Fig. 15.15**). Important causes of compressive optic neuropathy include neoplasm (including optic nerve sheath or skull base meningioma, pituitary adenoma, and craniopharyngioma), sinus lesions, bony processes (such as fibrous dysplasia), enlarged extraocular muscles (as in Graves disease ophthalmopathy), or aneurysms (**Fig. 15.16**). Meningiomas of the optic nerve

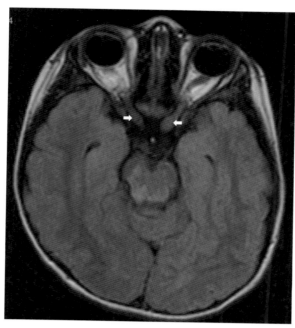

Fig. 15.17 Axial fluid-attenuated inversion recovery (FLAIR) MRI in a patient with bilateral optic nerve gliomas (juvenile pilocytic astrocytomas) *(white arrows)*. The patient had stigmata of type 1 neurofibromatosis. *(Reprinted with permission from Prasad et al., 2010.)*

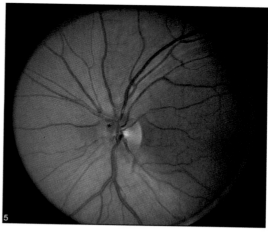

Fig. 15.18 Fundus photograph of the left eye in a patient with Leber hereditary optic neuropathy. Visual acuity was 20/200. Note hyperemia with appearance of slight nasal disc swelling *(asterisk)*. *(Reprinted with permission from Prasad et al., 2010.)*

sheath occur primarily in women and can cause acuity loss associated with either disc swelling or atrophy.

Primary optic nerve neoplasms include benign juvenile pilocytic glioma in children and (rarely) malignant glioblastoma in adults (**Fig. 15.17**). Juvenile pilocytic astrocytoma is often associated with neurofibromatosis type 1 and may be managed conservatively with frequent ophthalmological examination through adolescence (Listernick et al., 2007). When clinical or radiographic progression is detected, chemotherapy should be first-line therapy, followed by radiation and rarely surgery. Malignant optic nerve glioblastoma is much rarer, affects adults, and has a considerably worse prognosis (Spoor et al., 1980). Other neoplastic conditions include lymphoma, leukemia, carcinomatous meningitis, and optic nerve metastasis. Almost any form of carcinoma can metastasize to the optic nerve; breast and lung carcinomas are the most common.

Optic neuropathy may occur as a delayed effect of radiation therapy. It can occur with or without disc edema and can sometimes be difficult to distinguish from tumor recurrence (Danesh-Meyer, 2008). Radiation optic neuropathy is suggested by exposure (typically 50-Gy dosage), characteristic 6- to 24-month time lag to symptoms, and accompanying radiation changes in proximal tissues. Progression occurs over weeks to months, and spontaneous recovery is rare. Corticosteroids may help by reducing edema in the affected optic nerve.

Visual loss in a patient with known or suspected cancer raises the possibility of a paraneoplastic optic neuropathy or retinopathy (Damek, 2005). In paraneoplastic optic neuropathy, evidence of other neurological dysfunction is common, and the antibody most commonly identified is directed toward collapsin response mediator protein 5 (CRMP5).

Paraneoplastic retinopathies, on the other hand, include cancer-associated retinopathy (with antibodies to recoverin protein) and melanoma-associated retinopathy (with antibodies to rod ganglion cells).

Leber hereditary optic neuropathy (LHON) is a subacute, sequential, maternally inherited optic nerve disorder in which 80% to 90% of affected persons are males in the second or third decade of life (see Chapter 14) (Man et al., 2002; Newman, 2005). Although true disc edema is not present, the optic disc may appear hyperemic and mildly swollen in the acute phase; nevertheless, fluorescein angiography should confirm the absence of capillary leakage. Circumpapillary telangiectatic vessels, frequently present in the peripapillary nerve fiber layer, are an important clue to the diagnosis (**Fig. 15.18**). These early funduscopic changes also may be noted in presymptomatic eyes. As the condition progresses, the discs become atrophic. Because fibers mediating the pupillary light reflex may be selectively spared, the light reflex may be preserved despite significant visual loss. Genetic diagnosis of LHON is based on the identification of related mitochondrial DNA mutations (see Chapter 63). Most patients have permanent vision loss, although a minority will experience some recovery of vision. The prognosis depends upon the specific mutation harbored; patients with mtDNA mutation T14484C are more likely to have spontaneous recovery than patients with mutations G11778A or G3460A (Newman, 2005). At present, no effective treatment for this condition is available (Chinnery and Griffiths, 2005).

Direct traumatic optic neuropathy (TON) may include nerve avulsion or transection and is easily recognized by the relevant history of injury (Sarkies, 2004) (**Fig. 15.19**). Fundus examination may reveal extensive intraocular hemorrhages. On the other hand, posterior indirect traumatic optic neuropathy will present with visual loss in the absence of significant fundus abnormalities; it may result from shearing forces and subsequent edema within the optic canal. Up to half of these patients may improve spontaneously (Sarkies, 2004). There is weak evidence that corticosteroid therapy may be helpful within the first 8 hours, but no other medical or surgical interventions have proven effective (Yu Wai Man and Griffiths, 2005; Yu Wai Man and Griffiths, 2007).

A description of other uncommon causes of unilateral optic disc edema that occasionally can have a unilateral presentation will be discussed next.

Bilateral Optic Disc Swelling
Papilledema

The term *papilledema* refers specifically to optic disc swelling secondary to increased ICP. Disc swelling in papilledema results from blockage of axoplasmic flow in nerve fibers, increasing the volume of axoplasm in the optic disc (Hayreh, 1977). Although papilledema is typically bilateral, it can be asymmetrical, based on anatomical differences in the meningeal covering of the intracranial optic nerves that can lead to differences in transmitted pressure. On the basis of the chronicity and fundus appearance, papilledema can be divided into four stages: early, fully developed (acute), chronic, and atrophic. The acute phase of papilledema is strongly suggested by a mismatch between a markedly swollen disc and relatively spared optic nerve function, particularly central visual acuity.

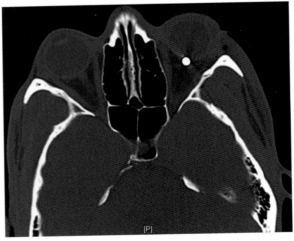

Fig. 15.19 Axial CT scan *(bone windows)* from a patient with direct left traumatic optic neuropathy due to avulsion by a BB pellet. *(Reprinted with permission from Prasad et al., 2010.)*

The most common visual field defects encountered in patients with early or acute papilledema are enlargement of the physiological blind spot, concentric constriction, and inferior nasal field loss. When acute papilledema is accompanied by decreased acuity (and often metamorphopsia), fluid typically extends within the retina to the macula itself.

In early papilledema, swelling is most prominent at the superior and inferior poles of the optic disc where the nerve fiber layer is thickest. With further development of papilledema, swelling encompasses the disc surface more uniformly, and the degree of disc elevation increases (**Fig. 15.20**). The retinal veins may distend slightly, and the disc may appear mildly hyperemic. These vascular changes result from nerve fiber swelling causing compression of capillaries and venules, leading to venous stasis and dilation, formation of microaneurysms, and finally disc and peripapillary splinter hemorrhages (see **Fig. 15.20**). Correspondingly, in fluorescein angiography, fluorescence may be absent during the retinal arterial phase as a result of delayed circulation caused by disc swelling. Dilated capillaries, microaneurysms, and flame-shaped hemorrhages may appear in the arteriovenous phase, and fluorescein may leak from dilated capillaries in the venous phase. Retinal cotton-wool spots may occur secondary to ischemia in the nerve fiber layer. Spontaneous venous pulsations usually are absent once the ICP exceeds 18 cm H_2O. Although papilledema typically is bilateral, it can be asymmetrical because of differences in transmitted pressure related to anatomical variation in the meningeal covering of the intracranial and intracanalicular optic nerves.

The disc appearance changes as papilledema becomes chronic, usually after weeks to months. The nerve fiber layer may appear pale and take on a gliotic appearance as a result of optic atrophy and astrocytic proliferation (**Fig. 15.21**). Hemorrhages are less prominent (and often have resolved completely). The disc takes on a "champagne cork" appearance in which small, glistening white bodies (pseudodrusen) result from extruded axoplasm after prolonged stasis. Shunt vessels due to compensatory dilation of preexisting communications between the retinal and ciliary circulation begin to appear.

If increased ICP and papilledema persist, optic nerve axons become damaged, and visual field loss develops. At this stage, optic disc swelling lessens, and pallor develops (atrophic papilledema). Finally, patients with end-stage papilledema exhibit optic nerve atrophy (disc pallor) without evidence of swelling.

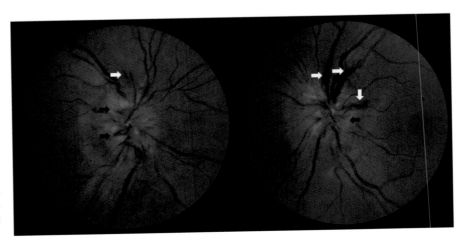

Fig. 15.20 Fundus photographs in a patient with acute papilledema. Note that swelling of the peripapillary nerve fiber layer causes an obscured view of underlying retinal vessels *(black arrows)*. Splinter hemorrhages, which also suggest true papilledema rather than pseudopapilledema, are seen *(white arrows)*. *(Reprinted with permission from Prasad et al., 2010.)*

Chronic atrophic papilledema, unlike the acute phase, is often characterized by loss of visual acuity with severely constricted visual fields.

Papilledema due to increased ICP can be the consequence of numerous processes. An expanding mass lesion such as a brain tumor, cerebral edema due to stroke, or intracranial hemorrhage will increase ICP, particularly in a younger patient without age-related brain atrophy. Compression of the ventricular system in the posterior fossa is particularly likely to cause papilledema. Venous sinus thrombosis is another common cause, especially in pregnancy and other states of hypercoagulability. Cryptococcal meningitis is the infectious disorder most commonly associated with significant papilledema.

Pseudotumor cerebri, or idiopathic intracranial hypertension, can lead to disc swelling and progressive visual loss (Friedman, 2004). The condition is most common in obese women, but modest weight gain (by 5%-15%) even in non-obese women is a risk factor for disease. Additional risk factors are the use of tetracycline derivatives or vitamin A, and when present, these agents should be discontinued. Weight loss can be imperative in the management of pseudotumor cerebri. In the short term, treatment with acetazolamide can improve symptoms and reduce optic disc swelling. In refractory cases, optic nerve sheath fenestration or cerebrospinal fluid (CSF) shunting may be indicated.

Malignant Hypertension

A marked elevation in blood pressure may produce bilateral optic disc swelling indistinguishable from papilledema (Hayreh, 1977). Peripapillary cotton-wool spots also are a prominent feature in patients with malignant hypertension. Encephalopathic signs are common but not always present. Disc edema tends to develop at a lower blood pressure in patients with renal failure than in those without renal disease.

Diabetic Papillopathy

Diabetic papillopathy is a rare cause of bilateral (or sometimes unilateral) disc swelling in patients with type 1 diabetes (Barbera et al., 1996). This entity is distinct from typical NAION in that there is often bilateral, simultaneous optic nerve involvement. Often visual loss is minimal, with the exception of an enlarged physiological blind spot. Disc edema may be accompanied by marked capillary telangiectasias overlying the disc surface (**Fig. 15.22**). Neuroimaging and lumbar puncture may be necessary to distinguish this condition from papilledema. The pathogenesis is unclear but may relate to a mild impairment of blood flow causing disc swelling without infarction of the optic nerve head (as in the case of premonitory NAION). In many cases, the optic disc edema resolves without residual visual deficit.

Other Causes

Anemia, hyperviscosity syndromes, pickwickian syndrome, hypotension, and severe blood loss are less common causes of bilateral optic disc swelling. The clinical setting generally provides clues to the diagnosis. In addition, any of the entities described under unilateral optic disc edema, particularly the infiltrative disorders, rarely can cause bilateral disc swelling. In children, optic neuritis commonly is bilateral and often is associated with bilateral papillitis (disc swelling). Bilateral ischemic optic neuropathies should prompt immediate evaluation for giant cell (temporal) arteritis in patients older than 55 years. Although most toxic optic neuropathies manifest with normal-appearing optic discs, disc edema is characteristic of methanol poisoning and also may occur in patients with ethambutol toxicity.

Pseudopapilledema

In patients with pseudopapilledema, visible optic disc drusen (hyaline bodies) may be present. Even when disc drusen are not apparent, the distinction between true disc swelling and pseudopapilledema can frequently be made on the basis of fundus examination findings (**Table 15.1**). The most important distinguishing feature is the clarity of the peripapillary

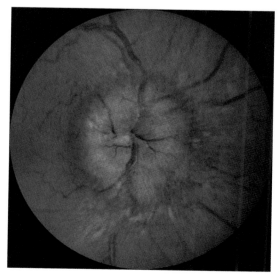

Fig. 15.21 Fundus photograph of the right eye of a patient with chronic papilledema. Note pale, gliotic "champagne-cork" disc appearance, without retinal hemorrhages. *(Reprinted with permission from Prasad et al., 2010.)*

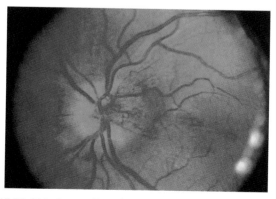

Fig. 15.22 Diabetic papillopathy in a 17-year-old girl. Note the telangiectatic vessels on the disc surface. *(Reprinted with permission from Beck, R.W., Smith, C.H., 1988. Neuro-Ophthalmology: A Problem-Oriented Approach. Little, Brown, Boston.)*

nerve fiber layer. In patients with true disc edema, the nerve fiber layer is hazy, obscuring the underlying retinal vessels, whereas in pseudopapilledema, this layer can remain distinct. In addition, the presence of spontaneous venous pulsations (SVPs) supports the diagnosis of pseudopapilledema, although SVP can be absent in pseudopapilledema as well. Although subretinal hemorrhages may be present in patients with pseudopapilledema (particularly in the setting of optic disc drusen), splinter hemorrhages are characteristic of true papilledema. Finally, fluorescein angiography will show leakage from vessels in papilledema, which is not seen in pseudopapilledema (Davis and Jay, 2003).

Optic Disc Drusen

Optic disc drusen, which constitute a common cause of pseudopapilledema, refer to calcium deposits within the optic nerve head. Although etiology is unclear, drusen may result from axonal degeneration from altered axoplasmic flow, particularly in the setting of a small optic canal (Auw-Haedrich et al., 2002). In children, disc drusen tend to be buried, whereas in adults, they often are visible on the disc surface (**Figs. 15.23 and 15.24**). The progression from buried to surface drusen in individual patients has been well documented. The prevalence of optic disc drusen is approximately 2% within the general population, and they can be bilateral in two-thirds of cases. Optic disc drusen are much more common in caucasian patients than in African Americans and may be genetic, inherited in an autosomal dominant pattern with incomplete penetrance.

Patients with optic disc drusen generally do not complain of visual symptoms, although rarely a patient may experience transitory visual obscurations similar to those described by patients with true papilledema. Although patients may be unaware of a visual field defect, such deficits are common, occurring in approximately 70% of eyes with visible disc drusen and in 35% of those with pseudopapilledema but no visible drusen (Auw-Haedrich et al., 2002). The scotoma probably results from nerve fiber layer thinning and axonal dysfunction caused by the drusen. The visual field defects, therefore, generally follow a nerve fiber bundle distribution, most commonly affecting the inferior nasal visual field. Enlargement of the blind spot and generalized field constriction also may occur. Progression of visual field defects in the setting of drusen is well documented. In addition, visual field loss in the setting of optic disc drusen occurs secondary to hemorrhage, superimposed ischemic optic neuropathy, or an associated retinal degeneration. Visual acuity loss associated with drusen is rare, however, and should prompt an evaluation for alternative causes.

Optic Neuropathies with Normal-Appearing Optic Discs

Many optic neuropathies manifest initially with a completely normal disc appearance; these are classified as retrobulbar optic neuropathies. The disc appearance is normal because the pathological process is posterior to the lamina cribrosa. As with the swollen disc, the differential diagnosis depends on whether optic nerve involvement is unilateral or bilateral.

Table 15.1	**Differentiation of Early Papilledema and Pseudopapilledema**	
Feature	**Papilledema**	**Pseudopapilledema**
Disc color	Hyperemic	Pink, yellowish pink
Disc margins	Indistinct early at superior and inferior poles, later entire margin	Irregularly blurred, may be lumpy
Vessels	Normal distribution, slight fullness; spontaneous venous pulsations absent	Emanate from center, frequent anomalous pattern, ± spontaneous venous pulsations
Nerve fiber layer	Dull as a result of edema, which may obscure blood vessels	No edema; may glisten with circumpapillary halo of feathery light reflections
Hemorrhages	Splinter	Subretinal, retinal, vitreous

Reprinted with permission from Beck, R.W., Smith, C.H., 1988. Neuro-Ophthalmology: A Problem-Oriented Approach. Little, Brown, Boston.

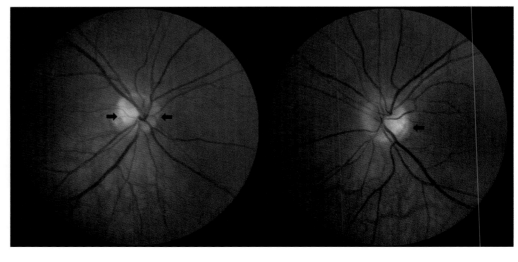

Fig. 15.23 Fundus photographs in a patient with pseudopapilledema. There is a "lumpy-bumpy" disc appearance due to visible disc drusen *(black arrows)*. Note that retinal vessels are not obscured by nerve fiber layer edema. Spontaneous venous pulsations may also indicate pseudopapilledema. *(Reprinted with permission from Prasad et al., 2010.)*

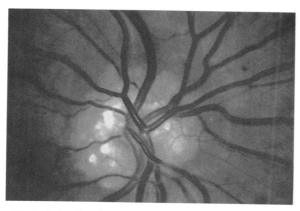

Fig. 15.24 Optic disc drusen in a 50-year-old man. *(Reprinted with permission from Beck, R.W., Smith, C.H., 1988. Neuro-Ophthalmology: A Problem-Oriented Approach. Little, Brown, Boston.)*

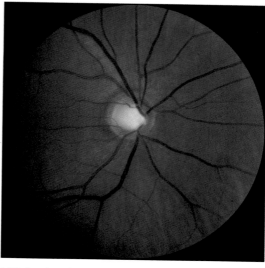

Fig. 15.25 Fundus photograph of the right eye in a patient with glaucoma. The cup-to-disc ratio has increased to approximately 0.7. The intraocular pressure was 29 mm Hg before treatment. *(Reprinted with permission from Prasad et al., 2010.)*

Unilateral Presentations

The most common causes of unilateral retrobulbar optic neuropathy are optic neuritis and compressive lesions. The time course of vision loss usually is helpful in distinguishing between these two entities. No definite way exists to differentiate these disorders on examination, but the detection of a superior temporal field defect in the fellow eye (a junctional scotoma) is highly suggestive of a compressive lesion affecting the anterior optic chiasm and the posterior optic nerve, involving the decussating fibers (termed *Willebrand knee* or *genu*). Posterior (retrobulbar) ischemic optic neuropathy (PION) may occur in patients with giant cell arteritis, other vasculitides, or severe blood loss (Chang and Miller, 2005; Hayreh, 2004). For practical purposes, no retrobulbar correlate to NAION exists.

Bilateral Presentations

Bilateral optic neuropathies in which the optic discs appear normal include nutritional optic neuropathy (including tobacco-alcohol amblyopia), vitamin B$_{12}$ or folate deficiencies, toxic optic neuropathy (from heavy metals), drug-related optic neuropathy (due to chloramphenicol, isoniazid, ethambutol, and others), and inherited optic neuropathies. When these conditions are chronic, optic atrophy may ensue. Other diagnostic considerations in this category include bilateral compressive lesions and bilateral retrobulbar optic neuritis. Finally, posterior indirect traumatic optic neuropathy can result from shearing forces and subsequent edema within the optic canal.

Optic Neuropathies with Optic Atrophy

Any optic neuropathy that produces damage to the optic nerve may result in optic atrophy. Compressive lesions characteristically will cause progressive visual loss and optic atrophy. The presence of gliotic changes suggests that the disc was previously swollen.

Glaucomatous optic neuropathy is easily distinguished from optic neuritis, since it occurs in the setting of elevated intraocular pressure and optic disc cupping (**Fig. 15.25**) (Jonas and Budde, 2000). However, angle closure glaucoma may present with painful acute visual loss, resembling the features of optic neuritis. Distinguishing characteristics include the severity of pain (which can be excruciating) and a red eye with an enlarged, nonreactive pupil. Normal-tension glaucoma is more difficult to recognize but will present with optic disc cupping and progressive field constriction, despite normal intraocular pressures; many of these patients have a fairly benign natural history (Anderson et al., 2001).

Dominantly inherited optic atrophy typically presents with insidious asymmetrical visual loss in childhood (Newman, 2005). These patients often have a striking disc appearance, with pallor and excavation of the temporal portion of the disc (**Fig. 15.26**). The disorder is due to mutations of the OPA1 gene, with autosomal inheritance and variable penetrance. The OPA gene product is believed to target the mitochondria and support membrane stability. Because over 90 different pathogenic OPA1 mutations have been described, a simple DNA test does not exist as it does for LHON.

Optic atrophy also occurs as a consequence of disorders of the retina, optic chiasm, and optic tract. In patients with optic tract lesions, there is often temporal pallor of the ipsilateral disc and so-called bow-tie atrophy, with both nasal and temporal pallor of the contralateral disc. Acquired geniculocalcarine lesions (posterior to the optic tract) do not produce disc pallor, although congenital lesions may lead to optic atrophy through transsynaptic degeneration.

Congenital Optic Disc Anomalies

Congenital optic nerve anomalies (in addition to optic disc drusen, as discussed earlier in this chapter) include a tilted optic disc and optic nerve dysplasia. Visual loss associated with a congenital disc anomaly can range from total blindness to minimal dysfunction.

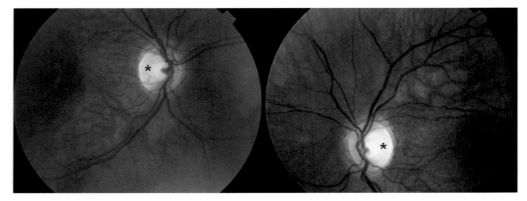

Fig. 15.26 Fundus photographs in a patient with dominant optic atrophy. Note extreme temporal pallor, with excavated appearance *(asterisks)*. *(Reprinted with permission from Prasad et al., 2010.)*

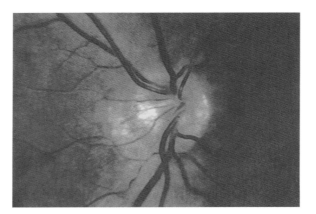

Fig. 15.27 Tilted optic disc. The disc in the fellow eye had a similar appearance.

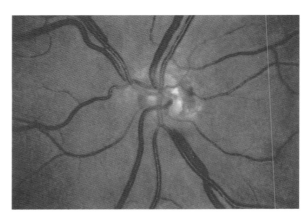

Fig. 15.28 Optic nerve hypoplasia. *(Reprinted with permission from Beck, R.W., Smith, C.H., 1988. Neuro-Ophthalmology: A Problem-Oriented Approach. Little, Brown, Boston.)*

Tilted Optic Disc

A tilted optic disc usually is easily recognizable on fundus examination. The disc may appear foreshortened on one side, and one portion may appear elevated, with the opposite end depressed (**Fig. 15.27**). Often the retinal vessels run in an oblique direction. Tilted optic discs are of neurological importance in that they usually are bilateral and may be associated with temporal field loss, thus mimicking a chiasmal syndrome. However, differentiation from chiasmal disease generally is possible because visual field defects in patients with tilted discs typically do not respect the vertical meridian.

Optic Nerve Dysplasia

Of the several types of optic nerve dysplasia, optic nerve hypoplasia is the most common (Taylor, 2007). In this condition, the optic disc appears small and surrounded by choroid and retinal pigment changes that resemble a double ring (**Fig. 15.28**). The abnormality may be unilateral or bilateral. In most cases, no specific cause is identifiable. The frequency of optic nerve hypoplasia appears to be increased in children of mothers who had diabetes mellitus or ingested antiepileptic drugs, quinine, or lysergic acid diethylamide (LSD) during pregnancy. De Morsier syndrome (septo-optic dysplasia) is characterized by developmental abnormalities of structures

sharing an embryological forebrain derivation, including bilateral optic nerve hypoplasia, absent septum pellucidum, and pituitary gland dysfunction (classic growth hormone deficiency) (Taylor, 2007). Optic nerve aplasia, or complete absence of the optic discs, is extremely rare.

Optic nerve coloboma is more common than optic nerve hypoplasia and results from incomplete closure of the fetal fissure (**Fig. 15.29**). It may occur as an isolated finding or as part of a congenital syndrome including Aicardi syndrome and trisomy 13. Another type of congenital anomaly, the optic pit, is manifested as a small grayish area, usually located in the inferior temporal portion of the optic disc. In some optic nerve dysplasias, the disc appears enlarged. This is true of the so-called morning glory disc in which a large whitish concavity is surrounded by pigmentation that resembles a morning glory flower. This appearance occurs because defective closure of the embryonic fissure is followed by growth of glial tissue and vascular remnants.

Retinal Disorders

Retinal Arterial Disease

Retinal arterial disease can manifest as a central retinal artery occlusion, branch retinal artery occlusion (CRAO/BRAO), or

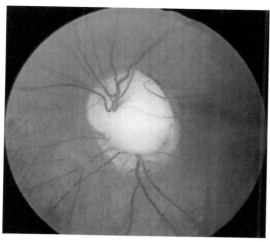

Fig. 15.29 Optic disc coloboma. *(Reprinted with permission from Beck, R.W., Smith, C.H., 1988. Neuro-Ophthalmology: A Problem-Oriented Approach. Little, Brown, Boston.)*

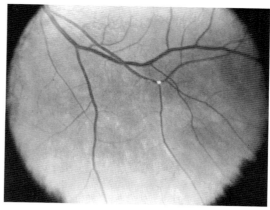

Fig. 15.31 Hollenhorst plaque at a retinal arteriole bifurcation. *(Reprinted with permission from Beck, R.W., Smith, C.H., 1988. Neuro-Ophthalmology: A Problem-Oriented Approach. Little, Brown, Boston.)*

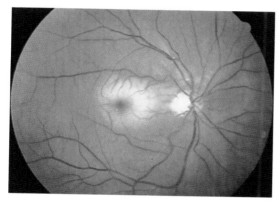

Fig. 15.30 Central retinal artery occlusion. Note the cherry-red spot in the center of the macula, with surrounding whitening of the retina.

amaurosis fugax (transient monocular visual loss). Carotid artery atherosclerotic disease is the most common cause; cardiac valvular disease also must be considered. Evaluation and treatment for retinal arterial disease are similar to those for stroke and cerebrovascular disease in general because the annual risk of stroke or death in patients with visible retinal emboli can be increased 10-fold to 8.5% compared with controls. Acute retinal artery occlusion (CRAO/BRAO) is characterized by retinal whitening (edema) secondary to infarction. In CRAO, these findings usually are more prominent in the posterior pole than they are in the periphery (**Fig. 15.30**). A marked narrowing of the retinal arterioles often is noted. Because the fovea (the center of the macula) receives its blood supply from the choroid and there are no overlying retinal ganglion cells, this area retains its normal reddish-orange color, producing the characteristic cherry-red spot. The retinal edema usually subsides fairly rapidly over days to weeks. After resolution, the retinal appearance typically returns to normal, although the prognosis for visual recovery generally is poor.

When present, retinal emboli most often are located at arteriolar bifurcations (**Fig. 15.31**). Visualization of retinal emboli is more common in BRAO than in CRAO. They take on a glistening or whitish or yellowish appearance and may be located on or near the optic disc or in the retinal periphery. The three major types of retinal emboli are (1) cholesterol (Hollenhorst plaques, most commonly from the carotid artery), (2) platelet-fibrin (most commonly from the cardiac valves), and (3) calcific (from either a carotid or cardiac source). It is difficult to accurately distinguish among these on the basis of fundus examination alone. With impaired blood flow after a CRAO, a portion of a retinal arteriole may take on a whitish appearance. This represents not an embolus, but rather stagnant lipid in the blood or changes in the arteriole wall.

Branch Retinal Artery Occlusions and Encephalopathy (Susac Syndrome)

Branch retinal artery occlusions and encephalopathy (Susac syndrome) is a rare disorder characterized by multiple branch retinal artery occlusions and neurological dysfunction (Gross and Eliashar, 2005; Susac, 2004). Susac syndrome most commonly affects women between the ages of 20 and 40 years. A viral syndrome may precede the development of ocular and neurological signs. The most prominent neurological manifestations are impaired mentation and sensorineural hearing loss. Cerebrospinal fluid in patients with Susac syndrome shows a mild lymphocytic pleocytosis and elevated protein. Antinuclear antibody (ANA) testing and cerebral arteriography are generally normal, but brain MRI most often demonstrates multiple areas of high signal intensity that resemble demyelinating plaques on T2-weighted images.

Ocular Ischemic Syndrome

Generalized ocular ischemia indicates involvement of both retinal and ciliary circulations in the eye. Signs of optic nerve and retinal ischemia may be present, as well as ophthalmoplegia and evidence of anterior segment ischemia (iris atrophy, loss of pupil reactivity, cataract formation, rubeosis iridis). Carotid artery occlusion or dissection and giant cell arteritis are the primary considerations in patients with ocular ischemia.

Retinal Vein Occlusion

Central or branch retinal vein occlusions rarely occur in patients younger than 50 years. The diagnosis is established clinically by the presence of characteristic retinal hemorrhages in the setting of acute vision loss. These occur diffusely in central retinal vein occlusion and focally in branch retinal vein occlusion (**Fig. 15.32**). Disc edema often is present and in some cases is the predominant fundus feature. In ischemic occlusion, treatment with panretinal photocoagulation can improve prognosis. No direct associations between retinal vein occlusion and carotid artery atherosclerotic disease are recognized. Patients require evaluation for vascular risk factors but generally do not require carotid imaging or ultrasound examination. In cases of bilateral retinal vein occlusion, evaluate the patient for hyperviscosity syndromes or hypercoagulable states.

Retinal Degenerations

Among the many diseases of retinal degeneration, several are associated with neurological disease. The cause of retinitis pigmentosa (RP) is degeneration of the retinal rods and cones. Rods are predominantly affected early in the course of RP, impairing night vision. Visual field loss occurs first in the midperiphery and progresses to severe field constriction. Pigmentary retinal changes that look like bony spicules are the hallmark of RP (**Fig. 15.33**). In some cases, however, pigment changes are not prominent, and the visual field loss may be mistaken for a neurological disorder. Even without the characteristic bony spicule–type changes, the diagnosis of RP can be made on the basis of the retinal thinning, narrowing of retinal arterioles, and waxy optic disc pallor. RP may be associated with Kearns-Sayre syndrome, Cockayne syndrome, Refsum syndrome, Batten disease, inherited vitamin E deficiency, and spinocerebellar ataxia type 7.

Retinal photoreceptor degenerations also can occur as a remote effect of cancer (the paraneoplastic retinopathies). These include cancer-associated retinopathy (CAR), which affects primarily rods and manifests with night blindness; cancer-associated cone dysfunction, which manifests as dyschromotopsia; melanoma-associated retinopathy, which has a relatively better prognosis; and others. Visual acuity in these conditions initially can range from normal to significantly impaired, typically with a rapid rate of deterioration. Arteriolar narrowing is a consistent finding, and pigmentary changes in the retina are variable. Electroretinography is markedly abnormal (showing reduced to extinguished rod and cone components), and antiphotoreceptor antibodies often can be identified in the serum. Treatment of the underlying malignancy typically does not improve vision, but immunosuppression with steroids can be effective.

Progressive cone dystrophies are retinal degenerations that commonly demonstrate autosomal dominant inheritance. Typically, vision loss develops in both eyes, beginning in adolescence and worsening over several years. Early in the course of cone dystrophy, the fundus may appear normal; with time, however, pigmentary changes develop in the macula, and electroretinography demonstrates characteristic reductions of the photopic response.

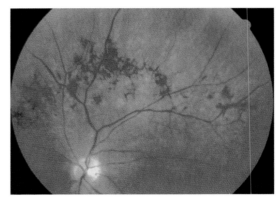

Fig. 15.33 Retinal findings in retinitis pigmentosa. Note prominent bony spicule changes in the retinal midperiphery.

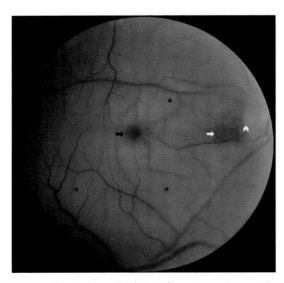

Fig. 15.32 Fundus photograph of the left eye in a patient with central retinal vein occlusion. Note mild disc swelling and hyperemia *(asterisks)*, engorgement of retinal veins *(black arrows)*, and intraretinal dot-and-blot hemorrhages *(white arrows)*. *(Reprinted with permission from Prasad et al., 2010.)*

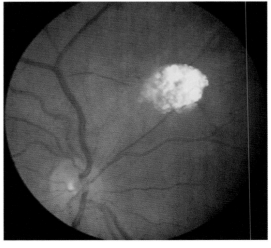

Fig. 15.34 Astrocytic hamartoma in a patient with tuberous sclerosis.

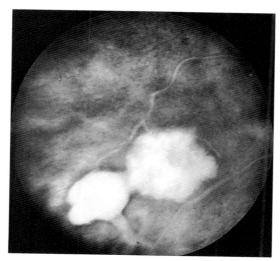

Fig. 15.35 Retinal angioma in a patient with von Hippel-Lindau disease.

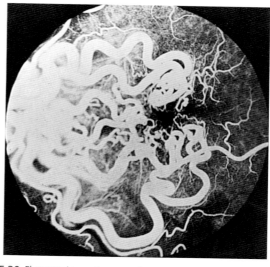

Fig. 15.36 Fluorescein angiogram of a racemose arteriovenous malformation in the retina in a patient with Wyburn-Mason disease.

Phakomatoses

Retinal findings are common in phakomatoses that affect the nervous system, particularly tuberous sclerosis and von Hippel-Lindau disease. Neurological features of phakomatoses are described in Chapter 65. In tuberous sclerosis, retinal astrocytic hamartomas are characteristic (**Fig. 15.34**). These usually are multiple and may appear either as a fullness in the retinal nerve fiber layer or as a nodular refractile lesion (mulberry type). Von Hippel-Lindau disease is characterized by the presence of one or more retinal angiomas that appear as reddish masses with a feeding artery and a draining vein (**Fig. 15.35**). Treatment with photocoagulation or cryotherapy may be necessary. Wyburn-Mason disease is characterized by racemose arteriovenous malformations in the retina (**Fig. 15.36**).

References

The complete reference list is available online at www.expertconsult.com.

Chapter 16

Pupillary and Eyelid Abnormalities

Janet C. Rucker

Pupillary Abnormalities

Pupil Anatomy and Neural Control

The size of the pupil is determined by the balance of action between two muscles embedded in the iris: the sphincter pupillae, primarily under parasympathetic control, and the dilator pupillae, primarily under sympathetic control. The sphincter is located circumferentially around the pupil and constricts the pupil on exposure to light. The dilator is situated radially and dilates the pupil in darkness. The resting tone of the pupil is primarily determined by the degree of baseline parasympathetic innervation. On exposure to light, the pupil constricts as a result of the pupillary light reflex (**Fig. 16.1**). The afferent limb of the light reflex originates in the retinal ganglion cells and travels via the optic nerve, chiasm, and optic tract to the dorsal midbrain pretectum just rostral to the superior colliculus, from which neuronal signals are relayed bilaterally to the paired parasympathetic Edinger-Westphal nuclei of the oculomotor nerve (Akert et al., 1980; Nester et al., 2010; Papageorgiou, Wermund, and Wilhelm, 2009). In primate studies, the pretectal olivary nucleus is identified as the primary relay between retinal ganglion cells and the Edinger-Westphal nuclei (see **Fig. 16.1**) (Kourouyan and Horton, 1997; Pong and Fuchs, 2000; Warwick, 1954). The efferent limb of the light reflex consists of the preganglionic parasympathetic fibers traveling from the Edinger-Westphal nuclei in both oculomotor nerves to the intraorbital ciliary ganglion and the postsynaptic, postganglionic short ciliary nerves carrying the parasympathetic innervation from the ciliary ganglion to the sphincter muscle (see Chapter 70 for a more extensive discussion of oculomotor nucleus and nerve anatomy). The pupillary near reflex consists of pupillary constriction as a response to viewing of a near target. Such miosis is a component of the near triad, along with lens accommodation and ocular convergence. The anatomic substrate of the pupillary near reflex is less well defined than that of the light reflex.

Sympathetic nerves destined for the dilator muscle consist of a chain of three neurons: first-, second-, and third-order neurons (**Fig. 16.2**). First-order neurons originate in the posterolateral hypothalamus and descend in the dorsolateral brainstem and in the intermediolateral cell column of the spinal cord to the thoracic level (T2). After the first-order neurons synapse in the spinal cord, second-order neurons exit to the paravertebral cervical sympathetic chain via the ventral horns. They ascend near the lung apex and then with the common and internal carotid arteries to reach the superior cervical ganglion in the neck at the angle of the jaw, where they synapse with the third-order neurons. At this point, sudomotor fibers related to facial sweating separate anatomically from those fibers serving pupillary dilation. From the superior cervical ganglion, third-order neurons continue their ascent with the carotid artery through the skull base and into the cavernous sinus, where they temporarily travel with the abducens nerve. They then join branches of the trigeminal nerve, with which they enter the orbital apex, bypass the ciliary ganglion, and reach the dilator muscle via long ciliary nerves (see **Fig. 16.2**).

Normal Pupil Phenomena

Hippus, or pupillary unrest, is a nonrhythmical, small-amplitude (<1 mm) variation in pupil size that occurs in healthy eyes after light stimulation and is not triggered by accommodation (Hunter et al., 2000; Thompson et al., 1971). After a light stimulus, the pupil constricts, redilates, and then oscillates. The role (if any) of these oscillations in pupillary or visual function is unclear.

Physiological anisocoria (also termed *central, simple,* or *benign anisocoria;* unequal pupils) occurs in up to 20% of the

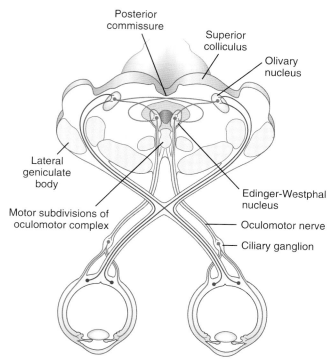

Fig. 16.1 Schematic diagram of the pupillary light reflex in the macaque monkey, showing the afferent limb via the retina, optic nerve, and chiasm; the midbrain connections between the pretectal olivary nuclei and the Edinger-Westphal nuclei; and the efferent limb via the oculomotor nerve and ciliary ganglion. For simplicity, a single neuron in the olivary nucleus is shown projecting to both Edinger-Westphal nuclei, and inputs from both olivary nuclei converge on a single neuron in the Edinger-Westphal nucleus. *(Courtesy J.C. Horton; republished with permission from Kourouyan, H.D., Horton, J.C., 1997. Transneuronal retinal input to the primate Edinger-Westphal nucleus. J Comp Neurol 381, 78.)*

Labels in figure: Posterior commissure; Superior colliculus; Olivary nucleus; Lateral geniculate body; Edinger-Westphal nucleus; Motor subdivisions of oculomotor complex; Oculomotor nerve; Ciliary ganglion

population; the difference is generally less than 0.5 mm, although it may occasionally be up to 1 mm. It should not be accompanied by abnormalities of pupillary light or near responses, nor should it be accompanied by ptosis.

With age, pupils become smaller and less reactive to light. Such pupils generally do not require diagnostic evaluation. Although not a normal condition, diabetes similarly affects the pupils sufficiently often as to make small and poorly reactive pupils "normal" in that clinical setting in the absence of any other pathological pupil state. Both parasympathetic and sympathetic pupillary dysfunction are reported in diabetes, and pupillary abnormalities are correlated with a number of other disease processes, including the presence of cardiovascular autonomic dysfunction, peripheral neuropathy, and retinopathy (Bremner and Smith, 2006; Bremner, 2009).

Afferent Pathological Conditions of the Pupils

The relative afferent pupillary defect (RAPD), or Marcus Gunn pupil, is a hallmark of optic nerve disease. It is a manifestation of a relative unilateral disruption of the afferent limb of the pupillary light reflex via the optic nerve and occurs as a result of the consensual and bilateral nature of the light reflex. When a light stimulus is applied to one eye, both pupils constrict as a result of the bilateral connections between

pretectal nuclei and the Edinger-Westphal nuclei. When the swinging flashlight test is performed to evaluate for RAPD, the light will be transmitted normally via one optic nerve and to a lesser extent by the diseased optic nerve. This results in the appearance of a brisk bilateral pupillary constriction when the light stimulus is applied to the normal eye and a lesser constriction with initial relative dilation when the light stimulus is transferred to the eye with the optic neuropathy, thus the RAPD. The greater the extent of retinal ganglion cell and optic nerve damage, the larger the relative dilation of the pupil will appear (Lagreze and Kardon, 1998). See Chapter 36 for a more detailed description and a table with step-by-step instructions on how to evaluate for an RAPD, and see Chapter 15 for an extensive discussion of optic nerve disease.

Efferent Pathological Conditions of the Pupils
Clinical Presentation and Examination

The medical history of a patient rarely begins with the statement "I noticed that I have unequal pupils." Most patients have anisocoria brought to their attention by a doctor, friend, or relative. Those who notice anisocoria themselves may confuse the diagnostician by giving a misleading account of the duration of the condition. Magnification of old photographs of the patient may prove helpful in this regard. Occasionally a patient has visual dysfunction caused solely by abnormal pupillary size. Photophobia and slow dark adaptation occur when a fixed, dilated pupil fails to protect the retina from increased illumination. Less often, a complaint of poor night vision (or dim daytime vision) may arise in patients with small, poorly reactive pupils; this symptom is caused by pupils not dilating normally, which decreases the light-gathering power of the eye in conditions of dim illumination.

The pupil examination (see Chapter 36 for additional discussion) of a patient being evaluated for a pupillary abnormality should begin with observation of the resting positions of the pupils in the ambient room light and of resting eyelid positions. If anisocoria is present, the degree of anisocoria in the light versus in the dark should be evaluated. Pupil evaluation in the dark is done by having the patient look straight ahead in a dark room while the examiner shines just enough light indirectly from below to allow visualization of the pupils. Assessment in the light versus in the dark will help determine which pupil, if either, is the pathological pupil. Anisocoria that is more pronounced in the light suggests that the large pupil is the abnormal pupil, because the small pupil will constrict normally to the light, enhancing the difference in size between the small pupil and the large, nonconstricting pupil. The differential diagnosis for this includes parasympathetic outflow damage (tonic pupil, oculomotor palsy), iris sphincter injury or ischemia, pharmacological pupil dilation, and excessive sympathetic activation. Anisocoria that is more pronounced in the dark suggests that the small pupil is the pathological pupil, because the large pupil will dilate normally in the dark, enhancing the difference in size between the large pupil and the small, nondilating pupil. A caveat to the suggestion that the small pupil is pathological in this situation is that the anisocoria will generally be slightly enhanced in the dark with physiological anisocoria, a normal situation in which neither pupil is pathological (Lam et al., 1987). The differential

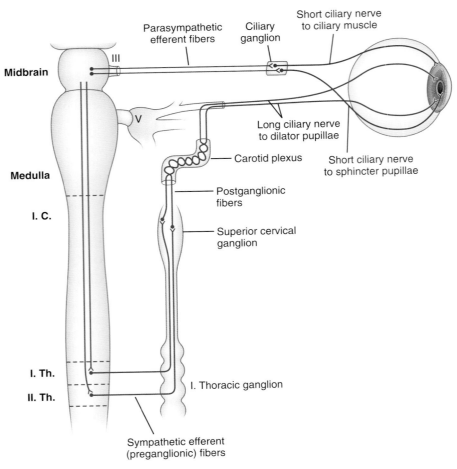

Fig. 16.2 Parasympathetic and sympathetic pathways for innervation of the sphincter pupillae and the dilator pupillae. *I. C.,* First cervical spinal cord segment; *II Th.,* second thoracic segment; *III,* oculomotor nerve; *V,* trigeminal nerve. *(Adapted from Gray, H., 1918. Anatomy of the Human Body, plate 840.)*

diagnosis for a pathologically small pupil includes sympathetic inhibition (Horner syndrome), local iris pathology such as inflammation, and parasympathetic stimulation (e.g., pharmacological stimulation).

The next step in the examination is evaluation of the direct and consensual pupillary light reflexes, followed by evaluation of the pupillary near response (Kasthurirangan and Glasser, 2006). The near response is best assessed by having the patient hold the thumb several inches in front of the eyes while looking across the room and then to have the patient shift and maintain gaze on the thumb. In certain abnormal conditions, the pupils may have light-near dissociation with poor direct light reflexes but relatively preserved constriction to near stimuli. Once the abnormal pupil is identified, pharmacological testing with a number of topical eye drops is often used for confirmation and assistance in localization (**Table 16.1**). The general method is application of a drop of the pharmacological agent into each eye, followed by reexamination of the pupils 30 to 45 minutes later. Sensitivity of accurate response detection is increased with before-and-after photographic documentation. Diagnostic use of topical pharmacological agents and additional helpful examination findings for each of the specific disorders are described in detail in the respective sections of this chapter covering the disorders and outlined in a systematic guideline in **Fig. 16.3**. The presence of a slight degree of ptosis in the eye with the small pupil may indicate sympathetic dysfunction; ptosis in the eye with the larger pupil may indicate oculomotor nerve dysfunction.

Careful examination of vision, ocular motility, facial strength and sensation, and ocular fundus should also be performed.

Anisocoria Greater in the Light
POSTGANGLIONIC PARASYMPATHETIC DYSFUNCTION—TONIC PUPIL

A tonic pupil is large and reacts poorly to light and slowly to near stimuli; after distance refixation, it exhibits a slow, tonic redilation (**Fig. 16.4**). After removal of the near stimulus, such tonic redilation transiently reverses the anisocoria, making the tonic pupil smaller than the normal pupil, because the normal pupil quickly redilates, and the tonic pupil does not (see **Fig. 16.4,** D). In the ophthalmology office, evaluation of a tonic pupil at the slit lamp reveals wormlike segmental constriction of some portions of the pupil and absent constriction of other portions. Because of parasympathetic denervation of the iris sphincter muscle, denervation supersensitivity may occur, and instillation of a dilute solution of the cholinergic agent, pilocarpine, may confirm the diagnosis (**Fig. 16.5**; see also **Table 16.1**). A 0.1% solution is often suggested, but false-positive results may be more frequent than with a 0.0625% solution (Ashker et al., 2008; Leavitt et al., 2002). Dilute pilocarpine will constrict the tonic pupil, but not a normal pupil or a dilated pupil from another cause such as oculomotor palsy or pharmacological toxicity. Solutions of pilocarpine less than 1% are not commercially available and must be prepared by dilution with preservative-free normal saline solution.

Table 16.1 Diagnostic Pupillary Eyedrop Testing

Testing	Mechanism of Action	Diagnostic Utility and Expected Response
ANISOCORIA GREATER IN THE LIGHT (ABNORMAL LARGER PUPIL)		
Dilute pilocarpine (0.0625% or 0.1%)	Parasympathomimetic; direct sphincter stimulation	Tonic pupil will constrict (denervation supersensitivity)
		Normal pupil and pupil affected by oculomotor palsy or pharmacological blockade will not respond
Pilocarpine (1%)	Parasympathomimetic; direct sphincter stimulation	Normal pupil and pupil affected by oculomotor palsy will constrict
		Pupil affected by pharmacological blockade will not respond
ANISOCORIA GREATER IN THE DARK (ABNORMAL SMALLER PUPIL)		
Cocaine (2% to 10%)	Inhibits norepinephrine reuptake at the sympathetic terminus	Horner pupil will not dilate
		Normal pupil will dilate
Hydroxyamphetamine (1%)	Induces third-order sympathetic neuron to release any stored norepinephrine	Preganglionic (first- or second-order neuron) Horner pupil will dilate
		Postganglionic (third-order neuron) Horner pupil will not dilate
Apraclonidine (0.5%)	Weak sympathetic agonist	Horner pupil will dilate (denervation supersensitivity)
		Normal pupil will not change or will constrict slightly

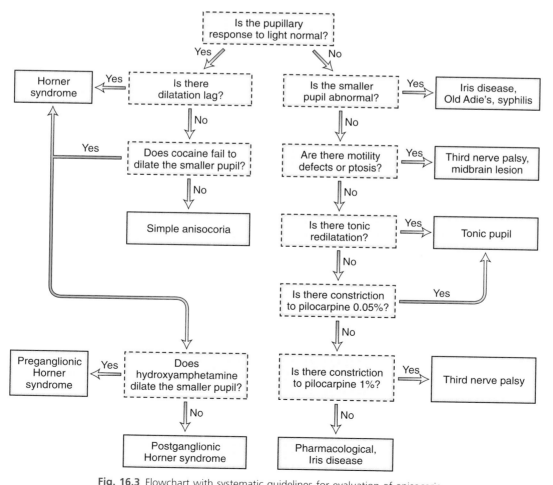

Fig. 16.3 Flowchart with systematic guidelines for evaluation of anisocoria.

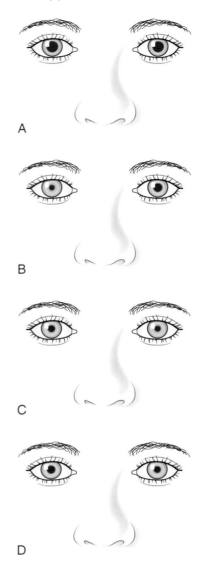

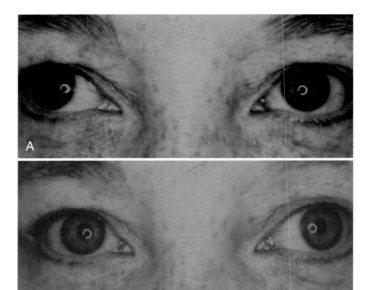

Fig. 16.5 Right tonic pupil. **A,** Anisocoria with larger right pupil prior to dilute pilocarpine administration. **B,** Thirty minutes after dilute pilocarpine, the right pupil is constricted and the left unchanged. Patient also has an unrelated congenital strabismus with an exotropia (outward deviation of the eyes) and full ocular motility without diplopia.

Fig. 16.4 Left tonic pupil. **A,** In darkness, anisocoria is minimal because the normal right pupil is dilated. **B,** In bright light, anisocoria is enhanced because the normal right pupil constricts, and the tonic pupil does not. **C,** A near stimulus results in constriction of the tonic pupil, demonstrating light-near dissociation. **D,** A few seconds after return of gaze to a distant target, the normal right pupil has redilated, and the tonic pupil remains small.

Tonic pupils result from damage to the intraorbital ciliary ganglion or short ciliary nerves from any etiology, including focal infectious (herpes zoster, syphilis) or noninfectious (giant cell arteritis) inflammation, malignant infiltration, paraneoplastic processes, and trauma. Tonic pupils may also be seen as a component of a systemic autonomic neuropathy (see Chapter 77) (Bremner and Smith, 2006; Yamashita et al., 2010), Guillain-Barré syndrome or its Miller Fisher variant, and botulism. Perhaps the most common and most easily recognizable tonic pupil is the benign Holmes-Adie pupil, which often presents with acute painless enlargement of the pupil and may be accompanied by complaints of photophobia and blurred near vision due to involvement of fibers serving the ciliary body for lens accommodation. In 80% of patients, the condition is unilateral. It is most common in healthy young women and is thought to be due to a viral ciliary ganglionitis. Additional examination findings may include decreased deep tendon reflexes and decreased corneal sensation. The affected pupil tends to become smaller over time and may even eventually become smaller than the unaffected pupil. Ross syndrome is the triad of tonic pupils, hyporeflexia, and segmental anhidrosis (Ross, 1958). It is unclear whether this syndrome is a variant of the Holmes-Adie syndrome or a mechanistically distinct disorder, but impaired thermoregulation is the distinguishing element (Nolano et al., 2006; Shin et al., 2000). Harlequin syndrome, failure of facial flushing to thermal or emotional stress, may also occur with tonic pupils and hyporeflexia, although Horner syndrome is more common (Bremner and Smith, 2008).

Preganglionic Parasympathetic Dysfunction—Oculomotor Palsy

Pupillary enlargement from oculomotor palsy may be accompanied by ocular motor deficits due to impairment of the oculomotor-innervated medial, inferior, and superior rectus and inferior oblique muscles, and by ptosis due to involvement of the levator superioris muscle. Isolated pupillary involvement may occur as an early sign of neurovascular compression by a posterior communicating artery aneurysm because the pupillary fibers are located superficially on the superomedial surface of the nerve. It may also be a sign of herniation of the temporal lobe uncus from increased intracranial pressure, known as *Hutchinson pupil* (Ropper, 1990). A fixed and dilated Hutchinson pupil on initial presentation of head trauma, stroke, or intracranial mass lesion is associated with 75% mortality (Clusmann et al., 2001). Although dilute pilocarpine (0.1%) does not typically result in constriction of the pupil in this situation, it should constrict after administration of 1% pilocarpine (see **Table 16.1**). This may help in differentiating isolated pupillary enlargement from an oculomotor palsy from pharmacological pupillary enlargement, because the pharmacological pupil should not constrict. See Chapter 70 for a complete discussion of oculomotor nerve anatomy and clinical lesions; Fig. 70.2 shows an example of oculomotor palsy.

Iris Sphincter Injury and Ischemia

Blunt trauma to the eye can damage the iris sphincter, causing mydriasis (pupillary enlargement) with poor pupillary constriction to both light and near stimuli. Tears at the pupillary margin may be evident. Immediately after injury, the pupil may be smaller than normal (spastic miosis), but after a few minutes, it becomes dilated and poorly reactive. This course of events may simulate uncal herniation. Iris ischemia may also cause mydriasis and poor pupillary reactivity. This may occur with acute angle closure glaucoma and ocular ischemic syndrome. Both situations are generally accompanied by poor vision and pain. Additional signs of acute glaucoma include corneal edema and ocular injection. The ocular ischemic syndrome arises in patients with marked stenosis of an internal carotid artery or narrowing of both internal and external carotid arteries on one side. Associated eye findings include neovascularization of the retina or iris (rubeosis iridis), iritis, ocular hypotony, and corneal edema. Some rare forms of iris degeneration, such as iris atrophy and Fuchs heterochromic iridocyclitis, cause pupillary dilation, often with irregularity of the pupillary outline. Eyes with local iris disease may not constrict to 1% pilocarpine, depending on the severity of pupillary sphincter involvement.

Pharmacological Mydriasis

Pharmacological mydriasis usually occurs after accidental or intentional instillation of anticholinergic agents such as atropine. Accidental mydriasis usually occurs by hand-to-eye contact in individuals who have contact with dilating agents; examples include use of a scopolamine skin patch for motion sickness, administration of eye drops to a family member with eye disease, or exposure to plants with parasympathetic blocking activity such as angel's trumpet (Havelius and Asman, 2002). Inadvertent administration of nebulized ipratropium into the eye via an ill-fitting face mask in a critically ill patient may result in unilateral mydriasis that mimics a Hutchinson pupil from intracranial hypertension and uncal herniation (Eustace et al., 2004). Pharmacologically dilated pupils tend to be larger than the dilated pupil of third cranial nerve palsy. Sympathomimetic agents, such as phenylephrine, cause mydriasis that is less extensive and prolonged than that caused by anticholinergic agents. Pharmacologically dilated pupils do not constrict after administration of 1% pilocarpine (see **Table 16.1**).

Anisocoria Greater in the Dark

HORNER SYNDROME

The classic Horner syndrome triad of sympathetic dysfunction consists of ipsilateral ptosis, miosis, and facial anhidrosis. The lesion may be anywhere along the three-neuron

sympathetic pathway (described in Pupillary Anatomy and Neural Control). Anhidrosis is only present with lesions of the first- or second-order (preganglionic) neurons because the fibers serving facial sweating take a pathway distinct from those destined for the pupillary dilator muscle after synapsing in the superior cervical ganglion. The ptosis results from impaired innervation of the Müller muscle, which contributes only slightly to maintenance of eyelid opening. As a result, the maximum ptosis possible from sympathetic dysfunction is only 1 to 2 mm. Apparent enophthalmos (an illusion of a smaller, "sunken" eye) due to palpebral fissure narrowing from involvement of the Müller muscle in combination with subtle elevation of the lower lid ("reverse" or "upside down" ptosis) from involvement of lower lid smooth muscle may occur. An additional finding on examination is dilation lag, the delayed dilation of the Horner pupil in darkness (Pilley and Thompson, 1975) (**Fig. 16.6**).

The differential diagnosis for Horner syndrome varies for a preganglionic lesion (first- or second-order neurons) versus a postganglionic (third-order neuron) lesion, and differentiation between the two will dictate the diagnostic approach. Determination of preganglionic versus postganglionic lesion can be made with pupillary diagnostic eye drops (Mughal and Longmuir, 2009). Hydroxyamphetamine (1%) is the drop most commonly used for this purpose. However, some diagnosticians prefer to utilize cocaine (2% to 10%) eye drops to confirm the presence of Horner syndrome rather than proceeding directly to hydroxyamphetamine to determine a preganglionic versus postganglionic lesion. Administration of both cocaine and hydroxyamphetamine cannot be done on the same day; at least 48 hours must separate the two diagnostic eye drop tests. From a practical standpoint, both medications are difficult to obtain. Cocaine is a controlled substance, must be kept under lock and key, and results in a positive urine toxicology screen for 2 days after ocular administration (Jacobson et al., 2001). Hydroxyamphetamine eye drops are no longer

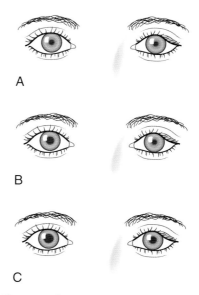

Fig. 16.6 Left Horner syndrome. **A,** Mild upper lid ptosis and miosis in room light. **B,** Anisocoria is increased at 5 seconds after lights are dimmed, owing to dilation lag of left pupil. **C,** Fifteen seconds after lights are dimmed, left pupil exhibits increased dilation compared to the image in **B.**

marketed in the United States but are usually obtainable from compounding pharmacies such as Leiter's Park Avenue Pharmacy, 1756 Park Avenue, San Jose, CA 95126 (www.leiterrx.com; phone 800-292-6773). Cocaine inhibits the reuptake of norepinephrine at the sympathetic terminus, thereby causing accumulation of norepinephrine that is continuously released from sympathetic nerve terminals (Kardon et al., 1990). The result is dilation of a normal pupil but impaired dilation in the sympathetically denervated pupil, with a resultant increase in anisocoria. Lack of dilation after cocaine administration occurs for both preganglionic and postganglionic Horner syndrome. Hydroxyamphetamine induces the third-order neuron to release any stored norepinephrine. It will dilate a normal pupil and a pupil with an intact third-order sympathetic neuron. Therefore, if pupillary dilation occurs in a Horner pupil, the lesion is localized to the preganglionic first- or second-order neurons. If pupillary dilation fails to occur, a third-order neuron Horner syndrome is likely (**Fig. 16.7,** *A-B*).

Apraclonidine, in a 0.5% solution, is a recent addition to the diagnostic armamentarium for Horner syndrome (Koc et al., 2005; Morales et al., 2000). It is an α-adrenergic agonist approved for lowering intraocular pressure during certain ophthalmologic surgical procedures. After bilateral administration of apraclonidine in a patient with Horner syndrome, there is reversal of the anisocoria caused by dilation of the Horner pupil and either constriction or no change in the normal pupil (**Fig. 16.8**). This occurs because apraclonidine is a weak α-1 agonist with no direct dilating activity in the normal pupil; the Horner pupil is dilated due to denervation supersensitivity. In addition to pupil dilation, the Horner-induced ptosis is resolved; however, this alone cannot be used to confirm diagnosis, because elevation of the eyelid may also be seen in normal eyes. Apraclonidine as a replacement for cocaine in the diagnosis of Horner syndrome is promising, but rigorous study is needed; it is unclear whether all interruptions of sympathetic outflow will result in denervation sensitivity and how much time is necessary for this to occur (Kardon, 2005). Positive apraclonidine testing is reported within 36 hours of lesion onset; however, false-negative testing is also reported up to 16 days after carotid dissection (Dewan et al., 2009; Lebas et al., 2010).

Any inflammatory, compressive, neoplastic, traumatic, or other lesion along the course of the three-neuron sympathetic pathway may cause Horner syndrome. Two lesions in particular deserve detailed description, owing to their clinical importance and potential ominous prognosis if left undetected. These are carotid dissection, with presentation as an isolated Horner syndrome, and the Pancoast tumor. Acute onset of a painful Horner syndrome leads to suspicion of a carotid

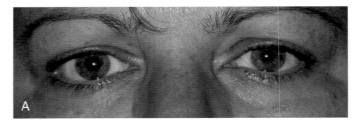
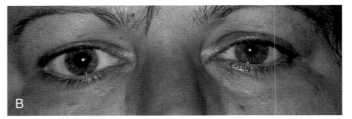
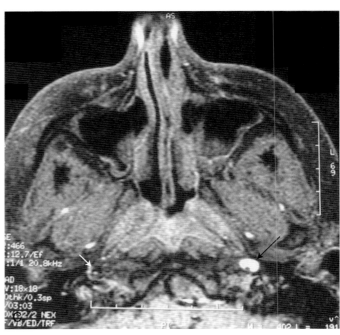

Fig. 16.7 Acute-onset, painful, left postganglionic third-order neuron Horner syndrome secondary to a left carotid dissection. **A,** Left miosis and slight ptosis. **B,** Failure of left pupil to dilate 30 minutes after 1% hydroxyamphetamine instillation, confirming the postganglionic location of the lesion. **C,** T1-weighted axial magnetic resonance image without gadolinium through the skull base, showing a left carotid dissection with a crescent of hyperintense blood in the wall of the artery, causing narrowing of the artery lumen (*black arrow*). The normal flow void of the right carotid artery is seen at the tip of the short white arrow.

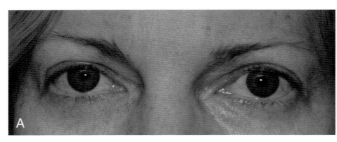
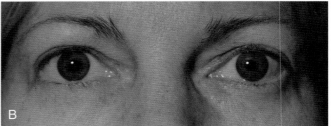

Fig. 16.8 A, Right Horner syndrome with mild right ptosis and anisocoria with a small right pupil. **B,** Forty minutes after administration of apraclonidine. Note reversal of anisocoria secondary to dilation of the Horner pupil and resolution of ptosis.

dissection until proven otherwise. Such presentation requires a very high degree of suspicion because it is often the intracranial precavernous portion of the carotid artery that is affected. It is not uncommon for this lesion to be missed on magnetic resonance angiography (MRA) and detected only by careful examination of non–contrast-enhanced axial T1-weighted magnetic resonance images (MRIs) through the base of the skull, looking for a crescent of hyperintense signal surrounding the carotid artery flow void (see **Fig. 16.7**, *C*). Treatment most typically consists of anticoagulation with heparin, followed by warfarin for 3 to 6 months, to minimize the risk of emboli from the dissected artery. A preganglionic Horner syndrome, particularly in a patient with a history of tobacco use, should prompt a search for a pulmonary apical neoplasm, or Pancoast tumor. Outside of these two clinical settings, the workup for Horner syndrome consists of neuroimaging of the affected sympathetic pathways: brain and spine (the entire cervical and first two thoracic segments) MRI with gadolinium for a preganglionic lesion, and brain MRI with gadolinium and MRA for a postganglionic lesion (Almog et al., 2010; Digre et al., 1992). In children, the majority of Horner syndromes are congenital; however, birth trauma, vascular malformations, carotid dissection, and neoplasm are also possible causes. The recommended evaluation in children includes neuroimaging and urinary catecholamine testing to screen for neuroblastoma (Smith et al., 2010).

Iritis (Iris Inflammation)

Acute inflammatory disease of the iris (iritis) may cause pupillary constriction. If inflammation persists, adhesions between the iris and the lens (posterior synechiae) may lead to pupillary irregularity and immobility. Usually the inflamed eye is red and the patient has photophobia. However, some chronic forms of iritis, such as sarcoid, can cause iris adhesions without these manifestations. Syphilis most commonly causes Argyll-Robertson pupils but may cause focal iris inflammation and degeneration. Infiltration of the iris by tumor or amyloid can also cause irregular pupils.

Episodic Anisocoria

Anisocoria may be intermittent. Physiological anisocoria can vary from week to week and occasionally from hour to hour. A rare condition known as *tadpole pupil* results from intermittent spasms of segments of the pupillary dilator muscle; often these patients have an underlying Horner syndrome (Thompson et al., 1983). A related phenomenon is oculosympathetic spasm associated with lesions of the cervical spinal cord.

Benign episodic unilateral mydriasis is a diagnosis of exclusion in which episodes of pupillary dilation last from minutes to a few days (Jacobson, 1995). Some patients have typical migraine headaches or a trigeminal autonomic cephalgia, but many patients have isolated monocular visual blurring or no symptoms at all (Antonaci et al., 2010). The frequency of episodes varies from a few per week to one every few years. Some patients appear to have parasympathetic insufficiency; others, sympathetic hyperactivity of the pupil, but no other neurological problems develop. Cyclical oculomotor palsy is a rare condition in which periodic oculomotor spasms occur in a patient with third cranial nerve palsy. During the spasms, the eyelid rises, the exotropic eye moves to the midline, and

the pupil constricts. In some cases, the spasms are limited to the pupil. Intermittent spasm of portions of the pupillary sphincter may occur in traumatic third cranial nerve paralysis and with aberrant oculomotor regeneration. Unilateral pupillary dilation and other pupillary signs can also occur during seizures, and rhythmic pupillary oscillation is reported in Creutzfeld-Jakob disease (Nagasaka et al., 2010).

Pupillary Light-Near Dissociation

The term *light-near dissociation* refers to pupils that have marked diminution of constriction to light, with a much better constriction to near stimuli. The differential diagnosis includes tonic pupils, Argyll-Robertson pupils, and the dorsal midbrain syndrome (Han et al., 2010). Tonic pupils were described earlier (Anisocoria Greater in the Light). Argyll-Robertson pupils are small and irregular. This condition is historically most commonly seen in the setting of syphilis, but currently diabetes is likely the most common etiology, although the pupils are not miotic. Localization of the lesion causing such pupils is unclear, but possibilities include the ciliary ganglion and the dorsal midbrain (Thompson and Kardon, 2006). The dorsal midbrain syndrome, or Parinaud syndrome (see Chapter 19) consists of impaired upgaze, convergence-retraction nystagmus, and lid retraction (Collier sign), in addition to pupillary light-near dissociation. It is generally due to pineal gland lesions or hydrocephalus. Light-near dissociation in this centrally mediated mechanism may be due to destruction of the dorsally located olivary pretectal nuclei involved in the pupillary light reflex (see Pupillary Anatomy and Neural Control), with relative sparing of the fibers serving the pupillary near response, which seem to approach the pupillomotor center from a more ventral pathway.

Eyelid Abnormalities
Eyelid Anatomy and Neural Control

The width of the palpebral fissure is determined by the activity balance of the orbicularis oculi muscles, the levator palpebrae superioris muscles, smooth muscle called *Müller muscle*, and periorbital and eyelid connective tissues. The orbicularis oculi is innervated by the facial nerve, the levator palpebrae superioris by the oculomotor nerve, and Müller muscle by the sympathetic nervous system. Activation of the orbicularis oculi results in eye closure. The levator palpebrae and, to a lesser extent, Müller muscle are responsible for maintaining eye opening. See Chapter 70 for a complete discussion of the anatomy of the facial and oculomotor nerves.

Pathological Conditions of the Eyelids
Clinical Presentation and Examination

Patients with abnormal eyelids may present complaining of a change in the physical appearance of one or both eyelids, or they may complain of symptoms related to impaired eyelid function such as dry or burning eyes, often a result of excessive eyelid opening or incomplete eyelid closure. In contrast, patients may be unaware of a problem but have had an asymmetrical eye appearance brought to their attention by an acquaintance or family member. Patients will often indicate that they have a "droopy eye" even if the eye with the smaller palpebral fissure is the normal eye and the widened eye is the pathological side. It is up to the examiner to determine which eye has an abnormal lid position. Familiarity with the resting position of the eyelids is essential to determine whether a pathological state exists.

Steps in the examination of the eyelids are summarized in **Box 16.1**. The normal palpebral fissure is between 12 and 15 mm. At rest, the upper eyelid normally covers the upper 1 to 2 mm of the iris, and the upper border of the lower eyelid just touches the lower border of the iris (**Fig. 16.9**). In an eye with mild upper lid retraction, the lid just touches the upper limit of the iris, or a small amount of sclera is visible between the iris and the upper lid margin (superior scleral show) (**Fig. 16.10**). With lower lid retraction, sclera is visible between the iris and the lower lid margin (inferior scleral show). Patients with factitious (voluntary) ptosis display contraction of the orbicularis oculi with wrinkling of the skin near the lid margin and a lowered eyebrow. An example of true upper lid ptosis is seen in **Fig. 16.10**. In an effort to elevate the lids, patients with bilateral ptosis often have associated frontalis contraction with eyebrow elevation. Proptosis (exophthalmos, or eye protrusion) can be evaluated by inspecting the globe position with respect to the orbital rim by looking tangentially across the orbital margin from above, below, or laterally.

Assessment of lid position in different gaze positions may reveal lid retraction on downgaze, which suggests lid lag from orbital disease such as thyroid ophthalmopathy or aberrant regeneration of the oculomotor nerve. The latter condition may also cause lid retraction on adduction (see **Fig. 70.2**, *A-B*). There are many potential lid abnormalities with neuromuscular junction disease such as myasthenia gravis, including increased ptosis or induction of ptosis with prolonged upgaze, Cogan sign, enhanced ptosis, and the peek sign. Cogan sign is induced by rapid return of the eyes to central position after sustained downgaze; the upper eyelid may elevate excessively, twitch, and then return to its ptotic position. Enhanced ptosis is increased ptosis in a less or nonptotic eyelid on manual elevation of the more ptotic lid. The peek sign is positive when prolonged eye closure increases orbicularis oculi weakness and causes lid separation and globe exposure despite initial complete eye closure. Incomplete gentle eye closure may also suggest facial weakness from causes other than myasthenia gravis, including facial nerve palsy or a myopathic process such as chronic progressive external ophthalmoplegia (CPEO). More subtle weakness of the orbicularis oculi muscles may be detected with forced eye closure (**Fig. 16.11**). Forced lid closure with rapid reopening is an excellent technique for evaluating hemifacial spasm, apraxia of lid opening, and blepharospasm—conditions that are often worsened by this maneuver. Patients with apraxia of lid opening contract their forehead and elevate their brows when asked to open their eyes, but the eyes remain closed. Patients with blepharospasm have persistent orbicularis oculi contraction after being asked to open their eyes.

The final step in evaluation is to look for abnormalities of the pupil and ocular motility and to perform a full neurological examination. Ophthalmological consultation may be helpful from a diagnostic standpoint if the etiology of the lid

---

Box 16.1 Clinical Examination of the Eyelids

Observe for at least 1 minute, looking for the following:
  Palpebral fissure asymmetry
  The resting position of each upper and lower eyelid relative to the iris edge
  Upper or lower lid retraction and scleral show
  Ptosis
  Proptosis (eye protrusion) or enophthalmos (inward or "sunken" eye)
  Eyelid edema or scarring
  Blink rate (normal is roughly 18 times per minute)
Assess lid position in different gaze directions
If ptosis is present, assess for worsening with prolonged upgaze
Observe gentle and forced lid closure
Examine for pupillary abnormalities, ocular motor abnormalities, and facial weakness

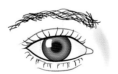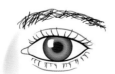

Fig. 16.9 Normal eyelid position. Upper lid covers the upper 1 to 2 mm of the iris. Lower lid just touches the lower edge of the iris.

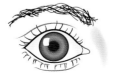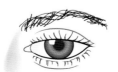

Fig. 16.10 Mild lid retraction with superior scleral show in right eye and ptosis in left eye.

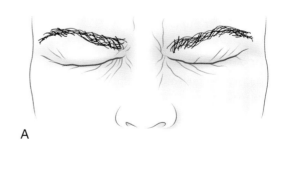

A

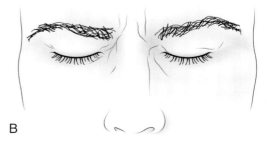

B

Fig. 16.11 Forced eyelid closure. **A,** Normal forced eyelid closure. **B,** Weak eyelid closure. Lashes remain visible.

abnormality is not readily apparent; it will also help ensure the corneal health of patients with lid abnormalities. After completion of these examination steps (outlined in **Table 16.2**), it should be possible to determine whether the abnormal palpebral fissure is the one that is too wide or the one that is too narrow, and to determine whether the dynamics of eyelid opening and closure are normal.

Pathologically Widened Palpebral Fissures

When the abnormal palpebral fissure is too wide, the differential diagnosis includes lid retraction from orbital disease (e.g., thyroid eye disease) or facial nerve dysfunction with resultant orbicularis oculi weakness (Bartley, 1996). Less common, but also to be considered in the differential diagnosis, are the stare and decreased blinking associated with parkinsonism; Summerskill sign, lid retraction associated with end-stage hepatic disease (Meadows et al., 2001); and Collier sign, or midbrain-induced lid retraction seen as a component of the dorsal midbrain syndrome. These conditions may result in exposure keratitis, causing the patient to complain of eye pain and blurred vision.

Patients with thyroid eye disease may be clinically and serologically hyperthyroid, hypothyroid, or euthyroid. In addition to the lid lag (higher-than-normal lid position in downgaze), thyroid eye disease is often accompanied by periorbital edema, conjunctival injection and chemosis, proptosis, eyelid retraction, lagophthalmos (inability to close the eye completely), and von Graefe sign (dynamic slowing of lid descent during eye movement from upgaze into downgaze). Diagnosis is confirmed by demonstration of enlarged extraocular muscles on orbital computed tomography or MRI and by the presence of thyroid-stimulating antibodies.

Lower lid retraction deserves special mention, because it may suggest a different differential when found in the absence of upper lid retraction. It may be congenital or mechanical due to lower lid laxity, but most often it is a sign of proptosis. As with upper lid retraction, thyroid eye disease is likely the most common cause, but it may appear to be spuriously retracted in three situations: (1) when the contralateral lower lid is elevated (as in Horner syndrome), (2) when the globe is elevated in conditions that cause hypertropia (e.g., fourth cranial nerve palsy), and (3) when the lower lid is weak from myasthenia gravis or facial nerve palsy.

Pathologically Narrowed Palpebral Fissures

When the abnormal palpebral fissure is too narrow, the differential diagnosis includes pseudoptosis and true ptosis (Figueiredo, 2010). Pseudoptosis may result from dermatochalasis (redundancy of eyelid skin) or contralateral lid retraction. True ptosis may be congenital or acquired via mechanical, myopathic, or neurogenic factors. Congenital ptosis can be caused by abnormalities of the levator muscle or its innervation and can be unilateral or bilateral. Additional congenital anomalies resulting in ptosis include trigeminal-levator synkinesis (Marcus Gunn jaw-wink phenomenon), in which unilateral ptosis occurs with jaw movements; Duane syndrome with paresis of abduction, adduction, (or both), associated with ptosis and globe retraction on attempted adduction; congenital oculomotor palsies; and congenital Horner syndrome (Demirci et al., 2010).

Acquired mechanical causes of ptosis include dehiscence of the levator aponeurosis secondary to aging (involutional blepharoptosis, or senile ptosis) or trauma and inflammation or infiltration of the lid with amyloid or malignancy (Klapper et al., 1998). Dehiscence of the levator aponeurosis is likely the most common cause of ptosis in the elderly and is accompanied by an elevated superior eyelid crease. Such ptosis typically worsens with downgaze (Olson and Putterman, 1995). The most common myopathic cause of ptosis is CPEO, which is most frequently a manifestation of a mitochondrial myopathy (see Chapter 63). CPEO may occur in isolation or as a component of a wider mitochondrial defect such as Kearns-Sayre syndrome, with pigmentary retinopathy and cardiac conduction defects. Oculopharyngeal muscular dystrophy and myotonic dystrophy are additional myopathic causes of ptosis. Myasthenia gravis is a frequent cause of acquired ptosis—either in isolation or accompanied by ocular motor defects or generalized weakness. Diagnosis is most reliably confirmed with acetylcholine receptor antibodies, a decremental response with electromyographic repetitive stimulation, or single-fiber electromyography. Neurogenic etiologies include Horner syndrome, oculomotor paresis, and occasionally, disease of the cerebral hemispheres (cerebral ptosis)—particularly right hemispheric lesions (Averbuch-Heller et al., 2002; Manconi et al., 2006) (**Table 16.2**). Rightward gaze deviation and upgaze paresis often accompany cerebral ptosis. Horner syndrome and oculomotor paresis are described in detail earlier in this chapter. Lower lid elevation may accompany upper lid ptosis in Horner syndrome and may occur secondary to enophthalmos (e.g., from orbital blowout fractures), local lid edema, excessive lid closure, or factitious ptosis.

Dynamic Eyelid Abnormalities

Dynamic lid abnormalities include blepharospasm, apraxia of lid opening, hemifacial spasm, myokymia, and myotonia.

Table 16.2 Lid Abnormalities Associated with Cerebral Hemisphere Lesions

Lid Abnormality	Pathological Findings
Unilateral ptosis	Contralateral hemisphere lesions; contralateral and ipsilateral hemisphere lesions
Bilateral ptosis	Bilateral frontal lobe lesions; unilateral and bilateral hemisphere lesions
Impairment of voluntary lid opening and closure	Dominant hemisphere or bilateral hemisphere lesions or basal ganglia disease
Impairment of voluntary and reflex lid opening (apraxia of lid opening)	Basal ganglia disease; bilateral hemisphere lesions; nondominant cerebral lesion
Difficulty maintaining lid closure (motor impersistence)	Nondominant hemisphere or bilateral hemisphere lesions
Difficulty maintaining lid opening (reflex blepharospasm)	Nondominant hemisphere or bilateral hemisphere lesions

Modified with permission from Nutt, J.G., 1977. Lid abnormalities secondary to cerebral hemisphere lesions. Ann Neurol 1, 149-151; and from Johnston, J.C., Rosenbaum, D.M., Picone, C.M., et al., 1989. Apraxia of eyelid opening secondary to right hemisphere infarction. Ann Neurol 25, 622-624.

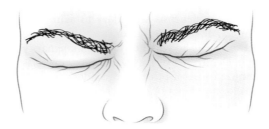

Fig. 16.12 Blepharospasm, involuntary forced eye closure.

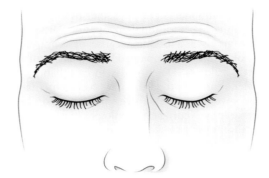

Fig. 16.13 Apraxia of lid opening. Elevated eyebrows and forehead contraction with persistent eye closure.

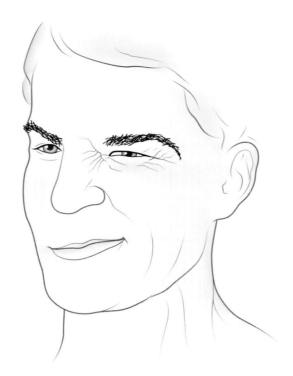

Fig. 16.14 Hemifacial spasm. Synchronous contraction of muscles innervated by the left facial nerve.

Blepharospasm consists of uncontrolled bilateral orbicularis oculi contraction causing eyelid closure (**Fig. 16.12**) (Etgen et al., 2006; Hallett, 2002). Secondary blepharospasm may occur as a result of photophobia from ocular disease such as dry eyes, corneal disease (abrasion, keratitis), and ocular inflammation. When the condition is bilateral with no associated ocular or neurological abnormalities, the diagnosis is benign essential blepharospasm, which is a focal dystonia. When there are dystonic movements of the lower face, jaw, tongue, or neck, the designation is oromandibular dystonia with blepharospasm (Meige syndrome), a segmental dystonia. When orbicularis contraction occurs only with lid manipulation or other stimulation, the term *reflex blepharospasm* is sometimes used. Most patients with parkinsonism have reflex blepharospasm, and all types of blepharospasm are made worse by lid manipulation and photophobia. Factitious (voluntary) blepharospasm is rare. The term *apraxia of lid opening* describes inappropriate inhibition of the levator palpebrae muscle that occurs in some patients with bilateral or nondominant cerebral lesions or in association with benign essential blepharospasm (**Fig. 16.13**) (Dewey and Marion, 1994; Krack et al., 1994).

Hemifacial spasm is characterized by paroxysmal, involuntary, synchronous contraction of all muscles innervated by the facial nerve on one side (**Fig. 16.14**) (see Chapter 70). Involuntary twitches of portions of the orbicularis oculi muscle (orbicularis myokymia) are common in normal individuals; these generally affect the lower eyelid. In facial myokymia, these muscular contractions involve other facial muscles. Occasionally, facial myokymia is associated with spastic paretic hemifacial contracture, a condition characterized by tonic contraction of facial muscles on one side with associated weakness of the same muscles. Facial myokymia may be unilateral or bilateral. This sign indicates brainstem disease; the most common causes are multiple sclerosis and brainstem neoplasm (usually gliomas), but Guillain-Barré syndrome and extraaxial neoplasms may be causal. Myotonia of lid closure may occur in myotonic dystrophy, hypothyroidism, and hyperkalemic (and more rarely, hypokalemic) familial periodic paralysis.

References

The complete reference list is available online at www.expertconsult.com.

Disturbances of Smell and Taste

Richard L. Doty

The senses of smell and taste play important roles in human safety, nutrition, and quality of life. In a study of 750 consecutive patients presenting to our center with chemosensory complaints, 68% reported altered quality of life, 46% reported changes in appetite or body weight, and 56% described adverse influences on daily living or psychological well-being (Deems et al., 1991a). In another study of 445 such patients, at least one hazardous event, such as food poisoning or failure to detect fire or leaking natural gas, was reported by 45.2% of those with anosmia, 34.1% of those with severe hyposmia, 32.8% of those with moderate hyposmia, 24.2% of those with mild hyposmia, and 19.0% of those with normal olfactory function (Santos et al., 2004). In a longitudinal study of 1162 older persons without dementia, mortality risk was 36% higher in those with low compared to high scores on a 12-item odor identification test after adjusting for such variables as sex, age, and education (Wilson et al., 2010). Of particular importance to the neurologist is the fact that chemosensory function can provide unique insight into neurological health. Thus, olfactory disturbances are among the early preclinical or presymptomatic signs of Alzheimer disease (AD) and sporadic Parkinson disease (PD) (Ross et al., 2008). Indeed, recent research suggests that a standardized odor identification test is as effective in detecting PD as a single-photon emission computed tomography (SPECT) scan employing [123I]ioflupane (DaTSCAN) (Deeb et al., 2010)

It is critical for the physician to realize that most complaints of decreased "taste" function reflect decreased olfactory function (Deems et al., 1991a). Flavor sensations such as cola, coffee, chocolate, strawberry, pizza, licorice, steak sauce, and vanilla depend upon stimulation of the olfactory receptors by molecules that enter the nasal pharynx during deglutition, a process called *retronasal olfaction*. Such "taste" sensations disappear when the olfactory epithelium is severely damaged, leaving intact only sensations from free nerve endings of the trigeminal nerve (CN V) and such taste bud–mediated sensations as sweet, sour, salty, bitter, and metallic. The ability to taste is much more resilient to pathological or trauma-related alterations than the ability to smell, largely reflecting the redundant innervation of the taste buds from multiple cranial nerves (i.e., CN VII, IX, X) (Deems et al., 1991a).

In this chapter, the anatomy and physiology of the olfactory and gustatory systems are reviewed, with an emphasis on pathophysiology. Chemosensory disturbances in diseases commonly encountered by the neurologist are described, along with means for patient assessment and symptom management.

Anatomy and Physiology

Olfaction

The olfactory receptor cells, which number around 6 million in the human, are located within a pseudostratified columnar neuroepithelium that also contains sustentacular or supporting cells, basal cells (the precursors of other cell types within the epithelium), and the poorly understood microvillar cells. This epithelium lines the cribriform plate and sectors of the superior septum, the middle turbinate, and the superior turbinate and is supported by a highly vascularized lamina propria that contains Bowman glands, the major source of the overlying mucus and enzymes that detoxify xenobiotic agents. It is into this mucus that each of the bipolar receptor cells projects 3 to 30 receptor-bearing cilia that interact with odorant molecules. These cells are unique, since they serve as both a receptor cell and a first-order neuron and can regenerate to some degree from basal cells after being damaged. Moreover, they exhibit the most diverse molecular phenotype of any neuron, expressing a wide range of receptor protein types and cell-surface antigens. A photomicrograph of the surface of the olfactory epithelium is shown in **Fig. 17.1**.

In the human, each receptor cell expresses only one of about 380 functional types of receptor proteins. Although roughly 950 genes express such receptor proteins, most of these genes are pseudogenes. Odor receptor genes are found in approximately 100 locations on all chromosomes except 20 and Y. Remarkably, the olfactory subgenome spans 1% to 2% of the total genomic DNA. Most single-chemical odorants stimulate more than one type of receptor, and overlap typically exists among the sets of receptors stimulated by various chemicals, implying complex across-fiber sensory coding at the periphery.

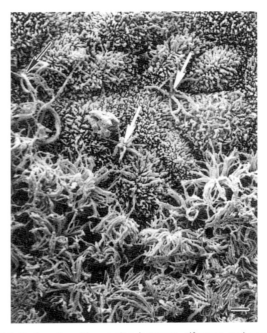

Fig. 17.1 Surface transition region between olfactory and respiratory epithelia. Bottom half displays olfactory epithelium; top half, respiratory epithelium. Arrows identify olfactory receptor cell dendritic endings with cilia. Bar = 5 μm. *(From Menco, B.Ph.M., Morrison, E.E., 2003. Morphology of the mammalian olfactory epithelium: form, fine structure, function, and pathology. In: Doty, R.L. (Ed.), Handbook of Olfaction and Gustation, second ed. Marcel Dekker, New York, pp. 32-97, with permission.)*

After coalescing into bundles (fila) within the lamina propria, the olfactory receptor axons traverse the foramina of the cribriform plate. These axons then distribute themselves across the surface of the olfactory bulb, a distinctly layered ovid structure composed of afferent and efferent nerve fibers, multiple interneurons, microglia, astrocytes, and blood vessels. The receptor cell axons selectively enter the sphere-like olfactory glomeruli located within an outer layer of the bulb. Those receptor cells expressing the same odorant protein converge onto the same glomerulus. The glomeruli number in the thousands in younger persons and are a defining feature of the olfactory system. With age, however, their number and integrity greatly decrease, being nearly absent in the elderly.

The activity of the primary output neurons of the olfactory bulb, the mitral and tufted cells, is modulated by many factors. In addition to being influenced directly by olfactory receptor cell activation, their membrane potentials are altered by numerous local interneurons and by centrifugal fibers. The most numerous cells of the olfactory bulb, the γ-aminobutyric acid (GABA)-ergic granule cells, can inhibit mitral and tufted cell activity via their connections with mitral cell secondary dendrites. These cells make up much of the core of the bulb and receive numerous inputs from central brain regions.

Unlike nearly all other central nervous system (CNS) neurons, the granule cells, as well as the largely dopaminergic periglomerular cells, undergo replacement over time (Altman, 1969). Astrocyte-like stem cells within the anterior subventricular zone of the brain generate large numbers of neuroblasts, some of which undergo restricted chain migration along the rostral migratory stream (Rousselot et al., 1994). This migration largely terminates within the granule cell layer of the olfactory bulb, from which some differentiating neuroblasts migrate more peripherally, thereby repopulating periglomerular cells. The architecture of the olfactory bulb, including its main cell types, is presented schematically in **Fig. 17.2**.

Central brain structures that receive the output axons of the mitral and tufted cells via the lateral olfactory tract include the anterior olfactory nucleus, the piriform cortex, the

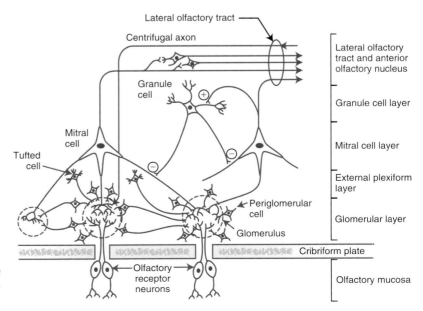

Fig. 17.2 Schematic of olfactory bulb structures, neurons, and layers. *(From Alloway, K.D., Pritchard, T.C., 2007. Medical Neuroscience. Hayes Barton, Raleigh, North Carolina, with permission.)*

anterior cortical nucleus of the amygdala, the periamygdaloid complex, and the rostral entorhinal cortex. These structures, collectively termed *primary olfactory cortex*, have reciprocal relations with one another and numerous other brain centers. For example, the entire length of the hippocampus receives fibers from the entorhinal cortex. Pyramidal cells from the anterior olfactory nucleus project to numerous ipsilateral and contralateral brain structures, the latter via the anterior commissure. While the olfactory system projects to cortical structures without initially synapsing in the thalamus, connections via the thalamus are present between primary (e.g., entorhinal) cortex and secondary (i.e., orbitofrontal) cortex.

The relative roles of central brain structures in odor perception are poorly understood. The piriform cortex appears to encode higher-order representations of odor quality, identity, and familiarity. This brain region also plays a role in odor learning and memory, as well as in coordinating information between olfaction, taste, and vision (Gottfried et al., 2002). The entorhinal cortex preprocesses information entering the hippocampus, whereas the amygdala seems to respond to the intensity of emotionally significant odors. The rostral regions of the orbitofrontal cortex are involved in odor memory, whereas the caudal regions are associated with odor detection. The processing of hedonic information about odors seems to occur within the orbitofrontal cortex, with pleasant odors activating the medial orbitofrontal cortex and unpleasant odors activating the lateral orbitofrontal cortex.

Gustation

Taste plays a critical role in identifying substances in foods and beverages, such as sugars and poisonous alkaloids, that promote or disrupt homeostasis. The taste receptor cells are found within the *taste buds*, small flask-like structures located on the surface of the oral epithelium (**Fig. 17.3**). These cells extend microvilli into the lumen of the bud near its apical opening, termed the *taste pore*. Like olfactory receptor cells, taste receptors die and become replaced at various intervals from basal cells within the bud.

Humans possess approximately 7500 taste buds, most of which are found on lingual protuberances called *papillae* (**Fig. 17.4**). Taste buds innervated by the chorda tympani division of the facial nerve (CN VII) are found on the fungiform papillae, which are most dense on the tip and lateral margins of the anterior tongue. The palatine branch of the greater superficial petrosal division of CN VII innervates the taste buds on the soft palate. Some taste buds found on the anterior foliate papillae, located on a sector of the tongue's posterior lateral margins, may also be innervated by branches of the chorda tympani nerve. Most foliate buds, as well as the buds on the circumvallate papillae—six to eight large structures that resemble flattened hills across the "chevron" of the posterior tongue—are innervated by the glossopharyngeal nerve (CN IX). Taste buds within the oral pharynx are supplied by the vagus (CN X) nerve. The small and somewhat pointed filiform papillae, which cover the entire tongue, harbor no taste buds. Although not involved in taste perception as such, the trigeminal nerve (CN V) participates in the formation of flavor via free nerve endings in the oral mucosa signaling sensations of touch, pain, and temperature. Thus, the fizziness of carbonated soft drinks and the warmth of coffee are dependent upon the stimulation of this nerve.

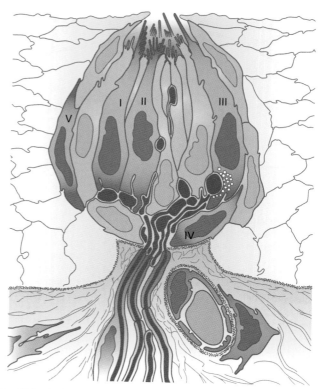

Fig. 17.3 Idealized drawing of longitudinal section of mammalian taste bud. Cells of type I, II, and III are elongated and form the sensory epithelium of the bud. These cells have different types of microvilli within the taste pit and may reach the taste pore. Type IV are basal cells, and type V are marginal cells. Synapses are most apparent at the bases of type III cells. The connecting taste nerves have myelin sheaths. *(From Witt, M., Reutter, K., Miller I.J., Jr. [2003] Morphology of the peripheral taste system. In: Doty, R.L., (Ed), Handbook of Olfaction and Gustation. NY: Marcel Dekker, pp. 651-677. The figure is on p. 663).*

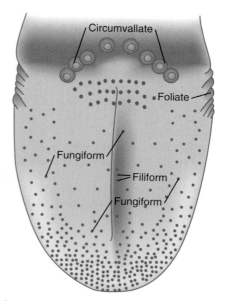

Fig. 17.4 Schematic representation of the tongue, demonstrating the relative distribution of the four main classes of taste papillae. Note that the fungiform papillae can vary considerably in size, and that they are more dense on the anterior and lateral regions of the tongue. *(Copyright © 2006, Richard L. Doty.)*

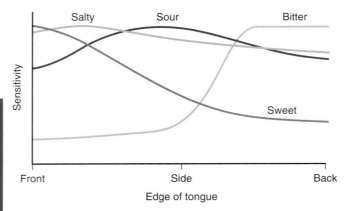

Fig. 17.5 Relative sensitivity of the edge of the tongue to the four classic taste qualities. Sensitivity reflects the reciprocal of the threshold value and is plotted as a ratio of maximal sensitivity = 1. Threshold data are from Hänig (1901). Note that all regions of the tongue that were evaluated were responsive to some degree to all stimuli, but that the anterior tongue was most sensitive to sweet, sour, and salty and least sensitive to bitter. The rear (base) of the tongue was relatively more sensitive to bitter. *(Adapted from Boring, E.G., 1942. Sensation and Perception in the History of Experimental Psychology. Appleton-Century Crofts, New York.)*

Individuals differ markedly in terms of the number and distribution of their taste buds. Although some physiology textbooks suggest that different regions of the tongue are responsible for the four basic taste qualities, this is an over-simplification of the facts. In general, the front of the tongue is more sensitive than other tongue regions to all taste qualities, although in the case of bitter, the back of the tongue is typically much more sensitive. The relative average sensitivity of tongue regions to the four prototypical taste qualities is shown in **Fig. 17.5**, although it must be emphasized that significant individual differences exist.

The specific receptors involved in sensing taste stimuli have now been identified (Hoon et al., 1999). A small family of three G protein–coupled receptors (GPCRs)—T1R1, T1R2, and T1R3—encode sweet and umami (monosodium glutamate–like) sensations. Bitter sensations are mediated by the T2R receptors, a family of about 30 GPCRs that are expressed on cells different from those that express the sweet and umami receptors. The salty sensation of sodium chloride arises from the entrance of Na^+ ions into the cells via specialized membrane channels such as the amiloride-sensitive Na^+ channel. Although sour taste has been suggested to depend upon a range of receptors, PKD2L1 is likely the primary sour taste receptor.

The nerves innervating the taste buds converge centrally onto the nucleus of the solitary tract of the brainstem. Although species differences exist, the afferent taste nerve fibers can be classified electrophysiologically into categories based upon their relative responsiveness to sweet, sour, bitter, and salty-tasting stimuli. In the hamster, for example, sucrose-best, HCl-best, and NaCl-best fibers have been observed (Frank et al., 1988). Despite the fact that fibers are generally "tuned" for rather specific stimuli, they can nonetheless respond to other stimuli. For example, a few sucrose-best fibers also respond to NaCl and HCl. NaCl-best fibers and HCl-best fibers are less tightly tuned than sucrose-best fibers, with more fibers responding to multiple classes of stimuli.

Fibers from the nucleus of the solitary tract project to a taste center within the upper regions of the ventral posterior nuclei of the thalamus via the medial lemniscus, a pathway connecting the brainstem to the thalamus. From here, information is sent to the amygdala and several cortical regions including the primary somatosensory cortex and the anterior insular cortex. Neurons within these regions respond to taste, touch, and in some cases odors.

The "taste code" interpreted by the brain depends on the specific neurons that are activated and the patterns of firing that occur both within and between these nerves. As with odors, the brain must remember what a particular tastant tastes like (e.g., sweet), and a matching or comparison of information coming from the taste pathways must be made at some point with the remembered sensation to allow for its recognition or identification. Higher brain regions play a significant role in establishing taste contrasts (e.g., something tasting more sour after prior experience with a sweet stimulus), inducing sensory fatigue, integrating multiple taste sensations, influencing taste hedonics, and integrating information from other senses to establish the experience of flavor.

Chemosensory Testing

Three general classes of sensory tests are available for quantifying human chemosensory function: psychophysical, electrophysiological, and psychophysiological (Doty, 2007). Psychophysical tests include tests where subjects make a conscious response, such as in tests of odor adaptation, detection, recognition, identification, discrimination, memory, hedonics, and suprathreshold scaling of various sensory dimensions. Electrophysiological tests measure minute stimulus-induced electrical changes from sensory receptors or the brain in the absence of verbal or other consciously overt subject responses. Included are summated electrical potentials from the surface of the olfactory epithelium (termed the *electro-olfactogram*), tongue, or scalp (changes in the electroencephalogram, such as event-related potentials or summated total power). Clinically, psychophysical tests have been most widely employed, in part due to reliability, practicality, and cost.

The most widely used psychophysical tests are those of identification and detection (Doty, 2007). In identification tests, a subject is typically asked to identify, usually from a list of alternatives, the quality of the sensation experienced when sniffing or tasting a stimulus. A response is required even if no sensation is perceived, a procedure called *forced-choice responding*. For example, in the most popular odor identification test, the University of Pennsylvania Smell Identification Test (UPSIT), the subject is provided with a series of 40 microencapsulated (scratch and sniff) odors and in each case asked to choose the name of the odor from four response alternatives (Doty et al., 1984b) (**Fig. 17.6**). The number of correct answers determines the degree of deficit and allows for both overall classification of function (i.e., normosmia, mild microsmia, moderate microsmia, severe microsmia, anosmia) and a relative percentile classification based upon age- and sex-related norms. Malingering can be discerned by improbable responses in the forced-choice situation, such as not correctly identifying any odors or otherwise identifying odors at a rate significantly below the expected chance performance of 25%. In an odor detection threshold test, a subject is typically presented with an odor and one or more blanks in random

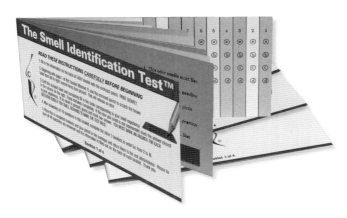

Fig. 17.6 Booklets of the University of Pennsylvania Smell Identification Test (UPSIT). The test comprises 4 booklets, each containing 10 microencapsulated scratch-and-sniff odorants that are released by a pencil tip. Associated with each odorant is a multiple-choice question about which of four possibilities is correct. Forced-choice answers are recorded on the last page of each booklet and assessed with a simple scoring key. *(Copyright © 2004, Sensonics, Inc., Haddon Heights, New Jersey. Reprinted with permission.)*

fashion and asked to identify which stimulus is stronger or otherwise discernable from the other stimuli. A common procedure is to present stronger stimuli when a miss occurs and weaker stimuli when a hit occurs, following a defined algorithm. This is termed a *staircase procedure*, and the *threshold* is defined as a set number of reversals of the staircase. With the exception of tests of hedonics and suprathreshold scaling, scores on tests of odor identification and detection, as well as discrimination and memory, are highly correlated, with the size of the correlations being dependent upon the less reliable of the intercorrelated tests (Doty et al., 1994). It is for this reason that a rather complete characterization of smell function can be obtained by simply using a reliable odor identification test.

Although very brief tests can be useful in screening, they have significant limitations. Short tests do not allow for the detection of malingering and are generally less sensitive than longer tests. As a general rule, the more trials contained in a test, the higher its reliability and sensitivity (Doty et al., 1995). Despite the fact that some very brief tests are reliable, their reliability is associated with less sensitivity and specificity, as brief tests can only clump patients into very broad dysfunction categories. This is analogous to the ability of a flashlight to determine blindness in a patient. While this may allow for accurate detection of absolute blindness, it does not allow for assessing varying degrees of less than total blindness.

Disorders of Olfaction

Olfactory loss can be total (anosmia) or less than total (hyposmia or microsmia). Strange and distorted smells, sometimes described as "chemical" or "garbage-like," can occur either in the absence of a stimulus (phantosmia, also called *olfactory hallucinations*) or when an odorant or warm air is smelled (dysosmia or parosmia). When a fecal-like character is present, this is often termed *cacosmia*. Most cases of dysosmia or phantosmia are due to neurological causes such as altered firing of the receptor cells during degeneration or regeneration,

although in some instances, bacterial infections within the nose or sinuses can produce foul smells that result in this condition. Olfactory agnosia, the inability to recognize odors by an otherwise intact olfactory system, may occur secondary to some brain lesions, although distinguishing this problem from other forms of dysfunction is challenging. Hypersensitivity to odorants (hyperosmia) has been reported, but many persons claiming hypersensitivity are experiencing dysosmias and show decrements in function upon testing. As with the other senses, olfactory dysfunction can be bilateral or unilateral.

Many factors influence the ability to smell: age, sex, smoking behavior, reproductive state, nutrition, toxic exposures, head trauma, and numerous diseases (**Table 17.1**). Men generally perform less well than women on olfactory tests. Age is a major correlate of smell dysfunction, with significant decrements occurring in over 50% of those between 65 and 80 years of age and in 75% of those 80 years of age and older (Doty et al., 1984a) (**Fig. 17.7**). Such losses help explain why many elderly find food distasteful and succumb to nutritional deficiencies and, in rare instances, natural gas poisoning.

The three most common causes of long-lasting or permanent smell loss of patients who present to smell and taste centers are, in order of frequency, upper respiratory infections, head trauma, and chronic rhinosinusitis (Deems et al., 1991a). Congenital, iatrogenic, and toxic chemical exposures are the next most common causes. These etiologies can result in permanent damage to the olfactory neuroepithelium, decreased number of receptor cells, and replacement of sensory epithelium with other types of epithelia. Susceptibility to such damage likely increases from reduction or inhibition of mucociliary transport by a range of factors including diet, drugs, disease, genetics, and age-related changes in nasal function and normal defense mechanisms.

Symptoms of the common cold and influenza are readily apparent to the patient, but it is important to remember that most viral infections are either entirely asymptomatic or so mild that they go unrecognized. Thus, during seasonal epidemics, the number of serologically documented influenza or arboviral encephalitis infections exceeds the number of acute cases by several hundred-fold (Stroop, 1995). For these and other reasons, many idiopathic cases of smell dysfunction likely reflect unrecognized viral infections. Smell dysfunction has been reported in rare instances following influenza vaccine inoculations (Fiser and Borotski, 1979). This may reflect a subtle but defining influence on an already compromised olfactory epithelium, although coincidental viral infection cannot be excluded from consideration. Under certain circumstances, some viruses can enter the brain after incorporation into the olfactory receptor cells, possibly catalyzing neurodegenerative disease (Doty, 2008). Such viruses as herpes simplex types 1 and 2, polio, the Indiana strain of wild-type vesicular stomatitis, rabies, mouse hepatitis, Borna disease, and canine distemper viruses are neurotropic for peripheral olfactory structures.

Loss of smell function from head trauma usually reflects coup-contrecoup movement of the brain that shears off the olfactory fila at the level of the cribriform plate (Doty et al., 1997). In most cases, scar tissue forms, precluding reconnection of axons from regenerating receptor cells. Fractures of the cribriform plate or other elements of the skull are rare in such cases and are not a prerequisite for the smell loss. In general,

Table 17.1 **Disorders and Conditions Associated with Compromised Olfactory Function, as Measured by Olfactory Testing**	
22q11 Deletion syndrome	Lubag
HIV/AIDS	Medications
Adenoid hypertrophy	Migraine
Adrenal cortical insufficiency	MS
Age	Multiple system atrophy
Alcoholism	Multi-infarct dementia
Allergies	Narcolepsy with cataplexy
AD	Neoplasms, cranial/nasal
ALS	Nutritional deficiencies
Anorexia nervosa	Obstructive pulmonary disease
Asperger syndrome	Obesity
Ataxias	OCD
Attention deficit/hyperactivity disorder	Orthostatic tremor
Bardet-Biedl syndrome	Panic disorder
Chemical exposure	PD
COPD	Parkinson dementia complex of Guam
Congenital	Pick disease
Creutzfeldt-Jakob disease	PTSD
Cushing syndrome	Pregnancy
Cystic fibrosis	Pseudohypoparathyroidism
Degenerative ataxias	Psychopathy
Diabetes	Radiation (therapeutic, cranial)
Down syndrome	REM behavior disorder
Epilepsy	Refsum disease
Facial paralysis	Renal failure/end-stage kidney disease
FTLD	Restless legs syndrome
Gonadal dysgenesis (Turner syndrome)	Rhinosinusitis/polyposis
Guamanian ALS/PD/dementia syndrome	Schizophrenia
Head trauma	Seasonal affective disorder
Herpes simplex encephalitis	Sjögren syndrome
Hypothyroidism	Stroke
HD	Tobacco smoking
Iatrogenesis	Toxic chemical exposure
Kallmann syndrome	Upper respiratory infections
Korsakoff psychosis	Usher syndrome
Leprosy	Vascular disorders (e.g., aneurysms, hemorrhages)
Liver disease	Vitamin B$_{12}$ deficiency

AD, Alzheimer disease; *AIDS,* acquired immunodeficiency syndrome; *ALS,* amyotrophic lateral sclerosis; *COPD,* chronic obstructive pulmonary disease; *FTLD,* frontotemporal lobar degeneration; *HD,* Huntington disease; *HIV,* human immunodeficiency virus; *MS,* multiple sclerosis; *OCD,* obsessive compulsive disorder; *PD,* Parkinson disease; *PTSD,* posttraumatic stress disorder; *REM,* rapid eye movement.

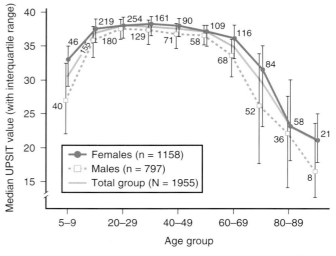

Fig. 17.7 Scores on the University of Pennsylvania Smell Identification Test (UPSIT) as a function of subject age and sex. Numbers by each data point indicate sample sizes. Note that women identify odorants better than men at all ages. *(From Doty, R.L., Shaman, P., Applebaum, S.L., et al., 1984a. Smell identification ability: changes with age. Science 226, 1441-1443. Copyright © 1984, American Association for the Advancement of Science.)*

the more severe the head trauma, the higher the likelihood that smell loss is present.

A major development in neurology is the discovery that a number of neurodegenerative diseases are associated with smell loss early in their course, most notably AD and PD. In most cases, the smell loss precedes the presentation of the classic clinical phenotype by several years. Interestingly, a number of disorders often confused with these two diseases are unaccompanied by meaningful olfactory dysfunction, making smell testing potentially useful as an aid in differential diagnosis. For AD, major affective disorder is an example (McCaffrey et al., 2000). For PD, such examples include progressive supranuclear palsy (PSP) (Doty et al., 1993), essential tremor (Busenbark et al., 1992), MPTP-induced parkinsonism (Doty et al., 1992), and vascular parkinsonism (Katzenschlager et al., 2004). The relative severity of olfactory dysfunction in a range of neurodegenerative diseases and in schizophrenia is shown in **Table 17.2**.

It is noteworthy that the olfactory loss is present in idiopathic rapid eye movement sleep behavior disorder (iRBD) as well as in PD, since individuals with iRBD frequently develop PD. The fact that rapid eye movement(REM) behavior disorder is seen not only in its idiopathic form but in association with narcolepsy led has led to findings that narcolepsy—independent of REM behavior disorder—is associated with a significant impairment in olfactory function (Buskova et al., 2010; Stiasny-Kolster et al., 2007). Orexin A, also called *hypocretin-1*, is significantly decreased or undetectable in the cerebrospinal fluid of patients with narcolepsy and cataplexy. The orexin-containing hypothalamic neurons project throughout the entire olfactory system (from the olfactory epithelium to the olfactory cortex) (Caillol et al., 2003). Thus, damage to these projections may potentially impair olfactory performance in narcoleptic patients. The intranasal administration of orexin A (hypocretin-1) to narcoleptic patients with cataplexy has been found to improve their olfactory function,

Table 17.2 Relative Degree of Olfactory Dysfunction in Various Neurological Diseases on an Arbitrary Scale

Disease	Relative Severity of Smell Loss
Idiopathic PD, AD, DLB, Guam PD-dementia complex, idiopathic rapid eye movement sleep behavior disorder	++++
HD, Down syndrome, PARK8 PD	+++
Multiple system atrophy (type-P), PARK1 PD, pallidopontonigral degeneration, drug-induced PD?, schizophrenia, semantic dementia?, X-linked dystonia-parkinsonism (Lubag), narcolepsy	++
Motor neuron disease, SCA2 PD, Friedreich ataxia, PARK3, corticobasal degeneration, FTD	+
Major affective disorder, essential tremor, vascular parkinsonism, MPTP-induced parkinsonism, idiopathic dystonia, SCA3 PD, PSP; PARK2	0

Modified and updated from Hawkes, C.H., Doty, R.L., 2009. The Neurology of Olfaction. Cambridge University Press, Cambridge, with permission.

Key: ++++ marked damage; + mild damage; 0 normal. Note that most of the values are based on relatively small patient numbers except for idiopathic PD.

AD, Alzheimer disease; *DLB,* dementia with lewy bodies; *FTD,* frontotemporal dementia; *HD,* Huntington disease; *PD,* Parkinson disease; *PSP,* progressive supranuclear palsy; *SCA,* spinocerebellar atrophy.

implying that mild olfactory impairment is not only a primary feature of this disorder but that CNS orexin deficiency could be a possible mechanism for this loss (Baier et al., 2008).

Disorders of Taste

As noted in the beginning of the chapter, most patients with complaints of taste loss have olfactory dysfunction, not taste dysfunction. This reflects the greater fragility of the olfactory system and the dependence of flavor sensations upon retronasal stimulation of this system. Impairment of whole-mouth gustatory function is rare outside of generalized metabolic disturbances, such as from diabetes, chronic renal failure, end-stage liver disease, thyroid disease, hypothyroidism, medications, and vitamin and mineral deficiencies. Nonetheless, taste perception can be altered by (1) viral invasion of one or more taste nerves, (2) the release of foul-tasting materials from the nasal and oral cavities secondary to medical conditions and oral appliances (e.g., rhinosinusitis, gingivitis, purulent sialadenitis), (3) transport problems of tastants to the taste buds (e.g., scaring of the lingual surface, mucosal drying, inflammatory conditions, infections), (4) damage to the taste buds (e.g., invasive carcinomas, local trauma), (5) damage to the taste nerves (e.g., chorda tympani damage from Bell palsy, middle ear infections or operations), and (6) damage to taste-related CNS structures from disorders such as multiple sclerosis, tumors, epilepsy, and stroke. Lesions caudal to the pons

produce ipsilateral deficits, whereas lesions within the pons proper can produce ipsilateral, contralateral, or bilateral deficits. Both ipsilateral and contralateral taste deficits have been noted in patients with lesions of the insular cortex, reflecting the bilateral representation of taste function at this level (Pritchard et al., 1999). Unlike CN VII, CN IX is relatively protected along its path, although iatrogenic interventions can result in CN IX injury (e.g., from tonsillectomy, bronchoscopy, laryngoscopy, radiation therapy), and this nerve is not immune to damage from tumors, vascular lesions, and infection. On rare occasion, epilepsy or migraine is associated with a gustatory prodrome or aura, and some tastes may actually trigger seizures or migraine attacks.

The influence of medications on taste function is well established. Over 250 medications have been implicated in taste dysfunction, including antineoplastic agents, antirheumatic drugs, antibiotics, and blood pressure medications (Doty et al., 2008). Terbinafine, a popular antifungal, can produce long-lasting loss of sweet, sour, bitter, and salty taste perception (Doty and Haxel, 2005). A recent double-blind study found that eszopiclone, a widely used sleep medication, induces a bitter dysgeusia in approximately two-thirds of individuals tested (Doty et al., 2009). This sensation was related to the time since drug administration, was stronger for women than for men, and correlated with both saliva and blood levels of the drug.

Clinical Evaluation of Taste and Smell

Etiology can usually be established from a clinical history that explores symptom nature, onset, duration, pattern of fluctuations, and potential precipitating events, such as upper respiratory infections that occurred prior to symptom onset. Information regarding head trauma, smoking habits, drug and alcohol abuse (e.g., intranasal cocaine, chronic alcoholism in the context of Wernicke and Korsakoff syndromes), exposures to pesticides and other toxic agents, and medical interventions are informative. The possibility of multiple or cumulative effects cannot be discounted. A determination of all the medications that the patient was taking before and at the time of symptom onset is important, as are comorbid medical conditions potentially associated with taste and smell impairment, such as renal failure, liver disease, hypothyroidism, diabetes, and dementia. Delayed puberty in association with anosmia (with or without midline craniofacial abnormalities, deafness, and renal anomalies) suggests the possibility of Kallmann syndrome. Recollection of epistaxis, discharge (clear, purulent, bloody), nasal obstruction, allergies, and somatic symptoms including headache or irritation have potential localizing value. Questions related to memory, parkinsonian signs, and seizure activity (e.g., automatisms, occurrence of black-outs, auras, déjà vu) should be posed. The possibility of malingering should be considered, particularly if litigation is involved. Intermittent smell loss usually implies an obstructive disorder, such as from rhinosinusitis or other inflammatory problem. Sudden smell loss alerts the practitioner to head trauma, ischemia, infection, or a psychiatric condition. Gradual smell loss can be a marker for the development of a progressive obstructive lesion, cumulative drug effects, or simply presbyosmia or presbygeusia. While losses secondary to head trauma are most commonly abrupt, in some cases the loss appears over time or only becomes apparent to the patient after a long interval.

In addition to quantitative sensory evaluation, which is key in defining the dysfunction, neurological and otorhinolaryngological (ORL) examinations, along with appropriate brain and nasosinus imaging, aid in evaluating patients with olfactory or gustatory complaints. In the case of olfaction, the neural evaluation should pay particular attention to possible skull base and intracranial lesions. The ORL examination should thoroughly assess the intranasal architecture and mucosal surfaces. Polyps, masses, and adhesions of the turbinates to the septum may compromise the flow of air to the olfactory receptors, since less than a fifth of the inspired air traverses the olfactory cleft in the unobstructed state. Blood serum tests may be helpful to identify such conditions as diabetes, infection, heavy metal exposure, nutritional deficiency (e.g., vitamin B_6, B_{12}), allergy, and thyroid, liver, and kidney disease.

Treatment and Management

Management of chemosensory disorders is condition specific. Optimism for prognosis is warranted for most patients with obstructive or inflammatory disorders (e.g., allergic rhinitis, glossitis, polyposis, intranasal or intraoral neoplasms) for which medical or surgical interventions are available. In cases of rhinosinusitis, for example, an oral taper of prednisone can initially be used to quell general inflammation, followed by topical administration of the nasal spray or drops in the inverted head position, such as the Moffett position (Canciani and Mastella, 1988), increasing the likelihood of the material reaching the olfactory epithelium. Candidiasis or other oral infections can be quelled with topical antifungal and antibiotic treatments. Some salty or bitter dysgeusias respond to chlorhexidine mouthwash, possibly as a result of its strong positive charge (Wang et al., 2009). Patients with excessive oral dryness, including dryness due to medications, often benefit from the use of mints, lozenges, or sugarless gum, as well as from oral pilocarpine or artificial saliva.

Medications that induce distortions of smell or taste can often be discontinued and other types of medications or modes of therapy substituted. Unfortunately, little empirical data are available for most drugs, and some drug-related effects on the taste system appear to be long lasting and not reversed by short-term drug discontinuance (Doty et al., 2008). There is suggestion that some antioxidants such as α-lipoic acid may be effectual in some cases of hyposmia, hypogeusia, dysosmia, dysgeusia, and burning mouth syndrome (Hummel et al., 2002), although strong scientific evidence for its efficacy is lacking. Despite being widely mentioned in the medical literature, zinc and vitamin A therapies offer unlikely benefit for olfactory disturbances except when frank deficiencies are present, although both of these agents may improve taste dysfunction secondary to hepatic deficiencies (Deems et al., 1991b). A recent report that theophylline improved smell function was not double blinded and lacked

a control group, failing to take into account that some meaningful improvement occurs without treatment (Henkin et al., 2009). Indeed, the percentage of patients reported to be responsive to the treatment was about the same as that noted by others to show spontaneous improvement over a similar time period. Similar issues are inherent in a recent claims of efficacy for acupuncture and transcranial magnetic stimulation. There are claims that some antiepileptics and antidepressants (e.g., amitriptyline) may be of value in treating some chemosensory disturbances, particularly following head trauma. However, in the case of amitriptyline, there is clear evidence that it can distort taste function, possibly from its anticholinergic effects (Schiffman et al., 1999). A recent study suggests that donepezil (acetylcholinesterase inhibitor) improved odor identification scores in patients with AD, and that such scores correlated with overall clinician-based impressions of change scales (CIBIC-plus), leading the authors to suggest that tests of smell identification function may be useful in assessing treatment responses to this medication (Velayudhan and Lovestone, 2009).

It is of interest that repeated exposure to odorants may in fact increase sensitivity to them in both animals and humans, providing a rationale for therapies in which multiple odors are smelled before and after going to bed (Hummel et al., 2009). However, double-blind studies with appropriate controls are needed to confirm the effectiveness of this approach. Importantly, spontaneous recovery over time occurs in some instances, providing hope to at least some patients. In a longitudinal study of 542 patients presenting to our center with smell loss from a variety of causes, modest improvement occurred over an average time period of 4 years in about half of the participants (London et al., 2008). Nonetheless, normal age-related function returned in only 11% of the anosmic and 23% of the hyposmic patients. The amount of dysfunction present at the time of presentation, not etiology, was the best predictor of prognosis. Other predictors were patient age and the time between dysfunction onset and initial testing.

An important but overlooked element of therapy comes from chemosensory testing itself. Confirmation or lack of conformation of loss is beneficial to patients, particularly ones who come to believe they may be "crazy" as a result of unsupportive medical providers or family members. Quantitative testing places the patient's problem into overall perspective, and if considerable function is present, patients can be informed of a more positive prognosis. It is extremely therapeutic for an older person to become aware that, while his or her smell function is not what it used to be, it still falls above the average of his or her peer group, a situation that happens, by definition, 50% of the time. It is unfortunate that many such patients are simply told by their physician they are getting old and nothing can be done for them, often exacerbating or leading to depression and decreased self-esteem.

References

The complete reference list is available online at www.expertconsult.com.

Chapter 18

Cranial and Facial Pain

J.D. Bartleson, David F. Black, Jerry W. Swanson

Headache is an exceedingly common symptom that affects virtually everyone at some time in their life. It is estimated that nearly half of the world's adult population has an active headache disorder (Robbins et al., 2010). Headache is one of the most common reasons for outpatient healthcare visits in the United States. Patients with head and/or face pain typically present for medical attention because the discomfort is severe, interferes with work and/or leisure activities, or raises the patient's or family's concern about a serious underlying cause.

Headache disorders are classified as primary or secondary (**Box 18.1**) (International Headache Society Classification Subcommittee, 2004). The primary headache disorders do not have an underlying structural cause, but all the primary headache disorders can be simulated by secondary conditions. The diagnosis of head and face pain depends on three elements: the history, neurological and general examinations, and appropriate investigations if needed. Treatment of headaches is discussed in Chapter 69.

History

The gold standard for diagnosis and management of headache is a careful interview and neurological and general medical examinations (De Luca and Bartleson, 2010). In the vast majority of patients with headache, the neurological and general examinations will be normal, so the diagnosis is based entirely on the history, and clinicians are well advised to spend most of their time interviewing the patient.

History-taking for head and face pain is similar to that for other presenting complaints, but several specific aspects should be addressed. The questions listed in **Box 18.2** are useful, and the discussion that follows illustrates some responses and their implications. Usually one begins by asking the patient to describe their symptoms or, alternatively, simply by asking how they can be helped. This approach allows patients to relax and say what they had planned to say. Usually the patient will speak for less than 2 minutes if not interrupted (Langewitz et al., 2002). Once the patient has had an opportunity to speak, directed but open-ended questions (see **Box 18.2**) can be asked.

Types of Headaches

Many individuals have more than one type of headache. It is valuable to establish this information at the beginning of the interview so each type of pain can be carefully delineated. A change in an established headache pattern can indicate a new condition.

Onset of Headaches

A stable headache disorder of many years' duration is almost always of benign origin. Migraine headaches often begin in childhood, adolescence, or early adulthood. A headache of recent onset obviously has many possible causes, including the new onset of either a benign or serious condition. "Recent onset" has been defined differently by various authors; the typical range is from 1 to 12 months. In general, the more recent the onset, the more worrisome. The "worst ever" headache, an increasingly severe headache, or change for the worse in an existing headache pattern all raise the possibility of an intracranial lesion. Headaches of instantaneous onset suggest

Box 18.1 International Classification of Headache Disorders, 2nd Edition

The Primary Headaches

Migraine
Tension-type headache
Cluster headache and other trigeminal autonomic cephalalgias
Other primary headaches:
- Primary stabbing headache
- Primary cough headache
- Primary exertional headache
- Primary headache associated with sexual activity:
  - Preorgasmic headache
  - Orgasmic headache
- Hypnic headache
- Primary thunderclap headache
- Hemicrania continua
- New daily-persistent headache

The Secondary Headaches

Headache attributed to head and/or neck trauma
Headache attributed to cranial or cervical vascular disorder
Headache attributed to nonvascular intracranial disorder
Headache attributed to substance or its withdrawal
Headache attributed to infection
Headache attributed to disorder of homeostasis
Headache or facial pain attributed to disorder of cranium, neck, eyes, ears, nose, sinuses, teeth, mouth or other facial or cranial structures
Headache attributed to psychiatric disorder

Cranial Neuralgias, Central and Primary Facial Pain and Other Headaches

Cranial neuralgias and central causes of facial pain
Other headache, cranial neuralgia, central or primary facial pain

Box 18.2 Useful Questions to Ask the Patient with Headache

- How many types of headache do you have?
- When and how did each type begin?
- If the headaches are episodic, what is the frequency and duration?
- How long does it take for your headaches to reach maximal intensity?
- How long do your headaches last?
- When do the headaches tend to occur, and what factors trigger your headaches?
- Where does your pain start, and how does it evolve?
- What is the quality and the severity of your pain?
- Is the pain steady or pulsating (throbbing), or both?
- Are there symptoms that herald the onset of your headache?
- What are they, when do they begin, and how long do they last?
- Are there symptoms that accompany your headaches?
- Do you get nauseated with your headaches?
- Does light and/or noise bother you a lot more when you have a headache than when you don't?
- Do your headaches limit your ability to work, study, or do what you need to do for at least 1 day?
- Does anything aggravate your pain (e.g., exertion)?
- Are your headaches getting better or worse, or are they about the same?
- What treatments have been used to treat the headaches, both acutely and preventively?
- What helps your pain?
- Is there a family history of headaches?
- What prior testing have you had?
- Do you have other medical or neurological problems?
- What do you think might be causing your headaches?
- How disabling are your headaches?
- Why are you seeking help now?

an intracranial hemorrhage, usually in the subarachnoid space, but also can be caused by intracerebral hemorrhage, cerebral venous thrombosis, arterial dissection, pituitary apoplexy, spontaneous intracranial hypotension, benign angiopathy of the central nervous system (CNS), acute hypertensive crisis, and idiopathic primary thunderclap headache (Ju and Schwedt, 2010). Onset of a new headache in patients older than 50 years raises suspicion of an intracranial lesion (e.g., subdural hematoma) or giant cell (temporal or cranial) arteritis (GCA). A history of antecedent head or neck injury should be sought; even a relatively minor injury can be associated with subsequent development of epidural, subdural, subarachnoid, or intraparenchymal hemorrhage and posttraumatic dissection of the carotid or vertebral arteries (Dziewas et al., 2003). However, posttraumatic headaches can occur following head injury in the absence of any significant pathology.

Frequency and Periodicity of Episodic Headaches

Migraine may be episodic or chronic. Chronic migraine, occurring 15 or more days per month, usually develops in individuals with a history of episodic migraine headaches.

Episodic migraine may become chronic with or without medication overuse.

Episodic cluster headaches typically occur daily for several weeks or months and are followed by a lengthy headache-free interval. Chronic cluster headaches occur at least every other day for more than 1 year. If there is no regular periodicity, it is useful to inquire about the longest and shortest periods of freedom between headaches. Having the patient monitor headache frequency, duration, intensity, triggers, and medication use on a headache calendar or in a diary is helpful in diagnosis and measuring response to treatment.

Temporal Profile

A chronic daily headache without migrainous or autonomic features is likely to be a chronic tension-type headache. Untreated migraine pain usually peaks within 1 to 2 hours of onset and lasts 4 to 72 hours. Cluster headache is typically maximal immediately (if the patient awakens with the headache in progress) or peaks within minutes (if it begins while awake). Cluster headaches can last 15 to 180 minutes (usually 45 to 120 minutes). Headaches similar to cluster but lasting only 2 to 30 minutes and occurring several times a day are typical of episodic or chronic paroxysmal hemicrania, both of which are more common in women and are prevented by indomethacin (Goadsby et al., 2010). Primary stabbing headaches ("ice-pick pains") are momentary, lasting only seconds. Stabbing pains are more common in patients with migraine and cluster headaches. Tension-type headaches commonly build up over hours and last hours to days to years. Headache that is daily and unremitting from onset, usually in patients without prior headaches, is classified as new daily-persistent headache and may have features suggestive of migraine or tension-type headache. A chronic, continuous, unilateral headache of moderate severity with superimposed attacks of more intense pain, associated with autonomic features, suggests the diagnosis of hemicrania continua, an indomethacin-responsive syndrome. Occipital neuralgia and trigeminal neuralgia manifest as brief shocklike pains, often triggered by stimulation in the territory served by the affected nerve. Occasionally a dull pain in the same nerve distribution persists longer, often after a series of brief, sharp pains. Short-lasting *u*nilateral *n*euralgiform headache with *c*onjunctival injection and *t*earing (SUNCT) is a rare syndrome consisting of paroxysms of first-division trigeminal nerve pain, lasting 5 to 240 seconds but occurring 3 to 200 times per day with the associated autonomic symptoms for which it is named (Goadsby et al., 2010)

Time of Day and Precipitating Factors

Cluster headaches often awaken patients from a sound sleep and may occur at the same time each day in an individual person. Hypnic headaches typically affect older patients and regularly awaken the patient at a particular time of night. Unlike cluster headaches, they are usually diffuse and not associated with autonomic phenomena (Donnet and Lanteri-Minet, 2009). Migraine headaches can occur at any time but often begin in the morning. A headache of recent onset that disturbs sleep or is worse on waking may be caused by increased intracranial pressure. Tension-type headaches typically are present during much of the day and often are more severe later in the day. Obstructive sleep apnea may be accompanied by the frequent occurrence of headache on awakening, as can medication-overuse headache ("rebound headache").

Patients with chronic recurrent headaches often recognize factors that trigger an attack. Migraine headaches may be precipitated by bright light, menstruation, weather changes, caffeine withdrawal, fasting, alcohol (particularly beer and wine), sleeping more or less than usual, stress and release from stress, certain foods and food additives, perfume and smoke, and others. Alcohol can trigger a cluster headache within minutes of ingestion. If bending, lifting, coughing, or Valsalva maneuver brings on a headache, an intracranial lesion, especially one involving the posterior fossa, must be considered. Exertional headache and headache associated with sexual activity both are worrisome. Although either can occur as a primary headache disorder unassociated with structural disease or can be associated with migraine, both types can also be due to subarachnoid hemorrhage and arterial dissection, both of which must be excluded with the first occurrence of such headaches. Intermittent headaches that are worsened by sitting or standing and improved by lying down are characteristic of a cerebrospinal fluid (CSF) leak. If there is no history of lumbar puncture, head trauma, or neurosurgical intervention, a spontaneous CSF leak may be the cause (Schievink, 2008). Lancinating face pain triggered by facial or intraoral stimuli occurs with trigeminal neuralgia. Glossopharyngeal neuralgia typically is triggered by chewing, swallowing, or talking, although cutaneous trigger zones in and about the ear are occasionally present.

Location

Asking the patient to outline the location of his or her pain with their finger can be very helpful. Trigeminal neuralgia is confined to one or more branches of the trigeminal nerve. The patient may be able to localize one or more trigger points on the face or in the mouth and then show how the pain spreads. Pain in the throat may be due to a local process or to glossopharyngeal neuralgia. Carotid artery dissection commonly presents with unilateral neck, face, and head pain, is frequently associated with an ipsilateral Horner syndrome, and often follows head or neck trauma.

Migraine commonly is unilateral and can be confined to the front or back of the head. Alternatively, the pain can start on one side and spread to the other or be global from onset. Cluster headaches are unilateral during an attack and typically are centered in, behind, or around one eye. Some patients' cluster headaches switch sides with different cluster periods, and a smaller number experience side shifts within a cluster period. The typical tension-type headache is generalized, although it may begin in the neck muscles and affect chiefly the occipital region or predominate frontally. When pain is localized to the eye, mouth, or ear, local processes involving these structures must be considered. Otalgia may be caused by a process involving the tonsil and posterior tongue. With chronic unilateral facial pain, an underlying lesion often cannot be identified. Occasionally, however, facial pain may be a symptom of nonmetastatic lung cancer (Eross et al., 2003).

Quality and Severity

The character and quality of the patient's pain can carry significance. In most cases, the type of pain can be designated as sharp, aching, or burning. Headaches may be steady or throbbing (pulsating) in character. It may be helpful to ask the patient to grade the severity of pain on a scale of 1 to 10. Patients who report their pain level is 20 are hurting but may be prone to exaggerate. Migraine pain often has a pulsating quality that may be superimposed on a more continuous pain. The pain of cluster headache characteristically is severe, boring, and steady and often is described as a "hot poker." SUNCT produces moderately severe pain in the orbital or temporal region and may be described as sharp and stabbing or (rarely) pulsatile. Tension-type headaches usually are described as a steady feeling of fullness, tightness, or pressure, or like a cap, band, or vise. Headaches caused by meningeal irritation, whether related to infectious meningitis or blood are typically severe. Trigeminal neuralgia is severe, brief, sharp, electric shock–like, or stabbing; pains can occur up to several times per minute, and a milder ache may persist between paroxysms of pain. Glossopharyngeal neuralgia pain is similar in character to that of trigeminal neuralgia.

Premonitory Symptoms, Aura, and Accompanying Symptoms

Some patients have premonitory symptoms that precede a migraine headache by hours. These can include psychological changes (e.g., depression, euphoria, irritability) or somatic symptoms (e.g., constipation, diarrhea, abnormal hunger, fluid retention, increased urination). The term aura refers to focal cerebral symptoms associated with a migraine attack. These symptoms typically last 20 to 30 minutes but can last 1 hour and usually precede the headache. At other times, the aura may continue into the headache phase or begin during the headache. Visual symptoms are most common and may consist of either positive (flickering lights, spots, or lines) or negative (scotomas or visual field loss) phenomena or both. The visual symptoms characteristically affect both eyes but can affect one eye alone. Other hemispheric symptoms, such as somatosensory disturbances (tingling and/or numbness) or dysphasic language disturbance, may occur with or without visual symptoms. Aura symptoms usually have a gradual onset and increase over minutes. If more than one symptom occurs (e.g., visual plus somatosensory), the onsets usually are staggered and not simultaneous. Patients can experience migraine aura without an associated headache. Positive symptoms, the slow spread of symptoms, and staggered onsets help differentiate migraine aura from focal symptoms caused by cerebrovascular disease.

Symptoms originating from the brainstem or both cerebral hemispheres simultaneously, such as vertigo, dysarthria, ataxia, auditory symptoms, diplopia, bilateral visual symptoms in both eyes, bilateral paresthesias, and decreased level of consciousness, may accompany basilar-type migraine. Migraine with aura that includes motor weakness can be due to familial hemiplegic migraine if there is a family history in at least one first- or second-degree relative, or due to sporadic hemiplegic migraine if there is no family history. It can be difficult for the patient to differentiate sensory loss from true weakness. Nausea, vomiting, photophobia, phonophobia, and osmophobia characteristically accompany migraine attacks. In addition, lacrimation, rhinorrhea, and nasal congestion can accompany migraine headache and mimic headache of sinus origin (Cady et al., 2005). Ipsilateral miosis, ptosis, lacrimation, conjunctival injection, and nasal stuffiness commonly accompany cluster headache; sweating and facial flushing on the side of the pain are much less common. Similar autonomic features also accompany episodic and chronic paroxysmal hemicrania and hemicrania continua. Even shorter attacks (5–240 seconds) with ipsilateral conjunctival injection and tearing suggest SUNCT (Goadsby et al., 2010). Horner syndrome is common in carotid artery dissection. In the setting of acute transient or persistent monocular visual loss, GCA and carotid dissection should be considered. Temporomandibular joint dysfunction includes jaw pain precipitated or aggravated by movement of the jaw or clenching of the teeth and is associated with reduction in the range of jaw movement, joint clicking, and tenderness over the joint. Headache accompanied by fever suggests an infection. Headache associated with persistent or progressive diffuse or focal CNS symptoms, including seizures, implies a structural cause. Purulent or bloody nasal discharge suggests an acute sinus cause for the headache. Likewise, a red eye raises the possibility of an ocular process such as infection or acute glaucoma. A history of polymyalgia rheumatica, jaw claudication, or tenderness of the scalp arteries in an older person strongly suggests GCA. Transient visual obscurations upon standing, usually pulsatile tinnitus, diplopia (especially for objects in the distance), and papilledema may be associated with increased intracranial pressure from any cause, including idiopathic intracranial hypertension (pseudotumor cerebri).

Aggravating Factors

The worsening of headache as a result of a cough or physical jolt suggests an intracranial element to the pain. Sufferers of cluster headache tend to endure their pain in an agitated state, pacing and moving about, whereas patients with migraine prefer to lie still. Precipitation or marked worsening of headache in the upright position suggests intracranial hypotension. Routine physical activity, light, sound, and smells typically aggravate migraine headaches.

Mitigating Factors

Rest, especially sleep, and avoidance of light and noise tend to benefit the migraineur. Massage, ice, or heat may reduce the pain associated with a tension-type headache. Local application of pressure over the affected eye or ipsilateral temporal artery, the local application of heat or cold, and (rarely) brief intense physical activity may alleviate the pain of cluster headache. Headache due to intracranial hypotension typically is helped by recumbency.

Family History of Headaches

Migraine often is an inherited disorder, and a family history of migraine (sometimes referred to as "sick headaches") is present in about two-thirds of patients. Tension-type headaches also can be familial. Cluster headache characteristically is not inherited. Familial hemiplegic migraine is a rare autosomal dominant variant of migraine with aura, wherein the aura includes hemiparesis lasting minutes to 24 hours.

Prior Evaluation

The patient should be asked about prior consultations and testing. If appropriate, the records and actual imaging studies can be obtained for review.

Prior Treatment

Response to treatment should be sought, including agents used to treat individual headache attacks and those used prophylactically. The dose and duration of each treatment should be reviewed. This information provides an opportunity to determine whether acute medications have been overused and whether prophylactic medications were optimized. A history of the use of caffeine-containing substances also should be elicited because they may cause or aggravate headaches through rebound withdrawal.

Disability

Baseline and follow-up assessment of headache-related disability is helpful in judging the effects of treatment and guiding headache therapy. The Migraine Disability Assessment Scale (MIDAS) is one useful validated clinical tool (Andrasik et al., 2005).

Patient Concerns and Reasons for Seeking Help

Headache pain can produce significant fear and anxiety regarding serious disease. The patient should be allowed to express any concerns so that each can be appropriately addressed.

The question of why the patient is seeking help may be obvious if the problem is of recent onset. If the problem is chronic, however, it can be useful to inquire why the patient has come for aid at this time. Red and yellow flags (see **Box 18.3**) help identify which patients are more likely to have a secondary cause of their pain.

Other Medical or Neurological Problems

A history of past and current medical and neurological conditions, injuries, operations, and medication allergies should be obtained. A list of all current medications and dietary supplements should be recorded. A number of medications can cause headache, including hormonal, cardiovascular, and gastrointestinal agents (De Luca and Bartleson, 2010).

Examination

The examination begins the moment the physician encounters the patient. Careful observation helps determine whether the patient appears ill, anxious, or depressed, and whether the history is reliable. A patient who is unable to give a reasonably coherent history should be suspected of having an abnormal mental status. Although typically the physical examination of the headache patient shows no abnormalities, findings on examination may yield important clues about the underlying cause.

Vital signs, especially blood pressure and pulse, should be assessed. Extremely high blood pressure can cause headache. If there is a question of fever, temperature should be measured. The body habitus should be noted. Patients with pseudotumor cerebri, typically young women, are usually obese. The general examination can include auscultation of the heart and lungs, palpation of the abdomen, and examination of the skin. A neurological examination, including examination of the mental status, gait, cranial nerves, reflexes, and motor and sensory systems, is essential. The skull and cervical spine should be examined. The skull should be palpated for lumps and local tenderness. The area over an infected sinus may be tender. Thickened, tender, irregular temporal arteries with a reduced pulse suggest GCA. In both migraine and tension-type headaches, the scalp may be tender. A short neck or low hairline suggests basilar invagination or a Chiari malformation. In an infant, bulging of the fontanelles suggests increased intracranial pressure, most commonly caused by hydrocephalus. Measuring head circumference is important in a child. The cervical spine also should be tested for tenderness and

mobility. Nuchal rigidity on passive neck flexion and Kernig sign indicate meningeal irritation.

Diagnostic Testing

In most cases, the history, together with the neurological and physical examinations, is all that is needed to make a diagnosis, especially in the patient with long-standing headaches. Migraine, tension-type headaches, and cluster headaches usually can be diagnosed with a high degree of certainty, and it is often possible to proceed directly to management.

In some situations, the diagnosis is uncertain, and additional diagnostic testing should be considered. The worrisome headache "warning flags" that increase the likelihood of a serious underlying intracranial process and often lead to additional testing are listed in **Box 18.3**. Red flags are

---

Box 18.3 Headache Warning Flags

Red Flags

- Head or neck injury
- New onset or new type or worsening pattern of existing headache
- New level of pain (e.g., worst ever)
- Abrupt or split-second onset
- Triggered by Valsalva maneuver or cough
- Triggered by exertion
- Triggered by sexual activity
  - Preorgasmic
  - Orgasmic
- Headache during pregnancy or puerperium
- Age > 50 years
- Neurological signs or symptoms
  - Seizures
  - Confusion
  - Impaired alertness
  - Weakness
  - Papilledema
- Systemic illness
  - Fever
  - Nuchal rigidity
  - Weight loss
  - Scalp artery tenderness
- Secondary risk factors
  - Cancer
  - Immunocompromised host
    - Human immunodeficiency virus (HIV)
    - On immunosuppressants
- Recent travel
  - Domestic
  - Foreign

Yellow Flags

- Wakes patient from sleep at night
- New onset side-locked headaches
- Postural headaches

From De Luca, G.C., Bartleson, J.D., 2010. When and how to investigate the patient with headache. Semin. Neurol. 30, 133–134. Used with permission.

more worrisome than yellow flags. Investigations for evaluation of the patient with headaches include almost all tests used in neurology and neurosurgery, as well as various medical studies. Selection of appropriate tests depends on the diagnostic formulation after the history and examination; indiscriminate use of batteries of tests is unwarranted.

Neuroimaging and Other Imaging Studies
Computed Tomography and Magnetic Resonance Imaging

Computed tomography (CT) and magnetic resonance imaging (MRI) are extremely useful tests in evaluating patients with headache. Tumors, hematomas, cerebral infarctions, abscesses, hydrocephalus, and many meningeal processes can be identified with CT and MRI. Abnormalities of the skull base, craniocervical junction, pituitary gland, meninges, and white matter are better seen with MRI. Advantages of CT over MRI include lower cost, a faster scan for those patients who either cannot remain still or are claustrophobic, compatibility with pacemakers and other implanted metal objects, and widespread availability. The iodinated contrast used in CT has been associated with allergic reactions and contrast-induced nephropathy. The contrast agent used in MRI is less likely to produce allergic reactions or renal damage, but it has been associated with nephrogenic systemic fibrosis, typically in patients with preexisting renal impairment. The imaging modality of choice to investigate various causes of headache is shown in **Box 18.4**.

CT can detect acute subarachnoid hemorrhage in at least 95% of patients if sufficient bleeding has occurred and the patient is scanned promptly. If findings on the CT scan are normal and the history is suggestive of recent subarachnoid hemorrhage, a lumbar puncture should be performed to assess for red blood cells and xanthochromia. CT can be helpful for evaluating abnormalities of the skull, orbit, sinuses, facial bones, and the bony cervical spine. Changes associated with intracranial hypotension are best shown with MRI and include enhancement of the pachymeninges, sagging of the brain, engorged veins, and subdural fluid collections (Schievink, 2008). The cervical spinal cord and exiting nerve roots are much better shown with MRI than with plain CT. Myelography with CT can be used to image the spine as an alternative to MRI. Magnetic resonance angiography is a noninvasive method that can demonstrate intracranial and extracranial vascular occlusive disease including large-vessel dissection, intracranial arteriovenous malformations, and aneurysms. CT angiography also can show arterial disease. Intracranial venous sinus thrombosis is best shown with magnetic resonance venography. For headache that is acute in onset or follows trauma, CT is the optimal imaging study to look for subarachnoid and other intracranial bleeding. For evaluation of patients with subacute and chronic headache, MRI is recommended (Sandrini et al., 2004). MRI is likely to reveal more than CT, but many of the abnormalities will be incidental, including asymptomatic cerebral infarctions, small aneurysms, and benign brain tumors (Vernooij et al., 2007).

Box 18.4 Imaging Modality of Choice to Investigate Causes of Headache

MRI Preferred

Vascular disease:
  Cerebral infarction
  Venous infarction
Neoplastic disease:
  Primary and secondary brain tumors (especially in posterior fossa)
  Skull base tumors
  Meningeal carcinomatosis and lymphomatosis
  Pituitary tumors
Infections:
  Cerebritis and brain abscess
  Meningitis
  Encephalitis
Other:
  Chiari malformation
  Cerebrospinal fluid hypotension with pachymeningeal enhancement and brain sag
  Foramen magnum and upper cervical spine lesions
  Pituitary apoplexy
  Rare encephalopathies and headache (CADASIL*, MELAS[†], SMART[‡])

CT Preferred

Fractures (calvarium)
Acute hemorrhage (subarachnoid, intracerebral)
Paranasal sinus and mastoid air cell disease

Draw between MRI and CT

MR angiography/CT angiography:
  Vasculitis (large and medium sized vessels)
  Intracranial aneurysms
  Carotid and vertebral artery dissections
MR venography/CT venography:
  Cerebral venous thrombosis

CT, Computed tomography; *MRI*, magnetic resonance imaging.
Copyrighted and used with permission of Mayo Foundation for Medical Education and Research.
*CADASIL – cerebral autosomal dominant arteriopathy with subcortical infarcts and leukoencephalopathy.
[†]MELAS – mitochondrial encephalomyopathy, lactic acidosis, and strokelike episodes.
[‡]SMART – strokelike migraine attacks after radiation therapy.

Plain Radiographs of the Skull, Sinuses, and Cervical Spine

Plain x-rays of the skull are unnecessary in the routine evaluation of patients with headache, but they can infrequently be useful in patients with an unusual bony abnormality found on physical examination or in the pediatric population where radiographs may answer the clinical questions without exposing the child to higher doses of radiation used with CT. Although plain radiographs of the sinuses can show infection, hemorrhage, fracture, or tumor, CT provides much greater definition and has become the test of choice for these conditions. The role of the cervical spine in causing headaches remains uncertain, but occipitonuchal pain may result from degenerative disk and joint disease of the mid- and upper cervical spine. Rheumatoid arthritis and ankylosing spondylitis can lead to craniocervical junction instability and pain. Tomographic images or CT may be needed to show bony changes in the upper cervical spine and craniocervical junction. Flexion and extension, odontoid, and pillar views of the cervical spine can help exclude ligamentous damage and fractures in patients with a history of head and neck injury. Congenital abnormalities of the cervical spine, such as the Klippel-Feil syndrome, may be associated with other disorders such as a Chiari malformation.

Temporomandibular Joint/Dental Imaging Studies

Panoramic x-ray examination, MRI, or CT of the temporomandibular joints may be helpful in selected patients. The presence of temporomandibular joint disease should not be taken as proof that the patient's headaches are related. Dental radiographs are useful if a dental origin for the pain is suspected.

Cerebral Angiography

Cerebral angiography is rarely needed in the initial investigation of headache. It can be helpful in confirming vascular disease including arterial dissections, arteriovenous malformations, intracranial aneurysms, and CNS vasculitis.

Myelography with Computed Tomography and Radioisotope Studies for Detection of Cerebrospinal Fluid Leaks

In addition to MRI of the brain and spine, myelography with CT and isotope cisternography (typically with indium-111) can be helpful in determining the presence and location of a spontaneous, posttraumatic, or postoperative CSF leak.

Cerebrospinal Fluid Tests

CSF examination can diagnose or exclude meningitis, encephalitis, subarachnoid hemorrhage, and leptomeningeal cancer and lymphoma. It can also document increased or decreased intracranial pressure and confirm the diagnosis of "*h*ea*d*ache and *n*eurological *d*eficits with CSF *l*ymphocytosis" (HaNDL) (Gomez-Aranda et al., 1997). Measurement of the opening CSF pressure should always be performed.

Electrophysiological Testing

Electroencephalography is not useful in the investigation of headache unless the patient also has a history of seizures, syncope, or episodes of altered awareness (Sandrini et al., 2004). There is no indication for use of evoked potentials in evaluating the patient with headache (Sandrini et al., 2004).

General Medical Tests

A few blood tests are important in the investigation of headache. Elevation of the erythrocyte sedimentation rate (ESR), often to 100 mm per hour or higher, is frequently seen in GCA. A normal ESR does not exclude the condition, because 4% of patients with positive findings on temporal artery biopsy have a normal ESR (Smetana et al., 2002). C-reactive protein and platelet count are also often elevated in patients with GCA. Rarely, episodic headaches associated with unusual behavior or impairment of consciousness can suggest an insulinoma, which is supported by elevated serum insulin and C-peptide levels in the face of a low or relatively low fasting glucose level. Levels of carboxyhemoglobin can be measured in patients complaining of early morning headaches during the home heating season, especially when several members of the same household are affected. Drug and alcohol screening may be helpful in certain patients. Thyroid function should be checked in patients with chronic headache, because hypothyroidism can present with headaches. Plasma and urine levels of catecholamines and metanephrines should be measured if a pheochromocytoma is suspected.

Rarely, cigarette smokers can present with face pain that includes the ear and is due to an underlying ipsilateral lung tumor without CNS involvement. Chest radiograph or CT of the chest can confirm the diagnosis (Eross et al., 2003).

Special Examinations and Consultations

In patients who wake from sleep with headache without other reason for awakening, polysomnography can be performed to look for a treatable sleep disorder such as sleep apnea.

Formal visual field testing can be useful. Tonometry can document elevated intraocular pressure in glaucoma, but unless the eye is red or the cornea is cloudy, glaucoma is an uncommon cause of head or even eye pain. These tests are routinely done by ophthalmologists, who also have the equipment and expertise to perform slit-lamp and other specialized examinations. If pain of dental or temporomandibular joint origin is suspected, an oral surgeon or dentist skilled in the detection and treatment of these disorders should be consulted. Diagnosis of tumors of the sinuses, nasopharynx, and neck, as well as inflammation of the sinuses, is aided by consultation with an otorhinolaryngologist. Temporal artery biopsy is performed to confirm or exclude GCA. In some selected cases (e.g., headaches as a manifestation of a chronic pain disorder or a history of drug abuse), psychiatric consultation may be helpful in diagnosis and management.

Further Observation

Sometimes a definitive diagnosis cannot be reached despite a careful history, thorough examination, and appropriate investigations. In such cases, further observation, with or without a trial of therapy, often reveals the diagnosis.

References

The complete reference list is available online at www.expertconsult.com.

Brainstem Syndromes

Michael Wall

Other chapters in this book that deal with symptoms emphasize history as the starting point for generating possibilities for the differential diagnosis. This list of diagnostic considerations is then refined during the examination. This chapter calls for a different approach. When the neurologist evaluates a patient with a brainstem disorder, often the most effective method of diagnosis is to organize the differential diagnosis around the objective physical findings, particularly in patients with an altered mental status such as coma. The symptoms are still integrated in the approach, but the physical findings take center stage.

Organization around physical findings is efficient because very specific neurological localization, which limits the diagnostic alternatives, often is possible. The long tracts of the nervous system traverse the entire brainstem in the longitudinal (rostrocaudal) plane. Cranial nerve nuclei and their respective cranial nerves originate and exit at distinct levels of the brainstem. This arrangement allows for exquisite localization of function based on the findings of the neurological examination.

The chapter begins with a discussion of the brainstem ocular motor syndromes, followed by descriptions of miscellaneous brainstem, brainstem stroke, diencephalic, and thalamic syndromes.

Ocular Motor Syndromes

Combined Vertical Gaze Ophthalmoplegia

Combined vertical gaze ophthalmoplegia is defined as paresis of both upward and downward gaze. Vertical gaze ophthalmoplegia is an example of a brainstem syndrome in which

the objective physical findings dictate the diagnostic approach to the problem. Symptoms of vertical gaze ophthalmoplegia, when present, are relatively nonspecific and usually occur in patients who have difficulty looking down, as required in reading, eating from a table, and walking down a flight of stairs. In addition, the patient's report of symptoms may be unobtainable because of mental status changes caused by dysfunction of the reticular formation that lies adjacent to the vertical gaze generator in the rostral midbrain (see Chapter 35).

The neurological examination discloses associated signs of the disorders listed in the differential diagnosis (see **Box 19.1**) (Graff-Redford et al., 1985). Coma may be associated with reticular system involvement. Long-tract signs and loss of pupillary reflexes are commonly associated. The syndrome of combined vertical gaze ophthalmoplegia is diagnosed when the ocular findings occur in isolation from long-tract signs.

With combined vertical gaze ophthalmoplegia, vertical saccades and pursuit are lost. This gaze limitation may be overcome by the oculocephalic (doll's head or doll's eye) maneuver, which tests the vestibulo-ocular reflex (VOR) (see Chapter 35). It is demonstrated by having the patient focus on an object and rotating the patient's head; a conjugate eye movement in the opposite direction is the expected response with this maneuver. The Bell phenomenon (reflex movement of the eyes up and out in response to forced eye closure) often is absent. Skew deviation (vertical malalignment of the eyes) may occur. Absence of convergence and loss of pupillary reactions to light are common.

The location of the lesion of combined vertical gaze ophthalmoplegia is the rostral interstitial nucleus of the medial longitudinal fasciculus (riMLF) for loss of vertical pursuit and

Box 19.1 Differential Diagnosis for Combined Vertical Gaze Ophthalmoplegia

Stroke:
  Ischemic
  Hemorrhagic
PSP
Corticobasal ganglionic degeneration
AVM
MS
Thalamic and mesencephalic tumors
Whipple disease
Syphilis
Vasculitis (e.g., systemic lupus erythematosus)
Metabolic disorders:
  Lipid storage diseases
  Wilson disease
  Kernicterus
Wernicke encephalopathy

AVM, Arteriovenous malformation; *MS*, multiple sclerosis; *PSP*, progressive supranuclear palsy.

Box 19.2 Differential Diagnosis for Dorsal Midbrain Syndrome

Pineal tumors
Stroke:
  Ischemic cerebrovascular disease
  Thalamic hemorrhage
Trauma
Hydrocephalus
MS
Transtentorial herniation
Congenital aqueductal stenosis
Metastatic tumors
Infections:
  Encephalitis
  Cysticercosis
Midbrain AVM
Stereotactic midbrain surgery
Metabolic disorders:
  Lipid storage disease
  Wilson disease
  Kernicterus
Wernicke encephalopathy

AVM, Arteriovenous malformation; *MS*, multiple sclerosis.

saccades (Leigh and Zee, 2006). **Box 19.1** lists the disorders involving the rostral mesodiencephalic region (for the differential diagnosis) that cause combined vertical gaze ophthalmoplegia (see Chapter 35). The most common causes of isolated combined vertical gaze ophthalmoplegia are stroke and progressive supranuclear palsy (PSP). In cortical-basal ganglionic degeneration, ocular motility findings are similar to those in PSP but are less severe. Whereas the supranuclear vertical gaze ophthalmoplegia may be prominent early in the course of PSP, obvious vertical and horizontal gaze restriction usually is a late finding in cortical-basal ganglionic degeneration (Rottach et al., 1996).

The diagnostic formulation varies with the age of the patient. Isolated combined vertical gaze ophthalmoplegia usually is due to infarction of the rostral dorsal midbrain. When onset is gradual instead of abrupt or if the patient is young, other disorders should be considered (see **Box 19.1**). In the elderly, PSP (see Chapter 66) is likely if the onset is gradual. PSP can be mimicked by the treatable Whipple disease (Averbuch-Heller et al., 1999). For Whipple disease, the movement disorder, oculomasticatory myorhythmia, is pathognomonic. Laboratory investigations used to evaluate combined vertical gaze ophthalmoplegia include computed tomography (CT) scan or, preferably, magnetic resonance imaging (MRI). Care should be taken not to overlook lesions inferior to the floor of the third ventricle. Lumbar puncture (LP), syphilis serology, erythrocyte sedimentation rate, and an antinuclear antibody test complete the evaluation when the cause is not obvious. Small-bowel biopsy should be considered if Whipple disease is a possible diagnosis. A polymerase chain reaction (PCR) assay of small-bowel biopsy specimen, cerebrospinal fluid (CSF), or other tissues for the 16S ribosomal ribonucleic acid (RNA) gene of *Tropheryma whippelii* appears to have both sensitivity and specificity for the diagnosis of Whipple disease (Lee, 2002).

Upgaze Paresis (Dorsal Midbrain or Parinaud Syndrome)

Another brainstem syndrome that often occurs without symptoms is the dorsal midbrain syndrome. When symptoms do occur, the patient has difficulty looking up and may have blurry distant vision caused by accommodative spasm.

The tetrad of findings in the dorsal midbrain syndrome are (1) loss of upgaze, which usually is supranuclear (loss of pursuit and saccades with preservation of the VOR); (2) normal to large pupils with light-near dissociation (loss of the light reaction with preservation of pupilloconstriction in response to a near target) or pupillary areflexia; (3) convergence-retraction nystagmus, in which the eyes make convergent and retracting oscillations after an upward saccade; and (4) lid retraction.

The location of the lesion causing the upgaze paresis of the dorsal midbrain syndrome is the posterior commissure and its interstitial nucleus (Leigh and Zee, 2006). The presence of the full syndrome implies a lesion of the dorsal midbrain (including the posterior commissure), a bilateral lesion of the pretectal region, or a large unilateral tegmental lesion.

The differential diagnosis is presented in **Box 19.2**. Other than the mild upgaze limitation that occurs with age, the most common cause of loss of upgaze is a tumor of the pineal region. The next most common causes are stroke and trauma. The upgaze palsy portion of the syndrome can be mimicked by any of several conditions: double elevator palsy, PSP, orbital causes such as thyroid ophthalmopathy and the bilateral Brown superior oblique tendon sheath syndrome, pseudo–dorsal midbrain syndrome secondary to myasthenia gravis (MG) or Guillain-Barré syndrome, and congenital upgaze limitation. Forced ductions (see Chapter 16) may be performed by grasping anesthetized sclera with forceps and moving the globe through its range of motion. The presence of restriction of movement with forced ductions implies a lesion within the orbit, as distinct from a midbrain lesion.

The diagnostic formulation for the dorsal midbrain syndrome varies with age. In children and adolescents, pineal region tumors usually are the cause. In young and middle-aged adults, the disorder is uncommon, and the cause may be trauma, multiple sclerosis (MS), or arteriovenous malformation (AVM). In the elderly, stroke and PSP are the most common causes.

The laboratory investigation needed to evaluate dorsal midbrain syndrome is MRI. If no tumor is present and an infectious or inflammatory cause is suspected, an LP should be performed.

Downgaze Paresis

Isolated downgaze paresis is uncommon. Symptoms, when they occur, are related to difficulty in reading, eating, and walking down stairs.

Neurological examination reveals loss of downward pursuit and saccades, although occasionally pursuit may be spared. The vertical oculocephalic maneuver may be normal or may disclose gaze limitation. Convergence may be lost, and gaze-evoked upbeat nystagmus may be present on upward gaze. In young patients, forced ductions should be evaluated for evidence of congenital downgaze limitation.

The site of the lesion for isolated downgaze paresis is bilateral involvement of the lateral portions of the riMLF. The main considerations in the differential diagnosis are ischemic stroke, PSP, and Whipple disease. Laboratory investigations to support the clinical diagnosis include CT or preferably MRI. Lesions may be detected in the rostral mesodiencephalic junction inferior to the floor of the third ventricle.

The diagnostic formulation for isolated downgaze limitation is uncomplicated. When acute in onset, this disorder usually is due to ischemic cerebrovascular disease. In an elderly patient with a progressive course, PSP should be considered.

Internuclear Ophthalmoplegia

Internuclear ophthalmoplegia (INO) is characterized by paresis of adduction of one eye, with horizontal nystagmus in the contralateral eye when it is abducted. It is due to a lesion of the MLF ipsilateral to the side of the adduction weakness.

Surprisingly, most patients with INO have no symptoms. The symptoms that may be associated with INO are diplopia, oscillopsia of one of the two images, and blurred vision. When diplopia is present, it is due to medial rectus paresis (horizontal diplopia) or skew deviation (vertical diplopia).

The MLF carries information for vertical pursuit and the vertical VOR. Consequently, other associated findings with MLF lesions are abnormal vertical smooth pursuit and impaired reflex vertical eye movements (doll's eye maneuver, Bell phenomenon). Voluntary vertical eye movements (pursuit and saccades) are unaffected. Gaze-evoked vertical nystagmus (usually on upgaze) and skew deviation may be present with the higher eye usually present on the side of the lesion. Skew deviation is a pure vertical ocular deviation that is not due to a cranial nerve palsy, orbital lesion, or strabismus but is caused by disturbed supranuclear input to the third and fourth

cranial nerve nuclei. It is thought to be due to unilateral damage to the otolith-ocular pathways or the pathways mediating the VOR (Zwergal et al., 2008).

Internuclear ophthalmoplegia, discussed further in Chapter 35, may occur as a false localizing sign. Brainstem compression due to subdural hematoma with transtentorial herniation and cerebellar masses may cause INO. Myasthenia gravis and Guillain-Barré syndrome also may simulate INO.

The diagnostic considerations are many and varied. Examination can differentiate a lesion of the MLF from a partial third cranial nerve palsy, MG, strabismus, or thyroid ophthalmopathy. The common causes of INO are stroke (including vertebral artery dissection) in older age groups and MS in the young. Keane's series (Keane, 2005) from a large inner-city hospital reveals that approximately one third of INO cases are due to stroke, one third to MS, and one third to other causes. The less common causes include trauma, herniation, infections, tumor, vasculitis, and surgical procedures.

Laboratory investigations that are performed to elucidate the cause include MRI. Thin cuts are often needed to find the lesion when INO is isolated. An edrophonium (Tensilon) test should be performed to evaluate for MG unless there are associated signs of obligatory brainstem dysfunction.

The diagnostic formulation for INO first necessitates accurate localization of the lesion. Limitation of adduction initially is formulated simply as an adduction deficit. It may be due to (1) a lesion of the midbrain or third cranial nerve disrupting innervation, (2) a disorder of the neuromuscular junction (MG), or (3) a lesion directly involving the medial rectus muscle.

Horizontal Gaze Paresis

Although there are no common symptoms of horizontal gaze paresis, this condition seldom occurs in isolation. Patients may complain of inability to see or to look to the side. Because supranuclear gaze pareses are conjugate by definition, diplopia does not occur.

On examination, with unilateral isolated involvement of the paramedian pontine reticular formation (PPRF), loss of ipsilateral saccades and pursuit is evident. However, full horizontal eye movements are demonstrated with the oculocephalic maneuver.

Lesions of the sixth cranial nerve nucleus cause horizontal gaze paresis with inability of the oculocephalic maneuver to overcome the gaze limitation. Although an associated ipsilateral peripheral facial palsy is usually associated from involvement of the fascicle of the seventh cranial nerve coursing over the sixth cranial nerve nucleus, cases of isolated horizontal gaze paresis caused by sixth nerve nuclear lesions have been reported (Miller et al., 2002). With bilateral lesions, loss or limitation of horizontal saccades and (usually) pursuit in both directions is characteristic. Gaze-paretic nystagmus may be present. In the acute phase, transient vertical gaze paresis and vertical nystagmus or upgaze paresis can occur. In the chronic phase, vertical eye movements are full, although nystagmus may be noted on upgaze.

The location of the lesion for horizontal gaze paresis is the frontopontine tract, mesencephalic reticular formation, PPRF, and sixth cranial nerve nucleus. The explanation of gaze palsy occurring with a nuclear lesion is given later in the chapter (see Syndromes Involving Ocular Motor Nuclei).

The diagnostic possibilities are varied. As with other ocular motility disorders, MG may cause gaze limitation that simulates a central nervous system (CNS) lesion. The diagnostic formulation varies with age, rapidity of onset, and associated clinical findings. For patients with an acute onset who are older than 50 years of age, cerebrovascular disease, ischemic or hemorrhagic, is a likely cause. With a subacute onset before the age of 50 years, a diagnosis of MS should be considered. Congenital cases usually are due to Möbius syndrome. Systemic lupus erythematosus (SLE), syphilis, and Wernicke encephalopathy should be considered for any acquired cases.

Laboratory investigations for horizontal gaze paresis should include MRI. If there are no obligatory signs of CNS dysfunction, MG has to be considered.

Global Paralysis of Gaze

The characteristic symptom of global paralysis of gaze is an inability to look voluntarily (saccades and pursuit) in any direction. Global paralysis of gaze rarely occurs in isolation, however, and signs and symptoms of involvement of other local structures usually are present.

The location of the lesion is the frontopontine tract for saccades, and the parieto-occipitopontine tract for pursuit, where they converge at the subthalamic and upper midbrain level (Thurtell and Halmagyi, 2008). The differential diagnosis for total ophthalmoplegia is given in **Box 19.3**. The common causes for this presentation are diseases outside the CNS, such as Guillain-Barré syndrome, MG, and chronic progressive external ophthalmoplegia (CPEO); for intraaxial lesions, considerations include stroke, Wernicke encephalopathy, and PSP.

The diagnostic formulation usually is concerned with extra-axial (cranial nerve, neuromuscular junction, or muscle) pathology, because isolated complete ophthalmoplegia is rarely caused by a brainstem lesion. Myasthenia gravis (sometimes in combination with thyroid ophthalmopathy), bilateral cavernous sinus metastases (Ebert et al., 2009), and Guillain-Barré syndrome are more likely possibilities if the onset is subacute. If the presentation is long-standing, slowly progressive,

---

Box 19.3 Differential Diagnosis for Total Ophthalmoplegia

Oculomotor apraxia
Guillain-Barré syndrome
MG
Thyroid ophthalmopathy (especially in combination with MG)
Chronic progressive external ophthalmoplegia syndromes
Wilson disease
Pituitary apoplexy
Botulism
Tetanus
PSP
Anticonvulsant intoxication
Wernicke encephalopathy
Acute bilateral pontine or mesodiencephalic lesions

MG, Myasthenia gravis; *PSP*, progressive supranuclear palsy.

---

and accompanied by eyelid ptosis, the CPEO syndromes, such as Kearns-Sayre syndrome, should be considered. In these extraaxial disorders, oculocephalic reflexes do not overcome the gaze limitations. PSP is a diagnostic possibility in the elderly, whereas Wernicke encephalopathy should be considered in alcoholics and nutritionally deprived patients. Whipple disease also can cause this rare clinical presentation.

Laboratory investigations for patients with global paralysis of gaze should include MRI. An edrophonium test is performed when MG is suspected. When botulism is suspected, electromyography with repetitive stimulation and serum assay for botulinum toxin should be performed.

One-and-a-Half Syndrome

The one-and-a-half syndrome is characterized by a gaze palsy on looking toward the side of the lesion, together with INO on looking away from the lesion. The common symptoms are diplopia, oscillopsia (the illusion that objects or scenes are oscillating), and blurred vision. Associated findings are skew deviation and gaze-evoked nystagmus on upgaze or lateral gaze, and less commonly on downgaze. Acutely, in the primary position there may be exotropia (one eye deviated outward). Other features may include limitation of upgaze, saccadic vertical pursuit, and loss of convergence.

The location of the lesion is the PPRF or sixth cranial nerve nucleus, with extension to involve the internuclear fibers crossing from the contralateral sixth cranial nerve nucleus, which causes the INO. Entities to consider in the differential diagnosis include MS, stroke, AVM, and tumor of the lower pons. A pseudo–one-and-a-half syndrome may occur with MG or Guillain-Barré syndrome. The diagnostic formulation for the one-and-a-half syndrome is similar to that for INO. Before the age of 50 years, the cause usually is MS; after age 50, it usually is cerebrovascular disease.

Appropriate laboratory investigations for the one-and-a-half syndrome are MRI and, if indicated, LP.

Syndromes Involving Ocular Motor Nuclei

Patients with lesions of the third or sixth cranial nerve nucleus not only present with accompanying long-tract signs but also show different ocular motility disturbances than with lesions of the third or sixth cranial nerve.

Third Cranial Nerve Nucleus

The common manifestations of nuclear third cranial nerve palsies are diplopia and ptosis. The signs present on the side of the lesion are weakness of the inferior and medial recti and the inferior oblique muscles. Upgaze limitation is present in both eyes because the superior rectus subnucleus is contralateral, and the axons cross within the nuclear complex. In addition, ptosis and dilated unreactive pupils may be present on both sides because the levator subnucleus and Edinger-Westphal nuclei are bilaterally represented.

To localize a lesion to the third cranial nerve nucleus, both eyes must have some involvement because of the bilateral representation. The superior rectus and levator of the eyelid, however, are bilaterally represented and thus cannot demonstrate single muscle involvement. In addition, because the medial rectus subnucleus is in the most ventral portion of the nucleus and all of the dorsal subnuclei send axons through it, single muscle involvement of the medial rectus may not be possible. The eyelid levator subnucleus may be spared because it is located at the dorsocaudal periphery of the nuclear complex.

Main considerations in the differential diagnosis are stroke (either ischemic or hemorrhagic), metastatic tumor, and MS. Of these diagnoses, only ischemic stroke is common. Disorders that simulate nuclear third cranial nerve palsy are MG, CPEO, thyroid ophthalmopathy, and Guillain-Barré syndrome.

The pertinent laboratory investigation for this syndrome is MRI, which usually demonstrates the ischemic cerebrovascular lesion. Once the proper localization has been made, the diagnostic formulation is straightforward.

Sixth Cranial Nerve Nucleus

The sixth cranial nerve nucleus has two populations of neurons. The abducens motor neurons terminate on the ipsilateral lateral rectus muscle. Internuclear neurons cross at the level of the sixth cranial nerve nucleus, join the MLF, and terminate on the medial rectus subnucleus of the third cranial nerve. Accordingly, a lesion of the sixth cranial nerve nucleus causes ipsilateral gaze palsy.

Patients with isolated horizontal gaze paresis usually are asymptomatic. If they do have symptoms, they complain of difficulty looking to one side. On examination, conjugate horizontal gaze paresis is present that is not overcome by an oculocephalic maneuver or caloric stimulation. This occurs because the fibers mediating this response, the VOR, synapse in the sixth cranial nerve nucleus. A peripheral seventh cranial nerve palsy invariably accompanies a lesion of the sixth cranial nerve nucleus. Considerations in the differential diagnosis include stroke (Miller et al., 2002), Wernicke encephalopathy, MS, and a tumor of the pontomedullary junction.

Laboratory investigations for evaluating a lesion of the sixth cranial nerve nucleus are MRI, possibly LP, and an edrophonium or prostigmine test for MG if there are none of the long-tract signs obligatory for intraaxial disease.

Other Brainstem and Associated Syndromes

Diencephalic Syndrome (Russell Syndrome)

The common symptoms of diencephalic syndrome are emaciation with increased appetite, euphoria, vomiting, and excessive sweating (Fleischman et al., 2005). Patients also may have an alert appearance with motor hyperactivity. Most cases occur in children younger than 3 years.

The differential diagnosis at this stage should encompass hyperthyroidism, diabetes mellitus, a tumor in the region of fourth ventricle, vein of Galen malformation, and a hypothalamic tumor. Most patients appear pale despite lack of anemia. Ophthalmological findings include optic atrophy and, less commonly, nystagmus.

Laboratory investigations for diencephalic syndrome may show an elevated serum growth hormone level that is incompletely suppressed by hyperglycemia. MRI usually demonstrates a hypothalamic mass lesion. Malignant cells may be present in the CSF, which are diagnostic. The CSF also may contain human chorionic gonadotropin in cases of germinomas. A lumbar puncture should not be performed if neuroimaging studies demonstrate a mass effect.

Thalamic Syndrome

Thalamic syndrome was first described by Dejerine and Roussy in 1906. The common symptoms of this syndrome are pain (thalamic pain), numbness, and hemisensory loss. The pain may be spontaneous or evoked by any form of stimulation. It often has a disagreeable and lasting quality. Patients also may complain of a distorted sense of taste. Right thalamic lesions appear to predominate.

On examination, a marked hemianesthesia is present which may be dissociated; that is, pain and temperature or light touch and vibration sense may be separately lost. Proprioceptive loss, often with astereognosis, is a usual feature. A transitory hemiparesis sometimes occurs.

The usual location of the lesion for this type of pain is the ventroposterolateral nucleus of the thalamus. In addition to the thalamus, thalamic-type pain can occur with lesions of the parietal lobe, medial lemniscus, and dorsolateral medulla (MacGowan et al., 1997). The differential diagnosis is between stroke and tumor. The diagnostic formulation depends on the rate of onset of symptoms, associated signs, and findings on neuroimaging studies. The apoplectic onset of symptoms implicates cerebrovascular disease. Gradual onset with progressive worsening of symptoms and signs is characteristic of brain tumor. Neuroimaging studies should confirm the clinical impression. The imaging modality of choice is MRI.

Tectal Deafness

The symptoms associated with tectal deafness are bilateral deafness associated with other related CNS symptoms such as poor coordination, weakness, or vertigo. The main considerations in the differential diagnosis for the deafness are conduction-type hearing loss, cochlear disorders, bilateral eighth cranial nerve lesions, tectal deafness, and pure word deafness.

On examination, deafness that usually spares pure tones is confirmed. Pure word deafness with lesions of the inferior colliculi has been reported (Vitte et al., 2002). Other brainstem signs, including the dorsal midbrain syndrome, often are associated. The location of the lesion is the inferior colliculi; the most common causes are trauma, stroke, or a tumor of the brainstem, cerebellum, or pineal region. The diagnostic formulation for hearing loss caused by lesions rostral to the cochlear nuclei is the presence of hearing loss characterized by sparing of pure tone, with marked deterioration when background noise distortion or competing messages are added. In addition, signs of damage to adjacent nervous system structures are present. Neuroimaging studies may confirm the diagnosis.

The pertinent laboratory investigations include MRI and an audiogram. Tests that reveal CNS auditory loss are distorted speech audiometry, dichotic auditory testing, and auditory brainstem evoked responses, although findings on the last test may be normal (Vitte et al., 2002).

Foramen Magnum Syndrome

Foramen magnum syndrome is characterized by upper motor neuron–type weakness and sensory loss in any modality below the head. Detecting this syndrome is important because it often is caused by benign tumors such as meningiomas or fibromas, which may be removed completely when detected early in their course. Its only manifestations may be those of a high spinal cord syndrome (see Chapter 24).

The common initial symptoms typically are neck stiffness and pain, which may radiate into the shoulder. Occipital headache also may be an early symptom. Other common symptoms are weakness of the upper or lower extremities, numbness (most commonly of hands or arms), clumsiness, and a gait disturbance.

Considerations in the differential diagnosis at this stage include cervical spondylosis, syringomyelia, MS, transverse myelitis, atlantoaxial subluxation, Chiari malformation, and foramen magnum or upper cervical cord tumor.

On examination, hemiparesis or quadriparesis and sensory loss are common. The loss of sensation may involve all modalities. It may be dissociated and capelike or may occur in a C2 distribution. Some patients have a hemisensory pattern below the cranium or involvement of only the lower extremities.

Pseudoathetosis resulting from loss of joint position sense may be an early sign. Atrophy of muscles of the upper extremities may occur at levels well below the lesion (e.g., intrinsic muscles of the hands). Electric shock–like sensations radiating down the spine, which may be transmitted into the extremities, may occur with neck flexion (Lhermitte sign). This phenomenon may occur with lesions of the posterior columns, most commonly MS. Lower cranial nerve palsies are less common. The presence of downbeat nystagmus in primary position or lateral gaze strongly suggests a lesion of the craniocervical junction. This sign may be missed unless the eyelids are manually elevated and the nystagmus is sought when the patient gazes laterally and slightly downward.

The differential diagnosis at this stage is focused on a foramen magnum or upper cervical cord tumor. The tumor type usually is meningioma, neurofibroma, glioma, or metastasis. Cervical spondylosis, MS, syringobulbia, and the Chiari malformation (often accompanied by a syrinx) are other diagnostic considerations. The definitive laboratory investigation for evaluation of the foramen magnum syndrome is MRI.

Patients with foramen magnum tumors may have a relapsing-remitting clinical course with features that simulate those of MS. Because many of these tumors are meningiomas, the clinician should be alert for patients at risk. Meningiomas occur with increased frequency in women in their childbearing years and increase in size during pregnancy. Cervical spondylosis usually is associated with a related radiculopathy and is not accompanied by downbeat nystagmus or lower cranial nerve abnormalities. Diagnosis requires a high index of suspicion early in the patient's course. Foramen magnum tumors are known to present difficult diagnostic problems because signs may be minimal despite a large tumor.

Syringobulbia

Syringobulbia is a disorder of the lower brainstem caused by progressive enlargement of a fluid-filled cavity that involves the medulla and almost invariably the spinal cord (syringomyelia). The symptoms and signs are primarily those of a disorder of the central spinal cord region (see Syringomyelia in Chapter 73).

The common symptoms of syringobulbia and syringomyelia are lack of pain with accidental burns, hand numbness, neck and arm pain, leg stiffness, and headache, together with oscillopsia, diplopia, or vertigo. On examination, signs of lower brainstem dysfunction are evident. Lower motor neuron signs of the ninth through twelfth cranial nerves may be present. Nystagmus, if present, is horizontal, vertical, or rotatory. Signs of a spinal cord lesion characteristically coexist. In the upper extremities, dissociated anesthesia of an upper limb or forequarter (i.e., loss of pain and temperature sensation with sparing of other modalities) may be noted. The sensory loss also may be in a hemisensory distribution. Absence of or decreased deep tendon reflexes in the upper extremities are the rule.

Spastic paraparesis, usually asymmetrical, may occur. Loss of facial sensation can occur in an onionskin pattern emanating from the corner of the mouth. Charcot (neuropathic) joints and trophic skin disorders may be features in long-standing cases. Horner syndrome and bowel and bladder disturbances are other occasional findings.

The lesion is located in a rostrocaudal longitudinal cavity from the medulla into the spinal cord. The cavity usually is located near the fourth ventricle or central canal of the spinal cord. The definitive laboratory investigation for syringobulbia is MRI, the most reliable and sensitive test to demonstrate a syrinx.

The main considerations in the differential diagnosis are an intrinsic central cord and lower brainstem lesion (syrinx, tumor, or trauma) and compressive foramen magnum syndrome caused by a tumor. Less likely causes are MS and spinal arachnoiditis.

The diagnostic formulation for syringobulbia is based on data from the history, examination, and laboratory evaluation. It usually is a disease of young adults, with a peak incidence in the third and fourth decades of life. Painless burns and dissociated segmental anesthesia of the upper extremities are of major diagnostic significance. A diagnosis of MS requires the presence of other noncontiguous lesions, oligoclonal bands in the CSF, and characteristic MRI findings. Tumors usually produce a more rapid course.

Brainstem Ischemic Stroke Syndromes

Vertebrobasilar ischemic lesions often have a rostrocaudal or patchy localization (**Fig. 19.1**), rather than the simplified transverse localization that usually is schematized (Kubik and Adams, 1946). In addition, all of the clinical features may not be explainable in anatomical terms; that is, clinicopathological correlation may not be precise.

The cardinal manifestations of brainstem stroke are involvement of the long tracts of the brainstem in combination

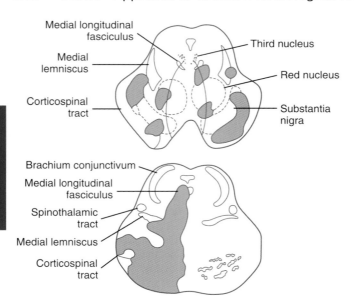

Fig. 19.1 A postmortem examination of a patient with embolism of the basilar artery. Note the rostrocaudal extension of the infarction, along with its patchy nature. *(Reprinted with permission from Kubik, C.S., Adams, R.D., 1946. Occlusion of the basilar artery: a clinical and pathological study. Brain 59, 73-121.)*

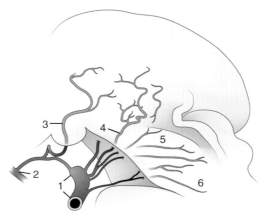

Fig. 19.2 Branches of the basilar communicating artery as seen in a sagittal section of the brainstem: thalamic polar (1), posterior communicating (2), posterior thalamosubthalamic paramedian (3), superior paramedian (4), inferior paramedian (5), and mesencephalic paramedian (6). *(Reprinted with permission from Percheron, G., 1976. Les artères et territoires du thalamus humain: II. Artères et territoires thalamiques paramédians de l'artère basilare communicante. Rev Neurol 132, 309-324.)*

with cranial nerve deficits. Crossed cranial nerve and motor or sensory long-tract deficits are characteristic. The cranial nerve palsy is ipsilateral to the lesion, and the long-tract signs are contralateral—hence the term *crossed*. Coma, ataxia, and vertigo, which are common with vertebrobasilar stroke, are uncommon with internal carotid artery circulation stroke. INO, unreactive pupils, lower motor neuron cranial nerve impairment, and ocular skew deviation, when caused by stroke, occur only with posterior circulation lesions. The same is usually true for nystagmus and most other ocular oscillations.

Another characteristic of vertebrobasilar ischemia is bilateral involvement of the long tracts. This can result in locked-in syndrome. This syndrome, usually caused by a lesion of the basis pontis, is characterized by quadriplegia with corticobulbar tract involvement and loss of the ability to produce speech. The reticular activating system is spared, so consciousness is preserved. Eye movements or blinking may be all that is left under voluntary control.

Another manifestation of bilateral lesions of the long tracts is pseudobulbar palsy. The symptoms resemble those that occur with lesions of the medulla (bulb). Cranial nerve nuclei have been disconnected from cortical input, however, which causes dysarthria, dysphagia, bilateral facial weakness, extremity weakness, and emotional lability. A more descriptive term for this syndrome is *supranuclear bulbar palsy*.

Blindness occurs with bilateral posterior cerebral artery occlusion and concomitant occipital lobe infarction.

Ischemic stroke syndromes are outlined next. These syndromes occur in isolation, as presented here, and in combination. The combinations can be medial, with lateral or often rostrocaudal extension. Several classic stroke syndromes, such as Wallenberg later medullary syndrome and Weber cerebral peduncle syndrome, exist. However, an investigation that looked prospectively at 304 cases of brainstem stroke found

1 of 24 named syndromes in only 20. About 20% of cases showed different unnamed crossed brainstem syndromes (Marx and Thomke, 2009).

Thalamic Stroke Syndromes

The blood supply of the thalamus is from the posterior cerebral, posterior communicating, basilar communicating (**Fig. 19.2**), and anterior and posterior choroidal arteries. Thalamic stroke syndromes are listed in **Table 19.1**. **Fig. 19.3** illustrates the five arterial territories of the thalamus.

Midbrain Stroke Syndromes

Ischemia of the midbrain is characterized by long-tract signs combined with involvement of the third and fourth cranial nerves (Bogousslavsky et al., 1994). Supratentorial (anterior circulation) stroke syndromes may manifest with midbrain signs when rostrocaudal deterioration occurs, causing transtentorial herniation. Classifications of the blood supply to the brainstem are numerous, and this variability is nowhere more apparent than in the midbrain.

Blood flows to the upper mesencephalon via perforating branches of the basilar communicating artery. The basilar communicating artery (P1 segment of the posterior cerebral artery or mesencephalic artery) connects the basilar artery with the posterior communicating artery. A simplified scheme used here divides the vascular territories into medial and lateral transverse regions.

The medial midbrain syndromes are characterized by an ipsilateral third cranial nerve palsy associated with a contralateral hemiparesis. Loss of the discriminative sensations (proprioception, vibration, and stereognosis) with involvement of the medial lemniscus may occur. The lateral syndromes are composed of contralateral loss of pain and temperature sensation and ipsilateral Horner syndrome and loss of facial sensation. Ataxia may occur on either side. Ischemic stroke syndromes of the mesencephalon are outlined in **Table 19.2**,

Table 19.1 Ischemic Stroke Syndromes of the Diencephalon

ANTEROLATERAL	LATERAL AND POSTERIOR INTERNAL CAPSULE
Common Symptoms	***Common Symptoms***

Contralateral weakness, vision loss
Confusion
Disorientation
Language disturbance
	Contralateral:
	  Hemiparesis
	  Numbness
	  Confusion

Signs	***Signs***

Contralateral:
  Hemiparesis
  Hemiataxia
  Hemisensory loss
  Homonymous hemianopia
Right-sided lesion: visuospatial abnormalities, hemineglect, nonverbal intellect affected
Left-sided lesion: disorientation, aphasia
	Contralateral:
	  Hemiparesis
	  Diminished pain and temperature
	  Dysarthria
	  Homonymous hemianopia; characteristically with a tongue of visual field spared along the horizontal meridian
	Memory impairment
	With right-sided lesions: visuoperceptual abnormalities

Arterial Territory Involved	***Arterial Territory Involved***
Thalamic polar (tuberothalamic) artery (see Figs. 19.2 and 19.3)	Anterior choroidal artery (see Fig. 19.3)
MEDIAL	**POSTEROLATERAL**
Common Symptoms	***Common Symptoms***

Disorientation and confusion
Coma with occlusion of mainstem variant
Visual blurring
	Contralateral:
	  Weakness
	  Numbness
	  Vision loss
	  Neglect
	  Confusion

Signs	***Signs***

Vertical gaze ophthalmoplegia
Loss of pupillary reflexes
Loss of convergence
Disorientation and confusion, stupor, coma, and various neuropsychiatric disturbances
	Contralateral:
	  Loss of touch, pain, temperature, and vibration sense (common)
	  Hemiparesis in some
	  Hemiataxia
	  Homonymous hemianopia
	Left hemispatial neglect
	Poor attention span

Arterial Territory Involved	***Arterial Territory Involved***
Posterior thalamosubthalamic paramedian artery (thalamic paramedian or deep interpeduncular profundus artery; (see Figs. 19.2 and 19.3)	Geniculothalamic artery (see Fig. 19.3)

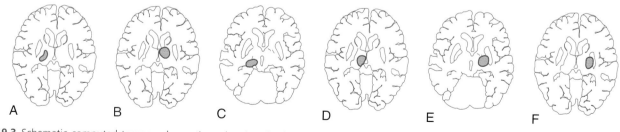

Fig. 19.3 Schematic computed tomography sections showing the five arterial territories of the thalamus. **A,** Geniculothalamic (inferolateral) artery territory. **B,** Anterior thalamosubthalamic paramedian (tuberothalamic) territory. **C,** Posterior choroidal territory. **D,** Posterior thalamosubthalamic paramedian territory. **E** and **F,** anterior choroidal territory. *(Modified with permission from Bogousslavsky, J., Regli, F., Uske, A., 1988. Thalamic infarcts: clinical syndromes, etiology and prognosis. Neurology. 38, 837-848.)*

and **Figs. 19.4** and **19.5** show the territories involved with occlusive and ischemic stroke syndromes in this area. Eponymic designations are given later in the text in Table 74.1. Mossuto-Agatiello (2006) identified a caudal paramedian midbrain syndrome with a distinctive clinical picture: bilateral cerebellar (truncal and gait) ataxia, eye movement disorders (nuclear third nerve palsy, INO), and palatal myoclonus.

Pontine Stroke Syndromes

The pons is supplied by numerous penetrating branches of the basilar artery. These arteries have little collateral supply; consequently, lacunar syndromes (see Chapter 51A) can occur (**Table 19.3**). These syndromes (**Figs. 19.6, 19.7, and 19.8**) may be clinically indistinguishable from lacunar

Table 19.2 Ischemic Stroke Syndromes of the Mesencephalon

MIDDLE MEDIAN MIDBRAIN SYNDROME	***Arterial Territory Involved***
Common Symptoms	Superior cerebellar artery

Contralateral:
  Weakness
  Ataxia
  Numbness
Ipsilateral:
  Eyelid ptosis
  Ataxia
  Diplopia
	INFERIOR MEDIAL MIDBRAIN SYNDROME (See Fig. 19.5)

	Common Symptoms
	Diplopia Contralateral weakness Clumsiness
Signs	***Signs***

Contralateral:
  Weakness
  Ataxia
  Supranuclear horizontal gaze paresis
Ipsilateral:
  Third cranial nerve palsy
  Nuclear
  Fascicular
Internuclear ophthalmoplegia
	Contralateral:
	  Fourth cranial nerve palsy
	  Ataxia (may be ipsilateral, depending on whether the lesion is before or after the crossing of the brachium conjunctivum)
	  Hemiparesis
	  Supranuclear horizontal gaze paresis (ipsilateral if below decussation in lower midbrain)
	Ipsilateral:
	  Internuclear ophthalmoplegia

Arterial Territory Involved	***Arterial Territory Involved***
Median and paramedian perforating ranches of the basilar or mesencephalic arteries	Median branches of the basilar artery
MIDDLE LATERAL MIDBRAIN SYNDROME (see Fig. 19.4)	**INFERIOR LATERAL MIDBRAIN SYNDROME (see Fig. 19.5)**
Common Symptoms	***Common Symptom***
Numbness: contralateral Clumsiness: ipsilateral	Contralateral numbness
Signs	***Signs***

Contralateral:
  Hemianesthesia
  Ataxia
Ipsilateral:
  Facial hemianesthesia (or contralateral)
  Horner syndrome
  Ataxia (if lesion is ventral to brachium conjunctivum)
	Contralateral:
	  Hemianesthesia
	Ipsilateral:
	  Hemianesthesia of face
	  Horner syndrome

	Arterial Territory Involved
	Superior cerebellar artery

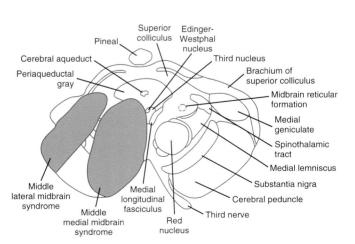

Fig. 19.4 Midbrain at the superior colliculus level, showing the medial and lateral territories involved with occlusive stroke syndromes in this area. *(Reprinted with permission from DeArmond, S.J., Fusco, M.M., Dewey, M.M., 1976. Structure of the Human Brain, second ed. Oxford University Press, New York.)*

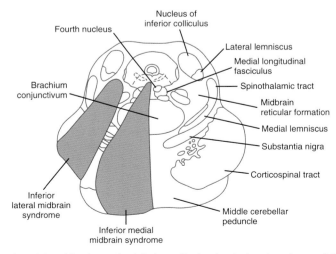

Fig. 19.5 Midbrain at the inferior colliculus level, showing the medial and lateral territories involved with ischemic stroke syndromes in this area. *(Reprinted with permission from DeArmond, S.J., Fusco, M.M., Dewey, M.M., 1976. Structure of the Human Brain, second ed. Oxford University Press, New York.)*

Table 19.3 Ischemic Stroke Syndromes of the Pons

SUPERIOR MEDIAL PONTINE SYNDROME (see Fig. 19.6)

Common Symptoms

Contralateral weakness
Clumsiness

Signs

On side of lesion:
    Ataxia
    Internuclear ophthalmoplegia
    Myoclonus of palate, pharynx, vocal cords
On side opposite lesion:
    Paralysis of face, arm, and leg

Arterial Territory Involved

Median branches of the basilar artery

SUPERIOR LATERAL PONTINE SYNDROME (see Fig. 19.6)

Common Symptoms

Clumsiness: ipsilateral
Contralateral numbness
Dizziness, nausea, vomiting

Signs

On side of lesion:
    Ataxia of limbs and gait, falling to side of lesion
    Horner syndrome
    Facial hemianesthesia
    Paresis of muscles of mastication
On side opposite lesion:
    Hemianesthesia (trigeminothalamic tract)
    Impaired touch, vibration, and position sense

Arterial Territory Involved

Superior cerebellar artery

MIDDLE MEDIAL PONTINE SYNDROME (see Fig. 19.7)

Common Symptoms

Contralateral hemiparesis
Ipsilateral clumsiness

Signs

On side of lesion:
    Ataxia of limbs
    Conjugate gaze paresis toward the side of the lesion
    Internuclear ophthalmoplegia
On side opposite lesion:
    Paresis of face, arm, and leg
    With bilateral lesions, locked-in syndrome may occur

Arterial Territory Involved

Median branches of the basilar artery

MIDDLE LATERAL PONTINE SYNDROME (see Fig. 19.7)

Common Symptoms

Numbness
Clumsiness
Chewing difficulty

Signs

Contralateral:
    Hemisensory loss
Ipsilateral:
    Ataxia of limbs
    Paralysis of muscles of mastication
    Impaired pain sensation over side of face
    Horner syndrome

Arterial Territory Involved

Long lateral branches of basilar artery

INFERIOR MEDIAL PONTINE SYNDROME (FOVILLE SYNDROME) (see Fig. 19.8)

Common Symptoms

Contralateral weakness and numbness
Facial weaknesses: ipsilateral
Diplopia

Signs

Contralateral:
    Paralysis of arm and leg
    Impaired tactile and proprioceptive sense over half the body
    Internuclear ophthalmoplegia
Ipsilateral:
    Paresis of conjugate gaze to side of lesion; to oculocephalic maneuver also if the sixth cranial nerve nucleus is involved
    One-and-a-half syndrome
    Nystagmus
    Diplopia on lateral gaze
    Lower motor neuron–type facial palsy

Arterial Territory Involved

Median branches of the basilar artery

INFERIOR LATERAL PONTINE SYNDROME (ANTERIOR INFERIOR CEREBELLAR ARTERY SYNDROME) (see Fig. 19.8)

Common Symptoms

Vertigo, nausea, vomiting
Oscillopsia
Deafness, tinnitus
Facial numbness
Dyscoordination

Signs

Contralateral:
    Impaired pain and thermal sense over half the body (may include the face)
Ipsilateral:
    Deafness
    Facial paralysis
    Ataxia
    Impaired sensation over face

Arterial Territory Involved

Anterior inferior cerebellar artery

syndromes due to lesions of the internal capsule. More extensive paramedian syndromes are accompanied by characteristic pontine findings. The findings may fluctuate (pontine warning syndrome) and in this situation may be treated by intravenous venous tissue plasminogen activator (Saposnik et al., 2008). Contralateral hemiparesis, ipsilateral ataxia, INO, and conjugate horizontal gaze paresis characterize the medial syndromes.

The lateral syndromes are distinguished by contralateral hemianesthesia and loss of discriminative sensation with ipsilateral Horner syndrome, facial hemianesthesia, and ataxia. Ipsilateral lower motor neuron–type facial paresis, sixth

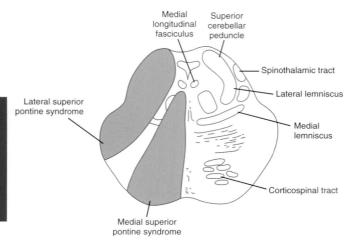

Fig. 19.6 Superior pontine level, showing the medial and lateral territories involved with occlusive stroke in this region. *(Reprinted with permission from Adams, R.D., Victor, M., 1993. Principles of Neurology, fifth ed. McGraw-Hill, New York.)*

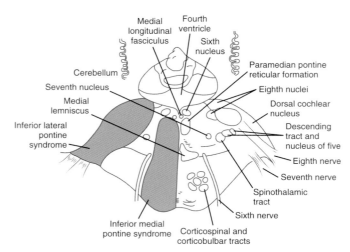

Fig. 19.8 Inferior pons at the level of the sixth cranial nerve nucleus, showing the medial and lateral territories involved with occlusive stroke in this area. *(Reprinted with permission from Adams, R.D., Victor, M., 1993. Principles of Neurology, fifth ed. McGraw-Hill, New York.)*

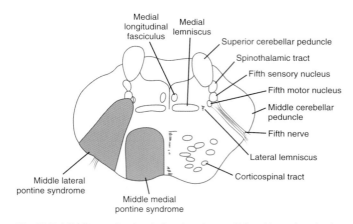

Fig. 19.7 Middle pontine level, showing the medial and lateral territories involved with ischemic stroke syndromes in this locality. *(Reprinted with permission from Adams, R.D., Victor, M., 1993. Principles of Neurology, fifth ed. McGraw-Hill, New York.)*

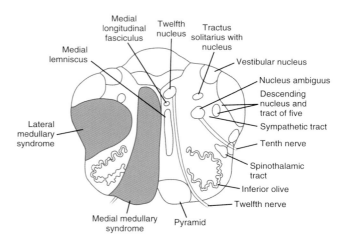

Fig. 19.9 Cross-section of medulla at the level of the inferior olivary complex, showing the medial and the more common lateral territory involved with ischemic stroke in this brainstem site. *(Reprinted with permission from Adams, R.D., Victor, M., 1993. Principles of Neurology, fifth ed. McGraw-Hill, New York.)*

cranial nerve paresis, deafness, and vertigo occur with inferior pontine lesions.

Medullary Stroke Syndromes

Medial medullary ischemia (**Fig. 19.9**) can cause crossed hypoglossal hemiparesis syndrome (**Table 19.4**). In addition, patients may have loss of discriminative-type sensation (position sense, graphesthesia, and stereognosis) when there is

associated medial lemniscus involvement. Kumral and associates (2002) have described four patterns of medial medullary stroke: (1) the most frequent, classic crossed hypoglossal hemiparesis syndrome, (2) sensorimotor stroke without lingual palsy, (3) pure hemiparesis, and (4) bilateral medial medullary stroke. Ocular motor findings often are prominent (Kim et al., 2005), with ocular contrapulsion, ocular tilt reaction, ipsilesional nystagmus (gaze-evoked, upbeating, and hemi-seesaw).

Table 19.4 Ischemic Stroke Syndromes of the Medulla

MEDIAL MEDULLARY SYNDROME (see Fig. 19.9)	**Signs**
Common Symptoms	Contralateral:
Contralateral weakness	Impaired pain sensation over half the body, sometimes
Dysarthria	including the face
Signs	Ipsilateral:
Contralateral:	Impaired sensation over half the face
Paralysis of arm and leg, sparing face	Ataxia of limbs, falling to side of lesion
Impaired tactile, vibratory, and proprioceptive sense over	Horner syndrome
half the body	Dysphagia, hoarseness, paralysis of vocal cords
Ipsilateral:	Diminished gag reflex
Paralysis with atrophy (late) of half the tongue	Loss of taste
Primary-position upbeat nystagmus	Other:
Arterial Territory Involved	Nystagmus:
Occlusion of vertebral artery or branch of vertebral or lower	Primary-position rotatory
basilar artery or anterior spinal artery	Gaze-evoked horizontal
LATERAL MEDULLARY SYNDROME (WALLENBERG SYNDROME) (see Fig. 19.9)	Downbeating on lateral gaze
	Ocular skew deviation
Common Symptoms	Hiccup
Ipsilateral facial pain and numbness	***Arterial Territory Involved***
Vertigo, nausea, and vomiting	Occlusion of any of five vessels may be responsible: vertebral;
Ipsilateral clumsiness	posterior inferior cerebellar; or superior, middle, or inferior
Diplopia, oscillopsia	lateral medullary artery
Numbness ipsilateral or contralateral to lesion	
Dysphagia, hoarseness	

Lateral medullary syndrome (Wallenberg syndrome; see **Fig. 19.9**) is one of the most dramatic clinical presentations in neurology (see **Table 19.4**). Long-tract signs (i.e., contralateral loss of pain and temperature sensation over half of the body, ipsilateral ataxia, ipsilateral axial lateropulsion [Eggers et al., 2009], Horner syndrome) are accompanied by involvement of the nuclei and fasciculi of cranial nerves V, VIII, IX, and X. Nystagmus often is present. The critical sign that distinguishes this from a lateral pontine syndrome is involvement of the nucleus ambiguus or its fasciculus and consequent weakness of the ipsilateral palate and vocal cord. It is increasingly found in the setting of vertebral artery dissection. (A more detailed discussion of stroke is presented in Chapter 51A.)

References

The complete reference list is available online at www.expertconsult.com.

Ataxic and Cerebellar Disorders

S.H. Subramony

The term *ataxia* denotes a syndrome of imbalance and incoordination involving gait, limbs, and speech and usually results from a disorder of the cerebellum and/or its connections. It appears to be derived from the Greek word *taxis*, meaning "order" (Worth, 2004). Ataxia can also result from a disturbance of proprioceptive input due to pathology along the sensory pathways (sensory ataxia). Evidence from anatomical connectivity studies suggest not only a motor function but also a potential cognitive role for the cerebellum (Strick et al., 2009). The clinical approach to patients with ataxia involves differentiating ataxia from other sources of imbalance and incoordination, distinguishing cerebellar from sensory ataxia, and designing an evaluation based on knowledge of various causes of ataxia and cerebellar disorders (Manto, 2009; Worth, 2004). This chapter describes the clinical features of ataxia and outlines a basic approach to patients with ataxia. A more detailed description of specific disorders can be found elsewhere in this book.

Symptoms and Signs of Ataxic Disorders

A few general statements can be made regarding cerebellar diseases. Lateralized cerebellar lesions cause ipsilateral symptoms and signs, whereas generalized cerebellar lesions give rise to more symmetrical symptomatology. Acute cerebellar lesions often produce severe abnormalities early but may show remarkable recovery with time. Recovery may be less optimal when the deep cerebellar nuclei are involved (Timmann et al., 2008). Chronic progressive diseases of the cerebellum tend to cause gradually declining balance with longer lasting effects. To some extent, signs and symptoms have a relation to the location of the lesions in the cerebellum (Stoodley and Schmahmann, 2010; Timmann et al., 2008). Ataxia of stance and gait are correlated with lesions in the medial and intermediate cerebellum: oculomotor features with medial, dysarthria with intermediate, and limb ataxia with lateral cerebellar lesions (Timmann et al., 2008). Stoodley and Schmahmann (2010) also point out that such lesion/symptom correlation can be extended to the proposed cognitive and limbic aspects of cerebellar function as well with anterior lobe lesions correlating with the traditional motor abnormalities and posterior lobe lesions with cognitive changes.

Symptoms in Patients with Ataxia
Gait Disturbances

Patients with cerebellar and sensory ataxia often present with abnormalities of gait. The initial symptoms may be a sense of insecurity while walking, especially when performing acts that require a bit more skill, such as turning or balancing on a narrow ledge. Even before gait becomes abnormal, patients may note problems with specialized skills such as skiing, bicycling, or climbing. Patients may report the sense of imbalance as dizziness, but the sensation is more like being on a boat rather than vertigo. Patients and family notice that the patient feels more secure with the feet progressively apart. An increase in imbalance when visual cues are removed suggests a sensory component to the ataxia.

Limb Ataxia

Ataxic diseases cause a variety of symptoms in the upper limbs, resulting from incoordination and tremor. Patients report clumsiness with activities such as writing, picking up objects, and buttoning. Movements tend to become slower. These symptoms are one-sided with lateralized lesions of the cerebellum.

Truncal Ataxia

Midline cerebellar lesions cause truncal ataxia. Patients may experience head tremor and truncal instability leading to oscillatory movements of the head and trunk while sitting or standing (titubation). They may need back support while sitting.

Dysarthria and Bulbar Symptoms

Ataxic diseases of cerebellar origin result in slurred speech and abnormalities of pitch and volume control (scanning speech). Dysphagia can result from incoordination of swallowing muscles, and patients report strangling and choking. Ineffectiveness of cough may also be a symptom.

Visual Symptoms

Patients may experience blurriness or a sense of environmental movements as a result of cerebellar ocular oscillations associated with cerebellar disease.

Symptoms in Sensory Ataxia

Patients with a sensory basis for ataxia usually do not experience dysarthria or visual symptoms. They may report other symptoms of sensory pathway disease such as paresthesias and numbness.

Neurological Signs in Patients with Cerebellar Ataxia

Gordon Holmes (1922, 1939) is often credited with the initial description of cerebellar deficits, although earlier works had reported on the effects of cerebellar lesions. Lesions of the cerebellum can cause deficits involving gait and stance, limb incoordination, muscle tone, speech, and the oculomotor system. They may also result in subtle cognitive deficits.

Stance and Gait

Patients with cerebellar disease initially experience an increase in body sway when the feet are placed together; the trunk moves excessively in the sideways direction (lateropulsion). With more severe disease, patients experience the increased sway even with normal stance and learn that balance is better with feet apart. Healthy persons usually have a foot spread of less than 12 cm during normal stance. Patients with cerebellar disease tend to have a much larger foot spread during quiet stance (Manto, 2002). In the clinic, one can detect even subtle problems with balance by asking the patient to do a tandem stance or stand on one foot; normal adults can do these maneuvers for at least 30 seconds. The Romberg test is usually positive in patients with cerebellar ataxia, although this tends to be more prominent in patients with proprioceptive or vestibular lesions. Many patients experience rhythmic oscillations of the trunk and head known as titubation. Severe truncal ataxia can also result in inability to sit upright without back support. Gait can be tested by asking the patient to walk naturally down a straight path. Ataxic gait is characterized by a widened base and an irregular staggering appearance resembling alcoholic intoxication. Overall, the speed of movements is not severely impaired, though patients may deliberately slow down to keep their balance. The steps are irregular, and the patient may lurch in unpredictable ways. Ataxic gait disturbance can be detected even earlier by testing tandem gait; patients with cerebellar lesions lose their ability to do heel-to-toe walking in a straight line.

Limb Incoordination

A number of clinical tests have been designed to test limb incoordination and the presence of tremor typically associated with cerebellar lesions. The finger-to-nose test involves repeatedly touching the tip of the nose and then the tip of the examiner's finger held just within reach of the patient's extended arm. The finger-chase test is done by asking the patient to follow the examiner's finger rapidly and accurately as the examiner moves his or her finger to a different location. Action tremor can be examined by placing the arms in the outstretched position and also by asking the patient to point the index fingers at each other at about chest level, separated by about 1 cm. Rapid alternating movements are examined by asking the patient to supinate and pronate the forearm in the unsupported position. This can also be done by having the patient alternately tap the palm and dorsum of one hand on the palm of the other (stationary) hand or on the thigh. Rebound is examined by allowing the patient to flex the elbow against the examiner's hand and then abruptly removing the resistance and assessing the ability to arrest the sudden flexion movement. The patient's face should be protected by the examiner's hand, as patients with severe cerebellar deficit would hit themselves in the face. In the lower limbs, the heel-to-shin maneuver is done by having the patient bring the heel of the leg being tested to the opposite knee and sliding it in a straight line down the anterior aspect of the tibia to the ankle. The foot should be nearly vertical while doing this. Having the patient rest the heel on the opposite knee for period of time can elicit tremor in the leg. The toe-to-finger test is done by asking the patient to touch the examiner's finger repeatedly with the great toe as the examiner moves the finger to a new position. Lower limb testing is best done in the supine position. These tests detect the following abnormalities in patients with ataxia.

DYSMETRIA

The term *dysmetria* refers to an inaccuracy of movement in which the desired target is either underreached (hypometria) or overreached (hypermetria). Dysmetria is evident in the finger chase and toe-to-finger tests. Holmes thought of dysmetria as a disturbance of the rate, range, and force of movement. Dysmetria is often increased by adding a mass to the hand.

KINETIC (INTENTION) TREMOR

Kinetic, or intention, tremor manifests as oscillations of the limb that occur during a voluntary movement intended to reach a target; the tremor often increases in amplitude as the target is reached. Kinetic tremor is typically seen with cerebellar lesions. The oscillations appear to result from instability at the proximal rather than distal portions of the limb and are typically perpendicular to the axis of motion. In contrast, patients with essential tremor who have no other cerebellar signs may exhibit an exaggeration of their tremor—primarily in the distal portions of the limbs—at the termination of a purposeful movement. The finger-to-nose and heel-to-shin maneuvers detect the kinetic tremor. Kinetic tremor is better evaluated when mass is added to the hand.

ACTION TREMOR

Cerebellar lesions can give rise to a postural tremor initiated by keeping the arms outstretched or pointing the fingers steadily at each other. In the legs, maintaining one heel on the opposite knee can bring out such a tremor.

OTHER TYPES OF TREMOR

Ataxic patients can exhibit an axial tremor involving the head and shoulders. Also, a severe tremor in the upper limbs that has both an intention and postural component can appear in cerebellar outflow tract disease. This has also been called a *rubral* or *wing-beating tremor*. This cerebellar outflow tremor is often seen in multiple sclerosis, Wilson disease, and midbrain strokes.

DYSDIADOCHOKINESIA

The term *dysdiadochokinesia* refers to irregularity of the rhythm and amplitude of rapid alternating movements. Simple tapping tasks such as the index finger on the thumb crease or the feet on the floor can also detect the disturbance in rhythm (dysrhythmokinesis).

Abnormalities of Muscle Tone and Strength

Although hypotonia can occur in acute cerebellar disease, it is not a major feature of most cerebellar diseases. The inability of patients to check forearm movement in the rebound test is often said to result from hypotonia but may have other explanations. Similarly, cerebellar lesions do not cause loss of strength in the traditional sense, but many patients experience problems with sustaining a steady force during sustained hand use (isometrataxia) (Manto, 2002).

Oculomotor Disturbances

Routine eye movement examination can detect most of the signs of cerebellar disease (Martin and Corbett, 2000). Fixation abnormalities are examined by asking the patient to maintain sustained gaze at the examiner's finger held about 2 feet in front. Then the patient is asked to follow the finger as it is moved slowly in all directions of gaze (pursuit). Eccentric gaze is maintained (at ≈ 30 degrees deviation) to check for nystagmus. Saccades are examined by having the patient shift gaze quickly between an eccentrically held finger and the examiner's nose in the middle. More sophistication can be brought to the clinical examination by looking at the vestibulo-ocular reflex, with the patient in a rotary chair and looking at an object that moves with the chair. A rotating striped drum is used to examine for optokinetic nystagmus (OKN), and Frenzel goggles can be used to remove fixation.

DISORDERS OF PURSUIT

Pursuit movements include fixation (pursuit at 0 degrees velocity). Small, 0.1- to 0.3-degree square-wave movements of the eyes are often seen even in normal individuals during fixation. *Square-wave jerks* are so named because in eye-movement recordings they appear as two saccades in opposite directions separated by a short period of no movement, giving a square appearance to the recording. Square-wave jerks exceeding 10 per minute are indicative of central nervous system disease, but they are not as specific for cerebellar ataxia as large-amplitude square-wave jerks. Square-wave jerks larger than 10 degrees in amplitude are called *macro–square-wave jerks*. Cerebellar disease also slows down pursuit

movements, requiring catch-up saccades to keep up with a moving target. Such saccadic intrusions and intrusions of square-wave jerks give a "ratchety" appearance to pursuit movement.

DISORDERS OF SACCADES

Saccade velocity is normal in cerebellar disease, but its accuracy is impaired so that both hypometric and hypermetric saccades are seen. Such saccades are followed by a corrective saccade in the appropriate direction (Munoz, 2002).

OTHER SACCADIC INTRUSIONS

Ocular flutter differs from square-wave jerks in that the back-and-forth horizontal saccades are not separated by an inter-saccade interval. *Opsoclonus* is characterized by continuous saccades in all directions in a chaotic fashion. Both ocular flutter and opsoclonus are associated with cerebellar disease, especially paraneoplastic or postinfectious syndromes.

NYSTAGMUS

Gaze-evoked nystagmus is elicited when eccentric gaze is maintained at about 30 degrees from the midline. There are repetitive drifts of the eyes toward midline, followed by saccades to the eccentric position. The fast phase of the nystagmus is always to the side of the eccentric gaze. This nystagmus is usually seen in cerebellar disease. When typical gaze-evoked nystagmus fatigues and reverses direction after a few seconds, it is called *rebound nystagmus*. Rebound nystagmus may also appear as a transient nystagmus in the opposite direction when the eye is returned to midline. Rebound nystagmus is also seen in cerebellar disease. *Downbeat nystagmus* is characterized by a rapid phase in the down direction in primary position of the eyes. Such downbeat nystagmus becomes more prominent with downgaze or gaze to the side. Downbeat nystagmus is typically seen in craniovertebral junction abnormalities such as Arnold-Chiari malformation, but it can also occur in some degenerative ataxias such as spinocerebellar ataxia type 6. Finally, upbeat primary position nystagmus can be seen in lesions of the anterior vermis.

VESTIBULO-OCULAR REFLEX

In a rotary chair, normal individuals can suppress the vestibular-ocular reflex (VOR) and keep their eyes on an object moving slowly with the chair. Patients with cerebellar disease cannot inhibit the VOR, so the eyes drift away from the object and make catch-up saccades as the chair is rotated.

Speech and Bulbar Function

Speech is evaluated by listening to patients' spoken words and asking them to speak standard phrases. Speech in cerebellar disease is characterized by slowness, slurring of the words, and a general inability to control the process of articulation, leading to unnecessary hesitations and stops, omissions of pauses when needed, and an accentuation of syllables when not needed. Also, there is a moment-to-moment variability in the volume and pitch of words and inappropriate control of the breathing needed for speech, causing a scanning dysarthria. Both speech execution and the motor programming of speech may be defective in cerebellar disease (Spencer and

Box 20.1 Acquired and Genetic Causes of Ataxia

Acquired Causes of Ataxia

Congenital: "ataxic" cerebral palsy, other early insults

Vascular: ischemic stroke, hemorrhagic stroke, AVMs

Infectious/transmittable: acute cerebellitis, postinfectious encephalomyelitis, cerebellar abscess, Whipple disease, HIV, CJD

Toxic: alcohol, anticonvulsants, mercury, 5FU, cytosine arabinoside, lithium

Neoplastic/compressive: gliomas, ependymomas, meningiomas, basal meningeal carcinomatosis, craniovertebral junction abnormalities

Immune: MS, paraneoplastic syndromes, anti-GAD, gluten ataxia

Deficiency: hypothyroidism, vitamin B_1 and B_{12}, vitamin E

Genetic Causes of Ataxia

Autosomal recessive: FA, AT, AVED, AOA 1, AOA 2, MIRAS, ARSACS, other newly defined autosomal recessive ataxias

Ataxia in other genetic diseases not traditionally classified as an "ataxia"

Autosomal dominant: SCA types 1 through 31, episodic ataxias (types 1, 2, others)

X-linked, including fragile X tremor-ataxia syndrome (FXTAS)

Mitochondrial: NARP, MELAS, MERRF, others including Kearns-Sayre syndrome

---

AOA, Ataxia with oculomotor apraxia; *ARSACS,* autosomal recessive spastic ataxia of Charlevoix-Saguenay;*AT,* ataxia telangiectasia; *AVED,* ataxia with vitamin E deficiency; *AVMs,* arteriovenous malformations; *CJD,* Creutzfeldt-Jakob disease; *FA,* Friedreich ataxia; *5FU,* 5 fluorouracil; *GAD,* glutamic acid decarboxylase; *HIV,* human immunodeficiency virus; *MELAS,* mitochondrial encephalopathy, lactic acidosis, stroke-like episodes; *MERRF,* myoclonus epilepsy with ragged red fibers; *MIRAS,* mitochondrial recessive ataxic syndrome; *MS,* multiple sclerosis; *NARP,* neuropathy, ataxia, and retinitis pigmentosa; *SCA,* spinocerebellar ataxia.

Table 20.1 Causes of Ataxia Related to Age at Onset

Age at Onset	Acquired	Genetic
Infancy	Ataxic cerebral palsy, other intrauterine insults	Inherited congenital ataxias (Joubert, Gillespie)
Childhood	Acute cerebellitis; cerebellar abscess; posterior fossa tumors such as ependymomas, gliomas; AVM; congenital anomalies such as Arnold-Chiari malformation; toxic such as due to anticonvulsants; immune related to neoplasms (opsoclonus-myoclonus)	FA; other recessive ataxias; ataxia associated with other genetic diseases; EA syndromes; mitochondrial disorders; SCAs such as SCA 2, SCA 7, SCA 13, DRPLA
Young adult	Abscesses; HIV; mass lesions such as meningiomas, gliomas, AVM; immune such as MS; Arnold-Chiari malformation; hypothyroidism; toxic such as alcohol and anticonvulsants	FA; SCAs, inherited tumor syndromes like von Hippel-Lindau syndrome
Older adult	Same as above plus "idiopathic" ataxia, immune related such as anti-GAD and gluten ataxia	More benign SCAs such as SCA 6

AVM, Arteriovenous malformation; *DRPLA,* dentate-rubral-pallidoluysian atrophy; *EA,* episodic ataxia; *FA,* Friedreich ataxia; *HIV,* human immunodeficiency virus; *MS,* multiple sclerosis; *SCA,* spinocerebellar ataxia (NOTE: SCA indicates a dominantly inherited ataxic disease).

Table 20.2 Causes of Ataxia Based on Onset and Course

Tempo	Acquired Diseases	Genetic Diseases
Episodic		Many inborn errors of metabolism; EA syndromes
Acute (hours/days)	Strokes, ischemic and hemorrhagic; MS; infections; parainfectious syndromes; toxic disorders	
Subacute (weeks/months)	Mass lesions in the posterior fossa; meningeal infiltrates; infections such as HIV, CJD; deficiency syndromes such B_1 and B_{12}; hypothyroidism; immune disorders such as paraneoplastic, gluten, and anti-GAD ataxia; alcohol	
Chronic	Mass lesions such as meningiomas; craniovertebral junction anomalies; alcoholic; idiopathic cerebellar and olivopontocerebellar atrophy; MSA	Most genetic disorders such as FA, AT, and other AR ataxias; SCAs

AR, Autosomal recessive; *AT,* ataxia telangiectasia; *CJD,* Creutzfeldt-Jakob disease; *EA,* episodic ataxia; *FA,* Friedreich ataxia; *GAD,* glutamic acid decarboxylase; *HIV,* human immunodeficiency virus; *MS,* multiple sclerosis; *MSA,* multiple system atrophy; *SCA,* spinocerebellar ataxia (dominantly inherited).

Box 20.2 Ataxias That Are Primarily Cerebellar, Cerebellar and Sensory, Primarily Sensory, and Associated with Spasticity

Cerebellar Ataxias

Most of the acquired lesions in Table 20.1; SCAs characterized by pure cerebellar ataxia (e.g., SCA 6, SCA 11, SCA 15)

Cerebellar-Sensory Ataxias

AT, AOAs, SCA 2, MJD, SCA 4, SCA 25

Sensory Ataxias

FA, AVED, acquired sensory ataxias related to "ataxic polyneuropathies" (e.g., paraneoplastic sensory neuropathy), Sjögren syndrome, diabetes, B$_6$ toxicity

Spastic Ataxias

SCA 1, MJD, SCA 7, SCA 8, some cases of FA, ARSACS

AOA, Ataxia with oculomotor apraxia; *ARSACS*, autosomal recessive spastic ataxia of Charlevoix-Saguenay; *AT*, ataxia telangiectasia; *AVED*, ataxia with vitamin E deficiency; *FA*, Friedreich ataxia; *MJD*, Machado-Joseph disease; *SCA*, spinocerebellar ataxia.

Table 20.3 Noncerebellar Neurological Signs or Symptoms That May Help in the Differential Diagnosis of Ataxia

Non-neurological Signs or Symptoms	Possible Diagnosis
Focal and lateralized brainstem deficits such as facial palsy, hemiparesis	Posterior circulation strokes, tumors, MS
Visual loss from optic atrophy/retinopathy	MS, FA, SCA 7, mitochondrial disease, Refsum disease, AVED
Papilledema, headache	Posterior fossa tumors, ataxia as "false localizing" sign
Internuclear ophthalmoplegia	Posterior circulation strokes, MS, some SCAs
Gaze palsies	Strokes, MS, NPC, MJD, SCAs 1, 2, 7
Ptosis, ophthalmoplegia	Strokes, MS, mitochondrial disease
Slow saccades/ocular apraxia	SCA 2, SCA 7, MJD, AT, AOA
Downbeat nystagmus	Arnold-Chiari malformation, basilar invagination, SCA 6, EA 2, lithium toxicity
Spasticity, upper motor neuron signs	Strokes, MS, tumors compressing brainstem, SCA 1, SCA 3, SCA 7, SCA 8; rarely FA
Basal ganglia deficits	Many SCAs like SCA 2, MJD, SCA 1, SCA 12, SCA 17; DRPLA, FXTAS, MSA, Wilson disease, Fahr disease
Tremor	SCA 12, SCA 15/16, FXTAS
Autonomic failure	Ataxic form of MSA, FXTAS
Deafness	Mitochondrial disease; superficial hemosiderosis
Epilepsy	Ataxia associated with anticonvulsants; DRPLA, SCA 7, SCA 10
Myoclonus	Mitochondrial disease, Unverricht-Lundborg disease, SCA 7 of early onset, SCA 14, sialidosis, ceroid lipofuscinosis, idiopathic (Ramsay-Hunt syndrome)
Palatal myoclonus	Alexander disease, SCA 20
Polyneuropathy	FA, AOA, AVED, SCA 2, MJD, SCA 1, SCA 4, SCA 25
Cognitive decline	Alcohol, MS, CJD, HIV, DRPLA, SCA 12, SCA 13, end-stage SCAs, superficial siderosis
Psychiatric features	SCA 12, SCA 17, SCA 27

NOTE: The above list is only a rough guide, and a precise diagnosis cannot be based on such phenotypic features alone. This is because phenotype can be variable, and the features indicated may not occur in all individuals with a particular disease. Also, for many of the disorders, the clinical features have been defined on the basis of limited clinical experience.

AOA, Ataxia with oculomotor apraxia; *AT*, ataxia telangiectasia; *AVED*, ataxia with vitamin E deficiency; *CJD*, Creutzfeldt-Jakob disease; *DRPLA*, dentatorubral-pallidoluysian atrophy; *EA*, episodic ataxia; *FA*, Friedreich ataxia; *FXTAS*, fragile X tremor ataxia syndrome; *HIV*, human immunodeficiency virus; *MJD*, Machado-Joseph disease; *MS*, multiple sclerosis; *MSA*, multiple system atrophy; *NPC*, Niemann Pick C; *SCA*, spinocerebellar ataxia.

Slocomb, 2007). Mild dysphagia is not uncommon in cerebellar disease. In children, a form of "cerebellar mutism" has been described after posterior fossa surgery. This is transient and followed by more typical cerebellar dysarthria.

Cognitive-Affective Features

A number of studies have suggested that cerebellar lesions can be accompanied by changes in cognitive and behavioral functions. Such changes have included defective executive function (often noted on the Wisconsin card sorting test) and defective visual and verbal memory and verbal fluency tasks. Acute cerebellar lesions may be accompanied by subtle language deficits, and a syndrome of cerebellar mutism has been noted in children with acute cerebellar lesions.

Neurological Signs in Patients with Sensory Ataxia

For patients with sensory ataxia, the major basis of ataxia is defective proprioception. Patients can be shown to have impaired position and vibration sense, and the deep tendon reflexes are often lost because of afferent fiber pathology. The Romberg test is positive. Many degenerative ataxic syndromes combine features of cerebellar and proprioceptive deficits in variable proportion.

Diagnostic Approach to Ataxia

Recognizing an ataxic basis for the patient's coordination problems and gait is usually easy. Other neural disorders that can give rise to similar problems with gait and dexterity—nerve and muscle disorders, spinal cord diseases, and basal ganglia diseases, for example—can usually be distinguished on the basis of physical signs alone.

Table 20.4 Systemic and Laboratory Features That May Be Useful in the Differential Diagnosis of Ataxia

Systemic Feature	Possible Diagnosis
Short stature	Mitochondrial disease, early CNS insults, AT
Conjunctival telangiectasia	AT
Cataracts	Marinesco-Sjögren syndrome, CTX
Cataplexy	NPC
KF rings	Wilson disease
Cervical lipoma	Mitochondrial disease
Abnormal ECG, Echocardiogram	FA, mitochondrial disease
Organomegaly	Niemann-Pick disease, LOTS, Gaucher disease, alcohol
Hypogonadism	Ataxia with hypogonadism (Holmes ataxia)
Myopathy	mtDNA mutations, CoQ10 deficiency
Diabetes	AT
Spine/foot deformity	FA, AT, AVED
Increased skin pigmentation	Adrenoleukodystrophy
Hematologic malignancy	AT
Sinopulmonary infections	AT
Tendon xanthomas	CTX
High CK	Mitochondrial disease, AOA
High α-fetoprotein	AT, AOA 2

AOA, Ataxia with oculomotor apraxia; *AT,* ataxia telangiectasia; *AVED,* ataxia with vitamin E deficiency; *CK,* creatine kinase; *CNS,* central nervous system; *CTX,* cerebrotendinous xanthomatosis; *ECG,* electrocardiogram; *FA,* Friedreich ataxia; *LOT,* late-onset Tay Sachs disease; *NPC,* Niemann Pick C disease.

Table 20.5 Brain Imaging Abnormalities That Can Serve to Differentiate the Ataxias

MRI Abnormality	Possible Diagnosis
Mass in the cerebellum/posterior fossa	Gliomas, meningiomas, abscess
Abnormal craniovertebral junction	Arnold-Chiari malformation, basilar invagination
Infarcts, vascular malformations	Ischemic lesions, AVM
Signal density change in the cerebellum	MS, acute cerebellitis
Signal density change in the MCP	FXTAS
Pure cerebellar atrophy	SCAs with pure cerebellar signs (e.g., SCA 5, SCA 6); idiopathic cortical cerebellar atrophy; toxic, deficiency, and autoimmune ataxias
Pontocerebellar atrophy	Many SCAs such as SCA 1, 2, and MJD; sporadic olivopontocerebellar atrophy; ataxic form of MSA
Cervical cord atrophy	FA, AVED
Cerebral white matter changes	Leukodystrophies presenting with ataxia, MS

AVED, Ataxia with vitamin E deficiency; *AVM,* arteriovenous malformation; *FA,* Friedreich ataxia; *FXTAS,* Fragile X tremor-ataxia syndrome; *MJD,* Machado-Joseph disease; *MS,* multiple sclerosis; *SCA,* spinocerebellar ataxia.

Some patients with bilateral frontal lobe lesions may have a gait disorder superficially resembling ataxia (Brun ataxia or frontal ataxia). However, limb and eye-movement signs of cerebellar disease are absent, and the gait abnormalities are out of proportion to the limb signs. Often the patient may experience a sense of being glued to the ground ("magnetic" gait). Other gait disorders associated with dystonia or chorea may also be occasionally mistaken for cerebellar ataxia.

Neurological examination also determines whether the ataxia is primarily cerebellar, primarily sensory, or a combination of both. This led Greenfield to classify ataxic disorders as spinal, cerebellar, or spinocerebellar in nature. Further diagnostic considerations and avenues for investigation are aimed at making a specific diagnosis (**Box 20.1**), and management is dependent on the diagnosis. This can be a daunting task,

especially when the disease appears to be "degenerative" in nature (i.e., associated with cerebellar atrophy). As an example, the Online Mendelian Inheritance in Man website lists more than 500 genetic disorders alone in which ataxia can occur. In the appropriate clinical setting when the initial diagnostic process (e.g., imaging studies) has been unfruitful, it may be important to educate the patient about the possibility of not being able to come to a specific diagnosis before embarking on an expensive process of laboratory studies. In patients with ataxia, many additional pieces of information may be useful in arriving at a diagnosis. These include age at onset (**Table 20.1**); the tempo of disease (**Table 20.2**); whether the ataxia is predominantly spinal, spinocerebellar, cerebellar, or associated with spasticity (**Box 20.2**); the presence or absence of noncerebellar neurological signs (**Table 20.3**); the occurrence of any distinctive systemic features (**Table 20.4**); and the nature of the imaging abnormalities (**Table 20.5**).

References

The complete reference list is available online at www.expertconsult.com.

Movement Disorders: Diagnosis and Assessment

Joseph Jankovic, Anthony E. Lang

The term *movement disorders* is often used synonymously with *basal ganglia* or *extrapyramidal diseases*. However, neither of those terms adequately encompasses all the disorders included under the broad umbrella of movement disorders. Movement disorders are neurological motor disorders manifested by slowness or poverty of movement (bradykinesia or hypokinesia, such as that seen in parkinsonian disorders) at one end of the spectrum and abnormal involuntary movements (hyperkinesias) such as tremor, dystonia, athetosis, chorea, ballism, tics, myoclonus, restless legs syndrome, stereotypies, akathisias, and other dyskinesias at the other. Although motor dysfunctions resulting from upper and lower motor neuron, spinal cord, peripheral nerve, and muscle diseases usually are not classified as movement disorders, abnormalities in muscle tone (e.g., rigidity, spasticity, stiff person syndrome), incoordination (cerebellar ataxia; see Chapters 20 and 74), and complex disorders of execution of movement denoted by the term *apraxia* (see Chapter 10) are now included among movement disorders.

The term *movement disorder* refers to a clinical sign for which there are many possible causes. In most fields of neurology, the recommended clinical approach is to determine where in the nervous system the disease process is located and what that process could be. When dealing with movement disorders, however, the first step is to define the most appropriate broad movement disorder class based on knowledge and recognition of phenomenology. Some abnormal movements may appear to be bizarre and therefore difficult to categorize. Despite attempts at uniformity in definition, classification errors are common. Inaccurate categorization occasionally has resulted in clinical, genetic, and epidemiological misinformation embedded in the literature. Video documentation is very useful in clarifying the phenomenology, thereby minimizing the risk of misdiagnosis.

Many movement disorders have no known or established cause. The classification of these disorders, sometimes called *essential* or *idiopathic movement disorders*, are now best classifiable as *primary movement disorders* and distinguished from those that are secondary to identifiable diseases. In the following sections, the emphasis is on historical and clinical features that help the clinician make this distinction. Family history, including ethnic origin (e.g., Ashkenazi Jewish) and parental consanguinity, often is helpful in arriving at a diagnosis. It is crucial to recognize that the symptoms in other family members may be different from those in the patient because of variability of gene expression and penetrance and because they may have an entirely different disorder. For example, some family members of patients with primary dystonia may have dystonic features, whereas others may have predominantly tremor. Additional problems that may hamper the acquisition of an adequate family history include adoption, uncertain paternity, and even the deliberate withholding of important family information. Denial of positive family history is particularly common in patients with Huntington disease (HD) and the genetic ataxias. An adult-onset disorder may not have been evident in a family member who died at an early age. It is particularly important to exclude Wilson disease (WD) because of the specific therapy available and the universally fatal outcome of the disease if left untreated (Lorincz, 2010).

Obtaining a history of birth and early developmental abnormalities is essential, especially emphasizing the possibility of anoxia or kernicterus. A history of encephalitis is important. Certain drugs and toxins have a strong potential for causing movement disorders, particularly drugs that block dopamine receptors. These include antipsychotic drugs, certain antiemetic drugs and other drugs used for various gastrointestinal (GI) disorders (e.g., metoclopramide, prochlorperazine, promethazine), calcium channel blockers (e.g., cinnarizine, flunarizine), central nervous system (CNS) stimulants (e.g., methylphenidate, cocaine), and dopaminergic drugs (e.g., levodopa).

Besides documenting the movement disorder, neurological examination should search for additional findings that would help indicate the secondary nature of the problem. General physical examination must be thorough. An extremely important component of the examination is a corneal evaluation, including slit-lamp examination, to exclude the presence of a Kayser-Fleischer ring, characteristic of WD (**Fig. 21.1**). The nature and extent of laboratory investigations depend on clinical suspicions. Without clues from the history and physical examination, however, very few specific or special investigations assist in diagnosing these patients.

Parkinsonism

The initial feature of many basal ganglia diseases is slowness of movement (bradykinesia) and paucity or absence of movement (akinesias), often associated with rigidity and tremor (Jankovic, 2007a). Some authors have used the term *hypokinesia* to describe a reduction in amplitude of movement. The combination of slowness and poverty of movement and increase in muscle tone explain many parkinsonian symptoms. The term *parkinsonism* is used to describe a syndrome manifested by a combination of the following six cardinal features: (1) tremor at rest, (2) bradykinesia, (3) rigidity, (4) loss of postural reflexes, (5) flexed posture, and (6) freezing (motor blocks). A combination of these signs is the basis to clinically define definite, probable, and possible parkinsonism. Diagnosis of definite parkinsonism requires that at least two of these features must be present, with one of them being resting tremor or bradykinesia; probable parkinsonism consists of resting tremor or bradykinesia alone; and possible parkinsonism includes at least two of the remaining four features. The four major characteristics of parkinsonism account for most of the described clinical abnormalities: tremor, rigidity, akinesia, and postural disturbances (forming the acronym *TRAP*).

The most common cause of idiopathic parkinsonism (akinetic-rigid syndrome) is Parkinson disease (PD). As a result of advances in genetics, many forms of idiopathic parkinsonism have been found to result from mutations in specific genes, such as those coding for α-synuclein (SNCA gene), parkin (PARK2 gene), leucine-rich repeat kinase 2 (LRRK2 gene), or PTEN-induced putative kinase 1 (PINK1 gene) protein (**Table 21.1**). Whereas some of the gene mutations (e.g., SNCA) are very rare causes of parkinsonism, PARK2 mutations account for up to 50% of all patients with early-onset parkinsonism, and LRRK2 mutations may account for a large proportion of cases in selected populations (e.g., North Africans, Ashkenazi Jews) (Dawson et al., 2010; Gandhi and Wood, 2010). Although less than 10% of all patients with PD have a genetic mutation, clinicians must learn about these genetic forms of parkinsonism not only to understand the pathogenic mechanisms better but also to learn how to interpret and use the increasingly available gene tests for genetic counseling (Tan and Jankovic, 2006). Because PD is idiopathic by definition, the notion of multiple Parkinson diseases is a consideration to draw attention to the different genetic causes of idiopathic parkinsonism. Besides genetic causes, there are many other causes of pure parkinsonism and of parkinsonism combined with other neurological deficits (parkinsonism-plus syndromes) (**Box 21.1**).

Motor Abnormalities

Early in the course of the disease, many patients with parkinsonism are unaware of any motor deficit. Often the patient's spouse comments on a reduction in facial expression (often misinterpreted as depression), a reduction in arm swing while walking, and a slowing of activities of daily living, most notably dressing, feeding, and walking. The patient may then become aware of a reduction in manual dexterity, with slowness and clumsiness interfering with activities. PD is typically asymmetrical, especially early in the course. A painful shoulder is one of the most common early symptoms of incipient unilateral rigidity and bradykinesia. This symptom, probably related to decreased arm swing and secondary joint changes or shoulder muscle rigidity, is often misdiagnosed as bursitis, arthritis, or a rotator cuff disorder. All recreational and work tasks, household chores, and self-care functions eventually become impaired. Handwriting often becomes slower and smaller (micrographia), with speed and size decreasing as the task continues. Eventually the writing may become illegible. Use of eating utensils becomes difficult, chewing is laborious, and choking while swallowing may occur. If the latter is an early and prominent complaint, one must consider bulbar

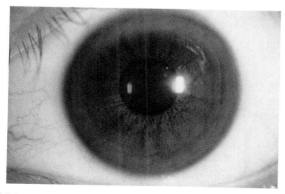

Fig. 21.1 Kayser-Fleischer ring. Note the golden-brown full-circumference ring, thickest and most readily seen between the 11 o'clock and 1 o'clock positions of the cornea.

Table 21.1 Genetic Causes of Parkinsonism

Disease	Inheritance	Gene Locus (Gene)	Protein
PARK1—typical PD	AD	4q21-23 (SNCA)	α-Synuclein
PARK2—juvenile parkinsonism, dystonia	AR	6q25.2-27 (PRKN, parkin)	Ubiquitin ligase
PARK3—typical PD	AD	2p13	Unknown
PARK4—parkinsonism, dementia, dysautonomia, postural tremor, LB, GCI	AD	4q21	α-Synuclein triplication
PARK5—PD	AD	4p14 (UCH-L1)	Ubiquitin cyclohydrolase A
PARK6—early-onset	AR	1p36 (PINK1)	(PTEN-induced kinase 1)
PARK7—early-onset	AR	1p36 (DJ-1)	DJ-1
PARK8—PD	AD	12p11.23-q13.11 (LRRK2)	LARRK2 (dardarin)
PARK9 (Kufor-Rakeb syndrome)—early-onset, spasticity, dementia, ophthalmoparesis, pallidal atrophy	AR	1p36 (ATP13A2)	Lysosomal type 5 P-type ATPase
PARK10—late-onset typical PD	AD	1p32	?
PARK11—middle-age	AD	2q36-37 (GIGYF2?)	GRB10-interacting gyf protein 2
PARK12—late-onset PD	X-linked	Xq21-q25	?
PARK13—late-onset typical PD	AD	2p12 (HtrA2)	Serine protease
PARK14—adult-onset dystonia-parkinsonism, subtype of NBIA	AR	22q13.1 (PLA2G6)	Phospholipase A2
PARK15—early-onset parkinsonian-pyramidal syndrome	AR	22q12-q13 (FBXO7)	F-box Protein7
PARK16	?	1q32	?

AD, Autosomal dominant; *AR*, autosomal recessive; *ATP*, adenosine triphosphate; *GCI*, glial cytoplasmic inclusions; *LB*, Lewy bodies; *NBIA*, neurodegeneration with brain iron accumulation; *PD*, Parkinson disease.

involvement in one of the parkinsonism-plus syndromes, such as progressive supranuclear palsy (PSP) and multiple system atrophy (MSA) (Stefanova et al., 2009; Williams and Lees, 2009) (**Table 21.2**). Dressing tasks such as fastening small buttons or getting arms into sleeves are often difficult. Hygiene becomes impaired. As with most other tasks, disability is greater if the dominant arm is more affected; shaving, brushing teeth, and other repetitive movements usually are affected the most.

Speech becomes slurred and loses its volume (hypophonia), and as a result, patients often must repeat themselves. Like gait, speech may be *festinating*; that is, it gets faster and faster (tachyphemia). A large number of additional speech disturbances may occur, including stuttering and *palilalia*, involuntary repetition of a phrase with increasing rapidity. Early, pronounced voice changes often indicate a diagnosis other than PD (e.g., palilalia is more commonly a feature of PSP and MSA). A harsher, nasal quality of the voice, which is quite distinctive from the hypophonic monotone of PD, also suggests the diagnosis of PSP. A higher-pitched quivering, "whiny" voice may suggest MSA, especially if it is associated with frequent sighing, respiratory gasps, laryngeal stridor, and other respiratory problems (Mehanna and Jankovic, 2010).

Another problem related to impairment of bulbar function is excessive salivation and drooling. Initially this may occur only at night, but later it can be present throughout the day, at times necessitating the constant use of a tissue or handkerchief.

Getting in and out of a chair or car and climbing in and out of the bathtub cause problems; patients often switch to showering. Many patients misinterpret these difficulties as resulting from "weakness." Generalized loss of energy and easy fatigability are also common complaints. Walking becomes slowed and shuffling, with flexion of the knees and a narrow base. When involvement is asymmetrical, one leg may drag behind the other. Stride then shortens, and turns include multiple steps (turning en bloc). Later, patients may note a tendency to advance more and more rapidly with shorter and shorter steps (festination), at times seemingly propelled forward with a secondary inadequate attempt to maintain the center of gravity over the legs. When this occurs, a nearby wall or an unobstructed fall may be the only method of stopping. Alternatively, the feet may seem glued to the floor, the so-called freezing phenomenon, or motor block. Early on, this is appreciated when the patient initiates walking (start hesitation), is turning (especially in an enclosed space), or attempts to walk through an enclosed area such as a doorway (an elevator door is a common precipitant). When combined with poor postural stability, prominent freezing results in the tendency to fall forward or to the side while turning. Later, impaired postural reflexes may cause falls without a propulsive or freezing precipitant. The early occurrence of falls suggests a diagnosis of PSP or other parkinsonian disorder rather than PD. Turning over in bed and adjusting the bedclothes often become difficult. Patients may have to sit up first and then turn, and later the spouse may have to help roll the person over or adjust position for comfort.

Box 21.1 Classification of Parkinsonism

I. Parkinson disease
   Parkinson disease—sporadic
   Parkinson disease—hereditary (see Table 21.1)
II. Multisystem degenerations ("parkinsonism plus")
   Progressive supranuclear palsy
   Multiple system atrophy (Shy-Drager syndrome):
      MSA-P (striatonigral degeneration)
      MSA-C (olivopontocerebellar atrophy)
   Lytico-Bodig disease, or amyotrophic lateral sclerosis and parkinsonism-dementia complex of Guam
   Corticobasal degeneration
   Progressive pallidal atrophy
   Parkinsonism-dementia complex
   Pallidopyramidal disease
III. Heredodegenerative parkinsonism
   Dopa-responsive dystonia
   Huntington disease
   Wilson disease
   Hereditary ceruloplasmin deficiency
   Neurodegeneration with brain iron accumulation (pantothenate kinase-associated neurodegeneration, also known as *Hallervorden-Spatz disease*)
   Olivopontocerebellar and spinocerebellar atrophies, including Machado-Joseph disease
   Frontotemporal dementia with parkinsonism (FTDP)
   Gerstmann-Sträussler-Scheinker syndrome
   Familial progressive subcortical gliosis
   Lubag (X-linked dystonia-parkinsonism)
   Familial basal ganglia calcification
   Mitochondrial cytopathies with striatal necrosis
   Ceroid lipofuscinosis
   Familial parkinsonism with peripheral neuropathy
   Parkinsonian-pyramidal syndrome
   Neuroacanthocytosis
   Hereditary hemochromatosis
   Neuroferritinopathy
   Aceruloplasminemia
IV. Secondary (acquired, symptomatic) parkinsonism
   Infectious: postencephalitic, acquired immunodeficiency syndrome, subacute sclerosing panencephalitis, Creutzfeldt-Jakob disease, prion diseases
   Drugs: dopamine receptor blocking drugs (antipsychotic, antiemetic drugs), reserpine, tetrabenazine, methyldopa, lithium, flunarizine, cinnarizine
   Toxins: MPTP, carbon monoxide, manganese, mercury, carbon disulfide, cyanide, methanol, ethanol
   Vascular: multi-infarct disease
   Trauma: pugilistic encephalopathy disease
   Other: parathyroid abnormalities, hypothyroidism, hepatocerebral degeneration, brain tumor, paraneoplastic, normal-pressure hydrocephalus, noncommunicating hydrocephalus, syringomesencephalia, hemiatrophy-hemiparkinsonism, peripherally induced tremor and parkinsonism, psychogenic

Cognitive, Autonomic, and Sensory Abnormalities

The complaints of patients with parkinsonism are not limited to the motor system, and a large variety of nonmotor symptoms, many of which are probably not directly related to dopaminergic deficiency, often emerge as the disease progresses. In many cases, they become more disabling than the classic motor problems (Lim et al., 2009) (see **Table 21.2**). Dementia occurs in a variety of parkinsonian syndromes (see Chapters 66 and 72). Depression is also a common problem, and patients often lose their assertiveness and become withdrawn, more passive, and less motivated to socialize. The term *bradyphrenia* describes the slowness of thought processes and inattentiveness often seen.

Complaints related to autonomic dysfunction are also common. In all parkinsonian syndromes, constipation is a common complaint and may become severe. However, fecal incontinence does not occur in PD unless the motor disability is such that the patient cannot maneuver to the bathroom, dementia is superimposed, or impaction has led to overflow incontinence. Bladder complaints such as frequency, nocturia, and the sensation of incomplete bladder emptying may occur. Urinary incontinence is especially suggestive of MSA. A mild to moderate degree of orthostatic hypotension is common in parkinsonian disorders, and antiparkinsonian drugs often aggravate the problem (see Chapter 71). If the autonomic features, particularly erectile dysfunction, sphincter problems, and orthostatic lightheadedness, occur early or become the dominant feature, one must consider the possibility of MSA (see Chapter 66). Impotence with early loss of nocturnal or morning erections and inability to maintain erection during intercourse is suggestive of MSA. The other symptom that may precede the onset of motor problems associated with several parkinsonian disorders, particularly PD, MSA, or dementia with Lewy bodies, is rapid eye movement (REM) sleep behavior disorder. One characteristic nonmotor feature of PD is excessive greasiness of the skin and seborrheic dermatitis, characteristically seen over the forehead, eyebrows, and malar area.

Visual complaints are usually not a prominent feature, with the following specific exceptions. In PD (and many other parkinsonian disorders), diplopia may occur during reading secondary to impaired convergence. Visual complaints sometimes occur in other parkinsonian disorders, particularly PSP (see Chapter 71). Oculogyric crises, which are sudden episodes of involuntary ocular deviation (most often up and to the side) in the absence of neuroleptic drug exposure, are virtually pathognomonic of parkinsonism after encephalitis lethargica, although they may occur in rare neurometabolic disorders as well. Sensory loss is not part of parkinsonism, although patients with PD may have poorly explained positive sensory complaints such as numbness and tingling, aching, and painful sensations that are sometimes quite disabling. Peripheral neuropathy suggests another disorder or an unrelated problem (e.g., diabetes mellitus), although recent evidence suggests a higher-than-expected incidence of peripheral neuropathy, possibly related to levodopa treatment and elevated methylmalonic acid levels (Toth et al., 2010).

Although a variety of neurophysiological and computer-based methods have been proposed to quantitate the severity of the various parkinsonian symptoms and signs, most studies rely on clinical rating scales, particularly the Unified

Table 21.2 Parkinsonian Syndromes: Differential Diagnosis

	PD	PSP	MSA-P	MSA-C	CBD	DLB	PDACG
Bradykinesia	+	+	+	±	+	±	+
Rigidity	+	+	+	+	+	±	+
Gait disturbance	+	+	+	+	+	±	+
Tremor	+	–	±	±	±	–	+
Ataxia	–	–	–	+	–	–	±
Dysautonomia	±	±	+	+	–	±	±
Dementia	±	+	±	–	±	+	+
Dysarthria or dysphagia	±	+	+	+	+	±	+
Dystonia	±	±	±	–	+	–	–
Eyelid apraxia	±	+	±	–	±	–	±
Limb apraxia	–	±	–	–	+	±	–
Motor neuron disease	–	–	±	–	–	–	+
Myoclonus	±	–	±	±	+	±	–
Neuropathy	–	–	–	±	–	–	–
Oculomotor deficit	–	+	–	+	+	±	±
Sleep impairment	±	±	±	±	–	±	–
Asymmetrical findings	+	±	±	–	+	–	–
L-dopa response	+	–	±	±	–	–	–
L-dopa dyskinesia	+	–	±	–	–	–	–
Family history	±	–	–	–	–	–	–
Putaminal T2 hypointensity	–	±	+	+	–	–	–
Lewy bodies	+	–	±	±	±	+	–

CBD, Corticobasal degeneration; *DLB*, dementia with Lewy bodies; *MSA-C*, multiple system atrophy, cerebellar type; *MSA-P*, multiple system atrophy, parkinsonian type; *PD*, Parkinson disease; *PDACG*, amyotrophic lateral sclerosis and parkinsonism-dementia complex of Guam; *PSP*, progressive supranuclear palsy.

Parkinson's Disease Rating Scale (UPDRS), Hoehn and Yahr staging scale, and Schwab and England Activities of Daily Living Scale (**Box 21.2**). Non-demented patients can reliably self-administer and complete the historical section of the UPDRS, now available in a revised version referred to as the *Movement Disorder Society (MDS)-UPDRS* (www.movementdisorders.org). The revision clarifies some ambiguities and more adequately assesses the nonmotor features of PD, which are among the most disabling symptoms, particularly in more advanced stages of the disease (Goetz et al., 2008). Some clinical research studies supplement the UPDRS by a more objective timed test such as the Purdue Pegboard Test and movement and reaction times. Many scales, such as the Parkinson's Disease Questionnaire-39 (PDQ-39) and the Parkinson's Disease Quality of Life Questionnaire (PDQL), attempt to assess the overall quality of life (Jankovic, 2008).

Onset and Course

As in other movement disorders, the age at onset of a parkinsonian syndrome is clearly important in considering a differential diagnosis. Although the majority of patients are adults, parkinsonism does occur in childhood (see **Box 21.1**). PD usually has a slow onset and very gradual progression (Jankovic, 2005). Generally, patients with early-onset PD and those with a tremor-dominant form tend to progress at a slower rate and are less likely to have an associated cognitive decline than those with postural instability and the gait difficulty form of PD. Other disorders (e.g., those due to toxins, cerebral anoxia, infarction) may present abruptly or progress more rapidly (resulting in so-called malignant parkinsonism) or may even improve spontaneously (e.g., those due to drugs, multiple infarcts, certain forms of encephalitis).

Examination and Clinical Signs

The diagnosis of parkinsonism often is immediately apparent on first contact with the patient. The facial expression, low-volume voice, tremor, poverty of movement, shuffling gait, and stooped posture provide an immediate and irrevocable first impression of parkinsonism. However, the physician must perform a detailed assessment, searching for any atypical features in attempting to distinguish between PD and other parkinsonian disorders. Loss of facial expression (*hypomimia*) often is an early sign of PD. But occasional patients have a wide-eyed, anxious, worried expression due to furrowing of the brow ("procerus sign") and deep facial folds, which strongly suggests PSP. Blink frequency usually is reduced, although *blepharoclonus* (repetitive spasms of the lids on gentle eye closure) and reflex blepharospasm (e.g., precipitated by shining

Box 21.2 **Unified Parkinson's Disease Rating Scale (UPDRS) Definitions of 0–4 Scale**

Mentation, Behavior, and Mood

1. Mentation
   0 = None.
   1 = Mild. Consistent forgetfulness with partial recollection of events and no other difficulties.
   2 = Moderate memory loss, with disorientation and moderate difficulty handling complex problems. Mild but definite impairment of function at home with need of occasional prompting.
   3 = Severe memory loss with disorientation to time and often place. Severe impairment in handling problems.
   4 = Severe memory loss with orientation preserved to person only. Unable to make judgments or solve problems. Needs much help with personal care. Cannot be left alone at all.

2. Thought disorder (caused by dementia or drug intoxication)
   0 = None.
   1 = Vivid dreaming.
   2 = "Benign."
   3 = Occasional to frequent hallucinations or delusions, without insight, could interfere with daily activities.
   4 = Persistent hallucinations, delusions, or florid psychosis. Not able to care for self.

3. Depression
   0 = Not present.
   1 = Periods of sadness or guilt greater than normal, never sustained for days or weeks.
   2 = Sustained depression (1 week or more).
   3 = Sustained depression with vegetative symptoms (insomnia, anorexia, weight loss, loss of interest).
   4 = Sustained depression with vegetative symptoms and suicidal thoughts or intent.

4. Motivation and initiative
   0 = Normal.
   1 = Less assertive than usual; more passive.
   2 = Loss of initiative or disinterest in elective (nonroutine) activities.
   3 = Loss of initiative or disinterest in day-to-day (routine) activities.
   4 = Withdrawn, complete loss of motivation.

Activities of Daily Living

5. Speech
   0 = Normal.
   1 = Mildly affected. No difficulty being understood.
   2 = Moderately affected. Sometimes asked to repeat statements.
   3 = Severely affected. Frequently asked to repeat statements.
   4 = Unintelligible most of the time.

6. Salivation
   0 = Normal.
   1 = Slight but definite excess of saliva in mouth; may have nighttime drooling.
   2 = Moderately excessive saliva with some drooling.
   3 = Marked excess of saliva with some drooling.
   4 = Marked drooling, needs constant tissue or handkerchief.

7. Swallowing
   0 = Normal.
   1 = Rare choking.
   2 = Occasional choking.
   3 = Needs soft food.
   4 = Needs nasogastric tube or gastrostomy tube feeding.

8. Handwriting
   0 = Normal.
   1 = Slightly slow or small.
   2 = Moderately slow or small; all words are legible.
   3 = Severely affected; not all words are legible.
   4 = The majority of words are not legible.

9. Cutting food
   0 = Normal.
   1 = Somewhat slow and clumsy, but no help needed.
   2 = Can cut most food, although clumsy and slow; some help needed.
   3 = Food must be cut by someone, but can still feed slowly.
   4 = Needs to be fed.

10. Dressing
    0 = Normal.
    1 = Somewhat slow but no help needed.
    2 = Occasional assistance with buttoning, getting arms in sleeves.
    3 = Considerable help needed, but can do some things alone.
    4 = Helpless.

11. Hygiene
    0 = Normal.
    1 = Somewhat slow, but no help needed.
    2 = Needs help to shower or bathe, or very slow in hygienic care.
    3 = Needs assistance for washing, brushing teeth, combing hair, going to bathroom.
    4 = Foley catheter or other mechanical aids.

12. Turning in bed
    0 = Normal.
    1 = Somewhat slow and clumsy, but no help needed.
    2 = Can turn alone or adjust sheets, but with great difficulty.
    3 = Can initiate but not turn or adjust sheets alone.
    4 = Helpless.

13. Falling
    0 = Normal.
    1 = Rare falling.
    2 = Occasionally falls, less than once per day.
    3 = Falls an average of once daily.
    4 = Falls more than once daily.

14. Freezing
    0 = None.
    1 = Rare freezing when walking; may have start hesitation.
    2 = Occasional freezing when walking.
    3 = Frequent freezing; occasionally falls from freezing.
    4 = Frequent falls from freezing.

15. Walking
    0 = Normal.
    1 = Mild difficulty. May not swing arms or may tend to drag leg.
    2 = Moderate difficulty, but needs little or no assistance.

Continued

Box 21.2 Unified Parkinson's Disease Rating Scale (UPDRS) Definitions of 0–4 Scale—cont'd

3 = Severe disturbance of walking; needs assistance.
4 = Cannot walk at all, even with assistance.

16. Tremor
0 = Absent.
1 = Slight and infrequently present.
2 = Moderate; bothersome to patient.
3 = Severe; interferes with many activities.
4 = Marked; interferes with most activities.

17. Sensory symptoms
0 = None.
1 = Occasionally has numbness, tingling, or mild aching.
2 = Frequently has numbness, tingling, or aching; not distressing.
3 = Frequent painful sensations.
4 = Excruciating pain.

Motor Examination

18. Speech
0 = Normal.
1 = Slight loss of expression, diction, or volume.
2 = Monotone, slurred but understandable; moderately impaired.
3 = Marked impairment; difficult to understand.
4 = Unintelligible.

19. Facial expression
0 = Normal.
1 = Minimal hypomimia; could be normal ("poker face").
2 = Slight but definitely abnormal diminution of facial expression.
3 = Moderate hypomimia; lips parted some of the time.
4 = Masked or fixed facies with severe or complete loss of facial expression; lips parted one-fourth inch or more.

20. Tremor at rest
0 = Absent.
1 = Slight and infrequently present.
2 = Mild in amplitude and persistent, or moderate in amplitude but only intermittently present.
3 = Moderate in amplitude and present most of the time.
4 = Marked in amplitude and present most of the time.

21. Action tremor
0 = Absent.
1 = Slight; present with action.
2 = Moderate in amplitude; present with action.
3 = Moderate in amplitude, with posture holdings as well as action.
4 = Marked in amplitude; interferes with feeding.

22. Rigidity (judged on passive movement of major points with patient relaxed in sitting position; cogwheeling to be ignored)
0 = Absent.
1 = Slight or detectable only when activated by mirror or other movements.
2 = Mild to moderate.
3 = Marked, but full range of motion easily achieved.
4 = Severe; range of motion achieved with difficulty.

23. Finger taps (patient taps thumb with index finger in rapid succession with widest amplitude possible, each hand separately)
0 = Normal.
1 = Mild slowing or reduction in amplitude.

2 = Moderately impaired; definite and early fatiguing; may have occasional arrests in movement.
3 = Severely impaired; frequent hesitation in initiating movements or arrests in ongoing movement.
4 = Can barely perform the task.

24. Hand movements (patient opens and closes hands in rapid succession with widest amplitude possible, each hand separately)
0 = Normal.
1 = Mild slowing or reduction in amplitude.
2 = Moderately impaired; definite and early fatiguing; may have occasional arrests in movement.
3 = Severely impaired; frequent hesitation in initiating movements or arrests in ongoing movement.
4 = Can barely perform the task.

25. Hand pronation-supination (pronation-supination movements of hands, vertically or horizontally, with as large an amplitude as possible, both hands simultaneously)
0 = Normal.
1 = Mild slowing or reduction in amplitude.
2 = Moderately impaired; definite and early fatiguing; may have occasional arrests in movement.
3 = Severely impaired; frequent hesitation in initiating movements or arrests in ongoing movement.
4 = Can barely perform the task.

26. Leg agility (patient taps heel on ground in rapid succession, picking up entire leg; amplitude should be about 3 inches)
0 = Normal.
1 = Mild slowing or reduction in amplitude.
2 = Moderately impaired; definite and early fatiguing; may have occasional arrests in movement.
3 = Severely impaired; frequent hesitation in initiating movements or arrests in ongoing movement.
4 = Can barely perform the task.

27. Arising from chair (patient attempts to arise from a straight back wooden or metal chair with arms folded across chest)
0 = Normal.
1 = Slow, or may need more than one attempt.
2 = Pushes self up from arms of seat.
3 = Tends to fall back and may have to try more than one time, but can get up without help.
4 = Unable to arise without help.

28. Posture
0 = Normal.
1 = Not quite erect, slightly stooped posture; could be normal for older person.
2 = Moderately stooped posture, definitely abnormal; can be slightly leaning to one side.
3 = Severely stooped posture with kyphosis; can be moderately leaning to one side.
4 = Marked flexion with extreme abnormality of posture.

29. Gait
0 = Normal.
1 = Walks slowly; may shuffle with short steps, but no festination or propulsion.
2 = Walks with difficulty, but needs little or no assistance; may have some festination, short steps, or propulsion.

Box 21.2 Unified Parkinson's Disease Rating Scale (UPDRS) Definitions of 0–4 Scale—cont'd

3 = Severe gait disturbance necessitating assistance.

4 = Cannot walk at all, even with assistance.

30. Postural stability (response to sudden posterior displacement produced by pull on shoulders while patient erect with eyes open and feet slightly apart. Patient is prepared.)

    0 = Normal.

    1 = Retropulsion, but recovers unaided.

    2 = Absence of postural response; would fall if not caught by examiner.

    3 = Very unstable; tends to lose balance spontaneously.

    4 = Unable to stand without assistance.

31. Body bradykinesia (combining slowness, hesitancy, decreased arm swing, small amplitude, and poverty of movement in general)

    0 = None.

    1 = Minimal slowness, giving movement a deliberate character; could be normal for some people; possibly reduced amplitude.

    2 = Mild degree of slowness, giving poverty of movement that is definitely abnormal; alternatively, some reduced amplitude.

    3 = Moderate slowness; poverty or small amplitude of movement.

    4 = Marked slowness; poverty or small amplitude of movement.

Complications of Therapy

Score these items to represent the status of the patient in the week before the examination.

Dyskinesias

32. Duration

    What proportion of the waking day are dyskinesias present? (historical information)

    0 = None

    1 = 1%-25% of day

    2 = 26%-50% of day

    3 = 51%-75% of day

    4 = 76%-100% of day

33. Disability

    How disabling are the dyskinesias? (historical information; may be modified by office examination)

    0 = Not disabling

    1 = Mildly disabling

    2 = Moderately disabling

    3 = Severely disabling

    4 = Completely disabling

34. Pain

    How painful are the dyskinesias?

    0 = No painful dyskinesia

    1 = Slight

    2 = Moderate

    3 = Severe

    4 = Marked

35. Presence of early morning dystonia (historical information)

    0 = No

    1 = Yes

Clinical Fluctuations

36. "Offs" duration

    What proportion of the waking day is the average duration of "offs" for the patient?

    0 = None

    1 = 1%-25% of day

    2 = 26%-50% of day

    3 = 51%-75% of day

    4 = 76%-100% of day

37. Are any medication?

    0 = No

    1 = Yes

38. Are any medication?

    0 = No

    1 = Yes

39. "Offs" sudden

    Do any of the "off" periods come on suddenly (i.e., over a few seconds)?

    0 = No

    1 = Yes

Other Complications

40. Anorexia, nausea, vomiting

    Does the patient have anorexia, nausea, or vomiting?

    0 = No

    1 = Yes

41. Sleep disturbances

    Does the patient have any sleep disturbances (e.g., insomnia or hypersomnolence)?

    0 = No

    1 = Yes

42. Symptomatic orthostasis

    Does the patient have symptomatic orthostasis?

    0 = No

    1 = Yes

Modified Hoehn and Yahr Staging

Stage 0 = No signs of disease

Stage I = Unilateral disease

Stage I.5 = Unilateral disease plus axial involvement

Stage II = Bilateral disease, without impairment of balance

Stage II.5 = Mild bilateral disease, with recovery on pull test

Stage III = Mild to moderate bilateral disease; some postural instability; physically independent

Stage IV = Severe disability; still able to walk or stand unassisted

Stage V = Wheelchair bound or bedridden unless aided

Modified Schwab and England Activities of Daily Living Scales

100%: Completely independent. Able to do all chores without slowness, difficulty, or impairment. Essentially normal. Unaware of any difficulty.

90%: Completely independent. Able to do all chores with some degree of slowness, difficulty, and impairment. Might take twice as long. Beginning to be aware of difficulty.

80%: Completely independent in most chores. Takes twice as long. Conscious difficulty and slowness.

Continued

Box 21.2 **Unified Parkinson's Disease Rating Scale (UPDRS) Definitions of 0–4 Scale—cont'd**

70%: Not completely independent. More difficulty with some chores. Takes three to four times as long to perform some. Must spend a large part of the day on chores.

60%: Some dependency. Can do most chores, but exceedingly slowly and with much effort. Errors; some impossible.

50%: More dependent. Help with half of chores, slower, etc. Difficulty with everything.

40%: Very dependent. Can assist with all chores, but few periods alone.

30%: With effort, now and then does a few chores alone or begins alone. Much help needed.

20%: Nothing alone. Can be a slight help with some chores. Severe invalid periods.

10%: Totally dependent, helpless. Complete invalid.

0%: Vegetative. Functions such as swallowing, bladder, and bowel are not functioning. Bedridden.

a light into the eyes or manipulating the lids) also may be seen. Spontaneous blepharospasm and apraxia of lid opening occur less often. Patients with apraxia of lid opening (not a true apraxia) often open their eyes using their hands, and once the eyes are fixated on an object, the eyelids remain open. Primitive reflexes, including the inability to inhibit blinking in response to tapping over the glabella (Myerson sign) and palmomental reflexes, are nonspecific and are commonly present in many parkinsonian disorders (Brodsky et al., 2004).

Various types of tremor, most notably resting and postural varieties, often accompany parkinsonian disorders. Patients should be observed with hands resting on their laps or thighs, and they should be instructed to hold their arms in an outstretched position or in a horizontal position with shoulders abducted, elbows flexed, and hands palms-down in front of their faces in the so-called wing-beating position. Resting tremor often reemerges after a period of quiescence in a new position (*re-emergent tremor*) (Jankovic, 2008). This re-emergent tremor may be wrongly attributed to postural tremor and lead to misdiagnosis as essential tremor. A true kinetic (intention) tremor, elicited by the finger-to-nose maneuver, is much less common in patients with PD and other parkinsonian disorders and usually indicates involvement of cerebellar connections. A jerky postural tremor indicative of additional myoclonus is suggestive of a diagnosis of MSA rather than PD. Head tremor (*titubation*) suggests a diagnosis other than PD, such as essential tremor, dystonic neck tremor, or a cerebellar tremor associated with the cerebellar form of MSA (MSA-C), spinocerebellar atrophy, or multiple sclerosis (MS).

Rigidity is an increase in muscle tone, usually equal in flexors and extensors and present throughout the passive range of movement. This contrasts with the distribution and velocity-dependent nature of spasticity. Paratonia (or Gegenhalten), on the other hand, increases with repetitive passive movement and attempts to get the patient to relax. It may be difficult to distinguish between milder forms of paratonia and rigidity, especially in the legs. Characteristically, the performance of voluntary movements in the opposite limb (e.g., opening and closing the fist or abduction-adduction of the shoulder) brings out rigidity, a phenomenon known as *activated rigidity* (Froment sign). Superimposed on the rigidity may be a tremor or cogwheel phenomenon. This, like the milder forms of rigidity, is better appreciated by placing one hand over the muscles being tested (e.g., placing the left thumb over the biceps and the remaining fingers over the triceps while flexing and extending the elbow with the right hand). The distribution of the rigidity

sometimes is helpful in differential diagnosis. For example, pronounced nuchal rigidity with much less hypertonicity in the limbs suggests the diagnosis of PSP, whereas an extreme degree of unilateral arm rigidity or paratonia suggests *corticobasal degeneration* (CBD) or *corticobasal syndrome* (CBS). The latter term is suggested for cases diagnosed clinically, as only 24% of such cases have pathologically proven CBD (Ling et al., 2010).

Akinesia and bradykinesia are appreciable on examination in several ways. Automatic movements normally expressed in conversation, such as gesturing with hands while speaking, crossing and uncrossing the legs, and repositioning the body in the chair diminish or are absent. The performance of rapid, repetitive, and alternating movements such as finger tapping, opening and closing the fist, pronation-supination of the forearm, and foot tapping is slow, with a gradual reduction in amplitude and eventual cessation of movement (*freezing*). In addition to fatiguing, there may be hesitation in initiating movement and arrests in ongoing movement. The severely afflicted patient may be barely able to perform the task. There is a tendency for rapid repetitive movements to take on the frequency of an accompanying tremor. In such cases, instruct the patient to slow the movement and attempt to complete it voluntarily. Watching the patient write is an important part of the examination. Observation may reveal great slowness and effort, even in someone with minimal change in the size of the script. In addition to micrographia, writing and drawing show a tendency to fatigue, with a further reduction in size as the task proceeds and a concomitant action tremor.

Postural disturbances are common in parkinsonian disorders. The head usually tilts forward and the body becomes stooped, often with pronounced kyphosis and varying degrees of scoliosis (Ashour and Jankovic, 2006). The arms become flexed at the elbows and wrists, with varying postural deformities in the hands, the most common being flexion at the metacarpophalangeal joints and extension at the interphalangeal joints, with adduction of all the fingers and opposition of the thumb to the index finger (*striatal hand*). Flexion also occurs in the joints of the legs. Variable foot deformities occur, the most common being hammer toe–like disturbances in most of the toes, occasionally with extension of the great toe (*striatal foot*), which may be misinterpreted as an extensor plantar response. Initially, abnormal foot posturing may be induced by action, occurring only during walking or weight bearing. The flexed or simian posture sometimes is extreme, with severe flexion at the waist (*camptocormia*) (Azher and Jankovic, 2005; Jankovic, 2010). Some patients, particularly those with MSA, exhibit scoliosis or tilted posture (*Pisa sign*). Despite the truncal flexion, the position of the hands in patients with PD often remains above the beltline because of flexion of the elbows. Occasional patients remain upright or even demonstrate a hyperextended posture. Hyperextension of the neck is particularly suggestive of PSP, whereas extreme flexion of the neck (head drop or bent spine) suggests MSA but also PD.

Postural instability is characteristic of parkinsonian disorders, particularly the postural instability and gait difficulty forms of PD, PSP, and MSA. As patients rise from a sitting position, poor postural stability, slowness, narrow base, and not repositioning the feet often combine to cause them to fall back into the chair "in a lump." PSP patients may "rocket" out of the chair inappropriately quickly, failing to recognize their inability to maintain stability on their feet. The PD patient may require several attempts, push off the arms of the chair, or need to be pulled up by an assistant. Gait disturbances in typical parkinsonism include lack of arm swing, shortened and later shuffling stride, freezing in the course of walking (especially at a door frame or when approaching a potential obstruction or a chair), and in more severe cases, propulsion and spontaneous falls (Jankovic, 2007a). In addition, walking often brings out or exacerbates a resting tremor. To assess postural instability, the physician performs the pull test. Standing behind the patient, the examiner pulls the patient backward by the shoulders (or by a hand on the sternum), carefully remaining close behind to prevent a fall. Once postural reflexes are impaired, there may be retropulsion or multiple backward steps in response to the postural perturbation. Later there is a tendency to fall en bloc without retropulsion or even normal attempts to recover or to cushion the fall.

In PD, the base of the gait is usually narrow, and tandem gait is performed well. When the gait is wide-based, a superimposed ataxia is a consideration, as is seen in MSA-C, although some of the spinocerebellar atrophies may present with parkinsonism and ataxia (see Chapter 72). Toe walking (*cock-walk*) is seen in some parkinsonian disorders (e.g., due to manganese poisoning), and a peculiar loping gait may indicate the rare patient with akinesia in the absence of rigidity, which may be one phenotype of PSP. The so-called magnetic foot, or marche à petits pas, of senility (also seen in multiple infarctions, Binswanger disease, and normal pressure hydrocephalus) more commonly results in a lower-body parkinsonism, typically associated with cerebrovascular disorders such as lacunar strokes. A striking discrepancy of involvement between the lower body and the upper limbs, with normal or even excessive arm swing, is an important clue to the diagnosis of vascular parkinsonism.

Differential Diagnosis

Although dementia commonly occurs in PD, this feature, particularly when present relatively early in the course, must alert the physician to other possible diagnoses (see Chapter 66), including the coincidental association of unrelated causes of cognitive decline (Galvin et al., 2006). Prominent eye movement disturbances are found in a number of conditions, including PSP, MSA-C, postencephalitic parkinsonism, and CBD. It is important to assess not only horizontal and vertical gaze (typically impaired in PSP) but also optokinetic nystagmus to note whether vertical saccadic eye movements (particularly as the optokinetic tape moves in upward direction) are impaired, as in PSP. The oculocephalic (doll's eye)

maneuver must be performed where ocular excursions are limited, seeking supportive evidence of supranuclear gaze palsy. Patients with PSP typically have trouble making eye contact because of disturbed visual refixation. As a result of persistence of visual fixation when PSP patients turn, their head turn lags behind their body turn. Obvious pyramidal tract dysfunction usually suggests diagnoses other than PD. An exaggerated grasp response indicates disturbance of the frontal lobes and the possibility of a concomitant dementing process. Occasionally a pronounced flexed posture in the hand may be confused with a grasp reflex, and the examiner must be convinced that there is active contraction in response to stroking of the palm. The abnormalities of rapid, repetitive, and alternating movements described earlier can be confused with the clumsy awkward performance of limb-kinetic apraxia (Zadikoff and Lang, 2005). More importantly, the abnormalities in performance of repetitive movement must not be confused with the disruption of rate, rhythm, and force typical of the dysdiadochokinesia of cerebellar disease. A helpful maneuver in testing for the presence of associated cerebellar dysfunction is to have the patient tap with the index finger on a hard surface. Watching and, in particular, listening to the tapping often allows a distinction to be made between the slowness and decrementing response of parkinsonism and the irregular rate and force of cerebellar ataxia. Testing for ideomotor apraxia, as seen in CBS, should also be performed by asking the patient to mimic certain hand gestures (intransitive tasks) such as the "victory sign" or the University of Texas "hook 'em horns sign" (extension of the second and fifth finger and flexion of the third and fourth finger) or to simulate certain activities (transitive tasks [using a tool or utensil]) such as brushing teeth and combing hair. However, in the later stages of many parkinsonian disorders, rigidity and other motor disturbances may make results of these tests difficult to interpret. In PD or MSA, the less affected limb may show mirror movements as the patient attempts to perform rapid repetitive or alternating movements with the most affected limb (Espay et al., 2005). On the other hand, in CBS, the most affected limb may mirror movements performed in the less affected limb. Some patients with parkinsonism and frontal lobe involvement exhibit signs of perseveration such as the *applause sign*, manifested by persistence of clapping after instructing the patient to clap consecutively three times as quickly as possible. Although initially thought to be characteristic of PSP, it is also present in some patients with other parkinsonian disorders (Wu et al., 2008).

The presence of other abnormal movements in an untreated patient may indicate a diagnosis other than PD. Seek stimulus-sensitive myoclonus by using light touch or pinprick in the digits and the proximal palm or the sole of the foot. Easily elicited and nonfatiguing myoclonic jerks in response to these stimuli may be seen not only in patients with CBS and MSA but also in patients with PD and dementia.

Despite a variety of sensory complaints, patients with PD do not show prominent abnormalities on the sensory examination, aside from the normal increase in vibration threshold that occurs with age. Cortical sensory disturbances suggest a diagnosis of CBS. Wasting and muscle weakness are not characteristic of PD, although later in the course of the disease, severely disabled patients show disuse atrophy and severe problems in initiating and maintaining muscle activation that are often difficult to separate from true weakness.

Combinations of upper and lower motor neuron weakness occur in several other parkinsonian disorders (see **Table 21.2**).

Assess autonomic function. At the bedside, this includes an evaluation of orthostatic changes in blood pressure and pulse (in supine position and at least 3 minutes after standing) and, in appropriate circumstances, the patient's response to the Valsalva maneuver, mental arithmetic, and the cold pressor test, among others. Finally, perform sequential examinations over time, carefully searching for the development of additional findings that may provide a clue to the diagnosis. Several parkinsonian syndromes present initially as pure parkinsonism; only later with disease progression do other signs develop.

Tremor

Tremor is rhythmic oscillation of a body part, produced by either alternating or synchronous contractions of reciprocally innervated antagonistic muscles. Tremors usually have a fixed frequency, although the rate may appear irregular. The amplitude of the tremor can vary widely, depending on both physiological and psychological factors. The basis of further categorization is the position, posture, and motor performance necessary to elicit it. A *rest tremor* occurs with the body part in complete repose, although when a patient totally relaxes or sleeps, this tremor usually disappears. Maintenance of a posture, such as extending the arms parallel to the floor, reveals a *postural tremor*; moving the body part to and from a target brings out an *intention tremor*. The use of other descriptive categories has caused some confusion in tremor terminology. *Action tremor* has been used for both postural and kinetic (also known as *intention*) tremors. Whereas a *kinetic tremor* is present throughout goal-directed movement, the term *terminal tremor* applies to the component of kinetic tremor that exaggerates when approaching the target. *Ataxic tremor* refers to a combination of kinetic tremor plus limb ataxia. **Box 21.3** provides a list of differential diagnoses for the three major categories of tremor and other rhythmic movements that occasionally are confused with tremor.

Common Symptoms

A description of symptoms occurs under the various categories of tremor. All people have a normal or physiological tremor demonstrable with sensitive recording devices. Two common pathological tremor disorders that are often confused are parkinsonian rest tremor and essential tremor. Although Chapter 71 discusses both conditions in detail, we discuss helpful distinguishing points here in view of the frequency of misdiagnosis.

Rest Tremor

A rest tremor occurs with the body part in complete repose and often dampens or subsides entirely with action. For this reason, patients with pure rest tremor experience greater social embarrassment than functional disability. Indeed, in some cases it is a family member or friend who first observes the tremor, which is noticeable to the patient only later. Alternatively, some patients complain of the sensation of trembling inside long before a rest tremor becomes overt. Early on, rest tremor may be intermittent and often precipitated only by anxiety or stress. The onset of most types of tremor is in the

---

Box 21.3 Classification and Differential Diagnosis of Tremor

Resting Tremors

PD
Other parkinsonian syndromes (less common)
Midbrain (rubral) tremor (Holmes tremor): rest < postural < intention
WD (also acquired hepatocerebral degeneration)
Essential tremor

Postural Tremors

Physiological tremor
Exaggerated physiological tremor; these factors can also aggravate other forms of tremor:
　　Stress, fatigue, anxiety, emotion
　　Endocrine: hypoglycemia, thyrotoxicosis, pheochromocytoma
　　Drugs and toxins: adrenocorticosteroids, β-agonists, dopamine agonists, amphetamines, lithium, tricyclic antidepressants, neuroleptics, theophylline, caffeine, valproic acid, alcohol withdrawal, mercury ("hatter's shakes"), lead, arsenic, others
Essential tremor (familial or sporadic)
Primary writing tremor and other task-specific tremors
Orthostatic tremor
With other CNS disorders:
　　PD (postural tremor, re-emergent tremor, associated essential tremor)
　　Other akinetic-rigid syndromes
　　Idiopathic dystonia, including focal dystonias
With peripheral neuropathy:
　　Charcot-Marie-Tooth disease (called the *Roussy-Levy syndrome*)
　　Other peripheral neuropathies
Cerebellar tremor
　　Intention tremors
Diseases of cerebellar outflow (dentate nuclei, interpositus nuclei, or both, and superior cerebellar peduncle):
　　MS, trauma, tumor, vascular disease, WD, acquired hepatocerebral degeneration, drugs, toxins (e.g., mercury), others
Miscellaneous rhythmic movement disorders
Psychogenic tremor
Rhythmic movements in dystonia (dystonic tremor, myorrhythmia)
Rhythmic myoclonus (segmental myoclonus, e.g., palatal or branchial myoclonus, spinal myoclonus), myorrhythmia
Oscillatory myoclonus
Asterixis
Clonus
Epilepsia partialis continua
Hereditary chin quivering
Spasmus nutans
Head bobbing with third ventricular cysts
Nystagmus

CNS, Central nervous system; *MS,* Multiple sclerosis; *PD,* Parkinson disease; *WD,* Wilson disease.

arms, often beginning asymmetrically. In the face, rest tremor usually affects the lips and jaw, and the patient may note a rhythmic clicking of the teeth. In the limbs, the tremor usually is most distally in the fingers (pill rolling) or may manifest by flexion-extension or a supination-pronation, oscillatory movement of the wrist and forearm, and flexion-extension movement of the ankle. In severe forms, it may be present more proximally, causing the entire body to shake. The presence of head tremor (titubation) should raise the possibility of essential tremor or of dystonic tremor associated with cervical dystonia or cerebellar outflow tremor, as is seen in patients with MS or posterior fossa disorders. Tremor in the legs, and especially in the feet while sitting, is usually caused by parkinsonian rest tremor. A history of progression from unilateral arm tremor to additional involvement of the ipsilateral leg suggests parkinsonism rather than essential tremor. Once the tremor has become noticeable to the patient, a variety of methods are used to conceal the movement, such as holding one hand with the other, sitting on the affected hand, or crossing the legs to dampen a tremulous lower limb. Many patients find that they can briefly abort the tremor.

Postural Tremor

In contrast to a pure rest tremor, postural tremors, especially with pronounced terminal accentuation, can result in significant disability. Many such patients are mistaken as having "bad nerves." People who perform delicate work with their hands (e.g., jewelers, surgeons) become aware of this form of tremor earlier than most. The average person usually first appreciates tremor in the acts of feeding and writing. Carrying a cup of liquid, pouring, or eating with a spoon often brings out the tremor. Writing is tremulous and sloppy, questioning the patient's signature on a check. The voice may be involved in essential tremor. Again, anxiety and stress worsen the tremor, and patients often notice that their symptoms are especially bad in public. The most common cause of postural tremor seen in movement disorders clinics is essential tremor (Jankovic, 2009).

Patients often adopt compensatory mechanisms to lessen the disability caused by tremor. Many give up certain tasks such as serving drinks and eating specific foods (e.g., soup), especially in public. When the tremor is very asymmetrical, patients often switch to using the less-affected hand for many tasks, including writing. Bringing a cup to the mouth becomes difficult; later, a straw is required. When writing, patients may use the other hand to steady the paper or the writing hand itself. Patients often switch from cursive to print, and the use of heavier or thicker writing instruments sometimes makes the script more legible. In some patients with parkinsonian disorders and severe rest tremor, the tremor may also be present while the patient holds an outstretched or wing-beating posture. This tremor usually occurs after a latency of several seconds, hence the term *re-emergent tremor*; in contrast, in essential tremor the tremor is evident immediately on taking up a new posture.

Other Types of Tremor

Various types of writing disturbances may combine with tremor. Primary writing tremor is one form of task-specific tremor that affects the writing act in isolation, with little or no associated postural or terminal tremor interfering with other acts. Dystonic writer's cramp can involve additional tremulousness on writing. Distinction is required from the voluntary excessive squeezing of the pen or pressing onto the page often seen in patients with essential tremor or primary writing tremor, which is attributable to their attempts to lessen the effect of tremor on writing. In addition, patients with postural tremor may consciously slow their writing to improve accuracy, but this is a voluntary compensatory mechanism not associated with the micrographia and fatigue that accompany parkinsonism.

Tremor in the head and neck, or titubation, occurs in isolation or combined with a postural tremor elsewhere, especially in the arms, as is seen in patients with essential tremor. When the head tremor is irregular and is associated with abnormal head posture and uneven contractions or hypertrophy of the neck muscles, the possibility of cervical dystonia requires consideration (dystonic tremor). Head tremor is rarely a source of physical disability but may create social embarrassment. Patients occasionally complain of a similar tremor of the voice. This is particularly noticeable to others who are listening to the patient on the telephone, and many ask the patient whether they are sad or have been crying.

Less often, patients with postural tremors note a similar tremor in the legs and trunk. The awareness of this form of tremor clearly depends on the activity performed. One form of postural tremor, orthostatic tremor, characteristically presents not as tremor but rather difficulty and insecurity on standing. It is associated with a 14- to 16-Hz tremor in the legs and trunk. This tremor typically subsides if the patient can walk about, lean against something, or sit down.

Other Clues in the History

Although patients with several different types of tremor may indicate that alcohol transiently reduces their shaking, a striking response to small amounts of alcohol is particularly characteristic of essential tremor (Mostile and Jankovic, 2010). Clues to the possible presence of factors aggravating the normal physiological tremor (see **Box 21.3**) require further inquiry.

Examination

In addition to clinical examination, various physiological, accelerometric, and other computer-based techniques can be employed to assess tremor, but a clinical rating scale usually is most practical, particularly in clinical trials. The Tremor Research Group (TRG) has developed a rating scale that can be used to quantitatively assess all types of tremor, particularly essential tremor, the most common type encountered in clinical practice (**Box 21.4**). The TRG Essential Tremor Rating Scale (TETRAS) is currently being validated and has been found to correlate well with quantitative computer-based systems (Mostile et al., 2010). Besides rest tremor, postural tremor, and kinetic limb tremor, examine patients for tremor of the head. With the patient seated or standing, head tremor may be evident as vertical ("yes-yes") nodding (*tremblement affirmatif*) or side-to-side ("no-no") horizontal shaking (*tremblement negatif*). There may be combinations of the two, with rotatory movements. Subtle head tremors may only be

Box 21.4 **Tremor Research Group Rating Scale**

Instructions for Completing The Observed Tremor Portion

1. Head tremor: Subject is seated upright. The head is observed for 10 seconds in midposition and for 5 seconds each during several provocative maneuvers. First the subject is asked to rotate his or her head to the maximum lateral positions slowly in each direction. The subject is then asked to deviate his or her eyes to the maximum lateral positions while the examiner gently touches the subject's chin.

0 = No tremor.
1 = Tremor seen or felt during provocative maneuvers.
2 = Mild tremor seen at midposition or moderate tremor seen with provocative maneuvers.
3 = Moderate tremor seen at midposition or severe tremor seen with provocative maneuvers.
4 = Severe tremor seen at midposition.

2a. Face tremor: Subject is seated upright and asked to smile and pucker his or her lips, each for 5 seconds. Tremor is specifically assessed for the lower facial muscles (excluding jaw and tongue) and upper face (eye closure).

0 = No tremor.
1 = Mild tremor seen only with active muscle contraction.
2 = Mild tremor seen at rest or moderate tremor seen with active muscle contraction.
3 = Moderate tremor seen at rest or severe tremor seen with muscle contraction.
4 = Severe tremor seen at rest.

2b. Tongue tremor: Subject is seated upright and asked to open his or her mouth for 5 seconds and then stick out his or her tongue for 5 seconds.

0 = No tremor.
1 = Mild tremor seen only with active muscle contraction.
2 = Mild tremor seen at rest or moderate tremor seen with active muscle contraction.
3 = Moderate tremor seen at rest or severe tremor seen with active muscle contraction.
4 = Severe tremor seen at rest.

2c. Jaw tremor: Subject is seated upright and asked to maximally open his or her mouth and clench the jaw for 5 seconds.

0 = No tremor.
1 = Mild tremor seen only with active muscle contraction.
2 = Mild tremor seen at rest or moderate tremor seen with active muscle contraction.
3 = Moderate tremor seen at rest or severe tremor seen with active muscle contraction.
4 = Severe tremor seen at rest.

3. Voice tremor: First assess speech during normal conversation; then ask subject to produce an extended "aaa" sound and "eee" sound for 5 seconds each.

0 = No tremor.
1 = Barely perceptible tremor only during provocative maneuver.
2 = Mild but clear tremor present with speaking.
3 = Moderate tremor (no voice breaks).
4 = Severe tremor (with voice breaks or unintelligible speech).

4. Arm tremor: Subject is seated upright. Tremor is assessed during four arm maneuvers (rest, forward horizontal reach posture, lateral "wing-beating" posture, and kinesis) for 5

seconds in each posture. Left and right arms may be assessed simultaneously. Amplitude assessment should be estimated using the maximally displaced point of the hand at the point of greatest displacement along any single plane. For example, the amplitude of a pure supination-pronation tremor, pivoting around the wrist, would be assessed at either the thumb or fifth digit.

a. Rest tremor. The subject should have his or her elbows on the arm rests. (If this is the previous assessment, no specific instructions should be given if the subject did not naturally assume an acceptable arm position for elbows on the arm rests, with hands resting freely.) Begin the second assessment only after the subject appears relaxed in the new position.

b. Forward outstretched postural tremor. Subject should bring his or her arms forward, slightly lateral to midline and parallel to the ground. The wrists should also be straight and the fingers slightly and comfortably abducted so that they do not touch each other.

c. Lateral "wing-beating postural" tremor. Subject abducts his or her arms parallel to the ground and flexes the elbows so that the two hands do not quite touch each other. The fingers are slightly and comfortably abducted so that they do not touch each other, with the pointer finger at shoulder height.

d. Kinetic tremor. Subject extends only his or her pointer finger, then touches a set object located at the same height (parallel to the ground) and slightly lateral to the midline. The subject then touches his or her own nose or chin and repeats this back-and-forth motion five times. Only the position along the trajectory of greatest tremor amplitude is assessed. This will typically be either at the nose or chin or at the point of full extent.

e. Tremor while walking: Have the patient walk a minimum of 6 m at a normal pace to and from the examiner, and observe his or her hands.

Rest tremor:

0 = No tremor.
1 = Tremor is barely visible or present only with mental provocation or reinforcement.
1.5 = Tremor is visible, but is < 1 cm amplitude.
2 = Tremor is 1–3 cm amplitude.
2.5 = Tremor is 3–5 cm amplitude.
3 = Tremor is 5–10 cm amplitude.
3.5 = Tremor is 10–20 cm amplitude.
4 = Tremor is > 20 cm amplitude.

Postural tremor:

0 = No tremor.
1 = Tremor is barely visible.
1.5 = Tremor is visible, but is < 1 cm amplitude.
2 = Tremor is 1-3 cm amplitude.
2.5 = Tremor is 3-5 cm amplitude.
3 = Tremor is 5-10 cm amplitude.
3.5 = Tremor is 10-20 cm amplitude.
4 = Tremor is > 20 cm amplitude.

Kinetic tremor:

0 = No tremor.
1 = Tremor is barely visible.
1.5 = Tremor is visible, but is < 1 cm amplitude.
2 = Tremor is 1-3 cm amplitude.

Box 21.4 Tremor Research Group Rating Scale—cont'd

2.5 = Tremor is 3-5 cm amplitude.
3 = Tremor is 5-10 cm amplitude.
3.5 = Tremor is 10-20 cm amplitude.
4 = Tremor is > 20 cm amplitude.
Tremor while walking:
0 = No tremor.
1 = Tremor is barely visible.
1.5 = Tremor is visible, but is < 1 cm amplitude.
2 = Tremor is 1-3 cm amplitude.
2.5 = Tremor is 3-5 cm amplitude.
3 = Tremor is 5-10 cm amplitude.
3.5 = Tremor is 10-20 cm amplitude.
4 = Tremor is > 20 cm amplitude.

5. Trunk tremor: Subject is comfortably seated in a chair and asked to flex both legs at the hips 30 degrees above parallel to the ground for 5 seconds. The knees are passively bent so that the lower leg is perpendicular to the ground. The legs are not allowed to touch. Tremor is evaluated around the hip joints and the abdominal muscles.
   0 = No tremor.
   1 = Tremor present only with hip flexion.
   2 = Obvious but mild tremor.
   3 = Moderate tremor.
   4 = Severe tremor.

6. Leg tremor action: Subject is comfortably seated and asked to raise his or her legs parallel to the ground with knees extended for 5 seconds. The legs are slightly abducted so they do not touch. Tremor amplitude is assessed at the end of the feet.
   0 = No tremor.
   1 = Barely perceptible tremor.
   2 = Obvious but mild tremor.
   3 = Moderate tremor; < 5 cm amplitude at any point.
   4 = Severe tremor; > 5 cm amplitude.

7. Leg tremor rest: Subject is comfortably seated with knees flexed and feet resting on the ground. Tremor amplitude is assessed at the point of maximal displacement.
   0 = No tremor.
   1 = Barely perceptible tremor.
   2 = Obvious but mild tremor.
   3 = Moderate tremor; < 5 cm amplitude at any point.
   4 = Severe tremor; > 5 cm amplitude.

8. Standing tremor: Subject is standing, unaided if possible. The internal malleoli are 5 cm apart. Arms are down at the sides. Tremor is assessed at any point on the legs or trunk.
   0 = No tremor.
   1 = Barely perceptible tremor.
   2 = Obvious but mild tremor.
   3 = Moderate tremor.
   4 = Severe tremor.

9. Spiral drawings: Ask the subject to draw the requested figures. Test each hand without leaving the hand or arm on the table. Use only a ballpoint pen.
   0 = Normal.
   1 = Slightly tremulous. May cross lines occasionally.
   2 = Moderately tremulous or crosses lines frequently.
   3 = Accomplishes the task with great difficulty. Figure still recognizable.
   4 = Unable to complete drawing. Figure not recognizable.

10. Handwriting: Have patient write "Today is a nice day."
    0 = Normal.
    1 = Mildly abnormal. Slightly untidy, tremulous.
    2 = Moderately abnormal. Legible, but with considerable tremor.
    3 = Markedly abnormal. Illegible.
    4 = Severely abnormal. Unable to keep pencil or pen on paper without holding down with the other hand.

11. Hold pencil approximately 1 mm above a point on a piece of paper for 10 seconds.
    0 = No tremor.
    1 = Tremor is barely visible.
    1.5 = Tremor is visible, but is < 1 cm amplitude.
    2 = Tremor is 1-3 cm amplitude.
    2.5 = Tremor is 3-5 cm amplitude.
    3 = Tremor is 5-10 cm amplitude.
    3.5 = Tremor is 10-20 cm amplitude.
    4 = Tremor is > 20 cm amplitude.

12. Pour water from one glass into another, using styrofoam coffee cups filled 1 cm from top. Rated separately for right and left hands.
    0 = Absolutely no visible tremor.
    1 = More careful than a person without tremor. No water is spilled.
    2 = Spills a small amount (<10%).
    3 = Spills large amount (10%-50%).
    4 = Unable to pour without spilling most.

appreciated when the examiner holds the patient's cranium while testing with the other hand for extreme lateral eye movements. Head tremors usually range from 1.5 to 5 Hz and are most commonly associated with essential tremor or cervical dystonia and with diseases of the cerebellum and its outflow pathways. A parkinsonian rest tremor may involve the jaw and lips. A similar tremor of the perioral and nasal muscles, the *rabbit syndrome*, has been associated with antipsychotic drug therapy but also occurs in PD. In many disorders, voluntary contraction of the facial muscles induces an action tremor. In addition, a postural tremor of the tongue often is present on tongue protrusion. In the case of tremors of head and neck structures, it is important to observe the palate at rest for the

slower rhythmic movements of palatal myoclonus (also called *palatal tremor*). Occasionally, tremor spares the palate, with similar movements affecting other branchial structures. Demonstration of a voice tremor requires asking the patient to hold a note as long as possible. Superimposed on the vocal tremulousness may be a harsh, strained quality or abrupt cessation of airflow during the course of maintaining the note, which suggests a superimposed dystonia of the larynx (*spasmodic dysphonia*).

A parkinsonian rest tremor is characteristically in the 4- to 6-Hz range. The frequency of postural arm tremors varies depending on cause and severity. Essential tremor usually is in the range of 5 to 10 Hz, with the greater-amplitude tremors

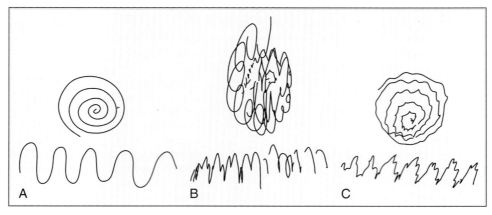

Fig. 21.2 Archimedes spiral and wavy-line drawings by the examiner **(A)** and by a patient with essential tremor **(B-C)**, in whom the tremor is asymmetrical and more evident in the right hand **(B)** than in the left hand **(C)**.

tending to be slower. Exaggerated physiological tremor has a frequency of 8 to 12 Hz. Many patients with parkinsonism demonstrate a combination of slower resting and faster postural tremors. Some patients with slower, larger-amplitude forms of essential tremor have a definite resting component.

A resting tremor in the limbs occurs even with the muscles in complete repose. Even a small amount of muscle activity, as may occur if the patient is somewhat anxious or the limb is not completely at rest, may bring out a higher-frequency action postural tremor. It is sometimes impossible to abate this postural tremor during a stressful office interview. Stress and concentration may bring out an occult resting tremor, such as the performance of serial sevens. Although a rest tremor characteristically subsides when the patient maintains a posture (e.g., holding the arms outstretched parallel to the floor), it may recur after a few seconds. As noted before, the re-emergent tremor that occurs after a latency of a few seconds (and sometimes as long as 1 minute) suggests an underlying parkinsonian disorder. Carrying out goal-directed movements, such as finger-to-nose testing, usually causes the tremor to dampen further or subside completely. On the other hand, a typical postural tremor associated with essential tremor usually occurs without latency after the initiation of a posture and may worsen further at the endpoints of goal-directed movement (*terminal tremor*). The slower kinetic tremor of cerebellar disease occurs throughout the movement but also worsens upon reaching the target. Occasionally, pronounced bursts of muscle activity in a patient with terminal tremor causes individual separate jerks, which give the impression of superimposed myoclonus. *Essential myoclonus* is an autosomal dominant disorder, and affected patients and their relatives have both jerklike myoclonus and postural tremor phenomenologically identical to essential tremor.

Having the patient point the index fingers at each other under the nose (without touching the fingers together or touching the face) with the arms abducted at the sides and the elbows flexed can demonstrate both distal tremor in the hands and proximal tremors. An example of proximal tremor is the slower wing-beating tremor of cerebellar outflow pathway disease, as may be seen in WD. Tremor during the course of slowly pronating and supinating the forearms with the arms outstretched or with forceful abduction of the fingers occurs

in patients with primary writing tremor. Holding a full cup of water with the arm outstretched often amplifies a postural tremor, and picking up the full cup, bringing it to the mouth, and tipping it to drink enhances the terminal tremor, often causing spillage. In addition to writing, one should have the patient draw with both hands separately. Useful drawing tasks include an Archimedes spiral, a wavy line from one side of the page to the other (**Fig. 21.2**), and an attempt to carefully draw a line or spiral between two well-defined, closely opposed borders. Another useful test designed to bring out position-specific tremor is the dot approximation test, in which the patient is instructed to be seated at the desk with elbow elevated and to hold the tip of the pen or pencil (for at least 10 seconds) as close as possible to a dot drawn on a sheet of paper without touching it. Many patients with action tremors note marked exacerbation of their tremor during this specific task.

In the legs, in addition to the standard heel-to-shin testing which brings out kinetic and terminal tremors, it may be possible to demonstrate a postural tremor by having the patient hold the leg off the bed and attempt to touch the examiner's finger with the great toe. With the legs flexed at the knees and abducted at the hips and the feet held flat on the bed, synchronous rhythmic 3-Hz abductions of the thighs may occur in patients with atrophy of the anterior vermis, as seen in alcoholic cerebellar degeneration.

On standing unsupported, patients with orthostatic tremor develop rapid, rhythmic contractions of leg muscles, causing the kneecaps to bob up and down. This dampens or subsides on walking. In contrast, cerebellar disease results in slower titubation of axial structures and the head, seen in the upright position. Often, observing the gait helps differentiate between upper-limb rest tremor and postural tremor that persists at rest as a result of stress. The former usually is clearly evident during walking, whereas the latter usually subsides. Obviously, observing additional features of the gait is helpful in making these distinctions as well.

Certain tremors persist in all positions. Disease in the midbrain involving the superior cerebellar peduncle near the red nucleus (possibly also involving the nigrostriatal fibers) results in the so-called midbrain, or rubral, tremor (*Holmes tremor*). Characteristically, this form of tremor combines features of the three tremor classes. It is often present at rest, increases with postural maintenance, and increases still further, sometimes to extreme degrees, with goal-directed movement. Tremor also may be a feature of psychiatric disease, representing a conversion reaction or even malingering. Usually, certain features are atypical or incongruous. This psychogenic tremor differs from most organic tremors in that the frequency is often quite variable, and concentration and distraction often abate the tremor instead of increasing it (Kenney et al., 2007; Thomas and Jankovic, 2010).

Dystonia

Dystonia is a disorder dominated by sustained muscle contractions, which often cause twisting and repetitive movements or abnormal postures (Jankovic, 2007b). The term *dystonia* is used in three major contexts: (1) to describe the specific form of involuntary movement (i.e., a physical sign), (2) to refer to a syndrome caused by a large number of different disease states, or (3) to refer to the idiopathic form of dystonia, in which these movements usually occur in isolation without additional neurological abnormalities (**Box 21.5**).

Dystonic movements may be slow and twisting or quite rapid, resembling the shock-like jerks of myoclonus. There may be additional rhythmic movements, especially when the patient actively attempts to resist the involuntary movement. If the patient relaxes, allowing the limb to move as it pleases, the abnormal dystonic posturing usually becomes evident, and the rhythmic dystonic tremor lessens. This position in which dystonic tremor ceases is the *null point*. A faster distal postural tremor similar to essential tremor is a common associated feature. The varied nature of these movements often causes the misdiagnosis of dystonia as some other type of movement disorder.

Another common error in diagnosis is the mislabeling of dystonia as hysteria. Stress and anxiety aggravate the movements, and rest and even hypnosis alleviate the movements. Patients often discover a variety of peculiar maneuvers (sensory tricks) that they can use to lessen or even completely abate the dystonic movements and postures (discussed in this chapter and in Chapter 71). The abnormal movements and postures may occur only during the performance of certain acts and not others that use the same muscles. An example of this action, *task-specific dystonia*, is involvement of the hand only in writing (writer's cramp or graphospasm) or playing a musical instrument, but not with other manual tasks such as using utensils. Dystonia of the oromandibular region only on speaking or eating is another example of task-specific dystonia, as is dystonia in legs and trunk that occurs only on walking forward but not on walking backward, climbing stairs, or running. On the other hand, some dystonias occur only during running (Wu and Jankovic, 2006). A final source of possible confusion with hysteria is the occurrence of dystonia after injury to the affected limb or after prolonged immobilization such as casting. Such peripherally induced dystonia, which is usually fixed rather than mobile, may be associated with a complex regional pain syndrome (previously referred to as *reflex sympathetic dystrophy*), depression, and personality changes and may occur on a background of secondary gain or litigation and other features of psychogenic dystonia (Gupta and Lang, 2009; Thomas and Jankovic, 2010).

Common Symptoms

Dystonia can affect almost all striated muscle groups. Common symptoms include forced eyelid closure (*blepharospasm*); jaw clenching, forced jaw opening, or involuntary tongue protrusion (oromandibular or lingual dystonia); a harsh, strained, or breathy voice (laryngeal dystonia or spasmodic dysphonia); and involuntary deviation of the neck in any plane or combination of planes (cervical dystonia or spasmodic torticollis). Other symptoms are spasms of the trunk in any direction, which variably interfere with lying, sitting, standing, or walking (axial dystonia); interference with manual tasks (often only specific tasks in isolation: the occupational cramps); and involvement of the leg, usually with inversion and plantar flexion of the foot, causing the patient to walk on the toes. All these disorders may slowly progress to the point of complete loss of voluntary function of the affected part. On the other hand, only certain actions may be impaired, and the disorder may remain focal in distribution. Chapter 71 deals with each of these forms of dystonia in more detail.

The age at onset and distribution of dystonia often are helpful in determining the possible cause. **Box 21.5** details the many causes of secondary dystonia. Whereas some patients with dystonia have "pure dystonia" without any other neurological deficit (*primary dystonia*), others have additional clinical features (*dystonia-plus syndrome*) such as parkinsonism, spasticity, weakness, myoclonus, dementia, seizures, and ataxia. Typically, childhood-onset primary dystonia (e.g., classic, Oppenheim, or DYT1 dystonia) begins in distal parts of the body (e.g., graphospasm, foot inversion) and spreads to a generalized dystonia. On the other hand, dystonia beginning in adult life usually is limited to one or a small number of contiguous regions such as the face and neck, remains focal or segmental, and rarely becomes generalized. Generalized involvement or onset in the legs in an adult usually implies the possibility of a secondary cause such as PD or some other parkinsonian disorder. Involvement of one side of the body (*hemidystonia*) is strong evidence of a lesion in the contralateral basal ganglia, particularly the putamen (Wijemanne and Jankovic, 2009). Most primary dystonias start as action dystonia occurring during some activity such as writing and walking or running, but consider peripheral or central trauma and psychogenic dystonia when the dystonia occurs at rest and consists of a fixed posture. A fixed posture maintained during sleep or anesthesia implies superimposed contractures or a musculoskeletal disturbance mimicking the postures of dystonia. Although rest and sleep lessens dystonia in many, some note a striking diurnal variation. The diurnal variation manifests with little or no dystonia on rising in the morning, followed by the progressive development of problems as the day goes on, sometimes to the point of becoming unable to walk late in the day. This diurnal variability strongly suggests a diagnosis of dopa-responsive dystonia. Important clues to dystonia causation are (1) the nature of symptom onset (sudden versus slow) and (2) its course, whether rapid or slow progression or episodes of spontaneous remission.

The family history must be reviewed in detail with the awareness that affected relatives may have limited or distinctly different involvement from that of the patient. The categorization of genetic dystonias according to loci is somewhat arbitrary, from DYT1 to DYT20 (Houlden et al., 2010; Müller, 2009). Obtaining a birth and developmental history is critical

Box 21.5 Etiological Classification of Dystonia

I. Primary dystonia
   A. Sporadic
   B. Inherited (all autosomal dominant)
      Classic (Oppenheim) dystonia (common in Ashkenazi Jews, DYT1, 9q34)
      Childhood- and adult-onset cranial-cervical-limb dystonia (DYT6, THAP1 mutation, 8p21–22)
      Adult-onset cervical and other focal dystonia (DYT7, 18p)
      Rapid-onset dystonia-parkinsonism, onset – adulthood, childhood (DYT12, Na+/K+-ATPase alpha3, ATP1A3; 19q13)
      Axial dystonia, oromandibular-laryngeal dystonia, parkinsonism unresponsive to levodopa, young-onset (DYT16, 2q31.2)
      Juvenile onset with torticollis, spreading to segmental and generalized dystonia (DYT17; 20p11.2-q13.12, autosomal recessive)
II. Secondary dystonia (dystonia-plus syndromes)
   A. Sporadic
      Parkinson disease
      Progressive supranuclear palsy
      Multiple system atrophy
      Corticobasal degeneration
   B. Inherited
      1. Autosomal dominant
         Dopa-responsive dystonia (DYT5, GTP cyclohydrolase I, 14q22.1, others)
         Myoclonus-dystonia (11q23, ε-sarcoglycan mutations, others)
         Alternating hemiplegia of childhood
      2. Autosomal recessive
         Dopa-responsive dystonia (11p11.5)
         Tyrosine hydroxylase deficiency (chromosome 21)
         Biopterin-deficient diseases
         Aromatic amino acid decarboxylase deficiency (dopamine agonist-responsive dystonia)
III. Heredodegenerative diseases (typically not pure dystonia)
   A. X-linked recessive
      Lubag (X-linked dystonia-parkinsonism, DYT3, Xq12–Xq21)
      Pelizaeus-Merzbacher disease
      Lesch-Nyhan syndrome
      Dystonia-deafness (Xq22)
      Deafness, dystonia, retardation, blindness
   B. Autosomal dominant
      Rapid-onset dystonia-parkinsonism
      Juvenile parkinsonism-dystonia
      Huntington disease (ITI5, 4P16.3)
      Spinocerebellar degenerations (SCA1–SCA8)
      Dentatorubral-pallidoluysian atrophy
      Neuroferritinopathy
      Hereditary spastic paraplegia with dystonia
      Thalamo-olivary degeneration with encephalopathy
   C. Autosomal recessive
      Wilson disease (Cu-ATPase, 13q14.3)
      Neurodegeneration with brain iron accumulation type 1 (PANK2, 20p12.3–p13)
      Aceruloplasminemia
      Hypoprebetalipoproteinemia, acanthocytosis, retinitis pigmentosa, and pallidal degeneration
      Ataxia-telangiectasia

Ataxia oculomotor apraxia 1 & 2
Associated with metabolic disorders:
   1. Amino acid disorders
      Glutaricacidemia
      Methylmalonicacidemia
      Homocystinuria
      Hartnup disease
      Tyrosinemia
      Glucose transporter-1 (GLUT-1) deficiency
   2. Lipid disorders
      Metachromatic leukodystrophy
      Ceroid lipofuscinosis
      Niemann-Pick disease type C (dystonic lipidosis, histiocytosis); defect in cholesterol esterification; caused by mutation in NPC1 gene 18q11) and HE1 gene (14q24.3)
      Gangliosidoses (GM1, GM2 variants)
      Hexosaminidase A and B deficiency
   3. Other metabolic disorders
      Biopterin-deficient diseases
      Triosephosphate isomerase deficiency
      Aromatic amino acid decarboxylase deficiency (dopamine agonist-responsive dystonia)
      Biotin-responsive basal ganglia disease
   D. Mitochondrial
      Leigh disease
      Leber disease
   E. Unknown inheritance
      Neuroacanthocytosis
      Rett syndrome
      Intraneuronal inclusion disease
      Infantile bilateral striatal necrosis
      Familial basal ganglia calcifications
      Hereditary spastic paraplegia with dystonia
      Deletion of 18q of a known specific cause
      Perinatal cerebral injury and kernicterus: athetoid cerebral palsy, delayed-onset dystonia
      Infection: viral encephalitis, encephalitis lethargica, Reye syndrome, subacute sclerosing panencephalitis, Creutzfeldt-Jakob disease, human immunodeficiency virus
      Other: tuberculosis, syphilis, acute infectious torticollis
      Drugs: l-dopa and dopamine agonists, dopamine receptor-blocking drugs, fenfluramine, anticonvulsants, flecainide, ergots, certain calcium channel blockers
      Toxins: magnesium, carbon monoxide, carbon disulfide, cyanide, methanol, disulfiram, 3-nitroproprionic acid, wasp sting
      Metabolic: hypoparathyroidism
      Paraneoplastic brainstem encephalitis
      Vitamin E deficiency
      Primary antiphospholipid syndrome
      Cerebrovascular or ischemic injury, Sjögren syndrome
      Multiple sclerosis
      Central pontine (and extrapontine) myelinolysis
      Brainstem lesions
      Spinal cord lesions
      Syringomyelia
      Brain tumor
      Arteriovenous malformation
      Head trauma and brain surgery (thalamotomy)

Box 21.5 **Etiological Classification of Dystonia—cont'd**

Lumbar stenosis
Peripheral trauma (with causalgia)
Electrical injury
IV. Other hyperkinetic syndromes associated with dystonia
   A. Tic disorders with dystonic tics
   B. Paroxysmal dyskinesias
      1. Paroxysmal kinesigenic dyskinesia (16p11.2–q12.1)
      2. Paroxysmal nonkinesigenic dyskinesia (2q33–35)
      3. Paroxysmal exertion-induced dyskinesia (16p12–q12)
      4. Paroxysmal hypnogenic dyskinesia (largely a frontal lobe seizure disorder with a gene localized to 20q13.2–13.3)
V. Psychogenic
VI. Pseudodystonia
   Atlanto-axial subluxation

Syringomyelia
Arnold-Chiari malformation
Trochlear nerve palsy
Vestibular torticollis
Posterior fossa mass
Soft-tissue neck mass
Congenital postural torticollis
Congenital Klippel-Feil syndrome
Isaacs syndrome
Satoyoshi syndrome
Stiff person syndrome
Dupuytren contractures
Trigger digits
Ventral hernia

in view of the frequency of dystonia after birth trauma, birth anoxia, and kernicterus. As with the other dyskinesias, seek a history of such features as previous encephalitis, drug use, and head trauma. There is also increasing support for the ability of peripheral trauma to precipitate various forms of dystonia, and occasionally this is combined with a complex regional pain syndrome, also called *reflex sympathetic dystrophy.*

Examination

Action dystonia is commonly the earliest manifestation of primary (idiopathic) dystonia. It is important to observe patients performing the acts that are most affected. Later, other tasks precipitate similar problems, the use of other parts of the body causes the dystonia to become evident in the originally affected site, and the dystonia may overflow to other sites. Still later, dystonia is periodically evident at rest, and even later the posturing may be persistent and difficult to correct passively, especially when secondary joint contractures develop. A significant deviation from this progression, particularly with the early appearance of dystonia at rest, should encourage the physician to search carefully for a secondary cause (see **Box 21.5**).

It is important to recognize the natural variability of dystonia, especially the effects of stress and anxiety. This is especially the case with blepharospasm, in which the increased concentration or anxiety associated with a visit to the doctor often reduces the severity of the problem. If only placing reliance on the degree of disability seen in the office, the physician may underestimate the severity of the blepharospasm and may misdiagnose the problem as hysterical.

Depending on the cause of the dystonia, several other neurological abnormalities may be associated. Consider WD in any patient with onset of dystonia before age 60 (Mak and Lam, 2008). Many secondary dystonic disorders (listed in **Box 21.5** and discussed in Chapter 71) result in additional psychiatric or cognitive disturbances, seizures, or pyramidal tract or cerebellar dysfunction. Ocular motor abnormalities suggest a diagnosis of Leigh disease, dystonic lipidosis, ataxia-telangiectasia, ataxia-oculomotor apraxia syndrome, HD, Machado-Joseph disease, or other spinocerebellar atrophies.

Optic nerve or retinal disease raises the possibility of Leigh disease, other mitochondrial cytopathies, GM2 gangliosidosis, ceroid lipofuscinosis, and neurodegeneration with brain iron accumulation (NBIA) (McNeill et al., 2008). One of the most common causes of NBIA is pantothenate kinase–associated neurodegeneration, previously called *Hallervorden-Spatz disease* (Schneider et al., 2009). Other causes include neuroferritinopathy, infantile neuroaxonal dystrophy, aceruloplasminemia, and PLA2G6-associated neurodegeneration. Lower motor neuron and peripheral nerve dysfunction occur with neuroacanthocytosis, ataxia-telangiectasia, ataxia-oculomotor apraxia syndrome, metachromatic leukodystrophy, Machado-Joseph disease, and other multisystem degenerations. Occasionally, prominent dystonic postures occur secondary to profound proprioceptive loss due to peripheral nerve, spinal cord, or brain lesions. The dystonia itself may cause additional neurological problems such as spinal cord or cervical root compression from long-standing torticollis, and peripheral nerve entrapment from limb dystonia. Also, independent of the cause, long-standing dystonic muscle spasms often result in hypertrophy of affected muscles (e.g., the sternocleidomastoid muscle in cervical dystonia).

Although the general medical examination must be thorough, it is usually unrevealing. As always, carefully seek the ophthalmological and systemic signs of WD. Abdominal organomegaly also may indicate a storage disease. Severe self-mutilation is typical of Lesch-Nyhan disease. Minor tongue and lip mutilation is seen in neuroacanthocytosis, in which orolingual action dystonia may be prominent (Walker et al., 2006). Oculocutaneous telangiectasia and evidence of recurrent sinopulmonary infections suggest ataxia-telangiectasia. Musculoskeletal abnormalities may simulate dystonia; rarely, dysmorphic features may serve as a clue to a mucopolysaccharidosis.

Chorea

The term *chorea* derives from the Greek *choreia*, meaning "a dance." This hyperkinetic movement disorder consists of irregular, unpredictable, brief, jerky movements that flow randomly from one part of the body to another (Jankovic, 2009). The term *choreoathetosis* describes slow chorea, typically seen in patients with cerebral palsy. Besides these disorders, there are numerous other causes of chorea (Cardoso et al., 2006), most of which are listed in **Box 21.6**.

Common Symptoms

Initially, patients often are unaware of the presence of involuntary movements, and the family may simply interpret the chorea as normal fidgetiness. The earliest patient complaints usually are those of clumsiness and incoordination, such as dropping or bumping into things. The limbs occasionally strike closely placed objects. In moderate to severe cases, patients may complain of abnormal involuntary jumping or jerking of the limbs and trunk. However, even when movements are overt, many patients deny their presence or only admit to being minimally aware of them. This discrepancy is particularly striking in the case of *tardive dyskinesia*, in which the patient often appears completely unaware of or indifferent to constant and severe movements of the mouth and tongue. Alternatively, it may be impossible to keep dentures in place, teeth may be ground or cracked, and there may be constant biting of the tongue or inner cheek. Take note that although the involuntary movements associated with tardive dyskinesia may superficially seem choreic, the muscle contractions are more predictable and repetitive, and the movements are more coordinated, often resembling seemingly purposeful motor acts such as chewing. *Stereotypies* are continuous, repetitive movements, which represent the most common phenomenology of tardive dyskinesia. Other causes of stereotypies, besides tardive dyskinesia, include autistic disorders and schizophrenia.

Other features often associated with chorea, particularly HD, include motor impersistence manifested by inability to maintain tongue protrusion (*trombone tongue*) and pendular reflexes, probably caused by motor hypotonia. Speech may be slurred, halting, and periodically interrupted, especially in HD, in which speech disturbances are severe and often do not correlate with the severity of chorea. Here, in addition to dysarthria, there is usually a reduction in the spontaneity and quantity of speech output. Problems with feeding result from a combination of limb chorea, which causes sloppiness, and swallowing difficulties, which can result in choking and aspiration. Eating is particularly difficult for patients with *neuroacanthocytosis* (previously termed *chorea-acanthocytosis*), in which severe orolingual dystonia (eating dystonia) can cause the tongue to push the food out of the mouth almost as quickly as the patient puts it in. Patients with this dystonia often place food at the back of the tongue and throw the head back to initiate swallowing. This lingual movement may resemble the orolingual stereotypy typically observed in patients with tardive dyskinesia or tardive dystonia. One form of choreic movement in patients with neuroacanthocytosis is continuous truncal bending and extending movements, giving the appearance of a "rubber man," most apparent while the patient is standing or walking. Disturbances of stance and gait can be an early complaint in patients with chorea. The patient may note a tendency to sway and jerk while standing and an unsteady, uneven gait often likened to a drunken stagger. Later still, added postural instability in HD results in falls.

Box 21.6 Etiological Classification of Chorea

Developmental and aging choreas
  Physiological chorea of infancy
  Cerebral palsy (anoxic), kernicterus
  Buccal-oral-lingual dyskinesia and edentulous orodyskinesia
  In older adults, senile chorea (probably several causes)
Hereditary choreas
  Huntington disease
  Benign hereditary chorea (TITF1 gene mutations)
  Neuroacanthocytosis
  Other central nervous system degenerations: olivopontocerebellar atrophy, Machado-Joseph disease and other spinocerebellar atrophies, ataxia-telangiectasia, ataxia oculomotor apraxia types 1 and 2, tuberous sclerosis of basal ganglia, pantothenate kinase-associated neurodegeneration, neurodegeneration with brain iron accumulation (Hallervorden-Spatz disease), neuroferritinopathy, "Huntington disease–like" disorders (e.g., PRNP, junctophilin or JPH3 mutations, SCA2, SCA17)
  Neurometabolic disorders: Wilson disease, Lesch-Nyhan syndrome, lysosomal storage disorders, amino acid disorders, Leigh disease, porphyria
Drugs: neuroleptics (tardive dyskinesia), antiparkinsonian drugs, amphetamines, cocaine, tricyclic antidepressants, oral contraceptives
Toxins: alcohol intoxication and withdrawal, anoxia, carbon monoxide, manganese, mercury, thallium, toluene
Metabolic
  Hyperthyroidism
  Hypoparathyroidism (various types)
  Pregnancy (chorea gravidarum)
  Hypernatremia and hyponatremia, hypomagnesemia, hypocalcemia
  Hypoglycemia and hyperglycemia (the latter may cause hemichorea, hemiballism)
  Acquired hepatocerebral degeneration
  Nutritional (e.g., beriberi, pellagra, vitamin B12 deficiency in infants)
Infectious and postinfectious
  Sydenham chorea
  Encephalitis lethargica
  Various other infectious and postinfectious encephalitis, Creutzfeldt-Jakob disease
Immunological
  Systemic lupus erythematosus
  Henoch-Schönlein purpura
  Others (rarely): sarcoidosis, multiple sclerosis, Behçet disease, polyarteritis nodosa
Vascular (often hemichorea)
  Infarction or hemorrhage
  Arteriovenous malformation, moyamoya disease
  Polycythemia rubra vera
  Migraine
  Following cardiac surgery with hypothermia and extracorporeal circulation in children
Tumors
Trauma, including subdural and epidural hematoma
Miscellaneous, including paroxysmal choreoathetosis

Respiratory dyskinesias may cause the patient to feel short of breath or unable to obtain enough air. Patients with involvement of the pelvic region may complain bitterly of thrusting and rocking movements in the lower trunk and pelvis. Respiratory and pelvic involvements are sources of complaint more often in tardive dyskinesia than in other choreic movement disorders.

Other Clues in the History

It is obvious from a review of **Table 21.8** that it is impractical to discuss additional historical clues for every cause of chorea. We therefore limit discussion here to a few practical and important points.

Age at onset and manner of progression vary depending on the cause. A helpful distinction made here is between benign hereditary chorea, associated with TITF1 gene (14q13.1-q21.1) mutation, and HD (Kleiner-Fisman and Lang, 2007). In the former, chorea typically begins in childhood with a slow progression and little cognitive change, whereas HD presenting in childhood is more often of the akinetic-rigid variety, with severe mental changes and rapid progression.

In most cases, the onset of chorea is slow and insidious. An abrupt or subacute onset is more typical of many of the symptomatic causes of chorea, such as Sydenham chorea, hyperthyroidism, systemic lupus erythematosus (SLE), cerebral infarcts, and neuroleptic drug withdrawal (withdrawal emergent syndrome) (Mejia and Jankovic, 2010). A pattern of remissions and exacerbations suggests the possibility of drugs, SLE, and rheumatic fever, whereas brief (minutes to hours) bouts of involuntary movement indicate a paroxysmal dyskinesia.

A recent history of streptococcal throat infection and musculoskeletal or cardiovascular problems in a child suggests a diagnosis of rheumatic (Sydenham) chorea (Cardoso et al., 2006). Rheumatic chorea tends to occur every 5 to 10 years in a community when a new population of children becomes susceptible to *Streptococcus* infection. One may obtain a previous history of rheumatic fever, particularly in women who develop chorea during pregnancy or while taking birth control pills. Chorea gravidarum may be more common in women with prior history of rheumatic chorea. The individual contractions in Sydenham disease are slightly longer (>100 msec) compared to those in HD (50 to 100 msec), and there are often associated features such as dysarthria, oculogyric deviations, "milkmaid's grip," obsessive-compulsive behavior and other features, including the prior history of streptococcal infection, that support the diagnosis of Sydenham disease.

In women, chorea during pregnancy or a history of previous fetal loss suggests the possibility of SLE with anticardiolipin antibodies, even in the absence of other features of collagen vascular disease. Symptoms isolated to one side of the body suggest a structural lesion in the contralateral basal ganglia. However, many patients who complain of unilateral involvement have abnormalities of both sides on examination.

A careful family history is crucial. The most common cause of inherited chorea is HD, which has fully penetrant autosomal dominant transmission (Frank and Jankovic, 2010). The family history can be misleading, however, because the clinical features of the disease in other family members may have been mainly behavioral, and psychiatric disturbances and the chorea hardly noticed.

Examination

The range of choreiform movements is quite broad, including eyebrow lifting or depression, lid winking, lip pouting or pursing, cheek puffing, lateral or forward jaw movements, tongue rolling or protruding, head jerking in any plane (a common pattern is a sudden backward jerk followed by a rotatory sweep forward), shoulder shrugging, trunk jerking or arching, pelvic rocking, and flitting movements of the fingers, wrists, toes, and ankles. Patients incorporate choreic jerks into voluntary movements, perhaps in part to mask the presence of the dyskinesia (so-called parakinesis).

Chorea often alters the performance of various tasks such as finger-to-nose testing and rapid alternating movements, causing a jerky, interrupted performance. Standing and walking often aggravate the chorea. Particularly in HD, the gait is irregular and lurching and has bizarre characteristics, not simply explained by increased chorea. The gait usually is wide-based despite the absence of typical ataxia. Patients may deviate from side to side in a zigzag fashion with lateral swaying and additional spontaneous flexion. In addition, the stride may be irregularly longer or shorter and the speed slowed, with some features similar to those of a parkinsonian gait, such as loss of arm swing, festination, propulsion, and retropulsion. One or both arms may flexed at the elbow as if holding a purse over the forearm.

Respiratory irregularities are common, especially in tardive dyskinesia, but are also present in other movement disorders (Mehanna and Jankovic, 2010). Periodic grunting, respiratory gulps, humming, and sniffing may be present in this and other choreic disorders, including HD. Other movement disorders often combine with chorea. Dystonic features probably are the most common and are seen in many conditions. Less common but well recognized are parkinsonism (e.g., with juvenile HD, neuroacanthocytosis, and WD), tics (e.g., in neuroacanthocytosis), myoclonus (e.g., in juvenile HD), tremor (e.g., in WD and HD), and ataxia (e.g., in juvenile HD and some spinocerebellar ataxias). Tone usually is normal to low. Muscle bulk is typically preserved, although weight loss and generalized wasting are common in HD. When distal weakness and amyotrophy are present, one must consider accompanying anterior horn cell or peripheral nerve disease, as in neuroacanthocytosis, ataxia-telangiectasia, Machado-Joseph disease, and spinocerebellar ataxias (see Chapter 72). Reduced tendon reflexes occur. On the other hand, chorea often results in hung-up and pendular reflexes, probably caused by the occurrence of a choreic jerk after the usual reflex muscle contraction.

Depending on the cause (see **Box 21.6**), several other neurological disturbances may be associated with chorea. In HD, for example, cognitive changes, motor impersistence (e.g., difficulty maintaining eyelid closure, tongue protrusion, constant handgrip), apraxias (especially orolingual), and oculomotor dysfunction are all quite common (see Chapter 71). *Milkmaid's grip*, appreciated as an alternating squeeze and release when the patient is asked to maintain a constant, firm grip of the examiner's fingers, probably is caused by a combination of chorea and motor impersistence.

Tardive Dyskinesia

Distinguish the usual movements seen in tardive dyskinesia from those of chorea. In contrast to the random and unpredictable flowing nature of chorea, tardive dyskinesia usually demonstrates repetitive stereotypical movements, which are most pronounced in the orolingual region (Mejia and Jankovic, 2010). These include chewing and smacking of the mouth and lips, rolling of the tongue in the mouth or pushing against the inside of the cheek (*bon-bon sign*), and periodic protrusion or flycatcher movements of the tongue. The speed and amplitude of these movements can increase markedly when the patient is concentrating on performing rapid alternating movements in the hands. Patients often have a striking degree of voluntary control over the movements and may be able to suppress them for a prolonged period when asked to do so. On distraction, however, the movements return immediately. Despite severe facial movements, voluntary protrusion of the tongue is rarely limited, and this act often dampens or completely inhibits the ongoing facial movements. This contrasts with the pronounced impersistence of tongue protrusion seen in HD, which is far out of proportion to the degree of choreic involvement of the tongue. Besides stereotypies, many other movement disorders are associated with the use of dopamine receptor blockers (**Table 21.3**).

Besides the impersistence typically seen in HD, several other clinical factors help distinguish between HD and tardive dyskinesia. Involuntary movements in tardive dyskinesia typically localize to the lower face, whereas in HD, irregular contractions of the frontalis muscles and associated elevation of the eyebrows is common. Despite the rocking movements of the pelvis, tapping of the feet, and shifting of the weight from side to side while standing (some of which may be caused by akathisia), the gait often is normal in patients with tardive dyskinesia, although a bizarre ducklike gait can be seen. This contrasts with the strikingly abnormal gait in many other choreic disorders, especially in HD.

Tardive dyskinesia caused by neuroleptic drugs such as the antipsychotics and other dopamine receptor blockers, particularly metoclopramide, is not the only cause of stereotypical oro-bucco-linguo-masticatory movements (Mejia and Jankovic, 2010). Other drugs, particularly dopamine agonists in PD, anticholinergics, and antihistamines, cause a similar form of dyskinesia. Multiple infarctions in the basal ganglia and possibly lesions in the cerebellar vermis result in similar movements. Older adults, especially the edentulous, often have a milder form of orofacial movement, usually with minimal lingual involvement. Here, as in tardive dyskinesia, inserting dentures in the mouth may dampen the movements, and placing a finger to the lips can also suppress them. Another important diagnostic consideration and source of clinical confusion is idiopathic oromandibular dystonia. Orofacial and limb stereotypies, often preceded by psychiatric symptoms, may be also seen in women with ovarian teratomas, and less frequently in males with testicular tumors, as part of anti-*N*-methyl-D-aspartate receptor (NMDAR) encephalitis (Florance et al., 2009).

Ballism

Ballism, or ballismus, is the least common of the well-defined dyskinesias. The name derives from the Greek word for "to throw," and the movements of ballism are high in amplitude, violent, and flinging or flailing in nature. As in chorea, they are rapid and nonpatterned. The prominent involvement of more proximal muscles of the limbs usually accounts for the throwing or flinging nature. Lower-amplitude distal movements also may be seen, and occasionally there is even intermittent prolonged dystonic posturing. Some authors emphasize the greater proximal involvement and the persistent or ceaseless nature of ballism in contrast to chorea. However, it is more likely that ballism and chorea represent a continuum rather than distinct entities. The coexistence of distal choreic movements, the discontinuous nature in less-severe cases, and the common evolution of ballism to typical chorea during the natural course of the disorder or with treatment all support this theory. Ballism usually confines to one side of the body, called *hemiballismus*. Occasionally, only one limb is involved (*monoballism*); rarely, both sides are affected (*biballism*) or both legs (*paraballism*).

Box 21.7 lists the various causes of hemiballism. These flinging movements often are extremely disabling to patients, who drop things from their hands or damage closely placed objects. Self-injury is common, and examination often reveals multiple bruises and abrasions. Additional signs and

---

Table 21.3 Neuroleptic-Induced Movement Disorders

Acute, Transient	Chronic, Persistent
Dystonic reaction	Tardive stereotypy
Parkinsonism	Tardive chorea
Akathisia	Tardive dystonia
Neuroleptic malignant syndrome	Tardive akathisia
	Tardive tics
	Tardive myoclonus
	Tardive tremor
	Persistent parkinsonism
	Tardive sensory syndrome

Modified from Jankovic, J., 1995. Tardive syndromes and other drug-induced movement disorders. Clin Neuropharmacol 18, 197-214.

Box 21.7 Causes of Ballism

Infarction or ischemia, including transient ischemic attacks; usually lacunar disease, hypertension, diabetes, atherosclerosis, vasculitis, polycythemia, thrombocytosis, other causes
Hemorrhage
Tumor
  Metastatic
  Primary
Other focal lesions (e.g., abscess, arteriovenous malformation, tuberculoma, toxoplasmosis, multiple sclerosis plaque, encephalitis, subdural hematoma)
Hyperglycemia (nonketotic hyperosmolar state)
Drugs (phenytoin, dopamine agonists in Parkinson disease)

symptoms depend on the cause, location, and extent of the lesion, which is usually in the contralateral subthalamic nucleus or striatum (see Chapter 71).

Tics

Tics are the most varied of all movement disorders. Patients with Tourette syndrome, the most common cause of tics, manifest motor, vocal, or phonic tics and a wide variety of associated symptoms (Jankovic, 2009). Tics are brief and intermittent movements (*motor tics*) or sounds (*phonic tics*). Motor tics typically consist of sudden, abrupt, transitory, often repetitive, and coordinated (stereotypical) movements that may resemble gestures and mimic fragments of normal behavior, vary in intensity, and repeated at irregular intervals. The movements are most often brief and jerky (clonic); however, slower, more prolonged movements (tonic or dystonic tics) also occur. Several other characteristic features are helpful in distinguishing this movement disorder from other dyskinesias. Patients usually experience an inner urge to make the movement or a local premonitory sensation, temporarily relieved by its performance. Tics are voluntarily suppressible for variable periods, but this occurs at the expense of mounting inner tension and the need to allow the tic to occur. Indeed, a large proportion people with tics, when questioned carefully, admit that they intentionally produce the movements or sounds that comprise their tics (in contrast to most other dyskinesias) in response to the uncontrollable inner urge or a premonitory sensation. **Box 21.8** provides examples of the various types of tics. Motor and phonic tics are divisible further as simple or complex. Simple motor tics are random, brief, irregular muscle twitches of isolated body segments,

particularly the eyelids and other facial muscles, the neck, and the shoulders. In contrast, complex motor tics are coordinated, patterned movements involving a number of muscles in their normal synergistic relationships. A wide variety of other behavioral disturbances may be associated with tic disorders, and it is sometimes difficult to separate complex tics from some of these comorbid disorders. These comorbid disturbances include obsessive-compulsive behavior, copropraxia (obscene gestures), echopraxia (mimicked gestures), hyperactivity with attentional deficits and impulsive behavior, and externally directed and self-destructive behavior, including self-mutilation. Some Tourette syndrome patients also manifest sudden and transitory cessation of all motor activity (*blocking tics*), including speech, without alteration of consciousness. These blocking tics are caused by either prolonged tonic or dystonic tics that interrupt ongoing motor activity such as speech (*intrusions*), or by a sudden inhibition of ongoing motor activity (*negative tic*).

Simple and complex phonic tics comprise a wide variety of sounds, noises, or formed words (see **Box 21.8**). The term *vocal tic* usually applies to these noises. However, because many of these sounds do not use the vocal cords, we prefer the term *phonic tic*. Although the presence of phonic tics is required for the diagnosis of definite Tourette syndrome, this criteria is artificial because phonic tics are essentially motor tics that result in abnormal sounds. Possibly the best-known (although not the most common) example of complex phonic tic is *coprolalia*, the utterance of obscenities or profanities. These are often slurred or shortened or may intrude into the patient's thoughts but not become verbalized (mental coprolalia) (Freeman et al., 2009).

Like most dyskinesias, tics usually increase with stress. In contrast to other dyskinesias, however, relaxation (e.g., watching television at home) often results in an increase in the tics, probably because the patient does not feel the need to suppress them voluntarily. Distraction or concentration usually diminishes tics, which also differs from most other types of dyskinesia. Many patients with idiopathic tics note spontaneous waxing and waning in their nature and severity over weeks to months, and periods of complete remission are possible. Many people with tics are only mildly affected, and many are even unaware that they demonstrate clinical features. This must be kept in mind when reviewing the family history and planning treatment. Finally, tics are one of the few movement disorders that can persist during all stages of sleep, although they usually subside in sleep.

Box 21.8 **Phenomenological Classification of Tics**

Simple Motor Tics

Eye blinking; eyebrow raising; nose flaring; grimacing; mouth opening; tongue protrusion; platysma contractions; head jerking; shoulder shrugging, abduction, or rotation; neck stretching; arm jerks; fist clenching; abdominal tensing; pelvic thrusting; buttock or sphincter tightening; hip flexion or abduction; kicking; knee and foot extension; toe curling

Simple Phonic Tics

Sniffing, grunting, throat clearing, shrieking, yelping, barking, growling, squealing, snorting, coughing, clicking, hissing, humming, moaning

Complex Motor Tics

Head shaking, teeth gnashing, hand shaking, finger cracking, touching, hitting, jumping, skipping, stamping, squatting, kicking, smelling hands or objects, rubbing, finger twiddling, echopraxia, copropraxia, spitting, exaggerated startle

Complex Phonic Tics

Coprolalia (wide variety, including shortened words), unintelligible words, whistling, panting, belching, hiccupping, stuttering, stammering, echolalia, palilalia (also mental coprolalia and palilalia)

Common Symptoms

Box 21.9 lists causes of tic disorders. Most are primary or idiopathic, and within this group, the onset almost always occurs in childhood or adolescence (Tourette syndrome). The male-to-female ratio is approximately 3:1. Idiopathic tics occur on a spectrum from a mild, transitory, single, simple motor tic to chronic, multiple, simple, and complex motor and phonic tics.

Patients and their families complain of a wide variety of symptoms (see **Box 21.8**). They may have seen numerous other specialists (e.g., allergists for repetitive sniffing, otolaryngologists for throat clearing, ophthalmologists for excessive eye blinking or eye rolling, and psychologists and psychiatrists for various neurobehavioral abnormalities). Often, someone

Box 21.9 Etiological Classification of Tics

I. Physiological tics
    A. Mannerisms
II. Pathological tics
    A. Primary
      Sporadic:
        1. Transient motor or phonic tics (<1 year)
        2. Chronic motor or phonic tics (>1 year)
        3. Adult-onset (recurrent) tics
        4. Tourette syndrome
      Inherited:
        1. Tourette syndrome
        2. Huntington disease
        3. Primary dystonia
        4. Neuroacanthocytosis
    B. Secondary ("tourettism")
      1. Infections: encephalitis, Creutzfeldt-Jakob disease, Sydenham chorea
      2. Drugs: stimulants, l-dopa, carbamazepine, phenytoin, phenobarbital, antipsychotics
      3. Toxins: carbon monoxide
      4. Developmental: static encephalopathy, mental thoughts but retardation, chromosomal abnormalities
      5. Other: head trauma, stroke, neurocutaneous syndromes, chromosomal abnormalities, schizophrenia, neuroacanthocytosis, degenerative disorders
III. Related disorders
    1. Stereotypies
    2. Self-injurious behaviors
    3. Hyperactivity syndrome
    4. Compulsions
    5. Excessive startle
    6. Jumping disease, latah, myriachit

Modified from Jankovic, J., 2001. Tourette's syndrome. N Engl J Med 345, 1184–1192.

close to the patient or a teacher suggests the diagnosis of Tourette syndrome to the family after learning about it in the media. Children may verbalize few complaints or feel reluctant to speak of the problem, especially if they have been subject to ridicule by others. Even young children, when questioned carefully, can provide the history of urge to perform the movement that gradually culminates in the release of a tic and the ability to control the tic voluntarily at the expense of mounting inner tension. Children may be able to control the tics for prolonged periods but often complain of difficulty concentrating on other tasks while doing so. Some give a history of requesting to leave the schoolroom and then releasing the tics in private (e.g., in the washroom). Peers and siblings often chastise or ridicule the patient, and parents or teachers, not recognizing the nature of the disorder, may scold or punish the child for what are thought to be voluntary bad habits (indeed, an older term for tics is *habit spasms*).

The history may include an exposure to stimulants for hyperactivity. Review the family history for the wide range of associated symptoms such as obsessive-compulsive behavior and attention deficit disorder. Additional neurological complaints, including other dyskinesias, suggest the possibility of a secondary cause of the tics.

Examination

In most patients with tics, the neurological examination is entirely normal. In patients with primary tic disorders, the presence of other neurological, cognitive, behavioral, and neuropsychological disturbances may simply relate to extension of the underlying cerebral dysfunction beyond the core that accounts for pure tic phenomena. Patients with secondary forms of tics (e.g., neuroacanthocytosis, tardive tics) may demonstrate other involuntary movements such as chorea, dystonia, and other neurological deficits (see **Box 21.8**). Careful interview stressing the subjective features that precede or accompany tics usually allows the distinction between true dystonia or myoclonus, and dystonic or clonic tics.

Despite bitter complaints by the family, it is common for patients to show little or no evidence of a movement disorder during an office appointment. Aware of this, the physician must attempt to observe the patient at a time when he or she is less likely to be exerting voluntary control, such as in the waiting room. If no movements have been witnessed during the interview, the physician should seemingly direct attention elsewhere (e.g., to the parents) while observing the patient out of the corner of the eye. The patient often releases the tics while changing in the examining room, particularly after suppressing tics during the interview. The physician should attempt to view the patient at this time or at least listen for the occurrence of phonic tics. If all else fails, ask the patient voluntarily to mimic the movements. This, in combination with associated symptoms such as urge, voluntary release, control, and the often varied and complex nature of the movements, usually is enough to provide the diagnosis, even if the physician never witnesses spontaneous tics in the office. Finally, ask the parents to provide home videos of the patient.

Myoclonus

Myoclonus is a sudden, brief, shocklike involuntary movement possibly caused by active muscle contraction (*positive myoclonus*) or inhibition of ongoing muscle activity (*negative myoclonus*). The differential diagnosis of myoclonus is broader than that of any other movement disorder (**Table 21.4**). To exclude muscle twitches, such as fasciculations caused by lower motor neuron lesions, some authors have insisted that an origin in the CNS be a component of the definition. Although the majority of cases of myoclonus originate in the CNS, occasional cases of brief shocklike movements clinically indistinguishable from CNS myoclonus occur with spinal cord or peripheral nerve or root disorders.

The clinical patterns of myoclonus vary widely. The frequency varies from single, rare jerks to constant, repetitive contractions. The amplitude may range from a small contraction that cannot move a joint to a very large jerk that moves the entire body. The distribution ranges from focal involvement of one body part, to segmental (involving two or more contiguous regions), to multifocal, to generalized. When the jerks occur bilaterally, they may be symmetrical or asymmetrical. When they occur in more than one region, they may be synchronous in two body parts (within milliseconds) or asynchronous. Myoclonus usually is arrhythmic and irregular, but

Table 21.4 Etiological Classification of Myoclonus

PHYSIOLOGICAL MYOCLONUS (NORMAL SUBJECTS)

Sleep jerks (hypnagogic jerks)
Anxiety-induced
Exercise-induced
Hiccup (singultus)
Benign infantile myoclonus with feeding

ESSENTIAL MYOCLONUS (NO KNOWN CAUSE AND NO OTHER GROSS NEUROLOGICAL DEFICIT)

Hereditary (phenotype may be pure myoclonus or myoclonus-dystonia)
Sporadic

EPILEPTIC MYOCLONUS (SEIZURES DOMINATE AND NO ENCEPHALOPATHY, AT LEAST INITIALLY)

Fragments of epilepsy
   Isolated epileptic myoclonic jerks
   Epilepsia partialis continua
   Idiopathic stimulus-sensitive myoclonus
   Photosensitive myoclonus
   Myoclonic absences in petit mal
Childhood myoclonic epilepsies
   Infantile spasms
   Myoclonic astatic epilepsy (Lennox-Gastaut syndrome)
   Cryptogenic myoclonus epilepsy
   Myoclonic epilepsy of Janz
Benign familial myoclonic epilepsy (Rabot syndrome)
Progressive myoclonic epilepsy: Baltic myoclonus (Unverricht-Lundborg syndrome)

SYMPTOMATIC MYOCLONUS (PROGRESSIVE OR STATIC ENCEPHALOPATHY DOMINATES)

Storage diseases
   Lafora body disease
   Lipidoses, such as GM2 gangliosidosis, Tay-Sachs disease, Krabbe disease
   Ceroid lipofuscinosis (Batten disease, Kufs disease)
   Sialidosis (cherry-red spot)
Spinocerebellar degeneration
   Ramsay Hunt syndrome (many causes)
   Friedreich ataxia
   Ataxia-telangiectasia
Basal ganglia degenerations
   Wilson disease
   Torsion dystonia
   Hallervorden-Spatz disease

   Progressive supranuclear palsy
   Huntington disease
   Parkinson disease
   Corticobasal degeneration
   Pallidal degenerations
   Multiple system atrophy
Mitochondrial encephalopathies, including myoclonic epilepsy and ragged-red fibers
Dementias
   Creutzfeldt-Jakob disease
   Alzheimer disease
Viral encephalopathies
   Subacute sclerosing panencephalitis
   Encephalitis lethargica
   Arbovirus encephalitis
   Herpes simplex encephalitis
   Postinfectious encephalitis
Metabolic
   Hepatic failure
   Renal failure
   Dialysis syndrome
   Hyponatremia
   Hypoglycemia
   Infantile myoclonic encephalopathy (polymyoclonus, with or without neuroblastoma)
   Nonketotic hyperglycemia
   Multiple carboxylase deficiency
Toxic encephalopathies
   Bismuth
   Heavy metal poisons
   Methyl bromide, dichlorodiphenyltrichloroethane
   Drugs, including L-dopa, tricyclic antidepressants
Physical encephalopathies
   Post hypoxia (Lance-Adams syndrome)
   Posttraumatic
   Heat stroke
   Electric shock
   Decompression injury
Focal central nervous system damage
   Post stroke
   Post thalamotomy
   Tumor
   Trauma
   Olivodentate lesions (palatal myoclonus)
   Spinal cord lesions (segmental or spinal myoclonus) disease

in some patients it is very regular (rhythmic), and in others there may be jerky oscillations that last for a few seconds and then fade away (oscillatory). Myoclonic jerks may occur spontaneously without a clear precipitant or in response to a wide variety of stimuli, including sudden noise, light, visual threat, pinprick, touch, and muscle stretch. Attempted movement (or even the intention to move) may initiate the muscle jerks (action or intention myoclonus). *Palatal myoclonus* is a form of segmental myoclonus manifested by rhythmic contractions of the soft palate. The rhythmicity has encouraged the alternative designation of *palatal tremor.* Symptomatic palatal myoclonus/tremor, usually manifested by contractions of the levator palatini, may persist during sleep; this form of palatal myoclonus usually is associated with some brainstem disorder. In contrast, essential palatal myoclonus/tremor consists of rhythmic contractions of the tensor palatini, often associated with a clicking sound in the ear, and disappears with sleep. Symptomatic but not essential palatal myoclonus often is

associated with hypertrophy of the inferior olive. Another term proposed for essential palatal tremor is *isolated palatal tremor,* with several different subtypes or causes possible, including tics, psychogenic, and volitional (Zadikoff et al., 2006).

Common Symptoms

As may be seen from the foregoing description and the long list of possible causes of myoclonus, the symptoms in these patients are quite varied. For simplification, we briefly review the possible symptoms with respect to four major etiological subcategories in **Table 21.4.**

Physiological forms of myoclonus occurring in normal subjects vary depending on the precipitant. Probably the most common form is the jerking most of us have experienced on falling asleep (*hypnagogic myoclonus,* or *jactitation*). This very familiar phenomenon is rarely a source of concern. Occasionally, anxiety- or exercise-induced myoclonus causes concern.

The history usually is clear, and there is little to find (including abnormal movements) when the patient is seen.

In the *essential myoclonus* group, patients usually complain of isolated muscle jerking in the absence of other neurological deficits (with the possible exception of tremor and dystonia). The movements may begin at any time from early childhood to late adult life and may remain static or progress slowly over many years. The family history may be positive, and some patients note a striking beneficial effect of alcohol (Mostile and Jankovic, 2010). Associated dystonia, present in some patients, also may respond to ethanol. Essential myoclonus and myoclonus dystonia are probably the same disorder.

Myoclonus occurring as one component of a wide range of seizure types is *epileptic myoclonus*. Many of these patients give a clear history of seizures as the dominant feature. Myoclonic jerks may be infrequent and barely noticeable to the patient or may occur frequently and cause pronounced disability. Myoclonus on waking in the morning or an increasing frequency of the myoclonic jerks may forewarn of a seizure soon to come. The clinical pattern of myoclonus in this instance also varies widely. Sensitivity to photic stimuli and other sensory input may be prominent. Occasional patients demonstrate isolated myoclonic jerks in the absence of additional seizure activity. In these cases, the family history may be positive for seizures, and the electroencephalogram (EEG) often demonstrates a typical centrencephalic seizure pattern that is otherwise asymptomatic (such as a 3-Hz spike-and-wave pattern). In others, myoclonus and seizures are equally prominent (the myoclonic epilepsies). These may or may not be associated with an apparent progressive encephalopathy (most often with cognitive dysfunction and ataxia) in the absence of a definable, underlying, symptomatic cause.

In the *disorders classified as causing symptomatic myoclonus*, seizures may occur, but the encephalopathy (either static or progressive) is the feature that predominates. Many different myoclonic patterns occur in this broad category. As can be appreciated from a review of **Table 21.4**, a plethora of other neurological and systemic symptoms may accompany the encephalopathy. Two clinical subcategories of this larger grouping are distinguishable to assist in differential diagnosis. In progressive myoclonic epilepsy, myoclonus, seizures, and encephalopathy predominate, whereas in progressive myoclonic ataxia (often called *Ramsay Hunt syndrome*), myoclonus and ataxia dominate the clinical picture, with less frequent or severe seizures and mental changes. Myoclonus may also originate in the brainstem and spinal cord. Spinal segmental myoclonus often is rhythmic and limited to muscles innervated by one or a few contiguous spinal segments. Propriospinal myoclonus is another type of spinal myoclonus that usually results in flexion jerks of the trunk.

Examination

Considering the varied causes, the possible range of neurological findings is wide. Alternatively, despite the complaint of abnormal movements, some patients with myoclonus (like those with tics and certain paroxysmal dyskinesias) have little to reveal on examination. This is particularly the case for the physiological forms of myoclonus and for those associated with epilepsy and some symptomatic causes. When myoclonus is clearly present on examination, the physician should try to characterize the movement, as outlined in this chapter. When the jerks are single or repetitive but arrhythmic, one must differentiate these movements from tics. Myoclonus usually is briefer and less coordinated or patterned. Furthermore, myoclonus is not associated with a premonitory urge or sensation. Rhythmic forms of myoclonus may be confused with tremors. Here, the pattern of movement is more one of repetitive, abrupt-onset, square-wave movements caused by contractions of the agonists, in contrast to the smoother sinusoidal activity of tremor produced by alternating or synchronous contractions of antagonist muscles. Rhythmic myoclonus usually is in the 1- to 4-Hz range, in contrast to the faster frequencies seen in most types of tremor. The oscillations of so-called oscillatory myoclonus may be faster. These are distinguishable by their bursting or shuddering nature, usually precipitated by sudden stimulus or movement, lasting for a few seconds and then fading away.

The distribution of the myoclonus is helpful in classifying the myoclonus and considering possible etiologies. Focal myoclonus may be more common in disturbances of an isolated region of the cerebral cortex. Segmental involvement, particularly when rhythmic, may occur with brainstem lesions (e.g., branchial or palatal myoclonus) or spinal lesions (spinal myoclonus) (Esposito et al., 2009). Multifocal or generalized myoclonus suggests a more diffuse disorder, particularly involving the reticular substance of the brainstem. When multiple regions of the body are involved, it is helpful to attempt to estimate whether movements are occurring in synchrony. It is sometimes difficult to do this clinically, and multichannel electromyographic (EMG) monitoring needed.

Throughout the examination, it is important to define whether the movements occur spontaneously or with various precipitants such as sudden loud noise, visual threat, perturbation, or a pinprick. Test several special-sense and somesthetic sensory inputs. In addition, it is important to evaluate the effects of passive and active movement. In the case of action or intention myoclonus, jerking occurs during voluntary motor activity, especially when the patient attempts to perform a fine motor task such as reaching for a target. This disturbance is often confused with severe ataxia. Action myoclonus may be evident in such activities as voluntary eyelid closure, pursing of lips or speaking, holding the arms out, finger-to-nose testing, writing, bringing a cup to the mouth, holding the legs out against gravity, heel-to-shin testing, and walking. In addition to the positive myoclonus that results from a brief active muscle contraction, negative myoclonus may occur. Although clinically these appear as brief jerks, causation is periodic inhibition of ongoing muscle activity and sudden loss of muscle tone.

The most common example of negative myoclonus is *asterixis*, which may be seen in liver failure (liver flap) and, to a lesser extent, in other metabolic encephalopathies and occasionally with focal brain lesions. The best-recognized location of asterixis is the forearm muscles, where it causes a flapping, irregular tremor-like movement with wrist extension. When mild and of low amplitude, this may be confused with 5- to 6-Hz postural tremor. A similar form of negative myoclonus accounts for the periodic loss of postural tone in axial and leg muscles in some patients with action myoclonus syndromes such as postanoxic action myoclonus. This results in a bobbing movement of the trunk while standing and may culminate in falls.

Miscellaneous Movement Disorders

Hemifacial spasm is a relatively common disorder in which irregular tonic and clonic movements involve the muscles of one side of the face innervated by the ipsilateral seventh cranial nerve. Unilateral eyelid twitching usually is the first symptom, followed at variable intervals by lower-facial muscle involvement. Rarely, the spasm affects both sides of the face, in which case the spasms are asynchronous on the two sides, in contrast to other pure facial dyskinesias such as cranial dystonia (Wu et al., 2010).

The term *akathisia* refers to a sense of restlessness and the feeling of a need to move. This was first used to describe what was thought to be a hysterical condition, and later the term was applied to the restlessness with inability to sit or stand still (motor impatience) seen in patients with idiopathic and post-encephalitic parkinsonism. The most common cause of the syndrome is as a side effect of major tranquilizing or anti-emetic drugs (neuroleptics) that act by blocking dopamine receptors. Akathisic movements appear to occur in response to the subjective inner feeling of restlessness and need to move, although some authors believe the subjective component is not necessary. The movements of akathisia are varied and complex. They include repetitive rubbing; crossing and uncrossing the arms; stroking the head and face; repeatedly picking at clothing; abducting and adducting, crossing and uncrossing, swinging, or up-and-down pumping of the legs; and shifting weight, rocking, marching in place, or pacing while sitting and standing. Occasionally, patients demonstrate a variety of vocalizations such as moans, grunts, and shouts. Akathisia can be an acute or delayed complication of antipsychotic drug therapy (acute akathisia and tardive akathisia, respectively). It also occurs in PD, secondary to selective serotonin reuptake inhibitors, and in certain confusional states or dementing processes.

Another disorder in which movements are secondary to the subjective need to move is the restless legs syndrome, perhaps the most common of all movement disorders, occurring in approximately 14% of women and 7% of men older than 50 years of age (Trenkwalder and Paulus, 2010). Unlike in akathisia, the patient with restless legs syndrome typically complains of a variety of sensory disturbances in the legs, including pins and needles, creeping or crawling, aching, itching, stabbing, heaviness, tension, burning, and coldness. Occasionally, similar symptoms occur in the arms. These complaints usually are experienced during recumbency in the evening and often are associated with insomnia. This condition commonly is associated with another movement disorder, periodic leg movements of sleep, sometimes inappropriately called *nocturnal myoclonus*. These periodic slow, sustained (1- to 2-second) movements range from synchronous or asynchronous dorsiflexion of the big toes and feet to triple flexion of one or both legs. More rapid myoclonic movements or slower, prolonged, dystonic-like movements of the feet and legs also may be present in these patients while awake, and these too may have a natural periodicity. Leg myoclonus or foot dystonia may also be the presenting feature of the stiff person syndrome.

Another uncommon but well-defined movement disorder of the lower limbs is painful legs and moving toes. Here, the patient typically complains of a deep pulling or searing pain in the lower limb and foot (a small proportion of patients have a painless variant) associated with continuous wriggling or writhing of the toes, occasionally the ankle, and less commonly more proximal muscles of the leg. Rarely, a similar problem is seen in the upper limb as well. In some cases, there is a history of root or nerve injury, and the examination may demonstrate evidence of peripheral nerve dysfunction.

Some dyskinesias occur intermittently rather than persistently. This is typical of tics and certain forms of myoclonus. Dystonia often occurs only with specific actions, but this is usually a consistent response to the action rather than a periodic and unpredictable occurrence. Some patients with dystonia have a diurnal variation (dopa-responsive dystonia) characterized by essentially normal motor function in the morning with emergence or worsening of dystonia as the day progresses, so that by the end of the day the patients are unable to ambulate because of severe generalized dystonia. A small group of patients with chorea or dystonia have bouts of sudden-onset, short-lived, involuntary movements known as *paroxysmal choreoathetosis* or, more appropriately, *paroxysmal dyskinesia* (**Box 21.10**). Certain features such as precipitants, duration, frequency, age of onset, and family history (see Chapter 71) characterize these disorders and sometimes help to separate them into diagnostic categories. Thus, paroxysmal dyskinesias may be categorized as kinesigenic (precipitated by voluntary movement such as arising from a chair or starting to run), nonkinesigenic, exertional, or nocturnal. In many cases, the movements are so infrequent that the physician never sees them, so a careful history is needed to determine the nature of the disorder, and having the patient provide a videotape of the events is often invaluable. There may be a family history of seizures or migraines. Increasing number of paroxysmal dyskinesias are being recognized as genetic channelopathies or mitochondrial disorders (Ghezzi et al., 2009). The glucose transporter-1 (GLUT-1) deficiency syndrome often results in paroxysmal exercise-induced dyskinesia as well as other clinical features (Leen et al., 2010; Pons et al., 2010). Periodic ataxias often are included in the group of paroxysmal movement disorders.

There are also disorders in which an abnormal or excessive response to startle occurs. In some patients, one simply finds an exaggerated startle response, which habituates poorly after repeated stimuli. In others, there is an abnormal response to the stimuli that normally evoke startle. Hyperekplexia, also

---

Box 21.10 Classification of Paroxysmal Dyskinesias

Paroxysmal kinesigenic dyskinesia
Paroxysmal nonkinesigenic dyskinesia
Paroxysmal exertion-induced dyskinesia
Paroxysmal nocturnal dyskinesia
Paroxysmal psychogenic dyskinesia; each category includes the following:
    Short-lasting (≤5 minutes)
        Idiopathic (familial or sporadic)
        Secondary
    Long-lasting (>5 minutes)
        Idiopathic (familial or sporadic)
        Secondary

known as *startle syndrome*, may be more akin to certain forms of myoclonus than to a normal startle response. Several other unusual disorders, first described in the 19th century together with Tourette syndrome, manifest excessive startle. Jumping disease (Jumping Frenchmen of Maine), latah, and myriachit also involve sudden striking out, echo phenomena, automatic obedience, and several other less common features. These disorders are quite distinct from Tourette syndrome and possibly represent culturally related operant-conditioned behavior rather than true neurological disease, although this point remains controversial.

Finally, psychogenic movement disorders characterized by abnormal slowness or excessive movements or postures that cannot be directly attributed to a lesion or an organic dysfunction in the nervous system are emerging as one of the most common groups of disorders encountered in movement disorder clinics (Gupta and Lang, 2009; Thomas and Jankovic, 2010). Derived primarily from psychiatric or psychological disorders, because of their rich spectrum of phenomenology and variable severity, psychogenic movement disorders present a major diagnostic and therapeutic challenge. Facilitating the diagnosis of psychogenic movement disorders are various clues that include somatic and psychiatric complaints and movement disorders whose phenomenology is incongruous with typical movement disorders. These include sudden onset (often related to some emotional or minor physical trauma), secondary gain, variable frequency of tremor, distractibility, and exaggeration of symptoms (**Box 21.11**).

Investigation of Movement Disorders

The nature and extent of the investigation of a patient presenting with a movement disorder vary depending on the clinical circumstances. When the historical and clinical features are typical of certain primary (idiopathic) disorders, further investigations may be unnecessary. Examples of these include normal physiological tremor and myoclonus, essential tremor (especially if familial), adult-onset focal dystonias, childhood tic disorders, and even PD. However, one must always be mindful of the possibility of additional occult aggravating factors superimposed on a known preexisting movement disorder. The reverse is also possible, in which the presumed cause is actually an aggravating factor or simply a coincidental association, particularly in the case of patients thought to have drug-induced disturbances. For example, chorea apparently caused by the birth control pill (or chorea gravidarum) may be a manifestation of underlying SLE. When dealing with presumed neuroleptic-induced movement disorders, it is important to consider the possibility that the antipsychotic drug given for initial psychiatric manifestations of a disease is now *causing* the movement disorder in question. HD and WD are two disorders in which this may occur.

The importance of excluding WD cannot be overemphasized. This includes slit-lamp examination, measurement of serum ceruloplasmin and copper, liver function tests, measurement of 24-hour urinary copper excretion and, if necessary, liver biopsy and genetic testing. Children, adolescents, and young adults presenting with parkinsonism, chorea, or a dystonic or myoclonic syndrome need additional careful hematological and biochemical assessment, as indicated in **Table 21.5**.

Box 21.11 Clues to the Presence of a Psychogenic Movement Disorder

Physical Factors

Movement Disorder
Abrupt onset
Incongruous movements
Inconsistent movements
Response to placebo or suggestion
Selective disability
Dramatic resolution
Maximum early disability
Deliberate slowing
Rhythmic shaking
Bizarre gait

Other Neurological Findings
Transient weakness
Sensory symptoms
Dizziness and fainting
"Seizures"
Convergence spasm
Bursts of verbal gibberish
Visual disturbances
Headache
Pain
Amnesia
Insomnia
Exhaustion

Multiple Somatizations
Self-inflicted injuries
Unwitnessed paroxysmal disorders

Psychiatric Problems

Depression
Anxiety disorder
Somatization disorder
Malingering
Factitious disorder

Predisposing Event

Trauma
Surgery
Major life event

Social Factors

Work-related injuries
Litigation
Relationship problems (spouse or children)
Physical abuse
Sexual abuse
Substance abuse
Secondary gain

Although in the majority of movement disorders, the diagnosis depends on recognizing typical clinical phenomena, diagnosis of certain movement disorders requires blood tests. Neuroacanthocytosis usually presents in adolescence or early adulthood with chorea, dystonia, tics, and progressive weakness; diagnosis requires demonstrating blood acanthocytes, elevated serum creatine kinase, and altered nerve conduction

Table 21.5 Investigation of Movement Disorders

Movement Disorder Investigation	A	C	B	D	T	M
Routine hematology (including sedimentation rate)	+	+	+	+	−	+
Routine biochemistry (including Ca2+, uric acid, liver function tests)	+	+	+	+	+	+
Serum copper, ceruloplasmin (with or without 24-hour urine Cu, liver biopsy, radiolabeled Cu studies)	++	++	−	++	+	+
Slit-lamp examination	++	++	−	++	+	+
Thyroid function	+	++	−	+	−	+
Antistreptolysin O test, anti-DNase B, antihyaluronidase	−	+	−	+	+	−
Antinuclear factor, LE cells, other immunological studies, anticardiolipin antibodies, Venereal Disease Research Laboratories test	+	++	+	+	−	+
Blood acanthocytes	+	+	−	+	+	+
Lysosomal enzymes	+	+	−	+	+	+
Urine organic and amino acids	+	+	−	+	−	+
Urine oligosaccharides and mucopolysaccharides	+	+	−	+	−	+
Serum lactate and pyruvate	+	+	−	+	−	+
DNA tests for gene mutations	+	+	−	+	−	+
Bone marrow for storage cells (including electron microscopy)	+	+	−	+	−	+
Electron microscopy of leukocytes; biopsy of liver, skin, and conjunctiva	+	+	−	+	−	+
Nerve or muscle biopsy	+	+	−	+	−	+
Oligoclonal bands	+	+	+	+	−	+
Computed tomography or magnetic resonance imaging	++	++	++	++	+	++
Electroencephalography	+	+	−	+	+	++
Electromyography and nerve conduction studies	+	+	−	+	+	+
Evoked potentials	+	+	−	+	−	++
Electroretinogram	+	+	−	+	−	+
Neuropsychological testing	+	+	−	−	+	−

Note: The extent of investigation depends on factors such as age of onset, nature of progression, and presence of historical or clinical atypical features suggesting a secondary cause of the movement disorder in question.

++, Very important or often useful; +, sometimes helpful; +, questionably helpful; —, rarely or never helpful. A, Akinetic rigid syndrome; B, hemiballism; C, chorea; D, dystonia; M, myoclonus; T, tics.

studies (Walker et al., 2006). Biochemical screening may also reveal evidence of hypoparathyroidism, which can cause calcification of the basal ganglia, resulting in several movement disorders. Hyperthyroidism, polycythemia rubra vera, and SLE are common enough causes of undiagnosed chorea in an adult to necessitate exclusion in all cases. Early clues are a history of recurrent fetal loss, a prolonged partial thromboplastin time, a false-positive VDRL (Venereal Disease Research Laboratories) test, and thrombocytopenia, which indicates the presence of antiphospholipid immunoglobulins such as the lupus anticoagulant and anticardiolipin antibodies. Consider Sydenham chorea in a child presenting with chorea of unknown origin, and obtain antistreptolysin O titer, antihyaluronidase, and electrocardiogram. In a patient with hemiballism, one should search for potential risk factors for vascular disease by measuring levels of blood sugar, hemoglobin, platelets, erythrocyte sedimentation rate, cholesterol, and triglycerides.

Genetic (deoxyribonucleic acid [DNA]) tests are increasingly being used in the evaluation of patients with familial and even sporadic PD and other movement disorders, but such testing should only be done with proper counseling, given the existing uncertainties, including incomplete penetrance and other difficulties interpreting such tests (Tan and Jankovic, 2006). Suspect an underlying cause in adults with generalized dystonia or dystonia beginning in the legs, and investigate accordingly. A test for DYT1 dystonia is available commercially, and some research laboratories perform tests for the ε-sarcoglycan (SGCE) gene responsible for the myoclonus-dystonia syndrome. Other DNA tests that may be helpful in the diagnosis of movement disorders include tests for HD, spinocerebellar atrophies, Friedreich ataxia and several other recessive ataxias, dentatorubral-pallidoluysian atrophy, pantothenate kinase–associated neurodegeneration (PKAN, formerly known as *Hallervorden-Spatz disease*), Unverricht-Lundborg disease, celiac disease (antigliadin antibodies), anti-GAD antibodies (stiff person syndrome), and antibodies for various paraneoplastic syndromes (Grant and Graous, 2009).

Imaging studies such as computed tomography (CT) and particularly magnetic resonance imaging (MRI) are useful in certain disorders. Most patients with hemidystonia have a definable lesion in the contralateral basal ganglia (most often the putamen). The cause of hemiballism or hemichorea is usually a structural lesion in the contralateral subthalamic nucleus or striatum. The cause is commonly a small lacunar infarction, so MRI typically is more successful than CT in localizing the lesion. A pattern of high signal in the striatum (especially the putamen) on T1 imaging is characteristic of hemiballism due to hyperosmolar non-ketotic hyperglycemia. In patients with parkinsonism, imaging must assess the possibility of hydrocephalus (either obstructive or communicating), midbrain atrophy (as in PSP), and cerebellar and brainstem atrophy (as in olivopontocerebellar atrophy). MRI clearly is much more effective in demonstrating these posterior fossa abnormalities than is CT. Atrophy of the head of the caudate nucleus occurs in HD, but it is not specific for this disorder and does not correlate with the presence or severity of chorea. Multiple infarctions, intracerebral calcification (better seen on CT), mass lesions (e.g., tumors, arteriovenous malformations), and basal ganglia lucencies (as seen in various disorders) may be found in patients with several movement disorders such as parkinsonism, chorea, and dystonia. In patients with striatonigral degeneration (one subcategory of MSA with prominent parkinsonism), T2-weighted and proton-density MRI scans often demonstrate a combination of striatal atrophy and hypointensity, with linear hyperintensity in the posterolateral putamen. T2-weighted gradient echo MRI often demonstrates hypointense putaminal changes (Brooks et al., 2009). The "hot cross bun" sign in the pons and hyperintensity in the middle cerebellar peduncles on fluid-attenuated inversion recovery (FLAIR) imaging also suggest MSA-C. The latter feature as well as additional supratentorial white-matter changes and atrophy also occur in the fragile X tremor ataxia syndrome (FRXTAS). Sagittal-view MRI in patients with PSP can show atrophy of the rostral midbrain tegmentum; the most rostral midbrain, the midbrain tegmentum, the pontine base, and the cerebellum appear to correspond to the bill, head, body, and wing, respectively, to form a "hummingbird" or "penguin" sign (although this is a rather late imaging feature). Further developments in MRI promise to improve our ability to differentiate between various degenerative disorders, especially if they are associated with characteristic pathological features. Examples are deposition of pigments or heavy metals. T1-weighted hyperintensity in the basal ganglia occur in hyperglycemia, manganese toxicity, hepatocerebral disease, WD, abnormal calcium metabolism, neurofibromatosis, hypoxia, and hemorrhage. Striatal T1-weighted hypointensity and T2-weighted hyperintensity suggest mitochondrial disorders. Striatal T2-weighted hypointensity, with hyperintensity of the mesencephalon sparing the red nucleus and the lateral aspect of the substantia nigra, gives the appearance of "face of the giant panda" sign, the typical MRI appearance of WD. T2-weighted MRI in PKAN typically shows hypointensity in the globus pallidus surrounding an area of hyperintensity, the "eye of the tiger" sign.

Magnetic resonance spectroscopy also holds promise for differentiating disorders with various neurodegenerative patterns or neurometabolic disturbances. Positron emission tomography (PET) using fluorodeoxyglucose, fluorodopa, and other radiolabeled compounds (e.g., demonstrating labeling of dopamine receptors) has shown reproducible changes in such conditions as HD and parkinsonian disorders. For example, F-dopa PET scans show reduced uptake in both the putamen and caudate in patients with atypical parkinsonism (e.g., PSP, MSA), whereas the caudate usually is preserved in patients with PD. The patterns of abnormalities seen may predict the underlying pathological changes and thus may be useful in differential diagnosis. Developments in single-photon emission computed tomography (SPECT) suggest that this will probably become a useful diagnostic tool in evaluating and diagnosing certain movement disorders. For example, SPECT study of the dopamine transporter (DAT) investigates parkinsonian disorders and helps differentiate these from other tremor disorders such as essential tremor. Finally, recent studies suggest that transcranial ultrasound demonstrating hyperechogenicity in the region of the substantia nigra compacta in PD may be a useful diagnostic tool.

Routine electrophysiological testing including EEG, somatosensory evoked potentials, EMG, and nerve conduction studies may provide supportive evidence of disease involving structures outside the basal ganglia. EMG analysis of the activity in various muscle groups studies most movement disorders, and the use of accelerometric recordings further documents tremor. Although these and other electrophysiological procedures have contributed to our understanding of the pathophysiology of movement disorders, they have been most crucial to the study of myoclonus. Here, EEG shows a variety of disturbances such as spikes, spike-and-wave patterns, and periodic discharges. Occasionally, spikes precede EMG myoclonic discharges, particularly if the myoclonus is associated with epilepsy. In the majority of cases, however, it is impossible to determine a correlation between spike discharges and myoclonic jerks by simple visual inspection. Special electrophysiological techniques averaging cortical activity that occurs before a myoclonic jerk (triggered back-averaging) may show focal contralateral central negativity lasting 15 to 40 msec, preceding the muscle jerk by 10 to 25 msec in the upper limbs and 30 to 35 msec in the legs. This is evidence of so-called cortical myoclonus, indicating that cortical activity results in the muscle jerks (although the primary pathology may not be in the cerebral cortex). In other forms of myoclonus that originate in subcortical areas, cortical discharges may be seen but are not time-locked in the same fashion to the jerks. In these cases, there may be generalized 25- to 40-msec negativity before, during, or after the muscle jerking. The muscle bursts seen on EMG typically are synchronous in antagonistic muscles and usually are less than 50 msec in duration. In one form of essential myoclonus, ballistic reflex myoclonus, the EMG bursts show alternating activity in antagonists that lasts 50 to 150 msec. With multichannel EMG recording, it may be possible to demonstrate the activation order of muscles. In cortical myoclonus, muscles activate in a rostrocaudal direction, with cranial nerve muscles firing in descending order before the limbs. In myoclonus originating from subcortical or reticular sources, it may be possible to show that the myoclonus propagates in both directions from a point source, up the brainstem, usually starting in muscles innervated by the eleventh cranial nerve, and down the spinal cord. In propriospinal myoclonus, the spread up and down the spinal cord occurs at a speed that suggests the involvement of a slowly conducting polysynaptic pathway. However, this pattern can also be mimicked voluntarily and may be present in psychogenic myoclonus.

Somatosensory evoked potentials and late EMG responses (C reflexes) often are enhanced in patients with myoclonus. Giant sensory evoked potentials occur in the hemisphere contralateral to the jerking limb in patients with cortical myoclonus. This is especially true in patients with focal myoclonus that is sensitive to a variety of sensory stimuli applied to the affected part (cortical reflex myoclonus). The cortical components of the sensory evoked potentials usually are not enhanced in subcortical or spinal myoclonus, but the latencies may be prolonged, depending on the location of the disease process. Electrophysiological studies are also useful in differentiating psychogenic from organic movement disorders, particularly in the case of myoclonus and tremor (Chen and Brashear, 2011).

In addition to blood and cerebrospinal fluid proteins, there are genetic, imaging, neurophysiological, and other biomarkers currently being investigated in attempts to diagnose presymptomatic or early disease (Wu et al., 2010). In caring for a patient with a movement disorder, the clinician must always keep an open mind to the possibility of finding a secondary cause. This should be the case even when the onset, progression, and clinical features of the movement disorder in question are typical of an idiopathic condition and the preliminary laboratory testing has not revealed another cause. Repeat thorough neurological examinations periodically in a search for clues that might indicate the need to pursue the investigation further.

References

The complete reference list is available online at www.expertconsult.com.

Gait Disorders

Philip D. Thompson, John G. Nutt

The maintenance of an upright posture and the act of walking are among the first, and ultimately the most complex, motor skills humans acquire. From an early age, walking skills are modified and refined. In later years, the interplay between voluntary and automatic control of posture and gait provides a rich and complex repertoire of motion that ranges from walking to running, hopping, dancing, and so on. The pattern of walking may be so distinctive that individuals can be recognized by the characteristics of their gait. Many diseases of the nervous system are identified by the disturbances of gait and posture they produce.

Physiological and Biomechanical Aspects of Gait

Humans assume a stable upright posture before beginning to walk. Mechanical stability when standing is based on musculoskeletal linkages between the trunk and legs. Dynamic equilibrium during walking is maintained by coordinated synergies of axial and proximal limb muscle contraction and a hierarchy of postural reflexes and responses. The latter include automatic righting reflexes keeping the head upright on the trunk, supporting reactions controlling antigravity muscle tone, anticipatory (feed-forward) postural reflexes occurring before limb movement, and reactive (feedback) postural adjustments counteracting body perturbations during movement. Postural responses are also modified by voluntary control according to the circumstances, such as rescue reactions to preserve the upright posture (a step or windmill arm movements), and protective reactions to prevent injury (an outstretched arm to break a fall). Postural reflexes and responses are generated by the integration of visual, vestibular, and proprioceptive inputs in the context of voluntary intent and ongoing changes in the environment in which the subject is moving. Once the trunk is upright and stable, locomotion can begin. The initiation of gait is heralded by a series of shifts in the center of pressure beneath the feet during the course of an anticipatory postural adjustment—first posteriorly, then laterally toward the stepping foot, and finally toward the stance foot to allow the stepping foot to swing forward. This sequence is then followed by the stereotyped stance, swing, and step phases of the gait cycle.

Anatomical Aspects of Gait

The neuroanatomical structures responsible for equilibrium and locomotion in humans are inferred from studies in lower species that suggest two basic systems. First, brainstem locomotor centers (Takakusaki, 2008) project through descending reticulospinal pathways into the ventromedial spinal cord. Stimulation of brainstem locomotor centers results in an increase in axial and limb muscle tone to assume an upright posture before stepping begins. Second, assemblies of spinal interneurons (central pattern generators or spinal locomotor centers) activate motoneurons of limb and trunk muscles in a patterned and repetitive manner to drive stepping movements and stimulate propriospinal networks that link the trunk and limbs to facilitate the synergistic coordinated limb and trunk movements of locomotion. In quadrupedal animals, spinal locomotor centers are capable of maintaining and coordinating rhythmic stepping movements after spinal transection. The cerebral cortex and corticospinal tract are not necessary for experimentally induced locomotion in quadrupeds but are required for precision stepping. The isolated spinal cord in humans can produce spontaneous movements, but it cannot generate rhythmic stepping or maintain truncal balance, indicating that brainstem and higher cortical connections are necessary for bipedal walking in humans. In monkeys, spinal stepping requires preservation of the descending ventromedial brainstem and ventrolateral spinal motor pathways. Lesions of the medial brainstem in monkeys interrupt descending reticulospinal, vestibulospinal, and tectospinal systems, resulting in dysequilibrium.

The control of posture and locomotion in humans may be mediated by similar networks, with an additional level of supraspinal control needed to maintain bipedal stance and the complex repertoire of gait. Frontal cortex, via corticospinal tract and the basal ganglia, provide the signals to brainstem locomotor centers such as the pedunculopontine and adjacent nuclei of the midbrain to increase postural tone and commence rhythmic stepping. The corticospinal tract also projects to spinal cord motoneurons, enabling precision foot movements for stepping or dancing. The parietal cortex integrates sensory inputs indicating where the individual is in space, the relationship to gravitational forces, the speed and direction of movement, and the characteristics of the terrain and environment. The cerebellum modulates the rate, rhythm, amplitude, and force of stepping and also contributes to the medial brainstem efferent system controlling equilibrium and truncal posture through projections from the flocculonodular and anterior lobes. Much of the automatic control of truncal posture and walking in humans must be derived from integration of these various functions at the highest levels of motor organization, but the precise details remain unknown.

History and Common Symptoms of Gait Disturbance

A detailed account of the patient's walking difficulty and its evolution provide the first clues to the underlying diagnosis. When evaluating the history, it is helpful to note the particular circumstances in which the walking difficulty occurs, the leg movements most affected, and any associated symptoms. Because disorders at many levels of the peripheral and central nervous systems give rise to difficulty walking, it is necessary to consider whether the problem is caused by muscle weakness, a defect of higher motor control, or imbalance due to cerebellar disease or proprioceptive sensory loss. Walking over uneven ground exacerbates most walking difficulties,

leading to tripping, stumbling, and falls. A ligamentous ankle strain or even a bony fracture may result from tripping, and falling may be the presenting symptom of a gait disorder. Fear of falling may lead to a variety of voluntary protective measures to minimize the risk of injury. In some patients, particularly the elderly, compensatory strategies and a fear of falling lead to a "cautious" gait that dominates the clinical picture. Often an individual is unaware of their gait abnormality, and family or friends note altered cadence, shuffling, veering, or slowness.

Weakness

Weakness of the legs may be described in several ways. Complaints of stiffness, heaviness, or "legs that do not do what they are told" may be the presenting symptoms of a spastic paraparesis or hemiparesis. Patients with spastic paraparesis frequently report that they drag their legs or that their legs suddenly give way, causing stumbling and falls.

Weakness of certain muscle groups may be described as difficulty performing particular movements during the gait cycle. Catching or scraping the toe on the ground and a tendency to trip may be the presenting symptom of hemiplegia (causing a spastic equinovarus foot posture) or foot drop caused by weakness of ankle dorsiflexion. Weakness of knee extension presents with a sensation that the legs will give way while standing or walking down stairs. Weakness of ankle plantar flexion interferes with the ability to stride forward, resulting in a shallow stepped gait. Weakness of certain movements may first become apparent in particular situations; for example, difficulty in climbing stairs or rising from a seated position is suggestive of a proximal myopathy.

Slowness and Stiffness

Slowness of walking is encountered in the elderly and in most gait disorders. Recent pooled analysis from nine selected cohorts has provided evidence that the speed of gait may correlate with longer survival in older adults (Studenski et al., 2011). Walking slowly is a normal reaction to unstable or slippery surfaces that cause postural insecurity and threaten balance. Similarly, those who feel their balance is less secure because of any musculoskeletal or neurological disorders walk slower. In Parkinson disease (PD) and other basal ganglia diseases, slowness of walking is due to shuffling with short, shallow steps. Difficulty initiating stepping when starting to walk (*start hesitation*) and when encountering an obstacle or turning (*freezing*) are common in more advanced stages of parkinsonian syndromes.

Difficulty rising from a chair or turning in bed and a general decline in agility may be clues to loss of truncal mobility in diffuse cerebrovascular disease, hydrocephalus, and extrapyramidal diseases. Axial muscle weakness due to peripheral neuromuscular diseases may also interfere with truncal mobility. Fatigue during walking accompanies muscular weakness of any cause and is a frequent symptom of the extra effort required to walk in upper motor neuron syndromes and basal ganglia disease.

The circumstances in which leg stiffness occurs when walking may be revealing. It is important to recognize that leg muscle tone in some upper motor neuron syndromes and dystonia may be normal when the patient is examined in the supine position but is increased during walking. An action dystonia of the foot is a common initial symptom of primary torsion dystonia in childhood. Stiffness, inversion, and plantar flexion of the foot and a tendency to walk on the toes may only become evident after walking some distance or running. Patients with dopa-responsive dystonia and prominent diurnal fluctuation typically develop symptoms in the afternoon. Exercise-induced dystonia of the foot when running may be the presenting symptom of PD.

Loss of Balance

Complaints of poor balance and unsteadiness are cardinal features of cerebellar ataxia and sensory ataxia (due to proprioceptive sensory loss). The patient with a cerebellar gait ataxia complains of unsteadiness, staggering, inability to walk in a straight line, and near falls. Turning and suddenly changing direction result in veering to one side or staggering as if intoxicated. Symptoms are exacerbated by an uneven support surface. A sensory ataxia presents with symptoms of unsteadiness when walking in the dark, because visual compensation for the proprioceptive loss is not possible. Patients with impaired proprioception and sensory ataxia complain of being uncertain of the exact position of their feet when walking. They may be unable to appreciate the texture of the ground beneath their feet and may describe abnormal sensations in the feet that give the impression of walking on a spongy surface or cotton wool.

Acute disturbances of balance and loss of truncal equilibrium occur in vascular lesions of the cerebellum, thalamus, and basal ganglia. Acute vertigo due to a peripheral vestibulopathy may also lead to a sensation of imbalance and a tendency to veer to one side.

Imbalance in basal ganglia disorders and subcortical cerebrovascular disease commonly occurs when turning while walking, stepping backwards, bending over to pick up something, or performing several tasks simultaneously, such as when walking and carrying an object.

Falls

Falls may be classified according to whether tone is retained ("falling like a tree trunk" or toppling) or is lost (collapsing falls). Loss of tone implies a loss of consciousness and is characteristic of syncope, faints, or seizures. Toppling falls are due to impaired postural reflexes and responses that control body sway. It is important to establish the circumstances in which falls occur and whether there are clear precipitants. Tripping may be due to foot drop or shallow steps, a tendency that may be exaggerated when walking on uneven ground. Proximal muscle weakness may result in the legs giving way. Unsteadiness and poor balance in an ataxic syndrome may lead to falls. Spontaneous falls, falls associated with postural adjustments, or falls that occur when performing multiple tasks suggest an impairment of automatic postural reflexes. In the setting of the early stages of an akinetic-rigid syndrome, spontaneous falls, especially backwards, are an important clue to diagnoses such as multiple system atrophy or progressive supranuclear palsy (Steele-Richardson-Olszewski syndrome) rather than PD. Tripping may also be a consequence of carelessness secondary to inattention, dementia, or poor vision.

Sensory Symptoms and Pain Associated with Gait Disorders

The distribution of any accompanying sensory complaints provides a clue to the site of the lesion producing walking difficulties. A common example is cervical spondylotic myelopathy with cervical radicular pain or paresthesias, sensations of tight bands around the trunk (due to spinal sensory tract compression), and a spastic paraparesis. Distal symmetrical paresthesias of the limbs suggest peripheral neuropathy. It is important to determine whether leg pain and weakness during walking are caused by the same focal pathology (a radiculopathy or neurogenic claudication of the cauda equina) or whether the pain is of musculoskeletal origin and is exacerbated by walking. Neurogenic intermittent claudication of the cauda equina should also be distinguished from vascular intermittent claudication in which ischemic muscle pain, typically affecting the calves, interrupts walking. Skeletal pain due to degenerative joint disease is aggravated by movement of the legs and often persists at rest (in contrast to claudication). The normal pattern of walking is frequently modified by joint disease (especially of the hip). Voluntary strategies to minimize pain by avoiding full weight bearing on the affected limb or by limiting its range of movement are a common cause of antalgic gait patterns.

Incontinence and Gait Disorders

A spastic paraparesis with loss of voluntary control of sphincter function suggests a spinal cord lesion. Parasagittal cerebral lesions such as frontal lobe tumors (parasagittal meningioma), frontal lobe infarction caused by anterior cerebral artery occlusion, and hydrocephalus should also be considered. Impairment of higher mental function and incontinence may be important clues to a cerebral cause of paraparesis. Urge incontinence is also common in parkinsonism and subcortical white-matter ischemia.

Examination of Posture and Walking

A scheme for the examination of posture and walking is summarized in **Box 22.1**. A convenient starting point is to observe the overall pattern of limb and body movement during walking. Normal walking progresses in a smooth and effortless manner. The truncal posture is upright, and the legs swing in a fluid motion with a regular stride length. Synergistic head, trunk, and upper-limb movement flow with each step. Observation of the pattern of body and limb movement during walking also helps the examiner decide whether the gait problem is caused by a focal abnormality (e.g., shortening, hip disease, muscle weakness) or a generalized disorder of movement, and whether the problem is unilateral or bilateral. After observing the overall walking pattern, the specific aspects of posture and gait should be examined (see **Box 22.1**).

Arising from Sitting

Watching the patient arise from a chair without using the arms informs about pelvic girdle strength, control of truncal movement, coordination, and balance. Inappropriate strategies in

Box 22.1 Examination of Gait and Balance*

Arising to Stand from Seated Position
Proximal muscle strength
Organization of truncal and limb movements
Stability
Stance base

Standing
Posture
Stance base
Body sway
Romberg test
Postural reflexes (pull test)

Walking
Initiation of stepping
Speed
Stance base
Step length
Cadence
Trajectory (shallow, shuffling or high stepping)
Associated trunk and arm movements
Posture

Turning While Walking
Number of steps to turn
Stabilizing steps
En bloc (truncal and limb movement)
Freezing

Other Maneuvers
Tandem walking
Walking backwards
Running
Walking on toes, heels

*To be considered in conjunction with general neurological examination.

Table 22.1 Summary of Clinical Features Distinguishing Different Types of Gait Ataxia

Feature	Cerebellar	Sensory	Frontal Lobe
Trunk posture	Leans forward	Stooped	Upright
Stance	Wide-based	Wide-based	Wide-based
Postural reflexes	Variable	Intact	Impaired
Initiation of gait	Normal	Normal	Start hesitation
Steps	Staggering, lurching	High-stepping	Short, shuffling
Speed	Normal, slow	Normal, slow	Very slow
Heel-to-toe	Unable	Variable	Unable
Turning corners	Veers away	Minimal effect	Freezing, shuffling
Romberg test	Variable	Positive; increased unsteadiness	Variable
Heel-to-shin test	Usually abnormal	Variable	Normal
Falls	Uncommon	Yes	Very common

which the feet are not positioned directly under the body or the trunk leans backwards while trying to stand up may be seen with frontal lobe disease.

Stance

The width of the stance base (the distance between the feet) during quiet arising from sitting, standing, and walking gives some indication of balance. Wide-based gaits are typical of cerebellar or sensory ataxia but also may be seen in diffuse cerebrovascular disease and frontal lobe lesions (**Table 22.1**). Widening the stance base is an efficient method of reducing body sway in the lateral and anteroposterior planes. Persons whose balance is insecure for any reason tend to adopt a wider stance and a posture of mild generalized flexion and to take shorter steps. Those who have attempted to walk on ice or other slippery surfaces will recognize this phenomenon. Eversion of the feet is another manner in which to increase stability and is particularly common in patients with diffuse cerebrovascular disease. Spontaneous sway, drift of the body in any direction, postural tremor, or ability to stay upright without touching furniture or assistance of another person are important clues.

Trunk Posture

The trunk is normally upright during standing and walking. Flexion of the trunk and a stooped posture are prominent features in PD. Slight flexion at the hips to lower the trunk and shift the center of gravity forward to minimize posterior body sway and reduce the risk of falling backward is common in many unsteady cautious gait syndromes. Neck and trunk extension is characteristic of progressive supranuclear palsy. Neck flexion occurs with weakness of the neck extensors in motor neuron disease and myasthenia and as a dystonic manifestation in multiple system atrophy and parkinsonism. An exaggerated lumbar lordosis, caused by hip-girdle weakness, is typical of proximal myopathies. Paraspinal muscle spasm and rigidity also produces an exaggerated lumbar lordosis in the stiff person syndrome. Tilt of the trunk to one side in dystonia is accompanied by axial muscle spasms, the most common being an exaggerated flexion movement of the trunk and hip with each step. Truncal tilt away from the affected side is observed in some acute vascular lesions of the thalamus and basal ganglia. Misperception of truncal posture and position results in inappropriate movements to correct the perceived tilt in the pusher syndrome, associated with posterolateral thalamic hemorrhages (Karnath et al., 2005). Acute vestibular imbalance in the lateral medullary syndrome leads to sway or tilt toward the side of the lesion (*lateropulsion*). Abnormal truncal postures occur in paraspinal myopathies that produce weakness of trunk extension and a posture of truncal flexion (*camptocormia*). Dystonia and parkinsonism also may alter truncal posture and lead to camptocormia or lateral truncal flexion (*Pisa syndrome*). Abnormal thoracolumbar postures also result from spinal ankylosis and spondylitis. A restricted range of spinal movement and persistence of the abnormal spinal posture when supine or during sleep are useful pointers toward a bony spinal deformity as the cause of an abnormal truncal posture. Truncal postures, particularly in the lumbar region, can be compensatory for shortening of one lower limb, lumbar or leg pain, or disease of the hip, knee, or ankle.

Postural Responses

Reactive postural responses are examined by sharply pulling the upper trunk backward or forward while the patient is standing. The pull should be sufficient to require the patient to step to regain their balance. This maneuver is referred to as the *pull test* (Hunt and Setni, 2006). The examiner must be prepared, generally by having a wall behind them, to prevent the patient from falling. A few short, shuffling steps backward (*retropulsion*) or a backwards fall after backward displacements, or forward (*propulsion*) after forward displacements, suggest impairment of postural righting (*reactive postural*) reactions. Falls after postural changes such as arising from a chair or turning while walking suggest impaired anticipatory postural responses. Falls without rescue arm movements or stepping movements to break the fall indicate loss of protective postural responses. Injuries sustained during falls provide a clue to the loss of these postural responses. A tendency to fall backward spontaneously is a sign of impaired postural reflexes in progressive supranuclear palsy and gait disorders associated with diseases of the frontal lobes.

Walking
Initiation of Gait

Difficulty initiating the first step (*start hesitation*) ranges in severity from a few shuffling steps, to small shallow steps on the spot without forward progress (*slipping clutch phenomenon*), to complete immobility with the feet seemingly glued to the floor (*magnetic feet phenomenon*). Patients may make exaggerated upper-body movements or alter the step pattern, such as stepping sideways or lifting the feet very high in an effort to engage their legs in motion. Start hesitation is occasionally seen in isolation in the syndrome of *gait ignition failure*. Magnetic feet suggest frontal lobe disease, diffuse cerebrovascular disease, or hydrocephalus. Start hesitation is commonly a feature of the "freezing gait" of PD when starting to walk and when walking has been interrupted by an obstacle of some sort. The small shuffling steps on the spot are often accompanied by trembling of the knees, standing on the toes, and forward tilt of the trunk.

Stepping

Once walking is underway, the length and trajectory of each step and the rhythm of stepping should be noted. Short, regular, shallow steps or shuffling and a slow gait are characteristic of the akinetic-rigid syndromes. Shuffling is most evident when starting to walk, stopping, or turning corners. Specifically examining these maneuvers may reveal a subtle tendency to shuffle. Once the person is underway, freezing may interrupt walking, with further shuffling and start hesitation. *Festination* (increasingly rapid, small steps) is common in PD but rare in other akinetic-rigid syndromes, which frequently are associated with poor balance and falls rather than festination. Unilateral loss of synergistic arm swing while walking is a valuable sign of early PD. A reduction in associated trunk movement and arm swing also may be evident in unilateral upper motor neuron and acute cerebellar syndromes. A slow gait also is seen in ataxic and spastic syndromes. Jerky steps of irregular rhythm and variable length and direction suggest ataxic or choreic syndromes. Subtle degrees of cerebellar ataxia may be unmasked by asking the patient to walk in a straight line heel-to-toe (tandem gait), to stand on one leg, or to walk and turn quickly. When vision is important in helping maintain balance, as in sensory ataxia caused by proprioceptive loss, the removal of vision greatly exaggerates the ataxia. This is the basis of the Romberg test, in which eye closure leads to a dramatic increase in unsteadiness and even falls in the patient with sensory ataxia. When performing the Romberg test, it is important that the patient be standing comfortably before eye closure and to remember that a modest increase in body sway is a normal response to eye closure. Distinctive leg postures and foot trajectories occur during stepping in sensory ataxia, foot drop, spasticity, and dystonia. It may be necessary to examine the patient running to identify an action dystonia of the legs in the early stages of primary torsion dystonia.

Turning

Turning while walking stresses balance much more than walking in a straight line and is often where gait abnormalities first appear. Slowing on turns may be the first abnormality in walking in a patient with PD. Multiple steps on turning are common in PD and diffuse cerebrovascular disease. An extra step or mild widening of the base on turning may herald the onset of ataxia.

More Challenging Tests of Walking

Tandem gait (walking heel-to-toe) is a good test for ataxia. Walking on toes and heels may bring out abnormal movements as well as deficits in the strength of dorsiflexion and plantar flexion of the ankle. Sometimes walking backwards or running may be informative.

Motor and Sensory Examination

After the patient has been observed walking, motor and sensory function in the limbs is examined with the patient sitting or supine to confirm the suspicions raised by the gait features. The size and length of the limbs should be measured in any child presenting with a limp. Asymmetry in leg size suggests a congenital malformation of the spinal cord or brain, or (rarely) local overgrowth of tissue. The spinal column should be inspected for scoliosis, and the lumbar region for skin defects or hairy patches indicative of spinal dysraphism.

Changes in muscle tone such as spasticity, lead-pipe or cogwheel rigidity, or paratonic rigidity (*gegenhalten*) point toward diseases of the upper motor neuron, basal ganglia, and frontal lobes, respectively. In the patient who complains of symptoms in only one leg, a detailed examination of the other leg is important. If signs of an upper motor neuron syndrome are present in both legs, a disorder of the spinal cord or parasagittal region is likely. Muscle bulk and strength are examined for evidence of muscle wasting and the presence and distribution of muscle weakness. Examination reveals whether the abnormal posture of the leg in a patient with foot drop

Box 22.2 Causes of Foot Drop and an Equinovarus Foot Posture When Walking

Peripheral nerve
  L5 radiculopathy
  Lumbar plexopathy
  Sciatic nerve palsy
  Peroneal neuropathy (compression)
  Peripheral neuropathy (bilateral)
  Anterior horn cell disease (motor neuron disease)
Myopathy
Scapuloperoneal syndromes
Spasticity
Dystonia
Sensory ataxia

(**Box 22.2**) is caused by spasticity or weakness of ankle dorsiflexors, which in turn may be due to anterior horn cell disease, a peripheral neuropathy, a peroneal compression neuropathy, or an L5 root lesion. Joint position sense should be examined for defects of proprioception in the ataxic patient or awkward posturing of the foot. Other signs such as a supranuclear gaze palsy, ataxia, and frontal lobe release signs should be sought where relevant.

Discrepancies on Examination of Gait

Several conditions are notable for producing minimal abnormal signs on physical examination of the recumbent patient, in striking contrast to the observed difficulty when walking. A patient with a cerebellar gait ataxia caused by a vermis lesion may perform the heel-to-shin test normally when supine but is clearly ataxic when walking. The finding of normal muscle strength, muscle tone, and tendon reflexes is common in dystonic syndromes in which an action dystonia causes abnormal posturing of the feet only when walking. A dystonic gait may be evident only when running or walking forward but not when walking backward. Gegenhalten (paratonia), with or without brisk tendon reflexes, may be the only abnormal sign in the legs of the recumbent patient with a frontal lobe lesion, hydrocephalus, or diffuse cerebrovascular disease who is totally unable to walk when standing. Such patients may be able to perform the heel-to-shin test and make bicycling movements of their legs when lying on a bed. A similar discrepancy can be seen in spastic paraplegia caused by hereditary spastic paraplegia, cerebral palsy (Little disease), or cervical spondylotic myelopathy, where only minor changes in muscle tone, strength, and tendon reflexes are evident during the supine examination, in contrast to the profound leg spasticity when standing and attempting to walk. The leg tremor of orthostatic tremor only appears during weight bearing.

Classification of Gait Patterns

The goal of classification is to arrange gait patterns into a scheme or order that reflects the physiological basis of human gait and helps the clinician recognize what levels of the nervous system are deranged. A scheme based on Hughlings Jackson's three orders of neurological centers—lower (simplest), middle, and higher (complex and integrative)—enables a classification according to function. Each center contributes sensory and motor function, but that of higher centers is more complex and dispersed within the nervous system.

Lower-Level Gait Disorders

Lower-level disorders have physical signs of neurological dysfunction such as weakness or sensory loss. Lower-level motor function and muscle contraction produce the force required for postural responses and locomotion. Lower-level motor dysfunction arises from muscle and peripheral nerve disease. Gaits that typify this category include foot drop or steppage gaits associated with distal weakness, usually due to neuropathy, and waddling gaits associated with proximal (usually myopathic) weakness. Lower-level sensory dysfunction arises from disorders of the three basic senses thought most important for gait and balance: proprioception, vision, and vestibular sensation. Lower-level sensory disorders arise from diseases affecting the peripheral transmission of these sensory modalities. Sensory ataxia results from deafferentation due to peripheral nerve, dorsal root ganglion, or posterior column lesions and is associated with loss of proprioception or joint position sense. Imbalance in acute peripheral vestibulopathies or visual impairment are other examples of lower-level sensory disorders.

Myopathic Weakness and Gait

Weakness of proximal leg and hip-girdle muscles interferes with stabilizing the pelvis and legs on the trunk during all phases of the gait cycle, and failure to stabilize the pelvis produces exaggerated rotation of the pelvis with each step (*waddling gait*). The hips are slightly flexed as a result of weakness of hip extension, and an exaggerated lumbar lordosis occurs. Weakness of hip extension interferes with the ability to stand from a squatting or lying position; patients may use their arms to push themselves up from a squatting position (*Gowers sign*). A myopathy is the most common cause of proximal muscle weakness, but neurogenic weakness of proximal muscles can also produce this clinical picture.

Neurogenic Weakness and Gait

Muscle weakness of peripheral nerve origin, as in a peripheral neuropathy, typically affects distal muscles of the legs and results in a *steppage gait*. The patient lifts the leg and foot high above the ground with each step because of weakness of ankle dorsiflexion and foot drop. When this clinical picture is confined to only one leg (unilateral foot drop), a common peroneal or sciatic nerve palsy or an L5 radiculopathy is the usual cause. Less common is foot drop caused by myopathic weakness, as in the scapuloperoneal syndromes. Weakness of ankle plantar flexion produces a shallow stepped gait. A femoral neuropathy, as in diabetes mellitus, produces weakness of knee extension and buckling of the knee when walking or standing. This may first be evident when walking down stairs. Progressive muscular atrophy in motor neuron disease or a quadriceps myopathy caused by inclusion body myositis may result in similar focal weakness.

Sensory Ataxia

Loss of proprioceptive input from the lower limbs deprives the patient of knowledge of the position of the legs and feet in space, the progress of ongoing movement, the state of muscle contraction, and finer details of the texture of the surface on which the patient is walking. Walking on uneven surfaces is particularly difficult. Patients with sensory ataxia adopt a wide base and advance cautiously, taking slow steps under visual guidance. During walking, the feet are thrust forward with variable direction and height. The sole of the foot strikes the floor forcibly with a slapping sound (slapping gait). The absence of visual information when walking at night or during the Romberg test leads to imbalance and falls. Lesions at any point in the sensory pathways that interrupt large-diameter proprioceptive afferent fibers produce this clinical picture. Peripheral neuropathies, posterior root or dorsal root ganglionopathies, and dorsal column lesions are typical etiologies.

Vestibular Imbalance, Vertigo, and Gait

Acute vestibular imbalance in the lateral medullary syndrome leads to sway, tilt, and veering toward the side of the lesion (*lateropulsion*). Acute peripheral vestibular disorders result in leaning and unsteady veering to the side of the lesion (and this is dependent on the position of the head). Paradoxically, running may be less affected by the acute vestibulopathy than walking. In general, patients with an acute vestibulopathy prefer to lie still to minimize the symptoms of acute vestibular imbalance. In chronic vestibular failure, gait may be normal, though unsteadiness can be unmasked during eye closure and with rotating the head side to side while walking.

Middle-Level Gait Disorders

Middle-level gait disorders are primarily motor dysfunctions and appear to be related to impaired modulation of force generated by the lower-level motor system. The middle-level motor disorders include: (1) spasticity from disruption of the corticospinal tracts, (2) ataxia arising from disturbances of the cerebellum and its connections, (3) hypokinetic gaits associated with parkinsonism, and (4) hyperkinetic gaits associated with chorea, dystonia, and other movement disorders.

Spastic Gait

Spasticity of the arm and leg on one side produces the characteristic clinical picture of a spastic hemiparesis. The arm is held adducted, internally rotated at the shoulder, and flexed at the elbow, with pronation of the forearm and flexion of the wrist and fingers. The leg is slightly flexed at the hip and extended at the knee, with plantar flexion and inversion of the foot. The swing phase of each step is accomplished by slight lateral flexion of the trunk toward the unaffected side and hyperextension of the hip on that side to allow slow circumduction of the stiffly extended paretic leg as it is swung forward from the hip, dragging the toe or catching it on the ground beneath. A minimum of associated arm swing occurs on the affected side. The stance may be slightly widened, and the speed of walking is slow. Balance may be poor because the hemiparesis interferes with corrective postural adjustments on the affected side. Muscle tone in the affected limbs is increased,

clonus may be present, and tendon reflexes are abnormally brisk, with an extensor plantar response. Examination of the sole of the shoe may reveal wear of the toe and outer borders of the shoe, suggesting that the spastic gait is of long standing. After identifying a spastic hemiparesis, determining the site at which the corticospinal tract is involved, determining the motor level, and confirmatory imaging with magnetic resonance imaging (MRI) of the brain (and where indicated, the spinal cord) should be the next steps in the diagnostic process.

Spasticity of both legs gives rise to a spastic paraparesis. The legs are stiffly extended at the knees, plantar flexed at the ankles, and slightly flexed at the hips. Both legs circumduct, and the toes of the plantar flexed feet catch on the floor with each step. The gait is slow and labored as the legs are dragged forward with each step. There is a tendency to adduct the legs, particularly when the disorder begins in childhood, an appearance described as *scissors gait*. The causes of a spastic paraparesis include hereditary spastic paraplegia, in which the arms and sphincters are unaffected and there may be little or no leg weakness, and other myelopathies. An indication of the extent and level of the spinal cord lesion can be obtained from the presence or absence of weakness or sensory loss in the arms, a spinothalamic sensory level or posterior column sensory loss, and alterations in sphincter function. Patients with paraparesis of recent onset should be investigated with MRI of the spinal cord to exclude potentially treatable causes such as spinal cord compression.

Occasionally, bilateral leg dystonia (*dystonic paraparesis*) mimics a spastic paraparesis. This typically occurs in dopa-responsive dystonia in childhood and may be misdiagnosed as hereditary spastic paraplegia or cerebral diplegia. Clinical differentiation between these conditions can be difficult. Brisk tendon reflexes occur in both, and spontaneous extension of a great toe in patients with striatal disorders may be interpreted as a Babinski response. Fanning of the toes and knee flexion suggest spastic paraplegia. Other distinguishing features include changes in muscle tone, such as spasticity in hereditary spastic paraparesis and rigidity in dystonic paraparesis. In young children, the distinction is important because a proportion of such patients can be treated successfully with levodopa (discussed in the following sections).

Cerebellar Ataxia

Disease of the midline cerebellar structures, the vermis, and anterior lobe produces loss of truncal balance, increased body sway, dysequilibrium, and gait ataxia. When standing, the patient adopts a wide-based stance; the legs are stiffly extended and the hips slightly flexed to crouch forward and minimize truncal sway. The truncal gait ataxia of midline cerebellar pathology has a lurching and staggering quality that is more pronounced when walking on a narrow base or during heel-to-toe walking. A pure truncal ataxia may be the sole feature of a midline (vermis) cerebellar syndrome and escape notice if the patient is not examined when standing, because leg coordination during the heel-to-shin test may be relatively normal when examined supine. Midline cerebellar pathologies also include masses, hemorrhage, paraneoplastic syndromes, and malnutrition in alcoholism. Patients with anterior lobe atrophy develop a 3-Hz anteroposterior sway of the trunk and a rhythmic truncal and head tremor (*titubation*) that is superimposed on the gait ataxia. This combination of truncal gait ataxia and truncal tremor is characteristic of some late-onset cerebellar degenerations affecting the anterior lobe.

Lesions of the cerebellar flocculonodular lobe (the vestibulocerebellum) exhibit multidirectional body sway, dysequilibrium, and severe impairment of body and truncal motion. Standing and even sitting can be impossible, although when lying down, results of the heel-to-shin test may appear normal, and upper-limb function may be relatively preserved.

Limb ataxia due to involvement of the cerebellar hemispheres is characterized by a decomposition of normal leg movement. Steps are irregular and variable in timing (*dyssynergia*), length, and direction (*dysmetria*). Steps are taken slowly and carefully to reduce the tendency to lurch and stagger. These defects are accentuated when attempting to walk heel to toe in a straight line. With lesions confined to one cerebellar hemisphere, ataxia is limited to the ipsilateral limbs, and there is little postural instability or truncal imbalance if the vermis is not involved. Vascular disease and mass lesions are generally responsible for hemisphere lesions.

Cerebellar gait ataxia is exacerbated by the rapid postural adjustments needed to change direction, turn a corner or avoid obstacles, and when stopping or starting to walk. Minor support, such as holding the patient's arm during walking, and visual compensation help the patient with a cerebellar ataxia reduce body sway. Eye closure may heighten anxiety about falling and increase body sway, but not to the extent observed in a sensory ataxia.

Episodic ataxias produce periods of impaired gait that typically last seconds to hours. Alcohol and drug use must be considered in the differential of episodic ataxias.

Spastic Ataxia

A combination of spasticity and ataxia produces a distinctive "springing or bouncing" gait. Such gaits are seen in multiple sclerosis, the Arnold-Chiari malformation, and hydrocephalus in young people. The gait is wide-based, and clonus precipitated by standing or walking aggravates the unsteadiness gives rise to a bouncing motion. Compensatory movements, made in an effort to regain balance, set up a vicious cycle of ataxic movements, clonus, and increasing unsteadiness, rendering the patient unable to stand or walk. Bouncing gaits must be distinguished from action myoclonus of the legs and cerebellar truncal tremors.

Hypokinetic (Parkinsonian) Gait

The most common hypokinetic-bradykinetic gait disturbance is that encountered in PD. In early PD, an asymmetrical reduction of arm swing and slight slowing in gait, particularly with turns, is characteristic. In more advanced PD, the posture is stooped, with flexion of the shoulders, neck, trunk, and knees. During walking, there is little associated or synergistic body movement. Arm swing is reduced or absent, and the arms are held immobile at the sides or slightly forward of the trunk. Tremor of the upper limbs frequently increases when walking, but parkinsonian tremor of the legs rarely affects walking. A characteristic feature of a parkinsonian gait is the tendency to begin walking with a few rapid, short, shuffling steps (start hesitation) before breaking into a more normal stepping pattern with small, shallow steps on a narrow base. Once underway, walking may be interrupted by shuffling or even cessation of movement (freezing) if an obstacle is encountered, when walking through doorways, or when attempting to undertake multiple tasks at once. These signs may be alleviated by levodopa treatment. In the long-term, levodopa therapy may induce dyskinesias, resulting in choreic and dystonic gaits as described later.

The posture of generalized flexion of the patient with PD exaggerates the normal tendency to lean forward when walking. To maintain balance when walking and avoid falling forward, the patient may advance with a series of rapid, small steps (festination). Retropulsion and propulsion are similar manifestations of a flurry of small, shuffling steps made in an effort to preserve equilibrium. Instead of a single large step, a series of small steps are taken to maintain balance. Freezing becomes increasingly troublesome in the later stages of PD, at which time sensory cues may be more useful in triggering a step than medication. The shuffling gait of PD that is responsive to levodopa characterizes the midlevel gait pattern. As the disease progresses, dysequilibrium and falls emerge that are features of a higher-level gait disorder (discussed later).

Choreic Gait

The random movements of chorea are accentuated and often most noticeable during walking. The superimposition of chorea on the trunk and leg movements of the walking cycle gives the gait a dancing quality owing to the exaggerated motion of the legs and arm swing. Chorea can also interrupt the walking pattern, leading to a hesitant gait. Additional voluntary compensatory movements appear in response to perturbations imposed by chorea. Chorea in Sydenham chorea or chorea gravidarum may be sufficiently violent to throw patients off their feet. Severe chorea of the trunk may render walking impossible. The chorea of Huntington disease usually causes a lurching, stumbling, and stuttering gait with frequent steps forward, backward, or to one side. Walking is slow, the stance may vary step to step but generally is wide-based, the trunk sways excessively, and steps are variable in length and timing. These characteristics may be misinterpreted as ataxia. Dystonic posturing such as hip or knee flexion and leg-raising movements commonly punctuate the stepping motion. Balance and equilibrium usually are maintained until the terminal stages of Huntington disease, when an akinetic-rigid syndrome may supervene. Neuroleptics such as haloperidol reduce chorea but do not improve gait in Huntington disease.

Dystonic Gait

Of all gait disturbances, dystonic syndromes produce some of the more bizarre and difficult diagnostic problems. The classic presentation of childhood-onset primary torsion dystonia is an action dystonia of a leg, with a sustained abnormal posture of the foot (typically plantar flexion and inversion) on attempting to run. In contrast, walking forward or backward or even running backward may be entirely normal at an early stage. An easily overlooked sign in the early stages is tonic extension of the great toe (the *striatal toe*) when walking. This may be a subtle finding but occasionally is so pronounced that a hole is worn in the toe of the shoe. With the passage of time, dystonia may progress to involve the whole leg and then become generalized.

More difficult to recognize are those dystonic syndromes that present with bizarre, seemingly inexplicable postures of the legs and trunk when walking. A characteristic feature common to dystonic gaits is excessive flexion of the hip when walking. Patients may hop or walk sideways in a crablike fashion, with hyperflexion of the hips producing an attitude of general body flexion in a simian posture, or a birdlike (peacock) gait with excessive flexion of the hip and knee and plantar flexion of the foot during the swing phase of each step. Many of these patients have been thought to be hysterical because of the unusual gait disturbance and because formal neurological examination is often normal when the patient is examined lying supine. Each of these gait patterns has been described in association with primary and secondary dystonic syndromes. Tardive dystonia following neuroleptic drug exposure may produce similar bizarre abnormalities of gait.

It is important to look for asymmetry in the assessment of childhood-onset dystonia. Symptomatic causes should be excluded in hemidystonic presentations, isolated leg dystonia in an adult, and early loss of postural responses and righting reflexes in association with a dystonic gait.

Dopa-responsive dystonia characteristically presents in childhood with walking difficulties and diurnal fluctuations in severity of dystonia. Typically the child walks normally in the early morning but develops increasing rigidity and dystonic posturing of the legs as the day progresses or after exercise; these difficulties may be relieved by a nap. Examination reveals a dystonic plantar flexion and inversion of the foot, with the additional feature of brisk tendon reflexes. Some of these patients respond dramatically to levodopa, so early recognition is important. Indeed, all children presenting with a dystonic foot or leg should have a therapeutic trial of levodopa before other therapies such as anticholinergic drugs are commenced.

Paroxysmal dyskinesias also may present with difficulty walking. Paroxysmal kinesigenic choreoathetosis may present with the sudden onset of difficulty walking as the result of dystonic postures and involuntary movements of the legs, often appearing after standing from a seated position. The attacks with this disorder are typically very brief, lasting a matter of seconds.

Mixed Movement Disorders and Gait

Many conditions, notably athetoid cerebral palsy, produce motor signs reflecting abnormalities at many levels of the nervous system, all of which interfere with and disrupt normal patterns of walking. These include spasticity of the legs, truncal and gait ataxia, dystonia, and dystonic spasms of the trunk and limbs. Difficulties arise in distinguishing this clinical picture from that of primary torsion dystonia, which may begin at a similar age in childhood. The patient with cerebral palsy usually has a history of hypotonia and delayed achievement of developmental motor milestones, especially truncal control (sitting up) and walking. Often there is a history of perinatal injury or birth asphyxia, but in a substantial proportion of patients, such an event cannot be identified. A major distinguishing feature is poor balance at an early age, which may be a contributing factor to the delay in sitting and later walking. As the child begins to walk, the first signs of dystonia and athetosis appear. The presence of spasticity and ataxia also help distinguish this condition from primary dystonia. Childhood neurodegenerative diseases may first manifest as a disorder of walking with a combination of motor syndromes. A

Box 22.3 Differential Diagnosis of Involuntary Movements of the Legs When Standing

Action myoclonus and asterixis of legs
Benign essential tremor
Orthostatic tremor
Cerebellar truncal tremor
Clonus in spasticity
Spastic ataxia
Parkinson disease

---

progressive course raises the possibility of a symptomatic or secondary movement disorder.

Tremor of the Trunk and Legs

Leg tremor in benign essential tremor is occasionally symptomatic, but leg tremor is generally overshadowed by tremor of the upper limbs. Trunk and leg tremor may contribute to unsteadiness in cerebellar disease (see cerebellar gait above). Orthostatic tremor has a unique frequency (16 Hz) and distribution, affecting trunk and leg muscles while standing. This rapid tremor produces an intense sensation of unsteadiness rather than shaking, which is relieved by walking or sitting down. Patients avoid standing still (e.g., in a queue) and may shuffle on the spot or pace about in an effort to avoid the unsteadiness experienced when standing still. Falls are rare. Examination reveals only a rippling of the quadriceps muscles during standing, and the rapid tremor is often only appreciated by palpation of leg muscles. Recording the patterns of electromyographic activity in leg muscles assists the differential diagnosis of involuntary movements of the legs when standing (**Box 22.3**).

Action Myoclonus

Postanoxic action myoclonus of the legs is often accompanied by negative myoclonus (*asterixis*) and severely disrupts normal postural control and any attempts to stand or walk. Repetitive action myoclonus produces jerky movements of the legs, throwing the patient off balance, and lapses of muscle activity between the jerks (negative myoclonus) cause the patient to sag toward the ground. This sequence of events gives rise to an exaggerated bouncing appearance, which the patient is able to sustain for only a few seconds before falling or seeking relief by sitting down. Difficulty walking is one of the major residual disabilities of postanoxic myoclonus. Many patients remain wheelchair bound as a result. The stance is wide-based, and there is often an element of cerebellar ataxia, although this may be difficult to distinguish from the effects of severe action myoclonus. Stimulus-sensitive cortical reflex myoclonus also may produce a similar disorder of stance and gait, with reflex myoclonic jerking of leg muscles, particularly the quadriceps, resulting in a bouncing posture.

Higher-Level Gait Disorders

Higher-level gait disorders are characterized by varying combinations of dysequilibrium, falls due to inappropriate or absent postural responses, and shuffling steps or freezing. In contrast to lower- and middle-level gait patterns, formal neurological examination fails to reveal signs that adequately explain the gait disturbance, though brisk reflexes and extensor plantar responses or depressed reflexes and minor distal sensory loss may be encountered. Slowness of sequential leg movement and poor control of truncal movement are often present. The stepping patterns are influenced by environmental cues that may facilitate stepping but may also may induce freezing of gait if present. The performance of multiple simultaneous tasks may precipitate freezing or falls.

There are many descriptions of similar gait patterns in the literature, often focusing on one element of the gait disturbance. Because of uncertainty about the pathophysiology of these clinical manifestations, there has been no agreement on the terminology used to describe them.

Hypokinetic Higher-Level Gait Patterns

With progression of PD, freezing of gait, dysequilibrium, and falls become increasingly troublesome and do not respond to increasing doses of levodopa. There is some evidence from clinical, imaging, and pathological studies to suggest that dysequilibrium is mediated via mechanisms other than dopaminergic deficiency, and subcortical cholinergic projections from the pedunculopontine nucleus have been implicated (Bohnen et al., 2009). Falls occur late in the course of PD, and a number of causes must be considered. These include festinating steps that are too small to restore balance, tripping or stumbling over rough surfaces because shuffling steps fail to clear small obstacles, and failure to step, with start hesitation and freezing. In each of these examples, falling stems from locomotor hypokinesia and a lack of normal-sized, rapid, compensatory voluntary movements. These falls are forward onto knees and outstretched arms (indicating preservation of rescue reactions). Other falls, in any direction, occur when changing posture or turning in small spaces and result from loss of postural and righting responses, either spontaneously when multitasking or after minor perturbations. It is also important to consider collapsing falls related to orthostatic hypotension, a common finding in PD.

Unlike the hypokinetic steps and flexed truncal posture, the loss of postural and righting responses generally does not respond to levodopa. Deep brain stimulation (DBS) of the subthalamic nucleus (STN) or the globus pallidus interna (GPi) may improve gait but also may worsen gait and may be associated with increased falls (Ferraye et al., 2008; Weaver et al., 2009). DBS in the region of the pedunculopontine nucleus is under investigation for disequilibrium and freezing of gait, with mixed results (Ferraye et al., 2010).

Similar slowness of leg movement and shuffling occurs in a variety of other akinetic-rigid syndromes (**Box 22.4**), the most common of which are multiple system atrophy, corticobasal degeneration, and progressive supranuclear palsy. A number of clinical signs help distinguish among these conditions (**Table 22.2**). In progressive supranuclear palsy, the typical neck posture is one of extension, with axial and nuchal rigidity rather than neck and trunk flexion as in PD. A stooped posture with exaggerated neck flexion is sometimes a feature of multiple system atrophy. A distinguishing feature of progressive supranuclear palsy and multiple system atrophy is the early appearance of falls due to loss of postural and righting responses, in comparison to the preservation of these

---

Box 22.4 Differential Diagnosis of an Akinetic-Rigid Syndrome and Gait Disturbance

Parkinson disease
Drug-induced parkinsonism
Multiple system atrophy
　　Striatonigral degeneration
　　Shy-Drager syndrome (idiopathic orthostatic hypotension)
　　Olivopontocerebellar atrophy
Progressive supranuclear palsy (Steele-Richardson-Olszewski Syndrome)
Corticobasal degeneration
Frontotemporal dementia
Creutzfeldt-Jakob disease
Cerebrovascular disease (Binswanger disease)
Hydrocephalus
Frontal lobe tumor
Juvenile Huntington disease
Wilson disease
Cerebral anoxia
Neurosyphilis

Table 22.2 Summary of Clinical Features Differentiating Parkinson Disease from Symptomatic Parkinsonism in Patients with an Akinetic-Rigid Gait Syndrome

Feature	Parkinson Disease	Symptomatic Parkinsonism
Posture	Stooped (trunk flexion)	Stooped or upright (trunk flexion/extension)
Stance	Narrow	Often wide-based
Initiation of walking	Start hesitation	Start hesitation, magnetic feet
Steps	Small, shuffling	Small, shuffling
Stride length	Short	Short
Freezing	Common	Common
Leg movement	Stiff, rigid	Stiff, rigid
Speed	Slow	Slow
Festination	Common	Rare
Arm swing	Minimal or absent	Reduced or excessive
Heel-to-toe walking	Normal	Poor (truncal ataxia)
Postural reflexes	Preserved in early stages	Absent at early stage
Falls	Late (forward, tripping)	Early and severe (backward, tripping, or without apparent reason)

---

reactions in PD until later stages of the illness. There also may be an element of ataxia in these akinetic-rigid syndromes that is not evident in PD. Falls occur in 80% of patients with progressive supranuclear palsy and can be dramatic, leading to injury. The disturbance of postural control in progressive supranuclear palsy is coupled with impulsivity due to frontal executive dysfunction that leads to reckless lurching movements during postural changes, such as sitting or arising, and toppling falls. Accordingly, the patient who presents with falls and an akinetic-rigid syndrome is more likely to have one of these variants of parkinsonism rather than PD. Finally, the dramatic response to levodopa that is typical of PD does not occur in these variants of parkinsonism, although some cases of multiple system atrophy respond partially for a short period.

In addition to the advanced hypokinetic disorders discussed previously, frontal lobe tumors (glioma or meningioma), anterior cerebral artery infarction, obstructive or communicating hydrocephalus (especially normal-pressure hydrocephalus), and diffuse cerebrovascular disease (multiple lacunar infarcts and Binswanger disease) also produce disturbance of gait and balance. These pathologies interrupt connections between the frontal lobes and other cortical and subcortical structures. The clinical appearance of the gait of patients with such lesions varies from a predominantly wide-based ataxic gait to an akinetic-rigid gait with slow, short steps and a tendency to shuffle. It is common for a patient to present with a combination of these features. In the early stages, the stance base is wide, with an upright posture of the trunk and shuffling when starting to walk or turning corners. There may be episodes of freezing. Arm swing is normal or even exaggerated, giving the appearance of a "military two-step" gait. The normal fluidity of trunk and limb motion is lost. Examination reveals normal voluntary upper-limb and hand movements and a lively facial expression. This "lower-half parkinsonism" is commonly seen in diffuse cerebrovascular disease. The *marche à petits pas* of Dejerine and Critchley's atherosclerotic parkinsonism refer to a similar clinical picture. Patients with this clinical syndrome commonly are misdiagnosed as having PD. The normal motor function of the upper limbs, retained arm swing during walking, upright truncal posture, wide-based stance, upper motor neuron signs including pseudobulbar palsy, and the absence of a resting tremor distinguish this syndrome from PD. In addition, the lower-half parkinsonism of diffuse cerebrovascular disease does not respond to levodopa treatment (see **Box 22.4**). Walking speed in subcortical arteriosclerotic encephalopathy is slower than in cerebellar gait ataxia or PD (Ebersbach et al., 1999). Slowness of movement and the lack of heel-to-shin ataxia distinguish the wide-based stance of this syndrome from that of cerebellar gait ataxia (see **Table 22.1**).

As the underlying condition progresses, the unsteadiness and slowness of movement become more pronounced. There may be great difficulty initiating a step, as if the feet were glued to the floor (magnetic feet). Attempts to take a step require assistance, with the patient seeking the support of nearby objects or persons. There may be excessive upper-body movement as the patient tries to free the feet to initiate walking. Once walking is underway, steps may be better, but small, shuffling, ineffective steps (freezing) reemerge when the patient tries to turn. Such patients rarely exhibit the festination of PD, but a few steps of propulsion or retropulsion may be taken. Postural and righting reactions are impaired and eventually lost. Falls are common and follow the slightest perturbation. In contrast, these patients are often able to move the legs with greater facility when seated or lying supine than when standing. Stepping, walking, or bicycling leg movements are possible when lying or seated but not when standing. This apparent discrepancy may reflect an inability to stand secondary to dysequilibrium, which in turn reflects poor truncal control. Impaired truncal mobility with truncal imbalance commonly appears in the advanced stages of a frontal gait disorder, so patients are unable to stand or turn over when lying in bed. Walking then becomes impossible, and even simple leg movements are slow and clumsy when lying down. Paratonic rigidity (gegenhalten) of the arms and legs is common. Tendon reflexes may be brisk, with extensor plantar responses. Grasp reflexes in the hands and feet may be elicited. Urinary incontinence and dementia frequently occur. Investigation of the brain with MRI reveals the majority of conditions causing this syndrome, such as diffuse cerebrovascular disease, cortical atrophy, or hydrocephalus.

Some patients display fragments of this clinical picture. Those with the *syndrome of gait initiation failure* exhibit profound start hesitation and freezing, but step size and rhythm are normal once walking is underway. Sensory cues may facilitate stepping. Balance while standing or walking is normal. These findings are similar to those seen with walking in PD, but speech and upper-limb function are normal, and there is no response to levodopa. Brain imaging results are normal. The cause of this syndrome is unknown, but the slowly progressive evolution of symptoms suggests a degenerative condition. Occasionally, isolated episodic festination with truncal flexion is encountered. Others complain of a loss of the normal fluency of stepping when walking; a conscious effort is required to maintain a normal stepping rhythm and step size. These symptoms may be associated with subtle dysequilibrium, manifesting as a few brief staggering steps to one side or a few steps of retropulsion after standing up, turning quickly, or making other rapid changes in body position. Finally, some elderly patients experience severe walking difficulties that resemble those described in frontal lobe disease. The history in these syndromes is one of gradual onset, without stroke-like episodes or identifiable structural or vascular lesions of the frontal lobes or cerebral white matter on imaging. The cause of these syndromes is unknown. The criteria for normal pressure hydrocephalus are not fulfilled, there are no signs of parkinsonism, levodopa is ineffective, and there is no evidence of more generalized cerebral dysfunction, as occurs in Alzheimer disease. Indeed, it is rare for patients with Alzheimer disease to develop difficulty walking until the later stages of the disease.

Elderly Gait Patterns, Cautious Gaits, and Fear of Falling

Healthy, neurologically normal elderly people tend to walk at slower speeds than their younger counterparts. The slower speed of walking is related to shorter and shallower steps with reduced excursion at lower limb joints. In addition, stance width may be slightly wider than normal, and synergistic arm and trunk movements are less vigorous. The rhythmicity of stepping is preserved. These changes give the normal elderly gait a cautious or guarded appearance. Factors contributing to a general decline in mobility of the elderly include degenerative joint disease, reducing range of limb movement, and decreased cardiovascular fitness, limiting exercise capacity. The changes in gait pattern of the elderly also provide a more secure base to compensate for a subtle age-related deterioration in balance.

In unselected elderly populations, a more pronounced deterioration in gait and postural control is evident. Steps are shorter, stride length is reduced, and the stance phase of walking is increased, leading to a reduction in walking speed. These changes are most marked in those who fall.

Elderly patients with an insecure gait characterized by slow short steps, en bloc turns, and falls often have signs of multiple neurological deficits such as peripheral motor (mild proximal) weakness, subtle sensory loss (mild distal light touch and proprioceptive loss, blunted vestibular or visual function), and even mild spastic paraparesis due to cervical myelopathy, without any one lesion being severe enough to explain the walking difficulty. The cumulative effect of these multiple deficits may interfere with perceived stability and equilibrium. Along with musculoskeletal disorders, postural hypotension, and loss of confidence (especially after falls), these factors contribute to a cautious gait pattern. In this situation, brain imaging is valuable to look for subcortical white-matter ischemia (especially in the frontal lobes and periventricular regions) that correlates with imbalance, increased body sway, falls, and cognitive decline (Baezner et al., 2008).

A cautious gait is a normal response related to the perception of impaired or threatened balance, as exemplified by walking on a slippery icy surface, and accordingly should be interpreted as compensatory and not specific for any level of the gait classification. Due account must be taken of the fear of falling that frequently accompanies gait difficulties. This may lead to a marked loss of confidence when walking and a cautious or protected gait. Such patients may be unable to walk without support. They hold onto furniture, lean on walls, and avoid crowded or open spaces because of a fear of falling. The gait may improve dramatically when support is provided. A formal program of gait retraining may help restore confidence and improve the ability to walk.

Perceptions of Instability and Illusions of Movement

A number of syndromes have been described in which middle-aged individuals complain of unsteadiness and imbalance associated with "dizziness," sensations or illusions of semicontinuous body motion, sudden brief body displacements, or body tilt. In some, the symptoms develop in open spaces where there are no visible supports (*space phobia*). Others develop sensations in particular situations such as on bridges, stairs, and escalators or in crowded rooms, leading to the development of phobic avoidance behavior and the *syndrome of phobic postural vertigo* (Brandt, 1996). Prolonged illusory swaying and unsteadiness after sea or air travel is referred to as the *mal de débarquement syndrome*. Past episodes of a vestibulopathy may suggest the possibility of a subtle semicircular canal or otolith disturbance, but a disorder of vestibular function is rarely confirmed in these syndromes. A fear of falling, anxiety, and related complaints are common accompaniments. These symptoms must be distinguished from the physiological "vertigo" and unsteadiness accompanying visual vestibular mismatch or conflict when observing moving objects, focusing on distant objects in large panoramas, or looking upward at moving objects.

Reckless Gait Patterns

Reckless gaits are those in which patients do not recognize their instability and take many risks that result in falls and injuries. This may occur in dementias such as Alzheimer disease and vascular dementias where there are often problems with gait as well as cognition. The most striking examples of reckless gaits, however, are patients with frontal dementias such as progressive supranuclear palsy and frontotemporal dementias when patients are impulsive and do not adapt their mobility to their precarious balance.

Hysterical and Psychogenic Gait Disorders

The wide range of abnormalities of gait seen in lesions of different parts of the nervous system make hysterical and psychogenic gaits among the most difficult to diagnose. The hallmark of hysterical gait paralysis is the inability to use one or both legs when walking, but normal synergistic movements of the affected leg(s) when the patient is examined while lying down or observed when changing position. This discrepancy is further illustrated by the *Hoover sign* in the patient with an apparently paralyzed leg when examined supine. As the patient lifts the normal leg, the examiner places a hand under the "paralyzed" leg and feels the presence (and strength) of synergistic hip extension. The apparent severe weakness of hysterical paresis often presents little disability or inconvenience in some patients; others with hysterical paraplegia are confined to bed and may even develop contractures from lack of leg movements.

A gait disorder is one of the more common manifestations of a psychogenic or hysterical movement disorder. The typical gait patterns encountered include transient fluctuations in posture while walking; knee buckling without falls; excessive slowness and hesitancy; a crouched, stooped, or other abnormal posture of the trunk; complex postural adjustments with each step; exaggerated body sway or excessive body motion especially brought out by tandem walking; and trembling, weak legs (Hayes et al., 1999). The more acrobatic hysterical disorders of gait indicate the extent to which the nervous system is functioning normally and is capable of high-level coordinated motor skills to perform various complex maneuvers. Suggestibility, variability, improvement with distraction, and a history of sudden onset or a rapid, dramatic, and complete recovery are other features of psychogenic gait (and movement) disorders. One must be cautious in accepting a diagnosis of hysteria, however, because a bizarre gait may be a presenting feature of primary torsion dystonia, and unusual truncal and leg postures may be encountered in truncal and leg tremors. Finally, higher-level gait disorders often have a disconnect between the standard neurological exam and the gait pattern.

Musculoskeletal Disorders and Antalgic Gait

Skeletal Deformity and Joint Disease

Degenerative osteoarthritis of the hip may produce leg shortening in addition to mechanical limitation of leg movement at the hip, giving rise to a waddling gait or a limp. Leg shortening with limping in childhood may be the presenting feature of hemiatrophy due to a cerebral or spinal lesion. Such walking difficulties between ages 1 and 5 years are the most common mode of presentation of spinal dysraphism. On examination, a variety of additional abnormalities may be detected, including lower motor neuron signs in the legs and sensory loss with trophic ulcers of the feet. Occasionally, upper motor neuron signs, such as a brisk knee reflex, are present in the same limb. Lumbosacral vertebral abnormalities (spina bifida), bony foot deformities, and a cutaneous hairy patch over the lumbosacral region are clues to the diagnosis. In adult life, spinal dysraphism (diastematomyelia with a tethered cord) may first become symptomatic after a back injury, with the development of walking difficulties, leg and lower back pain, neurogenic bladder disturbances, and sensory loss in a leg. Imaging of the spinal canal reveals the abnormality.

Painful (Antalgic) Gaits

Most people at one time or another experience a limp caused by a painful or an injured leg. Limps and gait difficulties due to joint disease, bone injury, or soft-tissue injury are not usually accompanied by muscle weakness, reflex change, or sensory loss. Limitation of the range of movement at the hip, knee, or ankle joints to reduce pain leads to short steps with a fixed leg posture. Hip disease causes a variety of gait adjustments; it is important to examine the range of hip movements (while supine) and any associated pain during passive movements of the hip in a patient with a gait disorder. Pain due to intermittent claudication of the cauda equina is most commonly caused by lumbar spondylosis and, rarely, by a spinal tumor. Diagnosis is confirmed by spinal imaging. It may be difficult to distinguish this syndrome from claudication of the calf muscles secondary to peripheral vascular disease. Examination of the patient after inducing the symptoms by exercise may resolve the issue by revealing a depressed ankle jerk or radicular sensory loss, with preservation of arterial pulses in the leg. Other painful conditions affecting the spine or lower limbs can obviously affect gait. Even such benign disorders as plantar fasciitis alter gait patterns.

References

The complete reference list is available online at www. expertconsult.com.

Hemiplegia and Monoplegia

Karl E. Misulis

Anatomy and Pathophysiology

Accurate neurological diagnosis begins with anatomical localization. Many disorders have diffuse localizations, but hemiplegia and monoplegia are likely to be due to focal structural lesions and are therefore easier to localize. Imaging studies often are confirmatory of the structural lesion, but clinical localization must precede and direct the imaging studies.

Hemiplegia and monoplegia are motor symptoms and signs, but associated sensory abnormalities are an aid to localization, so these are discussed when appropriate. Sensory deficit syndromes are discussed in more depth in Chapter 28. Motor power begins with *volition*, the conscious effort to initiate movement. Lack of volition does not produce weakness but rather results in akinesia. Projections from the premotor regions of the frontal lobes to the motor strip result in activation of corticospinal tract (CST) neurons. The descending fibers pass through the internal capsule and the cerebral peduncles, and then remain in the ventral brainstem before crossing in the medulla at the pyramidal decussation. Most of the CST crosses at this point, although a small subset of CST axons remains uncrossed until these axons reach the spinal segmental levels. Descending CST axons project to the spinal cord segments, where the fibers exit the CST and enter the spinal gray matter. Here, motoneurons are activated that then conduct action potentials via the motor axons to the muscle to produce muscle contraction.

Localization begins with identification of weakness. Differentiation is made among the following distributions:

- Generalized weakness
- Monoplegia
- Hemiplegia
- Paraplegia

Only hemiplegia and monoplegia are discussed in this chapter.

Hemiplegia
Cerebral Lesions

Cerebral lesions constitute the most common cause of hemiplegia. Lesions in either cortical or subcortical structures may be responsible for the weakness (**Table 23.1**).

Cortical Lesions

Cortical lesions produce weakness that is more focal than the weakness seen with subcortical lesions. **Fig. 23.1** is a diagrammatic representation of the surface of the brain, showing how the body is mapped onto the surface of the motor sensory cortex; this is the *homunculus*. The face and arm are laterally represented on the hemisphere, whereas the leg is draped over the top of the hemisphere and into the interhemispheric fissure.

Small lesions of the cortex can produce prominent focal weakness of one area, such as the leg or the face and hand, but hemiplegia—paralysis of both the leg and the arm on the same side of the body—is not expected from a cortical lesion unless the damage is extensive. The most likely cause of cortical hemiplegia would be a stroke involving the entire territory of the internal carotid artery.

INFARCTION

Both cortical and subcortical infarctions can produce weakness, but cortical infarctions are more likely than subcortical infarctions to be associated with sensory deficits. Also, many cortical infarctions are associated with what is called a *cortical*

Table 23.1 Cerebral Lesions		
Lesion Location	Symptoms	Signs
Motor cortex	Weakness and poor control of the affected extremity, which may involve face, arm, and leg to different degrees	Incoordination and weakness that depends on the location of the lesion within the cortical homunculus; often associated with neglect, apraxia, aphasia, or other signs of cortical dysfunction
Internal capsule	Weakness that usually affects the face, arm, and leg almost equally	Often associated with sensory impairment in same distribution
Basal ganglia	Weakness and incoordination on the contralateral side	Weakness, often without sensory loss; no neglect or aphasia
Thalamus	Sensory loss	Sensory loss with little or no weakness

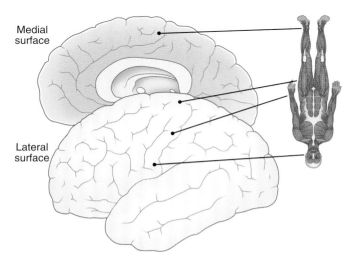

Medial surface

Lateral surface

Fig. 23.1 Representation of the body on the motor cortex. Face and arms are represented laterally, and legs are represented medially, with cortical representation of the distal legs bordering on the central sulcus.

sign—neglect with nondominant hemisphere lesions and aphasia with dominant hemisphere lesions. Unfortunately, this distinction is not absolute because subcortical lesions also occasionally can produce these signs.

Initial diagnosis of infarction usually is made on clinical grounds. The abrupt onset of the deficit is typical. Weakness that progresses over several days is unlikely to be caused by infarction, although some infarcts can show worsening for a few days after onset. Progression over days suggests demyelinating disease or infection. Progression over weeks suggests a mass lesion such as tumor or abscess. Progression over seconds to minutes in a marching fashion suggests either epilepsy or migraine; not all migraine-associated deficits are associated with concurrent or subsequent headache.

Computed tomography (CT) scans often do not show infarction for up to 3 days after the event but are performed emergently to rule out mass lesion or hemorrhage. Small infarctions may never be seen on CT. Magnetic resonance imaging (MRI) is superior in showing both old and new infarctions; diffusion-weighted imaging (DWI) on MRI distinguishes recent infarction from old lesions.

Middle Cerebral Artery

The middle cerebral artery (MCA) supplies the lateral aspect of the motor sensory cortex, which controls the face and arm. On the dominant side, speech centers also are supplied—the Broca area (expression) in the posterior frontal region and the Wernicke area (reception) on the superior aspect of the temporal lobe.

Cortical infarction in the territory of the MCA produces contralateral faciobrachial hemiparesis, usually associated with other signs of cortical dysfunction such as aphasia with left hemisphere lesions or neglect with right hemisphere lesions. Weakness is much more prominent in the arm, hand, and face than in the leg. Hemianopia sometimes is seen, especially with large MCA infarctions, as a result of infarction of the optic radiations. MCA infarction is suspected with hemiparesis plus cortical signs of aphasia or neglect. Confirmation is with imaging.

Anterior Cerebral Artery

The anterior cerebral artery (ACA) supplies the inferior frontal and parasagittal regions of the frontal and anterior parietal lobes. This region is responsible for leg movement and is important for bowel and bladder control. Infarction in the ACA distribution produces contralateral leg weakness. The arm may be slightly affected, especially the proximal arm, with sparing of hand and face. In some patients, both ACAs arise from the same trunk, so infarction produces bilateral leg weakness; this deficit can be mistaken clinically for myelopathy and is in the differential diagnosis for suspected cord infarction or other acute myelopathy.

ACA infarction is suggested by a clinical presentation of unilateral or bilateral leg weakness and CST signs. Confirmation is with MRI; cord imaging should be considered in all patients with bilateral leg weakness when no other cause can be demonstrated.

Posterior Cerebral Artery

The posterior cerebral arteries (PCAs) are the terminal branches of the basilar artery. They supply most of the occipital lobes and the medial aspect of the temporal lobes. PCA infarction is not expected to produce weakness but produces contralateral hemianopia, often with memory deficits due to bilateral hippocampal infarction.

The clinical diagnosis of PCA infarction may be missed because an examiner may not look for hemianopia in a patient who otherwise presents only with confusion. Visual complaints may be vague or nonexistent.

PCA infarction is suggested by a clinical presentation of acute confusion or visual disturbance, or both. A finding of hemianopia is supportive evidence. Imaging can show not only the area of infarction but also the location of the vascular defect—unilateral or bilateral PCA or basilar artery.

Subcortical Lesions

Subcortical lesions are more likely to produce equal weakness of the contralateral face, arm, and leg (hemiplegia) than cortical lesions because of the convergence of the descending axons in the internal capsule. The compact nature of the internal capsule makes it the most likely location for a hemiplegia. The internal capsule is a particularly common location for lacunar infarctions and also can be affected by hemorrhage in the adjacent basal ganglia or thalamus. Weakness of sudden onset is most likely to be the result of infarction, with hemorrhage in a minority of cases. Demyelinating disease is characterized by a subacute onset. Tumors are associated with a slower onset of deficit and can get quite large in subcortical regions before the patient presents for medical attention.

INFARCTION

Infarction usually is a clinical diagnosis but can be confirmed by CT or MRI scans, as discussed earlier (see Cortical Lesions). Infarction manifests with acute onset of deficit, although the course may be one of steady progression or stuttering. Lacunar infarctions are more likely than cortical infarctions to be associated with a stuttering course.

Lenticulostriate Arteries

Lenticulostriate arteries are small penetrating vessels that arise from the proximal MCA and supply the basal ganglia and internal capsule. Infarction commonly produces contralateral hemiparesis with little or no sensory involvement. This is one cause of the *syndrome of pure motor stroke*, which can also be due to a brainstem lacunar infarction (Lastilla, 2006).

Thalamoperforate Arteries

Thalamoperforate arteries are small penetrating vessels that arise from the PCAs and supply mainly the thalamus. Infarction in this distribution produces contralateral sensory disturbance but also can cause movement disorders such as choreoathetosis or hemiballismus; hemiparesis is not expected.

DEMYELINATING DISEASE

Demyelinating disease comprises a group of conditions whose pathophysiology implicates the immune system.

Multiple Sclerosis

Multiple sclerosis (MS) manifests with any combination of white-matter dysfunction. Hemiparesis can develop, especially if large plaques affecting the CST fibers in the hemispheres are present. Hemiparesis is even more likely with brainstem or spinal demyelinating lesions, because smaller lesions can produce more profound deficits in these areas. The diagnosis

is suggested by the progression over days plus a prior history of episodes of relapsing and remitting neurological deficits. Episodes of weakness that last for only minutes are likely not to be due to demyelinating disease but rather to transient ischemic attack (TIA) or migraine equivalent.

Diagnosis is based on clinical grounds for most patients, but the finding of areas of increased signal intensity on MRI T2-weighted images is suggestive for MS. Active demyelinating lesions often show enhancement on gadolinium-enhanced T1-weighted images. Cerebrospinal fluid (CSF) examination usually is performed and can give normal findings or show elevated protein, a mild lymphocytic pleocytosis, or oligoclonal bands of immunoglobulin G (IgG) in the CSF.

Acute Disseminated Encephalomyelitis

Acute disseminated encephalomyelitis (ADEM) is a demyelinating illness that is monophasic but in other respects manifests like a first attack of MS (Wingerchuk, 2006). This entity sometimes is called *parainfectious encephalomyelitis*, although the association with infection is not always certain. Symptoms and signs at all levels of the central nervous system (CNS) are common, including hemiparesis, paraplegia, ataxia, and brainstem signs. Diagnosis is based on clinical grounds, because MRI scans cannot definitively distinguish between MS and ADEM. CSF examination may show a mononuclear pleocytosis and elevation in protein, but these findings are neither always present nor specific. Even the presence or absence of oligoclonal IgG in the CSF cannot differentiate between ADEM and MS. Patients who present clinically with ADEM should be warned of the possibility of having recurrent events indicative of MS.

Progressive Multifocal Leukoencephalopathy

Progressive multifocal leukoencephalopathy (PML) is a demyelinating disease caused by reactivation of the JC virus, usually seen in immunodeficient patients. Predisposed patients include those with acquired immunodeficiency syndrome (AIDS), leukemia, lymphoma, tuberculosis, and sarcoidosis. Visual loss is the most common presenting symptom and weakness the second. MRI scan shows multiple white-matter lesions. CSF examination either reveals no abnormality or shows a lymphocytic pleocytosis or elevated protein, or both. Brain biopsy is required for specific diagnosis, although JC virus deoxyribonucleic acid (DNA) can be detected in the CSF by polymerase chain reaction (PCR) assay in most patients.

PML is suggested when a patient with immunodeficiency presents with subacute to chronic onset of neurological deficits and multifocal white-matter lesions on MRI.

MIGRAINE

Migraine can be divided into many subdivisions, including the following:

- Common migraine
- Classic migraine
- Basilar migraine
- Complicated migraine
- Hemiplegic migraine
- Migraine equivalent

All but common migraine can cause hemiplegia (Black, 2006). *Common migraine* is episodic headache without aura; by definition, there should be no deficit. *Classic migraine* is episodic headache with aura, most commonly visual. *Basilar migraine* is episodic headache with brainstem signs including vertigo and ataxia; this variant is a disorder mainly of childhood. *Complicated migraine* is that in which the aura lasts for hours or days beyond the duration of the headache. *Hemiplegic migraine*, as its name suggests, is characterized by paralysis of one side of the body, typically with onset before the headache; this variant often is familial. *Migraine equivalent* is characterized by the presence of episodic neurological symptoms without headache.

Migrainous infarction features sustained deficit plus MRI evidence of infarction that had developed from the migraine. Definitive diagnosis is problematic because patients with migraine have a higher incidence of stroke not associated with a migraine attack, so the onset of the deficit with this variant should resemble classic or complicated migraine, rather than the acute deficit of most strokes.

The diagnosis of migraine is suggested by the combination of young age of the patient with few risk factors, and a marching deficit that can be conceptualized as migration of spreading electrical depression across the cerebral cortex. Imaging often is necessary to rule out hemorrhage, infarction, and demyelinating disease.

SEIZURES

Postictal contralateral hemiplegia or hemiparesis can occur in patients with a unilateral hemispheric seizure disorder. This situation is identified by history and slowing on the electroencephalogram (EEG) contralateral to the side of weakness.

TUMORS

Tumors affecting the cerebral hemispheres commonly present with progressive deficits including hemiparesis. Coordination deficit commonly develops before the weakness. Cortical dysfunction is commonly present, such as aphasia with dominant hemisphere lesions and neglect. Other signs of expanding tumors may include headache, seizures, confusion, and visual field defects.

Tumor should be suspected in a patient with progressive motor deficit over weeks, especially with coexistent seizures or headache. MRI with contrast enhancement is more sensitive than CT for identification of tumors.

ALTERNATING HEMIPLEGIA OF CHILDHOOD

Alternating hemiplegia of childhood is a rare condition characterized by attacks of unilateral weakness, often with signs of other motor deficits (e.g., dyskinesias, stiffness) and oculomotor abnormalities (e.g., nystagmus) (Zhang et al., 2003). Attacks begin in young childhood, usually before age 18 months; they last hours, and deficits accumulate over years. Initially, patients are normal, but with time, neurological deficits including motor deficits and cognitive decline become obvious. A benign form can occur on awakening in patients who are otherwise normal and do not develop progressive deficits; this entity is related to migraine. Diagnostic studies often are performed, including MRI, electroencephalography, and angiography, but these usually show no abnormalities. Alternating hemiplegia is suggested when a young child presents with episodes of hemiparesis, especially on awakening, not associated with headache.

HEMICONVULSION-HEMIPLEGIA-EPILEPSY SYNDROME

In young children with the rare condition called *hemiconvulsion-hemiplegia-epilepsy syndrome*, unilateral weakness develops after the sudden onset of focal seizures. The seizures are often incompletely controlled. Neurological deficits are not confined to the motor system and may include cognitive, language, and visual deficits. Unlike alternating hemiplegia, the seizures and motor deficits are consistently unilateral, although eventually the unilateral seizures may become generalized. Imaging findings may be normal initially, but eventually atrophy of the affected hemisphere is seen (Freeman et al., 2002). CSF analysis is not specific, but a mild mononuclear pleocytosis may develop because of the CNS damage and seizures. Rasmussen encephalitis is a cause of this syndrome.

Brainstem Lesions

Brainstem lesions producing hemiplegia are among the easiest to localize because associated signs of cranial nerve and brainstem dysfunction are almost always present.

Brainstem Motor Organization

Fig. 23.2 shows the anatomical organization of the motor systems of the brainstem. Discussion of the complex anatomical organization of the brainstem can be simplified by concentrating on some important functions:

- Appendicular motor and sensory function
- Appendicular coordination
- Facial motor and sensory function
- Ocular motor function
- Descending sympathetic tracts

Motor pathways descend through the CST to the pyramidal decussation in the medulla, where they cross to innervate the contralateral body. Lesions of the pons and midbrain above this level produce contralateral hemiparesis, which may involve the contralateral face. Rostral lesions of the medulla produce contralateral weakness, whereas more caudal medullary lesions produce ipsilateral cranial nerve signs with a contralateral hemiparesis and sensory deficit.

Sensory pathways from the nucleus gracilis and nucleus cuneatus cross at about the same level as the motor fibers of the CST, so deficits in light touch and position sense tend to parallel the distribution of the motor deficit. By contrast, the spinothalamic tracts have already crossed in the spinal cord and ascend laterally in the brainstem. Accordingly, lesions of the lower medulla may produce contralateral loss of pain and temperature sensation and ipsilateral loss of touch and position sense. Lesions above the mid-medulla produce a contralateral sensory defect of all modalities similar to that from cerebral lesions, yet the clues to brainstem localization can include the following:

- Ipsilateral facial sensory deficit from a trigeminal lesion
- Ipsilateral hemiataxia from damage to the cerebellar hemispheres or nuclei

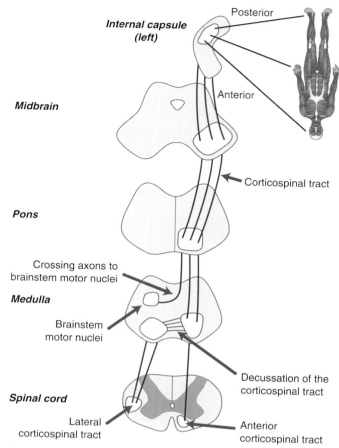

Fig. 23.2 Brainstem motor organization, beginning with internal capsule. Corticospinal tract remains topographically organized throughout brainstem and spinal cord, although isolated lesions below cerebral cortex are unlikely to produce topographically specific damage.

- Ocular motor weakness from any of multiple lesion locations
- Ipsilateral Horner syndrome from damage of the descending sympathetic tracts

Common Lesions

Table 23.2 shows some of the important lesions of the brainstem and their associated motor deficits. Brainstem lesions usually are due to damage to the penetrating branches of the basilar artery. Patients present with contralateral weakness along with other deficits that help localize the lesion. Hemiataxia often develops and can be mistaken for hemiparesis, so careful examination is essential. Demyelinating disease and tumors are the other most common causes of brainstem dysfunction.

Spinal Lesions

Spinal lesions can produce hemiplegia sparing the face, although they mostly will cause bilateral deficits typical of myelopathy. A spinal cord lesion should be suspected in a patient with bilateral weakness, bowel or bladder control deficits, and back pain.

Spinal Hemisection (Brown-Séquard Syndrome)

Spinal hemisection seldom is seen in clinical practice. Components of the syndrome occasionally are identified, however. This entity is usually associated with intradural tumors, trauma, inflammatory conditions such as demyelinating disease, and occasionally spinal infarction. Spondylotic myelopathy, disk disease, and most extradural tumors typically produce symmetrical deficits. Patients with the spinal hemisection syndrome present with weakness ipsilateral to and below the lesion. In addition, segmental motor loss may be seen with involvement of the motoneurons at the level of the lesion. Sensory abnormalities include loss of pain and temperature contralateral to and below the lesion. Position sense may be affected ipsilateral to the lesion.

Transverse Myelitis

Transverse myelitis is an acute myelopathic process that is presumed to be autoimmune in origin. Patients present with motor and sensory deficits below the lesion, usually in the form of a paraplegia. The abnormalities typically are bilateral but may be asymmetrical. MRI may show enhancement in the spinal cord, which has an appearance that differs subtly from that in involvement in MS. CSF analysis is nondiagnostic.

Transverse myelitis is a clinical diagnosis. The primary differential diagnosis is between MS and neuromyelitis optica (NMO); assessment to identify the latter includes measurement of titers of NMO antibodies in the plasma, which probably should be done in all patients with transverse myelitis.

Spinal Cord Compression

Spinal cord compression usually is due to disk protrusion, spondylosis, or acute trauma, but neoplastic and infectious causes should always be considered (Shedid and Bonzel, 2007). Disc disease and spondylosis typically are in the midline, so bilateral findings are expected. Extradural tumors also usually produce bilateral findings. Intradural tumors may produce unilateral deficits and occasionally can manifest as Brown-Séquard syndrome.

Lesions below the cervical spinal cord would produce not hemiplegia but rather monoplegia of a lower limb or paraplegia. Spondylosis with cord compression produces lower motor neuron (LMN) weakness at the level of the lesion and CST signs below the level of the lesion. Spinal cord compression resulting in paralysis should be evaluated as quickly as possible with MRI. Myelography should be considered if MRI is not urgently available.

Spinal Cord Infarction

Anterior spinal artery infarction usually causes paraparesis and spinothalamic sensory loss below the level of the lesion; dorsal column function is preserved. Rarely, one segmental branch of the anterior spinal artery can be involved with unilateral spinal cord damage and monoparesis or hemiparesis. Spinal cord infarction is suggested when a patient presents with paraparesis or paraplegia of acute onset, and MRI does not show cord compression or bilateral ACA infarction.

Table 23.2 Brainstem Lesions

Named Disorder	Lesion Location	Signs
MIDBRAIN		
Weber syndrome	CN III, ventral midbrain, CST	Contralateral hemiparesis, CN III palsy
Benedikt syndrome	CN III, ventral midbrain, CST, red nucleus	Contralateral hemiparesis, third nerve palsy, intention tremor, cerebellar ataxia
Top-of-the-basilar syndrome	Occipital lobes, midbrain oculomotor nuclei, cerebral peduncle, medial and temporal lobe, thalamus	Contralateral hemiparesis, cortical blindness, oculomotor deficits, memory difficulty, contralateral sensory deficit
PONS		
Millard-Gubler syndrome	CN VI, CN VII, ventral pons	Contralateral hemiparesis, CN VI and CN VII palsies
Clumsy hand syndrome	CST, CN VII	Contralateral hemiparesis, dysarthria, often with facial weakness
Pure motor hemiparesis (due to pons lesion)	Ventral pons	Contralateral hemiparesis with corticospinal tract signs
Ataxic hemiparesis (due to pons lesion)	CST, cerebellar tracts	Contralateral hemiparesis with impaired coordination
Foville syndrome	CN VII, ventral pons, paramedian pontine reticular formation	Ipsilateral CN VII palsy, contralateral hemiparesis, gaze palsy to the side of the lesion
MEDULLA		
Medial medullary syndrome	CST, medial lemniscus, hypoglossal nerve	Contralateral hemiparesis, loss of position and vibratory sensation, ipsilateral tongue paresis
Lateral medullary syndrome	Spinothalamic tract, trigeminal nucleus, cerebellum and inferior cerebellar peduncle, vestibular nuclei, nucleus ambiguus	*No hemiparesis* usually produced, but hemiataxia may be mistaken for hemiparesis; dysphagia, hemisensory loss, face weakness, Horner syndrome are common

CN, Cranial nerve; *CST*, corticospinal tract.

Peripheral Lesions

Peripheral lesions are not expected to produce hemiplegia. A pair of peripheral lesions affecting an arm and leg on the same side, however, may occasionally masquerade as hemiplegia. Differentiation depends on identification of the individual lesions as being within the distribution of one nerve, nerve root, or plexus division. The tendon reflexes are likely to be depressed in patients with peripheral lesions, rather than increased as with CST lesions.

Amyotrophic lateral sclerosis can produce weakness of one limb, followed by weakness of the other limb on the same side, with progression over months or even years. Usually the combined presence of upper motor neuron (UMN) and LMN involvement without sensory changes assists in making the diagnosis. If the predominant involvement is UMN in type, the picture can look like that of a progressive hemiparesis.

Mononeuropathy multiplex can manifest as separate lesions affecting individual limbs; involvement of an arm and leg on the same side can give the impression of hemiparesis. Diabetes is the most common cause, but other causes include leprosy, vasculitis, and predisposition to pressure palsies. Diagnosis is by electromyography (EMG), which can differentiate mononeuropathies from polyneuropathy (Misulis, 2003). Radiculopathy would not give hemiparesis but is a consideration in the differential diagnosis for monoplegia (see Radiculopathies, later in this chapter).

Functional Hemiplegia

Functional or psychogenic weakness includes both conversion reaction and malingering. In conversion reaction, the patient is not conscious of the nonorganic nature of the deficit, whereas in malingering, the patient is making a conscious effort to fool the examiner. Some secondary gain for the patient, either psychological or economic, is a factor with both types. In malingering, the secondary gain usually is more obvious and may be disability payments, litigation, family attention, or avoidance of stressors or tasks. Clues to functional weakness include the following:

- Improvement in strength with coaching
- Give-way weakness
- Inconsistencies in examination—for example, inability to extend the foot but able to walk on toes
- Hoover sign (when the patient lies supine on the bed and lifts one leg at a time, the examiner should feel effort to press down with the opposite heel if the leg is truly paralyzed; failure to do so constitutes the Hoover sign)
- Paralysis in the absence of other signs of motor system dysfunction, including tone and reflex changes

Diagnosis of functional weakness is based on inconsistencies on examination and elimination of the possibility of organic disease. Functional weakness should be diagnosed with caution. It is easy to dismiss the patient's complaints after an inconsistent feature is seen, especially if some secondary gain is obvious. Unfortunately, a patient with organic problems may have a functional overlay, which may exaggerate otherwise subtle clinical findings.

If functional weakness is suspected, some diagnostic testing often is required to rule out neurological disease, although such investigations should be kept to a minimum. Prescription of multiple tests and treatments may serve to reinforce the presumed presence of disease, thereby augmenting illness behavior. Psychological evaluation and treatment can be key to successful management. Nevertheless, functional deficit probably is overdiagnosed, so the examiner should remain alert for organic disease.

Monoplegia

Cerebral Lesions

Cerebral lesions more commonly produce hemiplegia than monoplegia, but isolated limb involvement can occasionally occur, especially with cortical involvement. The arm segment of the motor-sensory cortex lies on the lateral aspect of the hemisphere adjacent to the sylvian fissure. Subcortical lesions are less likely than cortical lesions to produce monoplegia because of the dense packing of the fibers of the CST in the internal capsule. The internal capsule generally is organized with the arm segments represented anteriorly in the capsule relative to the leg sections. Infarction in the distribution of the lenticulostriate arteries, however, usually affects both divisions.

Infarction

The arm region of the motor cortex is supplied by the MCA. Infarction of a branch of the MCA can produce isolated arm weakness, although facial involvement and cortical signs are expected—language deficit with left hemisphere lesions and neglect with right hemisphere lesions (Paciaroni et al., 2005). With more extensive lesions, visual fields can be abnormal because of infarction of the optic radiations. Mild leg weakness also can occur with medial cortical involvement of the infarct. The leg segment of the cortex lies in the parasagittal region and is supplied by the ACA. ACA infarction produces weakness of the contralateral leg.

Transient Ischemic Attack

Episodic paralysis of one limb sometimes is due to TIA. Evaluation for vascular disease usually is indicated. The main considerations in the differential diagnosis are migraine and seizure. Abrupt onset and absence of positive motor symptoms argue in favor of TIA.

Migraine

Migraine can produce sensation that marches along one limb, usually the arm. This marching pattern differs from the abrupt onset of stroke. Involvement of only the leg is unusual. The headache phase typically begins as the neurological deficit is resolving. Weakness can develop as part of the migraine aura, but this is much less likely than sensory disturbance. Of note, not all migrainous weakness is followed by headache.

Seizure

Seizure classically produces positive motor symptoms with jerking or stiffness. Focal seizures rarely can produce negative motor symptoms including paralysis. In such cases, the seizure can be impossible to diagnose without EEG, so EEG may be indicated in selected patients with focal weakness. Ictal paralysis can have abrupt onset and offset and can even resemble negative myoclonus.

Focal seizure activity may be suggested by subtle twitching or disturbance of consciousness associated with the episodes. In comparison with TIAs, seizures usually are more frequent and have a shorter duration. Lastly, postictal weakness of one limb can occur.

Multiple Sclerosis

Multiple Sclerosis can produce monoplegia secondary to a discrete white-matter plaque in the cerebral hemisphere, but because it is a subcortical disease, hemiparesis is more common. The corticospinal tracts are somatotopically organized, so monoparesis is theoretically possible. Onset of symptoms is subacute. MS is considered when a patient with neurological deficit is found to have multifocal lesions on clinical examination or MRI.

Tumors

Tumors deep to the cortex rarely produce monoplegia because the involvement is not sufficiently discrete to affect only one limb. Cortical involvement makes single-limb involvement more likely. Parasagittal lesions often produce leg involvement, which initially can be unilateral. Meningiomas often arise from one side of the falx, so they predominantly affect the opposite leg, initially with weakness, incoordination, and CST signs. With progression, bilateral symptoms develop.

Bilateral leg weakness with CST signs can be due to either cerebral or spinal lesions, although single leg deficit is only rarely due to a spinal cause. Metastatic tumors often are found at the gray/white junction; in this location, they can produce focal cortical damage. Early on, the lesion may be too small to produce other neurological symptoms, but with increasing growth, it is more likely to produce focal seizures. Tumor is suspected with insidious progression of focal deficit, especially if combined with headache or seizures.

Brainstem Lesions

Brainstem lesions seldom produce monoplegia because of the tight packing of the fibers of the CSTs in the brainstem. Unilateral cerebellar hemisphere lesions may produce appendicular ataxia, which is most obvious in the arm, although this should be distinguished from monoparesis by the absence of weakness or CST signs.

Spinal Lesions

Spinal lesions can produce weakness from segmental damage to nerve roots or CSTs. Weakness at the level of the lesion is in a radicular distribution and may be associated with muscle atrophy and loss of segmental reflexes. Weakness below the lesion can be unilateral or bilateral and is associated with CST signs.

Peripheral Lesions

Peripheral lesions usually produce monoparetic weakness in the distribution of a single nerve, nerve root, or plexus. A few conditions, such as amyotrophic lateral sclerosis and focal spinal muscular atrophy, may produce weakness in a mono-melic (monoplegic) distribution.

Pressure Palsies

Intermittent compression of a peripheral nerve can produce transient paresis of part of a limb. The patient may think the entire limb is paralyzed, but detailed examination shows that the paresis is limited to a nerve distribution. Recovery from the weakness usually occurs so rapidly that examination often is not possible before the improvement. Predisposition to pressure palsies can be seen in two main circumstances: on a hereditary basis and in the presence of peripheral polyneuropathy.

HEREDITARY NEUROPATHY WITH PREDISPOSITION TO PRESSURE PALSIES

Hereditary neuropathy with predisposition to pressure palsies is associated with episodic weakness and sensory loss associated with compression of isolated nerves. This disorder is inherited as an autosomal dominant condition. Nerve conduction studies may show distal slowing of conduction velocities in affected nerves. NCVs also may be reduced in asymptomatic gene carriers (Chance, 2006).

PRESSURE PALSIES IN POLYNEUROPATHY

Patients with polyneuropathy may have an increased susceptibility to pressure palsies. Areas of demyelination are more likely to have a depolarizing block produced by even mild pressure.

Mononeuropathies

Table 23.3 shows some important peripheral nerve lesions of the arm. **Table 23.4** shows some important peripheral nerve lesions of the leg.

Table 23.3 Peripheral Nerve Lesions of the Arm

Lesion	Clinical Findings	Electromyography Findings
MEDIAN NEUROPATHY		
Carpal tunnel syndrome	Weakness and wasting of abductor pollicis brevis if severe; sensory loss on palmar aspect of first through third digits	Slow median motor and sensory NCV through the carpal tunnel; denervation of abductor pollicis brevis if severe
Anterior interosseous syndrome	Weakness of flexor digitorum profundus, pronator quadratus, flexor pollicis longus	Denervation in flexor digitorum profundus, flexor pollicis longus, pronator quadratus
Pronator teres syndrome	Weakness of distal median-innervated muscles; tenderness of pronator teres	Slow median motor NCV through proximal forearm denervation of distal median-innervated muscles
Compression at the ligament of Struthers	Weakness of distal median-innervated muscles	As for pronator teres syndrome, with the addition of denervation of pronator teres
ULNAR NEUROPATHY		
Palmar branch damage	Weakness of dorsal interossei; no sensory loss	Normal ulnar NCV; denervation of first dorsal interosseus but not abductor digiti minimi
Entrapment at Guyon canal	Weakness of ulnar intrinsic muscles; numbness over fourth and fifth digits	Slow ulnar motor and sensory NCV through wrist
Entrapment at or near the elbow	Weakness of ulnar intrinsic muscles; numbness over fourth and fifth digits	Slow ulnar motor NCV across elbow, denervation in first dorsal interosseus, abductor digiti minimi, and ulnar half of flexor digitorum profundus
RADIAL NEUROPATHY		
Posterior interosseus syndrome	Weakness of finger and wrist extensors; no sensory loss	Denervation in wrist and finger extensors; sparing of the supinator and extensor carpi radialis
Compression at the spiral groove	Weakness of finger and wrist extensors; triceps usually spared; sensory loss on dorsal aspects of first digit	Slow radial motor NCV across spiral groove; denervation in distal radial-innervated muscles; triceps may be affected with proximal lesions

NCV, Nerve conduction velocity.

Table 23.4 Peripheral Nerve Lesions of the Leg

Lesion	Clinical Findings	Electromyography Findings
Sciatic neuropathy	Weakness of tibial- and peroneal-innervated muscles, with sensory loss on posterior leg and foot	Denervation distally in tibial- and peroneal-innervated muscles
Peroneal neuropathy	Weakness of foot extension and eversion and toe extension	Denervation in tibialis anterior; NCV across fibular neck may be slowed
Tibial neuropathy	Weakness of foot plantar flexion	Denervation of gastrocnemius
Femoral neuropathy	Weakness of knee extension; weakness of hip flexion if psoas involved	Denervation in quadriceps, sometimes psoas

NCV, Nerve conduction velocity.

MEDIAN NERVE

The most common median neuropathy is carpal tunnel syndrome, but other important anatomical lesions including anterior interosseus syndrome and pronator teres syndrome have been described.

Carpal Tunnel Syndrome

Carpal tunnel syndrome is the most common mononeuropathy. The median nerve is compressed as it passes under the flexor retinaculum at the wrist. Patients present with numbness on the palmar aspect of the first through the third digits. Forced flexion or extension of the wrist commonly exacerbates the sensory symptoms. Weakness of the abductor pollicis brevis may develop in advanced cases.

This condition would not normally be considered in the differential diagnosis for monoparesis, but because the patient can complain of weakness that is more extensive than the actual deficit, it is considered here. Nerve conduction studies show slow motor and sensory velocities through the carpal tunnel. EMG shows denervation in the abductor pollicis brevis muscle with severe disease.

Anterior Interosseus Syndrome

The anterior interosseous nerve is a branch of the median nerve in the forearm that supplies some of the forearm muscles. Damage can occur distal to the elbow, producing a syndrome that essentially is purely motor. Weakness of finger flexion is prominent. Affected muscles include the flexor digitorum profundus to the second and third digits (the portion to the fourth and fifth digits is innervated by the ulnar nerve). The distal median nerve entering the hand is unaffected because the anterior interosseous nerve arises from the main trunk of the median nerve.

Diagnosis is suspected by weakness of the median nerve–innervated finger flexors, with sparing of the abductor pollicis brevis and ulnar nerve–innervated flexors. EMG can confirm the diagnosis, but because this entrapment is not commonly looked for by many electromyographers, study of the appropriate muscles must be specifically requested.

Pronator Teres Syndrome

The median nerve distal to the elbow can be damaged as it passes through the pronator teres muscle. All median-innervated muscles of the arm are affected except for the pronator teres itself. The clinical picture is that of an anterior interosseous syndrome plus distal median neuropathy. The pronator teres may be tender, and palpation may exacerbate some of the distal pain.

ULNAR NERVE

Ulnar entrapment is most common near the elbow and at the wrist. Entrapment at the elbow produces weakness of the ulnar-innervated intrinsic muscles. Weakness of long flexors of the fourth and fifth digits also can develop. When the entrapment is at the wrist, the weakness is isolated to the intrinsic muscles of the hand, and more proximal muscles are unaffected. Although most of the intrinsic muscles of the hand are ulnar innervated, a few are median innervated and are unaffected in ulnar neuropathy.

The diagnosis of ulnar neuropathy is suggested when a patient complains of pain or numbness on the ulnar aspect of the hand. Additional findings that support this diagnosis include weakness and wasting of the intrinsic muscles of the hand, which is especially easy to see in the first dorsal interosseous.

RADIAL NERVE PALSY

Radial neuropathy is most commonly seen above the elbow, such that wrist and finger extensors are mainly affected. The triceps also can be affected. Radial nerve palsy is most commonly due to a pressure palsy in alcoholic intoxication. Peripheral neuropathy makes the development of pressure neuropathy of the radial nerve more likely.

FEMORAL NEUROPATHY

Femoral neuropathy can occur at the origin of the nerve from the lumbar plexus secondary to compression by intraabdominal contents (fetus or neoplasm), but we also have seen it from damage incurred during angiography or surgery. Patients present with pain in the thigh and weakness of knee extension. They usually report that the leg "gives out" during walking or that they cannot get out of a chair without using their arms. Examination may show quadriceps weakness, but this muscle group is so strong that the examiner may not be able to detect the deficit. Lower leg muscles must be examined to ensure that muscles in the sciatic distribution are normal. Diagnosis is confirmed by EMG showing denervation confined to the femoral nerve distribution. Unfortunately, electrical signs of denervation may not be obvious for up to 4 weeks after the injury.

SCIATIC NEUROPATHY

Sciatic neuropathy can have multiple causes, including acute trauma and chronic compressive lesions. The term *sciatica* describes pain in the distribution of the sciatic nerve in the back of the leg. It usually is due to radiculopathy (see Radiculopathies, later). An intramuscular injection into the sciatic nerve rather than the gluteus muscle is an occasional cause of sciatic neuropathy, which is characterized by initial severe pain followed by a lesser degree of pain and weakness.

Piriformis syndrome is a condition in which the sciatic nerve is compressed by the piriformis muscle. This is a difficult diagnosis to make, requiring demonstration of increased pain on tensing the piriformis muscle by flexing and adducting the hip. Piriformis syndrome should be considered in patients presenting with symptoms and signs referable to the sciatic nerve but with no evident cause seen on imaging of the lumbar spine and plexus.

Diagnosis of sciatic neuropathy is considered when a patient presents with pain or weakness of the lower leg muscles. EMG can confirm the distribution of denervation. Nerve conduction studies usually are normal. MRI of the lumbosacral plexus occasionally is needed to look for tumors and other causes of sciatic nerve or plexus compression.

PERONEAL NEUROPATHY

Peroneal neuropathy can develop from a lesion at the fibular neck, the popliteal fossa, or even the sciatic nerve in the thigh. The peroneal division of the sciatic nerve is more susceptible to injury than the tibial division, so incomplete sciatic injury affects predominantly the peroneal nerve–innervated muscles. The peroneal nerve innervates the tibialis anterior, extensor digitorum brevis, and peroneus muscles. In addition, the peroneal division innervates the short head of the biceps femoris in the distal posterior thigh. This is an important muscle to remember because distal peroneal neuropathy spares this muscle, whereas a proximal sciatic neuropathy, a peroneal division lesion, or a radiculopathy is expected to cause denervation not only in the tibialis anterior but also the short head of the biceps femoris (Marciniak et al., 2005).

Radiculopathies

Radiculopathy produces weakness of one portion of a limb. Common radiculopathies are summarized in **Table 23.5**. Complete paralysis of all of the muscles of an arm or leg is not caused by radiculopathy, other than in traumatic avulsion of the nerve roots, which may occur in the upper limbs with distraction injuries of the arm from the neck. Roots serving arm power include chiefly C5 to T1. Roots serving leg power are chiefly L2 to S1. A lesion at the L5 level often elicits a complaint of weakness of the entire limb because of the foot drop, which interferes with gait. Reflex abnormalities often are present early in a radiculopathy and are a manifestation of the sensory component. Motor deficits develop with increasingly severe radiculopathy.

Diagnosis of radiculopathy can be facilitated by EMG, which is an aid to localization and helps determine whether acute changes are developing. MRI shows the structural cause of a definite radiculopathy in most patients, although the diagnostic yield in patients with back pain without clear radicular symptoms is far less (see Chapters 29 and 30). Many

Table 23.5 Radiculopathies

Level	Motor Deficit	Sensory Deficit
CERVICAL RADICULOPATHY		
C5	Deltoid, biceps	Lateral upper arm
C6	Biceps, brachioradialis	Radial forearm and first and second digits
C7	Wrist extensors, triceps	Third and fourth digits
C8	Intrinsic hand muscles	Fifth digit and ulnar forearm
T1	Intrinsic muscles of the hand, especially APB	Axilla
LUMBAR RADICULOPATHY		
L2	Psoas, quadriceps	Lateral and anterior thigh
L3	Psoas, quadriceps	Lower medial thigh
L4	Tibialis anterior, quadriceps	Medial lower leg
L5	Peroneus longus, gluteus medius, tibialis anterior, extensor hallucis longus	Lateral lower leg
S1	Gastrocnemius, gluteus maximus	Lateral foot and fourth and fifth digits

APB, Abductor pollicis brevis.

surgeons still consider myelography followed by CT scanning to be more sensitive than MRI for detecting structural defects, although it is not performed as a first-line investigation because of the invasive nature of the procedure.

Radiculopathy should be suspected when a patient presents with pain radiating down one arm or leg, especially if neck or low back pain corresponding to the level of the deficit is a feature as well. Motor and sensory symptoms and signs should conform to one nerve root distribution.

Plexopathies

BRACHIAL AND LUMBAR PLEXITIS (OR PLEXOPATHY)

Brachial plexitis is an acute neuropathic syndrome of presumed autoimmune etiology. Patients present with shoulder and arm pain followed by weakness as the pain abates. Eventual functional recovery is the rule, although this takes months and occasionally is incomplete. Brachial plexitis is somewhat more common than lumbosacral plexitis. The upper plexus, C5 and C6, most commonly is affected, although the lower plexus can be involved. Lumbosacral plexitis has a clinical course similar to that with brachial plexitis.

A diagnosis of plexitis is considered when a patient presents with single limb pain and weakness that does not follow a single root or nerve distribution. MRI appearance of the region is normal unless neoplastic infiltration has occurred.

Findings on nerve conduction studies may be normal distally in the limbs, but F-waves will be slowed or absent. EMG findings may be normal initially, but eventually this study shows denervation in the distribution of the affected portion of the plexus.

Differentiation of plexitis from radiculopathy is accomplished on the basis of not only the more extensive deficits in patients with plexitis but also the time course of pain followed by weakness as the pain abates; this pattern is not expected in patients with radiculopathy. EMG of paraspinal muscles at the level of involvement will show denervation changes in a radiculopathy but not in a plexopathy. Sensory nerve action potentials may be lost distally in a plexopathy, but not in a radiculopathy, because of its preganglionic location, leaving the distal branches of the sensory neurons intact.

NEOPLASTIC PLEXUS INFILTRATION

The brachial and lumbar plexuses are in proximity to the areas that can be infiltrated by tumors, including those involving the lymph nodes, lungs, kidneys, and other abdominal organs. The first symptom of tumor infiltration usually is pain. Weakness and sensory loss are less common symptoms. Neoplastic plexus compression or infiltration manifests as a progressive painful monoparesis. Limb movements that stretch the plexus elicit pain, and the patient tends to hold the limb immobile to avoid exacerbating the pain.

Neoplastic infiltration of the brachial plexus usually involves the lower plexus, C8 to T1. Lung cancer and lymphoma are the most common tumors to cause this. Horner syndrome can develop with lower brachial plexus involvement. The main consideration in the differential diagnosis is radiation plexopathy. The diagnosis is suspected on the basis of the severe pain and weakness. EMG often shows denervation that spans single nerve and root distributions. Detailed knowledge of the plexus anatomy is essential during examination and EMG. MRI usually shows the infiltration or compression of the plexus.

RADIATION PLEXOPATHY

Radiation therapy in the region of the plexus can produce progressive dysfunction. The upper brachial plexus is especially susceptible because of the lesser amount of surrounding tissues to attenuate the radiation. Symptoms are dysesthesias and weakness. The dysesthesias may be associated with discomfort but seldom are described as painful. This absence of pain is one key to differentiation from neoplastic plexus infiltration, which typically is quite painful.

Diagnosis is suspected in the clinical setting of progressive painless weakness in a patient with cancer who has received radiation to the region. MRI is essential to rule out tumor infiltration. EMG shows denervation, which is not a differentiating feature, but myokymia is more commonly seen in patients with radiation plexopathy than in those with neoplastic infiltration.

PLEXOPATHY FROM HEMATOMAS

Hematomas can develop adjacent to and compress the brachial and lumbosacral plexuses, producing motor and sensory findings. Brachial plexus hematomas are usually from bleeding disorders or instrumentation such as central line placement. Lumbosacral plexus hematomas also can develop from coagulopathies, including that associated with anticoagulant treatment, and after procedures such as abdominal surgery or femoral arterial catheterization. In the latter circumstance, blood leaking from the puncture site can flow proximally, and a substantial amount of blood may be lost without a clinically obvious hematoma.

Hematomas interfere with the function of the peripheral nerves and plexus by blocking conduction. The prognosis generally is good so long as the plexus or nerve has not been directly injured, because the condition usually is neurapraxia rather than neurotmesis, and conduction usually is restored when the blood is resorbed. Large hematomas should be evacuated if severe plexus damage is present.

PLEXUS TRAUMA

A history of trauma makes the etiology of the plexopathy quite obvious. The main difficulty is in differentiating traumatic plexopathy from radiculopathy (nerve root avulsion) or peripheral nerve damage. Also, spinal cord damage must be considered because cord contusion and hematomyelia may manifest with weakness that is more prominent in one extremity. Motor vehicle accidents, childbirth, and occupational injuries are the most common causes of traumatic plexopathy. In many cases of plexus stretch, the mechanism is forced extension of the arm over the head or forced downward movement of the shoulder. Forced extension of the arm over the head damages the lower plexus, with the intrinsic muscles of the hand being especially affected (Klumpke palsy). Forced depression of the shoulder produces damage to the upper plexus, giving prominent weakness of the deltoid, biceps, and other proximal muscles (Erb palsy).

Trauma includes not only stretch injury but also penetrating injury such as knife and bullet wounds. Knife wounds can easily damage the brachial plexus but are much less likely to involve the lumbosacral plexus. Gunshot wounds may directly affect either the brachial or lumbosacral plexus, and the shock waves of high-velocity bullets may damage the plexus without direct contact. Unfortunately, the speed and extent of recovery from these types of injuries are poor.

Diagnostic studies should include imaging not only of the plexus but also of the adjacent spinal cord, looking for disk herniation, spondylosis, subluxation, or other anatomical deformity. Plain radiographs should be obtained to ensure skeletal integrity. MRI or CT of the region will visualize the soft tissues.

THORACIC OUTLET SYNDROME

Thoracic outlet syndrome is an overdiagnosed condition characterized by weakness of muscles innervated by the lower trunk of the brachial plexus. The motor axons in the lower trunk supply both the median- and ulnar-innervated intrinsic muscles of the hand. Finger and wrist flexors occasionally may be affected, causing marked impairments in use of the hand, which is not restricted to a single nerve distribution. This deficit must be differentiated from that due to a cortical lesion. Sensory loss is mainly in an ulnar distribution, because the sensory fibers of the median nerve ascend through the middle trunk rather than the lower trunk.

Diagnosis of thoracic outlet syndrome depends on demonstration of low-amplitude median and ulnar nerve compound motor action potentials and ulnar sensory nerve action potentials. Median sensory nerve action potentials are normal. CT or MRI of the plexus may be necessary to rule out infiltration by nearby tumor. Imaging of the neck and cervical spine occasionally reveals cervical ribs. These usually are asymptomatic, so their presence does not confirm the diagnosis of thoracic outlet syndrome.

DIABETIC AMYOTROPHY

Diabetic amyotrophy is one of the terms given to the syndrome of damage to the proximal lumbar plexus, serving mainly the femoral nerve, seen in diabetes mellitus. Patients present with weakness and pain in a femoral nerve distribution. Although a length-dependent diabetic peripheral neuropathy may be an accompanying feature, the femoral distribution symptoms and signs overshadow the other findings. Patients eventually improve, although the recovery often is prolonged and incomplete. It is difficult to study nerve conduction of the femoral nerve, so this test is diagnostically helpful only if results are normal. EMG usually shows denervation, although up to 4 weeks may pass before electrical signs of axonal dysfunction are seen.

Neuronopathies

Neuronal degenerations usually affect multiple individual nerve distributions and usually involve more than one limb. A few focal motor neuropathies, however, can produce single limb defects.

MONOMELIC AMYOTROPHY

Monomelic amyotrophy is a condition in which motoneurons of one limb degenerate; often the distribution suggests involvement of specific motoneuron columns in the spinal cord. It affects only one limb, usually an arm. The opposite limb can be affected to a much lesser extent. Pain and sensory loss are not features of this disorder. Progressive weakness develops over months to years and may eventually plateau without further worsening. Onset usually is in young adulthood, at the age of approximately 20 years, and men are predominantly affected. Diagnosis is confirmed by clinical presentation and EMG findings of active and chronic denervation without sensory abnormalities.

POLIOMYELITIS

Poliomyelitis is now uncommon but still occurs in some parts of the world. A poliomyelitis-like syndrome can result from viruses other than the poliovirus itself, including West Nile virus. The illness usually manifests with acute asymmetrical weakness after an initial phase of encephalitic symptoms including headache, meningeal signs, and possibly confusion or seizures. The paralysis may involve only one limb but more commonly is generalized. After recovery, only one limb may remain weak (monoparesis).

Pitfalls in the Differential Diagnosis for Hemiplegia and Monoplegia

Diagnosis of hemiplegia and monoplegia can always be a challenge, but identifying or localizing the underlying lesion can be especially difficult with certain clinical presentations. Some important points in the differential diagnosis with such presentations are considered next.

Focal Weakness of Apparently Central Origin
Focal Weakness That Appears to Be Central: Cerebral Cortex, Internal Capsule, Brainstem, or Spinal Cord?

Lesions in cerebral cortex, internal capsule, brainstem, and spinal cord all produce weakness due to CST dysfunction, with typical clinical findings. Note that acute lesions may not be associated with hyperreflexia and upgoing plantar response—these reflex alterations take time to develop.

Cerebral cortex lesions usually produce weakness that is most prominent in one region, such as arm, face, or leg, whereas internal capsule and brainstem lesions are more likely to produce equivalent dysfunction of the arm and leg. Cortical lesions often are associated with cortical deficits of aphasia or neglect, whereas lower lesions do not do this. Brainstem lesions commonly are associated with cranial nerve deficits, especially diplopia from disturbance of ocular motor centers. Vertigo and ataxia without weakness also suggest a brainstem lesion. Spinal cord lesions usually produce bilateral deficits below the level of the lesion, with both motor and sensory involvement. Structural lesions of the spine are almost always painful, although MS and transverse myelitis usually are not.

Focal Weakness That Appears to Be Central: Migraine, TIA, or Seizure?

Examination findings can be identical with migraine, TIA, and seizure, so clinical differentiation among these three insults rests on the history. TIA is characterized by an abrupt onset, with gradual recovery over the course of 5 minutes to 1 hour; deficits outside this time window argue in favor of alternative diagnoses—a TIA lasting hours is more likely to represent a small infarction with clinical resolution but persistent perfusion defect. The deficit of migraine evolves in keeping with the migration of spreading depression across the cerebral cortex—thus, over minutes the deficit marches from hand up arm to face, for example. Weakness with migraine usually precedes headache but may accompany headache or may even not be associated with headache in some instances. Seizure is a rare cause of transient weakness. Seizure is suggested by abrupt onset and offset of the deficit, and any associated symptoms of decreased response or twitching.

Weakness of the Hand and Wrist
Weakness in Intrinsic Muscles of the Hand: Median Nerve, Ulnar Nerve, Brachial Plexus, or Small Cerebral Cortical Lesion?

With weakness in the intrinsic muscles of the hand, the cause may be a lesion of the median nerve, ulnar nerve, brachial plexus, or cerebral cortex. Most of the intrinsic muscles of the hand are innervated by the ulnar nerve, so an isolated distal ulnar lesion produces profound loss of use of the hand. This lesion must be differentiated from a lateral frontocentral cerebral lesion, which if located in the hand region produces prominent loss of independent digit use. A median nerve lesion produces impaired hand function because of loss of function of the finger and wrist flexors more than of the intrinsic muscles of the hand. With stabilization of the hand, intact function of ulnar- and radial-innervated muscles can be demonstrated to rule out lesions at or above the plexus.

Lower brachial plexus lesions produce dysfunction of the median- and ulnar-innervated intrinsic muscles of the hand and also may affect the long finger flexors. This dramatic loss of function can be mistaken for central weakness, because the deficit spans peripheral nerve distributions. EMG usually documents the axonal damage.

A small cerebral cortical lesion can produce inability to use the hand, without signs of other deficit. Reflexes should be exaggerated, although acutely they may not be. The combination of cupping of the outstretched hand and pronator drift strongly suggest a central lesion. EMG cannot rule out a peripheral nerve lesion, because several weeks may be required before signs of axonal damage are evident on needle study. MRI of the brain is the most sensitive imaging study for evaluation of a small cerebral lesion.

Weakness of the Wrist: Radial Neuropathy or Small Cerebral Cortical Infarcts?

Radial neuropathy manifests with weakness of the wrist extensors, which if severe can result in destabilization of the intrinsic muscles of the hand and long finger flexors; these median- and ulnar-innervated muscles require opposition from radial-innervated extensors for proper function. Therefore, the deficit seems more extensive than would be expected on the basis of a radial lesion alone. A cerebral lesion is suggested; although cerebral lesions span neural distributions, wrist extension may be more obviously affected than grip or finger flexion.

Differentiation of radial neuropathy from a cerebral lesion depends on demonstration of intact median and ulnar nerve function by the examiner, following stabilization of the finger flexors and wrist. Also, corticospinal tract signs and other signs of cortical damage (aphasia or neglect) should be looked for in a patient with a possible cerebral infarct.

Leg Weakness
Peroneal Nerve Palsy or Paramedian Cerebral Cortical Lesion?

The underlying disorder in leg weakness may be peroneal nerve palsy or a lesion of the paramedian cerebral cortex. Peroneal nerve palsy results in weakness of foot dorsiflexion and eversion, with relative preservation of other motor functions. Small cerebral lesions of the leg region of the homunculus on the medial aspect of hemispheres can cause weakness that is most prominent in the same distribution as for a peroneal nerve palsy. Weakness of foot inversion suggests a cerebral lesion, because this is a tibial nerve function and not expected with peroneal palsy. EMG signs of denervation in the tibialis

anterior and other peroneal-innervated muscles indicate a peripheral rather than cerebral lesion. Cerebral lesions producing lower leg weakness usually cause upgoing plantar response and hyperactivity of the Achilles tendon reflex, despite little clinical evidence of gastrocnemius muscle involvement.

Cauda Equina Lesion, Myelopathy, or Paramedian Cerebral Cortical Lesion?

This chapter discusses monoplegia rather than paraplegia (see Chapter 24), but with leg weakness, it is important to differentiate between lower spinal cord dysfunction and cauda equina compression, between upper spinal cord involvement and cervical spondylotic myelopathy, and between these problems and midline cerebral lesions producing leg weakness.

Cauda equina lesions usually are due to acute disc herniations, spondylosis, or tumors in the lumbosacral spinal canal. The lumbar and sacral nerve roots are compressed, resulting initially in a depolarizing block but later axonal degeneration, which produces motor and sensory loss. With the syndromes of intermittent claudication of the cauda equina, repetitive nerve action potentials result in severe pain that is relieved by rest after only a few minutes and that may be accompanied by neurological dysfunction. Pain, sensory loss, and weakness typically are worsened by standing and relieved by flexing the lumbar spine.

Spondylotic myelopathy is compression of the spinal cord by degenerative spondylosis, usually in the cervical region. Compression of the corticospinal tracts produces weakness of the legs. Pain usually is near the level of the lesion, although the localizing value is not precise. Midline cerebral lesions produce unilateral or bilateral leg weakness, depending on the cause and exact location, with CST signs. Spine pain is not expected.

Differentiation among cauda equina, spinal cord, and cortical lesions can be tricky but in general the following rules apply:

- Bowel and bladder incontinence can develop with all three locations but is more common with cauda equina lesions.
- Cauda equina lesions are associated with depressed reflexes, whereas spinal cord and cerebral lesions are characterized by hyperactive reflexes and upgoing plantar responses.
- Sensory loss is more prominent with cauda equina lesions than with higher lesions.
- Pain in the spine is approximately at the level of the lesion, although the localization is not exact.

References

The complete reference list is available online at www.expertconsult.com.

Chapter 24

Paraplegia and Spinal Cord Syndromes

Bruce H. Dobkin, Leif A. Havton

Paraplegia may result from a variety of systemic and primary CNS medical conditions, as well as trauma at all segmental levels of the spinal cord (**Box 24.1**). A spinal cord syndrome may develop from extramedullary and intramedullary pathological processes (**Fig. 24.1**). Initial symptoms may be gradual in onset and progressive, including pain, dysesthesia, or subtle upper-or lower-extremity weakness. In other cases, such as an inflammatory myelitis, acute onset of severe motor, sensory, and autonomic deficits may develop without premonitory symptoms. Trauma from a cervical flexion-extension injury, for example, may produce a central cord injury of the lower cervical spinal cord with incomplete quadriparesis, whereas a complete transection injury at the lower thoracic spinal cord from a fall may result in complete paraplegia. Thus, both the rostrocaudal segmental level of disease involvement or trauma and completeness of the lesion in the transverse plane anticipate the person's impairments and disability. Details about the relationships between specific spinal cord segments and sensory dermatomes are reviewed in Chapter 28, and the segmental innervation of specific muscle groups are reviewed in Chapters 29 and 30. The sensorimotor clinical examination allows localization of the lesion (**Fig. 24.2**).

When examining a patient who presents with paraplegia, a careful neurological examination is critical for planning additional diagnostic workup and care. Identifying distinct spinal cord syndromes and determining the likely location of the underlying pathological process will guide subsequent imaging and electrodiagnostic studies. Structural information about the integrity of the spine may be obtained from radiographic plain films and computed tomography (CT) for bone pathology. Magnetic resonance imaging (MRI) and myelography are best to reveal cord pathology. A review of imaging of the spine is provided in Chapter 33A.

Acute and long-term care of patients is influenced by the clinical presentation, severity of neurological deficits, underlying pathology, and prognosis for gains over time. Patients presenting with an acute spinal cord syndrome after trauma show both early (days to 3 months) and late (up to 2 years) changes in their motor and sensory deficits (Fawcett et al., 2007). Both neurological improvements and clinical worsening may occur. When some sparing of sensation and movement is present in the first 72 hours after trauma, the prognosis for walking is rather good. Indeed, up to 90% of patients with a cervical central cord injury who have modest sensation and movement below the level of injury by 4 weeks after trauma will become functional ambulators (Dobkin et al., 2006). Thus, serial and careful neurological examinations are important to monitor the injury-related deficits, especially in the first weeks after onset. Rehabilitation of patients with paraplegia follows after the acute medical needs have been addressed. The aim is to promote as much functional independence as possible with and without assistive devices, decrease the risk of complications, and reintegrate the patient into home and community. Neurological rehabilitation for paraparesis after spinal cord syndromes is reviewed in Chapter 48.

Common Spinal Cord Syndromes

The clinical presentation of a spinal cord injury depends on whether the injury is complete or spares selected fiber tracts. A number of clinically characterized spinal cord syndromes may develop as a result of the involvement of different portions of the spinal cord gray and white matter.

Box 24.1 Differential Diagnosis of Diseases Affecting the Spinal Cord

Compressive Lesions

Non-Neoplastic

Trauma:
 Vertebral body fracture/dislocation
 Hyperextension injury
 Direct puncture, stab, or missile
Spondylosis:
 Cervical stenosis
 Lumbar stenosis
Intervertebral disk herniation
Infectious disorders (e.g., abscess, tuberculosis)
Inflammatory (e.g., rheumatoid arthritis, ankylosing spondylitis, sarcoid)
Hemorrhage:
 Epidural hematoma
 AVM
Syringomyelia
Congenital disorders
Arachnoid cysts
Paget disease
Osteoporosis

Neoplastic

Epidural
Intradural extramedullary (e.g., meningioma, neurofibroma, leptomeningeal metastasis)
Intramedullary

Noncompressive Myelopathies

Demyelinating (e.g., MS, ADEM)
Viral myelitis (e.g., varicella-zoster, AIDS–related myelopathy, human T-lymphotropic virus type I infection)
Vitamin B_{12} deficiency and other nutritional deficiencies
Infarction
Ischemia and hemorrhage from vascular malformations
Spirochetal diseases (syphilis and Lyme disease)
Toxic myelopathies (e.g., radiation-induced)
Autoimmune diseases (e.g., lupus, Sjögren syndrome)
Paraneoplastic
Neuronal degenerations
Acute and subacute transverse myelitis of unknown cause

ADEM, Acute disseminated encephalomyelitis; *AIDS*, acquired immunodeficiency syndrome; *AVM*, arteriovenous malformation; *MS*, multiple sclerosis.

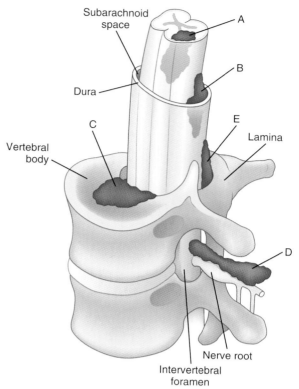

Fig. 24.1 Anatomical locations of spine metastases. **A,** Intramedullary metastasis may be located within the spinal cord. **B,** With leptomeningeal spread, metastasis is in the subarachnoid space and is extramedullary and intradural. **C-E,** Epidural metastases arise from extension of metastases located in one of the adjacent structures: vertebral column **(C)**, paravertebral spaces via the intervertebral foramina **(D)**, or rarely, the epidural space itself **(E)**. As these epidural metastases grow, they compress adjacent blood vessels, nerve roots, and the spinal cord, resulting in local and referred pain, radiculopathy, and myelopathy. *(Reprinted with permission from Byrne, T.N., 1992. Spinal cord compression from epidural metastases. N Engl J Med 327, 615 [Fig. 1].)*

Spinal Shock

Spinal shock refers to the period of depressed spinal reflexes caudal to an acute spinal cord injury; it is followed by emergence of pathological reflexes and return of cutaneous and muscle stretch reflexes (Ditunno et al., 2004). During the acute phase of spinal shock, paralysis of muscles, sensory impairment, and loss of autonomic function are present below the level of injury. Commonly, the first reflex to appear after a clinically complete spinal cord injury is the delayed plantar response. It is induced by stroking the plantar surface of the foot with a blunt instrument upward from the heel, along the lateral surface, and across the metatarsal heads. A delayed response consists of plantar flexion of the great toe and other toes, often detectable within the first hours after injury. When the delayed plantar response persists for more than 1 week, it is often associated with a severe spinal cord injury and a less favorable prognostic outlook for a significant functional recovery. The return of reflexes over days and weeks after the initial period of spinal shock appears to follow a general pattern, with cutaneous reflexes recovering before muscle stretch reflexes. Specifically, the bulbocavernosus and cremasteric reflexes commonly return before the ankle jerk, Babinski sign, and knee jerk.

Incomplete Lesions of the Spinal Cord
Unilateral Transverse Lesion

A hemisection lesion of the spinal cord causes a Brown-Séquard syndrome. A pure hemisection is unusual, but patients may show features of a unilateral lesion or hemisection. A Brown-Séquard lesion is characterized by ipsilateral weakness and loss of both vibration and position sense below the level of the injury. In addition, there is a loss of temperature and pain sensation below the level of the lesion on the contralateral side. As pain and temperature fibers extend rostrally a few segments before crossing the midline to enter the lateral

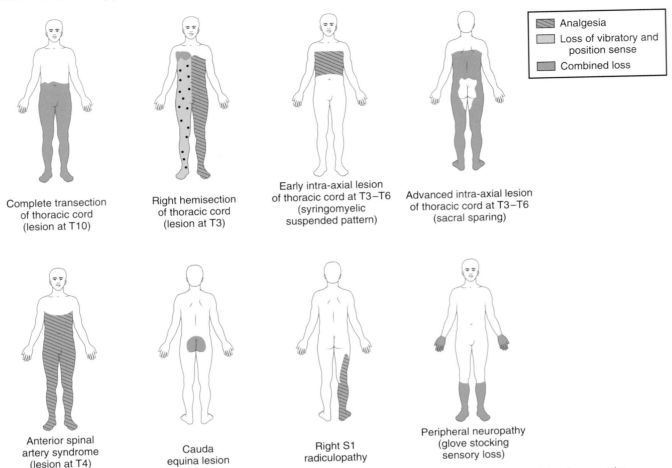

Fig. 24.2 Characteristic sensory disturbances found in various spinal cord lesions in comparison with peripheral neuropathy.

spinothalamic tract, the loss of pain and temperature sensory modalities extend rostrally on the contralateral side to a segmental level that is a few segments below the level of the lesion. In addition, at the segmental level of the hemisection injury, a limited patch of ipsilateral loss of pain and temperature in combination with a lower motor neuron weakness is often detected. A Brown-Séquard syndrome may be caused by a variety of etiologies but is commonly encountered after traumatic injuries, including bullet and stab wounds.

Central Cord Syndrome

Traumatic central cord syndrome is commonly characterized by the triad of (1) motor impairment that is disproportionately more severe in the upper than the lower extremities, (2) bladder dysfunction that usually includes urinary retention, and (3) sensory dysfunction of varying degrees. An international consensus group recently suggested that an upper- and lower-extremity difference of at least 10 motor score points, based on the Medical Research Council scale, can be considered as a quantitative addition to the commonly used qualitative criteria for making the diagnosis (van Middendorp et al., 2010). An additional clinical feature of the traumatic central cord syndrome is a dissociated sensory loss for pain and temperature, whereas vibration and position sense remain preserved. This sensory presentation may be explained by a direct

injury to intramedullary decussating fibers, which normally would ascend contralaterally as part of the spinothalamic tract. As a result, a capelike sensory deficit may be encountered in patients with a cervical level injury, but sensation within more caudal dermatomes would generally be spared (**Fig. 24.3**).

A traumatic central cord syndrome is mostly encountered in elderly patients who have suffered a relatively minor trauma in the form of a cervical hyperextension injury, commonly in the setting of an underlying cervical spondylosis. Falls and motor vehicle injuries are common etiologies. Syringomyelia or tumors may also produce a central cord syndrome.

Anterior Spinal Artery Syndrome

An anterior cord syndrome involves the anterior two-thirds of the spinal cord, sparing the posterior columns. The corticospinal and spinothalamic tracts are both affected. The syndrome is clinically characterized by paralysis and sensory impairments below the level of the lesion, with impaired sensation of pain and temperature; vibration sense and proprioception are preserved. Fiber tracts for autonomic control are also typically compromised, resulting in bladder, bowel, and sexual dysfunction. In the acute phase after injury, a spinal shock phase with decreased muscle tone and areflexia may present, followed by a gradual return of reflexes and hypertonicity and perhaps spasms.

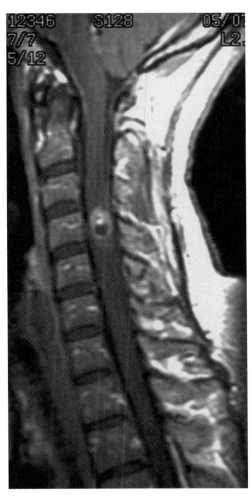

Fig. 24.3 Magnetic resonance image of the cervical spine showing a contrast-enhancing mass. Patient presented with a capelike sensory loss for pain and temperature. Resection of the mass revealed a glioma.

An anterior cord syndrome may be caused by trauma from central disk compression or a bone fragment, as well as a myelitis. Vascular occlusive causes are perhaps the most common etiology. For instance, the anterior cord syndrome may present as a spinal cord stroke from atherothrombotic or embolic occlusion of the anterior spinal cord artery. Invasive vascular and thoraco-abdominal surgical procedures may be complicated by impaired blood flow to the spinal cord, especially due to obstruction or hypoperfusion of the artery of Adamkiewicz near the T6 level. This may also follow surgery at the distal aorta and proximal iliac arteries with the use of aortic counter pulsation devices and, occasionally, from retroperitoneal hematomas or abscesses. Similarly, survivors of cardiac arrest and significant hypotensive episodes may demonstrate a mid-thoracic anterior cord ischemic syndrome, as the vascular supply near the T6 segment is particularly susceptible to distal field ischemia.

Anterior Horn and Pyramidal Tract Syndromes

Paralysis may be encountered in the setting of motor impairments in combination with relative sparing of sensory and autonomic functions, as seen in motor neuron disease including amyotrophic lateral sclerosis (ALS). Lower motor neuron weakness with atrophy and loss of reflexes is typically seen in combination with upper motor neuron weakness, signs of spasticity, and hyperreflexia. Different limbs may be affected to various degrees, but symptoms are progressive over the course of the disease. However, innervation of the external anal and urethral sphincters is normally preserved in ALS, with sparing of bladder and bowel functions.

Combined Posterior and Lateral Column Disease

A clinical syndrome characterized by development of a spastic ataxic gait pattern may be caused by lesions affecting the posterior and lateral white-matter tracts. Friedrich ataxia represents a genetic etiology, and vitamin B_{12} deficiency may result in subacute combined degeneration with spastic paretic gait and sensory ataxia. Dorsal horn and column injury alone may result from tabes dorsalis.

Characteristic Clinical Features of Lesions at Different Levels

Paralysis may be caused by lesions at any segmental level of the spinal cord from both intramedullary and extramedullary disease. The characteristic symptoms and signs affecting motor and sensory functions typically depend on the segmental level of injury.

Foramen Magnum and Upper Cervical Spine

When structural lesions are located in or adjacent to the foramen magnum, several different neurological patterns are possible. For example, brainstem signs may occur together with symptoms from a spinal cord injury. Involvement of the lower portion of the brainstem is suggested by speech impairments, including dysarthria and dysphonia, as well as by dysphagia. In addition, facial numbness and nystagmus may be detected in association with tumors or other structural lesions in the foramen magnum. When compression of the spinal cord occurs, long-tract signs may present from injury to the corticospinal tract with, for instance, a spastic hemiparesis or quadriparesis. A lower motor neuron injury component may also be detectable from lesions at the craniocervical junction and the foramen magnum, with upper extremity weakness, muscular atrophy, and decreased muscle stretch reflexes.

Several pathological processes and lesions may be present at the level of the foramen magnum and its immediate vicinity. These conditions include Arnold-Chiari malformations; traumatic injuries; rheumatoid arthritis; syringomyelia; vascular lesions such as thrombosis, dissection, or arteriovenous malformation; and a variety of tumors including meningiomas. Multiple sclerosis may also cause intramedullary lesions of the brainstem and the upper cervical spinal cord and selectively affect long white-matter tracts. Imaging studies, especially MRI, help determine the nature and precise anatomical location for pathological processes in the foramen magnum and upper cervical spine region.

Lesions affecting the uppermost portion of the cervical spine may be challenging to diagnose owing to a nonlocalizing symptom complex upon initial presentation. Pain is a common early symptom and may be localized to the neck or occipital region. At times, the pain may be aggravated by neck movement. When upper cervical nerve roots are compressed, a radicular pain may present in the corresponding dermatome. Irritation of the second cervical nerve root, for example, may present with a pain localized within the posterior aspect of the scalp, whereas an injury to the third and fourth nerve roots may induce pain that is projected to the neck or shoulder. A lower motoneuron injury presentation with upper extremity muscular weakness and atrophy may also be part of the clinical presentation. When the spinal cord is compressed by epidural or subdural space-occupying lesions, spastic weakness of upper and lower extremities typically follow.

An injury or disease process affecting the upper cervical spinal cord may also compromise breathing. Normal respiration requires functional use of the diaphragm muscle, which is innervated by the phrenic nerve. Motoneurons contributing to the phrenic nerve are located within the cervical spinal cord and contribute efferent axons to the C3-C5 ventral roots. Therefore, complete injuries affecting the spinal cord above the C3 segment will compromise the function of the diaphragm, and respiratory failure may follow.

Lower Cervical and Upper Thoracic Spine

Injuries to the lower part of the cervical spine and upper thoracic spine may be caused by extramedullary compression of nerve roots and the spinal cord or by an intramedullary disease process. The correlation between presenting symptoms and localization of the underlying lesion is most precise for the extramedullary pathological processes (e.g., tumors, herniated disks) that compress individual segmental nerve roots or spinal nerves. Intramedullary lesions may also present with pain, but the segmental localization is commonly less precise.

Extramedullary lesions typically first irritate segmental nerve roots and the spinal nerve, with radicular pain and sensory deficits typically following the corresponding dermatomal distribution. Similarly, motor deficits involve each myotome affected by the lesion. Muscle stretch reflexes may also provide helpful information with regard to the primary level of injury, as the affected segmental reflex is typically depressed or absent, and caudal reflexes are hyperactive. For instance, when a lesion is at the C4-C6 level, a radicular pattern of pain and sensory symptoms may typically involve the radial side of the arm, forearm, and hand. Motor deficits include weakness in elbow flexion. In addition, the biceps and brachioradialis muscle stretch reflexes may be depressed or absent, especially when the C5-C6 levels are involved.

In contrast, lesions at the C7-T1 level usually present with pain and sensory impairments over the ulnar side of the upper extremity, including the arm, forearm, and hand. Motor deficits related to affected myotomes commonly involve elbow extension, the intrinsic hand muscles, and the triceps reflex.

Lower and upper motoneuron signs may also be present in adjacent segments. If segmental nerve roots and the spinal cord are compressed by a herniated disk or space-occupying lesion at the C5-C6 level, for example, a decreased brachioradialis reflex may reflect a C6 radiculopathy, whereas a brisk and hyperactive finger flexor reflex reflects an upper motoneuron syndrome.

Thoracic Levels

Traumatic spinal cord injury at the thoracic level usually produces a complete lesion. The segmental level of injury is best determined by a careful sensory examination of dermatomes (Maynard et al., 1997). Useful clinical landmarks are the nipple line for the T4 dermatome and the umbilicus for the T10 dermatome. Pain may follow a radicular pattern around the chest or abdomen, corresponding to the segmental levels of injury. Sensory testing of pin, temperature, pressure, and light touch appreciation may determine the most caudal dermatome of normal sensation, as well as a zone of partial preservation. The sensory testing should include evaluation of dermatomes of the left and right side of the body, with comparisons of homologous levels. In addition to a combination of at-level pain, sensory deficits, and muscular weakness, autonomic dysfunction may develop from long-tract involvement and include urinary retention, bladder-sphincter dyssynergia, and bladder hyperreflexia.

Conus Medullaris and Cauda Equina

The conus medullaris of the spinal cord terminates approximately at the level of the L1 vertebra, although the precise location of the tip of the conus may show marked variability among subjects. This anatomical aspect of the spinal cord is important because spine trauma commonly takes place at the thoracolumbar junction, and the extent of such injuries is highly variable (Kingwell et al., 2008). Traumatic injuries to the conus medullaris usually result in weakness or paralysis of the lower extremities, absence of lower-extremity reflexes, and saddle anesthesia (**Fig. 24.4**). However, some patients with conus medullaris injuries exhibit a mixed upper and lower motoneuron syndrome. In contrast, a cauda equina injury

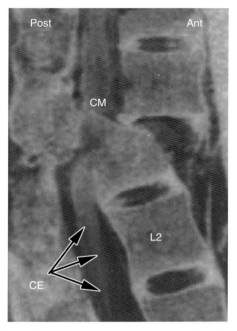

Fig. 24.4 Magnetic resonance imaging demonstrating the effects of trauma to the thoracolumbar portion of the spine with a crush injury of the cauda equina *(CE)* and conus medullaris *(CM)* portion of the spinal cord. Note T12/L1-level spine fracture and dislocation.

that lesions lumbosacral roots below the level of the conus medullaris is a pure lower motoneuron syndrome. Cauda equina injuries present with lower-extremity weakness, areflexia and decreased muscle tone, and variable sensory deficits. At least a third of these patients suffer considerable central pain. Affected limb and pelvic floor muscles develop flaccid weakness, and electromyography shows denervation after either a conus medullaris or cauda equina injury, especially following anatomically complete lesions.

Both conus medullaris and cauda equina injuries are associated with bladder, bowel, and sexual dysfunction (Pavlakis et al., 1983). Urodynamic evaluations typically demonstrate detrusor areflexia, and a rectal exam identifies a flaccid anal sphincter. In addition, the bulbocavernosus reflex is typically absent or diminished, and reflexogenic erection in males is commonly lost.

Imaging studies (e.g., plain radiographs, CT, MRI) identify structural pathology. Burst fractures and fracture dislocations are common injuries to the spinal column that result in neurological deficits suggesting a conus medullaris or cauda equina involvement. Following trauma to the thoracolumbar spine, imaging studies can be used to assess spinal stability and identify detailed aspects of spine fractures, including the presence and location of bone fragments, spinal canal encroachment, epidural hematomas, and herniated discs. A variety of treatment options exist (e.g., surgical stabilization of the spine, decompression of the conus medullaris and nerve roots).

A lumbar spinal stenosis due to a congenitally small-diameter spinal canal or central disk and spondylotic narrowing one or more levels below L1 may present with a subtle course. Over months to years, lower-extremity numbness or pain, usually in an L3-S1 single or multiradicular pattern, accompanies standing and walking, often gradually progressing to limit walking distance. Pain is commonly accompanied by weakness, but patients may not be aware of their deficit. Clinical insight into this diagnosis and level of cauda compression is gained by a manual muscle examination after a few minutes of being supine, followed by having the subject walk for about 500 feet, and then immediately retesting strength. Transient paresis often is found immediately after the walk and resolves within a minute or two.

Pain and Autonomic Dysfunction

In addition to motor and sensory impairments, pain is frequently associated with spinal cord injuries, along with autonomic impairments affecting bladder, bowel, sexual, and respiratory functions. The type and severity of autonomic dysfunction may vary and depend on location and severity of spinal cord injury. International spinal cord injury societies recently provided a practical system to document remaining autonomic function after a spinal cord injury (Alexander et al., 2009). These efforts are likely to increase our ability to communicate the effects of spinal cord injury on, for instance, cardiovascular, bladder, bowel, and sexual functions.

Pain Syndromes

Pain may originate from irritation, injury, or disease structures associated with the spine and present with a variety of pain syndromes. The symptoms of pain and their diagnostic features depend on the location of spine irritation and involved structures. Distinct pain syndromes may develop as a result of irritation or injury to the vertebral column, ligaments, the dura mater, nerve roots, and spinal cord. Neuropathic pain may take the form of *paresthesia* (abnormal but not unpleasant sensation that is either spontaneous or evoked), *dysesthesia* (an abnormal, unpleasant sensation that is spontaneous or evoked), *allodynia* (pain evoked by ordinary stimuli such as touch or rubbing), and *hyperalgesia* (an augmented response to a stimulus that is usually painful).

Local Pain

Localized neck or back pain may result from irritation or injury to innervated spine structures including ligaments, periosteum, and dura. The pain is typically deep and aching, may vary with a change in position, and often becomes worse from increased load or weight bearing on affected structures. Percussion or palpation over the spine may in some patients worsen the local pain. When the injured or diseased spine structures are irritated, secondary symptoms may develop and include muscle spasm and a more diffusely located pain.

Projected Pain

Irritation of or injury to the spine and associated structures may result in pain that can be projected to other parts of the body (e.g., a pathological process involving the facet joints may be experienced as pain in an upper or lower extremity). When a nerve root is irritated or injured, the projected pain represents a radicular pain. In contrast, when the spine itself is irritated, a nonradicular pain affecting a remote body part may develop as referred pain. Although both radicular pain and referred pain may be experienced as pain located at some distance from the source, the two forms of projected pain exhibit distinct features that aid diagnosis.

Radicular Pain

Radicular pain commonly has a sharp, stabbing quality and can often be exacerbated by activities that stretch the affected nerve root (e.g., straight leg raising or flexion of the neck). Other activities that may result in additional pressure on a nerve root, such as straining or coughing, may also increase the intensity and severity of radicular pain. Activities that decrease stretching of affected nerve roots, such as flexion of the hip and knee in cases of an S1 radiculopathy, tend to reduce radicular pain and discomfort. In addition to the symptoms of radicular pain, nerve root irritation and injury may also result in sensory and motor deficits following the same dermatome and myotome distribution as the affected nerve root. This helps localize the level of spinal cord injury that is causing paraplegia.

Pain after Spinal Cord Injury

Pain often accompanies injury to the spinal cord. Regardless of segmental level or completeness of injury, most patients with a traumatic spinal cord injury develop a clinically significant pain syndrome at some post-lesion time point (Waxman and Hains, 2006). Neuropathic pain after spinal cord injury may affect different locations. At-level pain affects the portions of the body that are innervated by the injured spinal cord segments. Below-level pain is located in body segments receiving innervation from the spinal cord caudal to the lesioned segments. Above-level pain is less common compared to the other two forms of postinjury pain but, when present, affects body segments innervated by spinal cord segments rostral to the site of spinal cord injury. Musculoskeletal sources of pain and pain with overuse of joints and soft tissues also are frequent but remedial sources of pain.

Pain developing after a spinal cord injury is commonly described as burning, pricking, or aching in quality. It can be experienced as deep or superficial in location. Some patients with spinal cord injury develop a severe and excruciating pain syndrome, which in many cases is difficult to treat and control symptomatically. In some patients, pain may be experienced below the segmental level of injury in body areas exhibiting complete loss of other types of sensation including touch, pressure, and proprioception. In such cases, pain in the lower extremities may be experienced after a thoracic spinal cord injury without noxious stimulation and without the patient being able to discriminate cutaneous or proprioceptive stimuli. The mechanisms for such painful phantom phenomena are not well understood but include dorsal horn, thalamic, and cortical adaptations to ordinary and noxious inputs.

Autonomic Dysreflexia

Injuries to the spinal cord that result in paraplegia from a lesion above T6 may also impair autonomic control and result in episodes of severe hypertension or hypotension (Blackmer, 2003). Autonomic dysreflexia represents an acute syndrome characterized by excessive and uncontrolled sympathetic output from the spinal cord. As a result, the blood pressure is suddenly and markedly elevated. Associated symptoms include headache; malaise; blurring of vision; flushed, sweaty skin above the level of injury; and pale, cool skin below it. An episode of autonomic dysreflexia can be triggered by any noxious stimulation below the segmental level of injury. Common triggers include bladder distension, constipation, rectal fissures, joint injury, and urinary tract infection. Autonomic dysreflexia may present soon after the initial injury but more commonly becomes symptomatic several months after the spinal cord injury. Prevention is the best approach. Treatment of acute symptoms targets removal of noxious stimuli and cautious lowering of the blood pressure.

Bladder Dysfunction

Normal bladder and bowel control depend on segmental reflexes involving both autonomic and somatic motor neurons, as well as descending and ascending tracts of the spinal cord (Fowler et al., 2008). As a result, bladder and bowel function may be impaired after an injury to any segmental level of the spinal cord. Different clinical syndromes develop depending on whether the injury or disease process affects the sacral spinal cord directly or higher segmental levels. Traumatic spinal cord injuries with paraplegia taking place above the T12 vertebra will interrupt spinal cord long-tract connections between supraspinal micturition centers in the brainstem and cerebral cortex and the sacral spinal cord. An upper motoneuron syndrome follows, with detrusor-sphincter dyssynergia caused by impaired coordination of autonomic and somatic motor control of the bladder detrusor and external urethral sphincter, respectively. Incomplete bladder emptying results. In addition, the upper motoneuron syndrome also includes detrusor hyperreflexia with increased pressure within the bladder. In contrast, injury to the T12 vertebra and below results in a direct lesion to the sacral spinal cord and associated nerve roots. A direct lesion to preganglionic parasympathetic neurons and somatic motoneurons of the Onuf nucleus located within the S2-S4 spinal cord segments results in denervation of pelvic targets. Injuries to both the conus medullaris and cauda equina present as a lower motoneuron syndrome characterized by weak or flaccid detrusor function. Urinary retention follows, with risk of overflow incontinence. The goal for all bladder care is to avoid retrograde urine flow, urinary tract infections, and renal failure. Management of both upper and lower motoneuron bladder impairment commonly includes clean intermittent bladder catheterizations. Chapter 38 discusses evaluation and treatment.

References

The complete reference list is available online at www. expertconsult.com.

Chapter 25

Proximal, Distal, and Generalized Weakness

David C. Preston, Barbara E. Shapiro

CHAPTER OUTLINE

Muscle weakness may be due to disorders of the central nervous system (CNS) or peripheral nervous system (PNS). The PNS includes the primary sensory neurons in the dorsal root ganglia, nerve roots, peripheral nerves, neuromuscular junctions, and muscles. Although not strictly peripheral, the primary motor neurons (anterior horn cells) in the brainstem and spinal cord are also conventionally included as part of the PNS. The neurological examination allows separation of the causes of weakness arising at these different locations. If the pattern of weakness is characteristic of upper motor neuron (UMN) dysfunction (i.e., weakness of upper-limb extensors and lower-limb flexors) together with hyperreflexia and extensor plantar responses, the weakness clearly is of CNS origin. Weakness with sensory loss may occur in both CNS

disorders and disorders of the nerve roots and peripheral nerves. Weakness without sensory loss may also occur from CNS disorders, but in the PNS, this pattern of weakness occurs in disorders of the anterior horn cell, neuromuscular junction, or muscle. Rarely in the PNS, peripheral motor fibers will be the site of pathology (e.g., as occurs in multifocal motor neuropathy with conduction block). Although fatigue often accompanies most disorders of weakness, marked fatigue, especially when involving the extraocular, bulbar, and proximal upper limb muscles, often indicates a disorder of the neuromuscular junction.

The motor unit is the primary building block of the PNS and includes the anterior horn cell, its motor nerve, terminal nerve fibers, and all their accompanying neuromuscular junctions and muscle fibers. This chapter concentrates on disorders of the motor unit and disorders that may also involve the peripheral sensory nerves. The pattern of weakness often localizes the pathological process to the primary neurons, nerve roots, peripheral nerves, neuromuscular junctions, or muscles. Muscle weakness changes functional abilities that are more or less specific to the muscle groups affected. Recognizable patterns of symptoms and signs often allow a reasonable estimation of the anatomical involvement. Identifying these patterns is the first step in the differential diagnosis of weakness, because certain disorders affect specific muscle groups. This chapter begins with a review of the symptoms and signs of muscular weakness with respect to the muscle groups affected. A discussion follows of the bedside examinations, functional examinations, and laboratory tests often used in evaluating patients with muscle weakness. The chapter concludes with an approach to the differential diagnosis of muscle weakness based on which muscle groups are weak, whether the muscle weakness is constant or fluctuating, and whether the disorder is genetic or acquired.

Clinical Presentation by Affected Region

General Considerations

As muscles begin to weaken, the associated clinical features depend more on which muscles are involved than on the cause of involvement. A complicating factor in evaluating weakness is the patient's interpretation of the term *weak*. Although physicians use this term to denote a loss of muscle power, patients tend to apply it more loosely in describing their symptoms. Even more confusing, many people use the words *numb* and *weak* interchangeably, so the clinician should not accept a complaint of weakness at face value; the patient should be questioned further until it is clear that weakness means loss of muscle strength.

If the patient has no objective weakness when examined, the clinician must rely on the history. In patients with weak muscles, a fairly stereotypical set of symptoms emerges according to which muscle groups are weak (discussed later in this section). The patient whose weakness is caused by depression or malingering has vague symptoms, avoids answering leading questions, and the stereotypical symptoms of weakness are seldom volunteered. Instead, these patients make such statements as "I have no strength to do the housework," "I just can't do (the task)," or "I can't climb the stairs because I get so tired and have to rest." When pressed regarding these symptoms, it soon becomes apparent that specific details are lacking. Patients who cannot get out of a low chair because of real weakness explain exactly how they have to maneuver themselves into an upright position (e.g., pushing on the chair arms, leaning forward in the seat, and bracing their hands against the furniture). The examiner should avoid providing patients with clinical details they appear to be searching for. Asking whether pushing on the arms of the chair is required to stand up provides the patient with key information that may later be used in response to the questions of baffled successive examiners. In addition, it often is difficult to differentiate true muscle weakness from apparent weakness that accompanies tendon or joint contractures or is secondary to pain. For example, patients with primary orthopedic conditions often complain of weakness. In these patients, however, pain with passive or active motion often is a prominent part of the symptoms.

In evaluating weakness, the first key task is to discern which muscle groups are affected. In this regard, it is helpful to consider the clinical presentation with involvement of specific body regions: ocular; facial and bulbar; neck, diaphragm, and axial; proximal upper extremity; distal upper extremity; proximal lower extremity; and distal lower extremity.

Ocular Muscles

Extraocular muscle weakness results in ptosis or diplopia. When looking in the mirror, the patient may notice drooping of the eyelids, or family and friends may point it out. It is important to keep in mind that ptosis occasionally develops in older patients as a consequence of aging (i.e., partial dehiscence of the levator muscles) or a sequela of ocular surgery (e.g., lens implantation for cataracts). To differentiate between acute and chronic ptosis, it helps to look at prior photographs. Because the ocular myopathies often are familial, examination of family members is useful. Bilateral ptosis may result in compensatory backward tilting of the neck to look ahead or upward. Rarely, this postural adaptation may lead to neck pain and fatigue as the prominent symptoms. In addition, true ptosis often results in compensatory contraction of the frontalis muscles to lessen the ptosis, resulting in a characteristic pattern of a droopy eyelid with prominent forehead furrowing produced by contraction of the frontalis muscle. Weakness of extraocular muscles may result in diplopia. Mild diplopia, however, may cause only blurring of vision, sending the patient to the ophthalmologist for new eyeglasses. It also is worth asking the patient whether closing one eye corrects the diplopia, because neuromuscular weakness is not among the causes of monocular diplopia.

Facial and Bulbar Muscles

Patients experience facial weakness as a feeling of stiffness or sometimes as a twisting or altered perception in the face (note that patients often use the word *numbness* in describing facial weakness). Drinking through a straw, whistling, and blowing up balloons all are particularly difficult tasks for these patients and may be sensitive tests for facial weakness, particularly when such weakness dates from childhood. Acquaintances may notice that the patient's expression is somehow changed. A pleasant smile may turn into a snarl because of weakness of the levator anguli oris muscles. In lower facial weakness, patients may have difficulty with drooling and retaining their saliva, often requiring them to carry a tissue in the hand—the so-called napkin sign—which often accompanies bulbar involvement in amyotrophic lateral sclerosis (ALS). A common observation in mild long-standing facial weakness, as with facioscapulohumeral (FSH) muscular dystrophy, is a tendency for the patient to sleep with the eyes open from weakness of the orbicularis oculi. Weakness of masticatory muscles may result in difficulty chewing, sometimes with a sensation of fatigue and discomfort, as may occur with myasthenia gravis (MG). Pharyngeal, palatal, and tongue weakness disturbs speech and swallowing. A flaccid palate is associated with nasal regurgitation, choking spells, and aspiration of liquids. Speech may become slurred or acquire a nasal or hoarse quality.

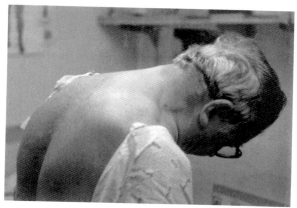

Fig. 25.1 Dropped head syndrome. With severe weakness of neck extensor muscles, patient no longer can extend the neck, and chin rests against chest.

In contrast with central lesions, no problem with fluency or language function is observed.

Neck, Diaphragm, and Axial Muscles

Neck muscle weakness becomes apparent when the patient must stabilize the head. Riding as a passenger in a car that brakes or accelerates, particularly in emergencies, may be disconcerting for the patient with neck weakness, because the head rocks forward or backward. Similarly, when the patient is stooping or bending forward, weakness of the posterior neck muscles may cause the chin to fall on the chest. A patient with neck-flexion weakness often notices difficulty lifting the head off the pillow in the morning. As neck weakness progresses, patients may develop the *dropped head syndrome*, in which they no longer can extend the neck, and the chin rests against the chest (**Fig. 25.1**). This posture leads to several secondary difficulties, especially with vision and swallowing.

Shortness of breath often develops when diaphragm muscles weaken, especially when individuals lie flat or must exert themselves. These symptoms can be mistakenly attributed to lung or heart disease. Severe diaphragmatic weakness leads to hypoventilation and carbon dioxide retention. This may first be manifested as morning headaches or vivid nightmares. Later, hypercapnia results in sedation and a depressed mental state. Rarely, axial and trunk muscles can be involved early in the course of a neuromuscular disorder. Weakness of the abdominal muscles may make sit-ups impossible. Focal weakness of the lower abdominal muscles results in an obvious protuberance that superficially mimics an abdominal hernia. Patients with weakness of the paraspinal muscles are unable to maintain a straight posture when sitting or standing, although they can do so when lying on the bed (so-called bent spine syndrome).

Proximal Upper Extremity

A feeling of tiredness often is the first expression of shoulder weakness. The weight of the arms is sufficient to cause fatigue. Early on, the patient experiences fatigue on performing sustained tasks with the hands held up, especially over the head. The most problematic activities include painting the ceiling, shampooing or combing the hair, shaving, and simply trying to lift an object off a high shelf.

Distal Upper Extremity

Hand and forearm weakness interferes with many common activities of daily living. Difficulty with activities that require dexterity, such as buttoning and using a zipper, is an early sign. With further decreased hand strength, other activities affected include opening a jar, turning on a faucet or the car ignition, using a key, holding silverware, writing, and opening a car door.

Proximal Lower Extremity

Weakness of the proximal lower extremity often is responsible for the earliest symptoms experienced by patients who develop weakness. Patients notice that they have difficulty arising from the floor or from a low chair and have to use the support of the hands or knees. Getting out of a bath or getting up from a toilet without handrails is particularly difficult. Older patients may attribute this limitation to arthritis or some similar minor problem. Walking becomes clumsy, and the patient may stumble. In descending stairs, people with quadriceps weakness tend to keep the knee locked and stiff. If the knee bends slightly as the weight of the body transfers to the lower stair, the knee may collapse. Greater problems with coming down stairs than with going up suggest quadriceps weakness, whereas the reverse is true for hip extensor weakness. Once patients with hip-girdle weakness are up and on level ground, they feel more secure. Family and friends, however, often will notice an obvious change in the affected person's gait. In patients with hip-girdle weakness, a waddling gait often develops because weakness of the hip abductors of the weight-bearing leg results in the hip's falling as the patient walks (*Trendelenburg gait*).

Distal Lower Extremity

Symptoms localized to deficits in the anterior compartment (i.e., peroneal muscle weakness) often constitute the first sign of weakness of the distal lower extremity. Weakness of the anterior tibial and ankle evertor muscles often results in tripping, even over small obstacles, and an increased tendency to repeatedly sprain the ankle. If the weakness becomes severe, a foot drop develops, and the gait incorporates a slapping component. To compensate for the foot drop, patients must raise the knee higher when they walk so that the sagging foot and toes clear the floor (*steppage gait*). Weakness of both anterior and posterior muscles of the lower leg often makes the stance unstable, which causes the patient to complain of poor balance. Isolated weakness of the posterior calf muscles makes standing on tiptoes impossible.

Bedside Examination of the Weak Patient

The neurological examination of patients with muscle weakness is the same as that used for patients with other neurological problems. Special attention to the observational and functional components of the evaluation, however, is particularly rewarding in the patient with weakness.

Observation

It is useful to spend a few moments observing the patient and noting natural posture and motion. When patients, particularly children, are aware of the examination, they often concentrate on performing as normally as possible. When unaware of scrutiny, their posture and movements may be more natural. At one time or another, we have heard the parent's exasperated cry, "He never does it that way at home." For example, ptosis may be obvious on inspection of the head and neck. The more severe the ptosis, the greater the patient's tendency to throw the head backward. The eyebrows are elevated and the forehead wrinkled in an attempt to raise the upper lids. This sometimes is so successful that ptosis is apparent only when the examiner smooths out the wrinkled forehead and allows the eyebrows to assume a more normal position. Psychogenic ptosis is easy to detect: the lower lid elevates with contraction of both parts of the orbicularis oculi muscles (i.e., blepharospasm) to accompany the lowered upper lid.

Weakness of the facial muscles present since childhood may give a smooth, unlined appearance to the adult face. In addition, facial expression diminishes or changes. A smile may become a grimace or a snarl, with eversion of the upper lip. The normal blink may slow, or eyelid closure may be incomplete so that the sclera is always visible. The normal preservation of the arch of the upper lip may be lost, and the mouth may assume either a tented or a straight-line configuration. Actual wasting of the facial muscles is difficult to see, but temporalis and masseter atrophy produce a characteristic scalloped appearance above and below the cheekbone. Because rearranging the hair style may cover the wasting, the examiner should make a conscious effort to check the upper portion of the patient's face. The tongue is inspected for atrophy and fasciculations. Inspecting the tongue at rest with the mouth open, looking for the random irregular twitching movements of fasciculations, is the best method. When the tongue is fully protruded, many patients have some normal quivering movements that can easily be mistaken for fasciculations. It is wise to diagnose fasciculations of the tongue only when there is associated atrophy.

Facial weakness causes the normal labial sounds (that of *p* and *b*) to be softened. The examiner with a practiced ear can detect other alterations of speech. Lower motor neuron (LMN) involvement of the palate and tongue gives the speech a hollow, nasal, echoing timbre, whereas UMN dysfunction causes the speech to be monotonous, forced, and strained. Laryngeal weakness also may be noticed in speech when the voice becomes harsh or brassy, often associated with loss of the glottal stop (the small sound made by the larynx closing, as at the start of a cough).

Weakness of the shoulder muscles causes a characteristic change in posture. Normally the shoulders brace back by means of the tone of the muscles, so the hands are positioned with the thumbs forward when the arms are by the side. As the shoulder muscles lose their tone, the point of the shoulder rotates forward. This forward rotation of the shoulder is associated with a rotation of the arm, so that the backs of the hands now are forward facing. Additionally, the loss of tone causes a rather loose swinging movement of the arms in normal walking. When shoulder weakness is severe, the patient may fling the arms by using a movement of the trunk, rather than lifting the arms in the normal fashion. In the most extreme example, the only way the patient can get the hand above the head on a wall is to use a truncal movement to throw the whole arm upward and forward so the hand rests on the wall, and then to creep the hand up the wall using finger movements. Atrophy of the pectoral muscles leads to the development of a horizontal or upward sloping of the anterior axillary fold. This is especially the case in facioscapulohumeral (FSH) muscular dystrophy. The examiner may observe *winging of the scapula*, a characteristic finding in weakness of muscles that normally fix the scapula to the thorax (i.e., the serratus anterior, rhomboid, or trapezius). As these muscles become weak, any attempted movement of the arm causes the scapula to rise off the back of the rib cage and protrude like a small wing. The arm and shoulder act as a crane—the boom of the crane is the arm, and the base is the scapula. Obviously, if the base is not fixed, any attempt to use the crane results in the whole structure's falling over. This is the operative mechanism with attempts to elevate the arm; the scapula simply pops off the back of the chest wall in a characteristic fashion. In the most common type of winging, the entire medial border of the scapula protrudes backward. In some diseases, particularly FSH muscular dystrophy, the inferomedial angle juts out first, and the entire scapula rotates and rides up over the back. This often is associated with a *trapezius hump*, in which the middle part of the trapezius muscle in the web of the neck mounds over the upper border of the scapula (**Fig. 25.2**). Note that when examining a slender person or a child, in whom prominent shoulder blades are common, the shoulder configuration returns to normal with forcible use of the arm, as in a push-up.

Muscle Bulk and Deformities

Assessment of muscle bulk looking for atrophy and hypertrophy is an important part of the neuromuscular examination. Prominent muscle wasting usually accompanies neurogenic disorders associated with axonal loss. However, severe wasting also occurs in chronic myopathic conditions. Wasting is best appreciated in the distal hand and foot muscles and around bony prominences. In the arm, wasting of the intrinsic hand muscles produces a characteristic hand posture in which the

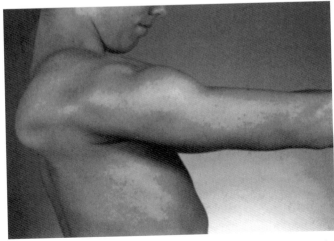

Fig. 25.2 Scapular winging of facioscapulohumeral muscular dystrophy is distinguished by prominent protrusion of inferior medial border of scapula. When viewed from the front, elevation of scapula under trapezius muscle produces characteristic *trapezius hump*.

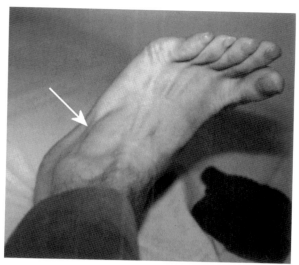

Fig. 25.3 The extensor digitorum brevis is a small muscle located on the lateral dorsum of the foot *(arrow)* that helps dorsiflex the toes. It often wastes early in neuropathic conditions but may become hypertrophied, as seen here, in proximal myopathic conditions.

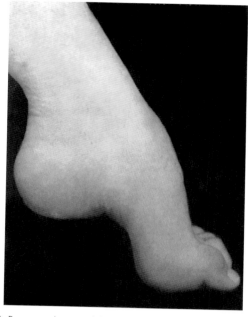

Fig. 25.4 *Pes cavus* is caused by intrinsic foot muscle weakness during early growth and development. This condition is recognized as a high arch, foreshortened foot, and hammer toes. It often is a sign that weakness has been present since early childhood and implies an inherited disorder in most patients.

thumb rotates outward so that it lies in the same plane as that of the fingers (the *simian hand*), and the interphalangeal joints flex slightly with slight extension of metacarpophalangeal joints (the *claw hand*). Wasting of the small muscles leaves the bones easily visible through the skin, resulting in the characteristic guttered appearance of the back of the hand. In the foot, one of the easier muscles to inspect is the extensor digitorum brevis, a small muscle on the lateral dorsum of the foot that helps dorsiflex the toes (**Fig. 25.3**). It often wastes early in neuropathies and anterior horn cell disorders. In myopathic conditions in which proximal muscles are affected more than distal muscles, the extensor digitorum brevis may actually hypertrophy to try to compensate for weakness of the long toe dorsiflexors above it.

Muscle mass of the leg is so variable among individuals that it is sometimes difficult to decide whether wasting of the muscles has occurred. Any marked asymmetry indicates an abnormality, but distinguishing a slender thigh from quadriceps muscle atrophy often is difficult. One way to try to distinguish these conditions is to ask the patient to tighten the knee as firmly as possible. The firm medial and lateral bellies of the normal quadriceps that bunch up in the distal part of the thigh just above the knee fail to appear in the wasted muscle. The same technique can be used to evaluate anterior tibial wasting. In a severely wasted muscle, a groove on the lateral side of the tibia (which normally is filled by the anterior tibial muscles) is apparent. A moderate degree of wasting is difficult to distinguish from thinness of the leg, but if the patient dorsiflexes the foot, the wasted muscle fails to develop the prominent belly seen in a normal muscle.

Abnormal muscle hypertrophy is uncommon but may be a key finding when present. Beyond the expected increase in muscle bulk that accompanies exercise, generalized muscle hypertrophy is a feature of *myotonia congenita* and *paramyotonia congenita*, giving the appearance of the extreme development typically seen in weight lifters. Hypertrophy is a common finding in the rare syndrome of *acquired neuromyotonia*, in which the continuous discharge of motor axons results in the

muscle effectively exercising itself. Exceptionally, hypertrophy occurs in some chronic denervating disorders, especially in the posterior calf muscle in S1 radiculopathies. Electromyography (EMG) in affected patients often reveals spontaneous discharges in these muscles (usually complex repetitive discharges) consequent to chronic denervation. By contrast, conditions exist in which muscle hypertrophy is not from true muscle enlargement but from infiltration of fat, connective tissue, and other material (i.e., pseudohypertrophy). *Pseudohypertrophy* occurs in calf muscles of patients with Duchenne and Becker muscular dystrophy, as well as in patients with limb-girdle muscular dystrophy, spinal muscular atrophy (SMA), and some glycogen storage disorders. Similarly, pseudohypertrophy occurs rarely in sarcoidosis, cysticercosis, amyloidosis, hypothyroid myopathy, and focal myositis. Palpable masses in muscles occur with muscle tumors, ruptured tendons, or muscle hernias.

Several bony deformities often provide important clues to the presence of neuromuscular conditions. Proximal and axial muscle weakness often leads to scoliosis. Intrinsic foot muscle weakness present from childhood often leads to the characteristic foot deformity of *pes cavus*, in which the foot is foreshortened with high arches and hammer toes (**Fig. 25.4**). Pes cavus is a sign that weakness has been present at least since early childhood and implies a genetic disorder in most patients. Likewise, a high-arched palate often develops from chronic neuromuscular weakness present from childhood.

Muscle Palpation, Percussion, and Range of Motion

Palpation and percussion of muscle provide additional information. Fibrotic muscle may feel rubbery and hard, whereas denervated muscle may separate into discrete strands that roll under the fingers. Muscle in inflammatory myopathies or rheumatological conditions may be tender to palpation, but severe muscle pain on palpation is unusual. An exception to this rule is in the patient experiencing an acute phase of viral myositis or rhabdomyolysis, whose muscles may be very sensitive to either movement or touch. Percussion of muscle may produce the phenomenon of *myotonia*, in which a localized contraction of the muscle persists for several seconds after percussion. Percussing the thenar eminence and watching for a delayed relaxation of the thumb abductors will best show this phenomenon. This defining characteristic of myotonic dystrophy and myotonia congenita is distinguishable from myoedema, which occasionally occurs in patients with thyroid disorders and other metabolic problems. In *myoedema*, the development of a dimple in the muscle, which then mounds to form a small hillock, follows the percussion.

In addition to its diagnostic value, the presence of muscle contracture across a joint may cause disability, even in the absence of weakness. Thus, an evaluation of range of motion at major joints is an important part of the clinical examination. A standard examination includes evaluation for contractures at the fingers, elbows, wrists, hips, knees, and ankles. At the hips, both flexion and iliotibial band contractures should be looked for.

Muscle Tone

The physiological origin of muscle tone is complex and outside the scope of this chapter. In examining the weak patient, however, muscle tone offers valuable information regarding the origins of the weakness. Variations from a normal muscle tone result in increased tone (*hypertonicity*) or decreased tone (*hypotonicity*). Increased tone results from the loss of CNS influences on the tonic contraction of muscle. Decreased tone usually implicates a problem with the proprioceptive or peripheral motor innervation of a muscle but also may result from an acute spinal cord or cerebral lesions. Patients usually do not complain directly of increased or decreased tone; for example, the spastic patient may complain of heaviness, stiffness, or slowness of movement.

Several methods are used to examine tone. First is the spontaneous posture of the extremities. With spasticity, the upper limbs often are in a fixed flexed posture, and affected muscles are firm to palpation. The examiner should attempt to relax the patient to allow free passive movement; helpful instructions may include statements such as "Don't try to help me do the work." Normally, resistance is the same throughout the range of motion and does not change with changes in the velocity of the movement. In a patient with spasticity, rapid passive displacement of the extremity results in increased resistance followed by relaxation (*clasp-knife phenomenon*). Resistance varies with the speed and direction of passive motion. Examination of tone in the legs should include supine examination, because with the patient in this position, the examiner easily accomplishes hip and knee flexion. In spasticity, the heel elevates off the examination table, while normally the heel remains in contact with the table. Hypotonia is the loss of normal tone and is felt as increased ease of passive movements during these maneuvers, or floppiness. In patients with severe hypotonia, the joints may be passively hyperextended.

Table 25.1 The Medical Research Council Scale for Grading Muscle Strength

Grade	Description
0	No contraction
1	Flicker or trace of contraction
2	Active movement with gravity eliminated
3	Active movement against gravity
4	Active movement against gravity and resistance
5	Normal power

Strength

Evaluation of individual muscle strength is an important part of the clinical examination. Many methods are available. Fixed myometry has become popular within the research community. This method uses a strain gauge attached to a rigid supporting structure, often integrated into the examining couch on which the patient lies. The patient then uses maximum voluntary contraction, quantitated in newtons (N). The merits of this method are debatable, and for the average clinician, the equipment expense is prohibitive.

In an office situation and in many clinical drug trials, manual muscle testing gives perfectly adequate results and is preferable to fixed myometry in young children. The basis is the Medical Research Council grading system, with some modification (**Table 25.1**). This method is adequate for use in an office situation, particularly if supplemented by the functional evaluation. A scale of 0 to 5 is used, in which 5 indicates normal strength. A grade of 5 indicates that the examiner is certain a muscle is normal and never used to compensate for slightly weak muscles. Muscles that can move the joint against resistance may vary quite widely in strength; grades of 4+, 4, and 4− often are used to indicate differences, particularly between one side of the body and the other. Grade 4 represents a wide range of strength, from slight weakness to moderate weakness, which is a disadvantage. For this reason, the scale has been more useful in following the average strength of many muscles during the course of a disease, rather than the course of a single muscle. Averaging many muscle scores smoothes out the stepwise progression noted in a single muscle. This may demonstrate a steadily progressive decline. A grade of 3+ is assigned when the muscle can move the joint against gravity and can exert a tiny amount of resistance but then collapses under the pressure of the examiner's hand. It does not denote the phenomenon of *sudden give-way*, which occurs in conversion disorders and in patients limited by pain. Grade 3 indicates that the muscle can move the joint throughout its full range against gravity, but not against any added resistance. Sometimes, particularly in muscles acting across large joints such as the knee, the muscle is capable of moving the limb partially against gravity but not through the full range of movement. A muscle that cannot extend the knee horizontally when the patient is in a sitting position but can extend the knee to within 30 to 40 degrees of horizontal is graded 3−. Grades 2, 1, and 0 are as defined in **Table 25.1**.

Although it is commendable and sometimes essential to examine each muscle separately, most clinicians test muscle groups rather than individual muscles. In our clinic, we test neck flexion, neck extension, shoulder abduction, internal rotation, external rotation, elbow flexion and extension, wrist flexion and extension, finger abduction and adduction, thumb abduction, hip flexion and extension, knee flexion and extension, ankle dorsiflexion and plantar flexion, and dorsiflexion of the great toe.

Fatigue

Fatigue is a common symptom in many neuromuscular disorders and many medical conditions. Anemia, heart disease, lung disease, cancer, poor nutrition, and depression are among the many disorders that can result in fatigue. In certain neuromuscular conditions, however, strength is normal at rest but progressively decays with muscle use. This clinical scenario most often characterizes the postsynaptic neuromuscular transmission disorders, especially MG. Repetitive or sustained muscle testing brings out true muscle fatigue. Always test fatigue in patients with suspected neuromuscular transmission disorder. Ptosis is provoked by sustained upgaze for 2 to 3 minutes. Counting out loud from 1 to 100 may result in slurred, nasal, or hoarse speech. Repetitive testing of the strength of shoulder abduction or hip flexion may result in progressive weakness in patients with MG.

Reflexes

In motor unit disorders, reflexes are either normal, reduced, or absent. ALS is the exception because both UMN and LMN dysfunction coexist, so hyperreflexia and spasticity often accompany signs of LMN loss. In neurogenic disorders with demyelination, reflexes are lost early in the disease, as occurs in Guillain-Barré syndrome, from blocking and desynchronization of muscle-spindle afferents and motor efferents. With disorders resulting in axonal loss, reflexes are depressed in proportion to the amount of loss. Because most axonal neuropathies predominantly affect distal axons, the distal reflexes (ankle reflexes) are depressed or lost early, and the more proximal ones remain normal. In myopathies, reflexes tend to diminish in proportion to the amount of muscle weakness. The same is true for postsynaptic neuromuscular transmission disorders. With presynaptic neuromuscular transmission disorders (e.g., Lambert-Eaton myasthenic syndrome), reflexes tend to be depressed or absent at rest but return to normal or at least improve after brief (10-second) periods of exercise.

Sensory Disturbances

Disorders of the motor unit generally are not associated with disturbances of sensation unless a second condition is superimposed. Motor neuron disorders, neuromuscular transmission disorders, and myopathies generally follow this rule. Among the few exceptions is the minor sensory loss in patients with X-linked spinobulbar muscular atrophy (Kennedy disease) and inclusion-body myositis, both of which may have coexistent degeneration of the peripheral nerves and dorsal root ganglion cells. In the paraneoplastic Lambert-Eaton myasthenic syndrome, patients often have minor sensory signs reflecting a more widespread paraneoplastic process.

Sensory deficits often accompany peripheral neuropathies that are predominantly motor and usually thought of as motor neuropathies. Such disorders include Guillain-Barré syndrome, Charcot-Marie-Tooth disease, and some toxic neuropathies (e.g., from lead). In these conditions, sensory abnormalities on examination or electrophysiological testing help identify the disorder as a neuropathy, thereby narrowing the differential diagnosis.

Peripheral Nerve Enlargement

Palpation of peripheral nerves may yield important information in several neuromuscular conditions. Diffusely enlarged nerves occur in some patients with chronic demyelinating peripheral neuropathies, especially Charcot-Marie-Tooth disease type 1, Dejerine-Sottas disease, and Refsum disease. In addition, focal enlargement occurs in nerve sheath tumors (neurofibromatosis) or with infiltrative lesions (e.g., amyloidosis, leprosy). Easily palpated nerves are the greater auricular nerve in the neck, the ulnar nerve at the elbow, the superficial radial sensory nerve as it crosses the extensors to the thumb distal to the wrist, and the peroneal nerve at the fibular head at the knee.

Fasciculations, Cramps, and Other Abnormal Muscle Movements

All limbs are examined to determine the presence or absence of fasciculations. A *fasciculation* is a brief twitch caused by the spontaneous firing of one motor unit. Fasciculations may be difficult or impossible to see in infants or obese patients. They can be present in normal people, so their presence in the absence of wasting or weakness is of no significance (benign fasciculations). Fasciculations that are widespread and seen on every examination may indicate denervating disease, particularly anterior horn cell disease. Mental or physical fatigue, caffeine, cigarette smoking, or drugs such as amphetamines exacerbate fasciculations.

In some patients who have been careful to avoid exposure to exacerbating factors, disease-related fasciculations may be absent or appear benign. This should be kept in mind during the evaluation. Abundant fasciculations may be difficult to differentiate from *myokymia*, which is a more writhing, bag of worms–like motion of muscle. Myokymia results from repetitive bursting of a motor unit (i.e., grouped fasciculations) and characteristically is associated with certain neuromuscular conditions (e.g., radiation injury, Guillain-Barré syndrome).

Similar to fasciculations, cramps may be benign or accompany several neuropathic conditions. A *cramp* is a painful involuntary muscle contraction. Cramps occur when a muscle is contracting in a shortened position. During a cramp, the muscle becomes hard and well defined. Stretching the muscle relieves the cramp. Superficially, a muscle contracture that occurs in a metabolic myopathy may resemble a cramp, although these two entities are completely different on electrophysiological testing. During a contracture, electrical silence is characteristic, whereas numerous motor units fire at high frequencies during a cramp.

Functional Evaluation of the Weak Patient

Walking

Alteration of gait may occur with weakness of the muscles of the hip and back, leg, and shoulder. In normal walking, when the heel hits the ground, the action of the hip abductors, which stabilize the pelvis, serves to counteract the shock. Thus in a sense, the hip abductors act as shock absorbers. Weakness of these muscles disturbs the normal fluid movement of the pelvis during walking, so when the heel hits the ground, the pelvis dips to the other side; bilateral weakness produces a waddle. Additionally, weakness of the hip extensors and back extensors makes it difficult for the patient to maintain a normal posture. Ordinarily the body is carried so that the center of gravity is slightly forward of the hip joint. To maintain an erect posture, the hip and back extensors are in continual activity. If these muscles become weak, the patient often throws the shoulders back so that the weight of the body falls behind the hip joints. This postural adjustment accentuates the lumbar lordosis. Alternatively, with pronounced weakness of the quadriceps muscles, the patient stabilizes the knee by throwing it backward. When the knee is hyperextended, it locks, deriving its stability from the anatomy of the joint rather than from muscular support. Finally, weakness of the muscles of the lower leg may result in a *steppage gait*, in which a short throw at the ankle midswing affects dorsiflexion of the foot. The foot then rapidly comes to the ground before the toes fall back into plantar flexion. Shoulder weakness is noted as the patient walks; the arms hang loosely by the sides and tend to swing in a pendular fashion rather than with a normal controlled swing.

Arising from the Floor

The normal method for arising from the floor depends on the age of the patient. The young child can spring rapidly to the feet without the average observer being able to dissect the movements. The elderly patient may turn to one side, place a hand on the floor, and rise to a standing position with a deliberate slowness. Despite such variability, abnormalities caused by muscle weakness are easily detectable. The patient with hip muscle weakness will turn to one side or the other to put the hand on the floor for support. The degree of turning is proportional to the severity of the weakness. Some patients must turn all the way around until they are in a prone position before they draw their feet under them to begin the standing process. Most people arise to a standing position from a squatting position, but the patient with hip extensor and quadriceps muscle weakness finds it easier to keep the hands on the floor and raise the hips high in the air. This has been termed the *butt-first maneuver*; the patient forms a triangle with the hips at the apex and the base of support provided by both hands and feet on the floor, and then laboriously rises from this position, usually by pushing on the thighs with both hands to brace the body upward. The progress of recovery or progression of weakness can be documented by noting whether the initial turn is greater than 90 degrees, whether unilateral or bilateral hand support is used on the floor and thighs, whether this support is sustained or transitory, and whether a butt-first maneuver is used. The entire process is known as the *Gower*

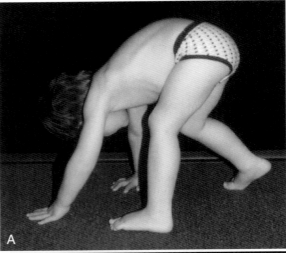

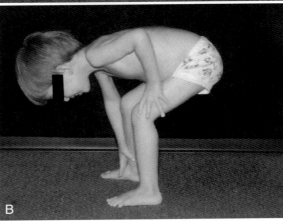

Fig. 25.5 Gower maneuver. **A,** Butt-first maneuver as hips are hoisted in the air. **B,** Hand support on the thighs.

maneuver, but it is useful to break it up into its component parts (**Fig. 25.5**).

Stepping Onto a Stool

For a patient with hip and leg weakness, stepping onto an 8-inch-high footstool is equivalent in difficulty to a normal person's stepping up onto a coffee table. This analogy is apt because the required maneuvers are similar in both cases. Whereas the patient with normal strength readily approaches a footstool and easily steps onto it, the patient with weakness often hesitates in front of the stool while contemplating the task. A curious little maneuver occurs, known colloquially as the *fast-foot maneuver.* Normal persons can easily take the weight of the body on one leg, straightening out the knee as they stand on the footstool. Patients with weakness feel unsafe. They like to get both feet under them before straightening the knees and rising to their full height. To accomplish this, they place one foot on the footstool. While the knee of this leg is still bent, they quickly transfer the other foot from the floor to the footstool and then straighten the knees. This gives the impression of a hurried transfer of the trailing foot from floor to footstool, hence the term *fast foot.* As the weakness increases, the pelvis may dip toward the floor as the leading leg takes up the strain and the patient's weight transfers from the foot on the floor to the foot on the stool, the so-called hip dip. Finally, if the weakness is severe, patients may either use hand support on the thighs or appear to gather themselves in and throw the body onto the footstool. Analysis of the various components—the hesitation, fast foot, hip dip, and throw—together with the presence or absence of hand support may provide a sensitive measure of changes in disease.

Psychogenic Weakness

An experienced examiner should be able to differentiate real weakness from psychogenic weakness. The primary characteristic of psychogenic weakness is that it is unpredictable and fluctuating. Muscle strength may suddenly give out when a limb is being evaluated. The patient has difficulty knowing the exact muscle strength expected and cannot adequately counter the examiner's resistance. This gives rise to a wavering, collapsing force. Tricks are useful to bring out the discrepancy in muscle performance. For example, if the weak thigh cannot lift off the chair in a seated position, then the legs should not swing up onto the mattress when being seated on the examining table. When the examiner suspects that weakness of shoulder abduction is feigned, the patient's arm is placed in abduction. With the examiner's hand on the elbows, the examiner can instruct the patient to push toward the ceiling. At first, the downward pressure is very light, and the patient is unable to move the examining hand toward the ceiling. However, the arm does not fall down either, and as the downward pressure is gradually increased, continued exhortation to push the examiner's hand upward results in increasing resistance to the downward pressure. The examiner ends up putting maximum weight on the outstretched arm, which remains in abduction. The logical conclusion is that the strength is normal. Patients do not realize this because they believe that because they did not move the examiner's hand upward, they must be weak.

Clinical Investigations in Muscular Weakness

In the investigation of diseases of the motor unit, the most helpful tests are measurement of the serum concentration of creatine kinase (CK), electrodiagnosis, and muscle biopsy. These are available to all physicians. Genetic testing increasingly provides definitive diagnosis. In addition, if facilities are available, exercise testing can provide useful information.

Serum Creatine Kinase

The usefulness of measuring the serum CK concentration in the diagnosis of neuromuscular diseases is in differentiating between neurogenic disease, in which normal or mild to moderate elevations of CK may be seen, and myopathies, in which the CK concentration often is markedly increased. Notable exceptions exist. CK concentrations may be elevated as high as 10 times normal in patients with spinal muscular atrophy and occasionally in those with ALS (see Chapter 74). Measurements of serial CK concentrations follow the progress of the disease. Problems have been recognized with both of these uses. Foremost is the determination of the normal level. A survey of 250 hospitals in Ontario, Canada, showed a surprising ignorance of the basic mechanisms involved in the test and

the way to derive normal values. Some hospital laboratories were unaware that race, gender, age, and activity level are important in determining normal values. Blood samples obtained from truly normal controls and not from inactive hospital patients not showing overt muscle disease show a higher normal serum CK concentration than would be anticipated. Furthermore, all studies on CK concentration show that gender and race affect values. A log transformation does much to convert this to a normal distribution curve, but even then, the results are not perfect.

In a survey of 1500 hospital employees, using carefully standardized methods, it was possible to detect three populations, each with characteristic CK values. The upper limits of normal (97.5th percentile) were as follows:

- Black men only: 520 U/liter
- Black women, non-black men: 345 U/liter
- Non-black women: 145 U/liter

The nonblack population included Hispanics, Asians, and Caucasians. Because expression of the upper limit is as a percentile of the mean, by definition, levels in 2.5% of the normal population will be above that. Although this does not seem like a large proportion, in a town of 100,000, 2500 people would have abnormal levels. The point is that the upper limit of normal CK concentration is not rigid and requires intelligent interpretation. Although the serum CK concentration can be useful in determining the course of an illness, judgment is required because changes in CK values do not always mirror the clinical condition. In treating inflammatory myopathies with immunosuppressive drugs or corticosteroids, a steadily declining CK concentration is a reassurance, whereas concentrations that are creeping back up again when the patient is presumably in remission may be concerning.

Serum CK concentrations are also useful to determine whether an illness is monophasic. A bout of myoglobinuria may be associated with very high concentrations of CK. The concentration then declines steadily by approximately 50% every 2 days. This pattern indicates that a single episode of muscle damage has occurred. Patients with CK concentrations that do not decline in this fashion or that vary from high to low on random days have an ongoing illness. Finally, exercise may cause a marked elevation in CK, which usually peaks 12 to 18 hours after the activity but may occur days later. CK concentrations are more likely to increase in people who are sedentary and then undertake unaccustomed exercise than in a trained individual.

Electromyography

The EMG is an operator-sensitive study, and an experienced electromyographer is essential to perform and interpret an EMG correctly. Chapter 32B discusses the principles of EMG. The EMG study may provide much useful information. An initial step in the assessment of the weak patient is to localize the abnormality in the motor unit: neuropathic, myopathic, or neuromuscular junction. Nerve conduction studies and needle electrode examination are particularly useful for identifying neuropathic disorders and localizing the abnormality to anterior horn cells, roots, plexus, or peripheral nerve territories (see Chapters 74 to 76). Repetitive nerve stimulation and single-fiber EMG can aid in elucidating disorders of the neuromuscular junction. Needle electrode examination may help distinguish between the presence of abnormal muscle versus nerve activity, depending on the presence of acute and chronic denervation, myotonia, neuromyotonia, fasciculations, cramps, and myokymia.

Muscle Biopsy

The use of muscle biopsy is important for establishing the diagnosis in most disorders of the motor unit. Histochemical evaluation is available at most hospitals and is particularly useful, and electron microscopy may provide a specific diagnosis. An important newer aspect of the muscle biopsy study is the analysis of the muscle proteins. Individual muscle proteins, including dystrophin, sarcoglycans, and other structural proteins may be missing in specific illnesses, and the diagnosis is often definitive with these analyses.

Chapter 83 reviews the details of muscle biopsy, but a word about the selection of the muscle to be biopsied is appropriate here. All biopsy procedures carry a risk of sampling error. Not all muscles are equally involved in any given disease, and it is important to select a muscle that is likely to give the most useful information. The gastrocnemius muscle, often chosen for muscle biopsy, is not ideal because it demonstrates a predominance of type 1 fibers in the normal person and often shows denervation changes caused by minor lumbosacral radiculopathy. In addition, it has more than its fair share of random pathological changes, such as fiber necrosis and small inflammatory infiltrates, even when no clinical suspicion of a muscle disease exists. For this reason, it is preferable to select either the quadriceps femoris or the biceps brachii if either of these muscles is weak. A biopsy should never be performed on a muscle that is the site of a recent EMG or intramuscular injection, because these procedures produce focal muscle damage. If such a muscle has to be biopsied, at least 2 to 3 months should elapse after the procedure before the biopsy is performed. In the patient with a relatively acute (duration of weeks) disease, it is wise to select a muscle that is obviously clinically weak. In patients with long-standing disease, it may be better to select a muscle that is almost normal to avoid an "end-stage" muscle. Sometimes an apparently normal muscle is biopsied. For example, in a patient who is suspected of having motor neuron disease and has wasting and weakness of the arms, with EMG changes of denervation in the arms but no apparent denervation of the legs, biopsy of the biceps muscle would show the expected denervation and would add no useful information. Biopsy evidence of denervation in a quadriceps muscle, however, would be consistent with widespread involvement, supporting the diagnosis of motor neuron disease. On the other hand, if biopsy of the quadriceps muscle yielded normal results, this would make the diagnosis of motor neuron disease less likely, because even strong muscles in patients with motor neuron disease usually show some denervation. Motor neuron disease is not usually an indication for biopsy unless the diagnosis is in question.

Genetic Testing

Chapter 40 covers the details of genetic testing and counseling. Genetic analysis has become a routine part of the clinical investigation of neuromuscular disease and in many situations has supplanted muscle biopsy and other diagnostic tests. This is a distinct advantage to the patient if a blood test can substitute for a muscle biopsy. The use of genetic testing for diagnosis in a specific patient implies that the genetic cause of a specific disease is established, and that intragenic probes are available that allow the determination of whether the gene in question is abnormal. Examples of such abnormalities are deletions in the dystrophin gene, seen in many cases of Duchenne muscular dystrophy, and the expansion of the triplet repeat in the myotonic dystrophy gene.

Linkage studies are useful when the gene has a known location, but tests for mutations of the gene itself are not available. The success of such studies depends on having probes that are close to the gene. With use of these closely situated probes, it often can be demonstrated that a person does or does not carry the part of the chromosome on which an involved gene must have occurred in another affected family member. For linkage studies to be successful, a sufficient number of family members both with and without the illness must be available for testing to allow an identification of the segment of the chromosome at fault. Hampering this type of study is the tendency of parts of the chromosome to become detached during meiosis and exchange with parts of another chromosome, a phenomenon known as *recombination*. The closer the probe is to the actual gene, the less likely recombination is to separate them. Genetic counseling based on linkage studies is less likely to be successful when only one or two patients with the illness and few family members are available. It is difficult to keep up with the mushrooming list of genes known to be associated with neuromuscular diseases, yet maintaining current knowledge is imperative if patients are to be provided with suitable advice. Useful references can be found in the journal, *Neuromuscular Disorders*, which carries a list of all known neuromuscular genetic abnormalities each month, and on the websites Online Mendelian Inheritance in Man (www.ncbi.nlm.nih.gov/omim/) and GeneTests-GeneClinics (http://www.ncbi.nlm.nih.gov/sites/GeneTests/).

Exercise Testing

Exercise testing may be an important part of the investigation of muscle disease, particularly in metabolic disorders. The two types of exercise tests used are forearm exercise testing and bicycle exercise ergometry. Forearm (grip) exercise protocols are designed to provide a test of glycolytic pathways, particularly those involved in power exercise. Incremental bicycle ergometry gives additional information regarding the relative use of carbohydrates, fats, and oxygen.

Forearm exercise testing is used in accordance with any of several schedules. The traditional method has been to have the patient grip a dynamometer repetitively, with a blood pressure cuff on the upper arm raised above systolic pressure. The necessity of the blood pressure cuff is now questionable. If the work performed by the patient is sufficiently strenuous, the cuff is unnecessary because the muscle is working at a level that surpasses the ability of bloodborne substances to sustain it. In addition, ischemic exercise may result in rhabdomyolysis in patients with defects in the glycolytic enzyme pathway.

After an adequate level of forceful exercise is maintained for 1 minute, samples of venous blood can be obtained at intervals after exercise to monitor changes in metabolites. In normal persons, the energy for such short-duration work derives from intramuscular glycogen. Thus, lactate forms when exercise is relatively anaerobic, as with strenuous activity. Additionally, serum concentrations of hypoxanthine and ammonia, as well as lactate, are elevated with short-duration strenuous activity. Patients with defects in the glycolytic pathways produce normal to excessive amounts of ammonia and hypoxanthine, but no lactate. Patients with adenylate deaminase deficiency show the reverse: neither ammonia nor hypoxanthine appears, but lactate production is normal. Patients who cannot cooperate with the testing and show poor effort produce neither high lactate nor ammonia concentrations.

In mitochondrial disorders and other instances of metabolic stress, the production of both lactate and hypoxanthine is excessive. More recently, a modified ischemic forearm test has been used as a sensitive and specific screen for mitochondrial disorders. During exercise in normal persons, mitochondrial oxidative phosphorylation increases 100-fold from that measured during rest. In mitochondrial disorders, the disturbed oxidative phosphorylation results in an impaired systemic oxygen extraction. In one study comparing 12 patients with mitochondrial myopathy, 10 patients with muscular dystrophy and 12 healthy subjects, measurement was made of cubital venous oxygen saturation after 3 minutes at 40% of maximal voluntary contraction of the exercised arm. Oxygen desaturation in venous blood from exercising muscle was markedly lower in patients with mitochondrial myopathy than in patients with other muscle diseases and healthy subjects. Measurement of serum lactate was not reliable at differentiating patients with mitochondrial myopathy from normal subjects.

Incremental bicycle ergometry allows the measurement of oxygen consumption and carbon dioxide production associated with varying workloads. The patient pedals a bicycle at a steady rate. The workload is increased every minute or two. Excessive oxygen consumption for a given work level suggests an abnormality in the energy pathway in muscle. In addition, the *respiratory exchange ratio* (RER)—the ratio of carbon dioxide produced to oxygen consumed—is characteristic for various fuel sources. Carbohydrate metabolism results in an RER of 1.0. Fat, on the other hand, has an RER of 0.7. The resting RER in normal persons is approximately 0.8. For complex reasons, at the end of an incremental exercise test in normal volunteers, the RER can be as high as 1.2. Patients with disorders of lipid metabolism often have an unusually high RER because they preferentially metabolize carbohydrates, whereas patients with disorders of carbohydrate metabolism may never increase RER to more than 1.0 because they preferentially metabolize lipids.

Differential Diagnosis by Affected Region and Other Manifestations of Weakness

Once the presence of weakness has been established by means of either the history or physical examination, the clinical features may be so characteristic that the diagnosis is obvious. At other times, the cause of the weakness may be less certain. **Fig. 25.6** displays an outline of diagnostic considerations based on

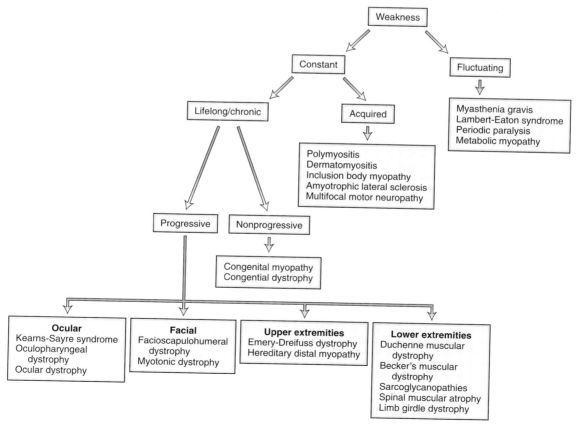

Fig. 25.6 Algorithm for the diagnostic approach to the patient with weakness.

the characteristics of the weakness, such as whether it is fluctuating or constant. This approach can be used in the differential diagnosis of weakness affecting specific body regions and with other manifestations of weakness, as described next.

Disorders with Prominent Ocular Weakness

In *oculopharyngeal muscular dystrophy*, slowly progressive weakness of the eye muscles, causing ptosis and external ophthalmoplegia, is associated with difficulty in swallowing. This disorder is inherited as an autosomal dominant condition, with symptom onset usually after the age of 50 years. Many patients also have facial weakness and hip and shoulder weakness. Swallowing difficulty may become severe enough to necessitate cricopharyngeal myotomy or gastrostomy tube placement; however, lifespan in this condition appears to be normal.

Kearns-Sayre syndrome is a distinctive collection of features including ptosis, external ophthalmoplegia, cardiac conduction defects, pigmentary degeneration of the retina, cerebellar ataxia, pyramidal tract signs, short stature, and mental retardation, with symptom onset before age 20 years. These findings accompany an abnormality of the mitochondria in muscle and other tissues. Kearns-Sayre syndrome usually is sporadic. It may be slowly progressive or nonprogressive. Other mitochondrial disorders also may include external ophthalmoplegia as a feature.

In addition, several other disorders may display prominent extraocular muscle involvement. Among these is *centronuclear myopathy*, one of the congenital myopathies. This condition is not restricted to the eye muscles and has prominent involvement of the limbs as well. External ophthalmoplegia of subacute progressive onset, with or without other bulbar and limb muscle involvement, may occur in variant forms of

Guillain-Barré syndrome (i.e., Miller Fisher syndrome) and in botulism. Finally, isolated ptosis or extraocular muscle weakness often is a presenting feature of MG and occasionally of Lambert-Eaton myasthenic syndrome.

Disorders with Distinctive Facial or Bulbar Weakness

The diagnosis of *FSH muscular dystrophy* may be delayed until early adult life. Weakness of the face may lead to difficulty with whistling or blowing up balloons and may be severe enough to give the face a smooth, unlined appearance with an abnormal pout to the lips (**Fig. 25.7, A**). Weakness of the muscles around the shoulders is constant, although the deltoid muscle is surprisingly well preserved and even pseudohypertrophic in its lower portion. When the patient attempts to hold the arms extended in front, winging of the scapula occurs that is quite characteristic. The whole scapula may slide upward on the back of the thorax. The inferomedial border always juts backward, producing the appearance of a triangle at right angles to the back, with the base of the triangle still attached to the thorax. In addition, a discrepancy in power often occurs between the wrist flexors, which are strong, and the wrist extensors, which are weak. Similarly, the plantar flexors may be strong, whereas the dorsiflexors of the ankles are weak. It is common for the weakness to be asymmetrical, with one side much less involved than the other (**Fig. 25.8**). Inheritance of the disorder is as an autosomal dominant trait, although mild forms of the illness often are asymptomatic.

Myotonic dystrophy type I is a common illness with distinctive features including distal predominance of weakness. Inheritance is as an autosomal dominant trait, but often the family history is negative because patients may be unaware that other family members have the illness. This is due to the

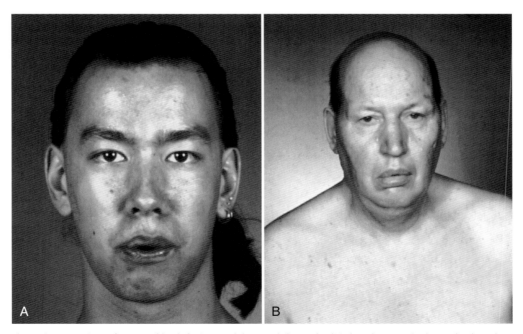

Fig. 25.7 Facial weakness is a prominent feature of both facioscapulohumeral dystrophy (FSH) and myotonic dystrophy, but characteristic features of each are so distinctive that the conditions are readily recognizable and not easily confused. **A,** Patient with FSH dystrophy is unable to purse the lips when attempting to whistle. **B,** Typical appearance of a patient with myotonic dystrophy is marked by frontal balding, temporalis muscle wasting, ptosis, and facial weakness. Related to FSH dystrophy is scapuloperoneal dystrophy, which has similar features but lacks the facial weakness.

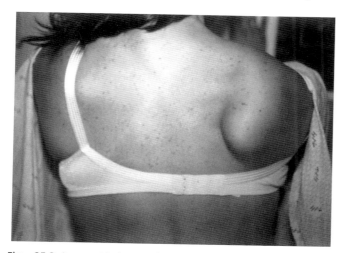

Fig. 25.8 Asymmetrical scapular winging in facioscapulohumeral muscular dystrophy.

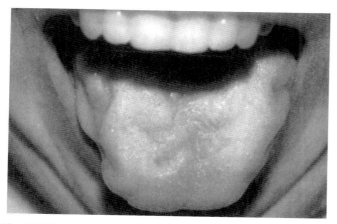

Fig. 25.9 Tongue atrophy in a patient with amyotrophic lateral sclerosis. *(Reprinted with permission from Katirji, B., Kaminski, H.J., Preston, D.C., et al., (Eds.), 2002. Neuromuscular Disorders in Clinical Practice. Butterworth Heinemann, Boston.)*

phenomenon of *anticipation*, whereby more severe syndromes appear in successive generations because of the expansion of the trinucleotide repeat. This diagnosis is suggested in any patient with muscular dystrophy and predominantly distal weakness. The neck flexors and temporalis and masseter muscles often are wasted. More characteristic than the distribution of the weakness is the long, thin face with hollowed temples, ptosis, and frontal balding (see **Fig. 25.7, B**). Percussion myotonia and grip myotonia occur in most patients after the age of 13 years. An EMG study can be diagnostic. Muscle biopsy usually is not necessary but may show characteristic changes. Genetic testing is now preferred to muscle biopsy for diagnosis of the disorder and is almost 100% accurate. The genetic defect is an amplified trinucleotide repeat in the 3′ untranslated region of the myotonin–protein kinase gene on chromosome 19.

A subset of patients with ALS present with isolated bulbar weakness of LMN type (i.e., progressive bulbar palsy) or UMN type (i.e., progressive pseudobulbar palsy). Frequently the condition shows a combination of UMN and LMN involvement. In these patients, dysarthria, dysphagia, and difficulty with secretions are the prominent symptoms. On examination, the tongue often is atrophic and fasciculating (**Fig. 25.9**), and the

jaw and facial reflexes are exaggerated. The voice often is harsh and strained as well as slurred, reflecting the coexistent UMN and LMN dysfunction. In patients with X-linked spinobulbar muscular atrophy (Kennedy disease), bulbofacial muscles also are prominently affected. Patients often have a characteristic finding of chin fasciculations.

Disorders with Prominent Respiratory Weakness

Disorders with prominent respiratory muscle weakness include inherited and acquired myopathies, disorders of the neuromuscular junction or peripheral nerves, motor neuronopathies, and CNS processes involving the brainstem or high cervical spinal cord. Adult-onset acid maltase deficiency (i.e., adult-onset Pompe disease), a glycogen storage disorder, frequently manifests with respiratory system–related symptoms of dyspnea or excessive daytime sleepiness, although proximal muscle weakness is present in most patients. Chronic progressive respiratory weakness occurs in Duchenne muscular dystrophy late in the course. In the intensive care unit (ICU) setting, critical illness myopathy may result in difficulty weaning from a ventilator, although limb muscles also are weak in this condition. Myasthenia gravis occasionally manifests with respiratory failure, although usually myasthenic crisis occurs in patients already known to have myasthenia. Botulism results in respiratory compromise when severe, but the onset usually is stereotypical, with oculobulbar weakness followed by descending weakness, aiding in diagnosis. Guillain-Barré syndrome is a frequent cause of neuromuscular respiratory failure, with subacute onset of ascending weakness and numbness as the most common presentation. ALS leads to respiratory muscle weakness, usually late in the course of the disease. The occasional patient with weakness in the ICU setting, however, is found to have ALS after evaluation for failure to wean from a ventilator. In a patient with limb and respiratory muscle weakness but normal bulbar muscle strength, the possibility of a high cervical cord lesion should be considered.

Disorders with Distinctive Shoulder-Girdle or Arm Weakness

In *Emery-Dreifuss muscular dystrophy*, clinical features include prominent early contractures of the elbows, posterior neck, and Achilles tendons, with atrophy and weakness of muscles around the shoulders, upper arms, and lower part of the legs. Cardiac conduction abnormalities are common, and acute heart block is a frequent cause of death.

Distal muscular weakness and atrophy are most common in neurogenic disorders. Among these is Charcot-Marie-Tooth disease, which usually manifests with distal weakness and wasting that starts in the distal lower limbs before involving the hands. ALS often begins as weakness and wasting in one distal limb. More important to identify, because it is treatable, is multifocal motor neuropathy with conduction block, a rare demyelinating polyneuropathy that may be confused clinically with ALS with LMN dysfunction. The initial features often are weakness, hyporeflexia, and fasciculations, especially of the hands. Clues to the diagnosis are a slow indolent course, weakness out of proportion to the amount of atrophy, and asymmetrical involvement of muscles of the same myotome but with a different peripheral nerve supply (e.g., weakness of ulnar nerve–innervated C8 muscles out of proportion to weakness of median nerve–innervated C8 muscles). Benign focal amyotrophy, also known as *Sobue disease* or *monomelic amyotrophy*, manifests with the insidious onset of weakness and atrophy of the hand and forearm muscles, predominantly in men between the ages of 18 and 22 years.

Distal muscular dystrophies that may manifest with upper-extremity complaints include myotonic dystrophy, discussed earlier, and *Welander myopathy*, a hereditary distal myopathy. Welander myopathy, transmitted as an autosomal dominant trait, has a predilection for the finger and wrist extensor muscles. Other hereditary distal myopathies typically present first in the lower extremities.

Insidious onset of weakness of the finger flexors with relative preservation of finger extensor strength is common in *inclusion-body myositis*, a condition that generally manifests after the age of 50 years. In patients with this disorder, however, weakness is also prominent in the lower extremities, especially the quadriceps.

Disorders with Prominent Hip-Girdle or Leg Weakness

Although patients with these disorders often have diffuse weakness including arm and shoulder-girdle weakness, hip and leg weakness brings them to medical attention.

The SMAs are hereditary neuronopathies manifesting with prominent proximal weakness. The atrophy results from the death of anterior horn cells in the spinal cord. This condition spares extraocular muscles, and reflexes are absent. The classification of the SMAs is by age at onset and severity; most forms share a defect in the survival motor neuron gene on chromosome 5q and are of autosomal recessive inheritance. Acute infantile SMA (*Werdnig-Hoffmann disease*) is a severe and usually fatal illness characterized by marked weakness of the limbs and respiratory muscles. Children with the intermediate form of SMA (chronic Werdnig-Hoffmann disease or spinal muscular atrophy type 2) also have severe weakness, rarely maintaining the ability to walk for more than a few years. The progression of the illness is not steady. The condition may plateau for some years, with periods of more rapid deterioration. Scoliosis is common. A fine tremor of the outstretched hands is characteristic. The chronic juvenile form of SMA (*Kugelberg-Welander syndrome*) begins sometime during the first decade of life, and patients walk well into the second decade or even into early adult life. Scoliosis is less common than in the infantile form. This condition is consistent with a normal lifespan. Finally, adult-onset SMA leads to slowly progressive proximal muscle weakness after the age of 20 years.

The inherited muscular dystrophies cause progressive, nonfluctuating weakness. Aside from the inherited distal muscular dystrophies discussed earlier in the chapter, other muscular dystrophies manifest with proximal muscle weakness. *Duchenne muscular dystrophy*, inherited as an X-linked recessive trait, is associated with an absence of dystrophin. Clinically, the combination of proximal weakness in a male child with hypertrophic calf muscles and contractures of the Achilles tendons gives the clue to the diagnosis. The serum CK concentration is markedly elevated. Although muscle biopsy is diagnostic, genetic testing is now preferred to confirm the diagnosis (see Chapter 40). The clinical features of *Becker muscular dystrophy* are identical except for later onset and slower progression. Cardiomyopathy also is a feature. Female carriers of the gene usually are free of symptoms but may present with limb-girdle distribution weakness or cardiomyopathy.

The limb-girdle dystrophies constitute a well-accepted diagnostic classification despite their clinical and genetic heterogeneity. Weakness begins in the hips, shoulders, or both and spreads gradually to involve the rest of the limbs and the trunk. Knowledge concerning the genetics of these disorders recently expanded (see Chapter 40), and genetic testing is now available for some limb-girdle dystrophies.

Severe early-onset limb-girdle dystrophy similar in phenotype to Duchenne muscular dystrophy, including calf hypertrophy, occurs in the *sarcoglycanopathies*. The cause is a deficiency in one of the dystrophin-associated glycoproteins (sarcoglycans α, β, γ, and δ). The inheritance pattern in these disorders is autosomal recessive, not X-linked, and the sarcoglycanopathies affect both genders equally. Cardiac involvement is rare, and mental retardation is not part of the phenotype. Another cause of a severe Duchenne-like phenotype is mutation of the FKRP gene, also inherited in an autosomal recessive manner.

With less severe limb-girdle phenotypes, several genetic causes have been recognized, and inheritance is both autosomal recessive and autosomal dominant. In general, the phenotype in the autosomal recessive group is clinically more severe, with earlier onset of weakness and more rapid progression.

Diagnostic evaluation of limb-girdle muscular dystrophies is rapidly evolving and covered in greater depth in Chapter 79. Genetic testing for dystrophin, sarcoglycans, and other genes may be appropriate before performance of muscle biopsy. If the appropriate genetic tests are uninformative, then muscle biopsy is indicated. The biopsy specimen will show dystrophic changes, separating limb-girdle dystrophy from other (inflammatory) myopathies and from denervating diseases such as SMA. Immunohistochemical analysis of dystrophic muscle may provide a specific diagnosis, but not in all cases. Unfortunately, many patients with limb-girdle muscular dystrophies do not receive a specific diagnosis.

With the exception of Welander myopathy, predominantly lower-extremity weakness is the usual presentation of hereditary distal myopathies. Among these disorders are the Markesbery-Griggs-Udd, Nonaka, and Laing myopathies, which affect anterior compartment muscles in the leg, and Miyoshi myopathy, which affects predominantly the posterior calf muscles.

In patients with inclusion-body myositis, the quadriceps and forearm finger flexor muscles often are preferentially involved. In some patients, this involvement may be asymmetrical at the onset. The other inflammatory myopathies—polymyositis and dermatomyositis—affect proximal, predominantly hip-girdle muscles in a symmetrical fashion. Although rare, the Lambert-Eaton myasthenic syndrome manifests with proximal lower-extremity weakness in more than half of patients, similar to a myopathy. Hyporeflexia and autonomic and sensory symptoms may suggest the diagnosis. EMG often is diagnostic.

Ascending weakness of subacute onset with hyporeflexia, usually with numbness, is the hallmark of Guillain-Barré syndrome. The examiner should take care to look for a spinal sensory level and UMN signs, because a spinal cord lesion can mimic this presentation. When present, bulbar weakness is helpful in the diagnosis. Respiratory weakness may result. As discussed earlier, multiple neuromuscular causes of weakness of subacute onset with respiratory failure are recognized.

Distal muscle weakness and atrophy are the hallmarks of neurogenic disorders. In both the demyelinating and axonal forms of Charcot-Marie-Tooth disease, the problem in the legs antedates that in the hands. In ALS, the weakness often is asymmetrical and may combine with UMN signs.

Disorders with Fluctuating Weakness

An important consideration in the differential diagnosis is whether the weakness is constant or fluctuating. Even constant weakness may vary somewhat in degree, depending on how the patient feels. It is well recognized that an individual's physical performance is better on days when they feel energetic and cheerful and is less optimal on days when they feel depressed or are sick. Such factors also can be expected to affect the patient with neuromuscular weakness. The examiner should make specific inquiries to determine how much variability exists. Does the strength fluctuation relate to exercise or time of day? Symptoms and signs provoked by exercise imply a disorder in the physiological or biochemical mechanisms governing muscle contraction. Pain, contractures, and weakness after exercise often are characteristic of abnormalities in the biochemistry of muscle contraction. Pathological fatigue is the hallmark of neuromuscular junction abnormalities.

Factors other than exercise may result in worsening or improvement of the disease. Some patients notice that fasting, carbohydrate loading, or other dietary manipulations make a difference in their symptoms. Such details may provide a clue to underlying metabolic problems. Patients with a defect in lipid-based energy metabolism are weaker in the fasting state and may carry a candy bar or sugar with them. The patient with hypokalemic periodic paralysis may notice that inactivity after a high-carbohydrate meal precipitates an attack.

The usual cause of weakness that fluctuates markedly on a day-to-day basis or within a space of several hours is a defect in neuromuscular transmission or a metabolic abnormality (e.g., periodic paralysis), rather than one of the muscular dystrophies. Most neurologists recognize that the cardinal features of MG are ptosis, ophthalmoparesis, dysarthria, dysphagia, and proximal weakness (see Chapter 78). On clinical examination, the hallmark of MG is pathological muscle fatigue. Normal muscles fatigue if exercised sufficiently, but in MG, fatigue occurs with little effort. Failure of neuromuscular transmission may prevent holding the arms in an outstretched position for more than a few seconds or maintenance of sustained upgaze. Frequently the patient is relatively normal in the office, making the diagnosis of myasthenia more difficult; the history and ancillary studies (assay for acetylcholine receptor antibodies, anti-MuSK antibodies, and EMG with repetitive stimulation or single-fiber EMG) must be relied on to establish the diagnosis.

In the Lambert-Eaton myasthenic syndrome, fluctuating weakness also may occur, but the fluctuating character is less marked than in MG. Weakness of the shoulder and especially the hip girdle predominates, with the bulbar, ocular, and respiratory muscles relatively spared. Exceptions to this latter rule have been recognized, and some presentations of Lambert-Eaton myasthenic syndrome mimic MG. Typically, reflexes are reduced or absent at rest. After a brief period of exercise, weakness and reflexes often are improved (facilitation), which is the opposite of the situation in MG. The electrophysiological correlate of this phenomenon is the demonstration of a marked incremental response to rapid, repetitive nerve stimulation or brief exercise. The underlying pathophysiology of Lambert-Eaton myasthenic syndrome is an autoimmune or paraneoplastic process mediated by anti–voltage-gated calcium channel antibodies; commercial testing for these antibodies is available.

Patients with periodic paralysis note attacks of weakness, typically provoked by rest after exercise (see Chapter 78). Inheritance of the primary periodic paralyses is as an autosomal dominant trait secondary to a sodium or calcium channel defect (see Chapter 64). In the hyperkalemic (sodium channel) form, patients experience weakness that may last from minutes to days; beginning in infancy to early childhood, the provocation is by rest after exercise or potassium ingestion. Potassium levels generally are high during an attack. In the hypokalemic (calcium channel) form, weakness may last hours to days, is quite severe beginning in the early teens, manifests more in males than in females, and the provocation is by rest after exercise or carbohydrate ingestion. Potassium levels generally are low during an attack.

Secondary hypokalemic periodic paralysis occurs in a subset of patients with thyrotoxicosis. The syndrome is clinically identical to primary hypokalemic periodic paralysis, except for the age at presentation, which usually is in adulthood. In both types of primary periodic paralysis, paralysis may be total, but with sparing of bulbofacial muscles. Respiratory muscle paralysis is rare in hypokalemic periodic paralysis. Patients with paramyotonia congenita also may experience attacks of weakness, especially in the cold. EMG with special protocols for exercise and cooling may be diagnostic; genetic testing also is available for these disorders.

Disorders Exacerbated by Exercise

Fatigue and muscle pain provoked by exercise, the most common complaints in patients presenting to the muscle clinic, often are unexplained. Diagnoses such as fibromyalgia (see Chapter 26) may confound the examination. Biochemical defects are being detected in an increasing number of patients with exercise-induced fatigue and myalgia. The metabolic abnormalities that impede exercise are disorders of carbohydrate metabolism, lipid metabolism, and mitochondrial function (see Chapter 79). The patient's history may give some clue to the type of defect.

Fatty acids provide the main source of energy for resting muscle. Initiation of vigorous exercise requires the use of intracellular stores of energy because bloodborne metabolites initially are inadequate. It takes time for the cardiac output to increase, for capillaries to dilate, and for the blood supply to muscle to be increased, and an even longer time to mobilize fat stores in the body in order to increase the level of fatty acids in the blood. Because muscle must use its glycogen stores for energy in this initial phase of heavy exercise, defects of glycogen metabolism cause fatigue and muscle pain in the first few minutes of exercise. As exercise continues, the blood supply increases, resulting in an increased supply of oxygen, glucose, and fatty acids. After 10 to 15 minutes, the muscle begins to use a mixture of fat and carbohydrate. The use of carbohydrate is not tolerated for long periods, however, because it would deplete the body's glycogen stores, potentially resulting in hypoglycemia. After 30 to 40 minutes of continued endurance exercise, the muscle is using chiefly fatty acids as an energy source. Patients with defective fatty acid metabolism easily tolerate the initial phase of exercise. With endurance exercise lasting 30 to 60 minutes, however, they may become incapacitated. Similarly, in the fasting state, the body is more dependent on fatty acids, which it uses to conserve glucose. Thus, the patient with a disorder of fatty acid metabolism may complain of increased symptoms when exercising in the fasting state. Ingestion of a candy bar may give some relief because this quickly boosts the blood glucose level. Patients with fatty acid metabolism defects often have well-developed muscles, because they prefer relatively intense, brief, power exercise such as weight lifting.

Disorders of mitochondrial metabolism vary in presentation. In some types, recurrent encephalopathic episodes occur, often noted in early childhood and resembling Reye disease (see Chapter 63). In other types, particular weakness of the extraocular and skeletal muscles is a presenting feature. In still other types, usually affecting young adults, the symptoms are predominantly of exercise intolerance. Defects occur in the electron transport system or cytochrome chain that uncouples oxygen consumption from the useful production of adenosine triphosphate (ATP). The resulting limit on available ATP causes metabolic pathways to operate at their maximum with even a light exercise load. Resting tachycardia, high lactic acid levels in the blood, excessive sweating, and other indications of hypermetabolism may be noted. This clinical picture may lead to an erroneous diagnosis of hyperthyroidism. It is essential always to measure the serum lactic acid concentration when a mitochondrial myopathy is suspected, even though the level is normal in some patients. In addition to lactate, ammonia and hypoxanthine concentrations also may be elevated.

Patients with suspected metabolic defects should undergo forearm exercise testing. A blood pressure cuff should not be used for the ischemic portion of the test, because this may be hazardous in patients with defects in the glycolytic pathway.

Disorders with Constant Weakness

With disorders characterized by constant weakness, the course is one of stability or steady deterioration. Without treatment, periods of sustained objective improvement or major differences in strength on a day-to-day basis are lacking. The division of this group of disorders into subacute and chronic also needs clarification. *Subacute* means that weakness appeared over weeks to months in a previously healthy person. In contrast, *chronic* implies a much less definite onset and prolonged course. Although the patient may say that the weakness came on suddenly, a careful history elicits symptoms that go back many years. This division is not absolute. Patients with polymyositis, usually a subacute disease, may have a slow course mimicking a muscular dystrophy. Patients with a muscular dystrophy may have a slow decrease in

strength but suddenly lose a specific function such as standing from a chair or climbing stairs and believe their deterioration to be acute in onset.

Acquired Disorders Causing Weakness

The usual acquired disorders that produce weakness are motor neuron diseases; inflammatory, toxic, or endocrine disorders of muscle; neuromuscular transmission disorders; and peripheral neuropathies with predominantly motor involvement. The first task is to determine whether the weakness is neuropathic, myopathic, or secondary to a neuromuscular transmission defect. In some instances this is straightforward, and in others it is very difficult. For instance, some cases of motor neuron disease with predominantly LMN dysfunction may mimic inclusion-body myositis, and Lambert-Eaton myasthenic syndrome may mimic polymyositis. If fasciculations are present, the disorder must be neuropathic. If reflexes are absent and muscle bulk is preserved, suspect a demyelinating neuropathy, although presynaptic neuromuscular junction disorders (e.g., Lambert-Eaton myasthenic syndrome) also show hyporeflexia with normal muscle bulk. The presence of sensory signs or symptoms, even if mild, may indicate a peripheral neuropathy or involvement of the CNS. Often, separating these conditions requires serum CK testing, EMG, and muscle biopsy.

ALS is the most common acquired motor neuron disease. Although peak age at onset is from 65 to 70 years, the disorder can occur at any adult age. It often follows a relatively rapid course preceded by cramps and fasciculations. Examination shows muscle atrophy and often widely distributed fasciculations. If the bulbar muscles are involved, difficulties with swallowing and speaking also are present. The diagnosis is relatively simple if unequivocal evidence of UMN dysfunction accompanies muscle atrophy and fasciculations. UMN signs include slowness of movement, hyperreflexia, Babinski sign, and spasticity. A weak, atrophic muscle associated with an abnormally brisk reflex is almost pathognomonic for ALS. The finding of widespread denervation on needle electrode examination in the absence of any sensory abnormalities or demyelinating features on nerve conduction testing supports the diagnosis. In all patients without bulbar involvement, it is important to rule out spinal pathology, because the combination of cervical and lumbar stenosis occasionally may mimic ALS with respect to clinical and electrophysiological findings.

In patients with only LMN dysfunction, it is essential to exclude the rare diagnosis of *multifocal motor neuropathy with conduction block*, a condition usually treatable with intravenous gamma globulin. Patients with multifocal motor neuropathy with conduction block usually have no bulbar features or UMN signs, and a characteristic finding includes demyelination (i.e., conduction block) on motor nerve conduction testing. Because the underlying pathophysiological process is conduction block, weakness usually is more severe than expected for the observed degree of atrophy. However, atrophy occurs, especially when the condition is of long duration.

Although most adults with motor neuron disease have ALS or one of its variants, sporadic forms of adult-onset SMA and especially X-linked spinobulbar muscular atrophy (Kennedy disease) can occur as well. In these cases, the progression of weakness is much slower, and UMN involvement is absent. Of importance, these latter cases, especially Kennedy disease, often have elevated CK levels in the range of 500 to 1500 U/liter.

If the patient has a myopathy, acquired and inherited causes should be considered. A discussion of the presentation of inherited myopathic disorders appears earlier in the chapter. Causes of acquired myopathies include inflammatory conditions and a large number of toxic, drug-induced, and endocrine disorders. Inflammatory myopathies include polymyositis, dermatomyositis, and inclusion-body myositis and often run a steadily progressive course, although some fluctuations occur, particularly in children. Onset of weakness in polymyositis and dermatomyositis is subacute, weakness is proximal, and serum CK levels usually are increased. If an associated rash is present, little doubt exists about the diagnosis of dermatomyositis. In its absence, polymyositis may be difficult to differentiate from any of the other causes of proximal weakness. Sometimes the illness occurs as part of an overlap syndrome in which fragments of other autoimmune diseases (e.g., scleroderma, lupus, rheumatoid arthritis) are involved. Polymyositis sometimes is difficult to differentiate from a muscular dystrophy, even after muscle biopsy; some inflammatory changes occur in muscular dystrophies, most notably in FSH muscular dystrophy. Other signs of systemic involvement such as malaise, transitory aching pains, mood changes, and loss of appetite are more common in polymyositis than in limb-girdle dystrophy.

Inclusion-body myopathy typically has a chronic, insidious onset. It occasionally mimics polymyositis but more often mimics ALS associated with LMN dysfunction. Clues to the diagnosis are male gender, onset after the age of 50 years in most patients, slower progression, and characteristic involvement of the quadriceps and long finger flexors. Some patients may have proximal muscle weakness, as in polymyositis, whereas others may have predominantly distal weakness mimicking that of ALS and other neuropathic conditions. Serum CK generally is elevated but occasionally may be normal. As with other chronic inflammatory myopathies, interpreting the EMG study may be difficult and requires an experienced examiner, because inclusion-body myopathy often shows a combination of myopathic and neuropathic features. Inclusion-body myopathy, unlike polymyositis, often is unresponsive to immunosuppressive therapy. Pathological features include rimmed vacuoles and intracytoplasmic and intranuclear filamentous inclusions.

Toxic, drug-induced, and endocrine disorders are always considerations in the differential diagnosis for acquired myopathies. Among toxins, alcohol is still one of the most common and may produce both an acute and a chronic myopathic syndrome. Several prescription medicines are associated with myopathies. Most prominent are corticosteroids, cholesterol-lowering agents (i.e., statins), and colchicine.

Although neuromuscular transmission disorders are always diagnostic considerations in patients with fluctuating symptoms, the Lambert-Eaton myasthenic syndrome may be an exception. It often manifests with progressive proximal lower-extremity weakness without fluctuations. Clues to the diagnosis include a history of cancer, especially small-cell lung cancer (although in many patients the myasthenic syndrome may predate the discovery of the cancer), hyporeflexia, facilitation of strength and reflexes after brief exercise, and coexistent autonomic symptoms, especially urinary and sexual dysfunction in men.

Sensory features separate peripheral neuropathies from disorders of the motor unit. The notable exception is multifocal motor neuropathy with conduction block, discussed earlier. Other neuropathies also may manifest with predominantly motor symptoms. Among these are toxic neuropathies (from dapsone, vincristine, or lead, or an acute alcohol-related neuropathy) and some variants of Guillain-Barré syndrome (especially the acute motor axonal neuropathy syndrome).

Lifelong Disorders

Most patients presenting to the neuromuscular clinic will have lifelong or at least very chronic, presumably inherited, disorders. These include inherited disorders of muscle (e.g., dystrophies, congenital myopathies), anterior horn cell (e.g., spinal muscular atrophies), peripheral nerves (e.g., Charcot-Marie-Tooth polyneuropathy), or very rarely, neuromuscular transmission (e.g., congenital myasthenic syndromes). In some of these disorders, the responsible genetic abnormality has been identified. An important point in the differential diagnosis is to determine whether the weakness is truly progressive. The examiner should ask questions until the progressive or nonprogressive nature of the disease is ascertained. The severity of the disease is not proof of progression. It is difficult to imagine that a 16-year-old girl confined to her wheelchair with spinal muscular atrophy and scoliosis and having difficulty breathing has a relatively nonprogressive disorder, but careful questioning may reveal no loss of function for several years. Furthermore, it is not sufficient to ask the patient in vague and general terms whether the illness is progressive. Questioning should be specific; for example, "Are there tasks you cannot perform now that you could perform last week (month, year)?" The examiner also must be alert for denial, which is common in young patients with increasing weakness. The 18-year-old boy with limb-girdle dystrophy may claim to be the same now as in years gone by, but questioning may reveal that he was able to climb stairs well when he was in high school, whereas he now needs assistance in college.

Lifelong Nonprogressive Disorders

Some patients complain of lifelong weakness that has been relatively unchanged over many years. Almost by definition, such disorders have to start in early childhood. Nonprogression of weakness does not preclude severe weakness. Later-life progression of such weakness may occur as the normal aging process further weakens muscles that have little functional reserve. One major group of such illnesses is the congenital nonprogressive myopathies, including central core disease, nemaline myopathy, and congenital fiber-type disproportion. The typical clinical picture in these diseases is that of a slender dysmorphic patient with diffuse weakness (**Fig. 25.10**). Other features may include skeletal abnormalities such as high-arched palate, pes cavus, and scoliosis, which are supportive of the presence of weakness in early life. Deep tendon reflexes are depressed or absent. Though unusual, severe respiratory involvement may occur in all these diseases. The less severe (non-X-linked) form of myotubular (centronuclear) myopathy is suggested by findings of ptosis, extraocular muscle weakness, and facial diplegia. Muscle biopsy usually provides a specific morphological diagnosis in the congenital

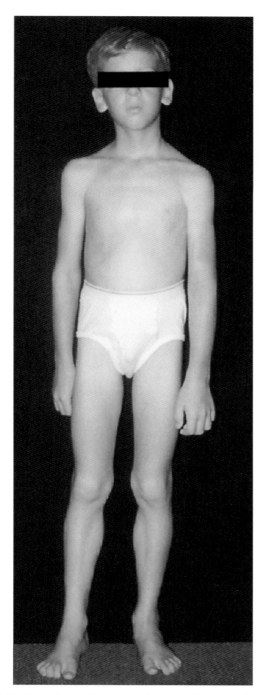

Fig. 25.10 The patient with a congenital myopathy is slender, without focal atrophy. Shoulder-girdle weakness is apparent from the horizontal set of the clavicles.

myopathies; specific genetic testing is now available for some congenital myopathies.

Several varieties of congenital muscular dystrophy (CMD) are recognized. The weakness in CMD manifests in the newborn period, with the affected child presenting as a floppy baby. Arthrogryposis may be present. The current classification is based on the presence or absence of associated structural CNS abnormalities. Such disorders without CNS defects constitute *classic CMD*. These disorders are subdivided into *merosin-positive* and *merosin-negative* disorders. Patients with classic CMD who are merosin-positive have the mildest phenotype. The disorders with CNS structural abnormalities are very severe; for example, characteristics of Fukuyama CMD include microcephaly, mental retardation, and seizures with severe disability. The serum CK concentration may be markedly elevated in CMDs. The muscle biopsy specimen shows dystrophic changes, and immunohistochemistry often provides a specific diagnosis.

Lifelong Disorders Characterized by Progressive Weakness

Most diseases in the category of lifelong disorders characterized by progressive weakness are inherited progressive disorders of anterior horn cells, peripheral motor nerve, or muscle. Among these are the spinal muscular atrophies, Charcot-Marie-Tooth polyneuropathies, and muscular dystrophies. Mild day-to-day fluctuations in strength may occur in these disorders, but the overall progression is steady (i.e., the disorder is slowly progressive from the start and remains that way); it will not suddenly change course and become rapidly progressive. As mentioned earlier, patients may experience long periods of stability when their disease is seemingly nonprogressive.

Traditional attempts to categorize disorders are based on whether the disorder is caused by anterior horn cell, peripheral motor nerve, or muscle disease, along with a specific pattern of muscle weakness. Certain characteristic patterns of weakness often suggest specific diagnoses. For example, the names of FSH and oculopharyngeal muscular dystrophies reflect their selective involvement of muscles. Today, all disorders are redefined and categorized in accordance with their specific genetic abnormality.

Other Conditions

No scheme of analysis is perfect in clinical medicine, and many exceptions to the guidelines provided earlier will exist. Most notable are disorders restricted to various parts of the body. The etiology for such localized illness is unclear, but examples are branchial myopathy and quadriceps myopathy, as well as the focal forms of motor neuron disease such as benign monomelic amyotrophy. These diseases often are "benign" in that they do not shorten life. The weakness may cause disability, although it usually is mild.

References

The complete reference list is available online at www.expertconsult.com.

Muscle Pain and Cramps

Leo H. Wang, Alan Pestronk

General Features of Pain

Pain is an uncomfortable sensation with sensory and emotional components. Short episodes of pain or discomfort localized to muscle are a universal experience. Common causes of short-term muscle discomfort are unaccustomed exercise, trauma, cramps, and systemic infections. Chronic muscle discomfort is also relatively common. In the population of the United States aged 25 to 74 years, 10% to 14% have chronic pain related to the joints and musculoskeletal system. Pain localized to muscle may be due to noxious stimuli in muscle or to referral from other structures including nerves, connective tissue, joints, and bone. Common syndromes with pain localized to muscle but no histological muscle pathology include fibromyalgia and small-fiber polyneuropathies. The referral of pain from other structures to muscle may involve stimulation of central neural pathways or secondary noxious contraction of muscle.

The best categorization of pain in muscle and other tissues is by temporal and qualitative features. Pain elicited by noxious stimulation of normal tissue has an early first phase perceived as sharp, well-localized, and lasting as long as the stimulus. A delayed second phase of pain follows that is dull, aching or burning, and more diffuse. Second-phase pain has both sensory and affective components and may predominate with visceral, muscle, and chronic pain. Pain from stimulation of diseased tissue is often associated with *hyperalgesia*, in which a noxious stimulus produces an exaggerated pain sensation, or with *allodynia*, pain induced by a normally innocuous stimulus. Neuropathic pain localized to muscle or other tissues is associated with increased afferent axon activity and occurs spontaneously or after peripheral stimuli.

Muscle Pain: Basic Concepts

Muscle pain is a neuropathic process. Pain generation involves activation of afferent axons, conduction of pain signals through the peripheral and central nervous systems (PNS, CNS), and central processing of varied properties of the afferent signals. The sensation of muscle pain probably represents a summation of afferent signals from a widespread area.

Nociceptor Terminal Stimulation and Sensitization

Stimuli of afferent axons can be chemical and mechanical. Increased levels of glutamate in muscle correlate temporally with the appearance of pain after exercise or experimental injections of hypertonic saline. Glutamate injection into muscle in humans both produces pain and sensitizes muscle afferents to other stimuli. Some mechanosensitive unmyelinated afferent axons in muscle are stimulated by acromelic acid-A, a kainoid mushroom toxin that produces long-lasting allodynia and burning pain when ingested. The injection of acid (H^+) into skeletal muscle elicits pain. Acid-sensing ion channel 3 (ASIC3) channels are expressed on sensory neurons innervating skeletal and cardiac muscle. H^+ ions may produce muscle pain by activating ASIC3 channels on afferent axons. ASIC3 channels may initiate the anginal pain associated with myocardial ischemia. Lactate, an anaerobic metabolite, probably does not play a primary role in directly stimulating muscle pain. Patients with myophosphorylase deficiency do not produce lactate under ischemia yet experience pain. Lactate may potentiate the effects of H^+ ions on ASIC3 channels in activating pain-related axons. Adenosine triphosphate (ATP), another metabolite, is present in increased levels in muscle interstitium during ischemic muscle contraction. Injection of ATP also elicits pain. Many peripheral nociceptors express ATP purinergic receptors, specifically $P2X_3$, $P2Y_2$, and $P2Y_3$. $P2X_3/P2X_{2/3}$ receptor antagonists can reverse the mechanical hyperalgesia that occurs with inflammation. Individual algogenic molecules only activate subsets of peripheral nociceptors. Combinations of protons, lactate, and other molecules synergistically activate the most sensory afferents in muscle tissue (Light et al., 2008).

DOI: 10.1016/B978-1-4377-0434-1.00026-8

Sensitization of nociceptive axon terminals is reduction of the threshold for their stimulation into the innocuous range. Sensitization of nociceptor terminals can have two effects on axons: (1) an increase in the frequency of action potentials in normally active nociceptors or (2) induction of new action potentials in a population of normally silent small axons that are especially prominent in viscera. Vanilloid receptors and tetrodotoxin-resistant sodium channels can play roles in the sensitization of nerve terminals. The heat and capsaicin receptor, transient receptor potential cation channel V1 (TRPV1) can be activated in strong acidic conditions. However, the main TRPV1 activator may be endogenous ligands such as oxidized metabolites of linoleic acid, which damaged myocytes potentially release. Factors released during damage or repetitive stimulation induce a reduction in the axon terminal thresholds in muscle. Substance P induces a low-frequency discharge in afferent axons that could contribute to spontaneous pain. Leukotriene D$_4$ may have a desensitizing effect on muscle nociceptors. The depression of muscle nociceptor activity by aspirin may reflect inhibition of the effects of prostaglandin E$_2$. Other endogenous substances proposed to play roles in activating or sensitizing peripheral nociceptive afferents include neurotransmitters (serotonin, histamine, glutamate, nitric oxide, adrenaline), neuropeptides (substance P, neurokinin 1, bradykinin, nerve growth factor [NGF], calcitonin gene-related peptide), inflammatory mediators (prostaglandins, cytokines), and potassium ions (Mizumura, 2009). GTP cyclohydrolase 1 (GCH1), a rate-limiting enzyme in the tetrahydrobiopterin synthetic pathway, may play a role in enhancing inflammatory and neuropathic pain sensitivity. Certain haplotypes of GCH1 are associated with reduced GCH1 activity and may be protective against pain in patients experiencing pain and normal healthy controls.

Nociceptive Axons

Many of the afferent nerve fibers that transmit painful stimuli from muscle (nociceptors) have small unmyelinated (free) axon terminals (Graven-Nielsen and Mense, 2001; Julius and Basbaum, 2001). These terminal axons (nerve endings) are mainly located near blood vessels and in connective tissue but do not contact muscle fibers. Free nerve endings have a small diameter (0.5 μm) with varicosities (expansions). They contain glutamate and neuropeptides. Noxious stimuli produce graded receptor potentials in nerve endings, with the amplitude dependent on strength of the stimulus. An action potential develops if the amplitude of the receptor potential is large enough to reach threshold. Action potentials arising in nociceptor terminals induce or potentiate pain by two mechanisms. *Centripetal conduction* to central branches of afferent axons brings nociceptive signals directly to the CNS. *Centrifugal conduction* of action potentials along peripheral axon branches causes indirect effects by invading other nerve terminals and causing release of glutamate and neuropeptides into the extracellular medium. These algesic substances can stimulate or sensitize terminals on other nociceptive axons.

Aδ-class (group III) and C-class (group IV) afferent axons play important roles in the conduction of pain-inducing stimuli from muscle to the CNS (Arendt-Nielsen and Graven-Nielsen, 2008). Blockade of both Aδ- and C-class axons eliminates the ability to detect acute noxious stimuli. Selective expression of sodium channel isoforms Na$_v$1.7, Na$_v$1.8, and Na$_v$1.9 occurs on axons and sensory ganglia in peripheral nerve pain pathways. Aδ-class nociceptive axons are thinly myelinated, conduct impulses at moderately slow velocities (3 to 13 m/sec), and have membrane sodium channels that are tetrodotoxin sensitive. Aδ axons are high-threshold mechanoceptors stimulated by strong local pressure and mediate rapid, acute, sharp (first-phase) muscle pain. Aδ-class axons probably mediate spontaneous pain and dysesthesias. C-class nociceptive axons are unmyelinated, conduct impulses at very slow velocities (0.6 to 1.2 m/sec), and have membrane sodium channels that are tetrodotoxin resistant. C-class axons in muscle are often polymodal, responding to a range of stimuli, but stimulus-specific axon terminals are also present. C fibers mediate somewhat delayed, diffuse, dull or burning (second-phase) pain evoked by noxious stimuli. Constituents of muscle nociceptor C axons include substance P, calcitonin gene-related peptide, and somatostatin. These constituents may place the nociceptive axons in a subgroup of C fibers that mediate hyperalgesia in response to inflammation. Aβ-class axons are large, myelinated, and conduct impulses at rapid velocities. They normally mediate innocuous stimuli, and stimulation may reduce the perception of pain. Inflammation or repetitive stimulation can sensitize Aβ axons, which then mediate mechanical allodynia in some tissues. Mediation of this "phenotypic switch" in Aβ axons may occur via up-regulation of neuropeptide Y and sprouting of terminals in the spinal cord from lamina III and IV into lamina II, with subsequent stimulation of ascending central pain pathways.

Central terminals of nociceptive axons from muscle end in lamina I in the dorsal horn of the spinal cord. Ascending central neurons with cell bodies in laminae I or II are stimulated by glutamate from the terminals of primary afferent axons and convey sensory pain modalities via a lateral nociceptive system that includes the contralateral spinothalamic tract, thalamic nuclei (Ren and Dubner, 2002), and somatosensory cortex. Some models suggest that tonic muscle pain may involve a medial set of central pathways including the ipsilateral insula and medial prefrontal regions (Thunberg et al., 2005). Transmission of affective features of pain may also involve medial pathways to the parabrachial nucleus, amygdala, thalamic intralaminar nucleus, and anterior cingulate gyrus. Interneurons and descending CNS pathways modulate afferent input, especially with chronic pain. Central sensitization to pain is associated with neurons containing substance P receptors. Glutamate acting at *N*-methyl-D-aspartate (NMDA) receptors is essential for the initiation of central sensitization and for the hyperexcitability of spinal cord neurons and persistent pain. Facilitation via descending CNS pathways may lead to allodynia and the maintenance of hyperalgesia. Decreased activation of inhibitory descending pathways is associated with increased opioid sensitivity and may provide a system of endogenous analgesia. There is enhanced net descending inhibition at sites of primary hyperalgesia associated with inflammation.

Pathological Conditions Producing Muscle Pain

Episodes of pain originating in muscle are commonly associated with exercise, inflammation, and trauma. Exercise can produce muscle pain via several pathways including exhaustion of fuel supply (with lack of training, vascular insufficiency [ischemia], or metabolic defects), cramps, or injury to muscle fibers or tendons. When muscle contracts while it is being stretched (eccentric contraction), damage and pain are especially likely. During exercise with eccentric contraction, the shearing forces on connective tissue may directly activate muscle nociceptors. Similar painful shearing forces occur during cramps, when the contracting segment stretches the remainder of the muscle. Delayed-onset muscle soreness (DOMS), a common syndrome after unaccustomed exercise, may be due to several factors including muscle fiber and connective tissue damage and inflammation. Pain with DOMS is associated with increased levels of glutamate in muscle. Muscle pain is especially prominent with fascial (connective tissue) damage.

In damaged muscles, tenderness, a decrease in pressure pain threshold, and pain with movement are due to sensitization of muscle nociceptors. The sensitized nociceptors have a lowered threshold of excitation and a greater response to noxious stimuli. With inflammation in muscle, pain at rest may be due to nociceptive axons that develop a raised level of background discharge. Mediators of this phenomenon could include algesic substances including substance P, bradykinin, and serotonin. The accumulation of algesic substances may relate to pain during muscle ischemia but probably not to lactate accumulation. Muscle pain may be associated with increased activity of group IV afferent axon activity. Eccentric exercise-induced mechanical hyperalgesia also involves centrally facilitated pain mechanisms. Muscle pain may produce increased discharges in motor neurons innervating agonist and antagonist muscles.

Fibromyalgia is a syndrome with diffuse chronic muscle pain and tenderness to palpation over trigger points. Central sensitization may underlie some of the symptoms of fibromyalgia and related syndromes of myofascial pain and stress-induced syndromes in which pain localizes to muscle, but without prominent physiological or morphological evidence of muscle damage (Bennett, 2005).

Clinical Features of Muscle Pain

General Features of Muscle Pain

In the clinical setting, patients describe muscle discomfort using a variety of terms: pain, soreness, aching, fatigue, cramps, or spasms. The perception of pain originating from muscle is as emanating from deep tissues. Chronic muscle pain may localize poorly, referred to or from another (usually deep) location, and be associated with autonomic and affective symptoms. The properties of muscle pain may reflect convergence of afferent axons from various tissues that mask identification of a specific location by higher centers. Pain with muscle cramps has an acute onset and short duration. Cramp pain is associated with palpable muscle contraction, and stretching the muscle provides immediate relief. Pain originating from fascia and periosteum has relatively precise localization. Cutaneous pain differs from muscle or fascial pain by its distinct localization and sharp, pricking, stabbing, or burning nature. Pain with small-fiber neuropathies is often present outside length-dependent distributions and may be located in proximal as well as distal regions. In fibromyalgia syndromes, it is common for patients to complain that fatigue accompanies their muscle discomfort. Depression is more common in patients with chronic musculoskeletal pain (18%) than in a population without chronic pain (8%).

Evaluation of Muscle Discomfort

The basis for the classification of disorders underlying muscle discomfort can be anatomy, temporal relation to exercise, muscle pathology, and the presence or absence of active muscle contraction during the discomfort (Kincaid, 1997; Pestronk, 2010). Evaluation of muscle discomfort typically begins with a history that includes the type, localization, inducing factors, and evolution of the pain; drug use; and mood disorders. The physical examination requires special attention to the localization of any tenderness or weakness. Accurate assessment of strength may be difficult in the presence of pain. The sensory examination is important because small-fiber sensory neuropathies commonly cause discomfort with apparent localization in muscle. A general examination is important to evaluate the possibility that pain may be arising from other tissues such as joints. Blood studies may include a complete blood cell count, sedimentation rate, creatine kinase (CK), aldolase, potassium, calcium, phosphate, lactate, thyroid functions, and evaluation for systemic immune disorders. Evaluate urine myoglobin in patients with a high CK and severe myalgias, especially when they relate to exercise. Electromyography (EMG) is a sensitive test for myopathy. A normal EMG can suggest that muscle pain is arising from anatomical loci other than muscle. Nerve-conduction studies may detect an underlying neuropathy, but objective documentation of small-fiber axonopathies can require quantitative sensory testing or skin biopsy with staining of distal nerve fibers. Magnetic resonance imaging, ultrasound, or radionuclide scans may reveal focal or diffuse anomalies in muscle, joints, or fascia that can be useful to guide biopsy procedures. Phosphorous magnetic resonance spectroscopy may become useful in evaluating and monitoring some metabolic myopathies, but its utility remains to be determined. Muscle ultrasound can be a useful and noninvasive method of localizing and defining types of muscle pathology. Muscle biopsy is most often useful in the presence of another abnormal test result such as a high serum lactate, aldolase, CK, or an abnormal EMG. However, important clues to treatable disorders such as fasciitis or systemic immune disorders (connective tissue pathology, perivascular inflammation or granulomas) may be present in muscle in the absence of other positive testing. Examination of both muscle and connective tissue increases the yield of muscle biopsy in syndromes with muscle discomfort. There is increased diagnostic yield from muscle biopsies if in addition to routine morphological analysis and processing, histochemical analysis includes staining for acid phosphatase, alkaline phosphatase, esterase, mitochondrial enzymes, glycolytic enzymes, C_{5b-9} complement, and MHC Class I. Measurement of oxidative enzyme activities can reveal causes of muscle discomfort or fatigue, even in disorders with no histopathological abnormalities. Ultrastructural examination of muscle rarely provides additional information in muscle pain syndromes.

Muscle Discomfort: Specific Causes

Muscle pain is broadly divisible into groups depending on its origin and relation to the time of muscle contraction. Myopathies may be associated with muscle pain without

Box 26.1 Myopathic Pain Syndromes*

Inflammatory:
  Inflammatory and immune myopathies:
    Systemic connective tissue disease
    Perimysial pathology: tRNA synthetase antibodies
    Fasciitis
    Childhood dermatomyositis
  Muscle infections:
    Viral myositis
    Pyomyositis
    Toxoplasmosis
    Trichinosis
Rhabdomyolysis ± metabolic disorder:
  Myophosphorylase: McArdle disease
  Phosphofructokinase
  Carnitine palmitoyltransferase II
  Mitochondrial myopathies
  Malignant hyperthermia syndromes
Other myopathies with pain or discomfort:
  Myopathy with tubular aggregates ± cylindrical spirals
  Myopathy with tubulin-reactive crystalline inclusions
  Myopathy with hexagonally cross-linked crystalloid inclusions
  Myoadenylate deaminase deficiency
  Neuromyopathy with internalized capillaries
  Myotonias: myotonic dystrophy 2; dominant myotonia congenita (occasional)
  Muscular dystrophies (occasional): Becker, limb-girdle dystrophy types 1A, 1C, 2D, 2H
  Selenium deficiency
  Vitamin D deficiency
  Toxic myopathy: eosinophilia myalgia, rhabdomyolysis
  Hypothyroid myopathy
  Mitochondrial disorders (fatigue or myalgias with exercise)
  Camurati-Engelmann syndrome (bone pain)
Drugs and toxins

_____

*Usual associated features: weakness, abnormal electromyogram.

associated muscle contraction (myalgias) (**Boxes 26.1** and **26.2**). Muscle pain during muscle activity (**Box 26.3**; also see **Box 26.2**) may occur with muscle injury, myopathy, cramps, or tonic (relatively long-term) contraction. Some pain syndromes perceived as arising from muscle originate in other tissues, such as connective tissue, nerve, or bone, or have no clear morphological explanation for the pain (**Box 26.4**).

Myopathies with Muscle Pain

Myopathies that produce muscle pain (see **Box 26.1**) are usually associated with weakness, a high serum CK or aldolase, or an abnormal EMG (Pestronk, 2010). Immune-mediated or inflammatory myopathies may produce muscle pain or tenderness, especially with an associated systemic connective tissue disease or pathological involvement of connective tissue (including myopathies with anti-tRNA synthetase antibodies). Pain is common in childhood dermatomyositis, immune myopathies associated with systemic disorders, eosinophilia-myalgia syndromes, focal myositis, and infections. Myopathies due to direct infections (e.g., bacterial,

viral, toxoplasmosis, trichinosis) are usually painful. Metabolic myopathies, including myophosphorylase and carnitine palmitoyltransferase (CPT) II deficiencies, typically produce muscle discomfort or fatigue with exercise and less prominently at rest. As a rule, disorders of carbohydrate utilization like myophosphorylase deficiency produce pain and fatigue after short, intense exercise, whereas lipid disorders (CPT II deficiency) cause muscle discomfort with sustained exercise. Rhabdomyolysis is usually associated with muscle pain and tenderness that can persist for days after the initial event. It may occur with a defined metabolic or toxic myopathy or sporadically in the setting of unaccustomed exercise, especially in hot weather. Rhabdomyolysis may produce renal failure—a life-threatening complication. Aggressively pursue diagnosis and treatment and avoid precipitating factors. Medications, including ε-aminocaproic acid and cholesterol-lowering agents, may produce a painful myopathy with prominent muscle fiber necrosis and a very high serum CK. Cholesterol-lowering agents more commonly produce a myalgia syndrome with no defined muscle pathology but can also produce rhabdomyolysis syndromes, especially in the setting of high serum drug levels. Muscular dystrophy and mitochondrial disorders are usually painless. Occasional patients with mild Becker muscular dystrophy or mitochondrial syndromes with minimal or no weakness may experience a sense of discomfort such as myalgias, fatigue, or cramps, especially after exercise. Hereditary myopathies with occasional reports of muscle discomfort or spasms in patients (or carriers) include limb-girdle dystrophy types 1A, 1C, 2D, 2H (sarcotubular myopathy), myotonic dystrophy type 2, and some mild congenital myopathies. Several myopathies defined by specific morphological changes in muscle but whose cause is unknown commonly have myalgias or exercise-related discomfort. These syndromes include tubular aggregates with or without cylindrical spirals, focal depletion of mitochondria, internalized capillaries, and adult-onset rod myopathies.

Muscle Cramps

Muscle spasms are abnormal involuntary muscle contractions. Muscle cramps (see **Box 26.3**) are localized, typically uncomfortable muscle contractions or spasms (Miller and Layzer, 2005). Characteristic features include a sudden involuntary onset in a single muscle or muscle group, with durations of seconds to minutes and a palpable region of contraction. Occasionally there is distortion of posture. Fasciculations often occur before and after the cramp. Cramps usually arise during sleep or exercise and are more likely to occur when muscle contracts while in a shortened position. Pain syndromes associated with cramps include discomfort during a muscle contraction and soreness after the contraction due to muscle injury.

Cramps, especially those in the calf or foot muscles, are common in normal people of any age. They may be more common in the elderly (up to 50%), at the onset of exercise, at night, during pregnancy, and with fasciculations. These types of cramps are usually idiopathic and benign. Cramps that occur frequently in muscles other than the gastrocnemius often herald an underlying neuromuscular disorder. The presence of fasciculations with mild cramps but no weakness usually represents a benign condition (benign fasciculation syndrome). When the muscle cramps are more disabling, the condition is the cramp-fasciculation syndrome. EMG is

Box 26.2 **Muscle Discomfort Associated with Drugs and Toxins**

Inflammatory myopathy:
  Definite:
    Hydralazine
    Penicillamine
    Procainamide
    1,1′-Ethylidinebis[tryptophan]
    Toxic oil syndrome
  Possible:
    Cimetidine
    Imatinib mesylate
    Interferon-α
    Ipecac
    Lansoprazole
    Leuprolide
    Levodopa
    Penicillin
    Phenytoin
    Propylthiouracil
    Sulfonamide
Rhabdomyolysis ± chronic myopathy:
  Alcohol
  ε-Amino caproic acid
  Amphetamines
  Cocaine
  Cyclosporine
  Daptomycin
  Hypokalemia
  Isoniazid
  Lipid-lowering agents*:
    Bezafibrate
    Clofibrate
    Fenofibrate
    Gemfibrozil
    Lovastatin
    Simvastatin
    Pravastatin
    Fluvastatin
    Atorvastatin
    Cerivastatin
    Nicotinic acid
    Red yeast rice
  Labetalol
  Lithium
  Organophosphates
  Propofol
  Snake venom
  Tacrolimus
  Zidovudine
Painful myopathy ± rhabdomyolysis:
  Colchicine

Emetine
Fenoverine
Germanium
Hypervitaminosis E
Taxenes
Zidovudine
Myalgia ± myopathy:
  All-trans-retinoic acid
  Azathioprine
  Bryostatin 1
  Captopril
  Cholesterol-lowering agents
  Ciguatoxin
  Corticosteroid withdrawal
  Cytotoxics
  Danazol
  Enalapril
  Gemcitabine
  Gold
  Interferon-α: 2a and 2b
  Isotretinoin
  Ketorolac
  Labetalol
  Methotrexate†
  Metolazone
  Mycophenolate mofetil
  Paclitaxel
  Retinoids
  Rifampin
  Spanish toxic oil
  Suxamethonium (succinylcholine)
  Vinca alkaloids
  Zimeldine
Cramps:
  Albuterol
  Anticholinesterase
  Bergamot (bergapten)
  Caffeine
  Clofibrate
  Cyclosporine
  Diuretics
  Labetalol
  Lithium
  Nifedipine
  Terbutaline
  Tetanus
  Theophylline
  Vitamin A

*Especially with concurrent cyclosporine A, danazol, erythromycin, gemfibrozil, niacin, colchicine.
†With concurrent pantoprazole.

Box 26.3 Cramps* and Other Involuntary Muscle Contraction Syndromes

Cramp syndromes:
  Ordinary:
    Common in normal individuals, especially gastrocnemius muscle, older age
    Pregnancy
  Systemic disorders:
    Dehydration: hidrosis, diuretics, hemodialysis
    Metabolic: low Na^+, Mg^{2+}, Ca^{2+}, glucose, uremia, cirrhosis
    Endocrine: thyroid (hyper- or hypothyroid), hypoadrenal, hyperparathyroid
  Ischemia
  Drug-induced
  Denervation, partial: motor neuron disease, spinal stenosis, radiculopathy
  Syndromes: cramp-fasciculation, Satoyoshi syndrome
Other contraction syndromes:
  Central disorders: stiff person syndrome, spasticity, tetanus, dystonia
  Peripheral nerve disorders: neuromyotonia, tetany, myokymia, partial denervation
  Muscle: contractures, myotonia, myoedema
Familial muscle contraction syndromes:
  Muscular dystrophy: Becker; LGMD 1C
  Myotonia: myotonia congenita, myotonic dystrophy
  Contractures:
    Brody syndrome: ATP2A1
    Glycogen disorders: phosphorylase deficiency
    Rippling muscle syndrome: CAV3
    HANAC: COL4A1
    Neuropathic
  Cramps: autosomal dominant:
    Schwartz-Jampel: Perlecan, LIFR
    Neuromyotonia and myokymia: KCNQ2; KCNA1
    Geniospasm
    Crisponi: CRLF1
Possible treatments for cramps and other muscle spasms:
  Normalize metabolic abnormalities
  Quinine sulfate, 260 mg qhs or bid
  Carbamazepine, 200 mg bid or tid
  Phenytoin, 300 mg daily
  Gabapentin, 300 mg qhs
  Tocainide, 200–400 mg bid
  Verapamil, 120 mg daily
  Amitriptyline, 25–100 mg qhs
  Vitamin E, 400 International Units daily
  Riboflavin, 100 mg daily
  Diphenhydramine, 50 mg daily
  Calcium, 0.5–1 g elemental Ca^{++} daily
  bid, Twice daily; *qhs*, daily at bedtime; *tid*, three times daily.

*Usual features: sudden involuntary painful muscle contractions (usually involve single muscles, especially gastrocnemius); local cramps in other muscles often associated with neuromuscular disease. Precipitants: muscle contraction, occasionally during sleep. Relief: passive muscle stretch, local massage.

Box 26.4 Pain Syndromes without Chronic Myopathy*

Pain of uncertain origin:
  Polymyalgia rheumatica
  Fibromyalgia
  Chronic fatigue syndrome
  Infections:
    Viral and postviral syndromes
    Brucellosis
  Endocrine
    Thyroid: increased or decreased
    Parathyroid: increased or decreased
  Familial Mediterranean fever
Pain with defined origin:
  Connective tissue disorders:
    Systemic
    Fasciitis
  Joint disease
  Bone: osteomalacia, fracture, neoplasm
  Vascular: ischemia, thrombophlebitis
  Polyneuropathy:
    Small-fiber polyneuropathies
    Guillain-Barré
  Radiculoneuropathy
  Central nervous system: restless legs syndrome, dystonias (focal)
Pain of muscle origin without chronic myopathy:
  Muscle ischemia: atherosclerosis, calciphylaxis
  Muscle overuse syndromes:
    Delayed-onset muscle soreness (DOMS)
    Cramps
  Drugs, toxins
  Muscle injury (strain)

*Usual features: muscle pain; may interfere with effort but no true weakness; present at rest, may increase with movement; muscle morphology and serum creatine kinase normal.

normal except for the presence of fasciculations. Slow, repetitive nerve stimulation provokes after-discharges of motor unit action potentials. Neurogenic disorders that produce partial denervation of muscles (e.g., amyotrophic lateral sclerosis, radiculopathies, polyneuropathies) can be associated with cramps, painful muscle spasms, or muscle discomfort. Other causes of cramps (see **Boxes 26.2** and **26.3**) include drugs and metabolic, neuropathic, and inherited disorders.

Muscle cramps are usually due to discharges originating in motor axons or nerve terminals. EMG during cramps demonstrates rapid, repetitive motor unit action potentials ("cramp discharges") at rates from 40 to 150 per second that increase and then decrease during the course of the cramp. CNS influences on cramps are minor and probably involve modulation of cramp thresholds. The EMG can distinguish cramps from other types of muscle contraction. Ultrasound imaging can visualize electrically silent muscle contractions or cramps.

Treatment of cramps and muscle contraction syndromes involves management of the underlying disorder or symptomatic trials of medications. Stretching affected muscles can relieve cramps. Active stretching, by contracting the antagonist, may be especially effective treatment because it evokes reciprocal inhibition. There is no clear benefit of prophylactic stretching on the frequency of cramps. Symptomatic treatment can reduce abnormal muscle contractions or the discomfort produced by the contractions. Quinine, tonic water, and related drugs can be effective in treating nocturnal muscle cramps, but side effects may outweigh benefits. Increased salt intake and magnesium lactate or citrate may help treat leg cramps during pregnancy.

Other Involuntary Muscle Contraction Syndromes

Diffuse muscle contraction syndromes, usually arising from the PNS or CNS (dystonias), often show widespread and continuous spontaneous motor unit fiber discharges. They may produce considerable discomfort. Causes are hereditary syndromes, CNS disorders, drugs, or toxins (see **Boxes 26.2** and **26.3**). Specific syndromes include stiff person syndrome, Isaac syndrome (neuromyotonia with contractions due to repetitively discharging motor units at high frequencies), Schwartz-Jampel syndrome, restless legs, and toxic disorders related to phencyclidine, amphetamine, tetanus, and strychnine. Tetany, typically associated with hypocalcemia or alkalosis, manifests with neuromyotonic-like discharges. Myokymic rippling of muscles shows recurring bursts of motor units at 30 to 80 Hz. In the postoperative period, a muscle contraction syndrome with fasciculations and myalgia often occurs after the use of succinylcholine (suxamethonium). Two diffuse contraction disorders, malignant hyperthermia and neuroleptic malignant syndromes, have not undergone a systematic evaluation by electrodiagnostic testing during episodes.

Muscle contractions originating from muscle include electrically active forms due to myopathy or myotonia and electrically silent contractures. *Myotonia* is repetitive firing of muscle fibers at rates of 20 to 80 Hz, with waxing and waning of the amplitude and frequency. Triggering the action potentials may be mechanical or electrical stimulation. Myotonic contractions are usually not painful. Patients with recessive myotonia congenita often note fatigue. *Muscle contractures* are active, painful muscle contractions in the absence of electrical activity. (The term is also used to describe fixed resistance to stretch of a shortened muscle due to fibrous connective tissue changes or loss of sarcomeres in the muscle). Contractures differ clinically from cramps, having a more prolonged time course, no resolution by muscle stretch, and occurrence only in an exercised muscle. Electrically silent muscle contractions occur in myopathies including myophosphorylase deficiency and other glycolytic disorders, Brody syndrome, rippling muscle disease, and hypothyroidism (myoedema). Exercise typically provokes prolonged and painful contractures in myophosphorylase deficiency.

Myalgia Syndromes without Chronic Myopathy

Pain originating from muscle, often acute, may occur in the absence of a chronic myopathy. Muscle ischemia causes a squeezing pain in the affected muscles during exercise. Ischemia produces pain that develops especially rapidly (within minutes) if muscle is forced to contract at the same time; the pain subsides quickly with rest. Cramps and overuse syndromes are associated with pain during or immediately after muscle use. DOMS occurs 12 to 48 hours after exercise and lasts for hours to days. Muscle contraction or palpation exacerbates discomfort. Serum CK is often increased. DOMS is most commonly precipitated by eccentric muscle contraction (contraction during muscle stretching) or unaccustomed exercise. The discomfort after eccentric contractions may be associated with repetitive overstretching of elastic noncontractile tissues. Exercise training typically protects against DOMS. Muscle fatigue after exercise, with reduced maximum levels of voluntary contraction, may occur via a disorder separate from DOMS involving disruption of excitation/contraction systems (Iguchi and Shields, 2010).

Polymyalgia syndromes (see **Box 26.4**) have pain localized to muscle and other structures. The pain may produce the appearance of weakness by preventing full effort. Typical of this type of "weakness" on examination is sudden reduction in the apparent level of effort, rather than smooth movement through the range of motion expected with true muscle weakness. Polymyalgic pain is often present at rest and variably affected by movement. Serum CK and EMG are normal. No major pathological change in muscle occurs unless the discomfort produces disuse and atrophy of type II muscle fibers. Muscle biopsies may also show changes associated with systemic immune disorders, including inflammation around blood vessels or in connective tissue. Polymyalgia syndromes can have identified causes including systemic immune disease, drug toxicity, and small-fiber polyneuropathies.

A series of clinical criteria define some syndromes of unknown pathophysiology associated with muscle discomfort (polymyalgia rheumatica, fibromyalgia, and chronic fatigue syndrome). *Polymyalgia rheumatica* usually occurs after age 50 years and manifests with pain and stiffness in joints and muscles, weight loss, and low-grade fever. The pain is symmetrical; involves the shoulder, neck, and hip girdle; and is greatest after inactivity and sleeping. Polymyalgia rheumatica can be associated with temporal arteritis and an elevated sedimentation rate (>40 mm/h). Pain improves within a few days after treatment with corticosteroids (prednisone, 20 mg/day). The diagnosis of *fibromyalgia* depends on a history of widespread musculoskeletal pain, most commonly around the neck and shoulders, and examination findings of excessive tenderness in predefined anatomical sites on the trunk and extremities. Patients also may note fatigue and disturbed sleep, headache, irritable bowel syndrome, and aggravation of symptoms by exercise, anxiety, or stress. The diagnosis of *chronic fatigue syndrome* requires symptoms of persistent and unexplained fatigue. Four or more symptoms must occur for the 6 months after the onset of fatigue, including impaired memory or concentration, sore throat, tender cervical or axillary lymph nodes, muscle pain, pain in multiple joints, new headaches, unrefreshing sleep, or malaise after exertion. Rest does not alleviate fatigue, which substantially compromises daily function. Chronic fatigue syndrome may improve spontaneously over time. Decreasing the central sensitization to pain is the focus of the pharmacological treatment of fibromyalgia and chronic pain. Medications include antidepressants such as tricyclics, selective serotonin reuptake inhibitors, selective norepinephrine reuptake inhibitors, and pregabalin. No clear evidence exists for the superiority of any one medication. Low-impact aerobic exercise training may reduce pain and pressure thresholds over tender points. Cognitive behavioral therapy may be useful. Controversial syndromes that include myalgias include myoadenylate deaminase deficiency, adjuvant breast disorders, Gulf War syndrome, and multiple chemical sensitivity.

Pain or discomfort localized to muscle may arise in other structures. For example, hip disease can suggest the misdiagnosis of a painful proximal myopathy with apparent leg weakness. In this situation, external or internal rotation of the thigh commonly evokes proximal pain. Radiological studies can confirm the diagnosis. Disorders of bone and joints, connective tissue, endocrine systems, vascular supply, peripheral nerves and roots, and the CNS may also present with discomfort localized to muscle.

References

The complete reference list is available online at www.expertconsult.com.

Hypotonic (Floppy) Infant

W. Bryan Burnette

Floppy, or hypotonic, infant is a common scenario encountered in the clinical practice of child neurology. It can present significant challenges in terms of localization and is associated with an extensive differential diagnosis (**Box 27.1**). As with any clinical problem in neurology, attention to certain key aspects of the history and examination allows correct localization within the neuraxis and narrows the list of possible diagnoses. Further narrowing of the differential is achievable with selected testing based on the aforementioned findings. Understanding the anatomical and etiological aspects of hypotonia in infancy necessarily begins with an understanding of the concept of tone. *Tone* is the resistance of muscle to stretch. Categorization of tone differs among authors, but assessment is performed with the patient at rest and all parts of the body fully supported; examination involves tonic or phasic stretching of a muscle or the effect of gravity. Tone is an involuntary function and therefore separate and distinct from strength or power, which is the maximum force generated by voluntary contraction of a muscle. Function at every level of the neuraxis influences tone, and disease processes affecting any level of the neuraxis may reduce tone. Although a comprehensive review of conditions associated with hypotonia in infancy is beyond the scope of a single chapter, this chapter considers the basic approach to evaluating the floppy infant and considers several key disorders.

Approach to Diagnosis

History

Several features of the history may point to a specific diagnosis or category of diagnoses leading to hypotonia, or may permit distinguishing disorders present during fetal development from disorders acquired during the perinatal period. Thoroughly investigate a family history of disorders known to be associated with neonatal hypotonia, especially in the mother or in older siblings. Certain dominantly inherited genetic disorders (e.g., myotonic dystrophy) are associated with *anticipation* (earlier or more severe expression of a disease in successive generations). Such disorders may be milder and therefore undiagnosed in the mother. A maternal history of spontaneous abortion, fetal demise, or other offspring who died in infancy may also provide clues to possible diagnoses. A history of reduced fetal movement is a common feature of disorders associated with hypotonia, and may indicate a peripheral cause (Vasta et al., 2005). A history of maternal fever late in pregnancy suggests in utero infection, while a history of a long and difficult delivery followed by perinatal distress suggests hypoxic-ischemic encephalopathy with or without accompanying myelopathy. Among the many potential causes of neonatal hypotonia, acquired perinatal injury is far more common than inherited disorders and is rarely overlooked. However, also consider the possibility of a motor unit disorder leading to perinatal distress and hypoxic-ischemic encephalopathy.

Physical Examination
General Features of Hypotonia

Assessing tone in an infant involves both observation of the patient at rest and application of certain examination maneuvers designed to evaluate both axial and appendicular musculature. Beginning with observation, a normal infant lying supine on an examination table will demonstrate flexion of the hips and knees so that the lower extremities are clear of the examination table, flexion of the upper extremities at the elbows, and internal rotation at the shoulders (**Fig. 27.1**). A hypotonic infant lies with the lower extremities in external rotation, the lateral aspects of the thighs and knees touching the examination table, and the upper extremities either

Box 27.1 Differential Diagnosis of the Floppy Infant

Cerebral Hypotonia

Chromosomal disorders:
   Prader-Willi Syndrome
Chronic nonprogressive encephalopathy
Chronic progressive encephalopathy
Benign congenital hypotonia

Combined Cerebral and Motor Unit Disorders

Acid maltase deficiency
Congenital myotonic dystrophy
Syndromic congenital muscular dystrophies
Congenital disorders of glycosylation
Lysosomal disorders
Infantile neuroaxonal dystrophy

Spinal Cord Disorders

Acquired spinal cord lesions
Spinal muscular atrophy
Infantile spinal muscular atrophy with respiratory distress
X-linked spinal muscular atrophy

Peripheral Nerve Disorders

Congenital hypomyelinating neuropathy/Dejerine-Sottas disease

Neuromuscular Junction Disorders

Juvenile myasthenia gravis
Neonatal myasthenia gravis
Congenital myasthenic syndromes
Infant botulism

Muscle Disorders

Congenital myopathies:
   Centronuclear myopathy
   Nemaline myopathy
   Central core disease
Nonsyndromic congenital muscular dystrophies:
   Merosin-deficient congenital muscular dystrophy
   Ullrich congenital muscular dystrophy
Other muscular dystrophies:
   Infantile facioscapulohumeral dystrophy

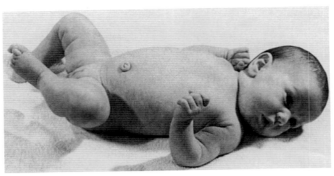

Fig. 27.1 Normal infant lying supine with legs flexed and arms adducted.

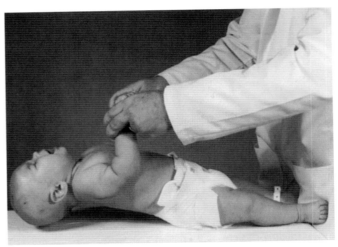

Fig. 27.2 Hypotonic infant demonstrating abnormal traction response, with excessive head lag and absence of flexion of arms and legs.

extended down by the sides of the trunk or abducted with slight flexion at the elbows, also lying against the examination table. Evaluation of the *traction response* is done with the infant in supine position; the hands are grasped and the infant pulled toward a sitting position. A normal response includes flexion at the elbows, knees, and ankles, and movement of the head in line with the trunk after no more than a brief head lag. The head should then remain erect in the midline for at least a few seconds. An infant with axial hypotonia demonstrates excessive head lag with this maneuver (**Fig. 27.2**), and once upright, the head may continue to lag or may fall forward relatively quickly. Absence of flexion of the limbs may also be seen and indicates either appendicular hypotonia or weakness. The traction response is normally present after 33 weeks postconceptional age. Vertical suspension is performed by placing hands under the infant's axillae and lifting the infant without grasping the thorax. A normal infant has enough power in the shoulder muscles to remain suspended without falling through, with the head upright in the midline and the hips and knees flexed (**Fig. 27.3, A**). In contrast, a hypotonic infant held in this manner slips through the examiner's hands, often with the head falling forward and the legs extended at the knees (see **Fig. 27.3, B**). Infants with axial hypotonia related to brain injury may also demonstrate crossing, or *scissoring*, of the legs in this position, which is an early manifestation of appendicular hypertonia. In *horizontal suspension*, the infant is held prone with the abdomen and chest against the palm of the examiner's hand. A normal infant maintains the head above horizontal with the limbs flexed, while a hypotonic infant drapes over the examiner's hand with the head and limbs hanging limply. Other examination findings in hypotonic infants include various deformities of the cranium, face, limbs, and thorax. Infants with reduced tone may develop occipital flattening, or *positional plagiocephaly*, as the result of prolonged periods of lying supine and motionless.

Localization

Once the presence of hypotonia in an infant is established, the next step in determining causation is localization of the abnormality to the brain, spinal cord, motor unit, or to

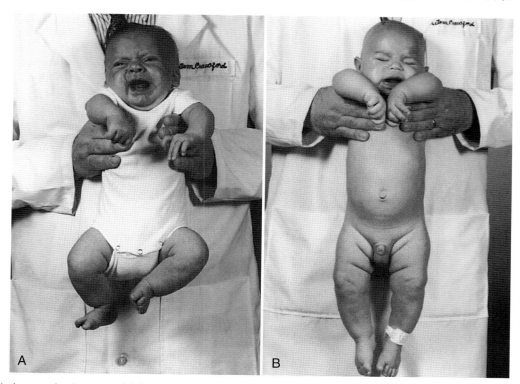

Fig. 27.3 A, Vertical suspension in a normal infant: arms adducted, upright position of head and shoulders maintained, flexion of legs. **B,** Ventral suspension in a hypotonic infant, with elevation of shoulders and arms (slip-through) and extension of legs.

multiple sites. A *motor unit* is a single spinal motor neuron and all the muscle fibers it innervates and includes the motor neuron with its cell body, axon, and myelin covering; the neuromuscular junction; and muscle. The major "branch point" at this stage of the assessment is whether the lesion is likely to be in the brain, at a more distal site, or at multiple sites.

The key features of disorders of cerebral function, particularly the cerebral cortex, are encephalopathy and seizures. Encephalopathy manifesting as decreased level of consciousness may be difficult to ascertain, given the large proportion of time normal infants spend sleeping. However, full-term or near-term infants with normal brain function spend at least some portion of the day awake with eyes open, particularly with feeding. Encephalopathy also manifests with excessive irritability or poor feeding, although the latter problem is rarely the sole feature of cerebral hemispheric dysfunction and may occur with disorders at more distal sites. Infants with centrally mediated hypotonia of many different etiologies frequently have relatively normal power despite a hypotonic appearance. Power may not be observable under normal circumstances because of a paucity of spontaneous movement, but it may be observable with application of a noxious stimulus such as a blood draw or placement of a peripheral intravenous catheter. Other indicators of central rather than peripheral dysfunction include *fisting* (trapping of the thumbs in closed hands), normal or brisk tendon reflexes, and normal or exaggerated primitive reflexes. Tendon reflexes should be tested with the infant's head in the midline and the limbs symmetrically positioned; deviations from this technique often result in spuriously asymmetrical reflexes. *Primitive reflexes* are involuntary responses to certain stimuli that normally appear in late fetal development and are supplanted

within the first few months of life by voluntary movements. Abnormalities of these reflexes include absent or asymmetrical responses, obligatory responses (persistence of the reflex with continued application of the stimulus), or persistence of the reflexes beyond the normal age range. Two of the most sensitive primitive reflexes are the Moro and asymmetrical tonic neck reflexes. The *Moro reflex* is a startle response present from 28 weeks after conception to 6 months postnatal age (Gingold et al., 1998). Quickly dropping the infant's head below the level of the body while holding the infant supine with the head supported in one hand and the body supported in the other readily elicits this reflex. The normal response consists of initial abduction and extension of the arms with opening of the hands, followed quickly by adduction and flexion with closure of the hands. The *tonic neck reflex* is a vestibular response and is present from term until approximately 3 months of age. The response is elicited by rotating the head to one side while the infant is lying supine. The normal response is extension of the ipsilateral limbs while the contralateral limbs remain flexed. Central disorders resulting in hypotonia may also be associated with dysmorphism of the face or limbs, or malformations of other organs. Various defects in O-linked glycosylation of α-dystroglycan, a protein associated with the dystrophin glycoprotein complex that stabilizes the sarcolemma, result in structural defects of the brain, eye, and skeletal muscle.

Disorders of the spinal cord leading to neonatal hypotonia are usually secondary to perinatal injury. Spinal cord injury may occur in the setting of a prolonged, difficult vaginal delivery with breech presentation, resulting in trauma to the spinal cord, or may result from hypoxic-ischemic injury to the cord concurrently with encephalopathy. In the latter case, hypotonia may initially be attributable to the encephalopathy. In cases of hypotonia resulting from spinal cord injury, diminished responsiveness to painful stimuli, sphincter dysfunction with continuous leakage of urine and abdominal distension, and priapism may provide clues to localization of the lesion.

The hallmark of disorders of the motor unit is weakness. Tendon reflexes are absent or reduced. Tendon reflexes reduced out of proportion to weakness usually indicate a neuropathy, often a demyelinating neuropathy, whereas tendon reflexes reduced in proportion to weakness are more likely to result from myopathy or axonal neuropathy. The motor unit is the final common pathway for all reflexes, and for this reason, primitive reflexes are depressed or absent in motor unit disorders. This phenomenon may hinder detection of central nervous system (CNS) abnormalities when lesions at both levels coexist. Other abnormalities related to motor unit disorders in infants include underdevelopment of the jaw (micrognathia), a high arched palate, and chest wall deformities, in particular pectus excavatum. Muscle atrophy may also occur but also occurs in cerebral disorders. Sensory function is not assessable in detail in a neonate or young infant, particularly in the presence of encephalopathy, although reduced responsiveness to pinprick may provide clues to the presence of a polyneuropathy or spinal cord lesion in the setting of normal mental status. Some motor unit disorders may result in perinatal distress due to weakness and may result in a superimposed encephalopathy that confounds the localization of hypotonia.

Hypotonic infants may have reduced movement during fetal development, leading to fibrosis of muscles or of structures associated with joints, as well as foreshortening of ligaments. This results in restricted joint range of motion, or *contractures*. The term *arthrogryposis* refers to joint contractures that develop prenatally. The most common form of arthrogryposis is unilateral or bilateral clubfoot. The most severe end of this clinical spectrum is *arthrogryposis multiplex congenita*, or multiple joint contractures. The causes of this condition may be abnormalities of the intrauterine environment, motor unit disorders, or disorders of the CNS. Hypotonia in utero may also result in congenital hip dysplasia.

Diagnostic Studies

Selective laboratory testing allows confirmation of the clinical localization of hypotonia, and in many cases leads to identification of a specific diagnosis. In all cases, ancillary testing guided by historical features and examination findings has the greatest chance of yielding a diagnosis. Available modalities include various forms of neuroimaging; electrophysiological techniques including electroencephalography (EEG), nerve conduction studies (NCV), electromyography (EMG), and repetitive nerve stimulation; muscle and nerve biopsy; and other laboratory studies such as serum creatine kinase (CK), metabolic studies, and genetic studies.

Neuroimaging

Neuroimaging studies, in particular magnetic resonance imaging (MRI), are most useful when suspecting structural abnormalities of the CNS. T1-weighted images most readily detect congenital malformations of the brain and spinal cord, while T2-weighted images and various T2-based sequences reveal abnormalities of white matter and show evidence of

ischemic injury. Specialized techniques such as MR spectroscopy may show evidence of mitochondrial disease (Matthews et al., 1993) or disorders of cerebral creatine metabolism (Frahm et al., 1994). When performing neuroimaging studies that require sedation on hypotonic infants, give particular consideration to airway management and other safety issues.

Electroencephalography

Electroencephalography may be informative when seizures are suspected either as a cause of unexplained encephalopathy or a result of a more global disturbance of brain function. EEG may also reveal evidence of underlying structural abnormalities and thus increase the pretest probability of a diagnostic finding on neuroimaging.

Creatine Kinase

Creatine Kinase catalyzes the conversion of creatine to phosphocreatine, which serves as a reservoir for the buffering and regeneration of adenosine triphosphate (ATP). It expresses in many human tissues, in particular smooth muscle, cardiac muscle, and skeletal muscle. The concentration of CK detectable in serum increases in any condition in which tissues expressing high levels of the enzyme undergo breakdown. Serum CK concentration may be elevated in congenital myopathies, congenital muscular dystrophies, or in spinal muscular atrophy, but levels may also be elevated transiently following normal vaginal deliveries or with perinatal distress. Conversely, serum CK is normal in some congenital myopathies and inherited neuropathies.

Metabolic Studies

Removal of low-molecular-weight toxic metabolites across the placenta typically prevents inborn errors of metabolism (e.g., amino acidopathies, organic acidurias, urea cycle defects, fatty acid oxidation defects, mitochondrial disorders) from causing in utero injury. More commonly, these disorders manifest in a previously healthy newborn who develops hypotonia, encephalopathy, or seizures within the first 24 to 72 hours after birth, after oral feeding begins and toxic intermediates begin to accumulate in the blood. Although detection of many disorders is by state-mandated newborn screens, these results may not be available before an affected infant becomes symptomatic. For this reason, newborns who develop hypotonia and encephalopathy after an unremarkable first few days of life should have enteral feedings held until metabolic studies such as blood ammonia level, plasma amino acid, acylcarnitine profile, and urine organic acids have definitively excluded an inborn error of metabolism. Because neonatal sepsis has a similar presentation, undertake investigation for infection with cultures of blood, urine, and cerebrospinal fluid in such cases; empirical antimicrobial therapy should be initiated while diagnostic studies are pending.

Nerve Conduction Studies and Electromyography

Nerve conduction studies and EMG are the studies of choice in a suspected motor unit disorder when other available clinical information does not suggest a specific diagnosis. The two techniques are complementary and always performed together. They allow distinction between primary disorders of muscle and peripheral nerve disorders when the two are indistinguishable on clinical grounds. Repetitive nerve stimulation (RNS) studies evaluate the integrity of the neuromuscular junction, abnormalities of which are not detectable with routine nerve conduction studies or EMG. The most commonly observed abnormality on low-rate (2-3 Hz) RNS studies of patients with various forms of myasthenia is a significant decrement, usually defined as 10% or greater, in the amplitude of the compound motor action potential (CMAP) between the first and fourth or fifth stimuli of a series. Single fiber EMG (SFEMG) is a highly specialized technique that evaluates the delay in depolarization between adjacent muscle fibers within a single motor unit, referred to as *jitter*. This modality is highly sensitive for neuromuscular junction abnormalities but has a low specificity and requires a cooperative patient. SFEMG with stimulation of the appropriate nerve has been described in pediatric patients (Tidwell and Pitt, 2007), but experience with this technique in infants is limited to a small number of centers. The utility of these neurophysiology studies is dependent on the skill and experience of the clinician performing the tests, as well as the precision of the question posed.

Muscle Biopsy

Muscle biopsy is integral to the diagnosis of certain inherited muscle disorders such as congenital myopathies, congenital muscular dystrophies, and metabolic myopathies and may also aid in the distinction between myopathies and motor neuron disorders. Give careful consideration to the site chosen for biopsy. Ideally, a muscle should be chosen that is moderately but not severely weak and that has not undergone needle EMG. Another important consideration is the quantity of tissue obtained. Obtain a sufficient quantity of tissue to rapidly freeze a portion for routine histochemical stains, submit additional tissue for specialized studies such as biochemical assays, electron microscopy, or genetic studies, and have additional tissue available to be stored for possible future studies. In practical terms, this usually entails obtaining at least three separate specimens weighing 1 to 1.5 g each. Although needle biopsy may procure an adequate sample in some cases, open biopsy is more likely to yield an appropriate amount of tissue, thereby avoiding the need for a second surgical procedure and its attendant risks. The value of muscle biopsy, as with neurophysiology studies, depends on the experience of the interpreting laboratory and the focus of the question asked by the referring clinician. In addition to these factors, proper handling of the tissue between the operating room and the receiving laboratory is a critical link in the chain of custody. This step is often the most difficult to control, but it requires attention equal to the other steps in the process in order to maximize the probability of obtaining a diagnostic sample and minimize the risk of subjecting the patient to a second procedure.

Nerve Biopsy

Nerve biopsy plays a more limited role in the diagnosis of hypotonia in infancy. It is nevertheless appropriate when a peripheral neuropathy is suspected on clinical grounds, but available testing fails to yield a diagnosis. The sural nerve is usually chosen because of its accessibility and the relatively minor deficit produced by its removal. Sural nerve biopsy is most likely to be informative in the setting of an abnormal response on nerve conduction studies. The limited choice of peripheral nerves available for biopsy confines use of this procedure to centers with considerable experience. Submit portions of the nerve for routine histochemical stains, paraffin-embedded sections, and thin plastic sections, the latter processed for light microscopy or electron microscopy.

Genetic Testing

In some cases of hypotonia in infancy, the combination of clinical history, examination, and ancillary testing points toward a specific genetic diagnosis. Genetic testing is commercially available for many conditions, and the number continues to expand rapidly. Consult one or more of the accessible resources such as the Internet-based Online Mendelian Inheritance in Man or GeneTests.org for the most current information on testing for specific disorders.

Serology

In cases of a suspected neuromuscular junction disorder such as myasthenia gravis, assays of antibodies directed against the sarcolemmal nicotinic acetylcholine receptor or muscle-specific kinase are commercially available. Autoimmune myasthenia gravis is rare in infancy, but absence of the antibodies is required for the diagnosis of a congenital myasthenic syndrome. Several forms of myasthenia gravis occur in infancy and are discussed in greater detail later in this chapter.

Specific Disorders Associated with Hypotonia in Infancy

Cerebral Disorders

Regardless of etiology, hypotonia is a common feature of disturbed function of the cerebral hemispheres in neonates and infants and, as previously noted, is frequently characterized by diminished tone that is disproportionate to the degree of weakness. Disorders of cerebral function in infancy are also frequently associated with concurrent axial hypotonia and appendicular hypertonia. Overall, central disorders are a far more common cause of hypotonia than motor unit diseases. Although a comprehensive listing of all such disorders is beyond the scope of a single chapter, a number of important categories of cerebral causes of hypotonia are considered here.

Chromosomal Disorders

Hypotonia is a prominent feature of many disorders associated with large- or small-scale chromosomal abnormalities. Such disorders also are frequently associated with a dysmorphic appearance of the face and hands. Among the most common of these disorders is *Prader-Willi syndrome*, which is caused by absence of the paternal PWS/Angelman syndrome region on chromosome 15 (Butler, Meaney, and Palmer, 1986).

Affected individuals often have profound hypotonia and poor feeding in infancy, suggesting a disorder of the motor unit or a combined cerebral and motor unit disorder. However, serum CK, EMG, muscle biopsy, and brain MRI are normal. The commonly recognized morphological features of almond-shaped eyes, narrow biparietal diameter, and relatively small hands and feet may not be readily apparent in early infancy. Approximately 70% of patients have a detectable small-scale deletion on chromosome 15 on high-resolution chromosomal analysis; DNA methylation studies reveal a pattern suggestive of exclusive maternal inheritance of this locus in 99%. Failure to thrive in infancy gives way in early childhood to hyperphagia and a characteristic pattern of behavioral abnormalities, intellectual disability, and hypogonadism.

Chronic Nonprogressive Encephalopathy

Chronic nonprogressive encephalopathy describes a clinical syndrome with many potential causes, including cerebral dysgenesis related to a genetic disorder, in utero infection, toxic exposure, inborn error of metabolism, or vascular insult. Perinatal brain injury resulting in a chronic encephalopathy is readily diagnosable and typically associated with a reduced level of consciousness and seizures. Hypoxic-ischemic brain injury in the newborn manifests with low Apgar scores, and lactic acidosis along with other indicators of injury to other vital organs is often present. Hypotonia related to ischemic brain injury usually gives way to spasticity. In cases of remote in utero injury or cerebral dysgenesis, hypotonia may be the only manifestation of the problem in the perinatal period. Clues to the presence of cerebral dysgenesis include malformations of other organs and abnormalities of head size or shape. In such cases, obtain an MRI of the brain, and a chromosomal anomaly should be sought with karyotype and chromosomal microarray analysis. The onset of hypotonia in a previously healthy neonate or infant is almost always cerebral in origin and may also relate to infection, vascular injury, or an inborn error of metabolism.

Chronic Progressive Encephalopathy

Chronic progressive encephalopathy more commonly presents with developmental regression than with hypotonia. Inborn errors of metabolism involving small molecules may cause this clinical presentation, but more frequently the cause is a disorder of lysosomal or peroxisomal metabolism leading to progressive accumulation of storage material in various tissues. These disorders frequently manifest with progressive facial dysmorphism, organomegaly, or skeletal dysplasia in addition to neurological decline.

Benign Congenital Hypotonia

Benign congenital hypotonia refers to infants with early hypotonia who later develop normal tone. It is a diagnosis made only in retrospect and has become less common in the era of high-resolution neuroimaging and genetic testing. Nevertheless, there remains a subset of children, often with a family history of a similarly affected parent or sibling who was undiagnosed. Intellectual disability of varying degrees frequently becomes apparent in later life.

Combined Cerebral and Motor Unit Disorders

Several genetic diseases manifest with abnormalities of both the brain and the motor unit. These conditions can present considerable diagnostic challenges.

Acid Maltase Deficiency

Acid maltase deficiency, an autosomal recessive deficiency of the lysosomal enzyme acid α-1,4-glucosidase, presents with a severe skeletal myopathy and cardiomyopathy and may also be associated with encephalopathy. Routine histochemical stains show accumulation of glycogen in lysosomal vacuoles and within the sarcoplasm. The diagnosis is confirmed with biochemical assay of enzyme activity in muscle or in cultured skin fibroblasts. Recombinant human enzyme is approved by the U.S. Food and Drug Administration (FDA) for replacement therapy, which can prolong survival (Kishnani et al., 2006).

Congenital Myotonic Dystrophy

Congenital myotonic dystrophy is an autosomal dominant disorder that typically presents in adolescence or early adulthood, but in some instances may be associated with profound hypotonia and weakness of the face and limbs in infancy. Approximately 25% of infants born to mothers with myotonic dystrophy are affected in this way, although the diagnosis in the mother may be unrecognized (Rakocevic-Stojanovic et al., 2005). Survivors of perinatal distress often have global developmental delay, with both intellectual impairment and motor disability throughout childhood, then develop myotonia and other characteristic symptoms of the muscular dystrophy as they approach puberty. To date, only myotonic dystrophy type 1, caused by abnormal expansion of a trinucleotide repeat within the gene, DMPK, has been associated with a congenital presentation. Genetic testing is commercially available.

Infantile Facioscapulohumeral Dystrophy

Facioscapulohumeral dystrophy (FSHD) is another dominantly inherited muscular dystrophy presenting most frequently in early adulthood, but which may have a congenital presentation. The genetic abnormality is contraction of a 3.3 kb repeat array at the D4Z4 locus. Those with the smallest integral number of repeats may have diffuse hypotonia and weakness in infancy and account for less than 5% of cases (Klinge et al., 2006). Affected infants may have cognitive impairment, epilepsy, and progressive sensorineural hearing loss. Serum CK is normal or mildly elevated. Family history may include a mildly affected parent, although cases also result from de novo mutations. Genetic testing is commercially available.

Syndromic Congenital Muscular Dystrophies

A group of congenital muscular dystrophies due to defects of O-linked glycosylation of dystroglycan, a component of the dystrophin-glycoprotein complex spanning the plasma membrane of skeletal myocytes, are associated with severe myopathy, a cerebral cortical malformation referred to as *cobblestone lissencephaly*, and ocular defects such as retinal dysplasia. In addition to profound hypotonia and weakness, affected infants often have intractable epilepsy. These diagnoses are suspected based on the characteristic constellation of abnormalities and have been clinically categorized as *Fukuyama congenital muscular dystrophy*, *Walker-Warburg syndrome*, and *muscle-eye-brain disease*. Thus far, six different causative genes have been identified (Muntoni et al., 2008), and there appears to be a far greater degree of phenotypic overlap among the different genotypes than was previously appreciated.

Congenital Disorders of Glycosylation

Congenital disorders of glycosylation are a group of recessively inherited defects in 21 different enzymes that modify N-linked oligosaccharides. Many forms present with hypotonia in infancy. The most common form, type Ia, results from a deficiency of the phosphomannomutase enzyme. In addition to hypotonia, affected infants may have hyporeflexia, global developmental delay, failure to thrive, seizures, and evidence of hepatic dysfunction, coagulopathy, and elevated thyroid-stimulating hormone (TSH). Characteristic examination findings include inverted nipples and an abnormal distribution of subcutaneous fat. Facial dysmorphism occurs but is not present in all cases. Brain MRI shows cerebellar hypoplasia. Analysis of transferrin isoforms in serum by isoelectric focusing reveals a characteristic pattern indicative of a defect in the early steps of the N-linked oligosaccharide synthetic pathway. Commercially available genetic testing identifies pathogenic sequence variants in 95% of affected individuals. Although cerebral dysfunction dominates the early clinical picture, some patients develop a demyelinating peripheral neuropathy in the first or second decade of life (Gruenwald, 2009).

Lysosomal Disorders

Certain defects of lysosomal hydrolases, in particular *Krabbe disease* and *metachromatic leukodystrophy*, result in progressive degeneration of both central and peripheral myelin (Korn-Lubetzki et al., 2003), producing both an encephalopathy and motor unit dysfunction (Cameron et al., 2004). Both disorders are associated with characteristic white matter abnormalities on brain MRI, and biochemical assays on peripheral blood of β-galactocerebrosidase in the case of Krabbe, and of arylsulfatase A in the case of metachromatic leukodystrophy confirm the diagnosis.

Infantile Neuroaxonal Dystrophy

Neuroaxonal dystrophy is a rare autosomal recessive disorder caused by mutations in the PLA2G6 gene, which encodes a calcium-independent phospholipase (Gregory et al., 2008). The classic form may present as early as 6 months of age with hypotonia, although psychomotor regression is more common, and progressive spastic tetraparesis and optic atrophy with visual impairment follow. Brain MRI shows bilateral T2 hypointensity of the globus pallidus, indicative of progressive iron accumulation, as well as thinning of the corpus callosum and cerebellar cortical hyperintensities. Nerve conduction studies show evidence of an axonal sensorimotor polyneuropathy with active denervation on EMG. The characteristic

pathological finding is of enlarged and dystrophic-appearing axons on biopsy of skin, peripheral nerve, or other tissue containing peripheral nerve. Commercially available genetic testing identifies abnormalities in approximately 95% of children with early symptom onset.

Spinal Cord Disorders

Disorders of the spinal cord leading to generalized hypotonia in infancy usually involve the cervical spine at a minimum but may involve the entire cord. They include both acquired processes and genetic syndromes.

Acquired Spinal Cord Lesions

Acquired spinal cord lesions relate to trauma sustained during delivery or occur as a part of the spectrum of hypoxic-ischemic encephalopathy. As previously noted, the highest risk of spinal cord injury occurs in vaginal deliveries with breech presentation, particularly when the head is hyperextended in utero. Herniation of the brainstem through the foramen magnum, as well as injury to the cerebellum, may also occur. Cervical spine injury may also occur in cephalic presentations with midforceps delivery, especially in cases of prolonged rupture of membranes. In both traction injury and hypoxic-ischemic injury, encephalopathy often dominates the early clinical picture and may obscure the extent of spinal cord dysfunction. Potential indicators in the acute phase include bladder distention with dribbling of urine and impaired sweating below the level of the lesion. Signs of spasticity gradually supplant early flaccid paraparesis. As mental status improves, the level and extent of motor impairment becomes apparent. MRI of the spine in the acute stage may show cord edema or hemorrhage, whereas imaging obtained later in the course may reveal cord atrophy.

Spinal Muscular Atrophy

Spinal muscular atrophy (SMA) is the most common inherited disorder of the spinal cord resulting in hypotonia in infancy, occurring with an incidence of approximately 1 in 10,000 live births per year. It is an autosomal recessive disorder in which the molecular defect leads to impaired regulation of programmed cell death in anterior horn cells and in motor nuclei of lower cranial nerves. Both populations of motor neurons are progressively lost, producing hypotonia and weakness of limb and truncal musculature, as well as bulbar dysfunction. In approximately 95% of cases, the genetic defect is homozygous deletion of the survival motor neuron 1 (SMN1) gene, which is located on the telomeric region of chromosome 5q13 (Ogino and Wilson, 2002). A virtually identical centromeric gene on 5q13, referred to as *SMN2*, encodes a similar but less biologically active product (Swoboda et al., 2005). While no more than two copies of SMN1 are present in the human genome, variable numbers of SMN2 copies are present. The protein product of SMN2 appears to partially rescue the SMA phenotype such that a larger SMN2 copy number generally results in a milder presentation and disease course.

Historically, SMA patients have been categorized into different phenotypes or syndromes based on age of presentation and maximum motor ability achieved. The disease results from a common genetic abnormality with a spectrum of phenotypic severity contingent upon modifying factors that include SMN2 copy number and other loci not yet identified. The classification of the most severely affected patients, with weakness and hypotonia evident at birth, is SMA type 0. These infants may have arthrogryposis multiplex congenita in addition to diffuse weakness of limb and trunk muscles, but facial weakness is usually mild if present. Perinatal respiratory failure causes death in early infancy. SMA type 1, also referred to as *Werdnig-Hoffmann disease,* is a designation given to infants who develop weakness within the first 6 months of life. These infants may appear normal at birth or may appear hypotonic. Facial expression is usually normal, and arthrogryposis is usually absent. Weakness is worse in proximal than in distal muscles and worse in the lower extremities, which may lead to suspicion of a congenital myopathy or muscular dystrophy. Further confounding the diagnosis is the presence of an elevated serum CK in a substantial portion of patients (Rudnick-Schoneborn et al., 1998), although CK rarely rises above 1000 U/L. In addition to limb weakness, affected infants demonstrate abdominal breathing due to relative preservation of diaphragm function as compared to abdominal and chest wall musculature. Needle EMG shows evidence of both acute and chronic denervation in the limbs and serves to distinguish this disorder from myopathies with a similar presentation.

Genetic testing is commercially available for SMN-related SMA. Among the 5% of patients without homozygous deletion of SMN1, most are compound heterozygotes with the characteristic deletion on one allele and a point mutation on the other. Parents of affected children are obligatory heterozygotes. The natural history of SMA is unique among anterior horn cell disorders in that the progression of weakness is most rapid early in the disease course and subsequently slows. Nevertheless, in the absence of supportive measures, median survival is 8 months, with death due to respiratory failure. Survivors have normal cognitive development. Several agents that act as histone deacetylase inhibitors increase the expression of SMN2 mRNA in vitro and in vivo, and among these agents, valproate, sodium phenylbutyrate, and hydroxyurea are currently or have recently been in clinical trials in SMA patients (Oskoui and Kaufmann, 2008).

Infantile Spinal Muscular Atrophy with Respiratory Distress Type 1

Infantile spinal muscular atrophy with respiratory distress type 1 (SMARD1), previously classified as a variant of SMA type 1, is a rare and distinct autosomal recessive anterior horn cell disorder. Unlike SMN-related SMA, affected infants develop early diaphragmatic paralysis and distal limb weakness that progresses to complete paralysis. Many have intrauterine growth restriction and are born with ankle contractures. Approximately one-third are born prematurely. Similar to SMN-related SMA, EMG and muscle biopsy reveal evidence of chronic active denervation. The causative gene encodes the immunoglobulin μ-binding protein 2 (IGHMBP2), for which testing is commercially available (Grohmann et al., 2001).

X-linked Spinal Muscular Atrophy

This rare X-linked anterior horn cell degenerative disorder shares a considerable degree of phenotypic overlap with SMN-related SMA. Distinctive features include polyhydramnios secondary to impaired fetal swallowing and arthrogryposis. Consider the diagnosis in any simplex case of a male infant with an SMA phenotype and normal SMN1 copy number. The only known causative gene encodes the ubiquitin-activating enzyme 1 (UBE1), for which testing is available on a research basis only (Ramser et al., 2008).

Peripheral Nerve Disorders

Polyneuropathies, both inherited and acquired, are a rare cause of infantile hypotonia. The two most common clinical designations for infantile polyneuropathies are *congenital hypomyelinating neuropathy* (CHN) and *Dejerine-Sottas disease* (DSD). In recent years, mounting evidence does not reveal that either entity is a monogenic disorder, nor are they clearly distinct from one another. Clinical features include hypotonia, distal or diffuse weakness, absent tendon reflexes, and evidence on nerve conduction studies of a demyelinating polyneuropathy. Traditionally, DSD was classified as hereditary motor and sensory neuropathy (HSMN) type III, but at least 4 genes associated with various demyelinating HMSN subtypes have been linked to the DSD and CHN phenotypes, including PMP22, MPZ, EGR2, and PRX (Plante-Bordenueve and Said, 2002). In general, patients with an infantile presentation are homozygotes or compound heterozygotes for mutations in the causative genes. The most common acquired autoimmune peripheral neuropathies, Guillain-Barré syndrome and chronic inflammatory demyelinating polyneuropathy (CIDP), occur rarely in the first year of life and typically present with weakness and hypotonia in a previously normal infant.

Neuromuscular Junction Disorders

Disorders of neuromuscular transmission resulting in hypotonia in infancy also feature varying degrees of weakness or fatigability. Appreciation of the latter is by fluctuating ptosis, weak suck, or premature discontinuation of oral feedings. Neuromuscular junction disorders presenting with hypotonia in infancy include juvenile myasthenia gravis, neonatal myasthenia gravis resulting from placental transmission of maternal antibodies against the fetal postsynaptic acetylcholine receptor, congenital myasthenic syndromes, and infant botulism.

Juvenile Myasthenia Gravis

Approximately 10% to 15% of cases of autoimmune myasthenia gravis due to endogenous production of antibodies directed against sarcolemmal nicotinic acetylcholine receptors or muscle-specific kinase occur in individuals younger than 16 years of age. The disorder is particularly rare in the first year of life (Andrews, 2004). The small number of infantile cases reported in the literature limits the conclusions drawn with respect to the occurrence of measurable antibody titers, treatment, and outcomes in this age group.

Neonatal Myasthenia

In approximately 15% of infants born to mothers with autoimmune myasthenia gravis, transitory symptoms of myasthenia occur in the neonatal period related to transfer of acetylcholine receptor antibodies across the placenta. Because the fetal nicotinic acetylcholine receptor is different from the adult form, the expression of myasthenic symptoms in newborns depends on the maternal production of antibodies against the fetal receptor. These antibodies are not active against the adult form of the receptor and therefore do not contribute to maternal symptoms. Likewise, antibodies against the fetal receptor are not detectable by commercially available assays. For these reasons, neither maternal symptom severity nor the maternal antibody titer predicts the likelihood or severity of neonatal myasthenic symptoms. As with juvenile myasthenia gravis, the predominant symptoms are ocular or bulbar, although generalized hypotonia or weakness may occur. Rarely, affected infants have arthrogryposis due to prenatal exposure to fetal antibodies, leading to prolonged immobility in utero. Affected infants may require respiratory support temporarily or may require symptomatic therapy with subcutaneous neostigmine prior to oral feeds to prevent fatigue and premature discontinuation of feeding. In a majority of cases, the symptoms resolve within the first month of life (Papazian, 1992).

Congenital Myasthenic Syndromes

Several genetic disorders of neuromuscular transmission have been identified as causing hypotonia; fluctuating or persistent weakness of ocular, bulbar, or limb muscles; or arthrogryposis in infancy. The basis of one widely used classification scheme of congenital myasthenic syndromes (CMS) is whether the abnormality occurs in the presynaptic motor nerve terminal, the synaptic cleft, or the postsynaptic sarcolemma. The cause of the presynaptic disorder is a defect in the enzyme choline acetyltransferase, which synthesizes the neurotransmitter, whereas the synaptic defect results from deficiency of the endplate cholinesterase. The causes of the postsynaptic disorders are various abnormalities of the structure, localization, or kinetics of the acetylcholine receptor. Inheritance of most CMS is autosomal recessive, except for the slow channel syndrome, which is autosomal dominant. The clinical presentation is similar to other forms of myasthenia occurring in infancy, although deficiencies of the presynaptic enzyme, choline acetyltransferase, and of the postsynaptic acetylcholine receptor–associated protein, rapsyn, are also associated with sudden episodes of apnea (Hantai et al., 2004). Infants with CMS have negative antibody studies and demonstrate a decremental response on RNS. Specialized electrophysiological testing on fresh muscle biopsy specimens has been useful as a diagnostic tool but is not widely available. Of the 10 different genes currently known to be associated with CMS, testing is commercially available for 7, while testing of the others is available on a research basis only. Most forms of CMS are treated with cholinesterase inhibitors and/or the potassium channel inhibitor, 3,4-diaminopyridine. However, cholinesterase inhibitors may exacerbate end-plate cholinesterase deficiency and slow-channel syndrome, while the latter may respond to fluoxetine (Harper et al., 2003). The natural history of CMS is highly variable even among patients with the same genotype.

Infant Botulism

Spores of the gram-positive anaerobe *Clostridium botulinum*, an organism found in soil and in some cases in contaminated foods, produce an exotoxin that prevents anchoring of acetylcholine-containing vesicles to the presynaptic nerve terminal of the neuromuscular junction, disrupting neuromuscular transmission and resulting in flaccid weakness. In adults, the cause of botulism is ingestion of the preformed toxin; the organism itself cannot survive in the acidic environment of the adult digestive tract. By contrast, infants who ingest spores may be colonized and develop botulism from in situ production of the toxin. Affected infants may present any time after 2 weeks of age and may have relatively greater involvement of bulbar than appendicular muscles. The characteristic finding on RNS is an increment in the CMAP with high-rate (50 Hz) stimulation (Cornblath et al., 1983). Diagnostic confirmation is obtained by testing a stool or enema specimen with a bioassay in mice inoculated against different strains of toxin. Aside from supportive measures, early administration of botulinum immune globulin shortens the course of the disease (Arnon et al., 2006). In most cases, treatment should be initiated based on the clinical suspicion and should not be delayed while awaiting results of the bioassay.

Muscle Disorders

Subsets of disorders that cause hypotonia in infancy relate to developmental or structural defects of myocytes and do not affect cerebral function. The *congenital myopathies* are developmental muscle disorders with distinctive features on muscle histology. Most are autosomal recessive or X-linked, although some are allelic with dominantly inherited conditions with later symptom onset. Common features include diffuse weakness and hypotonia with normal or mildly elevated serum CK, nonspecific myopathic abnormalities on EMG, and predominance of type I fibers on muscle histology. The diagnosis is contingent upon biopsy findings and in some cases can be confirmed with commercially available genetic testing. Cognition is usually normal, and there are no abnormalities of other organs. Weakness may be severe but is typically static or slowly progressive, and some affected infants show improved strength through the early childhood years. Treatment for these conditions is supportive. The nonsyndromic congenital muscular dystrophies also feature diffuse weakness and hypotonia and are often associated with significant elevations in serum CK. Although subcortical white matter abnormalities may be seen on brain MRI in affected patients, cognitive development is usually normal. Treatment of the disorders discussed in this section is largely supportive.

Congenital Myopathies
CENTRONUCLEAR MYOPATHY

Centronuclear myopathy has X-linked, recessive, and dominant forms due to defects in three different genes, although only the first two result in congenital weakness and hypotonia. X-linked centronuclear myopathy, caused by mutations in the MTM1 gene, affects male infants. Clinical features include facial weakness, ptosis, and ophthalmoplegia in addition to severe limb weakness. Affected infants may have macrocephaly, a thin face, and long digits. Serum CK is normal or mildly elevated, and EMG shows a nonspecific myopathic pattern. The characteristic findings on muscle pathology are the presence of large, single, centrally located nuclei in more than 5% of myofibers, and predominance of hypotrophic type I fibers

(Pierson et al., 2007). Mutations in the BIN1 gene result in a similar phenotype but with recessive inheritance (Nicot et al., 2007). A dominantly inherited form of centronuclear myopathy exists but presents beyond infancy.

NEMALINE MYOPATHY

At least six different genes have been associated with this disorder, all of which encode different components of thin filaments within the sarcomere. Inheritance may be recessive or dominant, and many cases are associated with de novo mutations. Characteristic of many forms is congenital weakness involving proximal limb muscles, the face, and extraocular muscles. Muscle biopsy reveals characteristic rod-shaped sarcoplasmic inclusions best visualized on Gomori trichrome staining of frozen muscle. The most common abnormality is in the gene encoding the skeletal muscle alpha actin (ACTA1), accounting for approximately 25% of cases. Genetic testing is commercially available for this gene, as well as four of the other known causative genes (Laing, 2007).

CENTRAL CORE DISEASE

The majority of individuals with central core disease have mild weakness, although congenital weakness with reduced fetal movement, arthrogryposis, and spinal deformities does occur. Sparing of the face and extraocular muscles is common. Histology of frozen muscle shows well-demarcated areas of absent staining by oxidative stains such as NADH-tetrazolium reductase. These areas tend to be centrally located within type I myofibers and run the entire length of the myofibers on longitudinal sections. The most common causative genetic abnormality affects the skeletal muscle ryanodine receptor 1 (RYR1), which mediates calcium release from the sarcoplasmic reticulum during excitation-contraction coupling. The disorder is allelic with susceptibility to malignant hyperthermia (Robinson et al., 2006). Some individuals have both phenotypes, others have only one of the two disorders. Both autosomal dominant and autosomal recessive inheritance of central core disease has been documented (Monnier et al., 2000).

Nonsyndromic Congenital Muscular Dystrophies

MEROSIN-DEFICIENT CONGENITAL MUSCULAR DYSTROPHY

The etiology of the most common nonsyndromic congenital muscular dystrophy is a recessively inherited deficit of α-2 laminin (merosin), a component of the dystrophin-associated glycoprotein complex in skeletal muscle. Affected infants are hypotonic, with weakness of face and limb muscles and arthrogryposis. Extraocular and bulbar muscles are not usually affected. Serum CK is highly elevated, and hypomyelination of cerebral white matter is apparent on brain MRI by 6 months of age. EMG is myopathic, and some infants also have evidence of peripheral myelin dysfunction on nerve conduction studies. Muscle biopsy shows evidence of a chronic necrotizing myopathy, and endomysial lymphocytic inflammation also occurs. Immunostaining demonstrates absence of skeletal muscle merosin. Sequencing of the LAMA2 gene is commercially available. Weakness is usually static. Epilepsy occurs at a higher rate in affected infants than in the general population, although cognition is usually normal (Herrmann et al., 1996).

ULLRICH CONGENITAL MUSCULAR DYSTROPHY

This autosomal recessive nonsyndromic congenital muscular dystrophy results from defects in the extracellular matrix protein, collagen VI. The presence of proximal joint contractures with striking hyperlaxity of distal joints in early life distinguishes it from other disorders in this category (Muntoni et al., 2002). Serum CK ranges from normal to 10 times the upper limit of normal. Reduced immunostaining of frozen skeletal muscle for collagen VI and production of the protein in cultured fibroblasts are diagnostic. Both assays, as well as genetic testing for abnormalities in the three different COL6A genes, are commercially available.

References

The complete reference list is available online at www.expertconsult.com.

Chapter 28

Sensory Abnormalities of the Limbs, Trunk, and Face

Karl E. Misulis

Clinical evaluation of sensory deficits is inherently more difficult than evaluation of motor deficits because of the subjective nature of the examination. Despite the best efforts of the clinician to make the sensory examination as precise as possible, inconsistency in the patient's responses is common, and the types of sensory abnormalities may differ greatly among patients. Nevertheless, identifying sensory deficits is important in localizing lesions.

Accurate localization begins with a foundation of detailed anatomy. Presence or absence of motor deficits are also aids to differentiating anatomical localization, so sensory data are always considered together with evidence of other neurological dysfunction.

Anatomy and Physiology

Sensory Transduction

Activation of sensory end organs produces a generator potential in the afferent neurons. If the generator potential reaches threshold, an action potential is produced that is conducted to the spinal cord by the sensory axons.

Sensory transducers are seldom directly affected by neuropathic conditions, although peripheral vascular disease can produce dysfunction of the skin sensory axons, and systemic sclerosis can damage skin sufficiently to produce a primary deficit of sensory transduction (**Table 28.1**).

Sensory Afferents

The rate of action potential propagation differs according to the diameter of the axons and depending on whether the fibers are myelinated or unmyelinated. In general,

nociceptive afferents are small myelinated and unmyelinated axons. Non-nociceptive afferents are large-diameter myelinated axons. Afferent fiber characteristics are shown in **Table 28.2**.

Spinal Cord Pathways

Sensory afferent information passes through the dorsal root ganglia to the dorsal horn of the spinal cord. Some of the axons pass through the dorsal horn without synapsing and ascend in the ipsilateral dorsal columns; these serve mainly joint position and touch sensations. Other axons synapse in the dorsal horns, and the second-order sensory neurons cross in the anterior white commissure of the spinal cord to ascend in the contralateral spinothalamic tract. Although this tract is best known for conduction of pain and temperature information, some non-nociceptive tactile sensation is conducted as well.

The dorsal column tracts ascend to the cervicomedullary junction, where axons from the leg synapse in the nucleus gracilis and axons from the arms synapse in the nucleus cuneatus. **Fig. 28.1** shows the ascending pathways through the spinal cord to the brain.

Brain Pathways
Brainstem

Axons from the nucleus gracilis and nucleus cuneatus cross in the medulla and ascend in the medial lemniscus (from a Greek word meaning "ribbon"). The spinothalamic tracts in the brainstem are continuations of the same tracts in the spinal cord and ascend lateral to the medial lemniscus in the brainstem.

Table 28.1 Sensory Receptors

Receptor	Type	Afferent Axon	Modality
Pacinian corpuscle	Multilayered capsule around a nerve terminal, producing a rapidly adapting mechanoreceptor	Large-diameter myelinated axons	Touch and vibration
Golgi tendon organ	Specialized organs in tendons near joints	Large-diameter myelinated axons	Joint position and rate of movement
Free nerve ending	Branched terminal endings of axons	Small myelinated and unmyelinated axons	Strong tactile and thermal stimuli, especially painful inputs
Merkel disk	Slowly adapting mechanoreceptor	Myelinated axons	Touch
Meissner corpuscle	Specialized quickly adapting mechanoreceptor	Myelinated axons	Touch
Krause end bulbs	Specialized terminal axon ending	Small myelinated axons	Thermal sensation
Muscle spindles	Specialized organ involving intrafusal muscle fibers and associated nerves	Large-diameter myelinated axons	Muscle length and contraction

Table 28.2 Sensory Afferents

Class (Older Terminology)	Diameter	Conduction Velocity	Modalities
Ia (Aα)	12-20 mm	70-100 m/sec	Proprioception (muscle spindles)
Ib (Aα)	12-20 mm	70-100 m/sec	Proprioception (Golgi tendon organs)
II (Aβ)	5-12 mm	30-70 m/sec	Touch and pressure from skin, proprioception from muscle spindles
III (Aδ)	2-5 mm	10-30 m/sec	Pain and temperature; sharp sensation; joint and muscle pain sensation
IV (C, unmyelinated)	0.5-2.0 mm	0.5-2.0 m/sec	Pain, temperature

NOTE: The terminology of sensory afferents has changed throughout the years. The older terminology, indicated in parentheses, spans motor and sensory modalities, so the newer classification presented here for sensory fibers should be used. The corresponding terminology is presented only for informational reference.

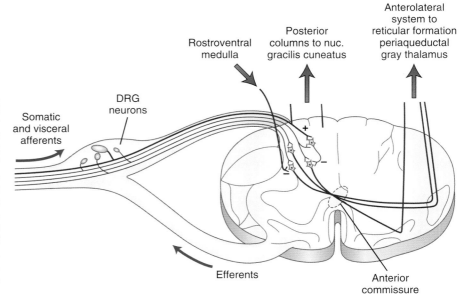

Fig. 28.1 Axial section of the spinal cord, showing dorsal and ventral roots forming a spinal nerve. Sensory afferents give rise to two major ascending pathways: the anterolateral system (nociceptive, serving thermal sensation primarily) and posterior columns (serving large-fiber modalities primarily including touch, vibration, and proprioception). Inhibitory input derives from descending fibers as well as collaterals, via interneurons, from mechanoreceptive fibers. Dashed circle indicates the anterior white commissure. *DRG,* Dorsal root ganglion. *(Modified with permission from Rizzo, M.A., Kocsis, J.D., Waxman, S.G., 1996. Mechanisms of paresthesiae, dysesthesiae, and hyperesthesiae: role of Na+ channel heterogeneity. Eur Neurol 36, 3-12.)*

Thalamus

Lesions of the thalamus rarely affect only a single region, but the functional organization characteristic of this structure may affect clinical findings. The ventroposterior complex is the main somesthetic receiving area and includes the ventroposterior lateral nucleus, which receives information from the body, and the ventroposterior medial nucleus, which receives sensory input from the head and face. Projections are to the primary somatosensory cortex on the postcentral gyrus. The posterior nuclear group receives nociceptive input from the spinothalamic tract and projects mainly to the secondary somesthetic region on the inner aspect of the postcentral gyrus, adjacent to the insula.

Cerebral Cortex

Classic neuroanatomical teaching presents a picture of the central sulcus bounded by the motor strip anteriorly and the sensory strip posteriorly. This division was derived largely from study of lower animals, in which the separation between these functions is marked. On ascending the evolutionary ladder, however, this division becomes less prominent, and many neurologists refer to the entire region as the *motor-sensory strip*. In general, sensory function is served prominently on the postcentral gyrus. The mapping of the cortex follows the same homunculus presented in Chapter 23 (see **Fig. 23.1**), with the head and arm portions located laterally on the hemisphere and the leg region located superiorly near the midline and wrapping onto the parasagittal cortex.

Sensory Abnormalities

Sensory perception abnormalities are varied, and the pattern of symptoms often is a clue to diagnosis:

- Loss of sensation (numbness)
- Dysesthesia and paresthesia
- Neuropathic pain
- Sensory ataxia

Patients often use the term *numbness* to mean any of a variety of symptoms. Strictly speaking, numbness is loss of sensation usually manifested as decreased sensory discrimination and elevated sensory threshold; these are negative symptoms. Some patients use the term *numbness* to mean weakness; others are referring to positive sensory symptoms such as dysesthesia and paresthesia.

Dysesthesia is an abnormal perception of a sensory stimulus, such as when pressure produces a feeling of tingling or pain. If large-diameter axons are mainly involved, the perception typically is tingling; if small-diameter axons are involved, the perception commonly is pain. *Paresthesia* is an abnormal spontaneous sensation similar in quality to dysesthesia. Dysesthesias and paresthesias usually are seen in localized regions of the skin affected by peripheral neuropathic processes such as polyneuropathy or mononeuropathy. These perceptual abnormalities also can be seen in patients with central conditions such as myelopathy or cerebral sensory tract dysfunction.

Neuropathic pain can result from damage of any cause to the sensory nerves. Peripheral neuropathic conditions result in failure of conduction of the sensory fibers, giving decreased sensory function plus pain from discharge of damaged nociceptive axons. The pathophysiology of neuropathic pain is interesting. Part of its basis is lowering of the membrane potential of the axons so that minor deformation of the nerve can produce repetitive action-potential discharges (Zimmermann, 2001). An additional feature with neuropathic conditions appears to be membrane potential instability, so that the crests of fluctuations of membrane potential can produce action potentials. Finally, cross-talk (ephaptic transmission) between damaged axons allows an action potential in one nerve fiber to be abnormally transmitted to an adjacent nerve fiber. These pathophysiological changes also produce exaggerated sensory symptoms including hyperesthesia and hyperpathia. *Hyperesthesia* is increased sensory experience with a stimulus. *Hyperpathia* is augmented painful sensation.

Sensory ataxia is the difficulty in coordination of a limb that results from loss of sensory input, particularly proprioceptive input. The resulting deficit may resemble cerebellar ataxia, but other signs of cerebellar dysfunction are seen on neurological examination.

Localization of Sensory Abnormalities

A general guide to sensory localization is presented in **Table 28.3**. Guidelines for diagnosis of these sensory abnormalities are summarized in **Table 28.4**. Details of specific sensory levels of dysfunction are discussed next.

Table 28.3 Sensory Localization

Level of Lesion	Features and Location of Sensory Loss
Cortical	Sensory loss in contralateral body restricted to portion of the homunculus affected by lesion. If entire side is affected (with large lesions), either the face and arm or the leg tends to be affected to a greater extent.
Internal capsule	Sensory symptoms in contralateral body which usually involve head, arm, and leg to an equal extent. Motor findings common, although not always present.
Thalamus	Sensory symptoms in contralateral body including head. May split midline. Sensory dysfunction without weakness highly suggestive of lesion of the thalamus.
Spinal transaction	Sensory loss at or below a segmental level, which may be slightly different for each side. Motor examination also key to localization.
Spinal hemisection	Sensory loss ipsilateral for vibration and proprioception (dorsal columns), contralateral for pain and temperature (spinothalamic tract).
Nerve root	Sensory symptoms follow dermatomal distribution.
Plexus	Sensory symptoms span two or more adjacent root distributions, corresponding to anatomy of plexus divisions.
Peripheral nerve	Distribution follows peripheral nerve anatomy or involves nerves symmetrically.

Table 28.4 Diagnosis of Sensory Abnormalities

Abnormality	Features	Lesion	Cause
Distal sensory deficit	Sensory loss with or without pain distal on the legs. Arms may also be affected	Peripheral nerve	Peripheral neuropathy
Proximal sensory deficit	Sensory loss on trunk, without limb symptoms	Neuropathy with predominantly proximal involvement	Porphyria, diabetes, other plexopathies
Dermatomal distribution of pain and/or sensory loss	Pain and/or sensory loss in the distribution of a single nerve root	Nerve root	Radiculopathy due to disc, osteophyte, tumor, herpes zoster
Single-limb sensory deficit	Loss of sensation on one entire limb that spans neural and dermatomal distributions	Plexus or multiple single nerves	Autoimmune plexitis, hematoma, tumor
Hemisensory deficit	Loss of sensation on one side of body. May be associated with pain. Face involved with brain lesions but not spinal lesions	Thalamus, cerebral cortex, or projections. Brainstem lesion, spinal cord lesion, lower lesions do not involve face	Infarction, hemorrhage, demyelinating disease, tumor, infection
Crossed sensory deficit: unilateral facial and contralateral body	Unilateral loss of pain and temperature sensation on contralateral body	Lesions of uncrossed trigeminal fibers and crossed spinothalamic fibers	Lateral medullary syndrome
Pain/temperature and vibration/ proprioception deficits on opposite sides	Unilateral loss of sensation on face, unilateral loss of vibration and proprioception on other side	Spinal cord lesion ipsilateral to vibration and proprioception deficit and contralateral to pain and temperature deficit	Disc protrusion, spinal stenosis, intraspinal tumor, transverse myelitis, intraparenchymal lesions are more likely to produce dissociated sensory loss.
Dissociated suspended sensory deficit	Loss of pain and temperature sensation on one or both sides, with normal sensation above and below	Syringomyelia in the cervical or thoracic spinal cord	Chiari malformation, hydromyelia, central spinal cord tumor, or hemorrhage
Sacral sparing	Preservation of perianal sensation, with impaired sensation in legs and trunk	Lesion of the cord, with mainly central involvement sparing peripherally located sacral ascending fibers	Cord trauma, intrinsic tumors of the cord

Peripheral Sensory Lesions

Lesions of peripheral nerves and the plexuses produce sensory loss that follows their peripheral anatomical distribution. Exact mapping of sensory deficit is commonly difficult because sensory testing is subjective. Also recognized are interindividual differences in sensory peripheral anatomy including distribution and overlap of sensory fields. Peripheral sensory loss produces a multitude of potential complaints. Clues to localization are as follows:

- Distal sensory loss and/or pain in more than one limb suggests peripheral neuropathy.
- Sensory loss in a restricted portion of one limb suggests a peripheral nerve or plexus lesion, and mapping of the deficit should make the diagnosis.
- Sensory loss affecting an entire limb seldom is due to a peripheral lesion, because even proximal plexus lesions rarely affect the entire limb. A central lesion should be sought.

Unfortunately, especially with peripheral lesions, a discrepancy between the complaint and the examination findings is common. The patient may complain of sensory loss affecting an entire limb when the examination shows a median or ulnar distribution of sensory loss. Alternatively, the patient may complain of sensory loss, but examination fails to reveal a sensory deficit. This discrepancy is more likely to be due to limitations of the examination than to malingering. Also, patients may have significant sensory complaints as a result of pathophysiological dysfunction of the afferent axons while the integrity and conducting function of the axons are still intact, so the examination will show no loss of sensory function.

Fig. 28.2 summarizes the peripheral nerve anatomy of the body, and **Fig. 28.3** shows the dermatomal distribution.

Spinal Sensory Lesions

Certain sensory syndromes suggest a spinal lesion:

- Sensory level on the trunk
- Dissociated sensory loss on the trunk or limbs, sparing the face
- Suspended sensory loss
- Sacral sparing

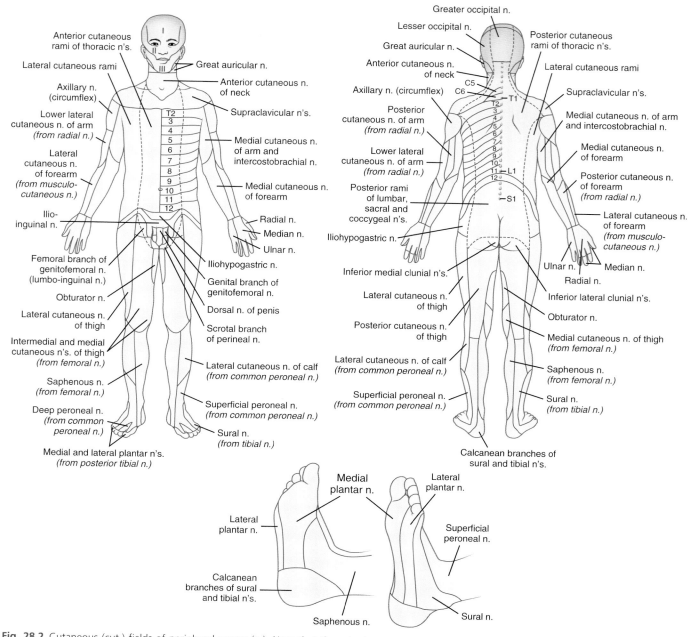

Fig. 28.2 Cutaneous (cut.) fields of peripheral nerves (n.). Note that thoracic dermatomes are innervated by primary anterior and posterior rami of spinal nerves from the respective level. Spinous processes of T1, L1, and S1 are indicated. *inf.,* Inferior; *lat.,* lateral; *med.,* median. *(Reprinted with permission from Haymaker, W., Woodall, B., 1953. Peripheral Nerve Injuries: Principles of Diagnosis. W.B. Saunders, Philadelphia.)*

Sensory level is a deficit below a certain level of the spinal cord segments. *Dissociated sensory loss* is disturbance of pain and temperature on one side of the body and of vibration and proprioception on the other side. The term also can be used to describe loss of one sensory modality (e.g., pain and temperature) with normality of the other sensory modality—in this instance, vibration and proprioception. *Suspended sensory loss* describes the clinical situation in which sensory loss involves a number of dermatomes while those above and below are spared. *Sacral sparing* is disturbance of sensory function in the legs, with preservation of perianal sensation.

Sensory Level

A spinal localization is suggested by loss of sensation below a certain spinal level (i.e., a sensory level). Loss of sensation in a myelopathic distribution without weakness and reflex abnormalities would be very unusual. Sensory symptoms with incipient myelopathy are more often positive than negative; the Lhermitte sign (electric shock–like paresthesias radiating down the spine and often into the arms and legs, produced by flexion of the cervical spine) is a common presentation of cervical myelopathy. Although the Lhermitte sign commonly is thought of as being associated with inflammatory

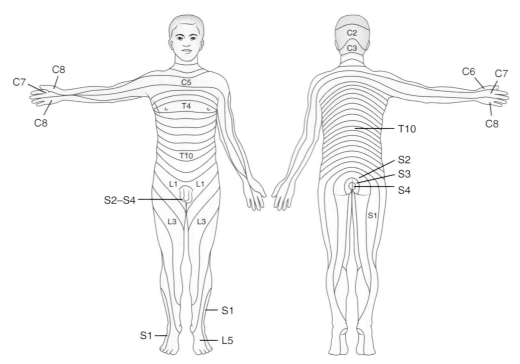

Fig. 28.3 Dermatomes: cervical (C), thoracic (T), lumbar (L), and sacral (S). Boundaries are not quite as distinct as shown here because of overlapping innervation and variability among individuals. *(Reprinted with permission from Martin, J.H., Jessell, T.M., 1991. Anatomy of the somatic sensory system. In: Kandel, E.R. (Ed.), Principles of Neural Science. Appleton & Lange, Norwalk, Conn.)*

conditions such as multiple sclerosis, it more commonly is seen with cervical spondylotic myelopathy and has been reported after radiation therapy affecting the cervical spinal cord and also even after cervical injections.

Although a spinal cord localization is suspected with a sensory level, the level of the sensory loss may be slightly different between the two sides; this finding does not indicate a second lesion. Also, a basic tenet of neurology for evaluation of spinal sensory levels is to look for a lesion not only at the upper level of the deficit but also higher. Magnetic resonance imaging (MRI) is the best noninvasive test for assessing sensory loss of spinal origin. Of note, demyelinating disease and other inflammatory conditions of the spinal cord may not be visualized on MRI, although if an inflammatory lesion is suspected, a contrasted study on a high-field scanner has greater diagnostic sensitivity (Runge, Muroff, and Jinkins, 2001).

Dissociated Sensory Loss

Pain and temperature fibers cross shortly after entering the spinal cord and ascend contralaterally in the spinothalamic tract, whereas vibration and proprioception fibers ascend uncrossed in the dorsal columns. Therefore, unilateral lesions of the spinal cord can produce loss of vibration and proprioception ipsilateral to the lesion and loss of pain and temperature sensation contralateral to the lesion. This dissociation of sensory loss is most prominent in patients with intrinsic spinal cord lesions such as tumors but can also be seen with focal extrinsic compression. MRI usually shows the spinal lesion. The level of the deficits is often not congruent because of intersegmental projection of the pain and temperature

axons in the posterolateral tract before synapsing on second-order neurons.

A second form of dissociated sensory loss can arise from selective lesions of the dorsal or ventral aspects of the cord. Anterior spinal artery syndrome produces infarction of the ventral aspect of the cord, sparing the dorsal columns, so deficit of pain and temperature is found below the level of the lesion, but vibration and proprioception are spared. A selective lesion of the dorsal columns is less likely, but predominant dorsal column deficits can occur in patients with tabes dorsalis, multiple sclerosis, subacute combined degeneration, or Friedreich ataxia, and occasionally in focal spinal cord mass lesions.

Suspended Sensory Loss

A third form of dissociated sensory loss with loss of pain and temperature sensation, sparing of touch and joint-position sensation (usually affecting the upper limbs), and normal sensation above and below the lesion is seen in syringomyelia (see Syringomyelia, later).

Sacral Sparing

Ascending spinal afferents are topographically organized, with caudal fibers peripheral to more rostral fibers. Therefore, central cord lesions can affect the higher fibers before the lower fibers, so sensory loss throughout the legs with sparing of perianal sensation may be found. In some patients with severe cord lesions, this preserved sensation may be the only neurological function below the level of the lesion. The cause usually is trauma, but intrinsic mass lesions also can produce this clinical picture.

Brainstem Sensory Lesions

Brainstem lesions uncommonly affect sensory function without affecting motor function. The notable exception is trigeminal neuralgia, characterized by lancinating pain without sensory loss in the distribution of a portion of the trigeminal nerve. The diagnosis is clinical, and MRI can serve to eliminate other possibilities.

Lateral medullary syndrome typically results from occlusion of the posterior inferior cerebellar artery and produces sensory loss on the ipsilateral face (from trigeminal involvement) plus loss of pain and temperature sensation on the contralateral body (from damage to the ascending spinothalamic tract). With this syndrome, however, the motor findings eclipse the sensory findings; these include ipsilateral cerebellar ataxia, bulbar weakness resulting in dysarthria and dysphagia, and Horner syndrome.

Medial medullary syndrome typically results from occlusion of a branch of the vertebral artery and is less common than lateral medullary syndrome. Patients have loss of contralateral position and vibration sensation, but again, the motor findings predominate, including contralateral hemiparesis and ipsilateral paresis of the tongue.

Ascending damage in the brainstem from vascular and other causes also can produce contralateral sensory loss, but as with the aforementioned syndromes, the sensory findings are trivial compared with the motor findings.

Cerebral Sensory Lesions

Thalamic Lesions

Pure sensory deficit of cerebral origin usually arises from damage to the thalamus. The thalamus receives vascular supply from the thalamoperforate arteries, which are branches of the posterior cerebral arteries, often with some contribution from the posterior communicating arteries. In some patients, both thalami are supplied by one posterior cerebral artery, so bilateral thalamic infarction can develop from unilateral arterial occlusion. Thalamic pain syndrome is an occasional sequela of a thalamic sensory stroke and is characterized by spontaneous pain localized to the distal arm and leg, exacerbated by contact and stress.

Cortical Lesions

Lesions of the postcentral gyrus produce more sensory symptoms than motor symptoms. Infarction of this region involving a branch of the middle cerebral artery can produce sensory loss with little or no motor loss. More posterior lesions may spare the primary modalities of sensation (pain, temperature, touch, joint position) but instead impair higher sensory function, with manifestations such as graphesthesia, two-point discrimination, and the perception of double simultaneous stimuli.

Common Sensory Syndromes

Some common sensory syndromes are outlined in **Table 28.5**. Many of these are associated with motor deficits as well.

Peripheral Syndromes

Sensory Polyneuropathy

The most common presenting complaint among patients with distal symmetrical peripheral polyneuropathy is sensory disturbance. The disturbance can be negative (decreased discrimination and increased threshold) or positive (neuropathic pain, paresthesias, dysesthesias), or both. Most neuropathies involve motor and sensory fibers, although the initial symptoms usually are sensory.

Nerve conduction studies can evaluate the status of the myelin sheath, thereby identifying patients with predominantly demyelinating polyneuropathies, including acute inflammatory demyelinating polyneuropathy (AIDP) and chronic inflammatory demyelinating polyneuropathy (CIDP). Electromyography (EMG) can demonstrate denervation and hence axonal damage, thereby identifying the motor involvement of many neuropathies with predominantly axonal features (Misulis and Head, 2002).

Cerebrospinal fluid (CSF) study is rarely performed for isolated neuropathy, but in patients with autoimmune demyelinating neuropathies, it will show increased protein levels. Increased cellularity suggests an inflammatory cause.

Muscle biopsy usually is performed for evaluation of myopathy but in neuropathy may show denervation and reinnervation. Nerve biopsy can show several of the important causes of neuropathy including inflammatory infiltrates, segmental demyelination, amyloid deposition, and axonal dropout. Nerve and muscle biopsy should be left to those who have expertise in performing the procedure and interpreting the data.

Diabetic Neuropathies

Diabetic sensory neuropathy affects mainly small myelinated and unmyelinated axons, thereby producing disordered pain and temperature sensation. The findings often appear to be a paradox to the affected patient: loss of sensation yet with burning pain. Pathophysiologically, this makes perfect sense. The damaged axons cannot carry the patterns of action potentials, which accounts for the loss of sensation, yet spontaneous action potentials from damaged nerve endings, plus increased susceptibility to discharge from mechanical stimuli, cause the perceived neuropathic pain.

Acquired Immunodeficiency Syndrome–Associated Neuropathies

Human immunodeficiency virus type 1 (HIV-1) infection can produce a variety of neuropathic presentations. One of the most common is a painful, predominantly sensory polyneuropathy (Robinson-Papp and Simpson, 2009). The diagnosis can be confirmed by nerve conduction studies, EMG, and the appropriate clinical findings. CSF analysis and biopsy usually are not necessary unless an HIV-1–associated vasculitis or infection (such as cytomegalovirus) is present.

Toxic Neuropathies

Some toxic neuropathies can be predominantly sensory. Such presentations most commonly are seen in patients with chemotherapy-induced peripheral neuropathy

Table 28.5 Common Sensory Syndromes

Syndrome	Localization	Sensory Features	Associated Findings
Acute inflammatory demyelinating polyneuropathy	Demyelinating lesion of peripheral nerves and roots	Dysesthesias and paresthesias that may be painful, along with sensory loss	Areflexia common early in the course; motor findings predominant
Sensory neuropathy	Axonal or neuronal damage involving predominantly sensory axons	Burning pain, often with superimposed dysesthesias and paresthesias	Reflexes often suppressed distally early in the course
Carpal tunnel syndrome	Compression of the median nerve at the wrist	Numbness on the thumb and index and middle fingers	Weakness and wasting of the abductor pollicis brevis may occur in severe cases
Ulnar neuropathy	Ulnar nerve compression, most likely near the elbow and at the wrist	Loss of sensation on the fourth and fifth digits	Weakness of the interossei often evident with advanced cases
Syringomyelia	Fluid-filled cavity that expands the spinal cord, damaging segmental neurons and white matter tracts	Loss of pain and temperature at the levels of the lesion (capelike distribution; suspended sensory loss); dissociated sensory loss (i.e., affecting spinothalamic sensation and sparing posterior column sensation)	Weakness at the levels of the lesion can develop with motoneuron damage; spasticity below the lesion can develop in severe cases
Thalamic infarction	Infarction of the territory of the thalamoperforate arteries	Sensory loss and sensory ataxia involving the contralateral body	Weakness may develop; aphasia or neglect suggesting cortical damage can rarely develop with involvement of thalamocortical connections
Thalamic pain syndrome	Previous sensory stroke in the thalamus produces neuropathic pain of central origin	Burning dysesthetic pain in the contralateral body, especially distally in the limbs	Other signs of the thalamic damage are typical, including sensory loss
Trigeminal neuralgia	Dysfunction of the trigeminal nerve root	Paroxysms of lancinating electric shock–like neuropathic pain is seen; no other cranial nerve abnormality and no weakness seen	No sensory loss or motor findings

(Gutiérrez-Gutiérrez et al., 2010). Although motor abnormalities do occur, the sensory symptoms eclipse the motor symptoms for most patients. Development of dysesthesias, burning, and loss of sensation is the characteristic presentation. The neuropathy can be severe enough to be dose limiting for some patients and may continue to progress for months after cessation of chemotherapy administration, after which time some recovery is expected.

Patients with neuropathy that develops during chemotherapy can be presumed to have toxic neuropathy. If the association is not clear, however, other possibilities should be considered, including paraneoplastic and nutritional causes. Atypical features of chemotherapy-induced neuropathy include appearance of symptoms after completion of the chemotherapy regimen and development of prominent neuropathy with administration of agents that are seldom neurotoxic.

Amyloid Neuropathy

Primary amyloidosis can produce a predominantly sensory neuropathy in approximately one third of affected patients (Simmons and Specht, 2010). Familial amyloid polyneuropathy is a dominantly inherited condition. Patients present with painful dysesthesias plus loss of pain and temperature sensation. Weakness develops later. Autonomic dysfunction is typical. Eventually the sensory loss can be severe enough to make the affected extremities virtually anesthetic. The diagnosis can be suspected on clinical grounds, and confirmation requires positive results on either DNA genetic testing or nerve biopsy. Findings on nerve conduction studies and the EMG are not specific.

Proximal Sensory Loss

Proximal sensory loss involving the trunk and upper aspects of the arms and legs is uncommon but can be seen in patients with porphyria or diabetes and in some patients with proximal plexopathies with a restricted distribution. Other rare causes of proximal sensory loss include Tangier disease, Sjögren syndrome, and paraneoplastic syndrome (Rudnicki and Dalmau, 2005). These neuropathic processes can be associated with pain in addition to the sensory loss. Motor deficit also is common, with weakness in a proximal distribution.

Patients with thoracic sensory loss also should be evaluated for thoracic spinal cord lesion, which may not always be associated with corticospinal tract signs.

Temperature-Dependent Sensory Loss

Leprosy can produce sensory deficits that predominantly affect cooler regions of the skin including the fingers, toes, nose, and ears (Wilder-Smith and Van Brakel, 2008). Temperature sensation initially is impaired, with subsequent involvement of pain and touch sensation in the cooler skin regions. The deficit gradually ascends to warmer areas, typically in a stocking-glove distribution, with frequent trigeminal and ulnar nerve involvement. The diagnosis of leprosy is suggested by these findings and can be confirmed by additional testing including assay for antibodies to phenolic glycolipid-I (PGL-I) and nerve biopsy.

Acute Inflammatory Demyelinating Polyradiculoneuropathy

Acute inflammatory demyelinating polyradiculoneuropathy (AIDP), or Guillain-Barré syndrome, is an autoimmune process characterized by rapid progression of inflammatory demyelination of the nerve roots and peripheral nerves. Patients present with generalized weakness that may spread from the legs upwards or occasionally from cranial motor nerves downwards. Sensory symptoms generally are overshadowed by the motor loss. Tendon reflexes are lost as the weakness progresses (Hughes and Cornblath, 2005).

The diagnosis of AIDP is suspected in a patient who presents with progressive weakness with areflexia. Nerve conduction studies can confirm slowing, especially proximally (F-waves are particularly affected). CSF analysis shows increased protein level without a prominent cellular response (*albuminocytological dissociation*).

Mononeuropathy

Of the many recognized mononeuropathies, the most common is carpal tunnel syndrome, with ulnar neuropathy a close second. Although not classically considered a mononeuropathy, radiculopathy can be considered to fall into this category because one peripheral nerve unit is affected.

CARPAL TUNNEL SYNDROME

Compression of the median nerve at the wrist produces sensory loss on the palmar aspects of the first through the third digits. Motor symptoms and signs can develop with increasing severity of the mononeuropathy, but the sensory symptoms predominate, especially early in the course. Weakness and wasting of the abductor pollicis brevis can develop (Bland, 2005).

Nerve conduction studies usually show slowing of sensory and motor conduction of the median nerve through the carpal tunnel at the wrist. The slowing is present when conduction elsewhere is normal or at least when the distal slowing is far out of proportion to the slowing from neuropathy elsewhere. The EMG findings usually are normal, but denervation in the abductor pollicis brevis may develop with severe disease. MRI or ultrasound examination of the distal median nerve sometimes is used, though neither of these studies is part of routine evaluation.

ULNAR NEUROPATHY

Ulnar neuropathy is commonly due to compression in the region of the ulnar groove. Patients present with numbness in the ulnar two fingers (fourth and fifth digits). Weakness of the interossei develops with advanced ulnar neuropathy in any location, but sensory symptoms predominate, especially early in the course (Cut, 2007).

Motor nerve conduction studies show slowing of conduction across the elbow or wrist—the two common sites for ulnar nerve entrapment. Findings on sensory nerve conduction studies also will be abnormal if the lesion is at the wrist. EMG can show denervation in the ulnar-innervated intrinsic muscles of the hand; the muscle easiest to examine and study is the first dorsal interosseous muscle.

RADIAL NEUROPATHY

Radial neuropathy is often due to compression of the nerve in the spiral groove. Prototypically, this is seen in patients with alcohol intoxication, although cases are not confined to this association. Damage to the radial nerve in the spiral groove results in damage to muscles innervated distally to the triceps. Patients typically present with wrist drop, and sensory symptoms are minimal. Compression of the radial nerve distally in the forearm near the wrist can produce sensory loss and dysesthesias on the radial side of the dorsum of the hand, and in this case there is no motor loss.

Diagnosis is suspected clinically from the wrist drop in the absence of weakness of muscles of the arm innervated by other nerves; note that examination of median and ulnar-innervated muscles can be difficult if the radial deficit is severe. Sensory findings, when present, are typical. Sensory findings in a radial nerve distribution without motor involvement suggests distal radial sensory nerve damage (e.g., from pressure, handcuffs, intravenous catheter insertion, or other local trauma).

Radiculopathy

Radiculopathy commonly produces pain or sensory loss, or both, in the distribution of one or more nerve roots. Motor symptoms and signs develop with increasing severity, but sensory symptoms (usually pain) may be present for years without motor symptoms. Reflex abnormalities are common in radiculopathy, but such changes should be considered a sensory finding rather than a motor finding. Prominent weakness would have to be present to suppress a reflex, whereas mild sensory dysfunction may suppress or abolish the reflex.

Table 28.6 presents clinical features of common radiculopathies. Although cervical and lumbar radiculopathies are discussed here, any level can be affected. Diabetic radiculopathy and herpes zoster commonly affect thoracic dermatomes, as well as cervical and thoracic dermatomes usually unaffected by spondylosis or disk disease.

Radiculopathy is best investigated using MRI. In patients younger than 45 years of age, the most common etiological disorder is disk disease. In older patients, spondylosis and osteophyte formation predominate. The latter is slower to progress and less likely to be associated with spontaneous remissions and exacerbations. EMG can be helpful to identify any axonal damage from radiculopathy, which may help determine the need, location, and timing of decompressive surgery.

Table 28.6 Radiculopathies

Nerve Root	Sensory Loss	Motor Loss	Reflex Abnormality
C5	Radial forearm	Deltoid, biceps	None
C6	Digits 1 and 2	Biceps, brachioradialis	Biceps
C7	Digits 3 and 4	Wrist extensors, triceps	Triceps
C8	Digit 5	Intrinsic hand muscles	None
L2	Lateral and anterior upper thigh	Psoas, quadriceps	None
L3	Lower medial thigh	Psoas, quadriceps	Patellar (knee)
L4	Medial lower leg	Tibialis anterior, quadriceps	Patellar (knee)
L5	Lateral lower leg	Peronei, gluteus medius, tibialis anterior, toe extension	None
S1	Lateral foot, digits 4 and 5, outside of sole.	Gastrocnemii, gluteus maximus	Achilles tendon (ankle)

Spinal Syndromes

Myelopathy

Myelopathy typically produces sensory loss, although the motor and reflex findings eclipse the sensory findings in most patients. Nevertheless, when a patient presents with back pain with or without leg weakness, a sensory level should be sought.

Some basic "pearls" regarding sensory testing in patients with suspected myelopathy follow:

- A defined line-like level is not expected.
- The sensory mapping is not as precise as that shown on dermatome charts.
- The sensory loss is seldom complete, which makes precise localization even more difficult.
- The sensory level may not be at the same level on the two sides of the body—a discrepancy of up to several levels can be seen.
- Look for dissociated sensory loss due to crossed projections of pain/temperature versus uncrossed touch/proprioception projections.
- Discrepancy in sensory level between posterior column and spinothalamic levels can occur because of intersegmental projections of the axons of the posterolateral (Lissauer) tract.
- The sensory level may be much higher than might be expected from motor examination or pain. This is because the lesion may be much higher than indicated by the levels of clinical findings, reinforcing the basic precept that the examiner must start from the level of the symptoms and look up!

Syringomyelia

Syringomyelia is the presence of a syrinx, or fluid-filled space, in the spinal cord that extends over several to many segments. This is most commonly associated with a Chiari malformation (Koyanagi and Houkin, 2010). The pathogenic theory is that partial obstruction to CSF flow plus pressure waves in the CSF result in rupture of the central canal into the parenchyma of the spinal cord, which then produces symptoms by mechanical effects. The mass effect of the syrinx produces damage to the fibers crossing in the anterior commissure that are destined for the spinothalamic tract, which conveys pain and temperature sensation. With more severe enlargement of the syrinx, damage to the surrounding ascending tracts may occur, affecting sensation below the level of the lesion. By the time this develops, segmental motoneuron damage and descending corticospinal tract damage are almost always present, and clinical signs of these changes can be seen.

Spinal Hemisection

The spinal hemisection syndrome (Brown-Séquard syndrome) is classically described as the result of surgical or traumatic hemisection of the cord, but this presentation is rarely if ever encountered in clinical practice. Below the level of the lesion, ipsilateral deficits in vibration and proprioception from dysfunction of the dorsal columns, as well as contralateral deficits in pain and temperature from damage to the spinothalamic tracts, are the characteristic findings. Ipsilateral weakness also is seen from damage to the corticospinal tracts.

The diagnosis is suggested by the clinical presentation. This is a condition that can easily be missed unless the examiner assesses individual sensory modalities. Merely testing for pinprick will not identify this syndrome. MRI usually is performed to look for inflammatory or structural causes of the condition.

Tabes Dorsalis and Related Disorders

Tabes dorsalis is due to involvement of the dorsal roots by late neurosyphilis. Patients present with sensory ataxia, lightning pains, and often a slapping gait. Tendon reflexes are depressed. Diagnostic confirmation is by serological testing (Marra, 2009).

Syphilitic myelitis is a rare complication of neurosyphilis, characterized by progressive weakness and spasticity. Motor symptoms dominate in this condition, with lesser sensory symptoms than with tabes dorsalis. MRI of the spine must be performed to look for other structural causes of myelopathy.

Brain Syndromes
Thalamic Infarction and Hemorrhage

Thalamic infarction typically produces contralateral hemisensory loss and is the main cause of a pure sensory stroke. All modalities are affected to variable degrees. The thalamus and its vascular supply are not organized so that specific portions of the sensory system are affected without dysfunction of other sensory systems and regions.

Computed tomography (CT) scanning is performed on an emergency basis in patients with sensory symptoms of sudden onset. This study can differentiate infarction from hemorrhage, which has implications for emergent medical management. MRI is usually performed subsequently to accurately delineate the location and nature of the lesion.

Thalamic Pain Syndrome (Central Post-Stroke Pain)

Thalamic pain syndrome is an occasional sequela to thalamic infarction that usually affects the entire contralateral body, from face through arm, trunk, and leg. The pain, mainly distal in the limbs, is present at rest but is exacerbated by sensory stimulation. The distribution of the pain may shift so that the pain is poorly localized (Nicholson, 2004). Sensory detection thresholds are increased. Involvement of the posterior ventrobasal region is thought to be necessary for production of thalamic pain.

In a patient with a known history of thalamic infarction, additional study usually is not needed when thalamic pain occurs. If the pain develops long after the infarction, however, repeated scanning is warranted to look for a new pathological process such as recurrent infarction, hemorrhage, or (less likely) tumor.

The term *central post-stroke pain syndrome* is increasingly used, since not all post-stroke pain syndromes are due to primary thalamic damage, although the thalamus is still felt to be an important part of the pathophysiology (Klit, Finnerup, and Jensen, 2009).

Trigeminal Neuralgia

Trigeminal neuralgia is a painful condition that produces lancinating pain in the distribution of part of the trigeminal nerve. This is prototypical neuropathic pain. Patients have paroxysms of pain that usually last for seconds. Sensory loss does not occur, so its presence encourages further search for other diagnoses. Imaging studies commonly are performed in the evaluation of trigeminal neuralgia but seldom are revealing.

Cortical Infarction

Infarction of the sensory cortex serving the face and arm is due to thromboembolism of branches of the middle cerebral artery.

Infarction in the anterior cerebral artery territory produces sensory loss affecting the leg. Motor symptoms and signs are usually present, as are sensory abnormalities; however, if the region of infarction is limited, the sensory findings may be much more prominent than the motor findings.

Functional (or Psychogenic) Sensory Loss

Functional sensory loss is less common than other positive functional neurological symptoms such as seizures or paralysis. In fact, it is easy to mistakenly ascribe a pattern of sensory loss to a nonanatomical cause when in fact true disease is present. Such misdiagnosis is particularly common with thalamic infarction and plexus dysfunction. Of note, embellished sensory or motor loss, although obvious to the examiner, may be superimposed on a real neurological deficit. The patient may be unintentionally helping the examiner yet essentially ruining the credibility of the report.

These cautionary notes should be borne in mind. In general, however, clinical presentations suggesting functional sensory loss include:

- Sensory loss exactly splitting the midline, with a minimal transition zone
- Circumferential sensory loss around the body or an extremity
- Failure to perceive vibration with a precise demarcation
- Loss of vision or hearing on the same side of the body as for the cutaneous sensory deficit
- Total anesthesia

The discrepancies in total anesthesia can be failure to perceive any sensory stimulus on an extremity that moves perfectly well. This degree of sensory loss would be expected to produce sensory ataxia. Another trap for a patient with psychogenic anesthesia of a limb involves tapping the limb while the patient's eyes are closed; consequent movement of the limb confirms the functional nature of the deficit. Third, if the anesthetic limb is an arm, examining for sensory abnormality while the arms are folded across the chest can be confusing for the malingering patient, especially if performed quickly.

References

The complete reference list is available online at www.expertconsult.com.

Arm and Neck Pain

Michael Ronthal

Evaluation of the patient with arm and/or neck pain is based on a careful history and clinical examination. Diagnosis of the common causes and a treatment plan can almost always be accomplished in the office before laboratory investigation, but further study may be required if the patient fails to improve or has other specific indications for imaging or electrical studies.

A useful approach is to consider the diagnosis in terms of pain-sensitive structures in the neck and upper limbs. These structures may be part of the nervous system or may involve joints. Neurological causes should be considered in terms of the innervation of the neck and arm, and non-neurological causes are based on dysfunction of the other anatomical structures of the arm or neck. Because nerve root irritation generates neck muscle spasm, this type of pain is usually lumped into the "neurological" category. Some essentially non-neurological conditions have neurological complications and are grouped in this chapter as "in-between" disorders.

Clinical Assessment

History
Neurological Causes of Pain
MUSCLE SPASM

Posterior cervical muscles in spasm trigger local pain that is aggravated by neck movement, and the diagnosis is supported by the finding of palpable spasm and tenderness. The pain may radiate upward to the occipital region and over the top of the head to the bifrontal area. It is usually described as constant, aching, or bursting, or as a tight band or pressure

sensation on top of the head. Pain with similar characteristics can be triggered by abnormalities of the facet joints, cervical vertebrae, and even intervertebral disc pathology.

Neck mobility is best assessed by testing for movement in each of the main planes of movement, flexion and extension, lateral flexion to the right and left, and rotation to the right and left. Normally in flexion, the chin can touch the sternum, and in rotation the chin can approximate the point of the shoulder.

CENTRAL PAIN

Dysfunction affecting the ascending sensory tracts in the spinal cord may generate pain or paresthesias in the arm(s) or down the trunk and lower limbs. An electric shock–like sensation provoked by neck flexion and spreading to the arms, down the spine, and even into the legs is thought to originate in the posterior columns of the cervical spinal cord (Lhermitte sign). Although the symptom is frequent in patients with multiple sclerosis (MS), it is nonspecific and simply indicates a pathological process in the cervical cord. Sharp, superficial, burning pain or itching points to dysfunction in the spinothalamic system, whereas deep, aching, boring pain with paresthesias of tightness, squeezing, or a feeling of swelling suggests dysfunction in the posterior column system. The sensory symptoms indicate the dysfunctional tract but are poor segmental localizers.

NERVE ROOT PAIN

If the pathology involves a nerve root, it is referred into the upper limb in a dermatome distribution. Brachialgia (arm pain) aggravated by neck movement, coughing, or sneezing suggests radiculopathy. When these aggravating features are present, one can be fairly certain the pain is radicular. Their absence, however, does not rule out a radicular source. Nerve root pain is classically lancinating in character, but it can also be just a dull ache in the arm.

PLEXUS PAIN

Peripheral pathology may involve the brachial plexus (**Fig. 29.1**) or individual nerves extending to the hand. Infiltrative or inflammatory lesions of the brachial plexus produce severe brachialgia radiating down the upper limb and also spreading to the shoulder region. Radiation to the ulnar two fingers suggests that the origin is in the lower brachial plexus, and radiation to the upper arm, forearm, and thumb suggests an upper plexopathy. Patients with a thoracic outlet syndrome complain of brachialgia and numbness or tingling in the upper limb or hand when working with objects above the head.

ULNAR NERVE PAIN

Ulnar nerve entrapment causes numbness or pain radiating down the medial aspect of the arm to the little and ring fingers. Symptoms are often worse at night when the patient sleeps with a flexed elbow, and they may interrupt sleep. Ulnar paresthesias are also triggered by pressure on the nerve when the patient rests the elbow on the arm of a chair or desk. Tapping on the nerve in the ulnar groove at the elbow may evoke a tingly electrical sensation in the little and ring fingers—Tinel sign.

MEDIAN NERVE PAIN

Median nerve entrapment in the carpal tunnel classically awakens the patient from sleep with numbness and tingling in the thumb, index, and middle fingers, which is relieved by "shaking out" the hand. Pain generated in the median nerve can be sharp and lancinating and radiates to the thumb, index,

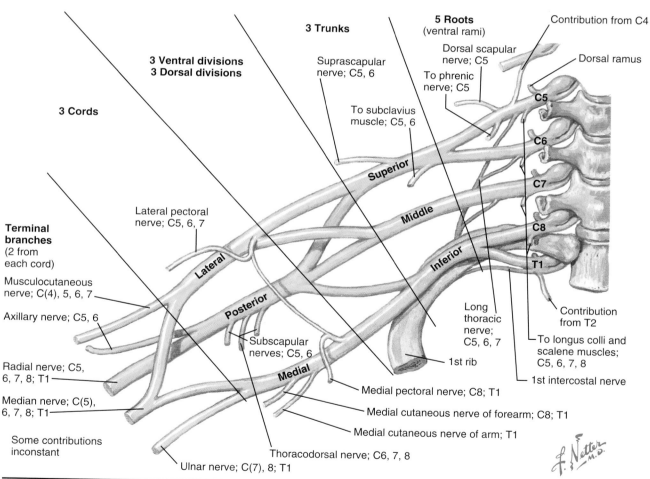

Supraclavicular Branches		Infraclavicular Branches		Infraclavicular Branches	
From plexus roots		*From lateral cord*		Ulnar	C(7), 8; T1
To longus colli and scalene muscles	C5, 6, 7, 8	Lateral pectoral	C5, 6, 7	Medial root of median	C8; T1
Dorsal scapular	C5	Musculocutaneous	C(4), 5, 6, 7	*From posterior cord*	
Branch to phrenic	C5	Lateral root of median	C(5), 6, 7	Upper subscapular	C5, 6, (7)
Long thoracic	C5, 6, 7	*From medial cord*		Lower subscapular	C5, 6
From superior trunk		Medial pectoral	C8; T1	Axillary (circumflex humeral)	C5, 6
Suprascapular	C5, 6	Medial cutaneous nerve of arm	T1	Thoracodorsal	C5, 6
To subclavius muscle	C5, 6	Medial cutaneous nerve of forearm	C8; T1	Radial	C5, 6, 7, 8

Fig. 29.1 Brachial plexus: schema. *(Netter illustration from www.netterimages.com © Elsevier Inc. All rights reserved.)*

and middle fingers. While entrapment at the wrist is common, occasionally the site of entrapment is at the elbow under the pronator muscle.

Non-Neurological Causes of Neck Pain and Brachialgia

Pain arising in muscle is deep, aching, and boring. In the cervical region, it is localized to the shoulders and sometimes radiates down the arm. If the patient is over 50 years of age, a sedimentation rate should be checked; if it is markedly elevated, the diagnosis of polymyalgia rheumatica should be considered. Patients with fibromyalgia may have pain in the neck, shoulders, and arms, with trigger spots or nodules that are exquisitely tender even to light pressure.

If pain is triggered or aggravated by movement of the upper limb, arthritis or tendonitis is the likely cause. Particular attention should be paid to these characteristics; pain on shoulder joint movement is unlikely to be neuropathic. The pain of epicondylitis may radiate down the forearm in a pseudoneuralgic fashion, but precipitation of pain by movement at the fingers or wrist indicates a rheumatological cause.

Examination

The physical examination is designed to localize a neurological deficit related to spinal cord, nerve roots, or peripheral nerves. Evaluation for non-neurological pathology is required because rheumatological problems often complicate a primarily neurological problem. A detailed knowledge of motor and sensory neuroanatomy is required for accurate localization.

Motor Signs

The examination begins with inspection. Particular attention is paid to atrophy of muscles of the shoulders, arms, and the small muscles of the hands. Fasciculations are often due to anterior horn cell disease, but they may be part of the neurology of cervical spondylosis and radiculopathy. Significant sensory signs would argue against anterior horn cell degeneration.

Muscles in the various myotomes must be tested individually. When there is unilateral weakness, the contralateral side can act as a control, but some standard measure of strength is necessary for accurate evaluation when bilateral weakness is present. If one can overcome the action of a patient's muscle by resisting or opposing its action close to the joint it moves, using an equivalent equipotent muscle of the examiner (fingers test fingers, whole arm tests biceps), then that muscle in the patient is, by definition, weak. The degree of weakness can be graded, and the 5-point (Medical Research Council [MRC]) grading scale is often used. Grade 5 represents normal strength. Grade 4 represents "weakness" somewhere between normal strength and the ability to move the limb only against gravity (grade 3). Grade 4 covers such a wide range of weakness that it is usually expanded. One simple expansion is into "mild, moderate, or severe." When the muscle can move the joint with the effect of gravity eliminated, it is graded at 2, and grade 1 is just a flicker of contraction.

The lower limbs must always be examined, even when the patient complains of symptoms only in the upper limbs. Evidence of a myelopathy as evidenced by the finding of sensory or motor dysfunction in the lower limbs, when combined with the presence of radicular signs in the upper limbs, indicates a spinal cord lesion in the neck.

The distribution of weakness is all important in localizing the problem to nerve root, plexus, peripheral nerve, muscle, or even upper motor neuron (central weakness). It is useful to use a simplified schema of radicular anatomical localization when evaluating nerve root weakness because overlap of segmental innervation of muscles can complicate the analysis (**Table 29.1**).

The thoracic outlet syndrome, or brachial plexus entrapment, is an overdiagnosed condition. Maneuvers designed to test for compromise of the neurovascular structures passing through the thoracic outlet are often difficult to interpret. In these maneuvers, the arm is extended at the elbow, abducted at the shoulder, and then rotated posteriorly. The examiner palpates the radial pulse while listening with a stethoscope over the brachial plexus in the supraclavicular fossa. The patient takes a deep inspiration and turns the head to one or the other side. Many normal individuals lose their radial pulse, but the emergence of a bruit does suggest at the least vascular entrapment (Adson test). The patient then exercises the hands held above the head with extended elbows—numbness, pain, or paresthesias, often with pallor of the hand, support the diagnosis (Roos test).

A distribution of weakness that does not conform to a clearly defined anatomical distribution of a single peripheral nerve in the upper limb suggests plexopathy. Upper plexus lesions cause mainly shoulder abduction weakness, and lower plexus lesions will affect the small muscles of the hand.

Sensory Signs

Skin sensation is tested in a standardized manner starting with pinprick appreciation at the back of the head (C2), followed by sequentially testing sensation in the cervical dermatomes, down the shoulder, over the deltoid, down the lateral aspect of the arm to the lateral fingers, and then proceeding to the medial fingers and up the medial aspect of the arm (**Fig. 29.2**).

Table 29.1 Segmental Innervation Scheme for Anatomical Localization of Nerve Root Lesions

Segment Level	Muscle(s)	Action
C4	Supraspinatus	First 10 degrees of shoulder abduction
C5	Deltoid Biceps/brachialis/brachioradialis	Shoulder abduction Elbow flexion
C6	Extensor carpi radialis longus	Radial wrist extension
C7	Triceps	Elbow extension
C7	Extensor digitorum	Finger extension
C8	Flexor digitorum	Finger flexion
T1	Interossei	Finger abduction and adduction
	Abductor digiti minimi	Little finger abduction

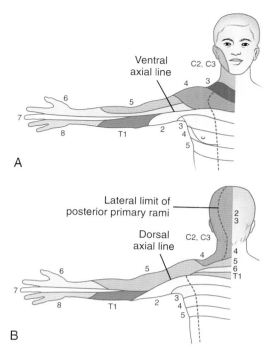

Fig. 29.2 Diagram of the dermatomes in the upper limbs. **A,** Anterior aspect. Although variability and overlap across the interrupted lines are evident, little or no overlap occurs across the continuous lines (i.e., dorsal and ventral axial lines). The examiner should routinely choose one spot in the "middle" of a dermatome and test at that point in all patients. C4 usually terminates at the point of the shoulder, T3 is almost always in the axilla, and T4 spreads across the chest so that C4 abuts T4 approximately at the nipple line. **B,** Posterior aspect.

The procedure is repeated with a wisp of cotton to test touch sensation and test tubes filled with cold and warm water to test temperature sensation. Vibration sense is rarely abnormal in the fingers. Position sense in the distal phalanx of a finger is tested by immobilizing the proximal joint and supporting the distal phalanx on its medial and lateral sides and then moving it up or down; the patient, with closed eyes, reports movement and its direction. Loss of position sense in the fingers usually indicates a very high cervical cord lesion.

Tendon Reflexes

Examination of the tendon reflexes helps localize segmental nerve root levels, but in cervical spondylosis, which is by far the most common underlying pathology, the reflexes are often preserved or even increased despite radiculopathy because of an associated myelopathy. An absent or decreased biceps reflex localizes the root level to C5, and an absent triceps reflex localizes the level to C6 or C7. An absent biceps reflex but with spread so that triceps or finger flexors contract is called an *inverted biceps jerk* and is strong evidence for C5 radiculopathy.

Non-Neurological Signs

The arm is passively abducted and internally and externally rotated at the shoulder. The complaint of pain on movement or at a point in the abductor arc indicates local shoulder joint pathology, usually shoulder tendonitis or pericapsulitis. The tendons anteriorly and at the lateral point of the shoulder may be tender to pressure. More diffuse tenderness anterior to the shoulder joint indicates bursitis. Tenderness over the medial or lateral epicondyle at the elbow indicates local inflammation, and pain on active or passive wrist or finger joint movement suggests tendonitis or arthritis.

Pathology and Clinical Syndromes

Spinal Cord Syndromes
Intramedullary Lesions

Primary intramedullary lesions may be neoplastic, inflammatory, or developmental. The most common presenting symptom of spinal cord tumor is pain, which is present in about two-thirds of patients, usually radicular in distribution, often aggravated by coughing or straining, and worse at night. A minority of patients show dissociated sensory signs (segmental loss of pin prick and temperature sensation with preserved light touch, vibration, and position sense) in the upper limbs to suggest central cord pathology. Long-tract signs in the lower limbs will ultimately develop. Magnetic resonance imaging (MRI) reveals swelling of the spinal cord. The most common tumors are glioma, lymphoma, and ependymoma.

Cervical myelitis presents with rapid onset of radicular and long-tract symptoms and signs and may be due to MS, postinfectious encephalomyelitis, or may be without an obvious cause (idiopathic).

Syringomyelia, a cystic intramedullary lesion of variable and unpredictable progression, may present with deep aching or boring pain in the upper limb, often characteristically referred to the ear. Asymmetrical lower motor neuron signs in the upper limbs, with dissociated suspended sensory loss (i.e., has an upper and lower border to the impairment of pin prick and temperature sensation), is very suggestive of a syrinx. However, the most common cause of intramedullary cord dysfunction is extrinsic spinal cord compression.

Extramedullary Lesions

Extramedullary lesions may result in any combination of root, central cord, and long-tract signs and symptoms. The most common cause of extrinsic nerve root and spinal cord compression is cervical spondylosis. This is a degenerative disorder of the cervical spine characterized by disc degeneration with disc space narrowing, bone overgrowth producing spurs and ridges, and hypertrophy of the facet joints, all of which can compress the cord or nerve roots. Hypertrophy of the spinal ligaments, with or without calcification, may contribute to compression. Hypertrophic osteophytes are present in approximately 30% of the population, and the incidence increases with age. The presence of such degenerative changes does not indicate that the patient has symptoms due to these changes; astuteness in diagnosis is necessary. Furthermore, the degree of bony change does not always correlate with the severity of the signs and symptoms it produces. This degenerative process is sometimes referred to as *hard disc* as opposed to an acute disc herniation or *soft disc* in which the onset is acute with severe neck pain and brachialgia. Patients with cervical spondylosis often awake in the morning with a painful stiff neck and diffuse nonpulsatile headache that resolves in a few hours.

The lesion is most commonly at C5/6 and C6/7, and focal signs are likely to be at these levels. Wasting and weakness of the small muscles of the hands, particularly weakness of abduction of the little finger, is also frequently seen. These signs localize to lower segmental levels, but there may be no observable anatomical change at those levels, and then they are referred to as *false localizers*. Restricted neck movement is always present with significant cervical spondylosis. Bladder dysfunction, indicated by frequency, urgency, and urgency incontinence or the finding of long-tract signs or symptoms, indicates the need for imaging of the cervical spine both to exclude other pathology and to define the severity of the spinal cord compression. Immobilization in a cervical collar often helps with the symptoms and signs of cervical spondylosis. The role of surgery in treatment is discussed in Chapter 75.

Extramedullary compression in the extradural space is usually due to primary or metastatic tumors. Of the primary tumors commonly encountered, a schwannoma produces signs and symptoms related to the nerve root on which it arises, and as it enlarges, progressive myelopathic dysfunction occurs. Plain radiographs of the cervical spine may demonstrate an enlarged intervertebral foramen, but MRI is diagnostic. A meningioma may present in a somewhat similar fashion but is more frequent in the thoracic region.

Epidural spinal cord compression due to metastatic malignancy presents initially with spine pain in over 90% of patients. Malignant bone pain is usually localized to the vertebra involved, and percussion tenderness is a good localizing sign, even in the neck. As the pathology spreads to the epidural space, radicular pain appears. Plain radiographs of the cervical spine may show bony pathology with preservation of disc spaces, and again, the imaging modality of choice is MRI. The whole spinal column should be scanned because the pathology is often at multiple sites and may be subclinical. Spinal cord compression due to metastatic disease is a neurological emergency requiring treatment with immediate high-dose steroids and local irradiation. Occasional patients are referred for surgery.

Epidural infection (abscess) may be either acute and pyogenic or more chronic when the organism is mycobacterial or fungal. Pyogenic epidural abscess usually presents acutely with fever, severe pain localized to a rigid neck, radicular pain, and rapidly progressing root and myelopathic signs. Sometimes the presentation is more subacute with less systemic evidence of infection. Imaging will usually reveal early destruction of the disc, with spread into the epidural space; only later is there spread to bone, with vertebral collapse. Optimal therapy is surgical decompression and evacuation combined with 6 to 12 weeks of appropriate antimicrobial therapy for pyogenic infections and more prolonged treatment for tuberculosis.

The differential diagnosis of a very rapidly progressing painful epidural lesion includes spinal epidural abscess and spinal subarachnoid, subdural, or epidural hemorrhage. The latter are usually associated with some form of coagulopathy or anticoagulant therapy and sometimes with vascular anomalies or trauma. The sudden onset of severe pain in the neck, with or without radicular pain, may be due to hemorrhage. Reversal of the coagulation deficit, if present, should be followed by decompression.

The sudden onset of pain at the back of the neck with associated posterior fossa signs suggests vertebral artery dissection. The diagnosis is easily made with MRI and fat suppression sequences.

Repetitive sudden shooting pains radiating from the occipital region to the temporal areas or vertex suggests the diagnosis of occipital neuralgia. There may be local tenderness over the greater or lesser occipital nerve, and a local injection of corticosteroid plus local anesthetic is both diagnostic and therapeutic. Failure to respond suggests that the craniovertebral junction area should be imaged.

Radiculitis

Herpes zoster may infect cervical sensory root ganglia. The pain is typically radicular, and the diagnosis becomes clear when, after 2 to 10 days, the typical vesicular rash appears. Motor involvement occasionally occurs, and when it does, it has a predilection for C5/6 segments. Myelitis with long-tract signs is seen in less than 1% of patients. If the pain lasts longer than 3 months after crusting of the skin lesions, postherpetic neuralgia has developed. The pain is described as constant, nagging, burning, aching, tearing, and itching, upon which are superimposed electric shocks and jabs. Treatment of postherpetic neuralgia pain is discussed in Chapters 69 and 75.

Brachial Plexopathy

Brachialgia and signs not respecting a single nerve root, associated with tenderness to palpation in the supraclavicular notch, should arouse suspicion of a brachial plexopathy.

Brachial Neuritis (Neuralgic Amyotrophy, Parsonage-Turner Syndrome)

Brachial neuritis is characterized by the abrupt onset of severe pain in one shoulder and arm, which is constant and unrelenting, worse at night, and rarely bilateral. The syndrome afflicts mainly young adult men. Within a week or so, muscle weakness, atrophy, and fasciculations are evident, mainly in the shoulder girdle but at times more distally and not in one particular myotome. There is usually little or no sensory loss despite the pain. Pathogenesis is thought to be autoimmune/inflammatory, and a number of antecedent inciting events have been described, including immunization, infections, and trauma. The syndrome is associated with autoimmune diseases and Hodgkin disease. There is no proven specific treatment, but a short course of corticosteroids is usually given. In general, treatment is supportive, and the pain often runs its course in 6 to 8 weeks. In some patients, recovery from paralysis can take up to a year, and occasionally there is some permanent mild weakness.

A subset of patients who have a familial history have recurrent attacks. Hereditary neuralgic amyotrophy is an autosomal dominant, and many have deletions of the PMP-22 gene in a portion of the distal long arm of chromosome 17.

Brachial Plexopathy in Cancer Patients

Plexopathy in patients with cancer, particularly those with breast cancer or lymphoma who have been irradiated, poses a problem: is this radiation plexopathy or malignant infiltration of the brachial plexus? Malignant infiltration is more likely to trigger severe brachialgia, a Horner syndrome, and to affect the lower plexus. Irradiation damage is less likely to cause severe pain and often affects the upper plexus. Both are slowly progressive, but radiation plexitis is more likely to be of longer duration. Electroneurophysiological studies (see Chapter 32B) are helpful; myokymia and fasciculations support the diagnosis of radiation plexitis. MRI for detecting infiltration with tumor has a sensitivity of 96%, a specificity of 95%, and positive predictive value of 95%. Occasionally a locally malignant, relentless, and recurrent schwannoma occurs in a plexus that has been irradiated many years before.

Thoracic Outlet Syndrome

Brachial plexus involvement as an entrapment syndrome in the thoracic outlet is rare. The very existence of this entrapment remains open to debate, partly because it is rare and difficult to diagnose, and partly because it has been used as a disability issue, often in the absence of proven pathology. Consequently, questions remain about diagnosis and the efficacy of surgical treatment. Entrapment may involve the plexus, the subclavian artery, or both. Sagging musculature with postural abnormalities including droopy shoulders and a long neck contribute to the predisposition for thoracic outlet syndrome.

A supernumerary cervical rib or simply an elongated transverse process of the seventh cervical vertebra may be seen on plain radiographs. The rib may articulate with the superior surface of the first true rib, or a fibrous band may extend from its tip or the tip of the abnormal transverse process connecting to the first true rib. The abnormal structure compresses the plexus, particularly when the upper limb is elevated above head level. Pain and paresthesias radiate to the ulnar side of the hand and fingers, and weakness of the intrinsic muscles of the hand secondary to lower plexus compression may be evident. Thoracic outlet maneuvers described earlier are generally considered to be unreliable but do raise suspicion. The examination may be normal, or there may be weakness of abductor digiti minimi and hypothenar sensory loss. Occasionally, the abductor pollicis brevis is particularly atrophic and weak.

The diagnosis is often one of exclusion; imaging of the cervical spine is normal, and nerve conduction studies below the clavicle are also normal. Venous and arterial anatomy can be studied by catheter angiography, Doppler flowmetry, or MR angiography and venography. Electrophysiological studies that show partial denervation of the small muscles of the hand and a decreased sensory nerve action potential amplitude from digit 5 are compatible with the diagnosis of thoracic outlet syndrome.

In all cases, a conservative approach should be tried initially. Postural exercises and thoracic outlet muscle strengthening exercises, instructions in proper sitting at work, and correction of unusual sleep positions should provide relief in 50% to 90% of patients, usually within 6 weeks. Failure of conservative treatment prompts consideration of a surgical opinion.

Suprascapular Nerve Entrapment

The suprascapular nerve may be entrapped or injured as it passes through the suprascapular notch (see Chapter 76). It is occasionally cut in the process of lymph node biopsy. The branch to the infraspinatus muscle can be entrapped at the spinoglenoid notch by a hypertrophied inferior transverse scapular ligament. The patient complains of deep pain at the upper border of the scapula, aggravated by shoulder movement, and there may be atrophy and weakness of the supra- and more commonly the infraspinatus muscles. The supraspinatus muscle accounts for the first 10 degrees of shoulder abduction, and the infraspinatus muscle externally rotates the arm.

Carpal Tunnel Syndrome

Carpal tunnel syndrome, the most common entrapment neuropathy, is more frequent in females. It is now accepted as an occupational hazard secondary to repetitive stress and occasionally is the presenting symptom of underlying systemic disease. The nerve is entrapped in the bony confines of the carpal tunnel, which is roofed by the transverse carpal ligament.

Pregnancy, diabetes, rheumatoid arthritis, hypothyroidism, sarcoidosis, acromegaly, and amyloid infiltration of the ligament are possible predisposing factors, and appropriate screening studies should be performed on all patients with carpal tunnel syndrome.

Numbness or pain radiates to the thumb, index, and middle fingers and often wakes the patient at night. At times there is diffuse brachialgia. Atrophy of the abductor pollicis brevis muscle may be marked, but the motor deficit is rarely the cause of disability. Significant sensory loss in median nerve distribution can be a handicap because of poor feedback when using the hand out of sight.

In advanced cases, examination reveals atrophy of the abductor pollicis brevis muscle, which produces a longitudinal furrow in the thenar eminence. There is weakness of thumb abduction. In theory there should also be weakness of the opponens, but patients recruit the long flexor tendons when testing opposition, so weakness is hard to identify. The palmar cutaneous nerve branch leaves the median nerve proximal to the flexor retinaculum and supplies the skin over the thenar eminence and proximal palm on the radial aspect of the hand. Hence, sensory loss secondary to dysfunction of the median nerve in the carpal tunnel, if present, is likely to involve the distal thumb, index, and middle fingers but not the thenar eminence, a diagnostic point helpful in localization of the lesion. The Phalen test is performed by holding the wrist in complete flexion, and the test is considered positive when numbness or tingling in a median nerve distribution is seen within 20 seconds, but the latency before the sensory symptoms occur can be up to a minute. Sensitivity is about 74% and the false-positive rate is about 25%. The Tinel sign, distal tingling on tapping the median nerve at the wrist, may be elicited. Confirmation of the diagnosis is provided by nerve conduction studies and electromyography (EMG); distal motor and sensory latencies are prolonged, and polyphasic reinnervation potentials are seen in the abductor pollicis brevis muscle. More extensive and expensive investigations are usually not warranted, but sonography and MRI have been utilized. Initial relief of the sensory symptoms can be obtained with the use of wrist splints, but patients with unremitting pain or significant motor and sensory signs, together with confirmatory nerve conduction studies, should be offered decompressive surgery. This is usually curative. The surgeon should always send the excised flexor retinaculum for histopathological examination to search for amyloid deposition.

Occasionally, carpal tunnel syndrome may be mimicked by entrapment of the median nerve more proximally at the elbow. Here it passes beneath the thick fascial band between the biceps tendon and the forearm fascia and then between the two heads of the pronator teres muscle. As the nerve passes between the heads of the pronator teres, it supplies that muscle as well as the flexor carpi radialis (which flexes and abducts the hand at the wrist) and the flexor digitorum superficialis (which flexes the fingers at the interphalangeal joints with the proximal phalanx fixed) muscles. After it passes between the two heads of the pronator teres muscle, it supplies the flexor pollicis longus muscle (which flexes the distal phalanx of the thumb with the proximal phalanx fixed), the flexor digitorum profundus muscle to the first and second digits (which flexes the distal phalanx with the middle phalanx fixed), and the pronator quadratus muscle (which pronates the forearm with the elbow completely flexed). Nerve conduction studies may localize the site of pathology, and the EMG precisely defines which muscles are involved.

Ulnar Entrapment at the Elbow

The ulnar nerve may be entrapped proximal to the epicondylar notch or as it passes through the cubital tunnel at the elbow, where a fibro-osseous canal is formed by the medial condyle, ulnar collateral ligament, and flexor carpi ulnaris muscle. Structural narrowing of the canal aggravated by occupational stress and a sustained flexion posture, especially when sleeping, and repetitive flexion/extension movements contribute to entrapment. Although numbness and tingling are more common than pain, both are referred to the hypothenar eminence and the little and ring fingers. A positive Tinel sign at the elbow over the ulnar nerve helps localize the site. In severe cases, there is wasting and weakness of the small muscles of the hand (excluding the abductor pollicis brevis and opponens muscles which are median innervated). There is decreased sensation over the palmar aspect of the ring and little finger, and there may be decreased sensation on the medial dorsal aspect of the hand and ulnar two fingers owing to involvement in the distribution of the dorsal branch of the ulnar nerve. In severe chronic cases, clawing of the fourth and fifth digits results from weakness of the third and fourth lumbrical muscles. Nerve conduction studies localize the area of entrapment. If the symptoms do not resolve by avoiding prolonged elbow flexion, and the physical signs are significant, surgical decompression should be considered (see Chapter 76).

Radial Nerve–Posterior Interosseus Nerve Syndrome

Having passed through the spiral groove of the humerus, the radial nerve pierces the lateral intermuscular septum to lie in front of the lateral condyle of the humerus between the brachialis and brachioradialis muscles. There it bifurcates to form the superficial branch, which provides sensory innervation to the lateral dorsal hand and the deep branch, referred to as the *posterior interosseus nerve*. This branch supplies the finger and thumb extensors and the extensor carpi radialis brevis muscle, which is of lesser importance for radial wrist extension (extensor carpi radialis longus is dominant, and its nerve supply comes off slightly more proximally, so radial wrist extension is spared in lesions of the posterior interosseus nerve). The deep branch passes through the fibrous edge of extensor carpi radialis muscle through a slit in the supinator muscle (arcade of Frohse). Entrapment of the posterior interosseous nerve produces symptoms similar to those of lateral epicondylitis—lateral arm pain or a dull ache in the deep extensor muscle area, which radiates proximally and distally and is increased with resisted active supination of the forearm. Extension of the elbow, wrist, and middle fingers against resistance increases the lateral elbow pain. Tenderness may be elicited over the posterior interosseous nerve just distal and medial to the radial head. Pain secondary to posterior interosseous entrapment is typically seen in manual laborers and occasionally in typists. The site of pathology is easily localized by EMG and nerve conduction studies, and surgical decompression is usually successful. Occasionally a neoplasm of the nerve causes the same symptoms, and some surgeons prefer MRI prior to surgery.

Complex Regional Pain Syndrome

Complex regional pain syndrome (CRPS) encompasses syndromes previously called *reflex sympathetic dystrophy* (RSD), *causalgia*, *shoulder-hand syndrome*, *Sudeck atrophy*, *transient osteoporosis*, and *acute atrophy of bone* (see Chapters 44, 76, and 77). By consensus, the syndrome requires the presence of regional pain and sensory changes following a noxious event. The pain is of a severity greater than that expected from the inciting injury and is associated with abnormal skin color or temperature change, abnormal sudomotor activity, or edema. *Type I CRPS* refers to patients with RSD without a definable nerve lesion, and *type II CRPS* refers to cases where a definable nerve lesion is present (formerly called *causalgia*). A soft-tissue injury is the inciting event in about 40% of patients, a fracture in 25%, and myocardial infarction in 12%.

The pathophysiology is unclear, but because many patients respond to sympathetic block and autonomic features are prominent, it has been suggested that there is an abnormal reflex arc that follows the routes of the sympathetic nervous system and is modulated by cortical centers. There is decreased sympathetic outflow to the affected limb, and autonomic manifestations previously ascribed to sympathetic overactivity are now thought to be due to catecholamine hypersensitivity. Significant emotional disturbances at the time of onset occur in many patients, and stress may be a precipitating factor.

Pain can be progressive, and three stages of progression have been described:

- Stage I: sensations of diffuse burning, sometimes throbbing, aching, sensitivity to touch or cold, with localized edema. Vasomotor disturbances produce altered skin color and temperature.
- Stage II: progression of soft-tissue edema, with thickening of skin and articular soft tissues and muscle wasting. This may last 3 to 6 months.
- Stage III: progression to limitation of movement, often with a frozen shoulder, contractures of the digits, waxy trophic skin changes, and brittle ridged nails. Plain radiographs show severe demineralization of adjacent bones.

Motor impairment is not necessary to make the diagnosis, but weakness, tremor, or dystonia are sometimes present.

The diagnosis is essentially clinical. Diffuse, severe, non-segmental pain with cyanosis or mottling, increased sweating and shiny skin, swollen nonarticular tissue, and coldness are characteristic. Hypersensitivity to pin prick may preclude precise sensory testing. There may be associated myofascial trigger points and tendonitis about the shoulder.

Autonomic testing may help with the diagnosis; the resting sweat output and quantitative sudomotor axon reflex test used together are 94% sensitive and 98% specific and are excellent predictors of a response to sympathetic block. Bony changes including osteoporosis and joint destruction may be seen. Bone scintigraphy is most sensitive in stage I and less useful in later stages. A stellate ganglion block may be useful both therapeutically and diagnostically (see Chapter 76).

These patients require a good deal of support as well as trials of symptomatic medication. Drugs that sometimes work are prazosin, propranolol, nifedipine or verapamil, guanethidine or phenoxybenzamine, and antidepressants. Bisphosphonates may prevent bone resorption and are also helpful with pain control. A trial of stellate ganglion block, which can be repeated if successful, is worthwhile. Sympathectomy has been used for progressive disease in patients who previously responded to sympathetic block.

"In-Between" Neurogenic and Non-Neurogenic Pain Syndrome—Whiplash Injury

"Whiplash is an acceleration-deceleration mechanism of energy transfer to the neck. It may result from rear-end or side impact motor vehicle collisions but can also occur during diving or other mishaps. The impact may result in bony or soft tissue injuries (whiplash injury), which in turn may lead to a variety of clinical manifestations (whiplash-associated disorders)."– Québec Task Force on Whiplash Associated Disorders (Spitzer et al., 1995).

Rear-end motor vehicle collisions are responsible for 85% of whiplash injuries, and about 1 million such injuries occur in the United States every year. Severe injuries can cause rupture of ligaments, avulsion of vertebral endplates, fractures, and disc herniations, often associated with cervical nerve root or spinal cord damage. The severity of injury can be graded:

- Grade I injuries: pain, stiffness, and tenderness in the neck—no physical signs
- Grade II injuries: grade I symptoms together with physical signs of decreased range of movement and point tenderness
- Grade III injuries: neurological signs are present—weakness, sensory loss, absent reflex or long-tract signs.

The prognosis is related to the severity of injury:

- Neck pain longer than 6 months after injury: grade I, 44%; grade II, 81%; grade III, up to 90%
- Headache longer than 6 months after injury: grade I, 37%; grade II, 37%; grade III, 70%

- In general, about 40% of patients report complete recovery at 2 years, and about 45% continue to have major complaints 2 years after the injury.

The cause of persistent symptoms in patients with minor injuries is unknown, and little evidence exists for a structural basis for chronic whiplash pain in this group. The difference between a trivial injury and one of more significance should be based on the presence or absence of neurological signs.

About 20% of patients complain of cognitive symptoms after whiplash; cognitive dysfunction is likely to be functional or malingering.

The influence of compensation and legal action in whiplash-associated disorders remains controversial. Two studies from Lithuania, where only a minority of car drivers are insured for personal injury, demonstrated both retrospectively and prospectively significantly less symptomatology than for similar accidents in the United States; at 1 year, no significant difference existed between collision and control groups. The Québec Task Force emphasizes that whiplash is essentially a benign condition, with the majority of patients recovering, but it is the refractory minority that accounts for an inordinate proportion of the costs.

Support, physical therapy, muscle relaxants, and antidepressants are the main therapeutic options, but if neurological signs are present, imaging of the cervical spine with MRI is indicated. Persistence of pain for more than 6 weeks should indicate referral to a more specialized service; often a multidisciplinary team approach is best.

Rheumatoid Arthritis of the Spine

Rheumatoid arthritis in the cervical spine involves all the synovial joints, but it is particularly dangerous when it involves the atlantoaxial articulation. Local inflammation and pannus formation cause pain on neck movement and rupture of the transverse ligament that holds the odontoid process in place. This may cause atlantoaxial subluxation. Pain is referred to the neck below the ear lobe, and there may be a high myelopathy or even sudden death. Spine radiographs show excessive space between the anterior arch of the atlas and the odontoid process.

Non-Neurological Neck/Arm Pain Syndromes

Patients with non-neurological causes for acute, subacute, or chronic neck and arm pain are frequently referred for neurological opinion. They may have no focal deficits or have minor nerve root or peripheral nerve signs that are incidental to their main complaint. Usually the clue to diagnosis is to be found in the history, where a good story of movement aggravating or triggering the pain signposts the cause.

Fibromyalgia and Myofascial Syndrome

Within this group of rheumatological disorders, fibromyalgia is considered to be the most common cause of generalized musculoskeletal pain in women between the ages of 20 and 55 years; its prevalence is approximately 2%. The pain may be initially localized to the neck and shoulders but can spread diffusely over the body. It may follow an episode of physical or emotional trauma or a flulike illness and be associated with depression and fatigue, which are present in more than 90% of cases. Many patients have a true sleep disorder. The only physical sign is muscle tenderness and the finding of "trigger spots," tender palpable nodules in the muscles. The diagnostic criteria are widespread musculoskeletal pain and excess tenderness in at least 11 of 18 predefined anatomic sites.

Myofascial pain is considered to be a localized form of fibromyalgia, with pain in one anatomic region, such as in the right or left neck and shoulder with local tenderness. The cause and pathology of the condition are unknown, and there is no specific treatment. Most patients are tried on muscle relaxants and antidepressants, with physical therapy and exercise. Failure to respond warrants a trial of trigger-point injections of corticosteroid in local anesthetic.

Polymyalgia Rheumatica

Polymyalgia rheumatica, usually seen in patients over the age of 50, presents with severe aching, pain, and tenderness in the neck and shoulder girdle muscles in association with a markedly elevated erythrocyte sedimentation rate. The condition responds dramatically to small doses of oral steroid. Some cases are associated with temporal arteritis. If there is weakness, one should consider the diagnosis of polymyositis, and the serum creatine kinase should be estimated.

Tendonitis, Bursitis, and Arthritis

SHOULDER

Pain triggered by shoulder joint movement suggests tendonitis, capsulitis, or an internal derangement of the joint. Flexion and elevation of the shoulder that evokes pain is often called the *impingement sign*. Patients with a painful arc syndrome often respond to local corticosteroid injections into the tender tendons. Tenderness anterior to the shoulder joint suggests bursitis, which also will usually respond to local corticosteroid injection. Weakness is said to indicate a rotator cuff tear, but pain on movement makes evaluation difficult, and MRI of the shoulder may be needed to establish the diagnosis. Acromioclavicular joint arthritis causes a more diffuse shoulder pain aggravated by arm elevation, and diagnosis will rest on radiographs of the shoulder joint. Nonsteroidal antiinflammatory medications help. Finally, in patients with marked limitation of shoulder joint movement such that the scapula moves en bloc with the arm and is associated with movement-evoked pain, a diagnosis of "frozen shoulder" or adhesive capsulitis is made. Treatment for adhesive capsulitis is not all that satisfactory. Analgesics and physical therapy help in a limited way; the course is likely to consist of many months of discomfort.

ELBOW

Epicondylitis

Pain in the elbow region triggered by clenching the fist (which tenses the extensor muscles and irritates their points of origin), or pain that increases with resisted finger and/or wrist extension and flexion suggests epicondylitis. Local tenderness will be found medially or laterally over the distal end of the humerus. Lateral epicondylitis is known as "tennis elbow," and medial epicondylitis as "golfer's elbow." Treatment with a firm elbow support can be supplemented by local corticosteroid injections. Occasionally these patients require surgery.

Olecranon Bursitis

Local tenderness and swelling at the point of the elbow, which can be extreme (Popeye joint), makes the diagnosis of olecranon bursitis. The condition may follow local irritation but can be part of gout and occasionally represents a pyogenic infection. The bursa should be aspirated for diagnosis.

WRIST

Tendonitis

Wrist tendonitis is diagnosed by finding local tendon tenderness and evoking a complaint of pain when the tendon in question is stretched. Thus, de Quervain tenosynovitis is diagnosed by finding tenderness over the radial aspect of the wrist and evoking pain by ulnar flexion, with the thumb held in the closed fist (Finklestein test). Splinting or casting and the use of local steroids usually resolves the process.

HANDS

In addition to the complaint of pain on finger joint movement, there may be swelling of the joints and inflammation, as indicated by rubor. Pain in the fingers, worse in the morning and not associated with numbness (as in carpal tunnel), suggests rheumatoid arthritis; frequently, spindling of the fingers or other joint deformity can be seen. Distal arthritis in the terminal interphalangeal joints suggests osteoarthritis or psoriatic arthropathy. Bony swelling of the terminal phalanges (Heberden nodes) is likely to be due to osteoarthritis, which can also cause local pain and tenderness.

Red, hot, painful extremities that are sensitive to heat suggest the diagnosis of erythromelalgia. This may represent abnormal sensitization of thermal receptors or abnormal platelet function and is sometimes associated with blood dyscrasias. Erythromelalgia usually responds to aspirin.

References

The complete reference list is available online at www.expetconsult.com.

Lower Back and Lower Limb Pain

Karl E. Misulis

Lower back pain is one of the most common reasons for neurological and neurosurgical consultation. The cost to society is huge, with estimates of up to $80 billion per year in direct and indirect healthcare costs and loss of productivity. In Switzerland, low back pain consumes 6.1% of the total healthcare budget and up to 2.3% of their GDP (Wieser et al., 2010). In many of the patients who present with lower back pain, the pain either developed or was exacerbated as a result of occupational activity. Lower limb pain is a common accompaniment to lower back pain but can occur independently.

The list of considerations in the differential diagnosis of lower back and lower leg pain is extensive and includes neural, bone, and non-neurological disorders. Although lower back pain usually is thought of as either neuropathic (specifically, radiculopathy-associated) or mechanical in origin, other possible sources of pain, including urolithiasis, tumors, and other intraabdominal processes, must be considered in the differential diagnosis.

Related Anatomy and Physiology

The lumbosacral spinal cord terminates in the conus medullaris at the level of the body of the L1 vertebra (**Fig. 30.1**). The motor and sensory nerve roots from the lumbosacral cord form the cauda equina. From there, the motor and sensory nerve roots unite at the dorsal root ganglion to form the individual spinal nerves. These anastomose in the lumbosacral plexus (**Fig. 30.2**), from which run the major nerves supplying the leg (**Table 30.1**).

Pain in the lower back can have many origins. A good beginning for the differential diagnosis is determining whether the leg also has pain. A complicating factor in this consideration is that local spine pain can be referred—that is, felt at a distance—because of the common nerve root innervation of the proximal spinal nerves and peripheral nerves supplying distal parts of the leg.

Causes of lower back pain without leg pain include:

- Ligamentous strain
- Muscle strain
- Facet pain
- Bony destruction
- Inflammation

Causes of lower back plus lower limb pain include:

- Radiculopathy
- Plexopathy

Important causes of leg pain without low back pain include:

- Sciatic neuropathy
- Femoral neuropathy
- Peroneal neuropathy
- Meralgia paresthetica
- Peripheral neuropathies

Isolated tibial neuropathy is uncommon. Individual peripheral nerve lesions usually are caused by local trauma, entrapment by connective tissue, or involvement with mass lesions.

Lower back pain occasionally is caused by non-neurological and nonskeletal lesions. Some of the most important causes are:

- Urolithiasis
- Ovarian cysts and carcinoma

DOI: 10.1016/B978-1-4377-0434-1.00030-X

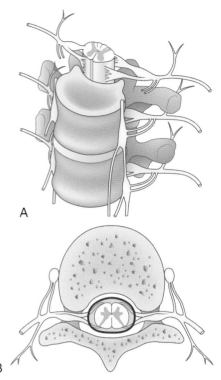

Fig. 30.1 Oblique **(A)** and axial **(B)** views of the spine showing anatomical relationships between neural and bone elements.

- Endometriosis
- Bladder or kidney infection
- Abdominal aortic aneurysm

Diagnosis

The first step in diagnosis is localization of the causative lesion. History and examination usually allow differentiation among mechanical, neuropathic, and non-neurological pain.

History and Examination

The history should focus first on features of the back and leg pain:

- Mode of onset
- Character
- Distribution
- Associated motor and sensory symptoms
- Bladder and bowel control
- Exacerbating and remitting factors
- History of predisposing factors (e.g., trauma, cancer, osteoporosis)

For example, the acute onset of lower back pain radiating down the leg suggests a lumbosacral radiculopathy. Onset with exertion suggests a herniated disk as a cause of the

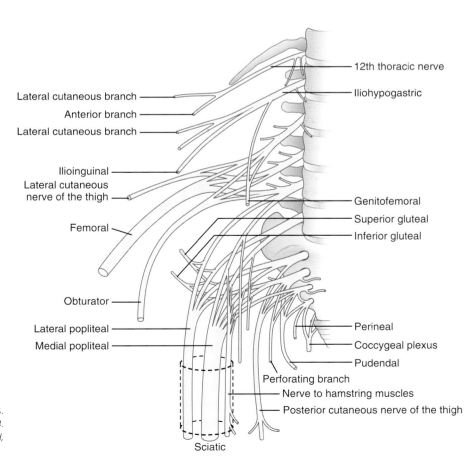

Fig. 30.2 Anatomy of the lumbosacral plexus. *(Reprinted with permission from Bradley, W.G., 1974. Disorders of the Peripheral Nerves. Blackwell, Oxford, p. 29.)*

Table 30.1 Motor and Sensory Function of Lumbosacral Nerves

Nerve	Origin	Motor Function	Sensory Function
Femoral	Lumbar plexus, L2-L4	Extension of knee, flexion of thigh	Anterior thigh
Saphenous	Distal sensory branch of femoral nerve	None	Inside aspect of lower leg
Lateral femoral cutaneous	Branch of lumbar plexus, L2-L3	None	Lateral thigh
Obturator	Lumbar plexus, L2-L4	Adduction of thigh	Medial aspect of upper thigh
Sciatic	Combined roots from lumbosacral plexus, partially separated into tibial and peroneal divisions	Foot plantar (tibial division) and dorsiflexion (peroneal division), foot inversion (tibial) and eversion (peroneal)	Lateral, anterior, and posterior aspects of lower leg and foot
Tibial	Lumbosacral plexus, L4-S3	Plantar flexion and inversion of foot	Posterior lower leg and sole of foot
Peroneal	Lumbosacral plexus, L5-S2	Dorsiflexion and eversion of foot	Dorsum of foot and lateral lower leg
Superficial peroneal	Distal sensory branch of peroneal nerve	None	Dorsum of foot
Sural	Cutaneous branches of peroneal and tibial nerves	None	Lateral foot to sole

radiculopathy. Onset following a motor vehicle accident also could be associated with a disk herniation, although contusion of a nerve root without ongoing compression is more common after this type of trauma. Progressive symptom development can be from any expanding lesion, such as a tumor or expanding disk extrusion.

Patients with lower back and leg pain usually have more symptoms than signs of neurological dysfunction. Therefore, if examination shows sensory and motor signs in a specific radicular or neural distribution, a detectable structural lesion is more likely.

The neurological examination is targeted to determine whether the symptoms are accompanied by abnormal neurological signs. General examination of the lower limb is important. Muscle groups that can be tested include:

- Hip-girdle muscles:
  - Hip flexors (psoas, sartorius)
  - Hip extensors (gluteus maximus, semitendinosus, semimembranosus, biceps femoris)
  - Hip adductors (adductor group: longus, brevis, magnus)
  - Hip abductors (gluteus medius, gluteus minimus, piriformis)
- Knee muscles:
  - Knee extension (quadriceps)
  - Knee flexion (semitendinosus, semimembranosus, biceps femoris)
- Ankle and foot muscles:
  - Foot plantar flexion (gastrocnemius)
  - Foot dorsiflexion (tibialis anterior)
  - Foot everters (peronei)
  - Foot inverters (tibialis posterior)
  - Toe extension (extensor digitorum)
  - Great toe extension (extensor hallucis longus)
  - Toe plantar flexion (flexor digitorum longus)
  - Great toe flexion (flexor hallucis longus)

Sensory examination should include the important nerve roots and peripheral nerve distributions: the femoral, peroneal, tibial, and lateral femoral cutaneous, lumbar roots L2-L5, and sacral root S1. Reflexes to be studied include the Achilles, patellar, and plantar reflexes.

Exacerbation of pain with some maneuvers also can be revealing. Stretch of damaged nerves results in increased pain by deforming the axon membrane, thereby increasing membrane conductance, depolarizing the nerve, and producing repetitive nerve pain action potentials. Straight leg raising augments pain in a lumbosacral radiculopathy. Hip extension exacerbates pain of upper lumbar radiculopathy or that due to damage to the upper parts of the lumbar plexus, such as from carcinomatous infiltration or inflammation.

Armed with the abnormalities recognized from this history and examination, the neurologist may come to a conclusion about the localization of the lesion. This knowledge narrows the differential diagnosis substantially.

Differential Diagnosis of Lower Back and Leg Pain

The differential diagnosis of lower back and leg pain can be addressed as shown in **Tables 30.2 through 30.5**. Classification into mechanical and neuropathic categories is useful to narrow the scope of diagnostic considerations. The possibility of non-neurological causes should always be kept in mind.

Some basic guidelines for the differential diagnosis of lower back and leg pain are as follows:

- Pain confined to the lower back generally is caused by a low back disorder.
- Pain confined to the leg usually is caused by a leg disorder, although neuropathic pain from lumbar spine disease can radiate down the leg without back pain in a minority of patients.

- Pain in both the low back and the leg usually is caused by lumbar radiculopathy or, less commonly, lumbosacral plexopathy.
- Clinical abnormalities confined to one nerve root distribution usually are caused by intervertebral disk disease or lumbosacral spondylosis producing radiculopathy.
- Clinical abnormalities that involve several nerve distributions usually are caused by plexus lesions, with cauda equina lesions being the alternative diagnosis.
- Bilateral lesions suggest proximal damage in the spinal canal affecting the roots of the cauda equina.
- Impairment of bladder control indicates either a cauda equina lesion or, less commonly, a bilateral sacral plexopathy.
- Presence of more than one lesion may complicate neurological localization.
- Non-neurological causes of lower back pain are possible and particularly include urolithiasis, abdominal aortic aneurysm, and other intraabdominal pathological processes.

- Multiple lesions can make the differential diagnosis more difficult. For example, radiculopathies at two or more levels may look like a plexopathy or peripheral neuropathic process.

Non-neurological causes of lower back pain include urolithiasis, ovarian cysts, endometriosis, pelvic carcinoma, bladder infection, and other retroperitoneal lesions including tumor, abscess, abdominal aortic aneurysm, and hematoma. These conditions produce pain that does not radiate unless neural structures are involved. Neural involvement in the abdomen and pelvis can produce radiating pain that can be clinically differentiated from radiculopathy only if multiple nerve roots are involved. Early involvement of bowel or bladder function together with abdominal pain suggests one of these non-neurological conditions.

Evaluation

Diagnostic evaluation of lower back and lower leg pain begins with proper clinical localization and classification of the complaint. Diagnostic tests are summarized in **Table 30.6** (Russo, 2006). The tests used depend on the clinical presentation, as discussed later (see Clinical Syndromes).

Magnetic Resonance Imaging

Magnetic resonance imaging (MRI) commonly is performed to assess the lumbosacral spine and lumbosacral plexus. It also can be used to evaluate the peripheral nerves in the pelvis and lower limbs.

MRI of the lumbosacral spine has the highest yield when the patient has back pain associated with radicular distribution of pain. Isolated back pain with no clinical symptoms or signs in the leg seldom is associated with significant findings on MRI. Intraspinal disorders that may not be revealed by MRI without contrast enhancement include neoplastic meningitis and some chronic infectious meningitides (Tan, Tsou, and Chee, 2002).

Techniques for MRI of the lumbosacral plexus and peripheral nerves have greatly improved, so this modality can reveal masses, infiltration, and some inflammatory lesions, but MRI can miss disorders that are without a structural defect.

Table 30.2 Classification of Lower Back and Lower Limb Pain

Type	Examples
Mechanical pain	Facet pain Bony destruction Sacroiliac joint inflammation Osteomyelitis Diskitis Lumbar spondylosis
Neuropathic pain	Polyneuropathy Radiculopathy from disk disease, zoster, and diabetes Mononeuropathy including sciatic, femoral, lateral femoral cutaneous, and peroneal neuropathies Plexopathy from cancer, abscess, hematoma, and autoimmune processes
Non-neurologic pain	Urolithiasis Retroperitoneal mass Ovarian cyst or carcinoma Endometriosis

Table 30.3 Differential Diagnosis of Lower Back and Leg Pain

Disorder	Clinical Features	Diagnostic Findings
Radiculopathy	Back pain radiating into leg in a dermatomal distribution. Sensory loss and motor loss are in a root distribution. Increased pain with coughing or straining.	Suspected when neuropathic pain radiates from back down into leg in a single root distribution. Disk or mass can be seen on MRI or CT. Zoster and diabetes can cause radiculopathy without abnormal studies.
Plexopathy	Back and leg pain with a neuropathic character, dysesthesias, burning, or electric sensation. Back pain can develop when cause is mass lesion in region of plexus.	Suspected when patient has leg pain in more than one peripheral nerve or root distribution. MRI of plexus or CT of abdomen and pelvis can show mass or hematoma.
Spinal stenosis	Pain in lower back, buttocks, and legs, especially with standing, walking, and lumbar spine extension.	MRI or CT shows obliteration of subarachnoid space.

CT, Computed tomography; *MRI*, magnetic resonance imaging.

Table 30.4 Differential Diagnosis of Isolated Lower Back Pain

Disorder	Clinical Features	Diagnostic Findings
Sacroiliac joint inflammation	Pain lateral to spine where sacrum inserts into top of iliac bone. Pain is exacerbated by movement and pressure but does not radiate down leg.	Clinical diagnosis. Radiographs can show degenerative changes in joint. Bone scan shows increased uptake in region.
Facet pain	Unilateral or bilateral paraspinal pain without radiation. Pain is increased by spine motion, especially extension.	Clinical diagnosis. Radiographs can show facet degeneration.
Ovarian cyst or cancer	Pain in hip and lower back, often but not always extending into lower quadrant. Bowel disturbance may develop with advanced disease.	Abdominal and pelvic CT shows mass lesion in ovary.
Endometriosis	Usually pelvic pain but occasionally pain in back and legs. Pain is often timed to menses.	Diagnosis suspected during pelvic exam. Vaginal ultrasound is supportive. Laparoscopy is diagnostic.
Retroperitoneal mass, abdominal aortic aneurysm, abscess, hematoma	Pain in back. May be bilateral to spine. May be associated with superimposed neuropathic pain in cases with plexus or proximal nerve involvement.	CT or MRI shows hematoma, aneurysm, eroding vertebral bodies, or abdominal mass.
Urolithiasis	Pain in upper to mid-back laterally that may radiate to groin. No radiation into leg.	Radiographs may show stones. Intravenous pyelography typically shows obstruction of flow. Contrasted abdominal CT usually shows the stone and obstruction.
Diskitis	Pain in lower back exacerbated by movement. Some patients may have radiation of pain to abdomen, hip, or leg.	MRI shows characteristic changes in disk and surrounding tissues.

Table 30.5 Differential Diagnosis of Isolated Leg Pain

Disorder	Clinical Features	Diagnostic Findings
Peroneal neuropathy	Loss of sensation on dorsum of foot. Weakness of foot and toe dorsiflexion.	Slowed nerve conduction velocity across region of entrapment, usually at fibular neck. EMG may show denervation in peroneal-innervated muscles, especially tibialis anterior, without involvement of short head of biceps femoris.
Femoral neuropathy	Pain and sensory loss in anterior thigh, often with weakness of quadriceps and suppression of knee reflex.	NCS can sometimes be performed but may be technically difficult. EMG may show denervation in a distribution limited to femoral nerve.
Piriformis syndrome	Pain from back or buttock down posterior thigh. Pain is exacerbated by sitting or climbing stairs. Stretch of piriformis (flexion and adduction of the hip) worsens pain.	Clinical diagnosis. Pain radiating down leg in a sciatic nerve distribution. Exacerbation of pain by flexion and adduction of hip. EMG and NCS may show proximal sciatic nerve damage.
Meralgia paresthetica (lateral femoral cutaneous nerve dysfunction)	Pain and loss of sensation of lateral femoral cutaneous nerve on lateral aspect of thigh.	Clinical diagnosis. NCS is difficult to perform on this nerve.
Claudication	Pain in thigh and lower leg with exertion. Pain does not occur with lumbar spine extension.	Suspected with exertional leg pain without back pain. Ultrasonography or angiography confirms arterial insufficiency.
Plexopathy	Back and leg pain that has a neuropathic character. Dysesthesias, burning, or electric sensation. Plexitis has no associated back pain.	Suspected when a patient has leg pain in more than one peripheral nerve distribution. MRI of plexus or CT of abdomen can show a structural lesion in some patients.
Radiculopathy	Pain largely in one dermatomal distribution. May be motor and reflex loss. Most patients have back pain, but not all.	Suspected with pain radiating down one leg with or without back pain. Best imaged by MRI or postmyelographic CT.

CT, Computed tomography; *EMG,* electromyography; *MRI,* magnetic resonance imaging; *NCS,* nerve conduction studies.

Table 30.6 Diagnostic Studies for Lower Back and Lower Limb Pain

Diagnostic Test	Advantages	Disadvantages
Magnetic resonance imaging (MRI)	Sensitive for identification of lumbar disk herniation, spinal stenosis, paravertebral mass in region of plexus, perineural tumors, and diskitis	May overemphasize structural lesions. May miss vascular lesions of spinal cord. Paravertebral disorders may be overlooked if they are not the focus of interest. Cannot be performed on patients with some implanted metallic and electrical devices.
Non-contrast computed tomography (CT)	Shows osteophytes and lateral disk herniations best. Can show bone fractures and extension of fragments into regions that may contain neural elements.	Cannot identify neural elements without intrathecal contrast. Disk herniations without bone involvement may be missed.
Myelography with postmyelographic CT	Many neurosurgeons consider this the definitive test for identification of lumbar disk herniation, osteophytes, and intervertebral foraminal stenosis. Postmyelographic CT should be routinely performed.	May miss far-lateral herniations. Is invasive with a small risk of serious adverse effects.
Nerve conduction studies (NCS) and electromyography (EMG)	Sensitive for identification of specific nerve root or peripheral neuropathic involvement	Patients may have clinically significant radiculopathy without EMG evidence of denervation (or vice versa if radiculopathy is old).
Diskogram	Can identify disk anatomy in comparison with bony and neural anatomy. May confirm disk level if it produces pain that reproduces patient's complaints.	Invasive test, but risk of serious complications is low. Seldom performed in routine practice.

Myelography and Postmyelographic Computed Tomography

With the advent of MRI, myelography has been performed less commonly. If adequate information is not obtained from non-invasive studies, myelography occasionally may be indicated.

Lumbar puncture is performed, and radiopaque dye is infused into the cerebrospinal fluid (CSF). Conventional radiographs are obtained as the dye is manipulated through the CSF pathways. Postmyelographic computed tomography (CT) is performed in most instances.

Nerve Conduction Studies and Electromyography

Nerve conduction studies (NCSs) and electromyography (EMG) are performed for two principal purposes: these studies are an important addition to peripheral nervous system examination in helping with localization, and EMG can determine whether a peripheral neuropathic lesion is associated with neuronal or axonal damage. Axonal damage seen with radiculopathy or entrapment neuropathy suggests consideration of surgical decompression. Of note, signs of denervation may not appear on EMG until up to 4 weeks after onset of axonal damage.

Entrapment neuropathy, or nerve root compression which can be responsible for lower limb pain, is likely to slow conduction velocity across the region of compression. Conduction velocities proximal and distal to the compression usually are normal, so conduction across the affected nerve segment must be studied.

Radiculopathy typically is associated with normal NCS findings in the peripheral branches of the nerves but with slowing of the F-wave. Absence of abnormalities on NCSs and EMG does not rule out the presence of a radiculopathy.

Mechanical lower back pain is associated with no EMG or NCS alterations, so these studies usually are not indicated unless symptoms or signs of neural involvement are present.

Radiography

Plain radiographs are obtained in patients with acute skeletal trauma and in almost all patients with isolated lower back pain. Among the potential findings are degenerative joint disease, vertebral body collapse, bony erosion, subluxation, and fracture. Radiographs of the pelvis and long bones also are obtained and may show fractures and destructive lesions.

Bone Scan

Bone scan is especially important for examining multiple bone regions in cases of suspected neoplastic bone involvement. Multifocal involvement makes a neoplastic cause more likely than an infectious cause for the destruction.

Clinical Syndromes

Lower Back and Leg Pain
Lumbar Spine Stenosis

Lumbar spine stenosis is a disorder that affects mainly late middle-aged and older adults. The cause is multifactorial, with disk disease, bony hypertrophy, and thickening of the ligamentum flavum being the most important. Some of the symptoms are undoubtedly caused by direct pressure of these tissues on the cauda equina and exiting nerve roots, but a major contributor appears to be compression of the vascular supply of the nerve roots. Standing is associated with extension of the lumbar spine, which causes anterior bulging of the ligamentum flavum that lies posteriorly. Compression of the vascular supply creates nerve root ischemia, which can produce severe pain and weakness with exertion.

A diagnosis of lumbar spine stenosis should be suspected in patients with leg pain that is exacerbated by standing and walking and relieved promptly by sitting. Lying down, especially in the prone position, may exacerbate the low back pain, again through lumbar extension, a feature that helps differentiate lumbar spine stenosis from lumbar radiculopathy.

Confirmation of the diagnosis is by MRI or CT of the lumbar spine, which shows obliteration of the subarachnoid space at the level of the lesion. The hypertrophied ligamentum flavum and osteophyte formation usually are evident on these studies. If doubt about the diagnosis exists, myelography with postmyelographic CT scanning can be performed, but this invasive test seldom is needed.

Treatment can be conservative in the absence of neurological deficits. Physical therapy and medications can help, but surgical decompression is often required. Weakness of the legs or sphincter disturbance indicates a need for decompression. Although good evidence supports the benefit of surgical decompression in at least the short term, it is not clear that complex spine surgery with instrumentation produces substantial improvement in outcome (Gibson and Waddell, 2005).

Cauda Equina Syndrome and Conus Medullaris Syndrome

Lesions of the lumbar spine can result in damage to the conus medullaris, cauda equina, or both. *Cauda equina syndrome* is compression of the nerve roots below the termination of the spinal cord. Nerve root dysfunction is due to direct compression by surrounding structures. Important causes include acute trauma, chronic degenerative bony disease with retropulsion of fragments into the spinal canal, lumbar disc disease, infections such as abscess, intraspinal and meningeal tumor, and intraspinal hematoma. This syndrome can be a rare complication of minor and major spinal procedures. Cauda equina syndrome usually develops as an insidious chronic process unless due to acute trauma. Symptoms can include back pain, leg pain, weakness and cramps in the legs. Sensory symptoms can be sensory loss as well as neuropathic pain. Sphincter disturbance is common, especially with progression.

Conus medullaris syndrome is due to damage to the terminus of the spinal cord above most of the cauda equina and therefore at a higher spinal level. Etiology can be compression from all the conditions listed above plus occasional infiltrating lesions of the conus medullaris itself, especially by tumor. Conus medullaris syndrome is usually more rapidly progressive, associated with earlier back pain and sphincter disturbance, and is more likely to be associated with preservation of some lower extremity reflexes, usually patellar.

MRI is the preferred diagnostic imaging method. If MRI cannot be performed, many causes of both syndromes can be identified on CT of the spine.

Lumbosacral Radiculopathy

Lumbosacral radiculopathy usually is caused by infringement on the neural foramen by either herniated disk material or osteophytes. Herniated disk is more common in young

Table 30.7 Lumbosacral Radiculopathy

Root	Motor Deficits	Sensory Deficits	Reflex Deficits
L2	Psoas, quadriceps	Lateral and anterior upper thigh	None
L3	Psoas, quadriceps	Lower medial thigh	Patellar (knee)
L4	Tibialis anterior, quadriceps	Medial lower leg	Patellar (knee)
L5	Tibialis anterior, peroneus longus, gluteus maximus	Lateral lower leg	None
S1	Gastrocnemii, gluteus maximus	Lateral foot, digits 4 and 5, outside of sole	Achilles (ankle)

patients; osteophyte formation is more common in older patients.

Patients present with back pain radiating down the leg in a distribution appropriate to the involved nerve root. The most common lumbosacral radiculopathy is of the S1 nerve root, produced by a lesion at the L5-S1 interspace. **Table 30.7** presents the typical motor, sensory, and reflex deficits associated with lumbosacral radiculopathy at individual levels.

The presence of lower back pain with radiating pain in a nerve root distribution points to a diagnosis of radiculopathy. Motor, sensory, and reflex deficits are not always present, so the diagnosis is suspected on the basis of symptoms without objective signs.

Confirmation of the diagnosis is by MRI, which can show disc protrusion or osteophyte encroachment with nerve root compression. MRI is the diagnostic procedure of choice for most surgeons, although postmyelographic CT is still occasionally used. Myelography with CT also may be used, especially in patients who cannot undergo MRI because of implanted electronic devices and metallic heart valves.

NCS findings usually are normal in patients with lumbosacral radiculopathy, although F-waves may be delayed in the affected root. EMG can reveal evidence of denervation in a nerve root distribution and usually can differentiate peripheral neuropathic processes from radiculopathy. This study also can determine whether denervation is present with radiculopathy.

Management of lumbosacral radiculopathy depends on the severity of symptoms, including pain and weakness. If the symptoms are mild, antiinflammatory agents may suffice. Muscle relaxants can produce short-term relief of muscle spasm and pain.

Surgical options for lumbosacral radiculopathy are considered when the patient has intractable pain refractory to conservative care; when weakness is prominent, especially if it is unresponsive to conservative management; and when sphincter disturbance is present. Sphincter disturbance caused by lumbar disk disease or spondylosis necessitates consideration of urgent surgery. Patients with such deficits should not be given a trial of conservative therapy.

An important management consideration is how long conservative treatment should be continued in patients with weakness before surgical options are considered. In general, weakness should prompt at least consideration of surgery. Patients may have mild and transient weakness that responds to conservative therapy, but if weakness is prolonged or severe, recovery is compromised.

Intractable pain without motor loss and with or without sensory loss can be treated surgically, but treatment effectiveness is limited.

Arachnoiditis

Arachnoiditis is inflammation of the arachnoid membranes surrounding the spinal cord. The inflammation can be caused by a number of processes including trauma to the spinal canal by injury or surgery, chronic compression of spinal nerves, chemicals such as intrathecal chemotherapy or contrast agents, blood products from subarachnoid hemorrhage, infections, or neoplasms. Some clinicians believe that arachnoiditis due to mechanical processes is overdiagnosed. Also, arachnoiditis has been attributed to some conditions for which causation is tentative at best, such as with some intrathecal contrast materials.

There is chronic inflammation of the motor and sensory nerve roots. The inflammation results in fibrinous adhesions between the membranes and nerve roots and between adjacent nerve roots.

Common symptoms include pain in the back and legs which typically has a neuropathic character. Sensory symptoms can be loss of sensation or dysesthesias. Muscle symptoms can include twitching and cramps, and in severe cases, weakness or even paralysis can develop.

Diagnosis of arachnoiditis is suspected in patients with low back and leg pain who have radiological studies which suggest the diagnosis; arachnoiditis is seldom a diagnosis of first consideration during initial evaluation. MRI shows thickened and clumped nerve roots. Careful examination of the imaging shows nerve roots adherent to each other and to the dura. When MRI cannot be performed, myelography can show the same overall appearance.

Diagnosis is confirmed by imaging, with MRI being the principal modality; myelography is typically used only if MRI cannot be performed. EMG can identify denervation spanning single root distributions and document motor dysfunction, but no EMG findings are specific for arachnoiditis. CSF analysis is performed if the differential diagnosis includes meningeal infection or tumor; neoplastic meningitis and chronic infections can produce a similar clinical and radiological appearance. CSF can be normal with noninfectious and non-neoplastic causes of arachnoiditis.

Treatment of arachnoiditis is dependent on the cause. For patients with arachnoiditis due to trauma, instrumentation, chronic nerve root compression, or other mechanical cause, treatment is symptomatic, involving medications and procedures for chronic neuropathic pain. Treatment is also symptomatic for patients with arachnoiditis due to resolved infections, previous chemical administration, or previous subarachnoid hemorrhage. Steroids are often administered to patients receiving some types of intrathecal chemotherapy to reduce the risk of arachnoiditis, although this is not completely protective.

Plexopathy
NEOPLASTIC LUMBOSACRAL PLEXOPATHY

Neoplasms affecting the lumbosacral plexus can be solid or infiltrating. Infiltrating tumors such as lymphoma usually are treated by radiation therapy, which commonly is followed by chemotherapy for the systemic cancer. Solid tumors affecting the lumbosacral plexus rarely can be completely surgically excised without producing severe damage to the plexus.

Diagnosis is suspected with pain and often weakness in a leg associated with a known neoplasm. In such patients, the differential diagnosis often includes plexus infiltration, compression, and radiation plexopathy. MRI of the lumbar spine and plexus may show plexus involvement by tumor. EMG can help with differentiation of radiation plexopathy from neoplastic infiltration (Jaeckle, 2010).

Radiation therapy is given initially. Pain often is relieved shortly after the radiation therapy has begun. During initial treatment, anticonvulsants can be used to relieve the neuropathic pain. Pure analgesics also may be used, and sustained-release opiate formulations are effective in treating this condition.

PLEXUS INJURY FROM RETROPERITONEAL ABSCESS

Retroperitoneal abscess usually is caused by peritonitis from gastrointestinal neoplasms or following surgery. Retroperitoneal abscess can affect the lumbosacral plexus. Patients present with abdominal and flank pain, often with overt signs of systemic infection, with fever, malaise, elevated white blood cell counts, and elevated C-reactive protein (CRP) concentration. The diagnosis is confirmed by CT of the abdomen. Management typically begins with surgical drainage followed by prolonged antibiotic treatment. Narcotics usually are needed for the pain of retroperitoneal abscess.

PLEXUS INJURY FROM RETROPERITONEAL HEMATOMA

Retroperitoneal hematoma usually is caused by a bleeding disorder, a pelvic fracture, or abdominal surgery. Occasionally, bleeding from the site of arteriography can result in tracking of blood into the region of the lumbosacral plexus, especially after thrombolytic therapy or anticoagulation. Hematoma has also been described in patients after lumbar plexus block and may be delayed (Aveline and Bonnet, 2004).

This diagnosis should be suspected in patients with leg motor and sensory symptoms who are at risk for intraabdominal hemorrhage; abdominal and leg pain are common. Confirmation of the diagnosis is by CT of the abdomen, which can show blood in the region of the plexus.

Treatment of plexus hematoma is supportive. Evacuation of the hematoma is seldom needed, and surgery commonly is reserved for patients with continued blood loss, which must be arrested.

Leg Pain without Lower Back Pain
Peripheral Nerve Syndromes

Peripheral nerve palsy is commonly the result of sustained compression. Peroneal palsy is the most common lower-extremity syndrome, usually caused by pressure at the fibular neck. Femoral neuropathy commonly results from intraabdominal causes and can be difficult to differentiate from upper-lumbar plexopathy.

The diagnosis of peripheral nerve palsy is clinical, with symptoms and signs confined to one neural distribution. Patients usually present with neuropathic pain and sensory loss. Dysesthesias and paresthesias in the affected distribution are common. Reflex abnormalities depend on the individual nerves affected.

Definitive treatment of peripheral nerve entrapment is surgical release. Surgery is not always necessary, and conservative management may be successful. Tumor compression of peripheral nerves can be treated surgically, but radiation therapy can shrink the tumor, thereby relieving pain. Conservative management includes physical therapy to maximize comfort and improve function, antiinflammatory agents and anticonvulsants to alleviate pain, and counseling on methods to avoid subsequent damage. The counseling should address prevention of nerve compression and nerve stretch. For example, to prevent peroneal nerve compression at the fibular neck, the patient can avoid pressure on the posterior knee while the leg is extended and also can avoid squatting with the knee acutely bent.

FEMORAL NEUROPATHY

The femoral nerve usually is injured in the pelvis as it passes beneath the inguinal ligament or in the leg. Intraabdominal disorders including mass lesions and hematoma are commonly implicated. Femoral artery puncture for angiography also may be a cause, either directly or via the resultant hematoma.

Patients present with weakness that is most easily detected in the psoas, because the quadriceps is so strong. Sensory loss is over the anterior thigh and medial aspect of the calf and has a saphenous nerve distribution (the terminal sensory branch of the femoral nerve). This distribution of sensory loss is helpful to differentiate femoral neuropathy from lumbar radiculopathy. The patellar reflex usually is depressed.

The diagnosis can be supported by EMG evidence of denervation in the quadriceps but not in the lower leg or posterior thigh muscles. The adductors are especially important to test because they are innervated by the same nerve roots as for the femoral nerve but instead are innervated by the obturator nerve. Normal EMG findings cannot rule out this diagnosis, because many patients do not have active or chronic denervation. NCS of the femoral nerve is difficult, especially in large patients, who are predisposed to development of femoral neuropathy.

Treatment is seldom surgical, except for the removal of a massive psoas or iliacus hematoma or mass lesion. Weight loss and avoidance of marked hip flexion can reduce the chance of persistent damage. Physical therapy will aid recovery of motor power. Femoral neuropathy usually resolves.

MERALGIA PARESTHETICA

Dysfunction of the lateral femoral cutaneous nerve commonly is caused by compression as it passes beneath the inguinal ligament. Obesity and pregnancy predispose to this disorder, as does intraabdominal surgery of a variety of types. Recent reports have even described soldiers with body armor having meralgia paresthetica. This problem is likely underdiagnosed and assumed to be a lumbar radiculopathy or atypical femoral neuropathy.

Meralgia paresthetica is the sensory syndrome of pain and sensory loss on the lateral thigh. Patients present with numbness and often pain on the lateral thigh. Motor deficits are not a feature. Meralgia paresthetica is differentiated from femoral neuropathy by the lateral distribution of the sensory findings and the absence of motor and reflex abnormalities.

Nerve conduction testing of the lateral femoral cutaneous nerve, although feasible, is technically difficult even in the best circumstances. It is even more difficult in obese patients, who are at particular risk for entrapment of the nerve.

Treatment is conservative. Weight loss usually is effective in preventing recurrence. Anticonvulsants and tricyclic antidepressants are effective for control of the neuropathic pain. A nerve block may be supportive of the diagnosis in patients unresponsive to conservative measures. Surgery is rarely performed, and controversy about its indications and effectiveness is ongoing (Harney and Patijn, 2007; Haim, et al., 2006).

SCIATIC NEUROPATHY

The sciatic nerve is most likely to be injured as it leaves the sciatic notch and descends into the upper leg. Compression can occur in patients in prolonged coma, especially those who are very thin. The sciatic nerve also is susceptible to injury from pelvic and sacral fractures, hip surgery or dislocation, needle injection injuries, and any penetrating injury.

Patients present with pain that usually is localized close to the level of the sciatic nerve lesion, although substantial radiation of the pain may be a feature. Loss of sensation is prominent below the knee, sparing the medial lower leg (the territory of the saphenous branch of the femoral nerve). Weakness can affect all muscles of the lower leg, but peroneal-innervated muscles are more likely to demonstrate weakness for two reasons. First, tibial-innervated foot extensors are so strong that substantial weakness would have to be present for weakness to be evident on examination. Second, the peroneal division of the sciatic nerve is more susceptible to compression injury than the tibial division, even high in the thigh.

Sciatic neuropathy is a clinical diagnosis, although the EMG can show evidence of denervation in sciatic-innervated muscles; signs of denervation may not be seen until 4 weeks after injury. NCS findings usually are normal, but F-wave study may show slowing.

Treatment of sciatic compression is supportive, with avoidance of recurrent compression. Tricyclic antidepressants and anticonvulsants commonly are used for the neuropathic pain. In some patients with acute sciatic injury, opiates are needed to deal with the pain in the short term. Surgical exploration and decompression are performed only in patients with clear evidence of a structural lesion such as neural or perineural tumor.

PIRIFORMIS SYNDROME

Piriformis syndrome is an uncommon condition in which the sciatic nerve is compressed by the piriformis muscle in the posterior gluteal area. Hypertrophy of the piriformis muscle and other anatomical variants predispose affected persons to development of the syndrome. This condition may affect not only the main sciatic trunk but also the superior gluteal nerve. The diagnosis and even existence of this as a singular condition is controversial (Halpin and Ganju, 2009).

Patients present with pain in the buttock that radiates down the leg and is exacerbated by adduction and flexion of the hip. Pain tends to be aggravated by prolonged sitting, climbing steps, and other maneuvers that irritate the piriformis muscle.

Piriformis syndrome is a clinical diagnosis. A patient with symptoms of sciatic neuropathy has typical clinical features on examination but no signs of radiculopathy or spinal stenosis on imaging. Spinal claudication can be confused with piriformis syndrome, so imaging of the spine usually is warranted. MRI neurography may show the lesion in many patients (Filler et al., 2005).

Piriformis syndrome usually is managed with antiinflammatory agents for acute exacerbations and with physical therapy, which can be tailored to address the specific problems and any associated limitations. Local injections of corticosteroids are given occasionally, but these are unlikely to produce long-term improvement. Surgical treatment is rarely performed, and controversy is ongoing about the indications and expected effectiveness of surgical treatment.

PERONEAL NEUROPATHY

Peroneal neuropathy commonly is caused by compression of the nerve as it passes from the popliteal fossa across the fibular neck into the anterior compartment of the lower leg. Patients often present with foot drop from weakness of the tibialis anterior muscle. The diagnosis is confirmed by NCSs and EMG, with slowing of peroneal nerve conduction across the region of entrapment, usually across the fibular neck. The EMG shows evidence of active and chronic denervation in many patients, in keeping with the axonal damage indicated by the foot drop (Marciniak et al., 2005).

Peroneal neuropathy may be secondary to prolonged bed rest, or it may result from hyperflexion of the knee, usually from an occupational activity. The condition also may accompany peripheral neuropathy, predisposing to pressure palsy, or may be the result of a fibrous band attached to the peroneus longus, predisposing to nerve compression (Dellon, Ebmer, and Swier, 2002). In addition, pressure in obstetrical stirrups, prolonged sitting with crossed legs, cast on the lower leg for sprain or fracture, and stretch and compression by the contracted tibialis anterior muscle in ballet dancers all have been implicated. A fibrous band beneath the superficial head of the peroneus longus is found in a much larger proportion of patients with peroneal entrapment than in normal persons.

POLYNEUROPATHY

Peripheral neuropathy is a common cause of lower-extremity pain. The differential diagnosis for this condition is broad in scope, as would be expected. Among the most common causes are diabetes mellitus, familial neuropathy, metabolic neuropathies, and vasculitis. Pain is the presenting manifestation and differs in character according to the type of neuropathy. Small-fiber neuropathies manifest with burning pain that often is worse in the evening. Large-fiber neuropathies manifest with dysesthesias and paresthesias, often with electric shock–like pains.

Diagnosis usually is confirmed by NCS and EMG. Axonal neuropathy is more common than demyelinating neuropathy. Occasionally, patients with a predominantly small-fiber sensory neuropathy have normal NCS findings. Laboratory studies for peripheral neuropathy typically are performed as outlined in Chapter 31.

Treatment is with tricyclic antidepressants or anticonvulsants. Amitriptyline commonly is used for patients with small-fiber neuropathic pain. Anticonvulsants are used predominantly for patients with large-fiber neuropathic pain. When patients have symptoms of both, treatment with gabapentin, pregabalin, or oxcarbazepine can be helpful. Combination therapy with a tricyclic and anticonvulsant may be beneficial. Pure analgesics occasionally are used on a nightly basis to assist with sleep (Singleton, 2005).

Plexopathy
LUMBOSACRAL PLEXITIS

Lumbosacral plexitis is similar to brachial plexitis, a presumed autoimmune process, but is less common. This entity is differentiated from radiculitis, which can be an inflammatory disorder of autoimmune or infectious origin (Tyler, 2008).

Management of idiopathic lumbosacral plexitis is supportive, with no medical intervention known to alter the course of the disease. Anticonvulsants commonly are used for pain management. Corticosteroids and high-dose intravenous immunoglobulin also are used occasionally, although it is not clear that their benefits outweigh the risks. Lumbosacral plexitis constitutes an indication for the use of pure opiates, because the duration of the pain usually is weeks rather than months. As the pain abates and the weakness is more prominent, the analgesics usually can be tapered and discontinued. Sustained-release opiates are especially helpful for patients with plexitis.

DIABETIC AMYOTROPHY

Diabetic amyotrophy is lumbosacral plexopathy occurring in persons with diabetes mellitus. The disorder is thought to be an inflammatory vasculopathy, with damage that probably is immune mediated. Patients present with pain in the hip and thigh associated with weakness of the quadriceps, psoas, and adductors. The plexopathy is more often unilateral than bilateral.

A diagnosis of diabetic amyotrophy is suggested by proximal pain and weakness in a patient with known diabetes. This disorder must be differentiated from lumbar radiculopathy and other structural lesions in the region of the plexus. NCSs and EMG show coexistent peripheral polyneuropathy denervation in proximal muscles including quadriceps, psoas, and adductors. MRI and CT do not show a structural lesion.

Treatment is symptomatic. Immune-modulating treatment with immunoglobulin may reduce the duration of the deficit but is not routinely administered. Most patients improve, although recovery is incomplete for most. The pain abates before recovery of muscle strength.

Herpes Zoster

With reactivation of varicella-zoster virus infection, the presenting symptom is pain in a single nerve root distribution. In most patients, a vesicular rash develops in the same cutaneous distribution, but the pain often begins before development of skin changes, and the skin changes are variable. Eventually the rash crusts over, leaving some pigmentary changes. The pain abates as the inflammation recedes, although the patient may be left with sensory or motor deficit. Weakness can be evident in muscle innervated predominantly by a single nerve root.

The diagnosis is based on clinical findings, and when the rash is present at onset, structural imaging usually is not necessary. NCSs and EMG often are not needed, but they may show denervation in affected muscles in cases with persistent nerve root damage. The differential diagnosis is broader in scope before development of the rash, and considerations include radiculopathy from other causes including disk disease and osteophytes.

Treatment with antiviral agents such as acyclovir or famciclovir should begin within 72 hours of symptom onset. Early treatment may help hasten recovery and reduce the incidence of postherpetic neuralgia. Corticosteroids often are used, and the chance of disseminated zoster is not appreciably higher in immune-competent patients. Corticosteroids reduce acute neuropathic pain and may decrease the incidence of postherpetic neuralgia. Use of corticosteroids is more important for zoster ophthalmicus than for lower-limb zoster.

Claudication of Leg Arteries

Arterial claudication is discussed here because it is an important element in the differential diagnosis of spinal stenosis. Vascular disease of the iliac arteries and terminal branches results in marginal perfusion of lower-limb muscles. Walking and other moderate activities exacerbate the ischemia, producing pain and weakness with exertion. The clinical picture may resemble that in spinal stenosis, but the lack of back pain with claudication, lack of exacerbation of leg pain with recumbent lumbar extension, and vascular changes in the leg are features that should be absent in spinal stenosis.

Claudication is diagnosed by vascular imaging. Ultrasound examination can be a good screening test, but angiography can provide a definitive diagnosis and in some patients can be the means for definitive treatment by angioplasty.

Lower Back Pain without Leg Pain
Mechanical Lower Back Pain

Mechanical lower back pain usually is caused by strain of paraspinal muscles and ligaments, with local inflammation. Muscle tears also may cause acute lower back pain. Therefore, mechanical lower back pain usually is a combination of bone, muscular, and connective tissue pain. Patients present with pain in the lower back without radicular symptoms and show no motor, sensory, or reflex abnormalities on examination. Any weakness or gait disturbance is due to pain and not neurological deficit.

Diagnosis is based on the clinical features and exclusion of other causes. In the absence of objective neurological deficits, spinal MRI usually is not needed initially, but radiography may be performed to look for bony fractures or erosion. NCSs and EMG usually are not needed. In the absence of signs of bony or neural destruction, conservative management may begin. If the patient does not respond to initial treatment, further study with MRI can be performed.

Mechanical lower back pain usually is treated by an initial period of rest of approximately 2 days, followed by an increase in activity. Physical therapy can be very helpful during this initial treatment period. After the initial treatment, self-help guidelines are followed to reduce the likelihood of recurrent lower back pain. Muscle relaxants can help reduce the tightness of the muscles, which impedes movement and can detract from successful physical therapy.

Patients who do not respond to conservative management may benefit from epidural blocks. Surgery for "bulging disks" occasionally is performed in patients who have clinically apparent mechanical back pain, but the likelihood of response is not high.

Facet Joint Pain Syndrome

Pain from the facet joints of the lumbosacral spine usually is not an isolated entity but rather a component of mechanical back pain. Pain results from long-term degenerative changes in the facet joints, usually caused by strain. Repetitive strenuous activity, excessive weight, and abnormal posture may predispose affected persons to the development of facet pain. Acute trauma to the back may produce active joint inflammation that can be self-limited.

Facet pain usually is lateral to the spine and exacerbated by extending the spine or bending toward the affected side. Facet pain often is bilateral. Prolonged sitting or walking up steps, as well as retaining one position for a prolonged time, tends to exacerbate the pain. Patients present with pain without motor, sensory, or reflex deficit unless radiculopathy or spinal stenosis is also present.

Results of diagnostic studies usually are normal. Chronic degenerative changes may be seen on radiographs, but with acute facet damage, even the radiographic appearance may be unremarkable.

Facet pain usually is treated with antiinflammatory agents and physical therapy. Avoidance of exacerbating activity usually is helpful. Facet blocks can be performed but often are not necessary, and effectiveness in terms of long-term relief is controversial (Varlotta et al., 2011). As part of physical therapy, traction can change the character of weight bearing on the joints. Physical therapy can strengthen paraspinal muscles and improve posture.

Lumbar Spine Osteomyelitis

Vertebral osteomyelitis is most common in the lumbar region and may develop as a sequela of trauma, urinary tract infection, respiratory infection, and other causes of sepsis. Patients present with lower back pain, which may develop weeks after the inciting infection has abated. Limitation of the motion of the spine and tightness of the paraspinal muscles are additional features. Local lumbar spine pain with tenderness to percussion is characteristic.

The diagnosis of vertebral osteomyelitis is suggested by lower back pain in a patient who has not received radiation therapy, associated with systemic signs of infection—fever, elevated CRP concentration, and elevated white blood cell count (An and Seldomridge, 2006). MRI shows changes in the vertebral body and often in adjacent psoas muscle. Radiographs show degeneration of the disk margin of the vertebral body and disk space narrowing. Needle biopsy can reveal the causative organism in most cases. Open biopsy usually is not necessary. The diagnosis can easily be missed initially, since it can occur in patients with preexisting lumbar spine pain, and inflammatory signs may not be marked early on (Mylona et al., 2009).

Treatment is with antibiotics and bed rest. Surgical débridement is needed in patients who do not respond to antibiotics.

Lumbar Spine Compression

Compression of the lumbar vertebral bodies occurs in the setting of acute trauma, osteoporosis, infection, or tumor. Presence of a tumor may predispose the lumbar vertebrae to collapse with minimal trauma or stress. Patients present with severe lower back pain, usually without radicular symptoms. If the collapse results in compression of the nerve roots by bone, radicular pain may develop in addition to the lower back pain. With compression of the cauda equina, diffuse weakness of the legs and sphincter disturbance can develop.

The diagnosis of lumbar spine compression is suggested by a clinical presentation of lower back pain that is exacerbated by movement, jarring, or certain postures such as bending or twisting. Radiographs and CT scans can easily show the associated bone destruction. Bone scan confirms the damage and can screen for other regions of damage. These studies, however, usually cannot pinpoint the cause of the compression. MRI is better able to make this differentiation, but it is not exact.

Treatment consists of immobilization of the fracture site, which may include bracing. Pure analgesics often are needed, especially at night. Corticosteroids should be avoided if the cause is osteoporotic but can be very helpful for malignant vertebral collapse. Malignant collapse usually is treated by radiation therapy; surgery is performed if the spine is unstable because of the destruction or in the absence of a known primary tumor in a patient with presumed neoplastic vertebral involvement. The benefits of acute surgical decompression for neoplastic cauda equina compression are controversial.

Lumbar Diskitis

Diskitis is an inflammatory process affecting the intervertebral disks of any level, often occurring in the lumbar spine. In adults, *Staphylococcus aureus* and mycobacteria are important causes, although the list of potential pathogens is large. The causative organism typically reflects the source from which the bacteria spread—for example, skin infection, urinary tract infection, or intestinal infection. Diskitis associated with recent lumbar surgery is likely to be caused by resistant bacteria. In children, diskitis is also usually due to *S. aureus*, but extraspinal manifestations of infection are less likely (Early, Kay, and Tolo, 2003).

Patients present with lower back pain with marked restriction of flexion of the spine, because flexion increases pressure on the disk and disk space. Patients with postoperative diskitis usually have systemic symptoms, but overt signs of infection with fever and chills may be absent.

A diagnosis of lumbar diskitis is suggested by the presence of severe lower back pain without a radicular component, with tenderness and spasm of the paravertebral muscles associated with willingness of the patient to flex the hips but not the spine (Mikhael et al., 2009). Erythrocyte sedimentation rate (ESR) and CRP concentration usually are increased. The diagnosis can be confirmed by MRI, which shows decreased signal intensity of the disk on T1-weighted images and increased signal intensity on T2-weighted images, often with changes in the end-plates of the adjacent vertebrae. Bone scan shows increased uptake in the region of the infected disk. Radiographs show disk space narrowing.

MRI is the most sensitive test for diskitis. Biopsy often is needed to identify an organism. Treatment begins with bed rest and antibiotics (Grados et al., 2007). Extensive surgery usually is not necessary; even tuberculous diskitis is successfully treated with antibiotics in more than 80% of cases (Bhojraj and Nene, 2002).

In some patients, diskectomy with fusion of the adjacent vertebral bodies may be required for relief of symptoms. Use of this management approach usually is restricted to adults; progression leading to surgery is less common in children.

References

The complete reference list is available online at www.expetconsult.com.

Part II

Neurological Investigations and Related Clinical Neurosciences

Laboratory Investigations in Diagnosis and Management of Neurological Disease

Robert B. Daroff, Gerald M. Fenichel, Joseph Jankovic, John C. Mazziotta

The history and examination are key to making the diagnosis in a patient with neurological disease (see Chapter 1). Laboratory investigations are becoming increasingly important in diagnosis and management, however, and are discussed in some detail in later chapters on the specific disorders. A test may be diagnostic (e.g., the finding of cryptococci in the cerebrospinal fluid [CSF] of a patient with a subacute meningitis, a low vitamin E level in a patient with ataxia and tremor, a low serum vitamin B_{12} level in a patient with a combined myelopathy and neuropathy).

Laboratory tests should be directed to prove or disprove the hypothesis that a certain disease is responsible for the condition in the patient. They should not be used as a "fishing expedition." Sometimes, a physician who cannot formulate a differential diagnosis from the clinical history and examination is tempted to order a wide range of tests to see what is abnormal. In addition to the high costs involved, this approach is likely to add to the confusion because "abnormalities" may be found that have no relevance to the patient's complaints. For instance, many patients are referred to neurologists to determine whether they have multiple sclerosis (MS) because their physicians requested magnetic resonance imaging (MRI) of the brain for some other purpose such as the investigation of headaches. If the MRI shows small T2-weighted abnormalities in the centrum semiovale (changes that are seen in a proportion of normal older adults and in those with hypertension and diabetes), the neuroradiologist will report that the differential diagnosis includes MS, despite the fact that the patient has no MS symptoms.

Moreover, neuroimaging modalities have expanded remarkably in the past decade, and the neurologist ordering these tests should be familiar with each one, so that appropriate sequences and methods are used to address the particular question presented by the patient's history. Also, because of the increasing use of pacemakers, deep brain stimulators, and other devices, the neurologist should be aware that certain precautions must be taken before MRI scans are ordered; in many instances, computed tomography (CT) scans or alternative investigations must be used to avoid potential danger to the patient.

Results of laboratory tests can be used to determine response to treatment. For instance, the high erythrocyte sedimentation rate (ESR) typical with cranial arteritis falls with corticosteroid treatment and control of the condition. A rising ESR as the corticosteroid dosage is reduced indicates that the condition is no longer adequately controlled and that headaches and the risk of loss of vision will soon return.

It is important to use laboratory tests judiciously and to understand their sensitivity, specificity, risks, and costs. The physician must understand how to interpret the hematological, biochemical, and bacteriological studies and the specific neurodiagnostic investigations. The latter studies include clinical neurophysiology, neuroimaging, and the pathological study of biopsy tissue. Knowledge of the various DNA tests available and their interpretation is critical before they are ordered; their results may have far-reaching implications not only for the patient but for all other family members. The neurologist also must have a working knowledge of several related disciplines that provide specific investigations to aid in neurological diagnosis. These include neuropsychology, neuro-ophthalmology, neuro-otology, uroneurology, neuro-epidemiology, clinical neurogenetics, neuroimmunology and neurovirology, and neuroendocrinology. Chapters 34 through 42 describe these disciplines and the investigations they offer.

Biopsy of skeletal muscle or peripheral nerve may be needed to diagnose neuromuscular diseases. A brain biopsy may be needed to diagnose a tumor, infection, vasculitis, or (rarely) degenerative disease of the nervous system.

The investigations used to diagnose neurological disease change rapidly. Genetic studies of DNA mutations in the blood now allow the diagnosis of Huntington disease (HD), a growing number of spinocerebellar ataxias and parkinsonian disorders, a form of autosomal dominant dystonia (DYT1), Duchenne and other muscular dystrophies, many forms of Charcot-Marie-Tooth disease, Rett syndrome, fragile X premutation, and a variety of other neurogenetic disorders (see http://www.ncbi.nlm.nih.gov/sites/GeneTests/?db=GeneTests; http://www.genetests.org; http://www.geneclinics.org; http://www.ncbi.nlm.nih.gov/entrez/query.fcgi?db=OMIM). Blood tests for human immunodeficiency virus infection (HIV), Lyme disease, and other infections and for various paraneoplastic syndromes affecting the nervous system also can be diagnostic. For example, three types of anti–Purkinje cell antibodies are recognized: anti-Yo (PCA-1), seen with tumors of breast, ovary, and adnexa; atypical anti–cytoplasmic antibody (anti-Tr or PCA-Tr), seen with Hodgkin disease and tumors of the lung and colon; and PCA-2, identified mostly with lung tumors. In addition, three antineuronal antibodies can be detected: anti-Hu (ANNA-1), seen in conjunction with encephalomyelitis, small cell lung tumor, and tumors of breast, prostate, and neuroblastoma; anti-Ri (ANNA-2), found with tumors of breast and ovary; and atypical anti-Hu, seen with tumors of lung, colon, adenocarcinoma, and lymphoma. Anti-CV2 (CRMP) antibody, expressed by oligodendrocytes, is associated with a syndrome of ataxia and optic neuritis and has been seen with small cell lung carcinoma. The role of antineuronal antibodies, such as those presumably directed to components of the basal ganglia, is not established and may be of doubtful pathogenic relevance.

Antibodies directed to a serum protein, Ma (anti-Ma1 and anti-Ma2), have been seen in patients with limbic encephalitis associated with testicular and other tumors. Antibodies directed to amphiphysin have been detected in patients with a cerebellar syndrome and small cell lung carcinoma. Antibodies against a glutamate receptor are seen in rare patients with a pure cerebellar syndrome associated with cancer and a variety of autoimmune diseases. Antibodies against glutamic acid decarboxylase (anti-GAD) have been seen in patients with the stiff person syndrome and in patients with ataxia in a setting of an autoimmune disease such as diabetes, thyroid disease, or vitiligo. Antigliadin antibodies are helpful in evaluating patients with unexplained ataxia. As a result of advances in laboratory technology, genetic, immunological, and other blood tests are expanding the ability of clinicians to confirm the diagnosis of an increasing number of neurological disorders, obviating more invasive studies.

MRI has replaced CT for most conditions, and MR angiography and venography have largely replaced conventional catheter-based blood vessel imaging studies. In general, older, more invasive tests are now used for therapy rather than diagnostics. For example, the diagnosis and cause of an acute stroke may be determined by MRI, but catheter angiography is used to deliver intraarterial tissue plasminogen activator (tPA) or perform embolectomies. The neurologist must know enough about each laboratory test to request it appropriately and to interpret the results intelligently. As a rule, it is inappropriate to order a laboratory test if the result will not influence diagnosis or management. Tests should be used to diagnose and treat disease, not to protect against litigation. When used judiciously, laboratory investigations serve both purposes; when ordered indiscriminately, they serve neither.

Diagnostic Yield of Laboratory Tests

When choosing tests, the neurologist must decide what information will help distinguish between the diseases on the differential diagnostic list. A test is justified if the result will confirm or rule out a certain disease or alter patient management, provided that it is not too risky or painful. A lumbar puncture (LP) is justified if the clinical picture is that of meningitis, when the test may both confirm the diagnosis and reveal the responsible organism. Culture and sensitivity testing should not be ordered on every sample of CSF sent to the laboratory, however, if meningitis is not in the differential diagnosis. Because the LP is invasive, with potential complications, it is not justified unless an abnormal finding will aid in the diagnosis. No test is justified unless the finding will influence the diagnostic process.

The physician should provide full clinical information and highlight the questions for which answers are being sought from the investigations. The electrophysiologist will look more carefully for evidence of denervation in a certain myotome if the patient has a syndrome suggesting herniation of that disk. The neuroradiologist will obtain additional views to search for evidence of a posterior communicating artery aneurysm if the neurologist reports a third nerve palsy in a patient with subarachnoid hemorrhage.

Interpretation of Results of Laboratory Investigations

Every biological measurement in a population varies over a normal range, which usually is defined as plus or minus 2 or 3 standard deviations (SDs) from the mean value; 2 SDs encompass 96%, and 3 SDs encompass 99% of the measurements from a normal population. Even with 3 SDs, 1 normal person in 100 has a value outside the normal range. Therefore, an abnormal result may not indicate the presence of a disease. It also is important to know the characteristics of the normal population used to standardize a laboratory test. Ranges that were normalized using adults are almost never correct for newborns and children. Ranges normalized using a hospitalized population may not be accurate for ambulatory people.

An abnormal test result may not be caused by the disorder under investigation. For example, an elevated serum creatine kinase (CK) concentration can result from recent exercise, electromyography (EMG) or intramuscular injection, liver disease, or myocardial infarction (MI), as well as from a primary muscle disease. A common problematic finding for pediatric neurologists is centrotemporal spikes on the electroencephalogram (EEG) in a child with headache or learning disability who has never had a seizure. The EEG should not have been ordered in the first place, and to give such a patient antiepileptic drugs would compound poor judgment in diagnosis with worse judgment in management.

The neurologist should personally review test results that are ordered. In most instances, the actual imaging studies should be reviewed in addition to the report, and when appropriate, the neuroradiologist should participate. Similarly, for neurologists experienced in pathology, biopsy findings may be reviewed with the neuropathologist. The neurologist who knows the patient may be of great help in interpreting imaging or pathological studies.

Risk and Cost of Investigations

If two different tests provide equivalent information, the physician should choose the one that causes less pain and risk to the patient. The costs of the two tests also should be considered. The diagnostic capability of two tests may not be identical, and the more expensive test may not be better. The cost of a test must be considered in the context of the total cost of the illness. An expensive test that shortens a hospital stay may be cost-effective. The selection of laboratory tests and the sequence in which performed are important components of good medical practice.

Risk-to-Benefit Analysis

The neurologist makes judgments about the risk-to-benefit ratio of tests every day. The following examples can help clarify the principles used in making these decisions.

Lumbar Puncture

The risks and benefits of LP must be weighed in every patient. The LP may yield a specific diagnosis such as subarachnoid hemorrhage or bacterial meningitis. It may help confirm the diagnosis, such as by showing raised intracranial pressure (ICP) in benign intracranial hypertension. The LP may yield information that is not specific but aids in confirming the diagnosis. A fourfold increase in the CSF protein concentration (without an increase in the cell count) suggests one of the following diagnoses: an acute or chronic inflammatory demyelinative polyradiculoneuropathy, schwannoma or meningioma within the CSF pathways, or spinal compression that obstructs the flow of CSF (Froin syndrome). A moderately increased number of lymphocytes, an increased g-globulin concentration, and oligoclonal bands in the CSF point to an immunological process in the central nervous system (CNS), such as MS.

LP carries significant risks, the most disastrous being cerebral or cerebellar herniation. The LP may suddenly release elevated CSF pressure produced by an expanding supratentorial lesion and may force the medial temporal lobe through the tentorium cerebelli to compress the midbrain. In the case of an expanding infratentorial lesion, it may cause the cerebellar tonsils to herniate through the foramen magnum and compress the cervicomedullary junction (see Chapter 50B). These herniations can be fatal, so never perform an LP in a patient with a possible space-occupying lesion without first examining the optic fundi for evidence of papilledema or consulting a recent head CT or MRI.

LP is justified in some situations despite increased ICP. The prime example is acute meningitis, in which CSF examination is essential to establish the diagnosis and identify the organism. Other risks associated with LP include the production of meningitis as a result of contamination of the needle, a post-LP headache (from low CSF pressure), a spinal epidural hematoma in a patient with a coagulopathy, and the later development of an implantation dermoid (if the needle is inserted without the trocar).

Cerebral Arteriography

The question of whether to request percutaneous cerebral arteriography (see Chapter 33B) entails analysis of the risks and benefits for each patient. In a patient with cerebrovascular disease, the study may show thrombotic or embolic occlusion of arteries and abnormalities of the arterial wall, including arteriosclerotic plaques, fibromuscular hyperplasia, medial dissection, and arteritis. It also may demonstrate an intracranial aneurysm or arteriovenous malformation (AVM). Any of these findings can clarify the diagnosis, treatment, and prognosis. Many of these diagnostic outcomes can be identified with advanced MRI or a combination of MRI, CT, and ultrasound strategies. Thus, it is critical that the attending neurologist have a specific hypothesis in mind before ordering such examinations, as well as understand the relative ability of noninvasive versus invasive tests to demonstrate specific abnormalities in the blood vessels. If treatment (e.g., aneurysm occlusion) can be combined with a diagnostic procedure (e.g., catheter angiography), this may also alter the decision-making outcome.

Invasive studies such as arteriography have risks. These include thrombosis of the artery at the site of puncture, dissection of the vessel wall, allergic reactions to contrast, and cerebral infarction from thrombosis, embolism, or dissection. The likelihood that a patient being considered for cerebral arteriography will experience a particular complication is influenced by patient-specific factors including age and the presence of arteriosclerosis and other diseases. Traditionally noninvasive tests such as MRI and CT can also have risks related to preexisting patient conditions (e.g., contrast for either procedure can damage the kidney in patients with prior renal disease or diabetes). These patient-specific probabilities of risk must be balanced against the potential benefits the angiographic information may provide, specifically the likelihood of demonstrating a treatable condition. The likelihood of risk also varies with the skill, experience, and judgment of the physician performing these procedures. As such, the neurologist requesting invasive procedures should have an accurate estimate of the physician-specific risk factors. The final decision will need to consider the combined risk probabilities, including both patient- and physician-specific factors.

Arteriography is definitely indicated in a previously healthy 55-year-old woman with an acute transient right hemiplegia and aphasia and a left carotid artery bruit, especially when carotid ultrasound and/or MRI studies suggest a 75% internal carotid artery stenosis. Invasive angiography clearly is not indicated in a 75-year-old woman with unstable congestive cardiac failure and advanced carcinoma of the breast who suffers a similar transient ischemic attack (TIA). Noninvasive techniques may be adequate for revealing the cause of the patient's symptoms, thereby avoiding the risks of catheter cerebral angiography. Carotid Doppler ultrasound and transcranial Doppler studies can be as reliable as angiography for demonstrating extracranial occlusive disease. MR angiography, a technique that images the main extracranial and intracranial vessels noninvasively, may obviate invasive angiography in patients with extracranial occlusive disease, AVMs or a family history of intracranial aneurysms.

Brain Biopsy

Brain biopsy carries significant risks that always necessitate discussion of the risk-to-benefit ratio with the patient and family. The four main situations in which a brain biopsy may be considered are intraparenchymal brain tumor, intraparenchymal infectious lesion, cerebral vasculitis, and in special circumstances, cerebral degenerative disease. The risk-to-benefit analysis is influenced by the availability of computer-assisted stereotactic technology to obtain a biopsy through a burr hole, reducing the risk of obtaining tissue for pathological and bacteriological study.

Open craniotomy for brain biopsy is significantly more risky. The patient's age, presence of other diseases, lesion location, and the patient's wishes all must be taken into account when open brain biopsy is considered. Hemorrhage, infection, post-biopsy epileptic seizures, and the production of a neurological deficit are the main risks associated with the procedure. The risk of a permanent neurological deficit is reduced if the biopsy specimen is from certain areas of the brain, such as the nondominant frontal or temporal lobes. The procedure carries a high risk of worsening the neurological deficit (unless that deficit is already total) if the lesion is located in the sensorimotor cortex, the Broca speech area, the internal capsule, or optic radiations.

The treatability of the possible cause of the disease is the crucial benefit to consider in the risk-to-benefit analysis. If the neuroimaging study suggests a malignant glioma, for which treatment is likely to be ineffective, biopsy alone may not be considered justified, although resection and tissue diagnosis would be. If it suggests a primary lymphoma of the brain, which is likely to respond to radiotherapy, then confirmatory biopsy may be recommended. If the differential diagnosis in a patient with acquired immunodeficiency syndrome includes toxoplasmosis or lymphoma, it may be reasonable to give anti-*Toxoplasma* therapy rather than perform a brain biopsy; biopsy would be needed only if the lesions do not respond to 2 to 3 weeks of treatment. **Figure 31.1** presents a risk-to-benefit analysis and prioritization of investigations for an 80-year-old man with possible cerebral degeneration.

Cost-to-Benefit Analysis

Cost-to-benefit analysis often presents the physician with an ethical dilemma. The patient and family want everything possible done, no matter what the cost. Society complains that healthcare costs are skyrocketing. Any effort at cost containment may place society's interests in conflict with those of the patient. MRI and MR angiography are safer procedures than arteriography for diagnosing an AVM but may be more costly. Where only limited funding is available for health care,

the money must be used to purchase the most cost-effective care for the greatest number of people. Clearly, physicians should acquaint themselves with the costs of the tests they order and practice cost-effective medicine.

Prioritization of Tests

The order in which tests are requested depends on their diagnostic specificity, sensitivity, availability, cost, and invasiveness. Therefore, most blood studies are performed before neuroimaging and LP. Sometimes a therapeutic trial is used as an investigation. For instance, in a patient with possible herpes simplex encephalitis, risk-to-benefit analysis indicates that EEG, MRI scan of the brain, and LP with polymerase chain reaction study of the CSF for herpes simplex are better than a brain biopsy. With typical changes of herpes simplex encephalitis and a response to a therapeutic trial of acyclovir, brain biopsy may be avoided.

Time may be used as an investigation. For example, a patient on a statin medication who experiences gradual-onset muscle weakness and myalgias would be better served by stopping the drug and observing whether the muscle symptoms resolve, rather than immediately performing a muscle biopsy.

Reliability of Laboratory Investigations

When a new laboratory test is developed, its sensitivity (the frequency with which the test is abnormal in patients with the particular disease) and specificity (the frequency with which the test is abnormal in people without the particular disease) must be determined. If a test is very sensitive but has poor specificity, it may not be useful for diagnosis. For instance, the ESR is very sensitive in cranial arteritis but is elevated in so many other conditions that it cannot be used to diagnose the condition. Of more use is a test that is highly specific, even if it has a lower sensitivity. The acetylcholine receptor antibody titer is raised in only about 60% of patients with myasthenia gravis, for example, but very rarely in normal people or those with other conditions. The specificity and sensitivity can be useful to quantitate the extent to which a test result makes a diagnosis of the disease more or less likely.

Decision Analysis

Diagnostic acumen and treatment success are the hallmarks of the experienced neurologist. This acumen can be taught and can be learned from years of practice. Decision analysis is a method developed to provide insight into the processes of diagnosis and management of a complex disease when often insufficient data are available. This method can help identify areas of uncertainty in currently accepted diagnostic and management methods. Decision analysis forces the clinician to make quantitative estimates of each of the many factors entering into a clinical decision and to calculate the risk-to-benefit ratio of each management decision. Decision analysis is an excellent teaching tool. Because crucial quantitative data often are not easily available, this necessitates a search for such data, either from the literature or through new research.

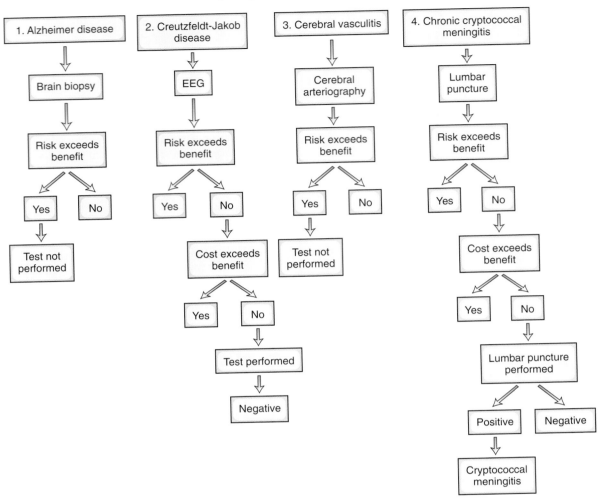

Fig. 31.1 Flowchart of the decision process involved in choosing investigations to elucidate the diagnosis in an 80-year-old man with a 3-month history of a progressive dementia. Considerations in the differential diagnosis included Alzheimer disease, Creutzfeldt-Jakob disease, cerebral vasculitis, and cryptococcal meningitis. A brain biopsy was not performed, and an electroencephalogram (EEG) did not show typical changes of Creutzfeldt-Jakob disease. The analysis suggests that arteriography is justified to look for a vasculitis, but the lumbar puncture revealed cryptococcal meningitis before angiography was performed.

Research Investigations and Teaching Hospitals

Because many of our readers are neurologists in training, here we briefly mention the use of investigations in teaching and research centers. Clinical research is closely regulated in most parts of the world, and research investigations cannot be performed until the protocol is approved by an institutional review board or an ethics-in-research committee. The peer review process is designed to ensure that the risks of the research study are justified, taking into account the patient's particular disease and the likely benefits of the research. The institutional review board ensures that the patient receives full information contained in an informed consent form and understands the risks of the study and what is likely to be learned from the research. Special policies and procedures also apply to minors, patients with cognitive dysfunction, those in emergency situations, or those with alterations in consciousness. No patient should be coerced, knowingly or unknowingly, into participating in a research procedure. Once the institutional review board gives permission for a research project, it continues to monitor the study to ensure that the research conforms to the protocol.

In a teaching hospital, the attending or consultant physician is legally and ethically responsible for the care provided to a patient by physicians in training. The attending neurologist must ensure that every investigation is justified for diagnostic and management purposes. All physicians are legally and ethically bound to ensure that the patient understands the reason for each investigation and gives informed consent. The neurologist in training must learn to use tests judiciously and not perform them simply for curiosity or education. The two-way discussion with more senior neurologists about the rationale, risk-to-benefit ratio, and cost-to-benefit ratio of each investigation is an important part of the learning process.

Patient Confidentiality

Some diagnostic tests, such as the DNA genetic test for HD and the test for HIV 1, necessitate prior counseling about the implications of these tests for possibly affected persons and their families. Results of such tests should be kept separate from the rest of the chart to maintain strict confidentiality for the patient. Physicians and their staff in the United States need to comply with the Health Insurance Portability and Accountability Act of 1996 (http://www.hhs.gov/ocr/hipaa).

Role of Laboratory Investigations in Neurological Disease Management

The standard neurological examination is designed more to detect abnormal function for diagnostic purposes than to quantify the neurological abnormalities. When possible, therefore, laboratory investigations are used to measure the response of the disease to treatment. Laboratory investigations usually are quantitative and may be helpful in managing disease. Generally, abnormal laboratory values return toward normal as a disease resolves or become increasingly abnormal as it worsens. The vital capacity in a patient with Guillain-Barré syndrome is an example of a measurement that improves as the disease improves. This is not always the case, however. In Duchenne muscular dystrophy, the serum CK concentration decreases as the disease worsens, because fewer muscle fibers remain to release enzyme into the serum. In myasthenia gravis, the patient's condition can go from minimal weakness to total paralysis unrelated to the titers of acetylcholine receptor antibodies in the blood. Therefore, monitoring laboratory values cannot always be used as an index of disease severity or response to treatment. Other limitations on the use of laboratory tests to monitor disease progression include sampling errors and test sensitivity and specificity.

Quantitative tools provide important information for measuring a patient's status objectively during the course of a disease. They can be as simple as visual acuity measurement, how many serial numbers from 1 to 100 a patient can count on a single breath, or the frequency and severity of headaches each month. Alternatively, they can be sophisticated measurements such as the force of maximum voluntary muscle contraction or the temperature perception threshold for an area of skin. They can be summated scores of semiquantitative assessments, such as the Kurtzke scale devised to follow the clinical course in patients with MS, the Norris score for amyotrophic lateral sclerosis, or the z-scores of muscle strength. Quantitative measures of neurological function allow much better assessment of the response of a disease to treatment than does the routine neurological examination.

II

Chapter 32A

Clinical Neurophysiology
Electroencephalography and Evoked Potentials

Ronald G. Emerson, Timothy A. Pedley

The techniques of applied electrophysiology are of practical importance in diagnosing and managing certain categories of neurological disease. Modern instrumentation permits selective investigation of various functional aspects of the central and peripheral nervous systems. The electroencephalogram (EEG) and evoked potentials are measures of electrical activity generated by the central nervous system (CNS). Despite the introduction of positron emission tomography (PET), functional magnetic resonance imaging (MRI), and magnetoencephalography (MEG), electroencephalography and evoked potential studies currently are the only readily available laboratory tests of brain physiology. As such, they generally are complementary to anatomical imaging techniques such as computed tomography (CT) or MRI, especially when it is desirable to document abnormalities that are not associated with detectable structural alterations in brain tissue. Furthermore, electroencephalography provides the only continuous measure of cerebral function over time.

This chapter is not intended as a comprehensive account of all aspects of electroencephalography and evoked potentials. Rather, the intent is to provide clinicians with an appreciation of the scope and limitations of these investigations as currently used.

Electroencephalography

Physiological Principles of Electroencephalography

The cerebral cortex generates EEG signals. Spontaneous EEG activity reflects the flow of extracellular space currents generated by the summation of excitatory and inhibitory synaptic potentials occurring on thousands or even millions of cortical neurons. Individual action potentials do not contribute directly to EEG activity. A conventional EEG recording is a continuous graph, over time, of the spatial distribution of changing voltage fields at the scalp surface that result from ongoing synaptic activity in the underlying cortex.

EEG rhythms appear to be part of a complex hierarchy of cortical oscillations that are fundamental to the brain's information processing mechanisms, including input selection and transient "binding" of distributed neuronal assemblies (Buzsaki and Draguhn, 2004). In addition to reflecting the spontaneous intrinsic activities of cortical neurons, the EEG depends on important afferent inputs from subcortical structures including the thalamus and brainstem reticular formation. Thalamic afferents, for example, probably are responsible for entraining cortical neurons to produce the rhythmic oscillations that characterize normal patterns like alpha rhythm and sleep spindles. An EEG abnormality may occur directly from disruption of cortical neural networks or indirectly from modification of subcortical inputs onto cortical neurons.

A scalp-recorded EEG represents only a limited, low-resolution view of the electrical activity of the brain. This is due in part to the pronounced voltage attenuation and "blurring" that occurs from overlying cerebrospinal fluid (CSF) and tissue layers. Relatively large areas of cortex have to be involved in similar synchronized activity for a discharge to appear on the EEG. For example, recordings obtained from arrays of microelectrodes penetrating into the cerebral cortex reveal a complex architecture of seizure initiation and propagation invisible to recordings from the scalp or even the cortical surface, with seizure-like discharges occurring in areas as small as a single cortical column (Schevon et al., 2008). Furthermore, potentials involving surfaces of gyri are more readily recorded than potentials arising in the walls and depths of sulci. Activity generated over the lateral convexities of the hemispheres records more accurately than does activity coming from interhemispherical, mesial, or basal areas. In the case of epileptiform activity, estimates are that 20% to 70% of cortical spikes do not appear on the EEG, depending on the region of cortex involved. Additionally, although the scalp-recorded EEG consists almost entirely of signals slower than approximately 40 Hz, intracranial oscillations of several hundred hertz may be recorded and, of clinical importance, have been associated with both normal physiological processes and seizure initiation (Schevon et al., 2009).

Such considerations limit the usefulness of electroencephalography. First, surface recordings are not useful to unambiguously determine the nature of synaptic events contributing to a particular EEG wave. Second, the EEG is rarely specific as to cause because different diseases and conditions produce similar EEG changes. In this regard, the EEG is analogous to findings on the neurological examination—hemiplegia caused by a stroke cannot be distinguished from that caused by a brain tumor. Third, many potentials occurring at the brain surface involve such a small area or are of such low voltage that they cannot be detected at the scalp. The EEG results then may be normal despite clear indications from other data of focal brain dysfunction. Finally, abnormalities in brain areas inaccessible to EEG recording electrodes (some cortical areas and virtually all subcortical and brainstem regions) do not affect the EEG directly but may exert remote effects on patterns of cortical activity.

Normal Electroencephalographic Activities

Spontaneous fluctuations of voltage potential at the cortical surface are in the range of 100 to 1000 mV, but at the scalp are only 10 to 100 mV. Different parts of the cortex generate relatively distinct potential fluctuations, which also differ in the waking and sleep states.

In most normal adults, the waking pattern of EEG activity consists mainly of sinusoidal oscillations occurring at 8 to 12 Hz, which are most prominent over the occipital area—the alpha rhythm (**Fig. 32A.1, A**). Eye opening, mental activity, and drowsiness attenuate (block) the alpha rhythm. Activity faster than 12 Hz beta activity normally is present over the frontal areas and may be especially prominent in patients receiving barbiturate or benzodiazepine drugs. Activity slower than 8 Hz is divisible into delta activity (1 to 3 Hz) and theta activity (4 to 7 Hz). Adults normally may show a small amount of theta activity over the temporal regions; the percentage of intermixed theta frequencies increases after the age of 60 years. Delta activity is not present normally in adults when they are awake but appears when they fall asleep (see **Fig. 32A.1, B**). The amount and amplitude of slow activity (theta and delta) correlate closely with the depth of sleep. Slow frequencies are abundant in the EEGs of newborns and young children, but these disappear progressively with maturation.

Common Types of Electroencephalographic Abnormalities

Focal Arrhythmic (Polymorphic) Slow Activity

Polymorphic slow activity is irregular activity in the delta (1 to 4 Hz) or theta (4 to 7 Hz) range, which when continuous has a strong correlation with a localized cerebral lesion such as infarction, hemorrhage, tumor, or abscess. Intermittent focal slow activity also may indicate localized parenchymal dysfunction but is less predictive than polymorphic slow activity.

Intermittent Rhythmic Slow Waves

Paroxysmal bursts of generalized bisynchronous rhythmic theta or delta waves usually indicate thalamocortical dysfunction and may be seen with metabolic or toxic disorders, obstructive hydrocephalus, deep midline or posterior fossa lesions, and also as a nonspecific functional disturbance in patients with generalized epilepsy. Focal bursts of rhythmic waves lateralized to one hemisphere usually indicate deep (typically thalamic or periventricular) abnormalities, often of a structural nature.

Generalized Arrhythmic (Polymorphic) Slow Activity

Diffuse disturbances in background rhythms marked by excessive slow activity and disorganization of waking EEG patterns arise in encephalopathies of metabolic, toxic, or infectious origin and with brain damage caused by a static encephalopathy.

Voltage Attenuation

Cortical disease causes voltage attenuation. Generalized voltage attenuation is usually associated with diffuse depression of function such as after anoxia or with certain degenerative diseases (e.g., Huntington disease). The most severe form of generalized voltage attenuation is electrocerebral inactivity, which is corroborative evidence of brain death in the appropriate clinical setting. Focal voltage attenuation reliably indicates localized cortical disease such as porencephaly, atrophy, or contusion, or an extra-axial lesion such as a meningioma or subdural hematoma.

Epileptiform Discharges

Epileptiform discharges are spikes or sharp waves that occur interictally in patients with epilepsy and sometimes in persons who do not experience seizures but have a genetic predisposition to epilepsy. Epileptiform discharges may be focal or generalized, depending on the seizure type.

Recording Techniques

The EEG recording methods in common use are summarized in the following discussion. Details can be found in the American Clinical Neurophysiology Society's Guidelines (2006).

A series of small gold, silver, or silver–silver chloride disks are symmetrically positioned over the scalp on both sides of the head in standard locations (the International Ten-Twenty

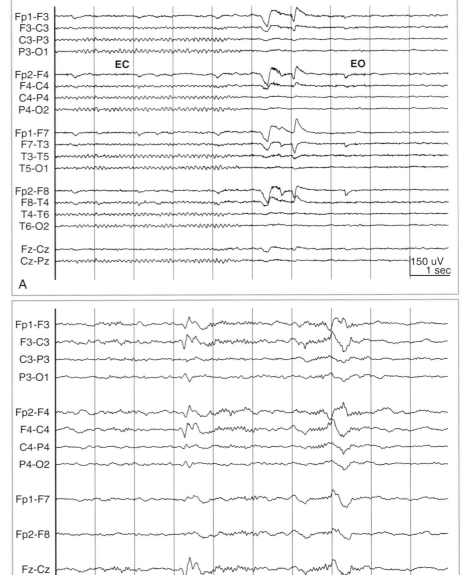

Fig. 32A.1 Samples of normal electroencephalographic recordings from two patients. **A,** Waking activity is characterized by a 9-Hz alpha rhythm that attenuates when the eyes are opened (EO) and resumes when the eyes are closed (EC). **B,** Stage 2 sleep is characterized by 2- to 5-Hz background activity, on which are superimposed vertex (V) waves and sleep spindles.

system). In practice, 20 or more channels of EEG activity are recorded simultaneously, each channel displaying the potential difference between two electrodes. Electrode pairs are interconnected in different arrangements called *montages* to permit a comprehensive survey of the brain's electrical activity. Typically, the design of montages is to compare symmetrical areas of the two hemispheres, anterior versus posterior regions, or parasagittal versus temporal areas in the same hemisphere.

A typical study is about 30 to 45 minutes in duration and includes two types of "activating procedures": hyperventilation and photic stimulation. In some patients, these techniques provoke abnormal focal or generalized alterations in activity that are of diagnostic importance and would

otherwise go undetected (**Fig. 32A.2**). Recording during sleep and after sleep deprivation, and placement of additional electrodes at other recording sites are useful in detecting specific kinds of epileptiform potentials. The use of other maneuvers depends on the clinical question posed. For example, epileptiform activity may occasionally activate only by movement or specific sensory stimuli. Vasovagal stimulation may be important in some types of syncope.

In the past, EEG recording instruments were simple analog devices with banks of amplifiers and pen-writers. In contrast, modern EEG machines make use of digital processing and storage, and the electroencephalographer interprets the EEG from a computer display rather than from paper. Technological advances have not fundamentally changed the principles

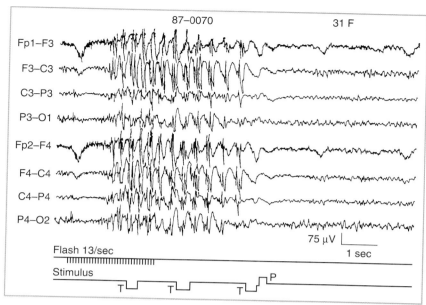

Fig. 32A.2 Intermittent stroboscopic light stimulation at 13 flashes per second elicited generalized bursts of 4- to 5-Hz spike-wave activity, termed a *photoparoxysmal (photoconvulsive) response.* The spike-wave paroxysm was associated with a brief absence, as documented by the patient's (P) inability to respond to a tone given by the technologist (T). Normal responsiveness returned immediately on cessation of the spike-wave activity. The remainder of the electroencephalogram was normal.

of EEG interpretation, but they have facilitated EEG reading. Early paper-based EEG systems required that all recording parameters—display gain, filter settings, and the manner in which scalp-recorded signals were combined and displayed (montages)—be fixed by the technologist at the time of recording. In contrast, digital EEG systems permit the electroencephalographer to adjust these settings at the time of interpretation. A given EEG waveform or pattern can be examined using a number of different instrument settings, including sophisticated montages (e.g., Laplacian montages), that were unavailable using traditional analog recording systems. Topographic maps can be useful to depict spatial relationships, displaying features of the EEG in a graphical manner similar to that for functional MRI (fMRI) or PET. For example, topographical maps can illustrate EEG voltage distributions over the scalp at a particular point in time (**Fig. 32A.3**) as well as the distributions of particular frequencies contained within the EEG. Although this flexibility does not change the interpretive strategies used to read an EEG, it does allow the electroencephalographer to apply them more effectively.

In addition to facilitating the standard interpretation of EEGs, mathematical techniques can also be used to reveal features that may not be apparent to visual inspection of raw EEG waveforms. For example, averaging techniques, useful in improving the signal-to-noise ratios of spikes and sharp waves, can reveal field distributions and timing relationships that are not otherwise appreciable. Dipole source localization methods have been used to characterize both interictal spikes and ictal discharges in patients with epilepsy and may contribute to localization of the seizure focus (Ebersole, 2000). Such methods are based on a number of critical assumptions that, if applied without recognition of their limitations, can result in anatomically and physiologically erroneous conclusions (Emerson et al., 1995), so caution is warranted in their use.

For patients undergoing long-term EEG recordings as part of the diagnosis or management of epilepsy, a time-locked digitally recorded video image of the patient is recorded simultaneously with the EEG. EEG data are often processed

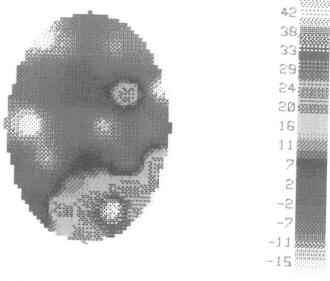

Fig. 32A.3 Frequency-domain topographical brain map obtained from a 32-channel bipolar electroencephalographic (EEG) recording. The patient was a 53-year-old man with hemodynamically significant left carotid stenosis. This map demonstrates an asymmetry over the occipital regions during eye opening, reflecting relative failure of left hemisphere alpha activity to attenuate normally. The color scale at the right reflects percentage change in EEG activity on going from the eyes-closed to the eyes-open state. *(Courtesy Dr. Bruce J. Fisch.)*

by software that can automatically detect most seizure activity. Similar systems are finding increased use in intensive care units (ICU), where EEG monitoring has become increasingly important in the management of patients with nonconvulsive seizure activity, threatened or impending cerebral ischemia, severe head trauma, and metabolic coma (Drislane et al., 2008; Friedman et al., 2009). In this setting, compressed spectrograms, which graphically summarize the frequencies present in several hours of EEG on a single screen, can help the electroencephalographer to rapidly pinpoint important changes in the EEG and sometimes spot patterns or trends that otherwise might go unnoticed (**Fig. 32A.4**) (Scheuer, 2002). It is important to emphasize that fully automated robust systems analogous to those employed for cardiac monitoring are not now available for EEG, and while various automated methods can be very useful, their proper use in clinical practice should be as adjuncts to standard EEG recording and interpretation. False positives and negatives are commonplace;

indeed, the very data reduction that makes such methods useful also makes them unsuitable for stand-alone application.

Clinical Uses of Electroencephalography

The EEG assesses physiological alterations in brain activity. Many changes are nonspecific, but some are highly suggestive of specific entities (epilepsy, herpes encephalitis, metabolic encephalopathy). The EEG also is useful in following the course of patients with altered states of consciousness and

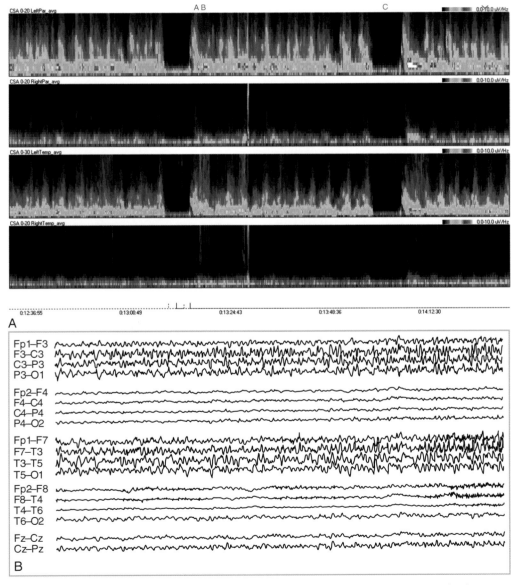

Fig. 32A.4 Frequency spectrograph depicting 2 hours of electroencephalographic (EEG) recording in a patient in focal status epilepticus. **A,** Upper two panels show activity in right and left parasagittal electrode derivations, respectively; lower two panels depict activity in temporal derivations. Time is represented on the horizontal axis. The vertical axis on each panel corresponds to frequency, from 1 Hz on the bottom to 20 Hz at the top. Colors indicate EEG voltage at a given frequency, from black for 0 mV/Hz to purple for 10 mV/Hz. This spectrograph shows bursts of relatively high-voltage, high-frequency *(green)* activity recurring approximately every 5 to 7 minutes, most prominent in the left parasagittal panel. This electroencephalogram (EEG) demonstrates a pattern of recurring electrographic seizures, as illustrated by representative EEG traces **B** and **C**, corresponding to points *a* and *b* on the spectrograph. Additionally, two quiescent periods with no activity *(black)* occur at most frequencies, corresponding to periods of postictal voltage depression, also illustrated in trace **D.**

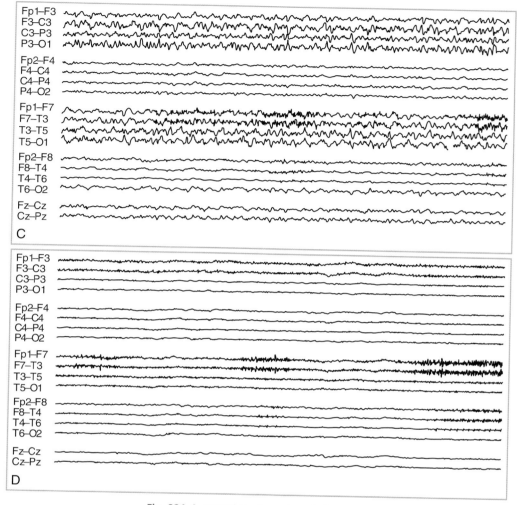

Fig. 32A.4, cont'd For legend see facing page.

may, in certain circumstances, provide prognostic information. It can be important in the determination of brain death.

Electroencephalography is not a screening test. It serves to answer a particular problem posed by the patient's condition, so providing sufficient clinical information helps design an appropriate test with meaningful electrographical clinical correlation. The request for this study should specifically state the question addressed by the EEG.

EEG interpretation should be rational and based on a systematic analysis that uses consistent parameters that permit comparisons with findings expected from the patient's age and circumstances of recording. Accurate interpretation requires high-quality recording. This depends on trained technologists who understand the importance of meticulous electrode application, proper use of instrument controls, recognition and (where possible) elimination of artifacts, and appropriate selection of recording montages to allow optimal display of cerebral electrical activity.

Epilepsy

The EEG usually is the most helpful laboratory test when a diagnosis of epilepsy is considered. Because the onset of seizures is unpredictable, and their occurrence is relatively infrequent in most patients, EEG recordings usually are obtained when the patient is not having a seizure. Fortunately, electrical abnormalities in the EEG occur in most patients with epilepsy even between attacks.

The only EEG finding that has a strong correlation with epilepsy is *epileptiform activity*, a term used to describe spikes and sharp waves that are clearly distinct from ongoing background activity. Clinical and experimental evidence supports a specific association between epileptiform discharges and seizure susceptibility. Only about 2% of nonepileptic patients have epileptiform EEGs, whereas as many as 90% of patients with epilepsy show epileptiform activity, depending on the circumstances of the recording and the number of studies obtained.

Nonetheless, interpretation of interictal findings always requires caution. Correlating most epileptiform discharges with the frequency and likelihood of recurrence of epileptic seizures is poor (Selvitelli et al., 2010). Furthermore, a substantial number of patients with unquestionable epilepsy have consistently normal interictal EEGs. The most convincing proof that a patient's episodic symptoms are epileptic is obtained by recording an electrographical seizure discharge during a typical behavioral attack. Although ictal EEG tracings greatly increase the sensitivity of the study in assessing the pathophysiology of specific behavioral episodes, the clinician must still be aware of limitations inherent in such recordings. (Videos showing actual EEG recordings obtained during seizures [Videos 32A.1 to 32A.3] are available at www.expertconsult.com.)

In addition to epileptiform patterns, EEGs in patients with epilepsy often show excessive focal or generalized slow-wave activity. Less often, asymmetries of frequency or voltage may be noted. These findings are not unique to epilepsy and are featured in other conditions such as static encephalopathies, brain tumors, migraine, and trauma. In patients with unusual spells, nonspecific changes on EEG should be weighed cautiously and are not to be considered direct evidence for a diagnosis of epilepsy. On the other hand, when clinical data are unequivocal, or when epileptiform discharges occur as well, the degree and extent of background EEG changes may provide information important for judging the likelihood of an underlying focal cerebral lesion, a more diffuse encephalopathy, or a progressive neurological syndrome. Additionally, EEG findings may help determine prognosis and aid in the decision to discontinue antiepileptic medication.

The type of epileptiform activity on EEG is helpful in classifying a patient's seizure type correctly and sometimes in identifying a specific epileptic syndrome (see Chapter 67). Clinically, generalized tonic-clonic seizures may be generalized from the outset or may be secondary to spread from a focus. Lapses of awareness with automatisms may be a manifestation either of a generalized nonconvulsive form of epilepsy (absence seizures) or of focal epileptogenic dysfunction (temporal lobe epilepsy). The initial clinical features of a seizure may be uncertain because of postictal amnesia or nocturnal occurrence. In these and similar situations, the EEG can provide information crucial to the correct diagnosis and appropriate therapy.

In generalized seizures of nonfocal origin, the EEG typically shows bilaterally synchronous diffuse bursts of spikes and spike-and-wave discharges (**Fig. 32A.5**). All generalized EEG epileptiform patterns share certain common features, although the exact expression of the spike-wave activity varies depending on whether the patient has pure absence, tonic-clonic, myoclonic, or atonic-astatic seizures. The EEG also may distinguish between primary and secondary generalized epilepsy. In the former instance, no cerebral disease is demonstrable, whereas in the latter, evidence can be found for diffuse brain damage. Typically, primary (idiopathic) generalized epilepsy is associated with normal or near-normal EEG background rhythms, whereas secondary (symptomatic) epilepsy is associated with some degree of generalized slow-wave activity.

Consistently focal epileptiform activity is the signature of partial (focal) epilepsy (**Fig. 32A.6**). With the exception of the benign focal epilepsies of childhood, focal epileptiform activity results from neuronal dysfunction caused by demonstrable brain disease. The waveform of focal epileptiform discharges is largely independent of localization, but a reasonable correlation exists between spike location and the type of ictal behavior. Anterior temporal spikes usually are associated with complex partial seizures, rolandic spikes with simple motor or

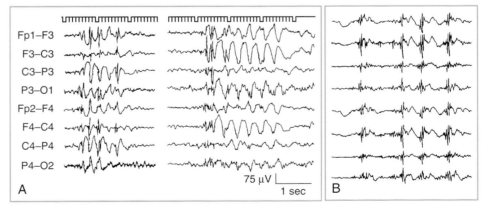

Fig. 32A.5 Examples of generalized spike-wave patterns from different patients with primary generalized (idiopathic) epilepsy. The patient in **A** had mainly tonic-clonic seizures, with occasional absence attacks. The patient in **B** had juvenile myoclonic epilepsy.

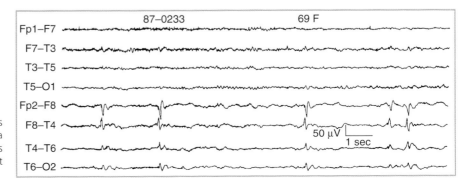

Fig. 32A.6 Focal right anterior temporal spikes occurring on the electroencephalogram of a 69-year-old woman with complex partial seizures after a stroke involving branches of the right middle cerebral artery.

sensory seizures, and occipital spikes with primitive visual hallucinations or diminished visual function as an initial feature.

In addition to distinguishing epileptiform from nonepileptiform abnormalities, EEG analysis sometimes identifies specific electroclinical syndromes. Such syndromes include hypsarrhythmia associated with infantile spasms (West syndrome) (**Fig. 32A.7**); 3-Hz spike-and-wave activity associated with typical absence attacks (petit mal epilepsy) (**Fig. 32A.8**); generalized multiple spikes and waves (polyspike-wave pattern) associated with myoclonic epilepsy, including so-called juvenile myoclonic epilepsy of Janz (see **Fig. 32A.5, B**); generalized sharp and slow waves (slow spike-and-wave pattern) associated with Lennox-Gastaut syndrome (**Fig. 32A.9**); central-midtemporal spikes associated with benign rolandic epilepsy (**Fig. 32A.10**); and periodic lateralized epileptiform discharges (PLEDs) associated with acute destructive cerebral lesions such as hemorrhagic cerebral infarction, a rapidly growing malignancy, or herpes simplex encephalitis (**Fig. 32A.11**) (Pohlmann-Eden et al., 1996). PLEDs may also reappear in patients with chronic structural lesions in the context of new metabolic derangements.

The increased availability of special monitoring facilities for simultaneous video and EEG recording and of ambulatory EEG recorders has improved diagnostic accuracy and the reliability of seizure classification. Prolonged continuous recordings through one or more complete sleep/wake cycles constitute the best way to document ictal episodes and should be considered in patients whose interictal EEGs are normal or nondiagnostic and in clinical dilemmas that are resolvable only by recording actual behavioral events. Although EEG documentation of an ictal discharge establishes the epileptic nature of a corresponding behavioral change, the converse is not necessarily true. Sometimes muscle or movement artifacts so obscure the EEG recording that it is impossible to know whether any EEG change has occurred. In these circumstances, postictal slowing usually is indicative of an epileptic event if similar slow waves are not present elsewhere in the recording and if the EEG recording subsequently returns to baseline. In addition, focal seizures not accompanied by alteration in consciousness occasionally have no detectable scalp correlate. On the other hand, persistence of alpha activity and absence of slowing during and after an apparent convulsive episode are inconsistent with an epileptic generalized tonic-clonic seizure.

Focal Cerebral Lesions

The use of electroencephalography to detect focal cerebral disturbances has declined because of the development and widespread availability of computerized anatomical imaging

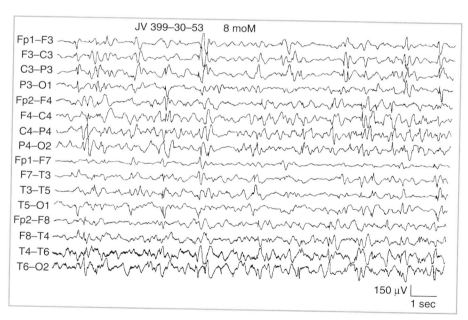

Fig. 32A.7 Electroencephalographic pattern termed *hypsarrhythmia* in a recording obtained in an 8-month-old boy with infantile spasms. Background activity is high-voltage and unorganized, with abundant multifocal spikes.

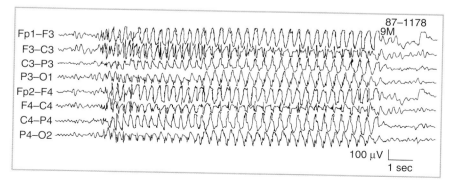

Fig. 32A.8 A 3-Hz spike-and-wave paroxysm on the electroencephalogram of a 9-year-old boy with absence seizures (petit mal epilepsy). During this 12-second discharge, the child was unresponsive and demonstrated rhythmic eye blinking.

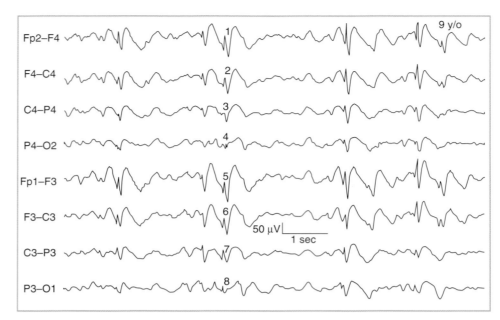

Fig. 32A.9 Generalized sharp-wave and slow-wave discharges on the electroencephalogram (EEG) of a 9-year-old child with mental retardation and uncontrolled typical absence, tonic, and atonic generalized seizures. This constellation of clinical and EEG features constitutes the Lennox-Gastaut syndrome.

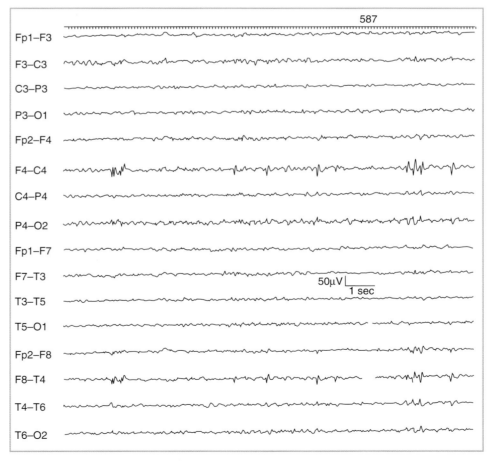

Fig. 32A.10 Electroencephalogram obtained during drowsiness in a 10-year-old boy with benign rolandic epilepsy. Stereotypical diphasic or triphasic sharp waves occur in the right central-parietal and midtemporal regions.

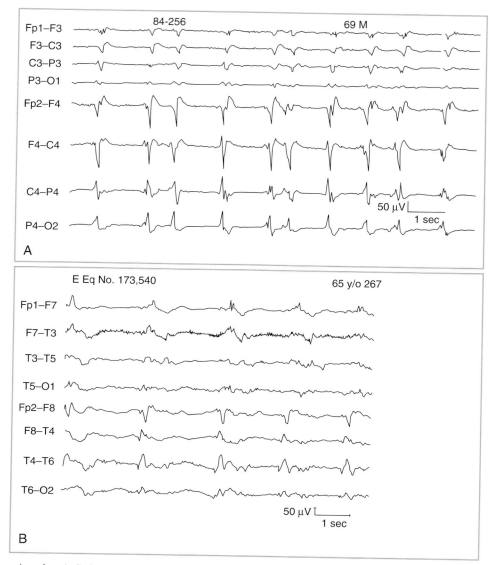

Fig. 32A.11 Two examples of periodic lateralized epileptiform discharges (PLEDs) on the electroencephalogram. **A,** Right parasagittal PLEDs in a 69-year-old man with severe brain damage caused by meningitis with multiple cerebral infarctions. **B,** A 65-year-old woman with herpes simplex encephalitis. PLEDs are bilateral but have a right-sided predominance.

techniques. Nonetheless, the EEG has a role in documenting focal physiological dysfunction in the absence of discernible structural pathology and in evaluating the functional disturbance produced by known lesions.

Focal delta activity is the usual EEG sign of a local disturbance. A structural lesion is likely if the delta activity is (1) present continuously; (2) shows variability in waveform, amplitude, duration, and morphology (so-called arrhythmic or polymorphic activity); and (3) persists during changes in wake/sleep states (**Fig. 32A.12**). The localizing value of focal delta activity increases when it is topographically discrete or associated with depression or loss of superimposed faster background frequencies. Superficial lesions tend to produce restricted EEG changes, whereas deep cerebral lesions produce hemispherical or even bilateral delta activity.

Bilateral paroxysmal bursts of rhythmic delta waves (**Fig. 32A.13**) with frontal predominance—once attributed to subfrontal, deep midline, or posterior fossa lesions—are actually nonspecific and seen more often with diffuse encephalopathies. Focal or lateralized intermittent bursts of rhythmic delta waves as the prominent EEG abnormality suggest a deep supratentorial (periventricular or diencephalic) lesion.

The character and distribution of the EEG changes caused by a focal lesion depend on its size, its distance from the cortical surface, the specific structures involved, and its acuity. A small stroke critically located in the thalamus may produce widespread hemispherical slowing and alteration in sleep spindles and alpha rhythm regulation. A lesion of the same size located at the cortical surface produces few if any EEG findings.

Single lacunae usually produce little or no change in the EEG. Similarly, transient ischemic attacks not associated with chronic cerebral hypoperfusion or imminent occlusion of a major vessel do not significantly affect the EEG outside the symptomatic period. Superficial cortical or large, deep hemispherical infarctions are usually associated with localized EEG abnormalities.

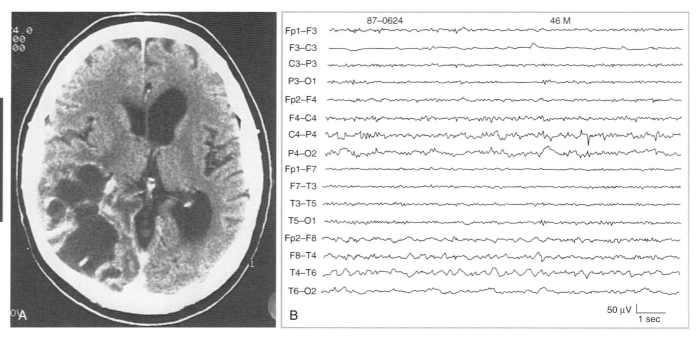

Fig. 32A.12 The patient was a 46-year-old man with a glioblastoma involving the right temporal and parietal lobes. **A,** Lesion is well demonstrated on this computed tomography scan of the brain. **B,** Electroencephalogram demonstrates continuous arrhythmic slowing over the right temporal and parieto-occipital areas. In addition, loss of the alpha rhythm and overriding faster frequencies are seen in corresponding areas of the left cerebral hemisphere.

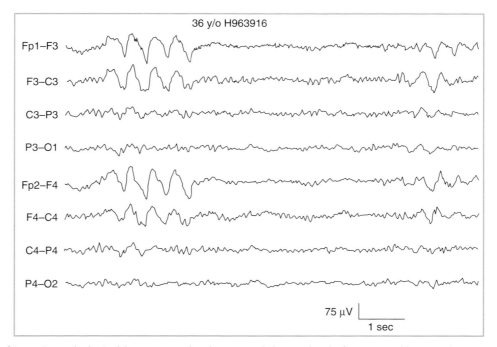

Fig. 32A.13 Bursts of intermittent rhythmic delta waves on the electroencephalogram (EEG) of a 36-year-old man with primary generalized epilepsy and tonic-clonic seizures. Generalized spike-wave activity occurred elsewhere in the EEG. Intermittent rhythmic delta waves are a nonspecific manifestation of the patient's generalized epileptic disorder. *(Courtesy Dr. Bruce J. Fisch.)*

Focal EEG changes (and other nonepileptiform abnormalities) are common in migraine. The likelihood of an abnormal EEG and the severity of the abnormality relate to the timing and character of the migraine attack. EEGs are more likely to be focally abnormal, with complicated rather than common migraine and during rather than between headaches. EEG changes seen with brain tumors are caused by disturbances in bordering brain parenchyma; tumor tissue is electrically silent. Focal EEG changes are caused by interference with patterns of normal neuronal synaptic activity, by destruction or alteration of the cortical neurons, and by metabolic effects caused by changes in blood flow, cellular metabolism, or the neuronal environment. Diffuse EEG changes are the consequence of increased intracranial pressure, shift of midline structures, or hydrocephalus. Electroencephalography is especially helpful in following the extent of cerebral dysfunction over time, in distinguishing between direct effects of the neoplasm and superimposed metabolic or toxic encephalopathies, and in differentiating among epileptic, ischemic, and noncerebral causes for episodic symptoms.

The role of electroencephalography in the management of patients with head injuries is limited. Transient generalized slowing is common after concussion. A persistent area of continuous localized slow-wave activity suggests cerebral contusion even in the absence of a focal clinical or CT abnormality, and unilateral voltage depression suggests subdural hematoma. Electroencephalography performed in the first 3 months after injury does not predict posttraumatic epilepsy.

Altered States of Consciousness

The EEG has a major role in evaluating patients with altered levels of consciousness. Because this study permits a reasonably critical assessment of supratentorial brain function, it complements the clinical examination in patients with significant depression of consciousness. Abnormalities typically are nonspecific with regard to etiology. In general, however, a correlation with the clinical state is good. Some findings are more suggestive of particular causes than of others and occasionally are prognostically useful as well. Specific questions the EEG may help to answer (depending on the clinical presentation) are the following:

- Are psychogenic factors playing a major role?
- Is the process diffuse, focal, or multifocal?
- Is depressed consciousness due to unrecognized epileptic activity (nonconvulsive status epilepticus)?

- What evidence, if any, points to improvement, despite relatively little change in the clinical picture?
- What findings, if any, assist in assessing prognosis?

Metabolic Encephalopathies

Metabolic derangements affecting the brain diffusely constitute one of the most common causes of altered mental function in a general hospital. Generalized slow-wave activity is the main indication of decreased consciousness. The degree of EEG slowing closely parallels the patient's mental status and ranges from only minor slowing of alpha-rhythm frequency (slight inattentiveness and decreased alertness) to continuous delta activity (coma). Slow-wave activity sometimes becomes bisynchronous and assumes a high-voltage, sharply contoured triphasic morphology, especially over the frontal head regions (**Fig. 32A.14**). These triphasic waves, originally considered diagnostic of hepatic failure, occur with equal frequency in other metabolic disorders such as uremia, hyponatremia, hyperthyroidism, anoxia, and hyperosmolarity. The value of triphasic waves is that they suggest a metabolic cause in an unresponsive patient.

Some EEG features increase the likelihood of a specific metabolic disorder. Prominent generalized rhythmic beta activity raises the suspicion of drug intoxication in a comatose patient. Severe generalized voltage depression indicates impaired energy metabolism and suggests hypothyroidism if anoxia and hypothermia can be excluded. A photoconvulsive response is seen more often with uremia than with other causes of metabolic encephalopathy. Focal seizure activity is common in patients with hyperosmolar coma.

Hypoxia

Hypoxia, with or without circulatory arrest, produces a wide range of EEG abnormalities depending on the severity and reversibility of the brain damage. EEGs obtained 6 hours or

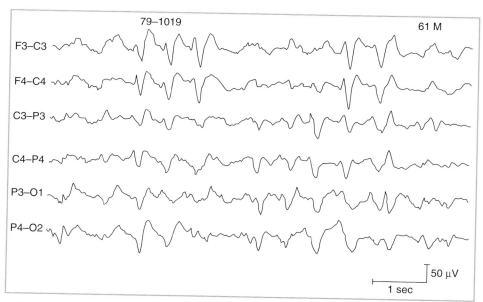

Fig. 32A.14 Triphasic waves on the electroencephalogram of a 61-year-old man with hepatic failure. *(Courtesy Dr. Bruce J. Fisch.)*

more after the hypoxic insult may show patterns that have prognostic value. Sequential EEGs strengthen the validity of such findings. EEG abnormalities associated with poor neurological outcome are alpha coma, burst suppression, and periodic patterns.

The term *alpha coma* refers to the apparent paradoxical appearance of monorhythmic alpha frequency activity in the EEG of a comatose patient; the EEG recording may appear normal to the inexperienced observer (**Fig. 32A.15**). In contrast with normal alpha activity, that seen with alpha coma is generalized, often maximal frontally, and unreactive to external stimuli.

The *burst suppression pattern* consists of occasional generalized bursts of medium- to high-voltage, mixed-frequency, slow-wave activity, sometimes with intermixed spikes, with intervening periods of severe voltage depression or cerebral inactivity (**Fig. 32A.16**). Massive myoclonic body jerks may accompany the bursts.

The *periodic pattern* consists of generalized spikes or sharp waves that recur with a relatively fixed interval, typically 1 or 2 per second (**Fig. 32A.17**). Sometimes the periodic sharp waves occur independently over each hemisphere. Myoclonic jerks of the limbs or whole body usually accompany a postanoxic periodic pattern.

The prognostic value of these patterns relates exclusively to the cause. Similar features are recognized with potentially reversible causes of coma including deep anesthesia, drug overdose, and severe liver or kidney failure.

Infectious Diseases

Of all infectious diseases affecting the brain, herpes simplex encephalitis is the one for which electroencephalography is most useful in initial assessment. Early and accurate diagnosis is important because the response to acyclovir is best when treatment is started early. Although establishing a definitive diagnosis requires brain biopsy, characteristic EEG changes in the clinical setting of encephalitis are helpful in selecting patients for early treatment and biopsy. The EEG result usually is abnormal and suggestive of herpes infection before CT lesions are recognized.

Viral encephalitis is expected to cause diffuse polymorphic slow-wave activity, and a normal EEG result raises doubt about the diagnosis. With herpes simplex encephalitis, a majority of patients show focal temporal or frontotemporal slowing that may be unilateral or, if bilateral, asymmetrical. Periodic sharp-wave complexes over one or both frontotemporal regions (occasionally in other locations and sometimes generalized) add additional specificity to the EEG findings (see **Fig. 32A.11, *B***). These diagnostic features usually appear between days 2 and 15 of illness and sometimes are detectable only with serial tracings.

Bacterial meningitis causes severe and widespread EEG abnormalities, typically profound slowing and voltage depression, but viral meningitis produces little in the way of significant changes. Although CT has replaced electroencephalography in evaluating patients with suspected brain abscess, focal EEG changes may occur in the early stage of

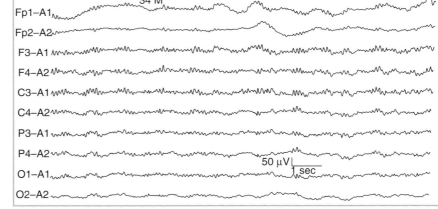

Fig. 32A.15 Alpha coma in a 34-year-old man with severe hypoxic-ischemic brain damage from subarachnoid hemorrhage with diffuse prolonged cerebral vasospasm. Unlike the normal alpha rhythm, the alpha range activity on the electroencephalogram of this comatose patient is widespread but maximal frontally, unreactive, and superimposed on low-voltage arrhythmic delta frequencies.

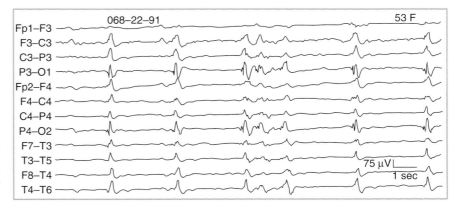

Fig. 32A.16 Burst suppression pattern on the electroencephalogram of a 53-year-old woman with anoxic encephalopathy following cardiorespiratory arrest. The patient died several days later. *(Courtesy Dr. Barbara S. Koppel.)*

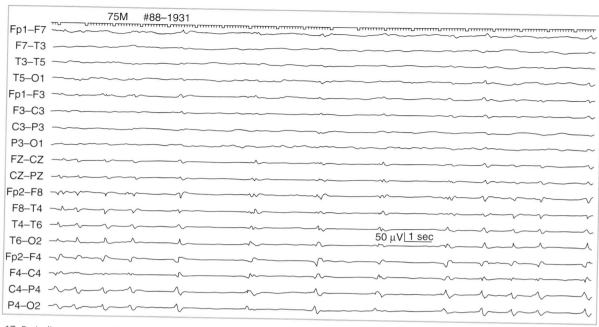

Fig. 32A.17 Periodic pattern on the electroencephalogram of a patient with anoxic encephalopathy following cardiorespiratory arrest. The patient was paralyzed with pancuronium because of bilateral myoclonus.

cerebritis before an encapsulated lesion is demonstrable on CT images.

EEG abnormalities usually resolve as the patient recovers, but the rate of resolution of clinical deficits and that of the electrographical findings may be different. It is not possible to predict either residual neurological morbidity or postencephalitic seizures by EEG criteria. An early return of normal EEG activity does not exclude the possibility of persistent neurological impairment.

Brain Death

The diagnosis of brain death rests on strict clinical criteria that, when satisfied unambiguously, permit a conclusive determination of irreversible loss of brain function. In the United States, the usual definition of brain death is irreversible cessation of all functions of the entire brain, including the brainstem. Because the EEG is a measure of cerebral—especially cortical—function, it has been widely used in association with clinical evaluation to provide objective evidence that brain function is lost. Several studies have demonstrated that enduring loss of cerebral electrical activity, termed *electrocerebral inactivity* or *electrocerebral silence*, accompanies clinical brain death and is never associated with recovery of neurological function. The determination of electrocerebral inactivity is technically demanding, requiring a special recording protocol. Specific criteria have been established by the American Clinical Neurophysiology Society.

Temporary and reversible loss of cerebral electrical activity is observable immediately after cardiorespiratory resuscitation, drug overdose from CNS depressants, and severe hypothermia. Therefore, accurate interpretation of an EEG demonstrating electrocerebral inactivity must take into account these exceptional circumstances. Chapter 48 summarizes the clinical criteria for establishing the diagnosis of brain death.

Aging and Dementia

Because the EEG is a measure of cortical function, theoretically it should be useful in the diagnosis and classification of dementia. The utility of single EEG examinations in evaluating patients with known or suspected dementing illnesses, however, is often disappointing. Two important reasons for this limitation are (1) problems in distinguishing the effects on cerebral electrical activity of normal aging from those caused by disease processes and (2) the absence of generally accepted quantifiable methods of analysis and statistically valid comparison measures.

With increasing age beyond 65 years, a slight reduction in alpha rhythm frequency and in the total amount of alpha activity is normal. Normal elderly persons also show slightly increased amounts of theta and delta activity, especially over the temporal and frontotemporal regions, as well as changes in sleep patterns. Early in the course of some dementing illnesses, no EEG abnormality may be apparent (this is the rule with Alzheimer disease), or the normal age-related changes may become exaggerated, differing more in degree than in kind.

In practice, the EEG can assist in the evaluation of suspected dementia by confirming abnormal cerebral function in patients with a possible psychogenic disorder and by delineating whether the process is focal or diffuse. Sequential EEGs usually are more helpful than a single tracing, and a test early in the course of the illness may provide more specific information than can be obtained later on. Overall, the degree of EEG abnormality shows good correlation with the degree of dementia.

EEG findings in Alzheimer disease are highly dependent on timing. The EEG initially is normal or shows an alpha rhythm at or just below the lower limits of normal. Generalized slowing ensues as the disease progresses. In patients with focal cognitive deficits, accentuation of slow frequency activity over the corresponding brain area may be a feature. Continuous

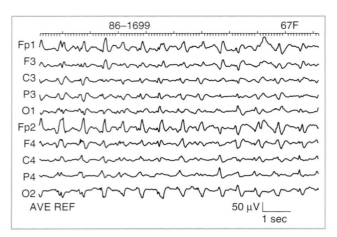

Fig. 32A.18 Periodic sharp-wave pattern on the electroencephalogram of a 67-year-old woman with Creutzfeldt-Jakob disease. Generalized bisynchronous diphasic sharp waves occur approximately 1.5 to 2.0 per second.

focal slowing is sufficiently unusual to suggest the possibility of another diagnosis. Prominent focal or bilateral independent slow-wave activity, especially if seen in company with a normal alpha rhythm, favors multifocal disease such as multiple cerebral infarcts. Sometimes a specific cause may be suggested. For example, an EEG showing generalized typical periodic sharp-wave complexes in a patient with dementia is virtually diagnostic of Creutzfeldt-Jakob disease (**Fig. 32A.18**).

Event-related evoked potentials have application in the study of dementia. These long-latency events (i.e., potentials occurring more than 150 msec after the stimulus) are heavily dependent on psychic and cognitive factors. Ideally, they measure the brain's intrinsic mechanisms for processing certain types of information and are potentially valuable in the electrophysiological assessment of dementia. The best known of the event-related potentials is the P300, or P3, wave. The place of these long-latency evoked potentials in the evaluation of dementia is still under investigation, but the pattern of electrophysiological abnormality may be helpful in distinguishing among types of dementia (Comi and Leocani, 2000).

Magnetoencephalography

Magnetoencephalography is a measure of brain function equivalent to electroencephalography in that the same neuronal sources that generate electrical activity also give rise to magnetic fields. However, MEG differs from EEG in several ways that have theoretical usefulness. The overlying CSF, dura, and skull substantially attenuate EEG potentials; these structures affect magnetic fields less. In addition, electroencephalography measures cortical current sources oriented in all directions but emphasizes radially oriented dipoles. Magnetoencephalography more accurately measures tangential dipoles that are parallel to the cortical surface.

Despite these differences, MEG recordings appear substantially similar to EEG recordings, and when interpreted by visual inspection, appear to have sensitivities for epileptiform activity similar to those of sleep-deprived EEGs (Colon et al., 2009). Although MEG may be potentially more

"patient-friendly" than EEG, because it does not require placement of electrodes on the scalp, its substantially greater cost has largely precluded its routine use. The main application of MEG has been to localize sources of evoked potentials and focal epileptiform activity, usually in consideration of epilepsy surgery. The limitations that apply to dipole source localization of EEG signals, however, apply similarly to MEG signals. For this reason, interpretation of MEG findings requires caution, and the technique is best viewed as an adjunct to established methods of localization such as intracranial electroencephalography (Cappell et al., 2006).

Evoked Potentials

Evoked potentials are electrical signals generated by the nervous system in response to sensory stimuli. The sensory system involved and the sequence of activation of different neural structures determine the timing and location of these signals. The choice of stimulus paradigms used in clinical practice is such that the responses the paradigms evoke are sufficiently stereotypical to allow the limits of normal to be clearly defined. Violation of these limits indicates dysfunction of the sensory pathways under study. The American Clinical Neurophysiology Society's Guidelines 9A to 9D provide an overview of recording methodology, criteria for abnormality, and limitations of use.

Because of their low voltage, evoked potentials generally are not discernible without computer averaging to differentiate them from ongoing EEG activity and other sources of electrical noise. Exceptions are the visual responses evoked by transient flash stimuli, which the routine EEG displays as photic driving. Typically, however, it is necessary to present the stimulus repeatedly, averaging the time-locked brain or spinal cord responses to a series of identical stimuli while allowing unrelated noise to average out.

In the clinical setting, evoked potential studies are properly an extension of the neurological examination. As with any neurological sign, they help reveal the existence and often suggest the location of neurological lesions. Evoked potentials, therefore, are most useful when they detect clinically silent abnormalities that might otherwise go unrecognized, or when they assist in resolving vague or equivocal symptoms and findings. Like electroencephalography, evoked potential studies are tests of function; the findings usually are not etiologically specific.

Visual Evoked Potentials

Cerebral visual evoked potentials (VEPs) are responses of the visual cortex to appropriate stimuli. Recording of the composite retinal response to visual stimuli, electroretinography, may be performed separately. Obtaining the cerebral VEP is accomplished by averaging the responses from occipital scalp electrodes generated by 100 or more sequential stimuli. Stimulus characteristics are critically important in determining the portion of the visual system to test by the VEP and the sensitivity of the test needed. Initial clinical applications of VEPs used a stroboscopic flash stimulus, but severely limiting the utility of the flash-evoked VEP are the great variability of responses among normal persons and its relative insensitivity to clinical lesions (**Fig. 32A.19**). Occasionally, flash VEPs may provide limited information about the integrity of visual pathways when the preferred pattern-reversal stimulus is not usable, as in infants or older patients unable to cooperate for more sensitive testing methods.

Normal Visual Evoked Potential

More sensitive and reliable responses are obtained using a pattern-reversal stimulus. The subject focuses on a high-contrast checkerboard of black and white squares displayed on a video or optical projection screen. The stimulus is the change of black squares to white and of white squares to black (pattern reversal). When appropriate check sizes are used (15 to 40 minutes of arc at the subject's eye), the VEP is generated primarily by foveal and parafoveal elements. Monocular full-field stimulation almost always is used, so the test is most sensitive to lesions of the optic nerve anterior to the chiasm. It is possible, however, to modify the stimulus presentation so that only selected portions of the visual field are stimulated, thereby permitting detection of postchiasmatic abnormalities as well. VEPs elicited by pattern-reversal stimuli show less intersubject variability than flash VEPs and are much more sensitive to lesions affecting the visual pathways.

A few investigators have further refined the pattern-shift stimulus by using a black-and-white sinusoidal grating rather than a checkerboard pattern. This adaptation appears to enhance test sensitivity by permitting selective stimulation of retinal elements responsive to specific spatial frequencies and of cortical elements sensitive to both spatial frequency and orientation.

A normal pattern-reversal VEP to full-field monocular stimulation is illustrated in **Fig. 32A.20**. The VEP waveform is deceptively simple. It is the sum of many waveforms generated simultaneously by various areas of the retinotopically organized occipital cortex. By selectively stimulating portions of the visual field, it is possible to dissect the full-field VEP wave into its component waveforms. For example, **Fig. 32A.21**, recorded from the same patient as in **Fig. 32A.20**, illustrates VEPs to right and left hemifield stimulation. It is apparent that the full-field VEP is the sum of the two hemifield responses. In principle, it is possible to divide the visual fields into progressively smaller and smaller components and to record the VEP to each independently.

The primary basis for interpretation of the VEP is measurement of the latency of the P100 component (the major positive wave having a nominal latency of approximately 100 msec in normal persons) after stimulation of each eye separately. After the absolute P100 latency for each eye is measured, the intereye P100 latency difference is determined. Comparison of these values with normative laboratory data will indicate the normal or abnormal nature of the response. Whenever possible, the clinical significance of the findings is interpreted in the context of other relevant clinical data.

Because optic nerve fibers from the temporal retina decussate at the chiasm, unilateral prolongation of P100 latency

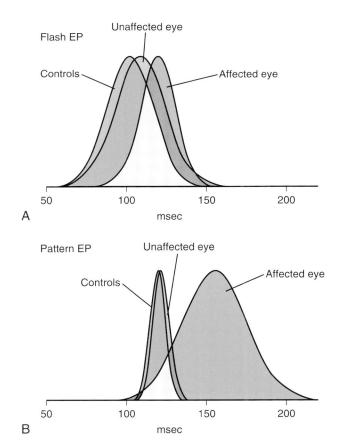

Fig. 32A.19 Distributions of latencies of the major occipital positivity to flash **(A)** and pattern-shift **(B)** stimulation in healthy control subjects and in the affected and unaffected eyes of patients with optic neuritis. The superior sensitivity of pattern-shift visual evoked potentials to demyelinating lesions is clearly demonstrated. *(Reprinted with permission from Halliday, A.M., 1982. The visual evoked potential in the investigation of diseases of the optic nerve, in: Halliday, A.M. (Ed.), Evoked Potentials in Clinical Testing. Churchill Livingstone, New York.)*

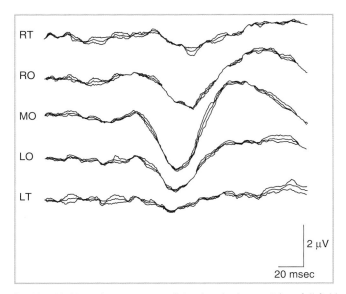

Fig. 32A.20 Normal pattern-reversal visual evoked potentials to full-field monocular stimulation. The MO electrode is in the posterior midline over the occiput. RO and RT are 5 and 10 cm, respectively, to the right of MO, and LO and LT are 5 and 10 cm, respectively, to the left of MO. All electrodes are referred to Fpz (a midline frontopolar electrode). The response is largest at MO and symmetrically distributed left and right of midline.

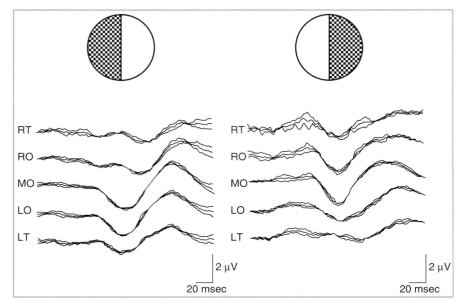

Fig. 32A.21 Normal pattern-shift visual evoked potentials to right and left hemifield stimulation of one eye. Same subject as in **Fig. 35A.20**. Partial-field responses are asymmetrical about the midline, with the largest positivities ipsilateral to the stimulated field.

after full-field monocular stimulation implies an abnormality anterior to the optic chiasm on that side. Bilateral lesions either anterior or posterior to the optic chiasm or a chiasmal lesion will cause bilateral delay of the P100, demonstrated by separate stimulation of each eye. Unilateral hemispherical lesions do not alter the latency of the full-field P100 (because of the contribution from the intact hemifield) but do alter the scalp topography of the response.

Visual Evoked Potentials in Neurological Disease

Acute optic neuritis is accompanied by marked attenuation or loss of P100 wave amplitude following pattern-reversal stimulation of the affected eye. After the acute attack, the VEP shows some recovery, but P100 latency usually remains prolonged, even with restoration of functionally normal vision. In patients with a history of optic neuritis, P100 latency typically is prolonged, but waveform amplitude and morphology often are relatively well preserved (**Fig. 32A.22**). Factors contributing to changes in P100 probably include the combined effects of patchy conduction block, areas of variably slowed conduction, temporal dispersion of the afferent volley in the optic nerve, loss of some components of the normal VEP, and the appearance of previously masked components.

Pattern-shift VEPs are abnormal in nearly all patients with a definite history of optic neuritis. More important, the pattern-shift VEP is a sufficiently sensitive indicator of optic nerve demyelination that it can reveal asymptomatic and clinically undetectable lesions. Thus, 70% to 80% of patients with definite multiple sclerosis (MS) but no history of optic neuritis or visual symptoms have abnormal VEPs. Many patients with abnormal VEPs have normal neuro-ophthalmological examination results.

Pattern-reversal VEPs are highly sensitive to demyelinating lesions but are not specific for MS. **Box 32A.1** provides a partial list of other causes of abnormal VEPs. VEPs may be helpful in distinguishing hysteria or malingering from blindness. A normal pattern-reversal VEP is strong evidence in

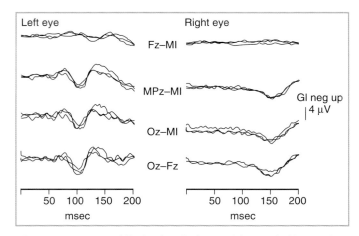

Fig. 32A.22 Pattern-shift visual evoked potentials recorded in a patient with right optic neuritis, illustrating marked delay of the P100 component from the right eye. As is typical with demyelinating optic neuropathies, the waveform is relatively preserved.

favor of psychogenic illness. Rare cases have been reported, however, in which essentially normal VEPs were present in cortical blindness because of bilateral destruction of Brodmann area 17, with preservation of areas 18 and 19, or bilateral occipital infarcts with preservation of area 17 (Epstein, 2000).

Brainstem Auditory Evoked Potentials

Brainstem auditory evoked potentials (BAEPs) are signals generated in the auditory nerve and brainstem after an acoustic stimulus. A brief stimulus, usually a sharp click, is given to one ear through an earphone while hearing in the opposite ear is masked with white noise to prevent its stimulation by transcranially conducted sound. The normal BAEP waveform consists of a series of waves that occur within the first 10 msec after the stimulus. The BAEP is extremely low-voltage (only ≈ 0.5 mV), and approximately 1000 to 2000 recordings typically have to be averaged to resolve the BAEP waveform.

Box 32A.1 Some Causes of Abnormal Visual Evoked Potentials

Ocular disease:
    Major refractive error
    Lens and media opacities
    Glaucoma
    Retinopathies
Compressive lesions:
    Extrinsic tumors
    Optic nerve tumors
Noncompressive lesions:
    Demyelinating disease
    Ischemic optic neuritis
    Nutritional and toxic amblyopias (including that due to pernicious anemia)
    Leber's hereditary optic atrophy
Diffuse CNS disease:
    Adrenoleukodystrophy
    Spinocerebellar degenerations
    PD

CNS, Central nervous system; *PD,* Parkinson disease.

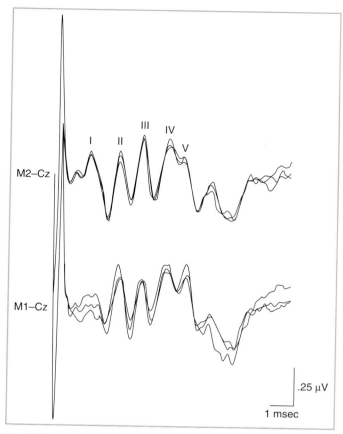

Fig. 32A.23 Normal brainstem auditory evoked potentials. Major waveform components are labeled with roman numerals and are discussed more fully in the text. M2 is an electrode over the mastoid process ipsilateral to the stimulated ear, in this case the right. Left and right mastoid electrodes are connected to an electrode at the vertex (Cz).

Normal Brainstem Auditory Evoked Potentials

Unlike VEPs, which are cortical responses, BAEPs are generated in or caudal to the mesencephalon. BAEPs are characteristically quite resistant to the effects of metabolic disturbances and pharmacological agents. Indeed, in the absence of anatomical lesions, BAEPs persist essentially unchanged into deep coma or in the presence of general anesthesia.

Fig. 32A.23 illustrates a normal BAEP recording. Summated neuronal activities in anatomical structures activated sequentially by the afferent sensory volley produce the components designated by roman numerals. Uncertainty exists regarding the relative contributions to the scalp-recorded BAEP of synaptic potentials occurring in nuclear structures and compound action potentials in fiber tracts. Although the following electroanatomical relationships may be somewhat oversimplified, they are useful for purposes of clinical localization. Wave I, corresponding to N1 of the electrocochleogram, represents the auditory nerve compound action potential, which arises in the distalmost portion of the nerve. The potential represented by wave II is generated mainly in the proximal eighth nerve but probably also includes a contribution from the intraaxial portion of the nerve and perhaps the cochlear nucleus as well. The wave III potential is generated in the lower pons in the region of the superior olive and trapezoid body. The generators of waves IV and V lie in the upper pons and the midbrain, as high as the inferior colliculus. Waves II and IV are inconsistently identified in some normal persons, so clinical interpretation of BAEPs is based primarily on latency measurements of waves I, III, and V. Despite decussation of brainstem auditory pathways at multiple levels, clinical experience indicates that unilateral BAEP abnormalities usually reflect lesions ipsilateral to the stimulated ear.

Brainstem Auditory Evoked Potentials in Neurological Disease

Auditory nerve pathology has several effects on the BAEP, related in part to the nature and size of the lesion. Findings range from prolongation of the I-III interpeak interval, to preservation of wave I with distortion or loss of later components, to loss of all BAEP components. Any of these abnormalities occur with acoustic neurinomas and other cerebellopontine angle tumors (**Fig. 32A.24**). In fact, the BAEP is perhaps the most sensitive screening test for acoustic neurinoma, detecting abnormalities in greater than 90% of the patients. The sensitivity of the test can be extended further by using a range of stimulus intensities and evaluating the effect on components of the BAEP (the latency intensity) (**Fig. 32A.25**).

In patients with focal brainstem lesions that impinge on the auditory pathways, the BAEP is abnormal and the type of abnormality reflects the lesion's location and extent. For example, **Fig. 32A.26** illustrates a BAEP recorded in a patient with a brainstem hemorrhage that involved the rostral two-thirds of the pons but spared the caudal third. Waves IV and V are absent, but waves I, II, and III are relatively normal.

BAEPs are normal when brainstem lesions do not involve auditory pathways, as is often the case in the locked-in syndrome produced by ventral pontine infarction, or with Wallenberg lateral medullary syndrome. By contrast, pontine gliomas nearly always produce abnormal BAEPs.

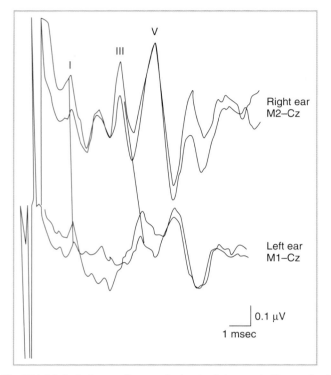

Fig. 32A.24 Brainstem auditory evoked potentials recorded in a patient with a left acoustic neurinoma. The I-III interval on that side is prolonged, and the overall response is not as well formed as that from the normal ear.

Nearly 50% of patients with definite MS have abnormal BAEP results. Of greater clinical importance, approximately 20% of patients with possible or probable MS have abnormal BAEPs even in the absence of clinical signs or symptoms referable to the brainstem. In such cases, abnormalities usually consist of absence or decreased amplitude of BAEP component waves, most often of waves IV and V, or increased III-V interpeak latency. Occasionally, prolongation of the I-III interpeak interval occurs, probably reflecting involvement of the central myelin that covers the proximal and immediately intraaxial portion of the auditory nerve.

BAEPs may document brainstem involvement in patients with nonfocal neurological disease, especially those affecting myelin, such as metachromatic leukodystrophy and adrenoleukodystrophy. In such diseases, BAEP testing also may show electrophysiological abnormalities in clinically asymptomatic heterozygotes.

BAEPs are useful to assess hearing in young children and in patients otherwise unable to cooperate with standard audiological testing. A latency intensity study, discussed previously, permits characterization of the response threshold for wave V as well as the relationship between wave V latency and stimulus intensity. Such testing allows estimation of hearing threshold and may distinguish between conductive and sensorineural types of hearing impairment. Brainstem audiometry, however, is not really a hearing test per se but rather a measure of the brainstem's sensitivity to auditory input. The BAEP is normal in the rare patient with deafness due to bilateral cortical lesions. On the other hand, patients with MS or a pontine glioma often have abnormal BAEP results but normal hearing (although their ability to localize sound accurately in space may diminish). One limitation to use of BAEPs to test hearing is that the brainstem must be intact, so that BAEP alterations reflect dysfunction in the peripheral hearing apparatus (Lueders and Terada, 2000).

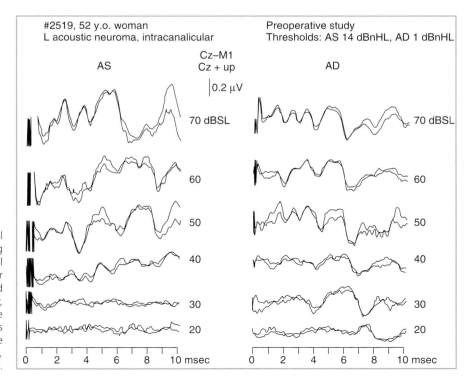

Fig. 32A.25 Brainstem auditory evoked potential wave V latency plots as a function of increasing stimulus intensity from 20 to 70 dBSL (decibel sound level) in a woman with a left intracanalicular acoustic neurinoma. Brainstem auditory evoked potentials at 70 dBSL are normal bilaterally, but responses at lower intensities are quite asymmetrical, and the response threshold is elevated on the left. Hearing thresholds are expressed in dBnHL, or dB hearing threshold. *AD,* Auris dextra (right ear); *AS,* auris sinistra (left ear).

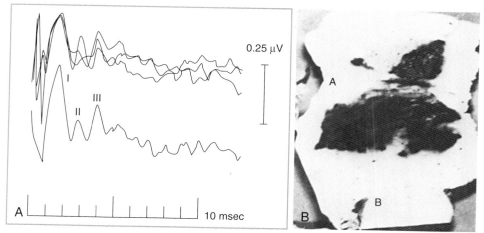

Fig. 32A.26 A, Brainstem auditory evoked potentials recorded in a patient with a brainstem hemorrhage sparing the lower third of the pons. Waves I, II, and III are preserved, but later components are lost. **B,** Coronal section through the pons; A is at the pontomesencephalic border, and B is at the pontomedullary border. *(Reprinted with permission from Chiappa, K.H., 1985. Evoked potentials in clinical medicine, in: Baker, A.B., Baker, L.H. (Eds.), Clinical Neurology. Harper & Row, New York.)*

Somatosensory Evoked Potentials

On electrical stimulation of a peripheral nerve, recordings from electrodes placed over the spine and scalp reveal a series of waves that reflect sequential activation of neural structures along the afferent somatosensory pathways. The dorsal column–lemniscal system is the major substrate of the somatosensory evoked potential (SEP), although other nonlemniscal systems such as the dorsal spinocerebellar tract have been shown to contribute to SEP generation. In clinical practice, SEPs usually are elicited by stimulation of the median nerve at the wrist, the common peroneal nerve at the knee, or the posterior tibial nerve at the ankle.

Normal Median Nerve Somatosensory Evoked Potentials

Fig. 32A.27 shows a normal SEP elicited by median nerve stimulation. The accompanying diagram indicates presumed generator sources for the various components of the SEP. An electrode at the Erb point ipsilateral to the stimulated arm registers the afferent volley as it passes through the brachial plexus. The Erb point potential serves as a reference point against which the latencies of subsequent components are measured. Electrodes over the midcervical dorsal spine record two potentials with independent but partially overlapping waveforms that reflect local activity in the spinal cord. The first of these, designated DCV (for dorsal column volley), is the afferent volley in the cuneate tract. The second, N13, reflects postsynaptic activity in the central gray matter of the cervical cord, generated by input from axon collaterals off the primary large-fiber afferents. A simultaneous potential of opposite polarity (P13) over the anterior neck accompanies the N13. Lesions that disrupt the central gray matter, such as syringomyelia, may selectively affect the N13/P13.

An electrode placed on the scalp away from the primary sensory area best records the SEP components generated in the brainstem. This electrode "sees" subcortical activity that is volume-conducted to the scalp surface. Generation of the P14 is in the cervicomedullary region, probably by the caudal medial lemniscus. Following the P14 is the N18, seen as a

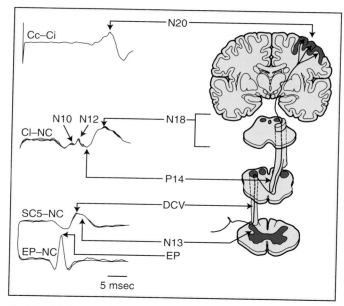

Fig. 32A.27 Presumed generator sources of median nerve somatosensory evoked potentials. Cc and Ci are central-parietal scalp locations contralateral (Cc) and ipsilateral (Ci) to the stimulated nerve. They are 2 cm posterior to the C3 and C4 placements of the International Ten-Twenty System. EP and SC5 are electrodes located over the Erb point and the spinous process of the fifth cervical vertebra, respectively. NC is a noncephalic (such as elbow) reference.

long-duration negative wave whose origin is uncertain but probably includes postsynaptic activity from multiple generators in the brainstem. **Fig. 32A.28** illustrates preservation of the P14 but loss of the N18 and all later waves in a patient with an arteriovenous malformation of the right pons. This pattern probably is the electrophysiological equivalent of functional transection of the medial lemniscus at a pontine level.

The initial cortical response to the afferent sensory volley is designated N20 and is best recorded by a scalp electrode placed directly over the primary sensory cortex contralateral to the stimulated side. The N20 waveform is a composite made

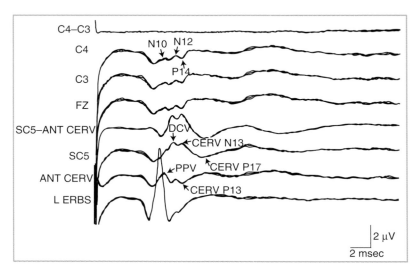

Fig. 32A.28 Left median nerve somatosensory evoked potentials recorded in a patient with a right pontine arteriovenous malformation. All components after P14 (cervicomedullary potential) are absent. Unless otherwise labeled, a right elbow reference was used.

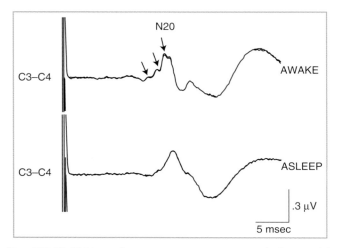

Fig. 32A.29 Right median nerve somatosensory evoked potentials recorded in a normal subject awake and then asleep after sedation with diazepam. Note the state-dependent change in morphology of the N20. Multiple small inflections present on the rising limb of N20 during wakefulness disappear during sleep.

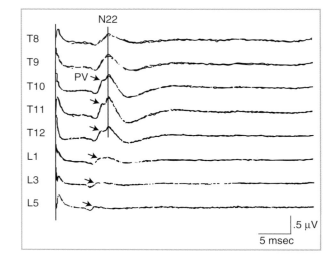

Fig. 32A.30 Recordings over the lumbar and lower thoracic spinal segments obtained after posterior tibial nerve stimulation. Recording electrodes are referenced to the iliac crest. Note increasing latency of the propagated volley (PV) and the appearance at T12 of a second stationary potential (N22). See text for further details.

up of signals from multiple generators within or close to the primary cortical receiving area. This can be demonstrated by selective stimulation of cutaneous and muscle-spindle afferent fibers in the median nerve, which are known to project to adjacent but distinct cortical regions, or by observation of state-dependent changes in the N20 (**Fig. 32A.29**). Sleep, for example, attenuates small inflections that are often present on the waking N20 wave, a phenomenon probably caused by downward modulation of some generators contributing to N20 and to alterations in thalamic input to cortex during sleep.

Normal Posterior Tibial Nerve Somatosensory Evoked Potentials

Somatosensory evoked potentials to posterior tibial nerve stimulation are in many ways analogous to median nerve SEPs. When the posterior tibial nerve is stimulated, recordings from electrodes over the lumbar spine show two distinct

potentials (**Fig. 32A.30**). One of these, PV, is produced by the afferent volley in the lumbar nerve roots and gracile tract, and the other, N22, is a summated synaptic potential generated in the gray matter of the lumbar cord. Because of its stability, fixed latency, and relatively high voltage, the clinical use of the N22 lumbar potential is as a reference point against which latencies of subsequent components are measured. Additionally, determination of the spinal level where N22 voltage is maximal provides an approximate indication of the position of the lumbar cord enlargement. This capability sometimes is clinically useful with suspected spinal cord tethering (**Fig. 32A.31**).

Subcortical activity from posterior tibial nerve stimulation consists of P31, seen on the EEG as a positive wave, followed by N34, seen as a long-duration negative wave (**Fig. 32A.32**). These components are analogous to the P14 and N18 occurring after median nerve stimulation and probably are generated by the afferent volley in the caudal medial

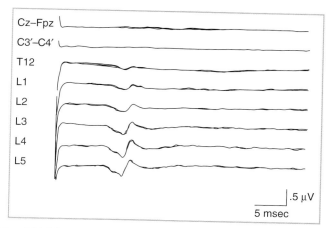

Fig. 32A.31 Posterior tibial nerve somatosensory evoked potentials recorded in a patient with a tethered spinal cord. The maximal amplitude of the lumbar potential, normally between T10 and T12, is caudally displaced. The cortical response also is absent. Unless labeled otherwise, an iliac crest reference was used.

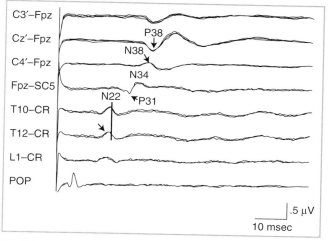

Fig. 32A.32 Normal posterior tibial somatosensory evoked potentials. The lower channel is a bipolar recording between two electrodes over the popliteal fossa.

lemniscus and by postsynaptic activity in the rostral brainstem, respectively.

The initial cortical response to posterior tibial nerve stimulation is a prominent positivity (P38) that is recorded from scalp electrodes placed at the vertex and central parasagittal regions, close to the cortical areas representing the leg (see **Fig. 32A.32**). This positive potential usually is maximal just lateral to the vertex, ipsilateral to the stimulated nerve. This apparently paradoxical localization of the P38 reflects the mesial location of the primary sensory area for the leg and foot within the interhemispherical fissure.

Somatosensory Evoked Potentials in Neurological Disease

Several different conditions that disturb conduction within the somatosensory system produce SEP abnormalities. These include focal lesions (tumors, strokes, cervical spondylosis) and diseases that affect the nervous system more diffusely (hereditary ataxias, subacute combined degeneration, vitamin E deficiency). Up to 90% of patients with definite MS have either upper- or lower-limb SEP abnormalities. Furthermore, an abnormal SEP occurs in 50% to 60% of patients with MS even in the absence of symptoms or signs referable to the large-fiber sensory system. Other diseases that affect myelin (e.g., Pelizaeus-Merzbacher disease, metachromatic leukodystrophy, adrenoleukodystrophy, adrenomyeloneuropathy) also produce SEP abnormalities. With adrenoleukodystrophy and adrenomyeloneuropathy, SEP abnormalities are demonstrable in heterozygotes.

Many lesions alter the SEP by producing a conduction delay or block. This results in prolonged interpeak latencies or in attenuation or even loss of one or more SEP components. Abnormally large SEPs involving exaggeration of cortical components occurring after N20 (from the median nerve) are characteristic of patients with progressive myoclonus epilepsy, some patients with photosensitive epilepsy, and children with late infantile ceroid lipofuscinosis (**Fig. 32A.33**) (Emerson and Pedley, 2003).

An important application of SEP is as an aid to prognosis in patients resuscitated following cardiopulmonary arrest. In that setting, bilateral absence of the N20 is accurately

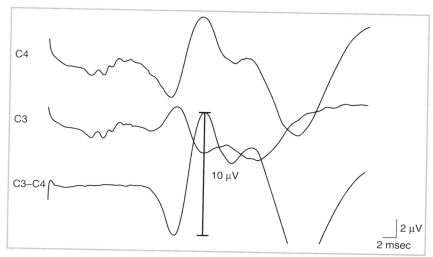

Fig. 32A.33 Recording from central-parietal scalp electrodes obtained after median nerve stimulation in a patient with cortical myoclonus. Marked exaggeration of later cortical components is evident. A noncephalic reference was used in the upper two tracings.

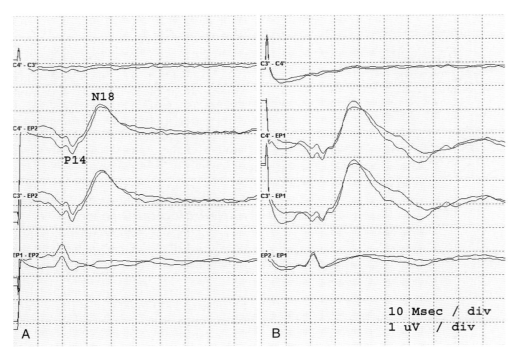

Fig. 32A.34 Left **(A)** and right **(B)** median nerve sensory evoked potentials (SEPs) recorded in a 45-year-old man with a history of a cardiomyopathy, 2 days following cardiopulmonary arrest and resuscitation. Erb point and subcortical (P14, N18) waves are present, but N20 is absent bilaterally *(top channel)*.

predictive of a poor neurological outcome (Wijdicks et al., 2006) (**Fig. 32A.34**).

Motor Evoked Potentials and Magnetic Coil Stimulation

It is possible to assess the functional integrity of the descending motor pathways using motor evoked potentials (MEPs). MEP studies generally entail stimulating the motor cortex and recording the evoked compound motor action potential over appropriate target muscles. The motor cortex may be stimulated either by directly passing a brief high-voltage electrical pulse through the scalp or by using a time-varying magnetic field to induce an electric current within the brain.

Whereas transcranial electrical stimulation is painful, magnetic coil stimulation is essentially painless. Therefore, use of transcranial electrical stimulation typically is restricted to intraoperative motor system monitoring in anesthetized patients, whereas magnetic stimulation generally is useful in studies of awake subjects and patients.

Direct electrical stimulation of the motor cortex produces a series of signals that are recordable from the pyramidal tract. The earliest wave, the D (direct) wave, results from direct activation of the pyramidal axons. Subsequent signals, the I (indirect) waves, probably reflect indirect transsynaptic activation of pyramidal cells. Transcranial electrical stimulation is capable of eliciting both D and I waves, but transcranial magnetic stimulation (TMS) generally elicits only I waves. For this reason, MEPs evoked by TMS occur at slightly greater latency and are less stable than those evoked by transcranial electrical stimulation.

It is possible to measure the central motor conduction time by subtracting the latency of the MEP elicited by cervical or lumbar stimulation from that obtained by TMS. For MEPs

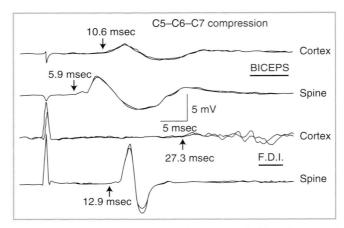

Fig. 32A.35 Motor evoked potentials (MEPs) recorded from biceps and first dorsal interosseous (FDI) muscles in a patient with cervical spondylosis producing C5-C7 spinal cord compression. MEPs recorded from biceps are normal after magnetic stimulation over both motor cortex and cervical spine. MEPs recorded from FDI are normal after stimulation over the cervical spine but are abnormally low voltage and polyphasic after cortical stimulation. *(Reprinted with permission from Maertens de Noordhout, A., Remade, J.M., Pepin, J.L., et al., 1991. Magnetic stimulation of the motor cortex in cervical spondylosis. Neurology. 41, 75-80.)*

elicited by TMS, this interval actually encompasses the time required for activation of cortical interneurons, transsynaptic activation of pyramidal neurons, and conduction of the efferent volley through the pyramidal tract and depolarization of the spinal motor neuron.

MEPs can provide information about motor pathways that complements data about sensory pathways obtained from SEPs. MEPs frequently are abnormal in patients with myelopathies caused by cervical spondylosis (**Fig. 32A.35**), in whom

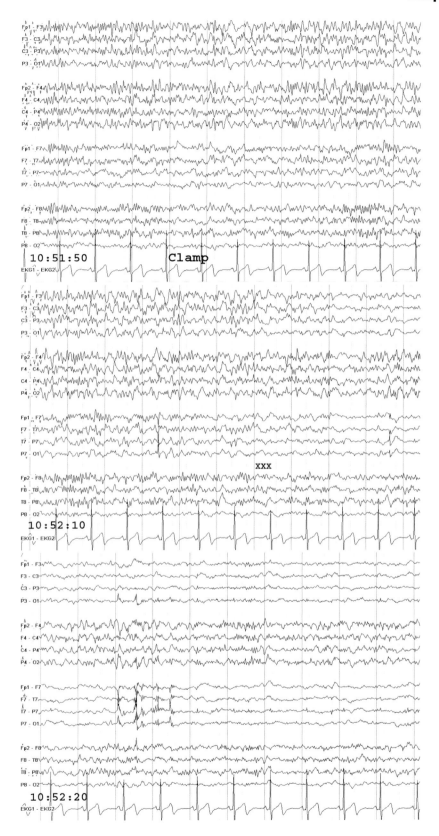

Fig. 32A.36 Intraoperative EEG monitoring in a 62-year-old patient with bilateral carotid stenosis during left carotid endarterectomy. Beginning approximately 22 seconds following clamping of the left internal carotid artery, there is prominent attenuation of EEG activity over the left hemisphere. Therefore, a temporary common carotid–to–internal carotid shunt was placed to maintain left hemisphere perfusion during removal of plaque and completion of the operation.

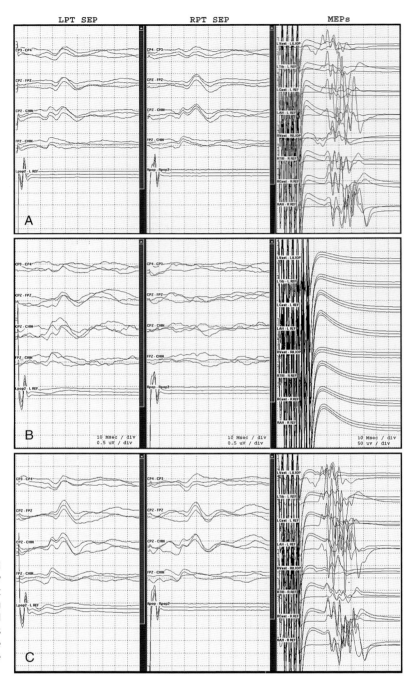

Fig. 32A.37 Intraoperative monitoring using posterior tibial SSEPs and transcranial electrical MEPs during spinal-deformity surgery in a 13-year-old girl with adolescent idiopathic scoliosis. Baseline recordings **(A)** were normal, but following instrumentation there is loss of the right SSEP and bilateral MEPs **(B)**. Upon removal of rods, responses return **(C)**. Rods were subsequently reinserted but adjusted to achieve a more modest correction; responses remained stable, and the patient was neurologically normal upon awakening.

they appear to be sensitive to early preclinical spinal cord compression. Often, delay occurs in patients with MS, and MEPs may be more sensitive to demyelinating lesions than VEPs or SEPs. In motor neuron disease, pyramidal tract conduction delays are demonstrable in patients without upper motor neuron signs.

MEPs also offer insights into the pathophysiology and evolution of disorders affecting the motor system. Patients with cerebral palsy may demonstrate enhanced MEPs in some muscle groups because of aberrant corticospinal projections. In Parkinson disease, MEP latencies are normal but may show increased amplitude, possibly because of spinal disinhibition or corticomotoneuronal hyperexcitability. MEPs have been used to study brain plasticity and to document cortical reorganization after spinal cord injury and amputation.

Transcranial magnetic coil stimulation provides a means of studying normal cortical physiology by transiently interrupting the regional function. Disruption of cortical processing produced by single or repetitive magnetic stimuli has been useful to study not only the function of the motor system but also cortical somatosensory, visual, and language processing function. Finally, proposed therapeutic uses for TMS include stroke, epilepsy, parkinsonism, dystonia, and depression (Rossini et al., 2010).

Intraoperative Monitoring

Electrophysiological monitoring is routinely used to assess the functional integrity of the brain and spinal cord during certain neurosurgical and orthopedic procedures. Such monitoring reduces neurological morbidity by detecting adverse effects at a time when prompt correction of the cause can avoid permanent neurological injury. In addition, monitoring may provide information about the mechanisms of postoperative neurological abnormalities and occasionally lead to changes in surgical approach or technique.

Monitoring can be done using EEG, sensory evoked potentials (usually BAEPs or SEPs), and MEPs. Which monitoring modality or combination of modalities is used depends on the type of surgery and the neural structures judged to be most at risk. Because neurological injury can occur suddenly and may be irreversible, the ideal monitoring method is one that detects impending, not permanent, damage. A certain percentage of false-positive results is therefore highly desirable. Experienced monitoring teams learn that small changes in recorded signals are common during surgery as a result of clinical and technical factors that have negligible effects on outcome. Other variables that affect electrical signals are the type of anesthesia, temperature, blood pressure, and neuromuscular blockade. Determining what constitutes a significant and reproducible change that warrants alerting the surgeon or anesthesiologist is a critical aspect of monitoring.

Patients occasionally experience a new postoperative neurological abnormality despite uneventful monitoring. A major neurological complication occurs only rarely, if at all, in a part of the nervous system monitored directly and accurately judged normal throughout the operation. More often, complications arise from involvement of structures not monitored directly (e.g., infarction of the ventral spinal cord when only dorsal column function was monitored using SEPs) or when a significant preexisting abnormality masks even moderate changes from baseline. Minor and usually transient neurological symptoms and signs (e.g., sensory dysesthesias, mild weakness, temporary neurogenic bladder) occur occasionally with stable intraoperative electrophysiological measures.

EEG monitoring is commonly used during carotid endarterectomy, embolization of cerebral arteriovenous malformations, and clipping or removal of some aneurysms. Monitoring is especially helpful in selecting patients for shunting during occlusion of the carotid artery (**Fig. 32A.36**). With monitoring, the rate of overall intraoperative major morbidity for endarterectomy should be reducible to 1%.

Monitoring auditory nerve function using BAEPs, with or without electrocochleography, is useful in any neurosurgical or neuro-otological procedure that risks injury to the eighth cranial nerve. Risk of hearing loss is minimized in patients with small, especially intracanalicular, acoustic neurinomas and other cerebellopontine angle tumors, as well as in patients undergoing microvascular decompression for hemifacial spasm or trigeminal neuralgia. Monitoring facial nerve function by recording compound nerve or muscle action potentials on direct stimulation of the intracranial portion of the seventh nerve has greatly reduced the incidence of permanent facial palsy after cerebellopontine angle surgery.

SEPs are in routine use to monitor baseline and spinal cord function during neurosurgical and orthopedic procedures. They provide useful and sensitive feedback information about the integrity of the dorsal column somatosensory system. MEPs are particularly sensitive to the effects of spinal cord ischemia, compression, distraction, and blunt trauma and are useful to monitor spinal cord function during surgical procedures (**Fig. 32A.37**). They complement SEPs in that SEPs may not detect surgical injuries limited to the lateral and anterior spinal cord (Mendiratta and Emerson, 2009).

References

The complete reference list is available online at www.expertconsult.com.

Clinical Neurophysiology
Clinical Electromyography

Bashar Katirji

Clinical electromyography is a distinct medical discipline that plays a pivotal role in the diagnosis of neuromuscular disorders (Katirji et al., 2002). The designations *clinical electromyography*, *electrodiagnostic examination*, and *electroneuromyography* are used interchangeably to encompass the electrophysiological study of nerve and muscle; the terms *needle electromyography* or *needle electrode examination* are reserved for the specific testing that involves needle electrode evaluation of muscle. Although many still refer to all such testing as simply *electromyography* (EMG), use of the word without a descriptor is discouraged because it can be confusing, often implying only the needle electrode part of the evaluation. For clarity, this chapter will refer to *clinical EMG* or *needle EMG* in the context of the discussion.

The clinical EMG examination is an important diagnostic tool that helps localize a neuromuscular problem at the motor neurons, nerve roots, peripheral nerves, neuromuscular junction, or muscle. It also helps establish the underlying process in these disorders and assess their management and prognosis. Electrodiagnostic testing provides the most valuable diagnostic information when the clinical assessment suggests a short list of differential diagnoses. The clinician should perform a detailed or focused neurological examination before referring the patient for a clinical EMG, which in turn serves as an independent procedure to provide an objective assessment of the peripheral nervous system (PNS) (Katirji, 2002). Patients with complex clinical pictures are best served by a neurological consultation prior to ordering electrodiagnostic testing.

The clinical EMG examination is composed of two main tests: nerve conduction studies (NCS) and needle EMG. These tests complement each other, and both often are necessary for a definite diagnosis. Additional electrodiagnostic procedures include assessment of F waves, H reflexes, and blink reflexes; repetitive nerve stimulation; and single-fiber EMG. A focused history and examination will help the electromyographer design the most appropriate electrodiagnostic study (Preston and Shapiro, 2005). The electromyographer must be proficient in using modern electrodiagnostic equipment and applying electrodiagnostic techniques, know the normal values for commonly and uncommonly examined nerve conduction studies and for motor unit action potentials (MUAPs) in different muscles, and be familiar with the specific and nonspecific electrodiagnostic findings in different neuromuscular disorders.

Nerve Conduction Studies
Principles

Electrical stimulation of nerve fibers initiates impulses that travel along motor, sensory, or mixed nerves and evoke a compound action potential. The three types of NCS are motor, sensory, and mixed. Analysis of the compound muscle action potential (CMAP), evoked by stimulating a nerve while recording from a muscle, indirectly assesses the conduction characteristics of motor fibers. Analysis of the sensory nerve action potential (SNAP) assesses the sensory fibers by stimulating a nerve and recording directly from a cutaneous nerve. Mixed NCS directly assess the sensory and motor fibers simultaneously by stimulating and recording from a mixed nerve and analyzing the mixed nerve action potential (MNAP). Use of standard NCS allows precise lesion localization and accurate characterization of peripheral nerve function.

Stimulators

Nerve conduction studies use two different kinds of surface (percutaneous) electric stimulators. *Constant voltage stimulators* regulate voltage output so that current varies inversely with the impedance of the system including the skin and subcutaneous tissues. *Constant current stimulators* change voltage according to impedance so that the amount of current that reaches the nerve is within the limits of skin resistance. As the current flows between the cathode (negative pole) and the anode (positive pole), negative charges accumulate under the cathode and positive charges under the anode, depolarizing and hyperpolarizing the nerve, respectively. In bipolar stimulation, both electrodes are over the nerve trunk, with the cathode closer to the recording site. Anodal conduction block of the propagated impulse may occur with inadvertent reversal of the cathode and anode of the stimulator. The cause of the block is hyperpolarization at the anode. This may prevent the nerve impulse evoked by the depolarization occurring under the cathode from proceeding past the anode.

Supramaximal stimulation of a nerve that results in depolarization of all available axons is a paramount prerequisite to accurate and reproducible NCS measurements. To achieve supramaximal stimulation, slowly increase current (or voltage) intensity until it reaches a level at which the recorded potential does not increase in size. Then increase the current an additional 20% to 30% to ensure the potential does not change further.

Recording Electrodes

Surface electrodes record the CMAP, SNAP, or MNAP. The advantages of surface recording are reproducible evoked responses that change only slightly with the position of the electrodes in relation to the recording muscle or nerve. In contrast, needle electrode recording registers only a small portion of the muscle or nerve action potentials; as a result, the evoked responses are variable and not reproducible, although they have less interference from neighboring discharges. Needle recordings improve the recording from small atrophic muscles or a proximal muscle not excitable in isolation. Most recording electrodes used in clinical practice are disk electrodes; ring electrodes are convenient for recording the antidromic sensory potentials from digital nerves over the proximal and distal interphalangeal joints.

Recording Procedure

A pre-pulse preceding the stimulus triggers the sweep on a storage oscilloscope. The amplifier sensitivity determines the size (amplitude) of the potential. Overamplification truncates the response, and underamplification prevents accurate measurements of the exact takeoff point from baseline. Digital averaging is very useful in recording low-amplitude SNAPs. Signals time-locked to the stimulus summate with averaging at a constant latency and appear as an evoked potential, distinct from the background noise. The signal-to-noise ratio increases in proportion to the square root of the trial number. For example, four trials give twice as big a response as a single stimulus, and nine trials give three times the amplitude. Modern instruments digitally indicate the latency and amplitude when the desired spot on the waveform is marked.

Motor Nerve Conduction Studies

The performance of motor NCS requires stimulating a motor or mixed peripheral nerve while recording the CMAP from a muscle innervated by that nerve. A pair of recording electrodes consists of an active lead, G1, placed on the belly of the muscle and a reference (indifferent or inactive) lead, G2, on the tendon (belly-tendon recording). The propagating muscle action potential, originating under G1 located near the motor point, gives rise to a simple biphasic waveform with an initial negativity. Initial positivity suggests incorrect positioning of the active electrode away from the motor end-plate zone or a volume-conducted potential from distant muscles activated by anomalous innervation or by accidental spread of stimulation to other neighboring nerves.

The nerve usually is stimulated, whenever technically feasible, at two or more points along its course. Shorter nerves such as the axillary, femoral, and facial nerves are stimulated at only one point, because the more proximal portions of the nerves are inaccessible. Otherwise, the nerve typically is stimulated distally near the recording electrode and more proximally to evaluate one or more proximal segments. Motor NCS evaluate several measurements (**Fig. 32B.1**):

CMAP amplitude: The usual measure of amplitude is from baseline to negative peak and expressed in millivolts. When recorded with surface electrodes, CMAP amplitude is a semiquantitative measure of the number of axons conducting between the stimulating and recording points. CMAP amplitude also depends on the relative conduction speed of the axons, the integrity of the neuromuscular junctions, and the number of muscle fibers that are able to generate action potentials.

CMAP duration: This measurement usually is the duration of the negative phase of the evoked potential and expressed in milliseconds. It is a function of the conduction rates of the various axons forming the examined nerve and the distance between the stimulation and recording electrodes. The CMAP generated from proximal stimulation is slightly longer in duration and of lower amplitude than that obtained from distal stimulation, as a result of temporal dispersion and phase cancellation (see forthcoming section).

CMAP area: This usually is limited to the negative phase area under the waveform and shows linear correlation with the product of amplitude and duration. Measurement is in millivolts per millisecond and requires electronic integration using computerized equipment. The ability to measure CMAP area has practically replaced the need to measure its duration.

Latencies: Latency is the time interval between nerve stimulation (shock artifact) and the CMAP onset. Expression of latency is in milliseconds and reflects the conduction rate of the fastest-conducting axon. Whenever technically possible, the nerve is stimulated at two points: a distal point near the recording site and a more proximal point; the measures obtained are the *distal latency* and *proximal*

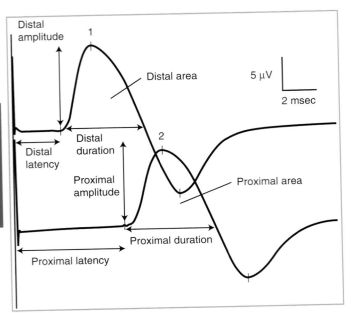

Fig. 32B.1 Motor nerve conduction study of the median nerve, revealing a typical compound muscle action potential (CMAP) with distal (wrist) and proximal (elbow) stimulations, showing the distal and proximal latencies and CMAP amplitudes, durations, and areas. The proximal CMAP has a lower amplitude (12.6 mV versus 11.3 mV) and area (37.3 mV/ms versus 34.50 mV/ms) than the distal CMAP because of temporal dispersion and phase cancellation. The proximal conduction velocity is calculated by measuring the distance of the elbow-to-wrist segment and using the following formula:

$$\text{Motor conduction velocity} = \frac{\text{Distance}}{\text{Proximal latency} - \text{Distal latency}}$$

So for the conduction velocity in this example, 210 mm/6.9 msec − 3.5 msec = 62 m/second.

latency, respectively. Both latencies depend mostly on the length of the nerve segment and, to a much lesser extent, on neuromuscular transmission time and propagation time along the muscle membrane.

Conduction velocity: This is a computed measurement of the speed of conduction expressed in meters per second. Measurement of conduction velocity allows comparison of the speed of conduction of the fastest fibers between different nerves and subjects, irrespective of the length of the nerve. The calculation requires measurement of the length of the nerve segment between distal and proximal stimulation sites. Measuring the surface distance along the course of the nerve estimates the nerve length; it should be more than 10 cm to improve the accuracy of surface measurement.

$$\text{Motor conduction velocity} = \frac{\text{Distance}}{\text{Proximal latency} - \text{Distal latency}}$$

As with latencies, motor conduction velocity measures the speed of conduction of the fastest axon. In contrast

with motor latency, however, motor nerve conduction velocity is a pure nerve conduction time, because neuromuscular transmission time and muscle fiber propagation time are common to both stimulation sites, and the latency difference between two points is the time required for the nerve impulse to travel from one stimulus point to the other.

Sensory Nerve Conduction Studies

Sensory axons are evaluated by stimulating a nerve while recording the transmitted potential from the same nerve at a different site. Therefore, SNAPs are true nerve action potentials. The measurement of antidromic sensory NCS requires recording potentials directed toward the sensory receptors. Obtaining orthodromic responses requires recording potentials directed away from these receptors. Sensory latencies and conduction velocities are identical with either method, but SNAP amplitudes generally are higher in antidromic studies. Orthodromic responses sometimes are low in amplitude, necessitating use of averaging techniques. Action potentials from distal muscles may obscure antidromic responses, because the thresholds of some motor axons are similar to those of large myelinated sensory axons. Fortunately, accurate measurement of SNAPs is still possible because the large-diameter sensory fibers conduct 5% to 10% faster than motor fibers. This relationship may change in disease states that selectively affect different fibers.

SNAPs may be obtained by several methods: (1) stimulating and recording a pure sensory nerve (such as the sural and radial sensory nerves); (2) stimulating a mixed nerve while recording distally over a cutaneous branch (such as the antidromic median and ulnar sensory responses), or (3) stimulating a distal cutaneous branch while recording over a proximal mixed nerve (such as in orthodromic median and ulnar sensory studies). Similar to their motor counterparts, sensory NCS record several measurements (**Fig. 32B.2**):

SNAP amplitude: This semiquantitatively measures the number of sensory axons that conduct between the stimulation and recording sites. The calculation is from the baseline to negative peak or from negative peak to positive peak, and expressed in microvolts. SNAP duration and area may be measured but are not useful because of significant temporal dispersion and phase cancellation (see later discussion).

Latencies: Sensory distal latencies are measured (in milliseconds) from the stimulus artifact to the peak of the negative phase (peak latency) or from the stimulus artifact to the onset of the SNAP (onset latency). A large shock artifact, a noisy background, or a wavy baseline may obscure onset latency. Although peak latency does not reflect the fastest-conducting sensory fibers, it is easily defined and more precise than onset latency.

Conduction velocity: This requires stimulation at a single site only because the latency consists of just the nerve conduction time from the stimulus point to the recording electrode. As with motor velocity, the calculation may be done using both distal and proximal stimulations. Only onset latencies (not peak latencies) are useful to calculate velocities to assess the speed of the fastest-conducting fibers.

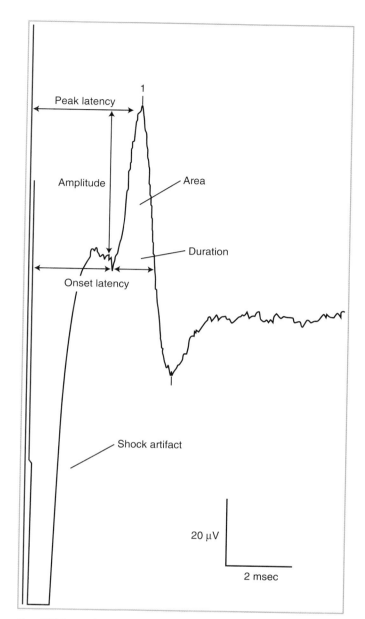

Fig. 32B.2 Antidromic median sensory nerve conduction study after stimulation at the wrist, revealing peak and onset latencies and sensory nerve action potential amplitude, duration, and area. The shock artifact interferes with accurate determination of onset latency, whereas peak latency is easily determined.

$$\text{Sensory conduction velocity}$$
$$= \frac{\text{Distance}}{\text{Onset latency}}$$
$$\text{or} = \frac{\text{Distance}}{\text{Proximal latency} - \text{Distal latency}}$$

Mixed Nerve Conduction Studies

Stimulating and recording from nerve trunks containing sensory and motor axons constitute mixed NCS. Often these tests require stimulating a nerve trunk distally and recording more proximally because large CMAPs contaminate the reverse by obscuring the lower-amplitude MNAPs. The MNAP may be of low amplitude or not elicitable when the nerve is deeply situated (as at the elbow or knee) because of tissue interposed between the nerve and the recording electrode. Therefore, MNAPs are limited to assessing mixed nerves in distal nerve segments in the hand or foot, such as the mixed palmar and mixed plantar studies used to evaluate carpal tunnel syndrome and tarsal tunnel syndrome, respectively.

Segmental Stimulation in Short Increments

Routine NCS are sufficient to localize the site of involvement in most patients with entrapment neuropathies. During evaluation of a focal demyelinating lesion, however, inclusion of the unaffected nerve segment in relatively long distal latency or conduction velocity calculation dilutes the effect of slowing at the injured site and decreases the sensitivity of the test. Therefore, incremental stimulation across a shorter nerve segment is useful to help localize an abnormality that might otherwise escape detection. Localization that is more precise entails "inching" the stimulus in short increments along the course of the nerve. The study of short segments provides better resolution of restricted lesions. For example, a nerve impulse may be found to conduct at a rate of 0.2 msec per 1.0 cm (50 m/sec). For a 1-cm segment, then, demyelination would double the conduction time to 0.4 msec/cm. In a 10-cm segment, normally covered in 2.0 msec, a 0.2-msec increase would constitute a 10% change, or approximately 1 standard deviation—well within the normal range of variability. However, the same 0.2-msec increase would represent a 100% change in latency if measured over a 1-cm segment. The large per-step increase in latency more than compensates for the inherent measurement error associated with stimulating multiple times in short increments.

The inching (or actually "centimetering") technique is particularly useful in assessing nerve conduction in patients with carpal tunnel syndrome or an ulnar neuropathy at the elbow or wrist (McIntosh et al., 1998). For example, stimulation of a normal median nerve in 1-cm increments across the wrist results in latency changes of approximately 0.16 to 0.21 msec/cm from midpalm to distal forearm (**Fig. 32B.3**). A sharply localized latency increase across a 1-cm segment indicates a focal abnormality of the median nerve (**Fig. 32B.4**). An abrupt change in waveform usually accompanies the latency increase across the site of compression.

Physiological Variability and Common Sources of Error

The major pitfalls in NCS usually involve technical errors in the stimulating or recording system (Kimura, 1997). Common errors include large stimulus artifact, increased electrode noise, submaximal stimulation, co-stimulation of adjacent nerve not under study, eliciting an unwanted potential from distant muscles, recording or reference electrode misplacement, and errors in measurement of nerve length and conduction time. Other errors are attributable to intertrial and physiological variability, which include the effects of temperature, age, the length of studied nerve, anomalous innervation, and temporal dispersion.

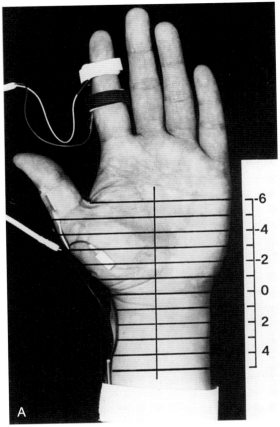

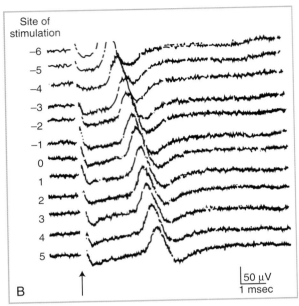

Fig. 32B.3 A, Twelve sites of stimulation in 1-cm increments along the length of the median nerve. The 0 level is at the distal crease of the wrist, corresponding to the origin of the transverse carpal ligament. Sensory nerve action potentials (SNAPs) and compound muscle action potentials are recorded from the second digit and abductor pollicis brevis, respectively. **B,** SNAPs in a normal subject recorded after stimulation of the median nerve at multiple points across the wrist. The site of each stimulus is indicated on the left. The latency changes increased linearly (approximately 0.16 to 0.21 msec) as the stimulus site was moved proximally in 1-cm increments. *(Reprinted with permission of the author and publisher from Kimura, J., 1979. The carpal tunnel syndrome: localization of conduction abnormalities within the distal segment of the median nerve. Brain 102, 619-635. By permission of Oxford University Press, Inc.)*

Temperature

Nerve impulse propagation slows by 2.4 m/sec, or approximately 5%, per degree centigrade from 38°C to 29°C of body temperature. Also, cooling results in a higher CMAP and SNAP amplitude and longer response duration, probably because of accelerated and slowed sodium channel inactivation (Rutkove et al., 1997). Therefore, a CMAP or SNAP with high amplitude and slow distal latency or conduction velocity should raise the suspicion of a cool limb. To reduce this type of variability, a plate thermistor measures skin temperature. This measurement correlates linearly with the subcutaneous and intramuscular temperatures. If the skin temperature falls below 33°C, warm the limbs by immersion in warm water or by application of warming packs or a hydrocollator. Adding 5% of the calculated conduction velocity for each degree below 33°C theoretically normalizes the result. The use of such conversion factors is based on evidence obtained in healthy persons, however, and may not be applicable in patients with abnormal nerves.

Age

Because myelination is incomplete at birth, nerve conduction velocities are half the adult values in full-term newborns; in 23- to 24-week premature newborns, velocities are

one-third the values for term newborns. They attain adult values at 3 to 5 years. Motor and sensory nerve conduction velocities tend to increase slightly in the arms and decrease in the legs during childhood up to the age of 19 years. Conduction velocities slowly decline after age 50, so the mean conduction velocity reduces by approximately 10% at 60 years of age.

Aging also diminishes SNAP and CMAP amplitudes, which decline slowly after age 60. SNAP amplitudes are affected more prominently, so much that normal upper limb SNAP amplitude drops to 50% by age 70, and lower limb SNAPs in many healthy persons older than 60 are low in amplitude or unevokable. Therefore, interpret absence of lower extremity SNAPs in older adults with caution; the finding is not necessarily abnormal without other confirmatory data.

Height and Nerve Segment Lengths

An inverse relationship between height and nerve conduction velocity suggests that longer nerves conduct slower than shorter nerves. For example, the nerve conduction velocities of the peroneal and tibial nerves are 7 to 10 m/sec slower than those of the median and ulnar nerves. The slightly lower temperature of the legs compared with the arms is not the entire

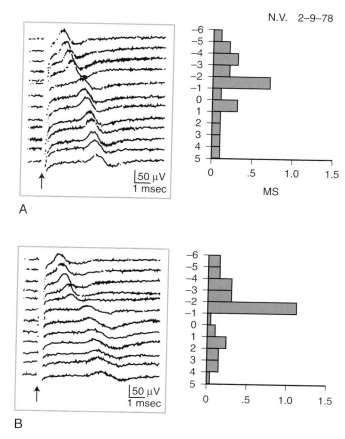

N.V. 2–9–78

A

B

Fig. 32B.4 Sensory nerve action potentials in a patient with bilateral carpal tunnel syndrome (see also **Fig. 35B.3** for settings). A sharply localized slowing was found from point –2 to point –1 in both hands, with a latency change measuring 0.7 msec on the left **(A)** and 1.1 msec on the right **(B),** compared with the other segments with normal latency changes of approximately 0.16 to 0.21 msec. Note also a distinct change in waveform of the sensory potential at the point of localized conduction delay. *(Reprinted with permission of the author and publisher from Kimura, J., 1979. The carpal tunnel syndrome: localization of conduction abnormalities within the distal segment of the median nerve. Brain 102, 619-635. By permission of Oxford University Press, Inc.)*

explanation. Possible factors accounting for the length-related slowing include abrupt distal axonal tapering, progressive reduction in axonal diameter, and shorter internodal distances. For similar reasons, nerve impulses propagate faster in proximal than in distal nerve segments. Adjustments of normal values are necessary for patients of extreme height; this usually is no more than 2 m/sec below the lower limit of normal.

Anomalies

Several anomalous peripheral innervations may influence interpretation of the electrodiagnostic study. Two of these variants, the Martin-Gruber anastomosis and the accessory deep peroneal nerve, have a significant effect on NCS.

MARTIN-GRUBER ANASTOMOSIS

In the Martin-Gruber anastomosis, anomalous fibers cross from the median to the ulnar nerve in the forearm. The communicating branches usually consist of motor axons supplying the ulnar innervated intrinsic hand muscles, particularly the first dorsal interosseous muscle, the hypothenar muscles (abductor digiti minimi), and the thenar muscles (adductor pollicis, deep head of flexor pollicis brevis), or a combination of these muscles. The Martin-Gruber anastomosis occurs in approximately 15% to 20% of the population and sometimes is bilateral. This anomaly manifests as a drop in the ulnar CMAP amplitude between distal and proximal stimulation sites (simulating the appearance of conduction block on ulnar NCS recording from the abductor digiti minimi or first dorsal interosseous). With distal stimulation (at the wrist), the CMAP reflects all ulnar motor fibers, whereas proximal stimulation activates only the uncrossed fibers, which are fewer in number. This anomaly can be confirmed by median nerve stimulation at the elbow, which evokes a small CMAP from the abductor digiti minimi or first dorsal interosseous, which is not present on median nerve stimulation at the wrist. When anomalous fibers innervate the thenar muscles, stimulation of the median nerve at the elbow activates the nerve and the crossing ulnar fibers, resulting in a large CMAP, often with an initial positivity caused by volume conduction of action potential from the ulnar thenar muscles to the median thenar muscles. By contrast, distal median nerve stimulation evokes a smaller thenar CMAP without the positive dip because the crossed fibers are not present at the wrist. In addition, the median nerve conduction velocity in the forearm is spuriously fast, particularly in the presence of carpal tunnel syndrome because the CMAP onset represents a different population of fibers at the wrist than at the elbow. Collision studies obtain an accurate conduction velocity by using action potentials of the crossed fibers (Sander et al., 1997).

ACCESSORY DEEP PERONEAL NERVE

About 20% to 30% of subjects have an anomalous deep peroneal nerve. It is a branch of the superficial peroneal nerve and usually arises as a continuation of the muscular branch that innervates the peroneus longus and brevis muscles. It passes behind the lateral malleolus and terminates in the extensor digitorum brevis (EDB) on the dorsum of the foot. During peroneal motor NCS recording from the EDB, the peroneal CMAP amplitude is larger-stimulating proximally than distally because the anomalous fibers are not present at the ankle. Stimulation behind the lateral malleolus confirms this anomaly, which yields a small CMAP that approximately equals the difference between the CMAP amplitudes evoked with distal and proximal peroneal nerve stimulations. Complete innervation of the EDB by the accessory deep peroneal nerve is rare but should be suspected if there is preservation of function in the EDB muscle (i.e., extension of lateral toes) in a patient with severe deep peroneal neuropathy (Kayal and Katirji, 2009).

PRE- AND POST-FIXED BRACHIAL PLEXUS

In most people, the brachial plexus arises from the C5 to T1 cervical roots. In some, the plexus origin shifts one level up (pre-fixed), arising from C4 to C8, and in others, one level down (post-fixed), originating from C6 to T2. These anomalies result in error in the precise localization of cervical root lesions based on myotomal and dermatomal representation. In pre-fixed plexus, the location of the cervical lesion is one level higher than concluded from findings on the clinical examination and electrodiagnostic studies. In contrast, with post-fixed plexus, the cervical root lesion is one level lower.

RICHE-CANNIEU ANASTOMOSIS

Riche-Cannieu anastomosis is a communication in the palm between the recurrent motor branch of the median nerve and the deep branch of the ulnar nerve. The result is dual innervation of some intrinsic hand muscles such as the first dorsal interosseous, adductor pollicis, and abductor pollicis brevis. Riche-Cannieu anastomosis is rather common but often is not clinically or electrophysiologically apparent. When this anomaly is prominent, denervation in ulnar muscles may follow a median nerve lesion, and vice versa. In addition, a complete median or ulnar nerve lesion may be associated with relative sparing of some median innervated muscles or ulnar innervated muscles in the hand.

Temporal Dispersion and Phase Cancellation

The CMAP, evoked by supramaximal stimulation, represents the summation of all individual MUAPs directed to the muscle through the stimulated nerve. Typically, as the stimulus site moves proximally, the CMAP slightly drops in amplitude and area and increases in duration. The cause is temporal dispersion in which the velocity of impulses in slow-conducting fibers lags increasingly behind those of fast-conducting fibers as conduction distance increases. With dispersion, a slight positive and negative phase overlap, and cancellation of MUAP waveforms is seen (**Fig. 32B.5**). The result of temporal dispersion and phase cancellation is a reduction of CMAP amplitude and area and prolongation of its duration.

Physiological temporal dispersion affects the SNAP more than the CMAP (**Fig. 32B.6**). This difference relates to two factors. The first relates to the disparity between sensory fiber and motor fiber conduction velocities. The range of conduction velocities between the fastest and the slowest individual human myelinated sensory axons is almost twice that for the motor axons (25 m/sec and 12 m/sec, respectively). The second factor is the difference in duration of individual unit discharges between nerve and muscle. With short-duration biphasic sensory spikes, a slight latency difference could line up the positive peaks of the fast fibers with the negative peaks of the slow fibers and cancel both (**Fig. 32B.7**). In longer-duration MUAPs, the same latency shift would only partially superimpose peaks of opposite polarity, and phase cancellation would be less of a factor.

Intertrial Variability

Principal factors contributing to an intertrial variability include errors in determining surface distance and measuring latencies and amplitudes of the recorded response. Amplitudes vary most, probably reflecting a shift in the recording site. NCS are more reproducible when administered by the same examiner because a significant degree of interexaminer difference exists.

Electrodiagnosis by Nerve Conduction Studies

Although both NCS and needle EMG are required in most patients to confirm an electrodiagnostic impression, certain neuromuscular disorders may be evident on NCS alone.

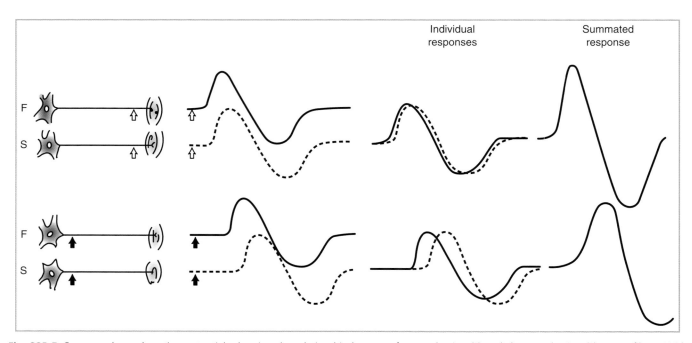

Fig. 32B.5 Compound muscle action potentials showing the relationship between fast-conducting (F) and slow-conducting (S) motor fibers. With distal stimulation (*top*), two unit discharges representing motor unit potentials sum to produce a muscle action potential twice as large. With proximal stimulation (*bottom*), motor unit potentials of long duration still superimpose nearly in phase despite the same latency shift of the slow motor fiber. Thus, a physiological temporal dispersion alters the size of the muscle action potential only minimally, if at all. Phase cancellation increases substantially when the latency difference between fast- and slow-conducting fibers is increased by a demyelinating neuropathy. This gives the false impression of motor conduction block. *(Reprinted with permission from Kimura, J., Machida, M., Ishida, T., et al., 1986. Relation between size of compound sensory or muscle action potentials and length of nerve segment. Neurology 36, 647-652.)*

MEDIAN NERVE STIMULATION

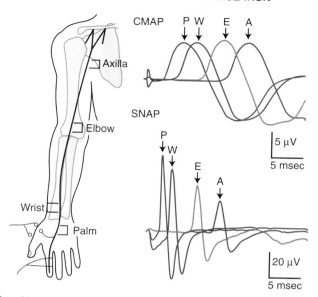

Fig. 32B.6 Simultaneous recordings of compound muscle action potentials (CMAPs) from the thenar eminence and sensory nerve action potentials (SNAPs) from index finger after stimulation of the median nerve at palm (P), wrist (W), elbow (E), and axilla (A). With progressively more proximal stimulation, CMAPs remained nearly the same; for SNAPs, however, both amplitude and the area under the waveform became much smaller.

Fig. 32B.7 Sensory nerve action potentials. A model for phase cancellation between fast-conducting (F) and slow-conducting (S) sensory fibers. With distal stimulation (*top*), two unit discharges sum in phase to produce a sensory action potential twice as large. With proximal stimulation (*bottom*), a delay of the slow fiber causes phase cancellation between the negative peak of the fast fiber and positive peak of the slow fiber, resulting in a 50% reduction in size of the summated response. *(Reprinted with permission from Kimura, J., Machida, M., Ishida, T., et al., 1986. Relation between size of compound sensory or muscle action potentials and length of nerve segment. Neurology 36, 647-652.)*

Focal Nerve Lesions

Peripheral nerve is composed of unmyelinated and myelinated axons surrounded by Schwann cells and a supporting tissue. Surrounding the unmyelinated axons are only the plasma membranes of Schwann cells. By contrast, wrapped around myelinated axons are multiple myelin layers that have a low capacitance and large resistance. Surrounding the myelinated axon is myelin, along with Schwann cells, except at certain gaps called the *nodes of Ranvier*, where sodium channels are highly concentrated and saltatory conduction occurs. Three supportive layers—the endoneurium, perineurium, and epineurium—are highly elastic and protect the myelin and axon from external pressure and tension surround nerves. Nerve fibers may be injured by a variety of mechanisms including compression, ischemia, traction, and laceration.

The classification of peripheral nerve lesions follows. In *neurapraxia (first-degree injury)*, distortion of myelin occurs near the nodes of Ranvier, producing segmental conduction block without wallerian degeneration. In *axonotmesis (second-degree injury)*, the axon is interrupted, but all the supporting nerve structures remain intact. In *neurotmesis*, the nerve injury is severe, resulting in complete disruption of the nerve with all the supporting structures (see Chapter 52D). Often, the neurotmesis category is divisible as follows: *third-degree injury*, with disruption of the endoneurium and with intact perineurium and epineurium; *fourth-degree injury*, with disruption of all neural elements except the epineurium; and *fifth-degree nerve injury*, with complete nerve transection resulting in complete discontinuity of the nerve. Electrodiagnostic studies alone cannot accurately distinguish among the five degrees of nerve injuries, but they can separate the first (neurapraxia) from the other types (Wilbourn, 2002).

DEMYELINATIVE MONONEUROPATHY

When focal injury to myelin occurs, conduction along the affected nerve fibers may alter. This may result in conduction slowing or block along the nerve fibers. The cause of conduction block is interruption of action potential transmission across the nerve lesion; it is the electrophysiological correlate of neurapraxia and usually results from loss of more than one myelin segment (segmental or internodal demyelination). Bracketing two stimulation points, one distal and one proximal to the site of injury, best localizes a nerve lesion with conduction block. With such lesions, stimulation distal to the lesion elicits a normal CMAP, whereas proximal stimulation evokes a response with reduced amplitude or fails to evoke any response, defined as partial or complete conduction block, respectively (**Fig. 32B.8, A**). Several limitations exist to the diagnosis of demyelinative conduction block:

1. Phase cancellation between peaks of opposite polarity may reduce CMAP size because of abnormally increased temporal dispersion. Such excessive desynchronization often develops in acquired demyelinative neuropathies. If the distal and the proximal responses have dissimilar waveforms, the discrepancy in amplitude or area between the two may be the result of phase cancellation rather than conduction block. Therefore, for a diagnosis of partial conduction block, findings should include a significantly lower CMAP amplitude and smaller

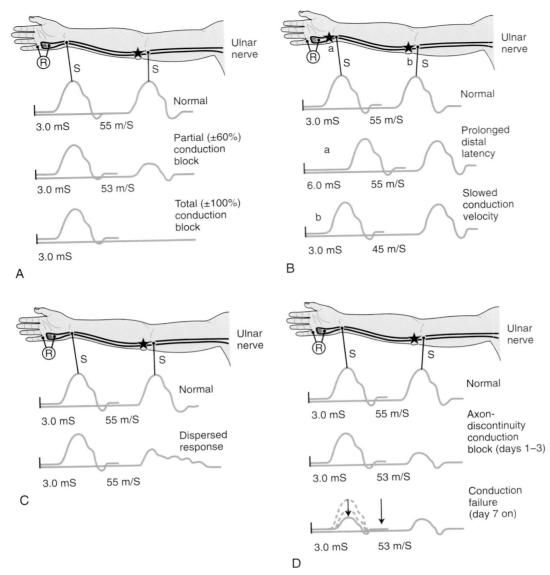

Fig. 32B.8 Findings on nerve conduction studies. **A,** Demyelinative conduction block. Note the proximal compound muscle action potential (CMAP) is either low in amplitude (partial block) or absent (complete block). **B,** Focal synchronized slowing of the distal nerve segment (a) or the proximal nerve segment (b). **D,** Axon loss (partial), studied early and late after nerve trauma. *R,* Recording; *S,* stimulation. *(Reprinted with permission from Wilbourn, A.J., 2002. Nerve conduction studies. Types, components, abnormalities and value in localization. Neurol Clin 20, 305-338.)*

CMAP area with stimulation proximal to the injury site than with the CMAP distal to it, and without any significant prolongation of CMAP duration. More than 50% decay of both the CMAP amplitude and area across the lesion usually is the criterion for definite conduction block.

2. Distal demyelinating lesions causing conduction block of the nerve segment between the most distal stimulating point and the recording site manifest as unelicitable or low CMAP amplitudes at both distal and proximal stimulation sites. This finding mimics the NCS seen with axonal degeneration.

3. The prominent temporal dispersion normally seen in evaluating SNAPs precludes the use of these potentials to diagnose conduction block.

4. Conduction block also may follow axonal loss before the completion of wallerian degeneration.

Focal slowing of conduction usually is the result of widening of the nodes of Ranvier (paranodal demyelination). Slowing, often synchronized, affects all large myelinated fibers equally. This results in prolongation of distal latency if the focal lesion is distal (see **Fig. 32B.8, B,a**), or slowing in conduction velocity if the focal lesion is proximal (see **Fig. 32B.8, B,b**). CMAP amplitude, duration, and area, however, are normal and do not change when the nerve is stimulated proximal to the lesion. Desynchronized slowing (differential slowing) occurs when conduction velocity reduces at the lesion site along a variable number of the medium or small nerve fibers (average- or slower-conducting axons). Here, the CMAP disperses with prolonged duration on stimulations proximal to the lesion. The speed of conduction along the injury site (latency or conduction velocity) is normal because of sparing of at least some of the fastest-conducting axons (see **Fig. 32B.8, C**). When synchronized and desynchronized slowing coexists, slowing of distal latency or conduction velocity accompanies the dispersed CMAP with prolonged duration.

AXON-LOSS MONONEUROPATHY

After acute focal axonal damage, the distal nerve segment undergoes wallerian degeneration. Characteristically, unelicitable or low CMAP amplitudes with distal and proximal stimulations are signs of complete or partial motor axonal loss lesions. The CMAP amplitudes provide a reliable estimate of the amount of axonal loss except in the chronic phase, in which reinnervation via collateral sprouting often increases the CMAP and gives a misleadingly low estimate of the extent of original axonal loss.

In partial axon-loss lesions, distal latencies and conduction velocities are normal or borderline. Selective loss of fast-conducting fibers associated with more than a 50% reduction in mean CMAP amplitude can slow conduction velocity up to 80% of normal value because the velocity represents the remaining slow-conducting fibers. Motor conduction velocity may slow to 70% of normal value with reduction of CMAP amplitude to less than 10% of the lower limit of normal.

Soon after axonal transection (i.e., for the first 48 hours), the distal axon remains excitable. Therefore, stimulation distal to the lesion elicits a normal CMAP, whereas proximal stimulation elicits a response with reduced amplitude, producing a conduction block pattern (see **Fig. 32B.8, D, middle panel**). This pattern is axonal noncontinuity, early axon loss, or axon-discontinuity conduction block. Soon, however, the distal axons undergo wallerian degeneration, and the distal CMAP decreases to equal the proximal CMAP (see **Fig. 32B.8, D, lower panel**). With wallerian degeneration, the distal CMAP decreases in amplitude starting 1 or 2 days after nerve injury and reaches its nadir in 5 to 6 days. In contrast, the distal SNAP lags slightly behind and reaches its nadir in 10 or 11 days (**Fig. 32B.9**). The difference between the decline of the SNAP and CMAP amplitudes after axon loss probably relates to neuromuscular transmission failure, which affects only the CMAP amplitude. Supporting this hypothesis is the fact that MNAPs recorded directly from nerve trunks follow the time course of SNAPs.

The study is repeated after 10 or 11 days, when degenerating axons have lost excitability, to distinguish between conduction block due to demyelination and that due to axon loss.

A reduction in amplitude of the evoked potential from stimulation above and below the lesion indicates axonal loss (see **Fig. 32B.8, D**). By contrast, if the distally evoked CMAP still has significantly higher amplitude than that of the proximally elicited response, this indicates partial segmental demyelination.

Identification of conduction block in the early days of axonal loss is extremely helpful in localizing a peripheral nerve injury, particularly the closed type in which the exact site of lesion is not apparent. Awaiting the completion of wallerian degeneration results in diffusely low or unevokable CMAPs (regardless of stimulation site), which does not allow accurate localization of the injury site. Needle EMG study is useful, but localization by this method is suboptimal (see later discussion).

PREGANGLIONIC (INTRASPINAL CANAL) LESIONS

Damage to the sensory axons in the nerve roots located proximal to the dorsal root ganglion does not affect the SNAP amplitude, because the peripheral sensory axons originating from the unipolar dorsal root ganglion neurons remain intact. Because the dorsal root ganglia usually are located outside the spinal canal and within the intervertebral foramina, axon-loss intraspinal canal lesions (such as radiculopathies or root avulsions) have no effect on SNAP amplitudes. However, these nerve root lesions often result in motor axon degeneration, reflected by abnormal needle EMG findings and, when severe, by low-amplitude CMAP. In contrast with intraspinal canal lesions that are preganglionic, axon-loss extraspinal lesions (such as plexopathies) are postganglionic and affect the CMAP as well as the SNAP amplitudes when mixed nerves undergo wallerian degeneration.

Generalized Polyneuropathies

Nerve conduction studies are essential in diagnosing peripheral polyneuropathies. They are very useful in confirming the diagnosis and establishing the types of fibers affected (large-fiber sensory, motor, or both). Of greatest importance, NCS often identify the primary pathological process of the various polyneuropathies: axonopathy (axonal loss) versus myelinopathy (segmental demyelination). This helps tremendously in identifying the cause of the polyneuropathy.

AXONAL POLYNEUROPATHIES

Axonal polyneuropathies produce length-dependent dying-back degeneration of axons. The major change on NCS is decrease of the CMAP and SNAP amplitudes, more marked

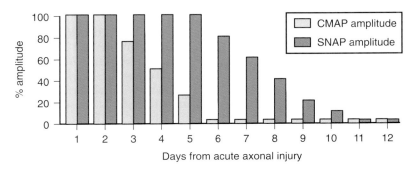

Fig. 32B.9 Distal compound muscle action potential (CMAP) and sensory nerve action potential (SNAP) amplitudes during wallerian degeneration after an acute axonal nerve injury. *(Reprinted with permission from Katirji, B., 2007. Electromyography in Clinical Practice: A Case Study Approach. Mosby, St. Louis.)*

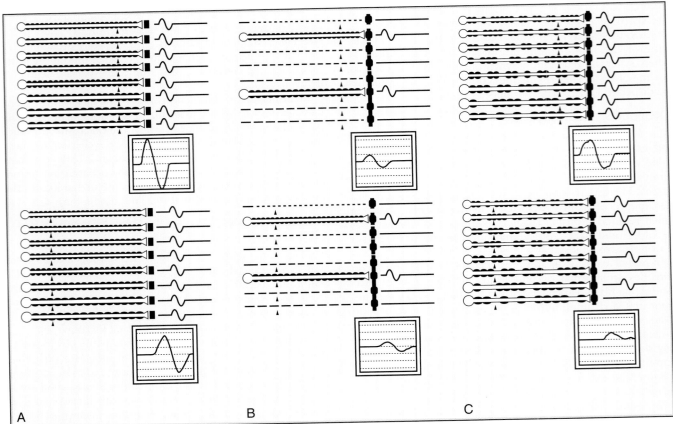

Fig. 32B.10 Computerized model of motor nerve conduction study of a peripheral nerve. **A,** Normal nerve. **B,** Nerve after axonal degeneration. **C,** Nerve with segmental demyelination. *(Reprinted with permission from Brown, W.F., Bolton, C.F. (Eds.), 1989. Clinical Electromyography. Butterworth Heinemann, Boston.)*

in the lower extremities. By contrast, conduction velocities and distal latencies usually are normal (**Fig. 32B.10, *B***). As with axon-loss mononeuropathies, selective loss of many fast-conducting fibers associated with more than a 50% reduction in CMAP amplitude can slow conduction velocity to 70% to 80% of normal value.

DEMYELINATING POLYNEUROPATHIES

The hallmark of demyelinating polyneuropathies is a widespread increase in conduction time caused by impaired saltatory conduction. Therefore, NCS findings are characterized by significant slowing of conduction velocities (less than 75% of the lower limit of normal) and distal latencies (>130% of the upper limit of normal). With distal stimulation, demyelination delays the distal latency, and there is usually moderate reduction of the CMAP amplitude because of abnormal temporal dispersion and phase cancellation. With proximal stimulation, the CMAP amplitude is lower, and the proximal conduction velocity markedly slows because the action potentials travel a longer distance, with increased probability for the nerve action potentials to pass through demyelinated segments (see **Fig. 32B.10, *C***). The proximal CMAP amplitude decay is the result of more prominent temporal dispersion and phase cancellation as well as possible conduction block along some fibers.

Nerve conduction studies further separates chronic demyelinating polyneuropathies into inherited and acquired polyneuropathies. Characteristic of demyelinating inherited polyneuropathies, such as Charcot-Marie-Tooth disease type I, is uniform slowing resulting in symmetrical abnormalities as well as the absence of conduction blocks. By contrast, acquired demyelinating polyneuropathies, such as chronic inflammatory demyelinating polyneuropathy, are often associated with nonuniform slowing that results in asymmetrical nerve conductions, even in the absence of clinical asymmetry. In addition, multifocal conduction blocks and excessive temporal dispersions at nonentrapment sites are characteristic of acquired demyelinating polyneuropathies.

In the most common form of Guillain-Barré syndrome, acute inflammatory demyelinating polyneuropathy, multifocal demyelination that fulfills the criteria for demyelination is evident in 35% to 50% of patients during the first 2 weeks of illness, compared with 85% by the third week (Al-Shekhlee et al., 2005; Albers et al., 1985). Two other suggestive nerve conduction findings in this disorder are abnormal upper extremity SNAPs with normal sural SNAPs, an unusual pattern in axonal length–dependent polyneuropathy, and diffuse absence of F waves with normal results on motor conduction studies, findings consistent with proximal peripheral nerve or spinal root involvement.

Needle Electromyographic Examination

Principles and Techniques

The motor unit consists of a single motor neuron and all the muscle fibers it innervates. A single motor unit consists of either type I or type II muscle fibers, but never both. All muscle fibers in one motor unit discharge simultaneously when stimulated by synaptic input to the lower motor neuron or by electrical stimulation of the axon. The ratio of muscle fibers per motor neuron (innervation ratio or motor unit size) is variable and ranges from 3:1 for extrinsic eye muscles to several thousand to 1 for large limb muscles. The smaller ratio generally is characteristic of muscles that perform fine gradations of movement. The distribution of a single motor unit's muscle fibers in a muscle is wide, with significant overlap between different motor units.

The muscle fiber has a resting potential of 90 mV, with negativity inside the cell. The generation of an action potential reverses the transmembrane potential, which then becomes positive inside the cell. An extracellular electrode, as used in needle EMG, records the activity resulting from this switch of polarity as a predominantly negative potential (usually triphasic, positive-negative-positive waveforms). When recorded near a damaged region, however, action potentials consist of a large positivity followed by a small negativity.

Concentric and Teflon-coated monopolar needle electrodes are equally satisfactory in recording muscle potentials, with little appreciable difference. Although monopolar needles are less painful, they require an additional reference electrode placed nearby, which often results in greater electrical noise caused by electrode impedance mismatch between the intramuscular active electrode and the surface reference disk.

The electromyographer first identifies the needle insertion point by recognizing the proper anatomical landmark and the activation maneuver for the sampled muscle. Needle EMG evaluation requires appreciation of the following technical considerations:

1. Inserting or slightly moving the needle causes insertional activity that results from needle injury of muscle fibers.
2. Moving the needle a small distance and pausing a few seconds assesses spontaneous activity in relaxed muscle. From a single cutaneous insertion, relocating the needle in four quadrants of the muscle completes the evaluations.
3. Minimal contraction assesses the morphology of several MUAPs measured on the oscilloscope or hard copy. The needle should be moved slightly (pulled back or moved deeper) if sharp MUAPs are not seen with minimal contraction.
4. Increasing the intensity of muscle contraction assesses the recruitment pattern of MUAPs. Maximal contraction normally fills the screen, producing the interference pattern.

An amplification of 50 μV per division best defines the insertional and spontaneous activity, whereas 200 μV per division is suited for voluntary activity. Most laboratories use oscilloscope sweep speeds of 10 to 20 msec per division for insertional, spontaneous, and voluntary activities.

Insertional and Spontaneous Activity
Normal Insertional and Spontaneous Activity

Brief bursts of electrical discharges accompany insertion and repositioning of a needle electrode into the muscle, slightly outlasting the movement of the needle. On average, insertional activity lasts for a few hundred milliseconds. It appears as a cluster of positive or negative repetitive high-frequency spikes, which make a crisp static sound over the loudspeaker.

At rest, muscle is silent, with no spontaneous activity except in the motor end-plate region, the site of neuromuscular junctions, which usually are located along a line crossing the center of the muscle belly. **Table 32B.1** lists normal and abnormal insertional and spontaneous activities (Katirji et al., 2002). Two types of normal end-plate spontaneous activity occur together or independently: end-plate noise and end-plate spikes (**Fig. 32B.11**).

END-PLATE NOISE (See Video 35B.1, available at www.expertconsult.com.)

The tip of the needle approaching the end-plate region often registers recurring irregular negative potentials, 10 to 50 μV in amplitude and 1 to 2 msec in duration. These potentials are the extracellularly recorded miniature end-plate potentials, non-propagating depolarizations caused by spontaneous release of acetylcholine quanta. They produce a characteristic sound on the loudspeaker much like that of a seashell held to the ear.

END-PLATE SPIKES (See Video 35B.2, available at www.expertconsult.com.)

End-plate spikes are intermittent spikes, 100 to 200 μV in amplitude and 3 to 4 msec in duration, firing irregularly at 5 to 50 impulses per second. Their characteristic waveform (initial negative deflection) and irregular firing pattern

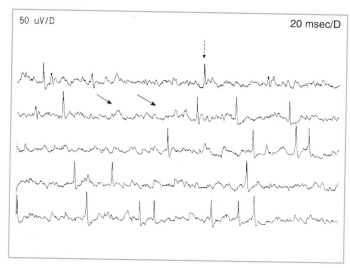

Fig. 32B.11 End-plate noise (*solid arrows*) and spikes (*dashed arrow*) representing normal insertional and spontaneous activities.

Table 32B.1 Insertional and Spontaneous Activity on Needle Electromyography

Potential	Source Generator and Morphology	Sound on Loudspeaker	Stability	Firing Rate	Firing Pattern
Endplate noise	Miniature endplate potentials (monophasic negative)	Seashell	—	20-40 Hz	Irregular (hissing)
Endplate spike	Muscle fiber initiated by terminal axonal twig (brief spike, diphasic, initial negative)	Sputtering fat in a frying pan	—	5-50 Hz	Irregular (sputtering)
Fibrillation (brief spike)	Muscle fiber (brief spike, diphasic or triphasic, initial positive)	Rain on a tin roof or tick-tock of a clock	Stable	0.5-10 Hz (occasionally up to 30 Hz)	Regular
Positive sharp wave	Muscle fiber (diphasic, initial positive, slow negative)	Dull pops, rain on a tin roof, or tick-tock of a clock	Stable	0.5-10 Hz (occasionally up to 30 Hz)	Regular
Myotonia	Muscle fiber (brief spike, initial positive, or positive wave)	Revving engine or dive bomber	Waxing and waning amplitude	20-150 Hz	Waxing and waning
Complex repetitive discharge	Multiple muscle fibers time-linked together	Machine	Usually stable, may change in discrete jumps	5-100 Hz	Perfectly regular (unless overdriven)
Fasciculation	Motor unit (motor neuron or axon)	Corn popping		Low (0.1-10 Hz)	Irregular
Myokymia	Motor unit (motor neuron or axon)	Marching soldiers		1-5 Hz (interburst), 5-60 Hz (intraburst)	Bursting
Cramp	Motor unit (motor neuron or axon)		—	High (20-150 Hz)	Interference pattern or several individual units
Neuromyotonia	Motor unit (motor neuron or axon)	Pinging	Decrementing amplitude	Very high (150-250 Hz)	Waning

Reprinted and revised with permission from Katirji, B., Kaminski, H.J., Preston, D.C., et al. (Eds.), 2002. Neuromuscular Disorders in Clinical Practice. Butterworth-Heinemann, Boston.

distinguish them from the regular-firing fibrillation potentials. Furthermore, they often are associated with end-plate noise and a sound on the loudspeaker like that of sputtering fat in a frying pan. The end-plate spikes are discharges of single muscle fibers generated by activation of intramuscular nerve terminals irritated by the needle. The similarity of the firing pattern of end-plate spikes to discharges of muscle spindle afferents suggests that they may originate in the intrafusal muscle fibers.

Abnormal Insertional and Spontaneous Activity

PROLONGED VERSUS DECREASED INSERTIONAL ACTIVITY

An abnormally prolonged (increased) insertional activity indicates instability of the muscle membrane, often seen in conjunction with denervation, myotonic disorders, or necrotizing myopathies such as inflammatory myopathies.

Insertional positive waves, initiated by needle movements only and identical to the spontaneous discharges, may follow the increased insertional activity, lasting a few seconds. This isolated activity usually signals early denervation of muscle fibers, such as occurs 1 to 2 weeks after acute motor axon loss. A marked reduction or absence of insertional activity suggests either fibrotic or severely atrophied muscle or functionally inexcitable muscle, such as during the paralytic attack of periodic paralysis.

FIBRILLATION POTENTIALS (See Videos 35B.3 and 35B.4, available at www.expertconsult.com.)

Fibrillation potentials are spontaneous action potentials of denervated muscle fibers. They result from reduction of the resting membrane potential of the denervated fiber to the level at which it can fire spontaneously. Fibrillation potentials, triggered by spontaneous oscillations in the muscle fiber membrane potential, typically fire in a regular pattern at a rate of 1 to 30 Hz. The sound they produce on the loudspeaker is crisp and clicking, reminiscent of rain on a tin roof or the tick-tock of a clock. Fibrillation potentials have two types of waveforms: brief spikes and positive waves. Brief spikes usually are triphasic with initial positivity (**Fig. 32B.12, A**). They range from 1 to 5 msec in duration and 20 to 200 μV in amplitude when recorded with a concentric needle electrode. Brief-spike fibrillation potentials may be confused with physiological end-plate spikes but are distinguishable by their regular firing

pattern and triphasic configuration with an initial positivity. Occasionally, placement of the needle electrode near the end-plate zone of a denervated muscle results in brief spikes, morphologically resembling end-plate spikes with an initial negativity. Positive waves have an initial positivity and subsequent slow negativity with a characteristic sawtooth appearance (see **Fig. 32B.12, B**). Making recordings near the damaged part of the muscle fiber (incapable of generating an action

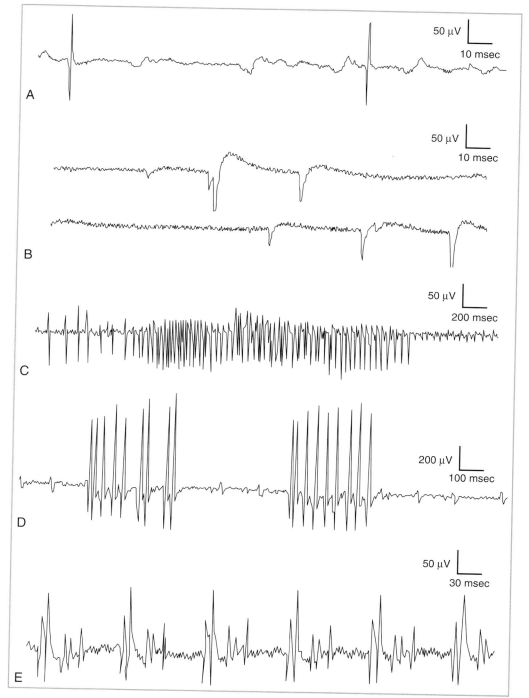

Fig. 32B.12 Abnormal insertional activities. **A,** Brief spike fibrillation potentials. **B,** Positive waves. **C,** Myotonic discharge. **D,** Myokymic discharge. **E,** Complex repetitive discharge. *(Reprinted with permission from Preston, D.C., Shapiro, B.E., 2005. EMG Waveforms. Butterworth Heinemann, Boston.)*

potential) accounts for the absence of a negative spike. Although usually seen together, positive sharp waves tend to precede brief spikes after nerve section, possibly because insertion of a needle in already irritable muscle membrane triggers the response.

Fibrillation potentials are the electrophysiological markers of muscle denervation. Based on their distribution, they are useful in localizing lesions to the anterior horn cells of the spinal cord, ventral root, plexus, or peripheral nerve. Insertional positive waves may appear within 2 weeks of acute denervation, but fibrillation potentials do not become full until approximately 3 weeks after axonal loss. Because of this latent period, their absence does not exclude recent denervation. In addition, late in the course of denervation, muscle fibers that are reinnervated, fibrotic, or severely atrophied show no fibrillation potentials. A numerical grading system (from 0 to 4) is the standard to semiquantitate fibrillation potentials. Their density is a rough estimate of the extent of denervated muscle fibers: 0, no fibrillations; +1, persistent single trains of potentials (less than 2 seconds) in at least two areas; +2, moderate number of potentials in three or more areas; +3, many potentials in all areas; +4, abundant spontaneous potentials nearly filling the oscilloscope.

Fibrillation potentials also occur in necrotizing myopathies such as the inflammatory myopathies and muscular dystrophies. The probable causes are (1) segmental necrosis of muscle fiber together with its central section (region of myoneural junction), leading to effective denervation of its distant muscle fiber segments as they become physically separated from the neuromuscular junction; (2) reduction of the resting membrane potential of partially damaged fibers to the level that allows spontaneous discharges to occur; and (3) damage to the terminal intramuscular motor axons, presumably by the inflammatory process, resulting in muscle fiber denervation. In disorders of the neuromuscular junction such as myasthenia gravis and botulism, fibrillation potentials are rare; when present, the explanation is a prolonged neuromuscular transmission blockade resulting in effective denervation of muscle fibers.

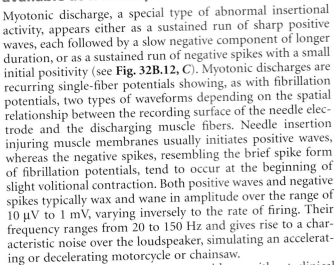

FASCICULATION POTENTIALS (See Video 35B.5, available at www.expertconsult.com.)

Fasciculation potentials are spontaneous discharges of a motor unit. They originate from the motor neuron or anywhere along its axon. Fasciculation potentials fire randomly and irregularly and undergo slight changes in amplitude and waveform from time to time, giving them a corn-popping sound on the loudspeaker. They have a much lower firing rate than that of voluntary MUAPs and are unaffected by slight voluntary contraction of agonist or antagonist muscles.

Fasciculation potentials are most common in diseases of anterior horn cells but also occur in radiculopathies, entrapment neuropathies, peripheral polyneuropathies, and the cramp fasciculation syndrome. Other causes are tetany, thyrotoxicosis, and overdose of anticholinesterase medication. In addition, they may occur in healthy people. No reliable method exists to distinguish "benign" from "malignant" fasciculation potentials, except that the benign discharges tend to fire more quickly, and grouped fasciculation potentials from multiple units are more common in motor neuron disease. Of greatest importance, the association of fasciculation potentials with fibrillation potentials or other neurogenic

MUAP changes constitutes strong evidence of a lower motor neuron (LMN) disorder.

MYOTONIC DISCHARGES (See Video 35B.6, available at www.expertconsult.com.)

Myotonic discharge, a special type of abnormal insertional activity, appears either as a sustained run of sharp positive waves, each followed by a slow negative component of longer duration, or as a sustained run of negative spikes with a small initial positivity (see **Fig. 32B.12, C**). Myotonic discharges are recurring single-fiber potentials showing, as with fibrillation potentials, two types of waveforms depending on the spatial relationship between the recording surface of the needle electrode and the discharging muscle fibers. Needle insertion injuring muscle membranes usually initiates positive waves, whereas the negative spikes, resembling the brief spike form of fibrillation potentials, tend to occur at the beginning of slight volitional contraction. Both positive waves and negative spikes typically wax and wane in amplitude over the range of 10 μV to 1 mV, varying inversely to the rate of firing. Their frequency ranges from 20 to 150 Hz and gives rise to a characteristic noise over the loudspeaker, simulating an accelerating or decelerating motorcycle or chainsaw.

Myotonic discharges may occur with or without clinical myotonia in the myotonic dystrophies (types I and II), myotonia congenita, myotonia fluctuans, and paramyotonia congenita. They also may accompany other myopathies such as acid maltase deficiency, colchicine myopathy, myotubular myopathy, and hyperkalemic periodic paralysis.

MYOKYMIC DISCHARGES (See Video 35B.7, available at www.expertconsult.com.)

Myokymia results from complex bursts of grouped repetitive discharges in which motor units fire repetitively, usually with 2 to 10 spikes discharging at a mean of 30 to 40 Hz (see **Fig. 32B.12, D**). Each burst recurs at regular intervals of 1 to 5 seconds, giving the sound of marching soldiers on the loudspeaker. Clinically, myokymic discharges often give rise to sustained muscle contractions, which have an undulating appearance beneath the skin ("bag of worms"). The origin of myokymic discharges probably is ectopic, in motor nerve fibers, and amplified by increased axonal excitability, such as after hyperventilation-induced hypocapnia.

Myokymic discharges in facial muscles are associated with brainstem glioma, multiple sclerosis, or Guillain-Barré syndrome. In limb muscles, myokymia may be focal, as with radiation plexopathies and carpal tunnel syndrome, or diffuse, as with Guillain-Barré syndrome, chronic inflammatory demyelinating polyneuropathy, gold intoxication, or Isaac syndrome.

COMPLEX REPETITIVE DISCHARGES (See Video 35B.8, available at www.expertconsult.com.)

A complex repetitive discharge results from the nearly synchronous firing of a group of muscle fibers. One fiber in the complex serves as a pacemaker, driving one or several other fibers ephaptically so that the individual spikes in the complex fire in the same order in which the discharge recurs. One of the late-activated fibers reexcites the principal pacemaker to repeat the cycle. The entire sequence recurs at slow or fast rates, usually in the range of 5 to 100 Hz. The discharge ranges from 50 μV to 1 mV in amplitude and up to 50 to 1000 msec in duration. The complex waveform contains several distinct spikes and remains uniform from one discharge to another (see **Fig. 32B.12, E**). These discharges typically begin abruptly, maintain a constant rate of firing for a short period, and cease as abruptly as they started when the chain reaction eventually blocks. They produce a noise on the loudspeaker that mimics the sound of a machine or a motorcycle.

Complex repetitive discharges are abnormal discharges but are less specific than other spontaneous discharges. They occur most often in myopathies but also occur in some neuropathic disorders such as radiculopathies. They most commonly accompany chronic conditions but are occasionally observed in subacute disorders. They also may occur in the iliacus or cervical paraspinal muscles of apparently healthy persons, probably implying a clinically silent neuropathic process.

NEUROMYOTONIC DISCHARGES (See Video 35B.9, available at www.expertconsult.com.)

Neuromyotonic discharges are extremely rare discharges in which muscle fibers fire repetitively with a high intraburst frequency (40 to 350 Hz), either continuously or in recurring decrementing bursts, producing a pinging sound on the loudspeaker. The discharges are more prominent in distal than proximal muscles, probably implicating the terminal branches of motor axons as the site of generation (Maddison et al., 2006). Many cases of neuromyotonia are associated with the syndrome of continuous motor unit activity or acquired neuromyotonia, an autoimmune antibody-mediated peripheral nerve potassium channelopathy (Hart et al., 1997). Other conditions that may be associated with neuromyotonia include anticholinesterase poisoning, tetany, and chronic spinal muscular atrophies.

CRAMP DISCHARGES (See Video 35B.10, available at www.expertconsult.com.)

A muscle cramp is a sustained involuntary muscle contraction. On needle EMG studies, cramp discharge consists of MUAPs usually firing at a rate of 40 to 60 Hz, with abrupt onset and cessation. Cramps most often occur in healthy people, but hyponatremia, hypocalcemia, myxedema, pregnancy, postdialysis state, and the early stages of motor neuron disease exaggerate their frequency. Clinically, cramps may resemble muscle contractures accompanying several metabolic muscle diseases, but characteristic of these contractures is complete electrical silence on the needle EMG.

Voluntary Motor Unit Action Potentials
MUAP Morphology

MUAP is the extracellular electrode recording of a small portion of a motor unit. The inherent properties of the motor unit and the spatial relationships between the needle and individual muscle fibers dictate the waveform. Slight repositioning of the electrode changes the electrical profile of the same motor unit. Therefore, one motor unit can give rise to MUAPs of different morphology at different recording sites. The amplitude, duration, and number of phases characterize the MUAP waveform.

AMPLITUDE

MUAP amplitude is the maximum peak-to-peak amplitude. It ranges from several hundred microvolts to a few millivolts with a concentric needle and is substantially greater with a monopolar needle. The amplitude of an MUAP decreases to less than 50% at a distance of 200 to 300 μm from the source and to less than 1% a few millimeters away. Therefore, the amplitude depends on the proximity of the tip of the needle electrode to the muscle fibers. Only a small number of individual muscle fibers located near the tip of the electrode determine the amplitude of an MUAP (probably less than 20 muscle fibers lying within a 1-mm radius of the electrode tip). In general, amplitude indicates muscle fiber density, not the motor unit territory.

DURATION (See Videos 35B.11 to 35B.13, available at www.expertconsult.com.)

MUAP duration reflects the activity from most muscle fibers belonging to a motor unit, because potentials generated more than 1 mm away from the electrode contribute to the initial and terminal low-amplitude portions of the potential. The duration indicates the degree of synchrony among many individual muscle fibers with variable length, conduction velocity, and membrane excitability. A slight shift in needle position or rotation influences duration much less than amplitude. MUAP duration is a good index of the motor unit territory and is the parameter that best reflects the number of muscle fibers in a motor unit. The measure of duration is from the initial deflection away from baseline to the final return to baseline. It normally ranges from 5 to 15 msec, depending on the sampled muscle and the age of the subject.

Long-duration MUAPs often are of high amplitude and are the best indicators of reinnervation, as seen with LMN disorders, peripheral neuropathies, and radiculopathies. They occur with increased number or density of muscle fibers or a loss of synchrony of fiber firing within a motor unit. Short-duration MUAPs often are of low amplitude. They occur in disorders associated with loss of muscle fibers, as seen with necrotizing myopathies (**Fig. 32B.13**).

PHASES (See Videos 32B.14 and 32B.15, available at www.expertconsult.com.)

A phase constitutes the portion of a waveform that departs from and returns to the baseline. The number of phases equals the number of negative and positive peaks extending to and from the baseline, or the number of baseline crossings plus one. Normal MUAPs have four phases or less. Approximately 5% to 15% of MUAPs, however, have five phases or more, and this may increase up to 25% in proximal muscles, such as the deltoid, gluteus maximus, and the iliacus. Increased polyphasia is an abnormal but nonspecific MUAP abnormality, since it occurs in both myopathic and neurogenic disorders. An increased number of polyphasic MUAPs suggests desynchronized discharge, loss of individual fibers within a motor unit, or temporal dispersion of muscle fiber potentials within a motor unit. Excessive temporal dispersion, in turn, results from differences in conduction time along the terminal branch of the nerve or over the muscle fiber membrane. In early reinnervation after severe denervation, the newly sprouting axons reinnervate only a few muscle fibers. Consequently, the MUAP also may be polyphasic, with short duration and low amplitude ("nascent" MUAP).

Some MUAPs have a serrated pattern characterized by several turns or directional changes without crossing the

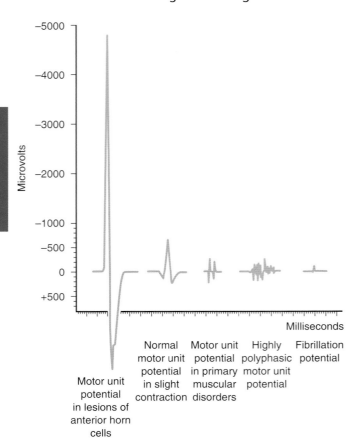

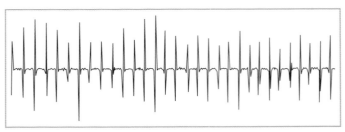

Fig. 32B.14 Motor unit action potential instability (moment-to-moment variation) in a patient with myasthenia gravis (recorded with a sweep speed of 100 msec/division and a sensitivity of 0.2 mV/division). Note the extreme amplitude variability of the activated single motor unit action potential. *(Reprinted with permission from Katirji, B., 2007. Electromyography in Clinical Practice: a Case Study Approach. Mosby, St. Louis.)*

Fig. 32B.13 Motor unit action potentials (MUAPs) in health and disease. *(Reprinted with permission from Daube, J., 1991. Needle electromyography in clinical electromyography. Muscle Nerve 14, 685-700.)*

baseline. This also indicates desynchronization among discharging muscle fibers. Satellite potential (linked potential or parasite potential) is a late spike of MUAP, which is distinct but time-locked with the main potential. It implicates early reinnervation of muscle fibers by newly formed collateral sprouts that usually are long, small, thinly myelinated, and slowly conducting. As the sprout matures, the thickness of its myelin increases and its conduction velocity increases. Hence, the satellite potential fires more closely to the main potential and may ultimately become an additional phase or serration within the main complex.

MUAP Stability

(See Video 32B.16, available at www.expertconsult.com.)
Motor units normally discharge semirhythmically, with successive MUAPs showing nearly identical configuration because all muscle fibers of the motor unit fire during every discharge. The morphology of a repetitively firing unit may fluctuate if individual muscle fibers intermittently block within the unit. Moment-to-moment MUAP variability indicates deficient neuromuscular transmission as recurring discharges deplete the store of immediately available acetylcholine (**Fig. 32B.14**). This instability occurs in neuromuscular junction disorders such as myasthenia gravis, the Lambert-Eaton myasthenic syndrome, and botulism, as well as in neurogenic disorders associated with recent reinnervation, such as motor neuron

disease, subacute radiculopathy, and polyneuropathy, and during the early stages of reinnervation in acute peripheral nerve injuries.

MUAP Firing Patterns

(See Videos 32B.17 and 32B.18, available at www.expertconsult.com.)
During constant contraction in a healthy person, initially only one or two motor units activate semirhythmically. The motor units activated early are primarily those with small type I muscle fibers. Large type II units participate later during strong voluntary contraction. Greater muscle force brings about not only recruitment of previously inactive units but also more rapid firing of already active units, with both mechanisms operating simultaneously (Erim et al., 1996).

Recruitment frequency is a measure of *motor unit discharge*, defined as the firing frequency (rate) at the time of recruiting an additional unit. In normal muscles, mild contraction induces isolated discharges at a rate of 5 to 10 Hz. This rate depends on the sampled muscle and the types of motor units studied. The reported ranges for healthy people and those with neuromuscular disorders overlap. Recruitment ratio is the average firing rate divided by the number of active units. This ratio normally should not exceed 5 : 1, for example, with three units each firing less than 15 Hz. Typically, when the firing frequency of the first MUAP reaches 10 Hz, a second MUAP should begin to fire; by 15 Hz, a third unit should fire, and so forth. A ratio of 10, with two units firing at 20 Hz each, indicates a loss of motor units. When motor unit loss is severe, intact residual motor units can increase their firing rate to a maximum of 30 to 50 Hz in most human skeletal muscles.

Activation is the central control of motor units that allows an increase in firing rate and force. Failure of descending impulses also limits recruitment, although here the excited motor units discharge more slowly than expected for normal maximal contraction. Thus, a slow rate of discharge (poor activation) in an upper motor neuron (UMN) disorder (such as stroke or myelopathy) or in volitional lack of effort (such as with pain, hysterical paralysis, or malingering) stands in sharp contrast to a fast rate of discharge in a LMN weakness (decreased recruitment). With greater contraction, many motor units begin to fire rapidly, making recognition of individual MUAPs difficult—hence the name *interference pattern*. Several factors influence the spike density and average amplitude of the summated response. These include descending input from the cortex, number of motor neurons capable of discharging, firing frequency of each motor unit, waveform of individual potentials, and phase cancellation. The causes of an incomplete interference pattern are poor activation and reduced recruitment. Methods to assess recruitment during maximum contraction include examination of the interference pattern or, during moderate levels of contraction, estimation of the number of MUAPs firing for the level of activation. Evaluating maximal contraction is most valuable in excluding mild degrees of decreased recruitment. In the extreme case when only few motor units fire rapidly, a picket fence–like interference pattern results.

In myopathy, low-amplitude, short-duration MUAPs produce a smaller force per motor unit than normal MUAPs. The instantaneous recruitment of many units is required to support a slight voluntary effort in patients with moderate to severe weakness (early recruitment). With early recruitment, a full interference pattern is attained at less than maximal contraction, but its amplitude is low because fiber density is below normal in individual motor units. In advanced myopathies with severe muscle weakness, loss of muscle fibers is so extensive that entire motor units effectively disappear, resulting in a decreased recruitment and an incomplete interference pattern, mimicking the recruitment pattern of a neurogenic disorder.

Electrodiagnosis by Needle Electromyography
Lower Motor Neuron Disorders

The first needle EMG change occurring after an acute LMN insult is an abnormal recruitment pattern. Recruitment frequency and ratio increase in lower motor neuron lesions,

because fewer motor units fire for a given strength of contraction. Furthermore, the interference pattern with maximal contraction decreases.

Insertional activity increases after the first week, and insertional positive waves may appear within 2 weeks after acute denervation. Spontaneous fibrillation potentials become apparent in all abnormal muscles after 3 weeks, however. Fasciculation potentials accompany electrical denervation changes in diseases of the anterior horn cells, roots, and peripheral nerves but do not have pathological significance when they appear alone. Limb myokymic discharges occur, usually with entrapments, radiation plexopathy, or Guillain-Barré syndrome. Complex repetitive discharges denote a chronic myopathy or radiculopathy, although they may occur with other LMN disorders, as well as in subacute disorders.

MUAPs are normal in morphology in the acute phase of denervation, but signs of reinnervation become apparent as early as 1 month later. Reinnervation causes first an increased number of MUAP turns and phases and later increased MUAP amplitude and duration. Amplitude generally reflects fiber density, whereas duration reflects motor unit territory. The expected MUAP from LMN lesions is a long-duration, high-amplitude, and polyphasic unit (**Fig. 32B.15**; see also **Fig. 32B.13**). The exception is in early reinnervation in which motor units acquire few muscle fibers, resulting in brief, small, polyphasic MUAPs ("nascent" MUAPs), mimicking a myopathic process.

RADICULOPATHIES

Needle EMG is the most sensitive and specific electrodiagnostic test for identifying cervical and lumbosacral radiculopathies, particularly those associated with axon loss. Needle EMG is useful for accurate localization of the level of

Lesion / EMG steps	Normal	Neurogenic lesion		Myogenic lesion		
		Lower motor	Upper motor	Myopathy	Myotonia	Polymyositis
1 Insertional activity	Normal	Increased	Normal	Normal	Myotonic discharge	Increased
2 Spontaneous activity		Fibrillation / Positive wave				Fibrillation / Positive wave
3 Motor unit potential	0.5-1.0 mv / 5-10 msec	Large unit / Limited recruitment	Normal	Small unit / Early recruitment	Myotonic discharge	Small unit / Early recruitment
4 Interference pattern	Full	Reduced / Fast firing rate	Reduced / Slow firing rate	Full / Low amplitude	Full / Low amplitude	Full / Low amplitude

Fig. 32B.15 A summary of characteristic findings on needle electromyography in normal subjects, patients with neurogenic lesions, and patients with myogenic lesions. Insertional activity is greater with lower motor neuron lesions and polymyositis and consists of myotonic discharges in myotonia. Spontaneous activity generally occurs with lower motor neuron disorders and inflammatory myopathy. Motor unit action potentials usually are large and polyphasic, with reduced recruitment in lower motor neuron conditions; in myopathies and polymyositis, motor units are small, with early recruitment. Interference pattern is reduced with both upper and lower motor neuron lesions, as well as in functional (nonorganic) weakness; however, firing rate is rapid in lower motor neuron lesions and slow with upper motor neuron lesions and functional (nonorganic) weakness (in which the rate may be irregular also). Interference pattern is full but of low amplitude in myopathic lesions. (*Reprinted from Kimura, J., 1989. Electrodiagnosis in Diseases of Nerve and Muscle: Principles and Practices, second ed. F.A. Davis, Philadelphia.Copyright 1989 by Oxford University Press, Inc. Used by permission of Oxford University Press, Inc.*)

the root lesion. Finding signs of denervation (fibrillation potentials, decreased recruitment, and long-duration, high-amplitude polyphasic MUAPs) in a segmental myotomal distribution (i.e., in muscles innervated by the same roots via more than one peripheral nerve), with or without denervation of the paraspinal muscles, localizes the LMN lesion to the root level (Wilbourn and Aminoff, 1998). In radiculopathies associated with axonal loss of proximal sensory fibers, the distal sensory axons do not degenerate, because the unipolar neurons of dorsal root ganglia and their distal axons usually escape injury. Hence, a normal SNAP of the corresponding dermatome ensures that the root lesion is within the spinal canal (i.e., proximal to the dorsal root ganglia). For example, in an L5 radiculopathy, the tibialis anterior (peroneal nerve) and tibialis posterior (tibial nerve) muscles often are abnormal on needle EMG, as may be those from the lumbar paraspinal muscles, but the superficial peroneal SNAP usually is normal.

PLEXOPATHIES

Plexopathies are lesions that involve extraspinal peripheral nerves. The diagnosis of brachial or lumbosacral plexopathies requires a solid knowledge of peripheral nerve anatomy. Brachial plexus anatomy is particularly complex, so that multiple NCS and muscle needle EMGs are needed for evaluation. An important task of the electrodiagnostic evaluation is to differentiate between lesions affecting the brachial plexus (postganglionic lesions) and those involving the roots (preganglionic lesions). This distinction is particularly important in brachial plexus traction injuries, which may mimic root avulsions (Ferrante and Wilbourn, 2002). In avulsions, the dorsal root ganglia remain intact, and their peripheral axons do not undergo wallerian degeneration. Therefore, root avulsions spare SNAPs, whereas SNAPs are low in amplitude or absent in brachial plexopathies when studied after the completion of wallerian degeneration (more than 10 days from injury).

MONONEUROPATHIES

Needle EMG is most useful in mononeuropathies caused by pure axonal loss and examined after the completion of wallerian degeneration. These lesions are not localizable by NCS because they are not associated with focal conduction slowing or conduction block, as seen with demyelinating mononeuropathies. NCS in axon-loss lesions often show low-amplitude or absent CMAPs and SNAPs following stimulations at distal and proximal sites, while distal latencies and conduction velocities are normal or slightly slowed.

The principle of localizing an axon-loss mononeuropathy by needle EMG is similar to manual muscle strength testing on clinical examination. Typically, the needle EMG reveals neurogenic changes (fibrillation potentials, reduced MUAP recruitment, and chronic neurogenic MUAP morphology changes) that are limited to muscles innervated by the involved nerve and located distal to the site of the lesion. Localization of axon-loss peripheral nerve lesions by needle EMG is suboptimal, however, because some nerves have very long segments from which no motor branches arise, such as the median and ulnar nerves in the arm or the common peroneal nerve in the thigh. In addition, needle EMG may falsely localize a partial nerve lesion more distally along the affected nerve because of fascicular involvement of nerve fibers or effective

reinnervation of proximally situated muscles (Wilbourn, 2002). An example is sparing of ulnar muscles in the forearm (flexor carpi ulnaris and ulnar part of flexor digitorum profundus) following an axon-loss ulnar nerve lesion at the elbow.

Needle EMG is particularly useful in assessing the progress of reinnervation occurring spontaneously or after nerve repair. MUAP recruitment and morphology help assess the process of muscle fiber reinnervation that occurs with proximodistal regeneration of nerve fibers from the site of the injury or collateral sprouting. Early proximodistal regeneration of nerve fibers in severe axon-loss lesions often manifests as brief, small, polyphasic (nascent) MUAPs. Collateral sprouting causes an increased number of MUAP turns and phases, followed by an increased duration and amplitude of MUAPs (Katirji, 2006).

PERIPHERAL POLYNEUROPATHIES

Widespread abnormalities on NCS are characteristic of polyneuropathies. The needle EMG depicts the temporal profile of the illness. In acute demyelinating polyneuropathies such as the Guillain-Barré syndrome, needle EMG during the acute phase of illness may show only reduced recruitment of MUAPs in weak muscles, with normal MUAP morphology and no spontaneous activity. In chronic demyelinating polyneuropathies such as chronic inflammatory demyelinating polyneuropathy, the needle EMG may show signs of mild axonal loss not always suspected on NCS, with fibrillation potentials and reinnervated MUAPs. In acute axon-loss polyneuropathy such as the axonal forms of Guillain-Barré syndrome or critical illness polyneuropathy, fibrillation potentials typically develop within 2 to 3 weeks, and reinnervated MUAPs become apparent after 1 to 2 months. In progressive axon-loss polyneuropathies, fibrillation potentials denote active denervation, while long-duration, high-amplitude polyphasic MUAPs confirm reinnervation. Both changes usually are symmetrical, follow a distal-to-proximal gradient, and are worse in the legs than in the arms. In chronic and very slowly progressive polyneuropathies, reinnervation may keep pace completely with active denervation, yielding few or no fibrillation potentials but reduced recruitment of reinnervated long-duration and high-amplitude MUAPs.

ANTERIOR HORN CELL DISORDERS

Needle EMG is the most important electrodiagnostic study to provide evidence of diffuse lower motor neuron degeneration in patients with motor neuron disease. The needle EMG often shows signs of active denervation (fibrillation potentials), active reinnervation (long-duration, high-amplitude polyphasic MUAPs and unstable MUAPs), and loss of motor units (reduced MUAP recruitment).

One disadvantage of needle EMG in motor neuron disease is that it evaluates only LMN degeneration; UMN degeneration requires clinical assessment. Therefore, clinical evaluation is the basis for diagnosing amyotrophic lateral sclerosis (ALS), with the electrodiagnostic studies playing a supporting role. The reasons to perform such studies in patients with suspected ALS are to (1) confirm LMN dysfunction in clinically affected regions, (2) detect evidence of LMN dysfunction in clinically uninvolved regions, and (3) exclude other pathophysiological processes such as multifocal motor neuropathy or chronic myopathy (Chad, 2002).

Although LMN degeneration in ALS may ultimately affect the entire neuraxis (brainstem and cervical, thoracic, and lumbosacral segments of spinal cord), participation in clinical trials requires early diagnosis. Lambert's initial criteria of fibrillation and fasciculation potentials detected in muscles of the legs and arms or in the limbs and the head were stringent. These criteria evolved into active and chronic denervation detected in at least three extremities or two extremities and cranial muscles (with the head and neck considered an extremity). The revised El Escorial criteria recommended that needle EMG signs of LMN degeneration be present in at least two of the four central nervous system regions (i.e., the brainstem, cervical, thoracic, and lumbosacral regions) (Brooks et al., 2000). Though rigid requirement of signs of chronic denervation and reinnervation as well as active denervation in the form of fibrillation potentials had been useful, recent consensus recommends including fasciculation potentials when seen in a muscle with chronic neurogenic changes as evidence equivalent in importance to the presence of fibrillation potentials (de Carvalho et al., 2008).

In patients with suspected motor neuron disease, NCS are useful mostly in excluding other neuromuscular diagnoses such as polyneuropathies. Sensory NCS findings usually are normal in anterior horn cell disorders, whereas motor NCS show normal results or low CMAP amplitudes consistent with LMN loss. Motor nerve conduction velocities are normal or slightly slowed but never below 70% of the lower limits of normal. Furthermore, the NCS do not show other demyelinating features such as conduction blocks, characteristic of multifocal motor neuropathy, a treatable disorder that may mimic LMN disease.

Upper Motor Neuron Lesions

In patients with UMN lesions, electrodiagnostic studies show normal insertional activity, no spontaneous activity at rest, and normal MUAP morphology. The only abnormality is a reduced interference pattern and a poor activation with a slow rate of motor unit discharge (see **Fig. 32B.15**). Recruitment measured by either recruitment frequency or ratio is normal. Nonphysiological weakness or poor effort produces a similar pattern, except that motor unit firing may be irregular.

Myopathic Disorders

Insertional activity usually is normal except in the late stage of muscular dystrophies, when it is reduced secondary to atrophy and fibrosis. Fibrillation potentials usually are absent, except in necrotizing myopathies such as inflammatory myopathies and muscular dystrophies (see Fibrillation Potentials). Random loss of fibers from the motor unit leads to a reduction of MUAP amplitude and duration (see **Fig. 32B.13**). Regeneration of muscle fibers sometimes gives rise to long-duration spikes and satellite potentials. Early recruitment is the rule because of the need for more motor units to maintain a given force in compensation for the small size of individual units (see **Fig. 32B.15**).

A disadvantage of the electrodiagnostic study of myopathies is that the needle EMG findings are not always specific enough to make a final diagnosis (**Table 32B.2**). Exceptions include conditions associated with (1) myotonia, such as the myotonic dystrophies, myotonia congenita, paramyotonia congenita, hyperkalemic periodic paralysis, acid maltase deficiency, and some toxic myopathies (such as from colchicine), and (2) fibrillation potentials, which occur in necrotizing myopathies such as inflammatory myopathies and progressive muscular dystrophies (such as Becker and Duchenne muscular dystrophies). Another disadvantage of the needle EMG is that findings either are normal or include subtle abnormalities in some myopathies, such as the metabolic and endocrine myopathies (Lacomis, 2002). Therefore, normal findings on the needle EMG do not exclude a myopathy.

In polymyositis and dermatomyositis, it is essential to recognize the changing pattern on the needle EMG at diagnosis, after treatment, and during relapse. Fibrillation potentials appear first at diagnosis or relapse and disappear early during remission. Abnormal MUAP morphology becomes evident later and takes longer to resolve. The presence of fibrillation potentials also is helpful in distinguishing exacerbation of myositis from a corticosteroid-induced myopathy (Wilbourn, 1993).

Specialized Electrodiagnostic Studies

F Wave

A supramaximal stimulus applied at any point along the course of a motor nerve elicits a small, late, motor response (F wave) after the CMAP (M response). The *F wave* derives its name from *foot*—the first recording was from the intrinsic foot muscles. The nerve action potential initiated during a motor nerve conduction study travels in two directions: distally (orthodromically) to depolarize the muscle and generate a CMAP, and proximally (antidromically), toward the spinal cord, to trigger an F wave. The long-latency F wave is a very small CMAP that results from backfiring of antidromically activated anterior horn cells, averaging 5% to 10% of the motor neuron pool. The F wave's afferent and efferent loops are the motor neuron, with no intervening synapse (Fisher, 2002). The F wave varies in latency, morphology, and amplitude with each stimulus because a different population of anterior horn cells backfires. Therefore, an adequate study requires that about 10 F waves be clearly identified (**Fig. 32B.16, *A***). Moving the stimulator proximally decreases the F wave latency because the action potential travels a shorter distance.

The F-wave minimal latency, measured from the stimulus artifact to the beginning of the evoked potential, is the most reliable and useful measurement and represents conduction of the largest and fastest motor fibers. The minimal F-wave latency depends on the length of the nerve studied (see **Fig. 32B.16, *B***). The most sensitive criterion of abnormality in a unilateral disorder affecting a single nerve is a minimum latency difference between the two sides or between two nerves in the same limb. Absolute latencies are useful only for sequential reassessment of the same nerve.

F-wave persistence is a measure of the number of F waves obtained for the number of supramaximal stimulations and usually is greater than 50%, except with stimulation of the peroneal nerve during recording in the EDB. The F-wave conduction velocity provides a better comparison between proximal and distal (forearm or leg) segments. F-wave

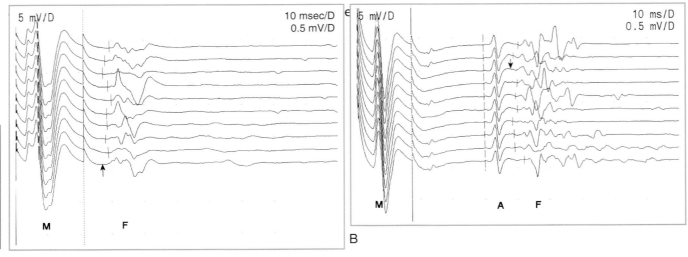

Fig. 32B.16 A, Normal F waves recorded from the hypothenar muscles after supramaximal stimulations of the ulnar nerve at the wrist. Ten consecutive traces are shown in a raster mode. Note the large M response and the significant variability of F-wave latencies (*vertical cursors*) and morphology. The minimum F-wave latency (*arrow*) is 28.5 msec. **B,** Normal F waves recorded from the abductor hallucis after supramaximal stimulations of the tibial nerve at the ankle. Ten consecutive traces are shown in a raster mode showing also the larger M response and the variability of F-wave latencies (*vertical cursors*) and morphology. Note that the minimum F-wave latency (*arrow*) is 48.5 msec owing to the greater length of the tibial nerve, compared with the ulnar nerve in **A.** Note also the presence of a simple A wave that precedes the F wave, with a constant morphology and latency (*dashed vertical line*).

Table 32B.2 Patterns of Needle Electromyographic Findings in Myopathies

Normal	Myopathic MUAPs with Fibrillation Potentials	Myopathic MUAPS Only	Fibrillation Potentials Only	Myopathic MUAPs and Myotonia	Myotonia Only
Metabolic myopathies: McArdle disease Tarui disease Brancher deficiency Debrancher deficiency CPT deficiency Carnitine deficiency Adenylate deaminase deficiency Mitochondrial myopathies: Kearns-Sayre syndrome MELAS MERRF Endocrine myopathies: Steroid (mild) Hypothyroid Hyperthyroid Hyperparathyroid Cushing Others: Fiber type disproportion Acute rhabdomyolysis Periodic paralysis*	Inflammatory myopathies: Polymyositis Dermatomyositis Inclusion body myositis Sarcoid myopathy HIV-associated myopathy Muscular dystrophies: Duchenne Becker Distal Others: Critical illness myopathy Myotubular myopathy Parasitic infections (trichinosis)	Muscular dystrophies: FSH Limb girdle Oculopharyngeal Congenital Congenital myopathies: Central core Nemaline rod Endocrine myopathies: Steroid (severe) Hypothyroid Hyperthyroid Hyperparathyroid Toxic myopathies: Alcohol Emetine	Inflammatory myopathies†: Polymyositis Dermatomyositis Sarcoid myopathy HIV-associated myopathy Others: Chloroquine	Myotonic dystrophies: DM1 DM2 Muscle channelopathies: Paramyotonia congenita Hyperkalemic periodic paralysis* Others: Acid maltase deficiency Myotubular myopathy Colchicine	Myotonia congenita Thomsen disease Becker disease Other myotonic disorders: Atypical painful myotonia Myotonia fluctuans

*, Between attacks; †, early or mild; *CPT,* carnitine palmitoyltransferase deficiency; *FSH,* facioscapulohumeral; *HIV,* human immunodeficiency virus; *McArdle disease,* myophosphorylase deficiency; *MELAS,* mitochondrial encephalomyopathy, lactic acidosis, and stroke-like episodes; *MERRF,* myoclonic epilepsy and ragged-red fibers; *MUAP,* motor unit action potential; *Tarui disease,* phosphofructokinase deficiency.
Reprinted with permission from Katirji, B., Kaminski, H.J., Preston, D.C., et al. (Eds.), 2002. Neuromuscular Disorders in Clinical Practice. Butterworth-Heinemann, Boston.

chronodispersion reflects the degree of scatter among consecutive F waves and can be determined by calculating the difference between the minimal and maximal F wave latencies; this measure indicates the range of motor conduction velocities in the nerve.

Prolonged F-wave minimal latencies occur in most polyneuropathies, particularly the demyelinating type. In the early phases of Guillain-Barré syndrome, findings on routine motor nerve studies may be normal except for prolonged or absent F responses, which imply proximal demyelination (Al-Shekhlee et al., 2005; Gordon and Wilbourn, 2001). F-wave latencies in radiculopathies have limited use. They may be normal despite partial motor axonal loss, and most muscles have multiple root innervations (Wilbourn and Aminoff, 1998).

A Wave

The A wave (axonal wave) is a potential seen occasionally during recording of F waves at supramaximal stimulation. The A wave follows the CMAP and often precedes, but occasionally follows, the F wave. The A wave may be seen in asymptomatic persons during studies of the tibial nerve. It may be mistaken for an F wave, but its constant latency and morphology differentiate it from the highly variable morphology and latency of the F wave (see **Fig. 32B.16, _B_**). A waves sometimes are seen in axon-loss polyneuropathies, motor neuron disease, and radiculopathies, whereas multiple or complex A waves often are associated with acquired or inherited demyelinating polyneuropathies. The exact pathway of the A wave is unknown; the constant morphology and latency of the A wave are best explained by the fixed point of a collateral reinnervating sprout or an ephapse between two axons.

H Reflex

The H reflex, named after Hoffmann for his original description, is an electrical counterpart of the stretch reflex elicited by a mechanical tap to the tendon. The group 1A sensory fibers and alpha motor neurons form the respective afferent and efferent arcs of this predominantly monosynaptic reflex. The H reflex and the F wave can be distinguished by increasing stimulus intensity. The H reflex is best elicited by a long-duration stimulus, submaximal to produce an M response (**Fig. 32B.17**), whereas the F wave requires supramaximal stimulus intensity. In contrast with the F wave, which can be elicited from any limb muscle, the H reflex from stimulating the tibial nerve while recording the soleus muscle (S1 arc reflex) is the most reproducible and commonly used in clinical practice. Absent H reflexes are very common although not specific in the early phases of Guillain-Barré syndrome (Al-Shekhlee et al., 2005; Gordon and Wilbourn, 2001) and in peripheral polyneuropathy. An asymmetrically absent or side-to-side latency difference greater than 1.5 msec or amplitude difference of more than 50% is common in S1 radiculopathy (Nishida et al., 1996).

Blink Reflex

The blink reflex generally evaluates the trigeminal and facial nerves and their connections in the pons and medulla. It has an afferent limb mediated by sensory fibers of the supraorbital

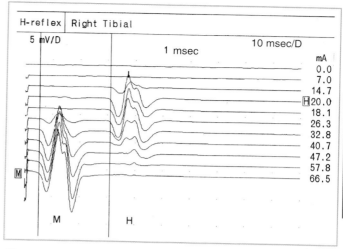

Fig. 32B.17 H reflex recorded from the soleus after stimulation of the tibial nerve at the knee. Shock intensity (in mA) was gradually increased to supramaximal stimulation (_right panel_). Note that the H reflex appeared with subthreshold level of stimulus (14.7 mA), followed by initial increase and subsequent decrease in amplitude with successive stimuli of progressively higher intensity. The H reflex disappeared with shocks of supramaximal intensity (66.5 mA), which elicited a maximal M response.

branch of the ophthalmic division of the trigeminal nerve and an efferent limb mediated by motor fibers of the facial nerve.

With two-channel recording, the blink reflex has two components: an early R1 and a late R2 response. The R1 response is present only ipsilateral to the stimulation and usually is a simple triphasic waveform with a disynaptic pathway between the main trigeminal sensory nucleus in the midpons and the ipsilateral facial nucleus in the lower pontine tegmentum. The R2 response is a complex waveform and is the electrical counterpart of the corneal reflex. It typically is present bilaterally, with an oligosynaptic pathway between the nucleus of the trigeminal spinal tract in the ipsilateral pons and medulla, and interneurons forming connections to the ipsilateral and contralateral facial nuclei.

The blink reflex is most useful in evaluating unilateral lesions such as facial palsy, trigeminal neuropathy, or a pontine or medullary lesion. With a facial nerve lesion, the R1 and R2 potentials are absent or delayed with supraorbital stimulation ipsilateral to the lesion, whereas the R2 response on the contralateral side is normal. With a trigeminal nerve lesion, the ipsilateral R1 and R2 and contralateral R2 are absent or delayed, whereas all responses are normal with contralateral stimulation. With a midpontine lesion involving the main sensory trigeminal nucleus or the pontine interneurons to the ipsilateral facial nerve nucleus, supraorbital stimulation on the side of the lesion results in an absent or delayed R1 but an intact ipsilateral and contralateral R2. Finally, with a medullary lesion involving the spinal tract and trigeminal nucleus or the medullary interneurons to the ipsilateral facial nerve nucleus, supraorbital stimulation on the affected side results in a normal R1 and contralateral R2 but an absent or delayed ipsilateral R2. In demyelinating polyneuropathies such as Guillain-Barré syndrome or type 1 Charcot-Marie-Tooth disease, a marked delay of all blink responses may occur, reflecting slowing of motor fibers or sensory fibers or both.

Repetitive Nerve Stimulation
Principles

Repetitive stimulation of motor or mixed nerves is performed to evaluate patients with suspected neuromuscular junction disorders, including myasthenia gravis, Lambert-Eaton myasthenic syndrome, botulism, and congenital myasthenic syndromes. The design and plans for repetitive nerve stimulation (RNS) depend on physiological factors inherent in the neuromuscular junction that dictate the type and frequency of stimulations used in the diagnosis of neuromuscular junction disorders. The CMAP obtained during routine NCS represents the summation of all muscle fiber action potentials generated in a muscle after supramaximal stimulation of all motor axons while recording via surface electrode placed over the belly of a muscle.

- A *quantum* is the amount of acetylcholine in a single vesicle, which is approximately 5000 to 10,000 acetylcholine molecules. Each quantum (vesicle) released results in a 1-mV change of postsynaptic membrane potential. This occurs spontaneously during rest and forms the basis of the miniature end-plate potential.
- The number of quanta released after a nerve action potential depends on the number of quanta in the *immediately available* (i.e., *primary*) store and the probability of release: $m = p \times n$, where m = the number of quanta released during each stimulation, p = the probability of release (effectively proportional to the concentration of calcium and typically about 0.2, or 20%), and n = the number of quanta in the immediately available store. In normal conditions, a single nerve action potential triggers the release of 50 to 300 vesicles (quanta), with an average equivalent to about 60 quanta (60 vesicles). In addition to the immediately available store of acetylcholine located beneath the presynaptic nerve terminal membrane, a *secondary* (or *mobilization*) *store* starts to replenish the immediately available store after 1 to 2 seconds of repetitive nerve action potentials. A *large tertiary* (or *reserve*) *store* also is available in the axon and cell body.
- The *end-plate potential* is the potential generated at the postsynaptic membrane after a nerve action potential. Because each vesicle released causes a 1-mV change in the postsynaptic membrane potential, this results in an approximately 60-mV change in the amplitude of the membrane potential.
- In normal conditions, the number of quanta (vesicles) released at the neuromuscular junction by the presynaptic terminal far exceeds the postsynaptic membrane potential change necessary to reach the threshold needed to generate a postsynaptic muscle action potential. This is the basis of the *safety factor*, which results in an end-plate potential that is always above threshold and able to generate a muscle fiber action potential. In addition to quantal release, other factors that contribute to the safety factor and the end-plate potential include acetylcholine receptor conduction properties, acetylcholine receptor density, and acetylcholinesterase activity (Boonyapisit et al., 1999).
- *Voltage-gated calcium channels* open after depolarization of the presynaptic terminal, leading to calcium influx.

Through a calcium-dependent intracellular cascade, vesicles dock into active release zones, releasing acetylcholine molecules. Calcium then diffuses slowly out of the presynaptic terminal in 100 to 200 msec. The rate at which motor nerves are repetitively stimulated dictates whether or not calcium accumulation plays a role in enhancing the release of acetylcholine. At slow rate of RNS (i.e., a stimulus every 200 msec or more; or a stimulation rate less than 5 Hz), the calcium role in acetylcholine release is not increased, and subsequent nerve action potentials reach the nerve terminal long after calcium has dispersed. By contrast, with rapid RNS (i.e., a stimulus every 100 msec or less; a stimulation rate greater than 10 Hz), calcium influx is greatly increased, and the probability of release of acetylcholine quanta increases.

Slow Repetitive Nerve Stimulation

The application of three to five supramaximal stimuli to a mixed or motor nerve at a rate of 2 to 3 Hz is the technique of slow RNS. This rate is low enough to prevent calcium accumulation but high enough to deplete the quanta in the immediately available store before the mobilization store starts to replenish it. Three to five stimuli are adequate for the maximal release of acetylcholine.

Calculation of the decrement with slow RNS entails comparing the baseline CMAP amplitude with the lowest CMAP amplitude (usually the third or fourth). The CMAP decrement is expressed as a percentage and calculated as follows:

$$\% \text{ Decrement} = \frac{\text{CMAP amplitude of 1st response} - \text{CMAP amplitude of 3rd or 4th response}}{\text{CMAP amplitude of 1st response}} \times 100$$

In normal conditions, slow RNS does not cause a CMAP decrement. Although the second through fifth end-plate potentials fall in amplitude, they remain above threshold (because of the normal safety factor) and ensure muscle fiber action potential generation after each stimulation. In addition, the secondary store begins to replace the depleted quanta after the first few seconds, with a subsequent rise in the end-plate potential. Therefore, all muscle fibers generate muscle fiber action potentials, and the CMAP does not change in size. In *postsynaptic neuromuscular junction disorders* (such as myasthenia gravis), the safety factor is reduced because fewer acetylcholine receptors are available. Therefore, the baseline end-plate potential reduces but usually is still above threshold. Slow RNS results in a decrease in end-plate potential amplitudes at many neuromuscular junctions. As end-plate potentials decline below the threshold, the number of muscle fiber action potentials produced declines, leading to a CMAP decrement (**Fig. 32B.18**). In *presynaptic neuromuscular junction disorders* (such as Lambert-Eaton myasthenic syndrome), the baseline end-plate potential is low, with many end-plates not reaching threshold. Therefore, many muscle fibers do not fire, resulting in low baseline CMAP amplitude (**Table 32B.3**). With slow RNS, further CMAP decrement occurs, caused by the further decline of acetylcholine release with the subsequent stimuli, resulting in further loss of many end-plate

Table 32B.3 CMAPs and RNS in Neuromuscular Junction Disorders

Neuromuscular Junction Defect	Prototype Disorder	CMAP	Slow RNS	Rapid RNS*
Postsynaptic	Myasthenia gravis	Normal	Decrement	Normal or decrement
Presynaptic	Lambert-Eaton myasthenic syndrome	Low	Decrement	Increment

*Or post brief-exercise CMAP.
CMAP, Compound muscle action potential; RNS, repetitive nerve stimulation.

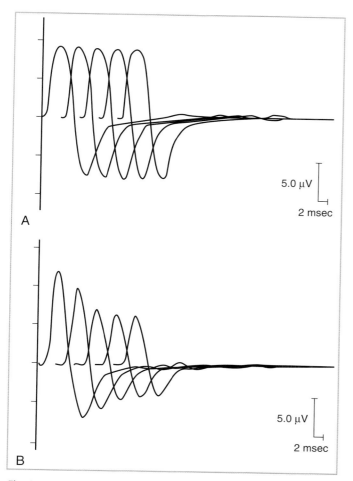

5.0 µV

2 msec

A

5.0 µV

2 msec

B

Fig. 32B.18 Slow (2-Hz) repetitive nerve stimulation in a healthy control subject **(A)** and in a patient with generalized myasthenia gravis **(B)** showing compound muscle action potential decrement. *(Reprinted with permission from Katirji, B., 2007. Electromyography in Clinical Practice: a Case Study Approach. Mosby, St. Louis.)*

potentials and muscle fiber action potentials (Katirji and Kaminski, 2002).

In patients with suspected myasthenia gravis, the diagnostic yield of slow RNS increases if the following recommendations are applied:

1. *Obtain slow RNS at rest and after exercise.* If a reproducible CMAP decrement (less than 10%) appears at rest, slow RNS should be repeated after the patient exercises for 10 seconds to demonstrate repair of the decrement (*posttetanic facilitation*). If no or equivocal (less than 10%) decrement occurs at rest, the patient should perform maximal voluntary exercise for 1 minute. Then, repeat slow RNS every 30 seconds afterward and for 3 to 5 minutes after exercise. Because the amount of acetylcholine released with each stimulus is at its minimum 2 to 5 minutes after exercise, slow RNS after exercise increases the chance of detecting a defect of neuromuscular transmission at the neuromuscular junction by demonstrating a worsening CMAP decrement (*postexercise exhaustion*).

2. *Record from clinically weakened muscles.* Most commonly used and technically feasible nerves for slow RNS are the median, ulnar, and spinal accessory nerves. The diagnostic sensitivity is clearly higher for slow RNS recording in proximal muscles than in distal muscles. Facial nerve repetitive stimulation is indicated in patients with oculobulbar weakness (Zinman et al., 2006), but this study is technically difficult and sometimes associated with a large stimulation artifact that renders waveform interpretation subject to error.

3. *Warm the extremity studied* (skin temperature should be above 32°C). This precaution decreases false-negative results, because cooling improves neuromuscular transmission and may mask the decrement.

4. *Discontinue cholinesterase inhibitors* for 12 to 24 hours (if clinically possible). This measure also decreases the false-negative rate with slow RNS.

Rapid Repetitive Nerve Stimulation

Rapid RNS is most useful in patients with suspected presynaptic neuromuscular junction disorders such as Lambert-Eaton myasthenic syndrome or botulism. The optimal frequency is 20 to 50 Hz for 2 to 10 seconds. A typical rapid RNS applies 200 stimuli at a rate of 50 Hz (i.e., 50 Hz for 4 seconds). Calculation of CMAP increment after rapid RNS is as follows:

$$\% \text{ Increment} = \frac{\text{CMAP amplitude of the largest response} - \text{CMAP amplitude of 1st response}}{\text{CMAP amplitude of 1st response}} \times 100$$

A brief (10-second) period of maximal voluntary isometric exercise is much less painful and has the same effect as that of rapid RNS at 20 to 50 Hz. Application of a single supramaximal stimulus generates a baseline CMAP. Then the patient performs a 10-second maximal isometric voluntary contraction, followed by another stimulus that produces the postexercise CMAP.

With rapid RNS or postexercise CMAP evaluation, two competing forces act on the nerve terminal. First, stimulation tends to deplete the pool of readily available synaptic vesicles. This depletion reduces transmitter release by reducing the number of vesicles released in response to a nerve terminal action potential. Second, calcium accumulates in the nerve terminal, thereby increasing the probability of synaptic vesicle release. In a normal nerve terminal, the effect of depletion of readily available synaptic vesicles predominates, so that with rapid RNS, the number of vesicles released decreases. The end-plate potential does not fall below threshold, however, because of the safety factor. Therefore, the supramaximal stimulus generates action potentials in all muscle fibers, and

no CMAP decrement occurs. In fact, rapid RNS or brief (10-second) exercise in normal subjects often leads to a slight physiological increment of the CMAP that does not exceed 40% to 50% of the baseline CMAP. The probable cause is increased synchrony of muscle fiber action potentials after tetanic stimulation (*posttetanic pseudofacilitation*).

In a presynaptic disorder such as Lambert-Eaton myasthenic syndrome, very few vesicles release, and many muscle fibers do not reach threshold, resulting in low baseline CMAP amplitude. With rapid RNS, the calcium concentrations in the nerve terminal increases high enough to enhance release of a sufficient number of synaptic vesicles to result in a larger end-plate potential that crosses threshold and is capable of action potential generation. This leads to many muscle fibers firing and results in a CMAP increment (see **Table 32B.3**). The increment often is higher than 200% in Lambert-Eaton myasthenic syndrome (**Fig. 32B.19**), with 10-second postexercise facilitation achieving the highest diagnostic sensitivity

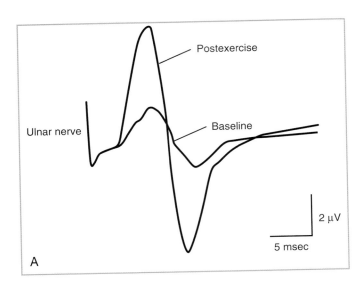

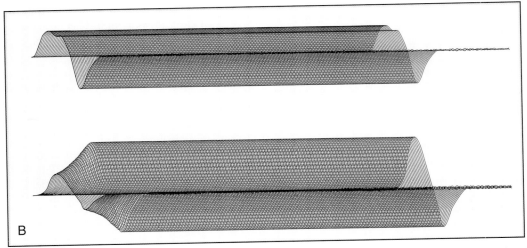

Fig. 32B.19 A, Baseline and compound muscle action potential (CMAP) after brief exercise (Postexercise) in a patient with Lambert-Eaton myasthenic syndrome. Note the significant CMAP increment (294%) after brief (10 seconds) exercise. **B,** Rapid (50-Hz) repetitive nerve stimulation in a control subject (*top*) and in a patient with Lambert-Eaton myasthenic syndrome (*bottom*). No CMAP increment is observed for the control subject, whereas a significant (250%) increment is apparent for the patient. (*Reprinted with permission from Katirji, B., 2007. Electromyography in Clinical Practice: a Case Study Approach. Mosby, St. Louis.*)

(Hatanaka and Oh, 2008). Patients with botulism have a less pronounced increment, ranging from 40% to 200%, due to the more severe neuromuscular blockade (Witoonpanich R et al., 2009). In a postsynaptic disorder such as myasthenia gravis, rapid RNS causes no change of CMAP, because the depleted stores are compensated by calcium influx. In severe postsynaptic blockade (such as during myasthenic crisis), the increased quantal release cannot compensate for the marked neuromuscular block, resulting in a drop in end-plate potential amplitude. Therefore, fewer end-plates reach threshold, and fewer muscle fiber action potentials are generated, resulting in CMAP decrement.

Single-Fiber Electromyography

The technical requirements for performing single-fiber EMG are as follows. First, a concentric single fiber needle electrode allows the recording of single muscle fiber action potentials. The small side port on the cannula of the needle serves as the pickup area. A single fiber needle electrode records from a circle of 300-mm radius, as compared with the l-mm radius of a conventional concentric EMG needle. Recent studies have shown no difference in sensitivity or specificity between the reusable single fiber and disposable concentric-needle electrodes (Sarrigiannis et al., 2006; Stålberg and Sanders, 2009). Second, the amplifier must have an impedance of 100 megohms or greater to counter the high electrical impedance of the small leadoff surface, the gain is set higher for single-fiber EMG recordings than for conventional EMG, the sweep speed is faster, and the filter should have a 500-Hz low frequency to attenuate signals from distant fibers. Third, an amplitude threshold trigger allows recording from a single muscle fiber, and a delay line permits viewing of the entire waveform even though the single-fiber potential triggers the sweep. Fourth, computerized equipment assists in data acquisition, analysis, and calculation.

Voluntary (recruitment) single-fiber EMG is a common method for activating muscle fibers. A mild voluntary contraction produces a biphasic potential with duration of approximately 1 msec and amplitudes that vary with the recording site. Single-fiber potentials suitable for study must have peak-to-peak amplitude greater than 200 μV, rise time less than 300 μsec, and a constant waveform. Rotate, advance, and retract the needle until a potential records meeting these criteria. Stimulation single-fiber EMG is a newer technique performed by inserting another monopolar needle electrode near the intramuscular nerve twigs and stimulating through it at a low current and constant rate. This method does not require patient participation and is therefore useful in children or on uncooperative or comatose patients. Single-fiber EMG is useful in assessing fiber density or in jitter analysis (see later discussion).

Fiber Density

Fiber density is calculated as the number of single-fiber potentials firing almost synchronously with the initially identified single-fiber potential. Increased muscle fiber clustering indicates collateral sprouting. Simultaneously firing single-fiber potentials within 5 msec after the triggering single-fiber unit are counted at 20 to 30 sites. For example, in the normal

extensor digitorum communis muscle, single fibers fire without nearby discharges in 65% to 70% of random insertions, with only two fibers discharging in 30% to 35%, and with three fibers discharging in 5% or fewer. Calculation of an average number of single muscle fiber potentials per recording site is possible. In conditions producing loss of the normal mosaic distribution of muscle fibers from a motor unit, such as following reinnervation, fiber density increases.

Jitter

Jitter is the variability of the time interval between two muscle fiber action potentials (a muscle pair) innervated by the same motor unit. It is the variability of the interpotential intervals between repetitively firing paired single fiber potentials (Stålberg and Trontelj, 1997) (**Fig. 32B.20**). Neuromuscular jitter can be determined by using a commercially available computer program. The program calculates the mean value of consecutive interval differences over a number of 50 to 100 discharges, as follows:

$$MCD = \frac{[IPI\ 1 - IPI\ 2] + [IPI\ 2 - IPI\ 3] + \ldots + [IPI\ (N-1) - IPI\ N]}{N-1}$$

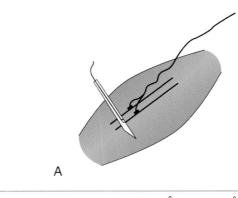

A

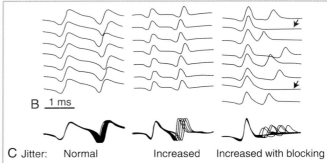

Fig. 32B.20 Voluntary single-fiber electromyographic jitter study. **A,** The jitter is measured between two single muscle fiber action potentials innervated by the same motor unit. Normal, moderately increased jitter is seen in a patient with myasthenia gravis, and greatly increased jitter with intermittent blocking (*arrows*) is evident in another patient with myasthenia gravis. The upper tracings **(B)** are shown in a raster mode, and the lower tracings **(C)** are superimposed. *(Reprinted from Stålberg, E., Trontelj, J.V., 1997. The study of normal and abnormal neuromuscular transmission with single fibre electromyography. J Neurosci Methods 74, 145-154, with permission from Elsevier Science.)*

MCD is the mean consecutive difference, IPI 1 is the interpotential interval of the first discharge, IPI 2 of the second discharge, and so on, and N is the number of discharges recorded.

Neuromuscular blocking is the intermittent failure of transmission of one of the two muscle fiber potentials. This reflects failure of one of the muscle fibers to transmit an action potential, owing to failure of the end-plate potential to reach threshold. Blocking is the extreme abnormality of the jitter, measured as the percentage of discharges of a motor unit in which a single-fiber potential does not fire. For example, in 100 discharges of the pair, if a single potential is missing 30 times, the blocking is 30%. In general, blocking occurs when the jitter values are significantly abnormal.

The expression of the results of single-fiber EMG jitter studies is by the mean jitter of all potential pairs, the percentage of pairs with blocking, and the percentage of pairs with normal jitter. Because jitter may be abnormal in 1 of 20 recorded potentials in healthy subjects, the study is considered to indicate defective neuromuscular transmission if the mean jitter value exceeds the upper limit of the normal jitter value for that muscle, if more than 10% of potential pairs (e.g., more than 2 of 20 pairs) exhibit jitter values above the upper limit of the normal jitter, or if any neuromuscular blocking is present.

Jitter analysis is highly sensitive but not specific. Although jitter often is abnormal in myasthenia gravis and other neuromuscular junction disorders, it also may be abnormal in a variety of neuromuscular disorders including motor neuron disease, peripheral neuropathies, and myopathies. Therefore, the diagnostic value of jitter must be considered in light of the patient's clinical manifestations and other electrodiagnostic findings.

References

The complete reference list is available online at www.expertconsult.com.

Clinical Neurophysiology
Transcranial Magnetic Stimulation

Young H. Sohn, Mark Hallett

At the beginning of the 1980s, Merton and Morton developed the first method of noninvasive brain stimulation, *transcranial electrical stimulation* (TES), and this had obvious clinical application. They used a single, brief, high-voltage electric shock and produced a relatively synchronous muscle response, the *motor evoked potential* (MEP). The latency of MEPs was compatible with activation of the fast-propagating corticospinal tract. It was immediately clear that this method would be useful for many purposes, but a problem with TES is that it is painful owing to simultaneous stimulation of pain fibers in the scalp. Five years later, Barker and colleagues demonstrated that it was possible to stimulate the brain (and nerves as well) using external magnetic stimulation (*transcranial magnetic stimulation*; TMS), with little or no pain. TMS is now commonly used in clinical neurology to study central motor conduction time. Depending on the stimulation techniques and parameters, TMS can excite or inhibit the brain activity, allowing functional mapping of cortical regions and creation of transient functional lesions. It is now widely used as a research tool to study aspects of human brain physiology including motor function and the pathophysiology of various brain disorders. Because TMS can influence the brain, there have been attempts to use it as therapy, particularly when used repetitively (*repetitive transcranial magnetic stimulation*, rTMS). Therapeutic investigations have included stroke rehabilitation, amelioration of movement disorders, and alleviation of pain and tinnitus, but effects demonstrated so far have generally been mild. There is currently only one therapeutic indication for rTMS: medically intractable depression (Padberg and George, 2009). In this situation it can be used as an alternative to electroconvulsive therapy (ECT) to induce a remission which would then be pharmacologically maintained.

Methods and Their Neurophysiological Background

For magnetic stimulation, a brief, high-current (usually several thousands amps within 200 µs) electrical pulse is produced in a coil of wire called the *magnetic coil*, which is placed above the scalp. A magnetic field is induced perpendicular to the plane of the coil. Such a rapidly changing magnetic field induces electric currents in any conductive structure nearby, with the flow direction parallel to the magnetic coil but opposite in direction. The magnetic field falls off rapidly with distance from the coil; with a 12 cm–diameter round coil, the strength falls by half at a distance of 4 to 5 cm from the coil surface. For this reason, stimulation is severely attenuated at deep sites. The electrical field induced by TMS is parallel to the surface, and horizontally oriented excitable elements such as the axon collaterals of pyramidal neurons and various interneurons are excited preferentially.

In experimental animals, a single electrical stimulus applied at threshold intensity to the motor cortex produces descending volleys in the pyramidal tract with the same velocity at intervals of about 1.5 ms. The first volley is termed the *D-wave* (D for direct wave), which is thought to originate from the direct activation of the pyramidal tract. The subsequent volleys are termed *I-waves* (I for indirect wave), presumed to be elicited by transsynaptic activation of the pyramidal tract via intrinsic corticocortical circuitry. TMS also produces both D- and I-waves in descending pyramidal neurons. In contrast to electrical stimulation that preferentially evokes D-wave first, TMS at threshold intensity often produces a corticospinal volley with I-waves but no early D-wave (Ziemann and Rothwell, 2000). This finding suggests that TMS activates pyramidal neurons indirectly through synaptic inputs but does not activate them directly, presumably because of the direction of its current flow. Standards for the use of TMS and review of side effects have been published (Rossi et al., 2009).

Stimulation Parameters
Central Motor Conduction Measurements

With TMS, it is possible to measure conduction in central motor pathways (*central conduction time*; CCT). CCT can be estimated by subtracting the conduction time in the peripheral nerves and neuromuscular junction from the total latency of MEPs measured at the onset of the initial deflection. *Peripheral motor conduction time* is currently measured through two methods: (1) F-wave recordings for the measurement of spine-to-muscle conduction time and (2) direct stimulation of the efferent roots and nerves over the spine. Magnetic stimulation on the posterior neck or the dorsal spine activates spinal roots at the level of the intervertebral foramen. Since the cervical roots are excited about 3 cm away from the anterior horn cell, magnetic stimulation of the roots is not an accurate measurement of CCT and may miss a proximal partial or complete block of impulse propagation. F-waves are usually elicited in the relaxed state by delivering supramaximal stimulation to the peripheral motor nerve at a site near the muscle under examination. The stimulus evokes an orthodromic volley in the motor nerves that produces a short latency response in the muscle (M wave). In addition, an antidromic volley travels back to the spinal cord, exciting the spinal motoneurons, and an efferent volley travels down to the motor nerve, causing a late excitation of the muscle known as the *F-wave*. Total peripheral motor conduction time can be estimated as: $(F + M - 1)/2$ (1 is the time due to the central delay at the level of α-motoneuron). Consequently, the CCT can be obtained as follows: MEP latency $- (F + M - 1)/2$. Using this method, the average CCT is about 6.4 ms for the thenar muscles and 13.2 ms for the tibialis anterior.

Motor Excitability Measurements
Motor Thresholds

Motor threshold (MT) represents the minimal stimulation intensity producing MEPs in the target muscle. This can be measured in resting (*resting motor threshold*, RMT) or contracting (*active motor threshold*, AMT) muscles. RMT is determined to the nearest 1% of the maximum stimulator output and is commonly defined as the minimal stimulus intensity required to produce MEPs of greater than 50 μV in at least 5 out of 10 consecutive trials. Here the MEP amplitudes are usually measured peak to peak. AMT is determined in the moderately active muscle (usually between 5% and 10% of the maximal voluntary contraction) and is defined as the minimum intensity that produces either MEPs of greater than 100 μV or silent period or MEPs of greater than 200 μV in at least 5 out of 10 consecutive trials. MT in resting muscle reflects the excitability of a central core of neurons, depending on the excitability of individual neurons and their local density. Since MT can be influenced by drugs that affect voltage-gated sodium and calcium channels, it may represent membrane excitability.

MEP Recruitment Curve

The *recruitment curve*, also known as the *stimulus response curve* or the *input-output curve*, is the growth of MEP size as a function of stimulus intensity. This underlying physiology is poorly understood but appears to involve neurons in addition to the core region activated at threshold. The slope of the recruitment curve is related to the number of corticospinal neurons that can be activated at a given stimulus intensity, mainly indirectly through corticocortical connections. The neurons that can be activated at a lower threshold are highly excitable neurons located in core regions of corresponding motor cortex, while neurons recruited at a higher intensity may have a higher threshold for activation, either because they are intrinsically less excitable or because they are spatially further from the center of activation by the magnetic stimulus. These neurons would be part of the "subliminal fringe." The changes in recruitment curve are usually more prominent with higher-intensity stimulations. This finding suggests that the recruitment curve may represent the excitability of less excitable or peripherally located neurons rather than highly excitable core neurons or the connections between them. The slope of the recruitment curve is increased by drugs that enhance adrenergic transmission (e.g., dextroamphetamine) and is decreased by sodium and calcium channel blockers and by γ-aminobutyric acid (GABA) agonists.

Silent Period and Long-Interval Intracortical Inhibition

The *silent period* (SP) is a pause in ongoing voluntary electromyography (EMG) activity produced by TMS (**Fig. 32C.1, A**). The SP is usually measured with a suprathreshold stimulus in moderately active (usually 5%–10% of maximal voluntary contraction) muscle. SP duration is usually defined as the interval between the magnetic stimulus and the first recurrence of rectified voluntary EMG activity (Chen et al., 1999; Curra et al., 2002). While the first part of the SP is due in part to spinal cord refractoriness, the latter part is entirely due to cortical inhibition (*cortical silent period*, CSP). If a second suprathreshold *test stimulation* (TS) is given during the SP following suprathreshold *conditioning stimulus* (CS) (usually 50–200 ms after the first stimulus), its MEP is significantly suppressed (*long intracortical inhibition*; LICI) (see **Fig. 32C.1, B**) (Chen et al., 1999; Curra et al., 2002). SP and LICI appear to assess GABA$_B$ function, although other drugs affecting membrane excitability or dopaminergic transmission also influence SP. Although LICI and SP share similar mechanisms, they may not be identical, because they are affected differently in various diseases (Berardelli et al., 1996).

Short-Interval Intracortical Inhibition and Intracortical Facilitation

Various inhibitory and excitatory connections in the motor cortex can be evaluated by TMS using a paired-pulse technique. A subthreshold CS preferentially excites interneurons, by which MEPs from a following TS are suppressed at *interstimulus intervals* (ISIs) of 1 to 5 ms (*short intracortical inhibition*; SICI for such inhibition at short intervals) or facilitated

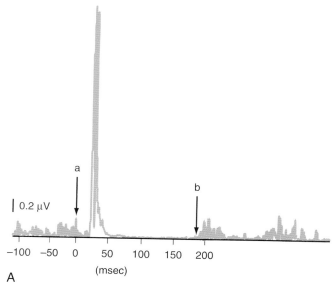

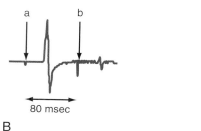

Fig. 32C.1 A, Rectified electromyography (EMG) recording of the first dorsal interosseus after single transcranial magnetic stimulation (TMS) under isometric contraction at 10% of maximal voluntary contraction. The silent period (SP) can be measured from TMS trigger (a) to reoccurrence of EMG activity (b). **B,** Paired-pulse TMS with suprathreshold conditioning stimulation. Test stimulation (b) with same stimulation intensity is applied at 80 ms after conditioning stimulation (a). MEP of test stimulation is significantly suppressed compared to conditioning stimulation. *LICI,* Long intracortical inhibition.

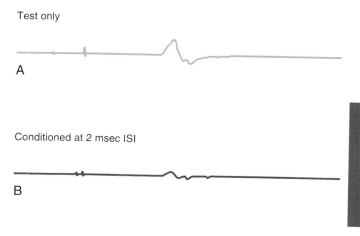

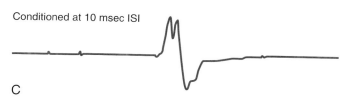

Fig. 32C.2 Paired-pulse transcranial magnetic stimulation with subthreshold conditioning stimulation. At 2 ms interstimulation interval (ISI) **(B)**, motor evoked potential (MEP) amplitude is significantly suppressed compared to test stimulation alone **(A)** (i.e., *short intracortical inhibition*, SICI). At 10 ms ISI, MEP amplitude is significantly increased **(C)** (i.e., *intracortical facilitation*, ICF).

at ISIs of 8-20 ms (*intracortical facilitation*; ICF) (**Fig. 32C.2**) (Ziemann, 1999; Ilic et al., 2002). SICI and ICF reflect interneuronal activity in the cortex. SICI is likely largely a GABAergic effect, especially related to GABA$_A$ receptors, whereas ICF is largely a glutamatergic effect. SICI can be divided into two phases, with maximum inhibition at ISI of 1 ms and 2.5 ms. SICI at 1 ms ISI is presumably caused either by neuronal refractoriness resulting in desynchronization of the corticospinal volley or by different inhibitory circuits; SICI at ISI of 2 ms or longer is most likely a synaptic inhibition.

The magnitude of SICI depends on the intensity of CS and TS. With a given CS, TS intensity variation results in a U-shaped variation of SICI magnitude, with a maximum inhibition at TS producing MEPs with peak-to-peak amplitude of around 1 mV. Variation of CS intensity at a given TS intensity also leads to a U-shaped change in SICI magnitude, with maximum SICI occurring at CS intensity around 90% AMT or 70% RMT. The low end of CS intensity producing SICI represents SICI threshold. Increased magnitude of SICI with CS above SICI threshold may indicate increasing recruitment

of inhibitory interneurons that contribute to SICI, and decreased magnitude of SICI with increased CS intensities above those producing maximum SICI may represent recruitment of facilitatory processes (presumably those mediating short-interval intracortical facilitation; see next section) that superimpose with SICI. Therefore, reduced SICI observed in various disease conditions may represent either a true reduction in SICI or enhanced facilitation or both. Measuring the low and high ends of CS producing SICI is now considered a more sensitive and informative method to assess neurophysiological changes occurring in various conditions than simply measuring the magnitude of SICI.

Short-Interval Intracortical Facilitation

Short-interval intracortical facilitation (SICF) is also known as *facilitatory I-wave interactions* and is measured in a paired-pulse TMS protocol. In contrast to SICI and ICF, however, SICF is elicited by a suprathreshold first stimulus and a subthreshold second stimulus, or two near-threshold stimuli. SICF is usually observed at discrete ISIs of 1.1 to 1.5 ms, 2.3 to 2.9 ms, and 4.1 to 4.4 ms. ISIs producing facilitatory response in SICF are about 1.5 ms apart, similar to the intervals of different I-waves, which suggests that SICF originates in those neural structures responsible for the generation of I-waves (Ziemann and Rothwell, 2000). The second pulse is thought to excite the initial axon segments of excitatory interneurons, which are depolarized by excitatory postsynaptic potentials from the first pulse without firing an action potential. GABA$_A$ agonists reduce SICF.

Short-Latency and Long-Latency Afferent Inhibition

Afferent inhibition can be measured by applying a conditioning sensory stimulus such as median nerve stimulation followed by a test stimulus over the contralateral motor cortex. MEP inhibition usually occurs at ISIs of approximately 20 ms (*short-latency afferent inhibition*, SAI) and 200 ms (*long-latency afferent inhibition*, LAI) (Chen, 2004). SAI is thought to be of cortical origin because the recordings of corticospinal volleys demonstrate a strong suppression of later I-waves, with unaffected earlier descending waves. SAI is reduced by the acetylcholine antagonist, scopolamine, suggesting that SAI can be used to test the integrity of cholinergic neural circuits. Accordingly, SAI is reduced in patients with Alzheimer disease and is improved with a single dose of rivastigmine, an acetylcholinesterase inhibitor. The mechanism mediating LAI is still unclear but is thought to be different from that of SAI.

Surround Inhibition

Surround inhibition (SI), suppression of excitability in an area surrounding an activated neural network, has been proposed to be an essential mechanism in the motor system, where it could aid the selective execution of desired movements. Using a self-triggered TMS technique in which TMS is set to be triggered by EMG activity from the activated muscle (agonist), MEPs of the surrounding muscles (i.e., muscles near the agonist but unrelated to its movement) are suppressed during the movement (up to 80 ms after EMG onset) despite enhanced

spinal excitability (Sohn and Hallett, 2004c). SI is reduced in patients with focal hand dystonia and may be altered in other disorders of human motor control such as Parkinson disease (PD).

Other Inhibitory Phenomena of the Motor Cortex

Interhemispheric inhibition (IHI) can also be assessed by TMS by applying a conditioning stimulus to the motor cortex, which suppresses MEPs produced by a test stimulus over the contralateral motor cortex at ISIs of between 6 and 50 ms (Di Lazzaro et al., 1999). IHI is thought to occur at the cortical level, although subcortical structures may also be involved. Long-latency IHI at ISIs between 20 and 50 ms is likely mediated by GABA$_B$ receptors.

Magnetic stimulation of the cerebellum, which can be performed using a double-cone coil, inhibits the MEPs produced by stimulation of the contralateral motor cortex 5 to 7 ms later (*cerebellar inhibition*, CBI) (Iwata and Ugawa, 2005). Cerebellar stimulation is thought to activate Purkinje cells in the cerebellar cortex, leading to inhibition of the deep cerebellar nuclei, such as dentate nucleus, which have a disynaptic excitatory pathway to the motor cortex via the ventral thalamus. CBI is reduced or absent in patients with cerebellar degeneration or lesions in the cerebellothalamocortical pathway.

Table 32C.1 summarizes the characteristics of different motor excitability measures using TMS.

Table 32C.1 Summary of Motor Excitability Measurements Using Transcranial Magnetic Stimulation

Measurement	Methods		ISIs (ms)	Proposed Mechanisms (Pharmacology)
	Conditioning	Test		
MT		Near threshold		Membrane excitability
RC		Suprathreshold		Recruitment of less excitable neurons
SP		Suprathreshold		GABA$_B$, GABA$_A$?, dopamine?
LICI	Suprathreshold	Suprathreshold	50-200	GABA$_B$
SICI	Subthreshold	Suprathreshold	1-6	GABA$_A$
ICF	Subthreshold	Suprathreshold	8-20	Glutamate
SICF	Suprathreshold/Near threshold	Subthreshold/Near threshold	1.1-1.5, 2.3-2.9, 4.1-5.0	GABA$_A$
SAI	Peripheral nerve	Suprathreshold	20	Acetylcholine
LAI	Peripheral nerve	Suprathreshold	200	
SI	Movement of unrelated muscle	Suprathreshold	0-80	GABA$_A$?
IHI	Opposite motor cortex	Suprathreshold	8-50	GABA$_B$?
CBI	Cerebellum	Suprathreshold	5-7	

CBI, Cerebellar inhibition; *GABA*, γ-aminobutyric acid; *ICF*, intracortical facilitation; *IHI*, interhemispheric inhibition; *ISI*, interstimulus interval; *LAI*, long-latency afferent inhibition; *LICI*, long-interval intracortical inhibition; *MT*, motor threshold; *RC*, recruitment curve; *SAI*, short-latency afferent inhibition; *SI*, surround inhibition; *SICF*, short-interval intracortical facilitation; *SICI*, short-interval intracortical inhibition; *SP*, silent period.

Clinical Applications

Since its introduction, TMS has been increasingly used to evaluate the underlying neurophysiological mechanisms in various neurological disorders (Curra et al., 2002; Chen, 2004; Sohn and Hallett, 2004b) (**Table 32C.2**). In addition, many studies have been performed to investigate the effect of various neurologically acting drugs on TMS measurements (Ziemann, 2004) (**Table 32C.3**), and these provide useful information about the mechanisms mediating various TMS techniques, as well as better understanding of the mechanism of these drugs. A report regarding the clinical diagnostic utility of TMS has been published by a committee of the IFCN (International Federation of Clinical Neurophysiology) (Chen et al., 2008).

Table 32C.2 Changes in Transcranial Magnetic Stimulation Measurements in Various Neurological Disorders

	MT	MEP/RC	SP	LICI	SICI	ICF	SAI	SI	CBI
Movement disorders:									
Parkinson disease	–		↓	↑/↓	↓	–	–	↓	–
Dystonia	–	↑	↓	↓/↑	↓	–	–	↓	
Huntington disease	–	↓	↑/–		↓	↑/↓	↓		
Paroxysmal kinesigenic dyskinesia	–	–	–	↓	–/↓	–		↑	
Other degenerative disorders:									
Alzheimer disease	↓/–	↑			↓	–	↓		
Cerebellar degeneration	↑		↑/–	↑	–	↓			↓
Amyotrophic lateral sclerosis	↑/–	↓	↓	↓	↓	–			–

↑, Increased; ↓, reduced; –, unchanged; *CBI*, cerebellar inhibition; *ICF*, intracortical facilitation; *IHI*, interhemispheric inhibition; *ISI*, Interstimulus interval; *LAI*, long-latency afferent inhibition; *LICI*, long-interval intracortical inhibition; *MEP*, motor evoked potential; *MT*, motor threshold; *RC*, recruitment curve; *SAI*, short-latency afferent inhibition; *SI*, surround inhibition; *SICF*, short-interval intracortical facilitation; *SICI*, short-interval intracortical inhibition; *SP*, silent period.

Table 32C.3 Acute Effects of Neurological Drugs on Transcranial Magnetic Stimulation Measurements

Drugs	MT	MEP/RC	CSP	LICI	SICI	ICF	SICF	SAI
Na$^+$ channel blockers	↑↑	=/↓	=		=/↓	=/↓	=	
GABA$_A$ agonists	=	↓↓	–/↑		↓↓/–	↓/–	↓	
GABA$_B$ agonists	–		↓	↓	↑	↓	–	
Glutamate (NMDA) antagonists	=	=	=		↑	↓	–	
Levodopa/dopamine agonists	=	=/↓	↑↑/–		↑↑/–	=	↓	
Dopamine antagonists	=	↑	=		=/↓	–/↑		
Norepinephrine agonists	=	↑	–		=/↓	↑↑		
Serotonin reuptake inhibitor	=	↑	–		↓	–		
Anticholinergics	–/↓	–/↑	=	↑	–/↓	–/↑		↓
Other drugs								
Ethanol	–	–	↑		↑	↓		
Gabapentin	=		↑↑		↑↑	↓↓		
Levetiracetam	–/↑	↓	–/↑		=	=		
Topiramate	–		–		↑			
Piracetam							↓	

↑, Increased; ↓, reduced; –, unchanged; ↑↑, ↓↓, =, indicate consistent observations in two or more studies; *CSP*, cortical silent period; *GABA*, γ-aminobutyric acid; *ICF*, intracortical facilitation; *LICI*, long-interval intracortical inhibition; *MEP*, motor action potential; *MT*, motor threshold; *NMDA*, N-methyl-D-aspartate; *RC*, recruitment curve; *SAI*, short-latency afferent inhibition; *SICF*, short-interval intracortical facilitation; *SICI*, short-interval intracortical inhibition; *SP*, silent period.

Movement Disorders

Parkinson Disease and Parkinson-Plus Syndromes

CCT is normal in Parkinson disease (PD) but can be prolonged in patients with multisystem atrophy (MSA) and progressive supranuclear palsy (PSP), which suggest a possible role of CCT measurements in patients with Parkinson-plus syndromes involving the pyramidal tracts. A reduction in SICI has been observed in various movement disorders regardless of the nature of the disturbances (Berardelli, 1999). In PD, reduced SICI is only observed at high CS intensities, suggesting increased facilitation rather than reduced inhibition (MacKinnon et al., 2005). In patients with corticobasal degeneration, SICI is often markedly reduced or turned into facilitation along with reduced IHI (Pal et al., 2008). SP is shortened in PD. Increased LICI has been noted in patients with PD and dystonia, but a recent study demonstrated a reduced LICI and reduced presynaptic inhibition in the motor cortex in PD (Chu et al., 2009). SAI is normal in patients with PD but is reduced in patients with MSA. LAI is reduced in PD, which is not affected by dopaminergic medications. SI is reduced or absent on the asymptomatic side of patients with unilateral PD (Shin et al., 2007). Dopaminergic drugs enhance SICI and prolong SP, whereas dopamine-blocking agents reduce SICI and increase ICF. These observations suggest that motor cortex excitability depends on the balance between different inhibitory mechanisms, some of which are under basal ganglia control. Several studies measured changes in TMS parameters after subthalamic nucleus deep brain stimulation (DBS). The SP is lengthened and ICF is enhanced after DBS, but no SP change was observed in another study. Reduced SAI, presumably associated with dopaminergic medications, and reduced LAI were restored by DBS.

Dystonia

In patients with focal dystonia, reduced SICI is not site specific and was also observed on unaffected sides in patients with upper-limb dystonia and in hand muscles of patients with cervical and facial dystonia. In patients with dystonia, shortening of SP is observed but only in dystonic muscles. In writer's cramp, decrease in LICI was observed in the symptomatic hand during muscle activation. Both SICI and LICI were found to be abnormal in psychogenic dystonia, which limits the value of these measures in differentiating organic from psychogenic disorders (Espay et al., 2006; Quartarone et al., 2009). SICI is normal in dopa-responsive dystonia (DYT5) (Hanajima et al., 2007). Recruitment curve, SP, SICI, LICI, ICF, and SICF were all normal in patients with myoclonus-dystonia (DYT15) (Li et al., 2008; van der Salm et al., 2009). In patients with focal dystonia, LAI is diminished or absent, but SAI is normal. SI is reduced or absent in patients with focal hand dystonia (Sohn and Hallett, 2004a) but may be extended in patients with paroxysmal kinesigenic dyskinesia (Shin et al., 2010).

Huntington Disease

Patients with Huntington disease (HD) have shown prolonged SP that correlates with the severity of chorea. However, preclinical and early-stage patients with HD showed normal SP,

normal or increased MT, normal SICI with slightly higher SICI threshold, enhanced ICF, and reduced SAI (Nardone et al., 2007; Schippling et al., 2009).

Other Neurodegenerative Disorders

In AD, motor cortical hyperexcitability was demonstrated by TMS, which included reduced MT, enhanced MEP, and reduced SICI. However, intracortical facilitation appeared normal as measured by ICF and SICF. Reduced MT was significantly correlated with the severity of cognitive impairments. SAI, representing cholinergic system function, is reduced in patients with AD and is reversed by the oral administration of cholinesterase inhibitors. Abnormal SAI in combination with a large increase in SAI after a single dose of anticholinesterase inhibitor may indicate a favorable response to these drugs. SAI was also found to be abnormal in patients with Lewy body dementia but is usually normal in frontotemporal dementia.

In patients with various types of cerebellar degeneration, MT, CSP and LICI are often increased. ICF is reduced without change in SICI, and CBI is usually reduced or absent. However, these changes are different among the various types of cerebellar degeneration (Schwenkreis et al., 2002). In patients with inherited cerebellar ataxia, reduced ICF can be more specific for spinocerebellar ataxia (SCA) 2 and 3, whereas prolonged CCT was found in patients with Friedreich ataxia and SCA 1, 2, and 6. The alterations in TMS measurement in patients with amyotrophic lateral sclerosis (ALS) are different according to the main lesions involved in the disease, but are usually increased MT and decreased MEP, CSP, LICI, and SICI. In some patients whose clinical manifestations are atypical, these TMS findings may help diagnose the disease.

Epilepsy and Antiepileptic Drugs

There are several different mechanisms for the genesis of epileptic seizures and for the modes of action of antiepileptic drugs (AEDs). TMS can be used to give information about these mechanisms by measuring cortical excitability. For example, motor threshold is decreased in untreated patients with idiopathic generalized epilepsy. On the other hand, in progressive myoclonic epilepsy, threshold is normal, but there is loss of cortical inhibition demonstrated with paired pulses at 100 to 150 ms and an increase in facilitation at 50 ms. Prolonged SP was found in idiopathic generalized epilepsy and also in partial motor seizures. Within 48 hours after a generalized tonic-clonic seizure, ICF is reduced but SICI is normal, presumably representing a protective mechanism against spreading or recurrence of seizures. Increased motor cortical excitability including reduced MT, increased ICF, and reduced SICI and LICI was observed in the 24 hours before a seizure; opposite changes in motor cortical excitability measures were seen in the 24 hours after a seizure (Badawy et al., 2009). SICI is reduced but ICF is normal in progressive or juvenile myoclonic epilepsy. LICI is also reduced in progressive myoclonic epilepsy and idiopathic generalized epilepsy. Weaker SICI and ICF in the hemisphere ipsilateral to seizure onset were found to have a predictive value for seizure attacks in the subsequent 48 hours in temporal lobe epilepsy patients with acute drug withdrawal (Wright et al., 2006). A long-term follow-up study in drug-naïve patients with generalized or partial epilepsy demonstrated that a decrease in cortical excitability such as increased MT and increased SICI and LICI after medication predicted a high probability of being seizure free after 1 year of treatment (Badawy et al., 2010).

Specific effects can be seen with various AEDs in normal subjects. AEDs that enhance the action of GABA (e.g., vigabatrin, gabapentin, lorazepam) increase SICI but have no effect on MT. In contrast, the AEDs blocking voltage-gated sodium or calcium channels (phenytoin, carbamazepine, lamotrigine) increase MT without significant effects on SICI (Ziemann et al., 1996). In addition to elucidating these mechanisms, TMS can potentially be used to quantify physiological effects in individual patients, and this may be more valuable in some circumstances than monitoring blood levels of AEDs.

Stroke

Several studies have attempted to correlate clinical recovery from stroke to the characteristics of MEPs. MEPs are often absent in severely affected stroke patients. In mildly affected patients, MEPs are usually of longer latency, smaller amplitude, and higher motor threshold. The presence of MEPs in the early stage of stroke is associated with a good functional recovery (Hendricks et al., 2002). Conversely, absence of MEPs in a paretic limb, with concomitantly increased MEP amplitudes in the unaffected limb, predicts poor recovery. In addition, the presence of ipsilateral MEPs in the paretic limb in response to the stimulation of the unaffected hemisphere is also associated with poor recovery. The recovery of MEP latency is highly correlated with return of hand function. Higher MT than normal is often associated with the signs of spasticity. Noninvasive mapping of the motor cortex can be carried out with TMS using the figure-of-eight-shaped coil. This technique has been used to evaluate cortical reorganization in various conditions. In stroke patients, it has been demonstrated that cortical reorganization of the motor output still occurs up to several months after insult. There is progressive enlargement of the motor maps of the recovering affected part. SICI is reduced in the affected hemisphere in the acute phase of a motor cortical stroke and remains reduced regardless of functional recovery. SICI also tends to be reduced in the unaffected hemisphere but subsequently returns to normal or can be greater than that in the affected hemisphere in patients showing good recovery. Enhanced SICI may lead to reduced activity in the unaffected hemisphere, which enhances activity of the affected hemisphere and promotes recovery.

Multiple Sclerosis

CCT measurement has been applied in the evaluation of patients with multiple sclerosis (MS), where there is frequent involvement of the corticospinal tract. Typically there is either a unilateral or bilateral prolongation of CCT consistent with demyelinating lesions in the corticospinal tract (Schmierer et al., 2002). Prolonged CCT is more pronounced in progressive MS than in relapsing-remitting MS. Similar to other evoked potential studies, MEPs vary considerably in latency, amplitude, and shape in patients with MS when they are measured consecutively. An increased MT is also frequently observed in patients with MS.

Cervical Myelopathy and Other Spinal Cord Lesions

Along with measurements of somatosensory evoked potentials, TMS is a useful tool for detecting cervical myelopathy. In patients with this disorder, MEPs as well as the MEP:CMAP ratio (compound muscle action potential), are usually reduced. CCT is prolonged, and their interside difference is increased. Simultaneous recordings from muscles innervated by different cord segments can help define the spinal level of a lesion. Prolonged CCT often correlates with the clinical severity and degree of cord compression observed with magnetic resonance imaging (MRI). In a study recruiting large numbers of patients with cervical myelopathy (Lo et al., 2004), the sensitivity of TMS in differentiating the presence and absence of MRI cord abnormality was 100%, and the specificity was around 85%. CCT measures of the muscles innervated by cranial nerves (e.g., trapezius, tongue) may help differentiate ALS from cervical myelopathy. Abnormal CCT to these muscles indicates high probability of ALS.

References

The complete reference list is available online at www.expetconsult.com.

Clinical Neurophysiology
Neuromodulation

Abhay Kumar, Ajay K. Pandey, Michael S. Okun

Many critical functions of the human body are controlled by the central and/or peripheral nervous systems. Certain disorders can disrupt normal, healthy functioning of either of these nervous systems and lead to clinically relevant symptoms. This chapter focuses on new developments in neuromodulatory strategies to combat nervous system dysfunction. As targets are identified for drug and device development, a new sense of hope has emerged among patients, families, and scientists alike. New breakthroughs have been made in targeting specific brain regions with neuropharmacological and neuromodulatory therapies.

Neuromodulation as a distinct specialty is a recent development in therapeutic and restorative management of nervous system disorders. Neuromodulation has evolved as an interdisciplinary area of medicine where collaborative efforts among experts from various fields have converged, with the common goal of designing, testing, and understanding the interface between engineered devices and the human brain in our attempts to treat human disease. To date, neuromodulatory electrical, chemical, and mechanical interventions have all been used in both animal models and humans. Neuromodulation is rapidly evolving and often parallels advances in technology.

Neuroscientists have defined *neuromodulation* as a dynamic process wherein a substance, usually a neurotransmitter, affects neuronal function by its action on the synapses and by modulating the response of the cell to other inputs, with potentially important behavioral implications. Neuromodulation has come to be more broadly defined as a process whereby the central, peripheral, or autonomic nervous system is electrically excited, inhibited, stimulated, modified, regulated, or therapeutically altered to achieve the desired effect (Krames et al., 2009). An ongoing dynamic process that affects targeted neural networks and utilizes electrical or neuropharmacological stimulation, neuromodulation may offer clinical outcomes that are potentially modifiable by simply adjusting stimulation parameters (Holsheimer, 2003). Other relevant terms that have been used to describe neuromodulation and its related techniques have included *neurostimulation, neuroaugmentation, neuroprosthetics, functional electrical stimulation* (FES), *assisted technologies,* and *neural engineering.* The International Neuromodulation Society has further defined neuromodulation "as a field of science, medicine and bio-engineering that encompasses both implantable and non-implantable technologies that may be electrical or chemical, and serve the purpose of improving quality of life and the overall functioning of humankind" (Sakas et al., 2007a).

Multiple specialties use neuromodulatory techniques for a variety of clinically relevant issues including augmentation of vision and hearing, cardiac pacing, and treating movement disorders, pain, epilepsy, stroke, depression, addiction, and gastrointestinal (GI) and urinary conditions. For more information on the history and classifications of neuromodulation, please go to www.expertconsult.com.

Applications of Neuromodulatory Devices

The human nervous system is composed of many complex and distinct neural networks. These networks may include chemical and electrical synapses, and they may communicate both within and between network structures. The structure and subsequently the behavior of these neural networks may be "shaped by the extrinsic as well as intrinsic neuromodulatory effects that include those of hormones and neurotransmitters" (Destexhe et al., 2004; Katz and Frost, 1996).

Table 32D.1 Classification of Neuromodulation Devices

Stimulation	Electrical (e.g., DBS, MCS, SCS, PNS, TENS) Pharmacological (e.g., infusion pumps)
Application	Neuroprosthesis (auditory, retinal implants, phrenic/sacral nerve stimulators) Neuro-orthosis
Purpose	Therapeutic (neurostimulators for breathing, bladder and bowel functions) Rehabilitation (neurostimulators for extremity functions)
Placement	Implanted and invasive (DBS) External and noninvasive (neurostimulators for extremity functions)
Control and directionality	Open-loop (VNS, DBS) Closed-loop (NeuroPace)
Effect on nervous system	Central nervous system (DBS) Peripheral nervous system (PNS)

DBS, Deep brain stimulation; *MCS*, motor cortex stimulation; *PNS*, peripheral nerve stimulation; *SCS*, spinal cord stimulation; *TENS*, transcutaneous electrical nerve stimulation; *VNS*, vagus nerve stimulation.

The classifications and applications of neuromodulation devices are summarized in **Table 32D.1**.

Neurostimulation devices may involve either the application of deep brain/spinal cord leads or surface leads, or alternatively they may use direct stimulation of the spinal cord and/or peripheral nerves. Precisely placed leads may be connected via an extension cable to a pulse generator and ultimately to some sort of power source (battery). This process has the potential to generate the necessary electrical stimulation and to (hopefully) provide clinically relevant benefits (Panescu, 2008). Signals can be excitatory, inhibitory, or both (e.g., excite fibers and inhibit cells) (Vitek, 2002).

Table 32D.2 offers a selected summary of the literature on deep brain stimulation (DBS) neuromodulation for movement and neuropsychiatric disorders, and **Table 32D.3** is a selected summary of the literature on non-DBS neuromodulation.

Extended versions of these tables are available online at www.ExpertConsult.com.

Motor Cortex Stimulation

Motor cortex stimulation (MCS) was utilized by Tsubokawa and colleagues, who originally presented this option as a possible safer alternative to DBS surgery in Dejerine syndrome (central thalamic pain syndrome) (Tsubokawa et al., 1991). It has been hypothesized that MCS induces antidromic activation of the sensory cortex, and this results in inhibition of the abnormal burst activity in a damaged and possibly deafferented sensory thalamus. Imaging studies "on" and "off" MCS have shown interesting blood flow changes within the ventrolateral (VL) tier of the thalamus, the medial thalamic regions, and the anterior cingulated cortex, orbitofrontal cortex, anterior insular cortex, and upper brainstem. Perhaps the most interesting aspect of post-MCS imaging has been the finding that blood flow does not seem to increase in the somatosensory cortex. Interpretations of this data have been variable, but the latest suggestions are that descending projections from the cortex to the thalamus can be activated and potentially lead to changes in basal ganglia pathophysiology within a loop responsible for both pain and emotional aspects of pain (Garcia-Larrea et al., 1999). It is thought that MCS may primarily stimulate γ-aminobutyric acid (GABA)-ergic interneurons that are found to be in parallel orientation to other layers of the cerebral cortex (Manola et al., 2007). Researchers have noticed that pain relief (≥40%-50% improvement on the visual analog scale) from MCS seems to be greatest in cases where the corticospinal tract is found to be relatively intact (Katayama et al., 1998). Interestingly, when MCS is applied, patients with paretic extremities and concomitant central pain problems may have noticeable benefits in motoric weakness, rigidity, and spasticity. These improvements can, in select cases, aid in improving rehabilitation potential (Katayama et al., 1998).

MCS has been applied in cases of pharmacoresistant trigeminal neuralgia, painful peripheral neuropathy, and certain spinal cord pathologies. A greater than 50% pain relief has been reported in various studies of patients with central and neuropathic pain (Katayama et al., 1998; Nguyen et al., 1999). Data from randomized controlled studies for any application of MCS are lacking, however. There appears to be a large placebo effect with the therapy, and it has been noted that the effects may wane over time (Fontaine et al., 2009; Lima et al., 2008). Motor cortex stimulation has been attempted for therapeutic treatment of Parkinson disease (PD) and multiple system atrophy (MSA), but to date, results have been disappointing (Gutierrez et al., 2009; Kleiner-Fisman et al., 2003).

Information on transcranial magnetic stimulation (TMS) can be found in Chapter 32C as well as in the online version of this chapter at www.ExpertConsult.com.

Deep Brain Stimulation

Over the last 2 decades, chronic DBS has become routine for several diagnoses in neurological practice (e.g., PD, dystonia, essential tremor) and has been used experimentally for selected neuropsychiatric indications (e.g., obsessive compulsive disorder [OCD], depression, Tourette syndrome [TS]). Interestingly, as early as the 1950s, temporary DBS electrodes were implanted into the septal region for pain control, and they were reported to have beneficial effects (Hamani et al., 2006). Over the ensuing years, there were various attempts at DBS, with most documented experiences revealing its usefulness in test stimulation prior to ablating brain lesions (Blomstedt and Hariz, 2010). In 1987 when Professor Benabid was operating on a chronic pain patient, he noticed that the patient's tremor improved during test stimulation, and he decided to chronically stimulate this patient. Over the ensuing 2 decades, multiple DBS placements into multiple brain regions for a variety of clinical indications have occurred (Awan et al., 2009).

High-frequency stimulation (HFS) has been thought to effect a basal ganglia network–wide change, acting as a sort of informational lesion (Birdno and Grill, 2008; McIntyre et al., 2004a; McIntyre et al., 2004b). Thus, PD computer model systems have been developed to attempt to elucidate

Table 32D.2 DBS Neuromodulation: Selected Summary of the Literature* (See Extended Online-Only Version)

Author	Site/ No.	Follow-up	Outcomes/Author Conclusions
PARKINSON DISEASE			
(Follett et al., 2010)	GPi (B/L): 152 STN (B/L): 147	2 years	Similar improvement in motor function with stimulation of either target. STN group: lesser medication requirement; more decline in visuomotor skills and level of depression compared to GPi group.
(Krack et al., 2003)	STN (B/L): 49	5 years	Improved motor function, dyskinesia and ADLs off medication. Worsened on medication: akinesia, speech, postural stability, freezing, and cognitive problems.
(Zahodne et al., 2009)	STN (U/L): 20 GPi (U/L): 22	6 months	U/L DBS in both STN and GPi improved QoL overall across several domains with greater improvements in GPi DBS reported. Decreased letter fluency in STN.
(Vesper et al., 2007)	STN (B/L):73	2 years	DBS of the STN is clinically as effective in elderly patients as in younger patients.
TREMOR			
(Hariz et al., 2008)	VIM: 38 (PD)	6 years	Tremor effectively controlled by DBS, with stable appendicular rigidity and akinesia. Axial scores worsened. Improvement in ADLs disappeared despite tremor control.
(Blomstedt et al., 2007)	VIM: 19 (ET)	7 years	Effective treatment for ET, but improvement diminishes over time.
DYSTONIA			
(Vidailhet et al., 2007)	GPi (B/L): 22	3 years	Motor improvement maintained 1 year postoperatively. Randomized study. Stopped in 3 patients, since no improvement.
(Coubes et al., 2004)	GPi (B/L): 31	2 years	Improvement in both DYT1 +/− mutation groups in overall functional as well as clinical scores at 2 years.
PAIN			
(Fontaine et al., 2010)	PH: 11 (CH)	1 year	Controlled phase failed to demonstrate superiority over sham stimulation. Open phase showed >50% improvement in 6 patients.
(Broggi et al., 2007)	PH: 16 (CH), 1: (SUNCT), 3: (AFP)	18 months	10/16 CH patients completely pain free; SUNCT patient responded; no benefit in AFP.
EPILEPSY			
(Fisher et al., 2010)	ANT: 110	2 years	54% patients with >50% seizure reduction at 2 years.
NEUROPSYCHIATRY			
(Greenberg et al., 2010)	VC/VS: 26 (OCD)	24-36 months	Two-thirds of patients improved; patients with more posterior target had more effective treatment.
(Goodman et al., 2010)	VC/VS: 6 (OCD)	1 year	4/6 patient responders; sham stimulation period for half the patients.
(Servello et al., 2008)	CM-Pfc, VO B/L: 18 TS	3-18 months	Variable, but overall good response.

AFP, Atypical facial pain; *ANT*, anterior nucleus of thalamus; *B/L*, bilateral; *CH*, cluster headache; *CM-Pfc*, centromedian-parafascicular; *DBS*, deep brain stimulation; *ET*, essential tremor; *GPi*, globus pallidus interna; *HT*, Holmes tremor; *OCD*, obsessive-compulsive disorder; *PD*, Parkinson disease; *PH*, posterior hypothalamus; *STN*, subthalamic nucleus; *SUNCT*, short-lasting unilateral neuralgiform headache attacks with conjunctival injection and tearing; *TS*, Tourette syndrome; *U/L*, unilateral; *VC*, nucleus ventrocaudalis of the thalamus; *VC/VS*, ventral capsule/ventral striatum; *VIM*, ventral intermediate thalamic nucleus.

*This table is a summary of some of the major neuromodulatory studies, but for space considerations, not all studies could be listed. We apologize to any authors who were excluded.

the mechanism of action of DBS (Birdno and Grill, 2008; McIntyre et al., 2004a; McIntyre et al., 2004b). HFS has been hypothesized to result in a decoupling of the cellular and axonal output within a thalamocortical relay circuit. The firing rates and patterns of the cell body may be suppressed, while the fibers and fibers of passage may be excited. DBS may ultimately effect a corticostriatopallido-thalamocortical (CSPTC) network and result in upstream as well as downstream changes within this complex basal ganglia network (McIntyre and Hahn, 2010). The specific effects of an electrical field are thought to reflect changes relative to the position and orientation of the axon to the actual DBS lead. Also, the electrical field is thought to exert trans-synaptic influences (McIntyre et al., 2004a; McIntyre et al., 2004b). The clinical benefits of DBS have been hypothesized to be due to more than just local neurotransmitter release (Stefani

Table 32D.3 **Non-DBS Neuromodulation: Selected Summary of the Literature* (See Extended Online-Only Version)**

Author	Indication	No.	Neuromodulation	Results
(Ghaemi et al., 2010)	Epilepsy	144	VNS	10/144 patients were seizure free >1 yr
(Colicchio et al., 2010)		135	VNS	89 patients had improvement. The seizure frequency reduction was significant in the group as a whole. Outcome best in children > adolescents > adults.
(Montavont et al., 2007)		50	VNS	~60% responders at 3 years of follow-up. Patients with generalized epilepsy and those with focal abnormality had useful palliation of seizures.
(Bajbouj et al., 2010)	Depression	74	VNS	At 24 months, >50% patients responded to treatment; 19 patients had complete remission.
(Nguyen et al., 1999)	Central and neuropathic pain	32	MCS	10/13 with central pain and 10/12 with neuropathic pain improved.
(Hosomi et al., 2008)	Intractable neuropathic pain	34	MCS	12/32 patients showed improvement in >/= 12-month follow-up.
(Sievert et al., 2010)	Traumatic thoracic spinal cord injury	10	SNM	Early SNM prevents detrusor overactivity and urinary incontinence.
(Brouwer and Duthie, 2010)	Fecal incontinence	55	SNM	Significant and sustained improvement in continence for the patient group as a whole during follow-up period.
(Powell and Kreder, 2010)	Painful bladder syndrome	39	SNM	Long-term benefit continued in 86% at a mean of 59.9 months.
(Kapural et al., 2010)	Chronic visceral abdominal pain	35	SCS	86% of patients had 50% pain relief.

*This table is a summary of some of the major neuromodulatory studies, but for space considerations not all studies could be listed. We apologize to any authors who were excluded.

MCS, Motor cortex stimulation; *SCS,* spinal cord stimulation; *SNM,* sacral neuromodulation; *VNS,* vagus nerve stimulation.

et al., 2005); however, several authors have argued that there is a collective effect and that transmitter release may be very important to the mechanism of action (Dostrovsky and Lozano, 2002; Lee KH et al., 2004; Vitek, 2002). Animal models of DBS have revealed increased extracellular concentrations of glutamate and GABA (Windels et al., 2003) and, most recently, adenosine and dopamine (Chang et al., 2009; Shon et al., 2010). Depolarization blockade, synaptic inhibition, and synaptic depression (McIntyre et al., 2004a; McIntyre et al., 2004b) have also been proposed to play a role in the potential mechanisms of action of DBS.

Selective placement of the DBS leads within different anatomical regions and different somatotopies may affect the neuronal network and, in the best possible cases, lead to improvement in clinical symptoms. For example, the placement of DBS electrodes in the ventralis intermedius nucleus of the thalamus for essential tremor may have an effect on an abnormal thalamocortical oscillatory loop and ultimately suppress tremor (Birdno et al., 2007). Similarly in PD, placement of a DBS lead in the ventralis intermedius may improve tremor; however, to affect bradykinesia and rigidity, one must either implant the ventralis oralis thalamic nucleus or, alternatively, either the subthalamic nucleus or globus pallidus internus (Mann et al., 2009; Oh et al., 2002).

DBS is a relatively simple technology. In its current form, it involves placement of a quadripolar (four contacts) lead into a specific and predetermined brain target. The lead is usually connected to a neurostimulator placed subcutaneously under the clavicle, although the battery can be placed in a multitude of regions. The neurostimulator can then be programmed or adjusted to tailor a setting to an individual patient. There are thousands of different combinations that may be chosen, and the voltage, frequency, and pulse width may be liberally changed. The optimal settings are patient and symptom specific, and they usually require that patients be reprogrammed frequently for the first 4 to 6 months and medications as well as stimulation monitored (Ondo et al., 2005; Rodriguez et al., 2007).

Each disorder or symptom considered for treatment with DBS should be carefully evaluated. Only a small fraction of any neurological or neuropsychiatric disorder may be eligible for this type of therapy. Most patients receiving DBS should be medication resistant, and they should undergo a complete multi-/interdisciplinary screening with a neurologist, psychiatrist, neuropsychologist, and neurosurgeon. Following screening, there should be a detailed interdisciplinary discussion about the goals of therapy (symptoms targeted, symptoms that will likely respond, symptoms not likely to respond). In cases of PD, patients should undergo an "off/on" levodopa medication challenge to determine which symptoms respond best to medication—these usually are the ones that respond best to stimulation (with the exceptions of tremor and dyskinesia). Risks and benefits of a potential DBS surgery, as well as the potential brain target(s), and unilateral versus bilateral DBS should all be carefully addressed in preoperative conversations with patients and families (Alberts et al., 2008; Kluger et al., 2009; Okun et al., 2004; Okun et al., 2007; Okun et al., 2009; Okun and Foote, 2004; Okun and Foote, 2009;

Rodriguez et al., 2007; Skidmore et al., 2006; Ward et al., 2010). There are many potential adverse events that may occur as a result of DBS, some of which may constitute emergencies (Morishita et al., 2010).

Depending on the region of the world and the preference of individual surgical teams, leads and batteries may be placed in a single setting or may be staged (separate operating room procedures). One lead, two leads, or in exceptional circumstances, more than two leads may be implanted in a single session. One recent review of DBS hardware-related complications cited lead migration, lead fracture, lead erosion/infection, and lead malfunction as common occurrences (Lyons et al., 2004; Oh et al., 2002). DBS surgically related and stimulation-related complications can occur and may include (but are not limited to) hemorrhage, infections, strokes, seizures, paresthesias, dysarthria, hypophonia, dystonia, mood worsening, suicide, and worsening of comorbidities. Difficulty with verbal fluency and anger seem to be common sequelae in PD patients (Blomstedt and Hariz, 2005; Blomstedt and Hariz, 2006; Hariz et al., 2008a; Okun et al., 2008a; Saint-Cyr and Albanese, 2006). DBS teams must differentiate between lesion effects, stimulation-induced effects, and transient versus permanent neurological dysfunction. More DBS and device-related studies are needed to prospectively document all adverse effects; this constitutes a critical weakness of many published series (Hariz et al., 2008b).

Parkinson Disease

Parkinson Disease is a complex disorder thought to be the result of extensive loss of neurons and their projections within motor and nonmotor basal ganglia circuitry (Alexander et al., 1986). A rationale for neuromodulatory therapy has been developed as a result of models of basal ganglia physiology. Perhaps the most famous model reveals loss of dopaminergic neurons in the substantia nigra pars compacta, with a resultant abnormal neuronal activity in both the direct and indirect basal ganglia circuitry. These changes are thought to result in the genesis of many of the motor symptoms of PD. Initial treatment of PD is usually with dopaminergic therapy, though over time, disease progression may lead to limitations in medical therapy including such symptoms as wearing off between doses, on/off fluctuations, and hyperkinetic dyskinesia. Subthalamic nucleus (STN) or globus pallidus interna (GPi) DBS have been used to neuromodulate basal ganglia pathways and restore important functions in selected patients (Pahwa et al., 2005; Weaver et al., 2009). Studies are underway to define the selection criteria and help tailor the procedure for individual patients. To date, STN and GPi DBS have shown similar motor outcomes, but STN DBS may allow for larger dopaminergic medication reductions, and GPi DBS may provide better dyskinesia suppression and a relatively safer risk/benefit profile (Anderson et al., 2005; Follett et al., 2010; Mikos et al., 2010; Okun and Foote, 2009; Zahodne et al., 2009). These conclusions, however, will need to be bolstered by randomized clinical studies.

Long-term efficacy of DBS in PD has been good overall, but in all cases, the disease progresses. An important guideline is that symptoms that respond to levodopa continue to respond to DBS, with the exceptions of tremor and dyskinesia, which may have persistent benefits (Krack et al., 2003; Schüpbach et al., 2005; Wider et al., 2008).

Dystonia

Dystonia results from co-contraction of agonist and antagonist muscles, and patients may experience involuntary repetitive movements that result in twisted and sometimes painful postures. Dystonia may be focal, segmental, or generalized based on the body region affected. Other classification systems use age of onset or etiology. The most studied dystonia syndrome has been DYT-1 genetic dystonia; when the DYT-1 gene is expressed prior to age 26, the disease manifests. In those who live asymptomatic past age 26, the mutation (which occurs in the torsin A gene and is due to deletion of the GAG code) remains clinically silent (a carrier state) (Bressman, 2003). This is a phenomenon referred to as *incomplete penetrance*.

Lesion surgery (pallidotomy and thalamotomy) have both been successfully employed for various primary and secondary dystonias (Lozano et al., 1995; Yoshor et al., 2001), though most centers prefer DBS because bilateral lesions may result in speech or cognitive issues (Hua et al., 2003; Ondo et al., 1998). DBS therapy is mainly performed in the pallidal (GPi) target, because stimulation in this region has provided a reasonable alternative to lesion therapy. Most DBS cases have responded best if the dystonia has been of primary origin, although selected secondary dystonias as well as tardive dystonia have had meaningful improvements in small series (Coubes et al., 1999; Kumar R et al., 1999; Kupsch et al., 2003; Tronnier and Fogel, 2000; Vercueil et al., 2001). There have been two large randomized trials to date that addressed primary generalized dystonia, and both short- and long-term outcomes have been promising (Coubes et al., 2004; Vidailhet et al., 2005; Vidailhet et al., 2007). Additionally, the number of indications has been expanding within dystonia (e.g., cerebral palsy), and the number of brain targets also continues to expand (e.g., STN).

One interesting and unique aspect of DBS for dystonia has been the phenomenon that in many cases, the effects seem to be delayed and appear gradually after stimulation initiation (weeks to months). It has been hypothesized that this phenomenon may be the result of neuroplasticity, but its true mechanism remains a mystery. The other evolving story in dystonia DBS has been the use of lower stimulation frequencies for selected cases (Alterman et al., 2007). Which cases may respond to lower frequencies remains an area of investigation.

Tremor

Tremor has been broadly defined as an involuntary and rhythmic oscillation of a body part and has been classified according to its etiology and/or characteristics (e.g., phenomenology, physiology, etc.). It has been hypothesized that physiological disturbances in the cerebellothalamic and pallidothalamic pathways may be the genesis of some but not all tremor subtypes. According to Deuschl et al. (2001), four pathophysiological mechanisms are proposed to result in tremor: mechanical oscillation of the extremity, reflex activation of the oscillation network, central oscillation, and a disturbance in the regulatory feed-forward or feedback loops of an oscillation network. The ventralis intermedius (VIM) nucleus of the thalamus, which takes its input from the cerebellum, forms a vital piece of this regulatory network and has been frequently targeted for high-frequency (≥100 Hz) DBS to address various medication refractory tremors, with the most common being essential tremor (Benabid et al., 1996). DBS therapy has been reported to have similar efficacy as thalamotomy (Schuurman et al., 2000), and it may have fewer short-term side effects but more long-term (device related) side effects when compared to lesion therapy. Although VIM DBS is preferred for pure essential tremor and certain cases of PD tremor, other cerebellothalamic and pallidothalamic pathways may be altered with DBS. For example, outflow (cerebellar/midbrain) tremor, posttraumatic tremor, and multiple sclerosis (MS) tremor have all been treated in small case series by either single or multiple leads in VIM, ventralis oralis posterior, or zona incerta (Foote and Okun, 2005; Foote et al., 2006; Papavassiliou et al., 2008). The exact target(s) for these more complex tremor disorders remain to be investigated.

Typically, unilateral VIM DBS has been employed to control medication-refractory tremor in a contralateral extremity. Unilateral DBS commonly results in side effects of ataxia and speech problems, and these issues may be more commonly encountered when bilateral DBS is used (Pahwa et al., 2006). Midline tremor, head tremor, and voice tremor seem to respond less consistently to DBS (Ondo et al., 2001). Longitudinal follow-up studies have revealed good long-term benefits, although there has been an emerging concern in the field about tolerance and disease progression (Blomstedt et al., 2007; Pahwa et al., 2006; Sydow et al., 2003; Zhang et al., 2010). Other indications such as cerebellar tremor, Holmes tremor, and MS tremor have had worse efficacy when compared to essential tremor, but these outcomes may change with the emergence of better targets, better technology, and multiple lead approaches.

Neuropsychiatric Disorders
Tourette Syndrome

Tourette syndrome (TS) is a complex neuropsychiatric disorder with a usual onset in childhood (mean age 7 years). The disorder is characterized most prominently by changing motor and vocal tics that must be present for at least 1 year and be marked by fluctuations in number, frequency, and complexity (Robertson, 2000). Patients frequently have associated behavioral abnormalities including anxiety, attention deficit hyperactivity disorder, self-injurious behavior, and obsessive-compulsive behavior, which may persist in their adult life even when motor and phonic tics decline or disappear (Jankovic, 2001; Leckman et al., 1998). Only a small minority of patients diagnosed with TS progress to disabling refractory tic disorder or to malignant TS that is unresponsive to medical and behavioral therapy (Cheung et al., 2007). Only a very select group of TS patients may be candidates for DBS.

Although the mechanisms that cause TS are unknown, abnormalities within the limbic and motor loops of the cortical-basal ganglia/thalamocortical circuitry that involve both dopaminergic and serotonergic neurotransmission likely contribute to the motor and behavioral manifestations in mild and severe TS cases (Albin and Mink, 2006; Wichmann et al., 2006). The centromedian-parafascicular (CM-PF) complex of the thalamus (Houeto et al., 2005), the GPi (both motor and non-motor territories), and the anterior limb of the internal capsule have all been targets for DBS therapy. To date, the GPi and the CM-PF seem to respond better than the anterior limb, but more careful studies, including characterization of individual targets, will be needed (Burdick et al., 2010; Flaherty et al., 2005; Maciunas et al., 2007; Porta et al., 2009; Servello et al., 2008; Shields et al., 2008; Visser-Vandewalle et al., 2003). The heterogeneity of patient populations and the small size of these studies have limited interpretation of reported successes and failures. Because of the special risks in this population, the Tourette Syndrome Association has published guidelines for selection of DBS candidates and for the preferred standardized outcome measures that should be employed if attempting these surgeries (Mink et al., 2006).

Depression

Severe refractory depression is much more common than any other potential patient group for DBS therapy. The loss of quality of life, the impact on lost work hours, and the suicide rate make neuromodulatory therapy an attractive alternative for a select group of these patients (Ward et al., 2010). DBS for medication-refractory depression remains investigational and should only be considered when medication, psychotherapy, and electroconvulsive therapy are not helpful, and when an institutional review board experimental protocol has been obtained. Experts have hypothesized that there is an abnormality in the corticostriatal-thalamic-cortical (CSTC) network in severely depressed humans, and that by lesioning or neuromodulating at specific nodes, clinical symptoms may be reduced (e.g., anterior cingulotomy, anterior capsulotomy, subcaudate tractotomy, limbic leucotomy). It has been reported that up to two-thirds of well-selected patients may benefit, but these data are highly preliminary and not inclusive of the entire population of depression patients (Greenberg et al., 2003). Neuromodulatory targets and outcomes have been rapidly emerging and may include subgenual cingulate gyrus/outflow tract, ventral capsule/ventral striatum, nucleus accumbens, and the inferior thalamic peduncle (Greenberg et al., 2010; Mayberg et al., 2005; Ward et al., 2010). To date, the most encouraging results have been achieved with area 25 (cingulate) and anterior limb internal capsule stimulation.

Obsessive-Compulsive Disorder

Another DBS indication that has recently emerged and received U.S. Food and Drug Administration (FDA) approval under a humanitarian device exemption has been OCD. OCD has been characterized by recurrent intrusive thoughts or obsessions that may produce overwhelming anxiety, relieved in some cases by indulgence in ritualistic compulsive behaviors. Functional neuroimaging has revealed hyperactivity within the ventral striatum (VS), medial thalamic region, and orbitofrontal cortex as a potentially abnormal network in this disorder. Patients who are refractory to medical treatment or behavioral approaches could be candidates for a neurosurgical intervention (Tye et al., 2009). Neurosurgical interventions have in the recent past involved lesioning of the anterior limb of the internal capsule (ALIC), cingulotomies, leucotomies, and other approaches (Ward et al., 2010). The idea underpinning early therapies was to create a disconnection between frontal lobe and basal ganglia circuitry to attempt to disrupt the abnormally firing neural network. Apathy and other irreversible complications resulted from early lesion approaches, and most were abandoned in favor of selective lesioning of the

VS or DBS. It has been reported that high-frequency DBS of the bilateral anterior limb of the internal capsule/nucleus accumbens region may achieve remission in more than 50% of well-selected patients (Goodman et al., 2010; Greenberg et al., 2010; Nuttin et al., 2008). Other brain areas that have been successfully targeted include the STN and the inferior thalamic peduncle (Mallet et al., 2008; Ward et al., 2010). It should be stressed that strong interdisciplinary teams including psychiatrists and psychologists should be employed to carefully screen and follow patients who undergo DBS for OCD, depression, and other neuropsychiatric disorders (Okun et al., 2005; Okun et al., 2008a).

Drug Addiction

Addiction is the behavior characterized by relentlessly seeking drugs despite knowledge of possible adverse consequences (Kreek, 2008). Addicts often relapse even after prolonged abstinence (Grant et al., 2004; Kalivas and Volkow, 2005; Substance Abuse and Mental Health Services Administration (SAMHSA), 2008). Imaging studies in humans have revealed that addiction seems to involve sudden surges in extracellular dopamine in limbic areas including the nucleus accumbens (NA) (shell and core) and dorsal striatum. The drug ingestion itself results in pleasurable effects (binge/intoxication stage). When abstaining, there seem to be changes in molecular targets of the specific drugs during an acute phase, and this leads to a proposed hypofunction of the dopamine pathways and may result in disrupted activity of frontal regions including dorsolateral prefrontal regions, cingulate gyrus, and orbitofrontal cortex (OFC) (withdrawal/negative affect stage). Prolonged drug abuse may result in reorganization of the reward and memory circuits and lead to increased sensitivity to various signals which may trigger relapse (craving stage) (Koob and Volkow, 2010). As an alternative to medical therapy, stereotactic neurosurgery-leucotomy (Knight, 1969), hypothalamotomy (Dieckmann et al., 1978), cingulotomy (Kanaka and Balasubramaniam, 1978), and ablation of the nucleus accumbens (Gao et al., 2003) have all been attempted in the past and shown some variable effectiveness. The irreversibility of lesions, the behavioral implications, and the trial designs of ablative procedures have led to uncertainty about their place in clinical practice (Stelten et al., 2008).

Subthalamic nucleus DBS in PD seemed to help with dopamine dysregulation syndrome (Witjas et al., 2005), and DBS in the accumbens seemed to help a single patient with OCD who was suffering from alcohol dependency (Kuhn et al., 2007). Preclinical studies involving DBS of the NA shell in mice (with cocaine-seeking behavior) seemed to reduce the craving for cocaine without affecting other functions. This data suggested that afferent and efferent neuronal activity in the NA may be inhibited or neuromodulated with DBS (Vassoler et al., 2008). Encouraging results from STN DBS and insular cortex DBS in animal models offer hope for this as a potential therapy (Forget et al., 2010; Rouaud et al., 2010).

Pain

Neuromodulatory approaches have been employed for persistent pain syndromes for more than half a century. Many initial studies focused on the hypothalamus as the treatment target, but in later studies, many regions emerged as potential targets for therapy, including various areas of the thalamus as well as periventricular (PV) and periaqueductal (PA) gray regions. PV/PA gray matter regions have been hypothesized to respond better to nociceptive pain, whereas targeting the sensory thalamus has been thought to be better for deafferentation pain (Levy et al., 1987). Neuromodulation has been specifically employed for pain due to phantom-limb, stroke, and anesthesia dolorosa (Bittar et al., 2005). Additionally, after it was appreciated by functional imaging that cluster headache and facial pain syndromes may be related to hypothalamic circuitry, neuromodulation of this region was attempted and has been reported successful in multiple cases (Leone et al., 2006). Follow-up performed for up to 2 years revealed improvement in 50% of patients with cluster headache (Bartsch et al., 2008; Broggi et al., 2007; Schoenen et al., 2005; Starr et al., 2007). A recent study, however, did not show as robust a benefit (Fontaine et al., 2010). Greater occipital nerve stimulation is a less invasive alternative being explored for refractory headaches (Burns et al., 2009).

Epilepsy

Epilepsy affects approximately 50 million people worldwide (Kale, 2002). Despite active antiepileptic drug (AED) development, up to 20% of patients suffer from poor seizure control even with optimal medical therapy (Devinsky, 1999). A subset of these patients may be candidates for anterior temporal lobectomy (ATL), which may result in 80% to 90% seizure freedom (Yoon et al., 2003). For the remaining patients, alternative therapies such as vagal nerve stimulation (VNS) have proven limited in efficacy, although some studies report remarkable improvements (see **Table 32D.3**). Given the tremendous success of DBS for the treatment of movement and neuropsychiatric disorders, clinicians have begun to explore the potential of electrical stimulation for the treatment of a select group of patients with medication-refractory epilepsy.

The process of empirical trials for epilepsy has to date resulted in the discovery of unlikely DBS targets, including the cerebellum and thalamic nuclei. Additionally, DBS for epilepsy has reinvigorated interest in the possibility of long-term, potentially positive neuronal changes that may occur secondary to chronic stimulation and may have benefits even when stimulation has ceased (e.g., batteries of devices burn out, closed-loop devices are employed). This idea of neuronal-level changes has been based in part on the phenomenon of secondary epileptogenesis in patients with long-term poorly controlled seizures. A challenge that DBS may be utilized to address is in repeated ictal insults that may be initiated from a single site and may eventually induce remote and independent ictal activity (Khalilov et al., 2003; Morrell, 1985; Wilder et al., 1969).

Despite recent FDA hearings for approval of DBS for epilepsy, the treatment remains investigational. The mechanisms by which DBS affects seizures or movement disorders are not completely understood. Some theorize that electrical stimulation results in the release of inhibitory neurotransmitters. Others posit that stimulation inactivates neurons via depolarization blockade, although most movement disorders experts agree this is likely not the mechanism of action. There are likely synaptic-level changes, neurochemical changes, and also neurophysiological changes underpinning the benefits of DBS

(Dostrovsky and Lozano, 2002; McIntyre et al., 2004a; Vitek, 2002). Recently it has been discovered that DBS may actually inhibit cells close to an electrical field and excite those farther from it. The timing of delivery of electrical stimulation is also an area of active research. Chronic stimulation with an "open-loop" system that responds to a cue (i.e., seizure) has been recently developed and has been referred to as "closed-loop" treatment (Fisher et al., 2010; Skarpaas and Morrell, 2009). Also, scheduled rather than chronic stimulation has been proposed. Multiple targets have been evaluated for DBS in epilepsy, with variable results. One of the reasons studies have reported variable results with the same DBS target may be that certain seizure types may respond differently to stimulation of a particular target. Multiple targets have been proposed and tried for epilepsy DBS (hippocampus, anterior nucleus, thalamus, CM nucleus, cerebellum, STN, etc.). Despite all the uncertainty, several trials have empirically demonstrated the efficacy of DBS for seizures, even in patients who have failed other therapies. These exciting results have fueled a number of studies designed to firmly establish DBS as an effective treatment for intractable epilepsy. In the largest controlled study of DBS for epilepsy (anterior nucleus stimulation) (Fisher et al., 2010), even though patients with a temporal lobe focus or foci had a significant reduction in seizure frequency, those with diffuse frontal, occipital, or parietal seizure foci failed to benefit. In contrast, STN DBS seems to be more effective in patients with seizures having a frontal focus or spread (Shon et al., 2005).

Closed-Loop Stimulation

Closed-loop devices are programmed to respond to detection of ictal or epileptiform discharges and abort impending seizures. An initial trial of closed-loop stimulation in eight patients with intractable epilepsy involved local closed-loop (n = 4) high-frequency electrical stimulation (HFES) directly to the epileptic focus in response to the abnormal electrocorticographic discharges detected by a seizure-detection algorithm. For patients (n = 4) with multiple remote seizure foci, closed-loop HFES was applied using the anterior nucleus of thalamus. There was significant decrease (>50%) in seizures during the experimental phase in both patient groups (Osorio et al., 2005). Similar experience in four patients (Kossoff et al., 2004) using an external responsive neurostimulator (eRNS; NeuroPace, Inc., Mountain View, California) has encouraged a multicenter trial of an implantable responsive neurostimulator (RNS) that continuously monitors electrographic activity from leads positioned near the seizure foci (up to two). An external programmer is used for detection and stimulation parameters and to retrieve recorded electrographic activity. The RNS delivers electrical stimulation to the seizure focus when it detects the epileptic activity (Skarpaas and Morrell, 2009). An initial feasibility study showed encouraging results, with 50% or greater reduction in 43% of patients with complex partial seizures and 35% reduction in all seizure types (n = 24). Patients with pharmacoresistant partial-onset epilepsy having more than three seizures every month over a period of 4 months were recruited for a randomized, double-blinded, multicenter, sham-controlled clinical trial, which was recently completed to establish safety and efficacy of the RNS system as an adjunctive therapy. Results of this trial should be announced soon (Clinicaltrials.gov NCT00264810).

Vagal Nerve Stimulation

Vagal nerve stimulation (VNS) is the only electrical stimulation–based therapy currently approved by the FDA for nonpharmacological treatment of partial-onset refractory epilepsy in adults and adolescents older than 12 years of age. It is also used in primary generalized epilepsies and in pediatric populations by some epileptologists. It is an open-loop device consisting of a pulse generator placed subcutaneously in the upper left chest. The generator delivers intermittent electrical stimulation via a bipolar lead to the cervical vagus nerve trunk. The electrical stimulation is adjusted based on patient tolerance and clinical response, and it can be modulated using a handheld magnet (Lulic et al., 2009). Although not clearly understood, the electrical stimulation to the vagus nerve involves the locus coeruleus–noradrenergic system and seems to result in modification of forebrain activity. Furthermore, norepinephrine and serotonin concentrations seem to change by modulation of the locus coeruleus and modulation of the raphe nuclei, respectively (George et al., 2010). Changes in concentrations of these neurotransmitters and enhanced activity in the brain regions associated with depression also may result in improved mood and cognition, as was reported in patients with VNS. The FDA approved the adjunctive application of VNS for treatment-resistant depression on the basis of studies (Rush et al., 2005) that showed better antidepressant effects in the VNS group (George et al., 2005; Rush et al., 2005); however, many experts dispute this antidepressant effect.

Common side effects from VNS include hoarseness, cough, paresthesias (that generally occur with delivery of stimulus), and headaches. Transient complications due to implantation of the VNS device include vocal cord injury, facial paralysis, and local infection. VNS is usually well tolerated, and results from retrospective studies suggest significant reduction in seizure frequency (Morris and Mueller, 1999; Murphy, 1999; Sakas et al., 2007b; Spanaki et al., 2004; Uthman et al., 2004).

Spinal Cord Stimulation

The rationale for spinal cord stimulation (SCS) for pain syndromes can be linked to the gate control theory of pain proposed by Melzack and Wall. In this theory, the wide dynamic range (WDR) neurons of the dorsal horn are thought to be abnormally excitable in neuropathic pain, and this may then be neuromodulated and inhibited by SCS. SCS may result in pre- and postsynaptic inhibition of the abnormal peripheral neurons responsible for maintaining excitability of the WDR cells. GABA-ergic function may be similarly augmented. SCS has been shown to result in the release of vasodilatory neurotransmitters and to have resultant reductions in sympathetic tone, especially when utilized for ischemic pain syndromes such as those resulting from angina and peripheral vascular disease (Kunnumpurath et al., 2009).

SCS has been the most commonly applied neuromodulatory approach in the treatment of spinal pain syndromes and especially in the failed back surgery syndrome (FBSS). FBSS can be diagnosed after recurrence of lower back/leg pain and follows a previously successful surgery. Although randomized control trials have revealed that SCS is more effective than conventional medical treatment for FBSS, with sustained pain relief over prolonged periods, the level of evidence remains moderate, and the experts remain somewhat skeptical, since the efficacy is in comparison to a failed treatment (Kumar K et al., 2007; Kumar K et al., 2008; Taylor, 2006). Treatment effects are shown to diminish in other patient populations (i.e., those with chronic complex regional pain syndrome) when followed over a 5-year period (Kemler et al., 2008). An interesting trial of thoracic SCS showed improvement in coughing and better breathing control in cervical spinal cord injury survivors, which would be helpful in improving their quality of life (DiMarco et al., 2009).

SCS can be a useful option when conventional medical therapies have failed. SCS requires a highly experienced team in both the operation and the follow-up programming and medical management. Patients and clinicians should carefully consider the risk/benefit ratio when considering SCS. There is a potential for adverse events including infection, bleeding, cerebrospinal fluid leak from dural puncture, and hardware-related failures (Kunnumpurath et al., 2009).

Transcutaneous Electrical Nerve Stimulation

Transcutaneous electrical nerve stimulation (TENS) has long been used as a means of analgesia in chronic pain, including neuropathic conditions. It has also been used in acute low back pain, labor pain, and postoperative pain. Electrodes can be applied to the skin to deliver modulated current output that can be varied according to different stimulus parameters (frequency, duration, amplitude) and by connecting to a battery-operated device. TENS inhibits the nociceptive C-fiber evoked responses within the dorsal horn by activating the large-diameter afferents (Fields and Levine, 1984). The effects of TENS are mediated by endorphins, and they also cause decreased levels of glutamate and increased release of GABA and serotonin (DeSantana et al., 2008).

While TENS has been popularly used in pain clinics, its application has not been substantiated by careful studies. A recent analysis by the Therapeutics and Technology Assessment Subcommittee of the American Academy of Neurology did not recommend TENS for treatment of chronic low back pain. There is, however, level B evidence supporting TENS for painful diabetic neuropathy (Dubinsky and Miyasaki, 2010).

Sacral Neuromodulation and Incontinence of Bowel and Bladder

Urinary urge incontinence results from the loss of voluntary control of voiding that may occur with aging and in neurological or inflammatory diseases that result in formation of reflex circuits mediated by C-fiber afferents. These afferents may be sensitized by bladder distension and trigger micturition reflexes. Bladder retention, on the other hand, usually results from persistent guarding reflexes that may be due to absent suprasacral pathways in spinal cord injury. There may be urethral-sphincteric relaxation blocks and detrusor contraction.

Sacral neuromodulation targets the somatic afferent axons in the spinal cord that modulate the voiding and continence reflex pathways (Leng and Chancellor, 2005). Direct inhibition of bladder preganglionic neurons, as well as inhibition of interneuronal transmission in the bladder reflex pathway, may suppress detrusor overactivity while inhibiting the guarding reflex. This may help with urinary retention and dysfunctional voiding (Leng and Chancellor, 2005).

Selection of patients should involve a careful history, physical examination, and review of a voiding diary (with evidence of having failed traditional measures) (Koldewijn et al., 1994; Scheepens et al., 2002). The surgical procedure usually involves a test stimulation staged percutaneous nerve evaluation prior to placement of a quadripolar electrode in a sacral foramen. When a DBS lead is placed, it is most commonly attached to S3.

Sacral neuromodulation is an FDA-approved treatment to improve urinary control. Long-term (≥2 years) follow-up of patients has revealed a reasonable success rate, with more than 50% improvement reported in 40% to 80% of patients (Oerlemans and van Kerrebroeck, 2008). With improvements in technology and expertise and low rates of complications, this approach appears to be an attractive option for patients, even for those with complete spinal cord injury (Sievert et al., 2010).

Additionally, outcome studies in patients with another disorder (fecal incontinence) followed for 2 years or more have been encouraging, with better than 80% reduction in incontinence episodes in 80% of patients (Kenefick, 2006; Melenhorst et al., 2007). Recent results showing improved bowel frequency in constipated patients have also raised this approach as an option in the most severe cases (Holzer et al., 2008; Kamm et al., 2010).

References

The complete reference list is available online at www.expertconsult.com.

Clinical Neurophysiology
Intraoperative Monitoring

Marc R. Nuwer

Neurophysiological intraoperative monitoring (IOM) uses electroencephalography (EEG), electromyography (EMG), and evoked potentials during surgical procedures to improve surgical outcome. When problems begin, these techniques warn the surgeon in time to intervene and correct the problem before it becomes worse or permanent. IOM methods also can identify neurological structures such as language cortex, so as to spare them from resection. A surgeon can rely on monitoring for reassurance about nervous system integrity, allowing the surgery to be more extensive than would have been safe without monitoring. Some patients are eligible for surgery with monitoring who may have been denied surgery in the past because of a high risk of nervous system complications. Patients and families can be reassured that certain feared complications are screened for during surgery. In these ways, monitoring extends the safety, range, and completeness of surgery.

Effective collaboration and communication is needed among surgeon, anesthesiologist, and neurophysiologist, who typically maintain communication throughout a specific procedure. An experienced electrodiagnostic technologist applies electrodes and ensures technically accurate studies. The interpreting neurophysiologist is either in the operating room or monitors continuously online in real time.

Techniques

Many intraoperative techniques are adapted from common outpatient testing: EEG, brainstem auditory evoked potential (BAEP), and somatosensory evoked potential (SEP) tests, for example. EEG is used for surgery that risks cortical ischemia, such as aneurysm clipping or carotid endarterectomy. BAEP is used for procedures around the eighth nerve or when the brainstem is at risk in posterior fossa procedures. SEP is widely used for many kinds of procedures in which the spinal cord, brainstem, or sensorimotor cortex is at risk.

Other techniques are more specific to the operating room. Transcranial electrical motor evoked potential (MEP) tests are evoked by several-hundred-volt electrical pulses delivered to motor cortex through the intact skull. Recordings are from extremity muscles. This monitors the corticospinal tracts during cerebral, brainstem, or spinal surgery. Electrocorticography (ECoG) measures EEG directly from the exposed cortex. This guides the resection to include physiologically dysfunctional or epileptogenic areas while sparing relatively normal cortex. Direct cortical stimulation applies very localized electrical pulses to cortex through a handheld wand. The electricity disrupts cortical function such as language, which can be tested in patients awake during portions of the craniotomy. Stimulation near motor cortex can produce movement. These techniques identify language or motor regions so they can be spared during resections. Similar direct nerve stimulation is used for cranial and peripheral nerves to locate them amid pathological tissue and check whether they still are intact. One version is stimulation at the floor of the fourth ventricle or during brainstem resection to identify tracts and nuclei of interest. For spinal procedures using pedicle screws, risk is incurred to the nerve roots or spinal cord during screw placement. To reduce that risk, EMG is monitored while electrical stimulation is delivered to the hole drilled in the spine or the screw as it is being placed. If the hole or screw errantly has broken through bone into the spinal or nerve root canal, stimulation will elicit an EMG warning of misplacement. In-depth descriptions of each procedure is beyond the scope of this chapter. The reader is referred elsewhere for extensive coverage of intraoperative neurophysiological techniques (Nuwer, 2008).

DOI: 10.1016/B978-1-4377-0434-1.00109-2

Spinal Cord Monitoring Techniques

SEP and MEP spinal cord monitoring is a good example of a common IOM technique. SEP electrical stimuli are delivered to the median nerve at the wrist or the posterior tibial nerve at the ankle. Stimuli are strong enough to evoke a muscle twitch at the thumb or foot muscles. Several hundred stimuli are delivered at about 5 per second. Averaged recordings are made at standardized surface locations over the spine and scalp. Small electrical potentials are recorded during the 25 to 45 msec after the stimulation, corresponding to transit of the axonal volley or synaptic events at the peripheral, spinal, brainstem, and primary sensory cortical levels. After establishing baseline values for typical peak latencies and amplitudes, this stimulation and recording is repeated every few minutes. MEP stimulating electrodes are placed on the scalp over motor cortex. Strong enough electrical pulses are delivered to discharge the axon hillock of motor cortex pyramidal cells. The resulting action potentials travel down corticospinal tracts and discharge spinal anterior horn cells. Recordings are made from limb muscles in the absence of neuromuscular blockage drugs; that EMG is seen at 25 to 45 msec after stimulation.

In uneventful spinal surgery, the measured peaks remain stable over time. When values change beyond established limits, the monitoring team warns the surgeon of an increased risk of neurological impairment. Which peaks are preserved and which are changed can localize the side level of impairment. Each of the four limbs is monitored. In thoracolumbar surgery, the median SEP nerve channels and upper extremity MEP channels serve as controls to separate systemic or anesthetic causes of change from thoracic or lumbar surgical reasons for change. Sometimes other nerves are stimulated for SEP. The ulnar nerve may be substituted for the median nerve during cervical surgery, so as to better cover the lower cervical cord. The peroneal nerve at the knee may substitute for the posterior tibial nerve at the ankle for elderly patients, diabetics, or others in whom a peripheral neuropathy may interfere with adequate peripheral conduction. Neuromuscular junction blockade is helpful to reduce muscle artifact in SEP but cannot be used if MEP also is monitored. Sometimes other incidental clinical problems are detected beyond the primary purpose of spinal cord, brainstem, or cortical region monitoring. For example, a developing plexopathy or peripheral nerve compression can be spotted by loss of the peripheral peak, which may be easily treated by repositioning an arm. Occasionally, changes warn of a systemic problem such as hypoxia secondary to a ventilation problem.

Interpretation

Interpretation of intraoperative neurophysiology includes two categories. One is *monitoring*, in which baseline findings are established and subsequent findings are compared to baseline. Alarm criteria are set in advance based on knowledge of how much change is acceptable without risk. The other category, *testing*, is decision making about structures and limits of resection. Testing is used in several ways. One is to identify a structure, such as finding the facial nerve within pathological tissue where it may be difficult to identify. Another is to identify motor or language cortex prior to a resection. A third example is identifying which cauda equina root is L5, which is S1, and which is S2, or which is the sensory or the motor portion of a root.

Monitoring

Monitoring interpretation uses latency and amplitude criteria for raising an alarm. A 50% SEP drop in recorded potentials raises an alarm. Latency increases of 10% raise an alarm. Latency measures take into account temperature effects, and amplitude measures take into account anesthetic effects from medication boluses or increased inhalation anesthetics. Technical problems can occur with electrodes themselves (e.g., becoming dislodged). Equipment can malfunction. Systemic factors such as hypotension or hypoxia can change EPs.

MEPs are judged more qualitatively. They either remain present or become absent. Some physicians raise an alarm if MEP amplitude decreases by more than 80% or latency increases by more than 10%.

For EEG, a 50% loss of fast activity is seen when cerebral blood flow drops below 20 mL/100 g/min. Still lower blood flow causes a 50% increase in slow activity. The third and worst degree of change is a 50% or more loss of signal amplitude that can progress all the way to an isoelectric state at 10 mL/100 g/min cerebral blood flow.

EMG monitoring observes for increased spontaneous activity. When a nerve is subject to excessive mechanical compression or ischemia, it often responds in a pattern referred to as a *neurotonic discharge*. Such a minute-long rapid firing is the same discharge as occurs when someone accidentally hits the ulnar nerve at the elbow and feels a minute-long painful sensation in the ulnar distribution. In the operating room, this warns of mechanical or ischemic nerve problems.

Testing

Interpretation of testing depends much more on the clinical question asked. For motor cortex identification with SEPs, the location is determined by identifying the postcentral primary somatosensory gyrus with median nerve SEP testing. The N20 peak is located with good precision, identifying the immediately anterior gyrus as motor cortex. For language localization, an awake patient is tested repeatedly with various oral and visual verbal and nonverbal tasks. Language active regions are those for which electrical stimulation disrupts the patient's ability to complete those tasks during the stimulation events. Corticospinal tracts in hemispheric white matter are identified by electrical stimulation with muscle recording. When 5 mA stimulation produces no motor responses, then the corticospinal tract is at least 5 mm from the site of stimulation; the general rule is 1 mm distance for each milliampere needed to elicit muscle responses. For cranial nerve nuclei, cranial nerves, or peripheral nerves, direct or nearby stimulation produces responses in appropriate muscles. The pattern of responses can separate structures (i.e., among L5, S1, and S2 roots). Motor roots and nerves require low stimulus intensity to provoke an EMG response, whereas sensory nerves or roots require a 10-fold or greater higher intensity to provoke a response through reflex pathways. That allows for identification of which root is motor and which is sensory.

Response to Change

The monitoring team quickly assesses whether a change is likely due to a technical, systemic, or surgical cause. Occasional transient significant changes occur without significant risk for postoperative neurological problems. Transient changes for a few minutes can occur without substantial risk of postoperative problems, especially if the neurophysiological findings return shortly to baseline. Risk of neurological complications is higher when changes remain through the end of the case. For example, a very high-risk situation is complete and permanent loss of EPs that previously had been normal and easily detected.

The surgeon reviews actions of the preceding 15 minutes that may have caused change. Surgical problems causing neurophysiological changes include direct trauma, excessive traction, excessive compression, stretching from spinal distraction, vascular insufficiency from compression, clamping, embolus or thrombus, and other clinical circumstances. Clamping a carotid during an endarterectomy commonly produces EEG changes within 15 seconds. Most other changes are cumulative over many minutes, leading to changes at many minutes after the offending action. Two factors compound that delay. Evoked potential recordings take 1 to several minutes to average and sometimes longer when electrocautery or other electrical noise is ongoing.

Many surgical or anesthetic actions can be taken. Remedial measures can be implemented depending on the recent surgical actions. The surgical maneuver underway can be paused, stopped, or reversed. Resection can be halted. A graft or fixation instrumentation can be removed or repositioned. If no recovery of EPs occurs within 20 minutes, the patient can be awakened on the operating table and told to move the legs ("wake-up test"). Blood pressure can be increased. Steroids sometimes are given, although the literature about their usefulness is controversial. A vascular shunt can be placed, clamped vessels can be unclamped, a clip can be adjusted, or transected aortic intercostal arteries can be reimplanted. Retractors can be repositioned. Spine distraction can be reduced. Causes can be sought through inspection and exploration for mechanical or hematoma nervous system impingement. Motor and language identified can be avoided during resection. Systemic or local hypothermia or barbiturate-induced coma can be implemented for nervous system protection. Lowering of cerebrospinal fluid pressure by free drainage can be used in some cases of spinal ischemia. Hemoglobin level can be increased by transfusion. Other interventions also are used.

Prediction of Deficits

Intraoperative monitoring is effective at preventing many postoperative neurological complications. Risks depend on severity and duration of IOM changes. Transient changes that revert to baseline within a few minutes are rarely accompanied by postoperative deficits. On many occasions, these represent clinically significant problems that are identified and corrected promptly and completely—the goal of monitoring. In other cases, transient changes are false alarms. Both are combined in outcome studies as "false-positive" monitoring events, since their causes cannot be directly separated. Outcomes studies show false positives in several percent of cases. Persistent changes of moderate degree are accompanied by a risk of new neurological postoperative impairment in about half of cases (Nuwer et al., 1995). Sometimes such postoperative neurological impairment is less than might have occurred if monitoring had not initiated interventions that partially corrected the problem. Severe monitoring changes often are

accompanied by postoperative neurological deficits. Some are due to intraoperative problems that were identified promptly but could not be completely corrected.

Anesthesia

Many inhalation anesthetics substantially affect cortical function (Sloan and Heyer, 2002). Agents commonly used attenuate or abolish cortical EP recordings. Limiting the inhalation anesthetic dose often produces satisfactory anesthesia compatible with monitoring. Boluses of centrally active medication are discouraged because they can cause transient IOM changes. Continuous-drip medication delivery is preferred. Much less susceptible to anesthetic effects are the nonsynaptic pathways such as peripheral nerve conduction techniques. Subcortical monosynaptic pathways are less affected than cortical polysynaptic pathways. For example, in SEP monitoring, brainstem peaks remain relatively robust despite inhalation anesthesia levels that nearly eliminate cortical peaks in the same pathway. MEPs tolerate inhalation anesthesia poorly, so most MEPs are carried out using total intravenous anesthesia with propofol, a centrally excitatory anesthetic agent, as opposed to the more inhibitory gas inhalation agents. Turning this effect around, anesthetic and drug effects can be monitored by the degree of evoked potential or EEG changes. When a barbiturate-induced cortically protective burst suppression state is desired, EEG is the primary tool to identify that sufficient depth has been achieved.

A surgical patient's core temperature may drop 1°C or more. Limb temperature may drop more. Axonal conduction velocity depends on is temperature, so peak latencies increase as temperature drops. Monitoring can help identify therapeutic temperature effects. When a hypothermia-induced cortically protective isoelectric state is desired, EEG is the primary tool to identify that sufficient depth has been achieved.

Clinical Settings

Box 32E.1 lists many clinical conditions and types of surgery for which IOM is used. Intracranial posterior fossa cases commonly use BAEP, SEP, and cranial nerve EMG monitoring. Typical applications are cerebellopontine angle and skull base tumor resection, brainstem vascular malformation and tumor resection, and microvascular decompressions (Møller, 1996). Intracranial supratentorial procedures include resections for epilepsy, tumors, and vascular malformations as well as for aneurysm clipping. These use a combination of EEG and SEP monitoring together with functional cortical localization with direct cortical stimulation and ECoG. Surgery of the carotid, aorta, or heart may use EEG to monitor hemispheric function or assess the need for shunting or adequacy of protective hypothermia (Plestis et al., 1997). Some also use or prefer SEPs for these vascular cases.

Spinal surgery is the most common setting for IOM. Disorders include cervical diskectomy and fusion for myelopathy, stabilization for deformities such as scoliosis, resection of spinal column or cord tumors, and stabilization of fractures. Both SEP and MEP often are used to assess the posterior columns and corticospinal tract functions. The use of MEP depends on the case, since it requires total intravenous anesthetic and incurs some movements during surgery. As a result, some spinal cases still are done with SEP alone. In cases

Box 32E.1 **Clinical Conditions Monitored During Surgery**

Epilepsy surgery
Cerebral tumor and vascular malformation resection
Intracranial aneurysm clipping
Movement disorders electrode placement
Mapping nerves, tracts, and nuclei during brainstem and cranial base surgery
Ear and parotid surgery near facial nerve
Thyroid and aortic arch surgery near laryngeal nerve
Carotid endarterectomy
Carotid balloon occlusion
Endovascular spinal and cerebral procedures
Spinal deformity correction
Spinal fracture stabilization
Spinal tumor resection
Cervical myelopathy decompression
Lumbar stenosis decompression and fusion
Tethered cord and cauda equina procedures
Dorsal root entry zone surgery
Brachial and lumbosacral plexus surgery
Peripheral nerve surgery
Cardiac and aorta procedures

involving pedicle screw placement, EMG is monitored to detect screw misplacement (Shi et al., 2003). Spinal cord monitoring also is used for cardiothoracic procedures of the aorta that jeopardize spinal perfusion (Jacobs et al., 2006). Peripheral nerve monitoring is carried out for cases risking injury to the nerves, plexus, or roots. Testing also can determine which segments of a nerve are damaged when performing a nerve graft.

Outcomes have been assessed most thoroughly for spinal cord surgery. In one large multicenter study of SEP IOM in 100,000 cases of spinal surgery, the rate of false-positive alarms was about 1%. The rate of false-negative cases was about 0.1%, which were those cases with postoperative neurological deficits in which monitoring did not raise an alarm. Some were minor transient changes, and others were neurological deficits that started during the hours or days postoperatively. The rate of major intraoperative changes missed by SEP monitoring was 0.063%. The risk of paraplegia was 60% less among the monitored cases when compared to historical and contemporaneous controls. That amounted to 1 case out of every 200 that did not have paraplegia when monitoring was used (Nuwer et al., 1995). To improve even further on these SEP IOM monitoring outcomes results, MEPs have been used more recently together with SEP for many spinal procedures. The expectation is that the rate of false-negative cases and postoperative neurological deficits will be reduced even further.

Summary

Intraoperative monitoring is used routinely to monitor the nervous system during procedures that present significant risk of brain, spinal cord, or nerve injury. Intraoperative testing is used to identify nerves and eloquent cortex and to define regions and structures for resection. Many different intraoperative procedures are now available, and they are applied in a wide variety of surgical procedures. Studies show significant improvement in patient outcome with monitoring.

References

The complete reference list is available online at www.exopertconsult.com.

Neuroimaging
Structural Imaging: Magnetic Resonance Imaging, Computed Tomography

Bela Ajtai, Eric Lindzen, Joseph C. Masdeu

Computed Tomography

Computed tomography (CT; other terms include *computer assisted tomography* [CAT]) has been commercially available since 1973. The term *tomography* (i.e., to slice or section) refers to a process for generating two-dimensional (2D) image slices of an examined organ of three dimensions (3D). CT imaging is based on the differential absorption of x-rays by various tissues. X-rays are electromagnetic waves with wavelengths falling in the range of 10 to 0.01 nanometers on the electromagnetic spectrum. X-rays can also be described as high-energy photons, with corresponding energies varying between 124 and 124,000 electron volts, respectively. X-rays in the higher range of energies, known as *hard x-rays*, are used in diagnostic imaging because of their ability to penetrate tissue yet (to an extent) also be absorbed or scattered differentially by various tissues, allowing for the generation of image contrast.

Owing to their high energy, x-rays are also a form of ionizing radiation, and the health risks associated with their use, although minimal, should always be accounted for in diagnostic imaging. The x-rays generated by the x-ray source of the CT scanner are shaped into an x-ray beam by a *collimator*, a rectangular opening in a lead shield. The beam penetrates the slab of tissues to be imaged, which will absorb/deflect it to a varying degree depending on their atomic composition, structure, and density (*photoelectric effect* and *Compton-scattering*).

The remaining x-rays emerge from the imaged slab and are measured by detectors located opposite the collimator. In fourth-generation CT scanners, the detectors are in a fixed position and the x-ray source rotates about the patient. As the beam of x-rays is transmitted through the imaged body part, sweeping a 360-degree arc for each slice imaged, the emerging x-rays are collected, then a computer analyzes the output of the detectors and calculates the x-ray attenuation of each individual tissue volume (voxel).

The degree of x-ray absorption by the various tissues is expressed and displayed as shades of gray in the CT image. Darker shades correspond to less attenuation. The attenuation by each voxel of tissue is projected on the flat image of the scanned slice as a tiny quadrilateral, generally square, called a *pixel* or picture element. Depending on the reconstruction matrix, a slice will be represented by more or fewer pixels, corresponding to more or less resolution. The shade of gray in each pixel corresponds to a number on an arbitrary linear scale, expressed as Hounsfield units (HU). This number varies between approximately −1000 and 3000+, with values of greater magnitude corresponding to tissues or substances of greater radiodensity, which are depicted in lighter tones. The −1000 value is for air, 0 is for water. Bone is greater than several hundred units, but cranial bone can be 2000 or even more. Fresh blood (with a normal hematocrit) is about 80 units, fat is −50 to −80. Tissues or materials with higher degrees of x-ray absorption, shown in white or lighter shades of gray, are referred to as *hyperdense*, whereas those with lower x-ray absorption properties are *hypodense*; these are relative terms compared to other areas of any given image.

By changing the settings of the process of transforming the x-ray attenuation values to shades on the grayscale, it is possible to select which tissues to preferentially display in the image. This is referred to as *windowing*. Utilizing a bone window, for instance, is very useful for evaluating fractures in cases of craniofacial trauma (**Fig. 33A.1**).

In CT, imaging contrast agents are frequently used for the purpose of detecting abnormalities that cause disruption of

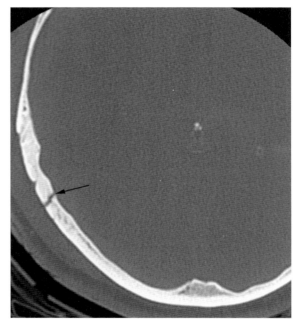

Fig. 33A.1 Computed tomography (CT) scan from a 32-year-old patient after a motor vehicle accident. Axial bone window CT image reveals a skull fracture *(arrow)*.

the blood-brain barrier (BBB) (e.g., certain tumors, inflammation, etc.). The damaged BBB allows for the net diffusion of contrast material into the site of pathology, where it is detected; this is referred to as *contrast enhancement*. Contrast materials used in CT scanning contain iodine in an injectable water-soluble form. Iodine is a heavy atom; its inner electron shell absorbs x-rays through the process of *photoelectric capture*. Even a small amount of iodine effectively blocks the transmitted x-rays so they will not reach the detector. The high x-ray attenuation/absorption will result in hyperdense appearance in the image. Other CT techniques requiring contrast administration are CT angiography, CT myelography, and CT perfusion studies.

More than 20 years ago, a fast-imaging technique called *spiral* (or *helical*) *CT scanning* was introduced to clinical practice. With this technique, the x-ray tube in the gantry rotates continuously, but data acquisition is combined with continuous movement of the patient through the gantry. The circular rotating path of the x-rays, combined with the linear movement of the imaged body, results in a spiral or helix-shaped x-ray path, hence the name. These scanners can acquire data rapidly, and a large volume can be scanned in 20 to 60 seconds. This technique offers several advantages, including more rapid image acquisition. During the short scan time, patients can usually hold their breath, which reduces/minimizes motion artifacts. Timing of contrast bolus administration can be optimized, and less contrast material is sufficient. The short scan time, optimal contrast bolus timing, and better image quality are very useful in CT angiography, where cervical and intracranial blood vessels are visualized. These images can also be reformatted as 3D views of the vasculature, which are often displayed in color and can be depicted along with reformatted bone or other tissues in the region of interest (**Fig. 33A.2**).

Superfast CT scanners have become available in the past 5 years. By multiplying by 4 the number of detectors, they can obtain 64 slices of an organ in a fraction of a second. They are particularly useful in cardiology and also allow for the acquisition of perfusion images of the entire brain. One shortcoming is a greater exposure to ionizing radiation per scan.

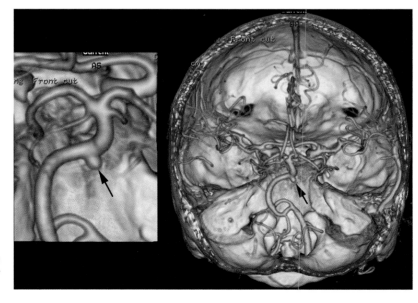

Fig. 33A.2 Computed tomography angiogram with 3D reconstruction. Reconstructed color images reveal a basilar artery aneurysm *(arrows)*.

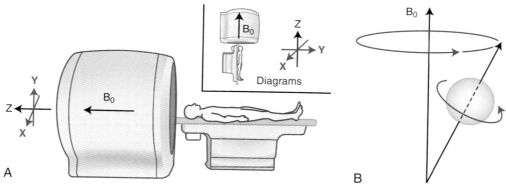

Fig. 33A.3 A, Magnetization in a magnetic resonance imaging scanner. Direction of external magnetic field is in the head-foot direction in the scanner. However, in diagrams that follow, the frame of reference is turned, so that the z direction is up *(inset)*. **B,** Precession. In an external magnetic field (Bo), protons spin around their own axis and "wobble" about the axis of the magnetic field. This phenomenon is called *precession*. (*A from Higgins, D., 2010. ReviseMRI. http://www.revisemri.com/questions/basicphysics/precession; **B** Reprinted with permission from Hashemi, R.H., Bradley, W.G., Lasanti, C.J., 2004. MRI—The Basics. 2nd ed. Lippincott Williams & Wilkins.)*

Magnetic Resonance Imaging

Basic Principles

Magnetic resonance imaging (MRI) is based on the magnetic characteristics of the imaged tissue. It involves creation of tissue magnetization (which can then be manipulated in several ways) and detection of tissue magnetization as revealed by signal intensity. The various degrees of detected signal intensity provide the image of a given tissue.

In clinical practice, MRI uses the magnetic characteristics inherent to the protons of hydrogen nuclei in the tissue, mostly in the form of water but to a significant extent in fat as well. The protons spin about their own axes, which creates a magnetic dipole moment for each proton (**Fig. 33A.3**). In the absence of an external magnetic field, the axes of these dipoles are arranged randomly, and therefore, the vectors depicting the dipole moments cancel each other out, resulting in a zero net magnetization vector and a zero net magnetic field for the tissue.

This situation changes when the body is placed in the strong magnetic field of a scanner (see **Fig. 33A.3, A**). The magnetic field is generated by an electric current circulating in wire coils that surround the open bore of the scanner. Most MRI scanners used in clinical practice are superconducting magnets. Here the electrical coils are housed at near–absolute zero temperature, minimizing their resistance and allowing for the strong currents needed to generate the magnetic field without undue heating. The low temperature is achieved by cryogens (liquid nitrogen or helium). Most clinical scanners in commercial production today produce magnetic fields at strengths of 1.5 or 3.0 tesla (T).

When the patient is placed in the MRI scanner, the magnetic dipoles in the tissues line up relative to the external magnetic field. Some dipoles will point in the direction of the external field ("north"), some will point in the opposite direction ("south"), but the net magnetization vector of the dipoles (the sum of individual spins) will point in the direction of the external field ("north"), and this will be the tissue's acquired net magnetization. At this point, a small proportion of the protons (and therefore the net magnetization vector of the tissue) is aligned along the external field (longitudinal magnetization), and the protons precess with a certain frequency.

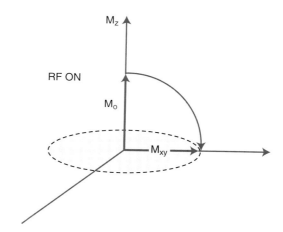

Fig. 33A.4 Flipping the net magnetization vector. When a 90-degree radiofrequency (RF) pulse is applied, the net magnetization vector of the protons (Mo) is flipped from the vertical (z) plane to the horizontal (xy) plane. *(Reprinted with permission from Hashemi, R.H., Bradley, W.G., Lasanti, C.J., 2004. MRI—The Basics. 2nd ed. Lippincott Williams & Wilkins).*

The term *precession* describes a proton spinning about its own axis and its simultaneous wobbling about the axis of the external field (see **Fig. 33A.3, B**). The frequency of precession is directly proportional to the strength of the applied external magnetic field.

As a next step in obtaining an image, a radiofrequency pulse is applied to the part of the body being imaged. This is an electromagnetic wave, and if its frequency matches the precession frequency of the protons, *resonance* occurs. Resonance is a very efficient way to give or receive energy. In this process, the protons receive the energy of the applied radiofrequency pulse. As a result, the protons flip, and the net magnetization vector of the tissue ceases transiently to be aligned with that of the external field but flips into another plane, thereby *transverse magnetization* is produced. One example of this is the 90-degree radiofrequency pulse that flips the entire net magnetization vector by 90 degrees to the transverse (horizontal) plane (**Fig. 33A.4**). What we detect in MRI is this transverse magnetization, and its degree will determine the *signal intensity*. Through the process of electromagnetic induction, rotating transverse magnetization in the tissue

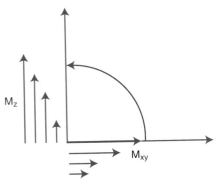

Fig. 33A.5 T1 and T2 relaxation. When the radiofrequency (RF) pulse is turned off, two processes begin simultaneously: gradual recovery of the longitudinal magnetization (Mz) and gradual decay of the horizontal magnetization component (Mxy). These processes are referred to as *T1* and *T2 relaxation*, respectively. *(Reprinted with permission from Hashemi, R.H., Bradley, W.G., Lasanti, C.J., 2004. MRI—The Basics. 2nd ed. Lippincott Williams & Wilkins.)*

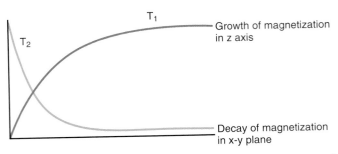

Fig. 33A.6 This diagram illustrates the simultaneous recovery of longitudinal magnetization (T1 relaxation) and decay of horizontal magnetization (T2 relaxation) after the RF pulse is turned off. *(Reprinted with permission from Hashemi, R.H., Bradley, W.G., Lasanti, C.J., 2004. MRI—The Basics. 2nd ed. Lippincott Williams & Wilkins.)*

induces electrical currents in *receiver coils*, thus accomplishing signal detection. Several cycles of excitation pulses by the scanner with detection of the resulting electromagnetic signal from the imaged subject are repeated per imaged slice. This occurs while varying two additional magnetic field gradients along the *x* and *y* axes for each cycle. Varying the magnetic field gradient along these two additional axes, known as *phase* and *frequency encoding*, is necessary to obtain sufficient information to decode the spatial coordinates of the signal emitted by each tissue voxel. This is accomplished using a mathematical algorithm known as a *Fourier transform*. The final image is produced by applying a gray scale to the intensity values calculated by the Fourier transform for each voxel within the imaging plane, corresponding to the *signal intensity* of individual tissue elements.

T1 and T2 Relaxation Times

During the process of resonance, the applied 90-degree radiofrequency pulse flips the net magnetization vectors of the imaged tissues to the transverse (horizontal) plane by transmitting electromagnetic energy to the protons. The radiofrequency pulse is brief, and after it is turned off the magnitude of the net magnetization vector starts to decrease along the transverse or horizontal plane and return ("recover or relax") toward its original position, in which it is aligned parallel to the external magnetic field. The relaxation process, therefore, changes the magnitude and orientation of the tissue's net magnetization vector. There is a decrease along the horizontal or transverse plane and an increase (recovery) along the longitudinal or vertical plane (**Fig. 33A.5**).

To understand the meaning of T1 and T2 relaxation times, the decrease in the magnitude of the horizontal component of the net magnetization vector and its simultaneous increase in magnitude along the vertical plane should be analyzed independently. These processes are in fact independent and occur at two different rates, T2 relaxation always occurring more rapidly than T1 relaxation (**Fig. 33A.6**). The *T1 relaxation time* refers to the time required by protons within a given tissue to recover 63% of their original net magnetization vector along the vertical or longitudinal plane immediately after completion of the 90-degree radiofrequency pulse. As an example, a

T1 time of 2 seconds means that 2 seconds after the 90-degree pulse is turned off, the given tissue's net magnetization vector has recovered 63% of its original magnitude along the vertical (longitudinal) plane. Different tissues may have quite different T1 time values (T1 recovery or relaxation times). T1 relaxation is also known as *spin-lattice relaxation*.

While T1 relaxation relates to the longitudinal plane, *T2 relaxation* refers to the decrease of the transverse or horizontal magnetization vector. When the 90-degree pulse is applied, the entire net magnetization vector is flipped in the horizontal or transverse plane. When the pulse is turned off, the transverse magnetization vector starts to decrease. The T2 relaxation time is the time it takes for the tissue to lose 63% of its original transverse or horizontal magnetization. As an example, a T2 time of 200 ms means that 200 ms after the 90-degree pulse has been turned off, the tissue will have lost 63% of its transverse or horizontal magnetization. The decrease of the net magnetization vector in the horizontal plane is due to dephasing of the individual proton spins as they precess at slightly different rates owing to local inhomogeneities of the magnetic field. This dephasing of the individual proton magnetic dipole vectors causes a decrease of the transverse component of the net magnetization vector and loss of signal. T2 relaxation is also known as *spin-spin relaxation*. Just like the T1 values, the T2 time values of different tissues may also be quite different. Tissue abnormalities may alter a given tissue's T1 and T2 time values, ultimately resulting in the signal changes seen on the patient's MR images.

Repetition Time and Time to Echo

As mentioned before, the amount of the signal detected by the receiver coils depends on the magnitude of the net magnetization vector along the transverse or horizontal plane. Using certain operator-dependent parameters, it is possible to influence how much net magnetization strength (in other words, vector length) will be present in the transverse plane for the imaged tissues at the time of signal acquisition. During the imaging process, the initial 90-degree pulse flips the entire vertical or longitudinal magnetization vector into the horizontal plane. When this initial pulse is turned off, recovery along the longitudinal plane begins (T1 relaxation). Subsequent application of a second radiofrequency pulse at a given time after the first pulse will flip the net magnetization vector that recovered so far along the longitudinal plane back to the transverse plane. As a result, we can measure the magnitude

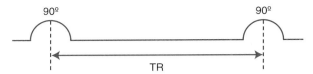

Fig. 33A.7 Repetition time. This pulse sequence diagram demonstrates the concept of repetition time (TR), which is the time interval between two sequential radio frequency pulses. *(Reprinted with permission from Hashemi, R.H., Bradley, W.G., Lasanti, C.J., 2004. MRI—The Basics. 2nd ed. Lippincott Williams & Wilkins.)*

of the net longitudinal magnetization that had recovered within each voxel at the time of application of the second pulse, provided that signal acquisition is begun immediately afterwards. The time between these radiofrequency pulses is referred to as *repetition time*, or TR (**Fig. 33A.7**). It is important to realize that contrary to the T1 and T2 times, which are properties of the given tissue, the repetition time is a controllable parameter. By selecting a longer TR, for instance, we allow more time for the net magnetization vector to recover before we flip it back to the transverse plane for measurement. A longer TR, because it increases the amount of signal that can potentially be detected, will also result in a higher signal-to-noise ratio, with higher image quality.

As described earlier, the other process that begins after the initial radiofrequency pulse is turned off is the decrease of net horizontal or transverse magnetization, owing to dephasing of the proton spins (T2 relaxation). *Time to echo* (TE) refers to the time we wait until we measure the magnitude of the remaining transverse magnetization. TE, just like TR, is a parameter controlled by the operator. If we use a longer TE, tissues with significantly different T2 values (i.e., different rates of loss of transverse magnetization component) will show more difference in the measured signal intensity (transverse magnetization vector size) when the signals are collected. However, there is a tradeoff. If the TE is set too high, the signal-to-noise ratio of the resulting image will drop to a level that is too low, resulting in poor image quality.

Tissue Contrast (T1, T2, and Proton Density Weighting)

By using various TR and TE values, it is possible to increase (or decrease) the contrast between different tissues in an MR image. Achieving this contrast may be based on either the T1 or the T2 properties of the tissues in conjunction with their proton density. Selecting a long TR value reduces the T1 contrast between tissues (**Fig. 33A.8**). Thus, if we wait long enough before applying the second 90-degree pulse, we allow enough time for all tissues to recover most of their longitudinal or vertical magnetization. Because T1 is relatively short, even for tissues with the longest T1, this is possible without resulting in excessively long scan times. Since after a long TR, the longitudinally oriented net magnetization vectors of separate tissue types are all of similar magnitudes prior to being flipped into the transverse plane by the second pulse, a long TR will result in little T1 tissue contrast. Conversely, by selecting a short TR value, there will be significant variation in the extent to which tissues with different T1 relaxation times will have recovered their longitudinal magnetization prior to being flipped by the second 90-degree pulse (see **Fig. 33A.8**). Therefore, with a short TR, the second pulse will flip

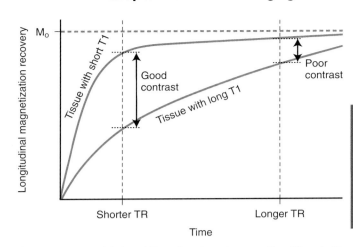

Fig. 33A.8 T1-weighting. When imaging tissues with different T1 relaxation times, selecting a short TR will increase T1 weighting, as the magnitudes of their recovered longitudinal magnetizations will be different. By selecting a longer TR, longitudinal magnetization of both tissues will recover significantly, and there will be a smaller difference between the magnitudes of their recovered magnetization vectors; therefore, the T1 weighting will be less.

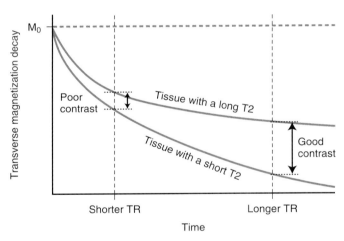

Fig. 33A.9 T2-weighting. In tissues with different T2 relaxation times, selecting a short TE will not result in much T2-weighting, because there is no major difference *yet* between the loss of their transverse magnetizations. However, by selecting a longer TE, we allow a significant difference to develop between the amount of transverse magnetization of the two tissues, so more T2-weighting is added to the image.

magnetization vectors of different magnitudes into the transverse plane for measurement, resulting in more T1 contrast between the tissues.

During T2 relaxation in the transverse plane, selecting a short TE will give higher measured signal intensities (as a short TE will not allow enough time for significant dephasing, i.e., transverse magnetization loss), but tissues with different T2 relaxation times will not show much contrast (**Fig. 33A.9**). This is because by selecting a short time until measurement (short TE) we do not allow significant T2-related magnitude differences to develop. If we select longer TE values, tissues with different T2 relaxation times will have time to lose different amounts of transverse magnetization, and therefore by

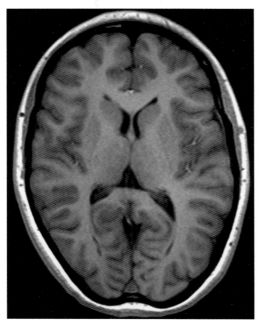

Fig. 33A.10 Axial T1-weighted image of a normal subject, obtained with a 3-tesla scanner.

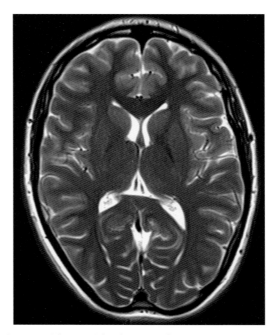

Fig. 33A.11 Axial T2-weighted image of a normal subject, obtained with a 3-tesla scanner.

the time of signal measurement, different signal intensities will be measured from these different tissues (see **Fig. 33A.9**). This is referred to as *T2 contrast.*

Based on the described considerations, selecting TR and TE values that are both short will increase the T1 contrast between tissues, referred to as *T1 weighting.* Selecting long TR and long TE values will cause increased T2 contrast between tissues, referred to as *T2 weighting.*

On T1-weighted images, substances with a longer T1 relaxation time (such as water) will be darker. This is because the short TR does not allow as much longitudinal magnetization to recover, so the vector flipped to the transverse plane by the second 90-degree pulse will be smaller with a lower resulting signal strength. Conversely, tissues with shorter T1 relaxation times (such as fat or some mucinous materials) will be brighter on T1-weighted images, as they recover more longitudinal magnetization prior to their proton spins being flipped into the transverse plane by the second 90-degree pulse (**Fig. 33A.10**). Among many other applications of T1-weighted images, they allow for evaluation of BBB breakdown: areas with abnormally permeable BBB show increased signal after the intravenous administration of gadolinium. Gadolinium administration is contraindicated in pregnancy. Breast-feeding immediately after receiving gadolinium is generally regarded to be safe (Chen et al., 2008). Renally impaired patients are susceptible to an uncommon but serious adverse reaction to gadolinium, *nephrogenic systemic fibrosis* (Marckmann et al., 2006).

On T2-weighted images, substances with longer T2 relaxation times (e.g., water) will be brighter because they will not have lost as much transverse magnetization magnitude by the time the signal is measured (**Fig. 33A.11**). The T1 and T2 signal characteristics of various tissues or substances found in neuroimaging are listed in **Table 33A.1**.

What happens if we select long TR and short TE values? With the longer TR, the T1 differences between the tissues

diminish, whereas the short TE does not allow much T2 contrast to develop. The signal intensity obtained from the various tissues, therefore, will mostly depend on their relative proton densities. Tissues having more proton density, and thereby larger net magnetization vectors, will have greater signal intensity. This set of imaging parameters is referred to as *proton density (PD) weighting.*

Magnetic Resonance Image Reconstruction

To construct an MR image, a slice of the imaged body part is selected, then the signal coming from each of the voxels making up the given slice is measured. Slice selection is achieved by setting the external magnetic field to vary linearly along one of the three principal axes perpendicular to the axial, sagittal, and coronal planes of the subject being imaged. As a result, protons within the slice to be imaged will precess at a Larmor frequency different from the Larmor frequency within all other imaging planes perpendicular to the axis along which the magnetic field gradient is applied. The *Larmor frequency* is the natural precession frequency of protons within a magnetic field of a given strength and is calculated simply as the product of the magnetic field, B_0, and the gyromagnetic ratio, gamma. The precession frequency of a hydrogen proton is therefore directly proportional to the strength of the applied magnetic field. The gyromagnetic ratio for any given nucleus is a constant, with a value for hydrogen protons of 42.58 MHz/T. In slices at lower magnetic strengths of the gradient, the protons precess more slowly, whereas in slices at higher magnetic field strengths, the protons precess more quickly. Based on the property of nuclear magnetic resonance, the applied radiofrequency pulse (which flips the magnetization vector to the transverse plane) will stimulate only those protons with a precession frequency that matches the frequency of the applied radiofrequency pulse. By selecting the frequency of the

Table 33A.1 MRI Signal Intensity of Some Substances Found in Neuroimaging

	T1-Weighted Image	T2-Weighted Image
Air	↓↓↓↓	↓↓↓↓
Free water/CSF	↓↓↓	↑↑↑
Fat	↑↑↑	↑
Cortical bone	↓↓↓	↓↓↓
Bone marrow (fat)	↑↑	↑
Edema	↓	↑↑
Calcification	↓ (Heavy amounts of Ca⁺⁺) ↑ (Little Ca⁺⁺, some Fe⁺⁺⁺)	↓
Mucinous material	↑	↓
Gray matter	Lower than in T2-WI	
White matter	Higher than in T2-WI	
Muscle	Similar to gray matter	Similar to gray matter
Blood products: • Oxyhemoglobin • Deoxyhemoglobin • Intracellular methemoglobin • Extracellular methemoglobin • Hemosiderin	Similar to background ↓ ↑↑ ↑↑ ↓	 ↑ ↓ ↑↑ ↓↓↓

CSF, Cerebrospinal fluid; *MRI,* magnetic resonance imaging; *T2-WI,* T2-weighted image.

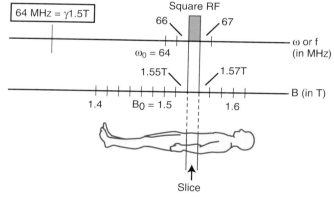

Fig. 33A.12 Slice selection gradient. Using a gradient coil, a magnetic strength gradient is applied parallel to the long axis of the subject's body in the scanner. As a result, the magnetic field is weakest at the feet and gets gradually stronger toward the head. In this example, magnetic field strength is 1.4T at the feet, 1.5T at the mid-body, and 1.6T at the head. Accordingly, protons in these regions will precess at different frequencies (ω): slowest in the feet and with gradually higher frequencies toward the head as the magnetic field gets gradually stronger. Since the radiofrequency (RF) pulse will resonate with those protons (and flip their magnetization vectors) that precess with the same frequency as that of the RF pulse, by selecting the frequency of the RF pulse, we can select which body region's protons to stimulate (i.e., which body slice to image). *(Reprinted with permission from Hashemi, R.H., Bradley, W.G., Lasanti, C.J., 2004. MRI—The Basics. 2nd ed. Lippincott Williams & Wilkins.)*

stimulating radiofrequency pulse during the application of the slice selection gradient, we can choose which protons (those with a specific Larmor frequency) to stimulate ("make resonate"), and thereby we can select which slice of the body to image (**Fig. 33A.12**).

After excitation of the slice to be imaged, using the slice selection gradient, the spatial coordinates of each voxel within the slice must be encoded to determine how much signal is coming from each voxel of that slice. This is achieved by means of two additional gradients that are orthogonal to each other within the imaging plane, known as the *frequency encoding gradient* and the *phase encoding gradient*. The phase encoding gradient briefly alters the precession frequency of the protons along the axis to which it is applied, thereby changing the relative phases of the precessing protons along this in-plane axis. The frequency encoding gradient, applied orthogonally to the phase encoding gradient within the imaging plane, alters the precession frequency of the protons along the axis to which it is applied, during the acquisition of the MRI signal. As a result of these encoding steps, each voxel will have its own unique frequency and its own unique phase shift, which upon repeating the acquisition with several incremental changes in the phase encoding gradient, will allow for deduction of the spatial localization of different intensity values for each voxel using a mathematical algorithm known as a *Fourier transform*. Phase encoding takes time; it has to be performed for each row of voxels in the image along the phase encoding axis. Therefore, the higher the resolution of the image along the phase encoding axis, the longer the time required to acquire the image for that slice of tissue.

In the online version of this chapter (available at www.expertconsult.com), there is a discussion of the nature and application of the following MRI sequences or techniques: spin echo and fast (turbo) spin echo; gradient-recalled echo (GRE) sequences, partial flip angle; inversion recovery sequences (FLAIR, STIR); fat saturation; echoplanar imaging; diffusion-weighted magnetic resonance imaging (DWI); perfusion-weighted magnetic resonance imaging (PWI); susceptibility-weighted imaging (SWI); diffusion tensor imaging (DTI); and magnetization transfer contrast imaging.

Structural Neuroimaging in the Clinical Practice of Neurology

Brain Diseases*

Brain Tumors

Epidemiology, pathology, etiology, and management of cancer in the nervous system are discussed in Chapters 52A-G. From the standpoint of structural neuroimaging, a useful anatomical classification distinguishes two main groups: intraaxial and extraaxial tumors. Intraaxial tumors are within the brain parenchyma, extraaxial tumors are outside the brain parenchyma (involving the meninges or, less commonly, the ventricular system). Intraaxial tumors are usually infiltrative with poorly defined margins. Conversely, extraaxial tumors, even though they often compress or displace the adjacent brain, are usually demarcated by a cerebrospinal (CSF) cleft or another tissue interface between tumor and brain parenchyma. For differential diagnostic purposes, intraaxial primary brain neoplasms can be further divided into the anatomical subgroups of supratentorial and infratentorial tumors (**Table 33A.2**).

*Please go to www.expertconsult.com for an extended version of this section.

For evaluation of brain tumors, the structural imaging modality of choice is MRI. Due to their gradual expansion and often infiltrative nature, most brain tumors are already visible on MRI by the time patients become symptomatic. Exceptions to this rule are tumors that tend to involve the cortex or corticomedullary junction, such as small oligodendrogliomas or metastases, which may cause seizures early, even before being clearly visible on noncontrast MRI. Meningeal involvement is also often symptomatic, for instance by causing headaches and confusion, but may not be appreciated on noncontrast images. Higher magnetic field strength (e.g., a 3-T scanner) and contrast administration (in double or triple dose if necessary) can improve detection of small or clinically silent neoplastic lesions.

Neuroimaging is particularly useful in the assessment of brain tumors. Unlike destructive lesions such as ischemic strokes, brain tumors often cause clinical manifestations that are difficult to interpret. Sometimes the clinical presentation may provide clues to localization—for example, a seizure is suggestive of an intraaxial tumor, whereas cranial nerve involvement tends to signal an extraaxial pathology. But edema, mass effect, obstructive hydrocephalus, and elevated intracranial pressure (ICP) can give rise to nonspecific

Table 33A.2 MRI Imaging Characteristics of Brain Tumors

Tumor	Typical Location, Appearance	Typical T1 Signal Characteristics	Typical T2 Signal Characteristics	Typical Enhancement Pattern
VENTRICULAR REGION				
Central neurocytoma	Intraventricular, at foramen of Monro	Isointense	Iso- to hyperintense	Variable, usually moderate and heterogeneous
Subependymal giant cell astrocytoma	Intraventricular, at foramen of Monro	Hypo- to isointense	Hyperintense with possible hypointense foci due to calcium	Intense
Choroid plexus papilloma	Intraventricular (lateral ventricle in children, fourth ventricle in adults) Calcification and hemorrhage may be present	Iso- to hypointense	Iso- to hyperintense	Intense
Subependymoma	Mostly fourth ventricle but can be third and lateral ventricles	Iso- to hypointense	Hyperintense	Mild or absent
INTRAAXIAL, MOSTLY SUPRATENTORIAL				
Ganglioglioma, gangliocytoma	Supratentorial, mostly temporal lobe. Solid and cystic	Solid portion isointense, cyst hypointense	Solid portion hypo-to hyperintense, cyst hyperintense	From none to heterogenous or rim
Pleomorphic xanthoastrocytoma	Cerebral cortex and adjacent meninges Has cystic portions	Hypo- or mixed intensity	Hyper- or mixed intensity	Solid portion and adjacent meninges enhance
Low-grade astrocytomas	Supratentorial in two-thirds of cases	Iso-to hypointense	Hyperintense	Grade II may enhance
Anaplastic astrocytoma	Frequently in frontal lobes	Iso- to hypointense	Hyperintense	Diffuse or ringlike
Oligodendroglioma	Supratentorial white matter and cortical mantle May exhibit cyst or calcification	Hypo- to isointense	Hyperintense; also typically hyperintense on DWI	Variable, patchy
Oligoastrocytoma	Similar to oligodendroglioma Calcification less common	Similar to oligodendroglioma	Similar to oligodendroglioma	Enhancement more common than in oligodendroglioma

Table 33A.2 MRI Imaging Characteristics of Brain Tumors—cont'd

Tumor	Typical Location, Appearance	Typical T1 Signal Characteristics	Typical T2 Signal Characteristics	Typical Enhancement Pattern
Gliomatosis cerebri	Throughout neuroaxis, typically starts in hemispheric white matter	Iso- to hypointense	Hyperintense	None in early stage, later multifocal
Glioblastoma multiforme	Frontal and temporal lobes, spreads along pathways such as corpus callosum	Mixed (edema, necrosis, hemorrhage)	Mixed (edema, necrosis, hemorrhage)	Intense, inhomogeneous, nodular or ringlike
Primary CNS lymphoma	Supratentorial or infratentorial In immunocompetent host, usually solitary at ventricular border; in immunocompromised, multiple in white matter	Iso- to hypointense	Iso- to hyperintense	Intense Typically ringlike in immunocompromised host
INTRAAXIAL, POSTERIOR FOSSA				
Pilocytic astrocytoma	Posterior fossa, sellar region Usually large cyst with mural nodule	Iso- to hypointense	Iso- to hyperintense	Solid component enhances intensely
Ependymoma	Fourth ventricle Cystic component	Iso- to hypointense	Iso- to hyperintense	Intense in solid portion, rim around cyst
Hemangioblastoma	Infratentorial Vascular nodule and cystic cavity	Hypo- to isointense, but can be mixed due to hemorrhage	Hyperintense, but can be mixed due to hemorrhage	Solid component enhances
Medulloblastoma	Arises from roof of fourth ventricle	Iso- to hypointense	Iso-, hypo-, or hyperintense	Heterogeneous
EXTRAAXIAL				
Esthesioneuroblastoma	Cribriform plate, anterior fossa	Isointense	Iso- to hyperintense	Heterogeneous
Meningioma	Falx, convexity, sphenoid wing, petrous ridge, olfactory groove, parasellar region, and the posterior fossa Calcification may be present	Iso- to slightly hypointense	Can be hypo-, iso-, or hyperintense	Intense, homogeneous
Schwannoma	CP angle, vestibular portion of cranial nerve VIII Cyst or calcification may be present	Iso- to hypointense	Iso- to hyperintense	Homogeneous
Neurofibroma	Arises from peripheral nerve sheath, any location	Iso- to hypointense	Hyperintense	Homogeneous
SELLA AND PINEAL REGIONS				
Pituitary adenoma	Sella, with potential supra- and parasellar extension	Hypo- or isointense	Hyperintense	Homogeneous, enhances in a delayed fashion (initially hypointense relative to the normally enhancing gland; on delayed images, hyperintense relative to the gland due to delayed contrast accumulation)
Craniopharyngioma	Suprasellar cistern, sometimes intrasellar Solid and cystic components	Iso- to hypointense Cyst has variable signal intensity	Solid and cystic component both hyperintense Calcification may be hypointense	Solid component enhances homogeneously
Pineoblastoma	Tectal area	Isointense	Iso- to hypo- to hyperintense	Moderate heterogeneous
Pineocytoma	Tectal area Well defined, noninvasive	Isointense	May be hypointense	Intense with variable pattern (central, nodular)
Germinoma	Tectal region	Variable, hypo- and hyperintense	Variable, hypo- and hyperintense	Intense

DWI, Diffusion-weighted imaging; MRI, magnetic resonance imaging.

symptoms (e.g., headache, visual disturbance, altered mental status), and false localizing signs may also appear, such as oculomotor or abducens nerve compression due to an expanding intraaxial mass.

Neoplastic tissues most commonly prolong the T1 and T2 relaxation times, appearing hypointense on T1 and hyperintense on T2-weighted images, but different tumors differ in this property, facilitating tumor identification on MRI. MRI is also very sensitive for detection of other pathologic changes that can be associated with tumors, such as calcification, hemorrhage, necrosis, and edema. The structural detail provided by MRI is useful for assessing involved structures and determining the number and macroscopic extent of the neoplasms, thereby guiding surgical planning or other treatment modalities.

Intraaxial Primary Brain Tumors

GANGLIOGLIOMA AND GANGLIOCYTOMA

Gangliogliomas (WHO grade I or II) are mixed tumors containing both neural and glial elements. *Gangliocytomas* (WHO grade I) are less common and contain well-differentiated neuronal cells without a glial component. Less commonly, gangliogliomas may exhibit anaplasia within the glial component and are classified as *anaplastic ganglioglioma* (WHO grade III). A rare type of gangliocytoma, dysplastic gangliocytoma of the cerebellum (also known as *Lhermitte-Duclos disease*) exhibits a characteristic "tiger-striped" appearance and is often present in association with Cowden disease, a phacomatosis.

The peak age of onset for gangliogliomas is the second decade. This tumor is usually supratentorial and is most commonly located in the temporal lobe. It is well demarcated, and a cystic component and mural nodule are often observed. Calcification is common.

On MRI (Provenzale et al., 2000) the solid component is usually isointense on T1 and hypo- to hyperintense on T2-weighted images. The cystic component, if present, exhibits CSF signal characteristics. The associated mass effect is variable. With contrast, various enhancement patterns are seen—homogenous or rim pattern—but no enhancement is also possible.

PILOCYTIC ASTROCYTOMAS

Pilocytic astrocytomas have two major groups: juvenile and adult. These tumors are classified as WHO grade I. Juvenile pilocytic astrocytomas are the most common posterior fossa tumors in children. The most common locations are the cerebellum, at the fourth ventricle, third ventricle, temporal lobe, optic chiasm, and hypothalamus (Koeller and Rushing, 2004). The appearance is often lobulated, and the lesion appears well demarcated on MRI. Hemorrhage and necrosis are uncommon. Areas of calcification may be present. The tumor usually exhibits solid as well as cystic components, with or without a mural nodule. The adult form is usually well circumscribed, often calcified, and typically exhibits a large cyst with a mural nodule. On MRI, the solid portions of the tumor are iso- to hypointense on T1 and iso- to hyperintense on T2-weighted images (Arai et al., 2006). The cystic component usually exhibits CSF signal characteristics. The associated edema and mass effect is usually mild, sometimes moderate. With gadolinium, the solid components (including the mural nodule) enhance intensely, but not the cyst, which rarely may show rim enhancement.

PLEOMORPHIC XANTHOASTROCYTOMA

Pleomorphic xanthoastrocytoma is a rare variant of astrocytic tumors. It is thought to arise from the subpial astrocytes and typically affects the cerebral cortex and adjacent meninges and may cause erosion of the skull. The most common location is the temporal lobe. It is classified as WHO grade II. It usually occurs in the second and third decades of life, and patients often present with seizures. On MRI (Tien et al., 1992) usually a well-circumscribed cystic mass appears in a superficial cortical location. A solid portion or mural nodule is often seen, and the differential diagnosis includes pilocytic astrocytoma and ganglioglioma. The signal characteristics are hypointense or mixed on T1, and hyperintense or mixed on T2-weighted images. With contrast, the solid portions and sometimes the adjacent meninges enhance. Calcification may be present. There is mild or no mass effect associated with this tumor.

LOW-GRADE ASTROCYTOMAS

Fibrillary astrocytomas, also termed *diffuse astrocytomas*, represent approximately 10% of all gliomas. Low-grade (WHO grade I and II) astrocytomas belong to this group (**Figs. 33A.17** and **33A.18**). These are well-differentiated tumors, usually arising from the fibrillary astrocytes of the white matter. Even though imaging may show a fairly well-defined boundary, these tumors are infiltrative and usually spread beyond their macroscopic border. Two-thirds of cases are supratentorial. A subgroup of these astrocytomas involves specific regions such as the optic nerves/tracts or the brainstem.

Low-grade astrocytomas are iso- or hypointense on T1-weighted images and hyperintense on T2-weighted images. Tissue expansion may be seen, and mass effect (if present) is generally modest. There is little to no associated edema. Fibrillary grade I astrocytomas do not enhance; grade II tumors may exhibit enhancement. The appearance of enhancement in a previously nonenhancing tumor is a worrisome sign of malignant transformation, often due to anaplastic astrocytoma.

ANAPLASTIC ASTROCYTOMA

Anaplastic astrocytoma is classified as grade III by the WHO grading system. It represents 25% to 30% of gliomas, usually appears between 40 and 60 years of age, and is more common in men. Anaplastic astrocytoma is a diffuse infiltrating tumor that often evolves from a well-differentiated astrocytoma as a result of chromosomal and gene alterations. It is most frequently found in the frontal lobes. On MRI, anaplastic astrocytomas appear as poorly circumscribed heterogenous tumors which are iso- to hypointense on T1-weighted and hyperintense on T2-weighted images, with associated hyperintensity in the surrounding white matter representing vasogenic edema. Foci of hemorrhage may be present but not too commonly. There is moderate mass effect associated with the lesions, and with contrast, a variable degree and pattern of enhancement is noted (diffuse or ringlike). This tumor is highly infiltrative, usually cannot be fully removed by surgery, and the median survival is 3 to 4 years.

OLIGODENDROGLIOMA

Oligodendroglioma accounts for 5% to 10% of all gliomas. It arises from the oligodendroglia that form the myelin sheath of the central nervous system (CNS) pathways.

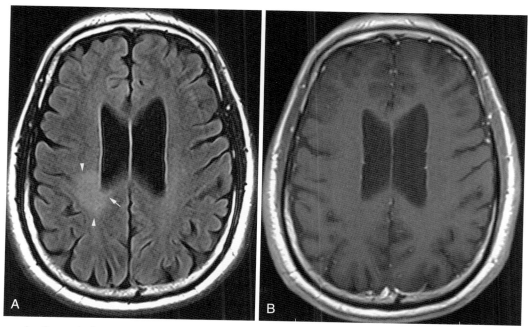

Fig. 33A.17 Low-grade glioma. **A,** On FLAIR image, a faint hyperintense lesion is seen *(arrowheads)* with somewhat blurred margins in the right corona radiata at the border of the lateral ventricle, extending minimally toward the corpus callosum *(arrow)*. **B,** On T1-weighted postcontrast image, this lesion does not enhance.

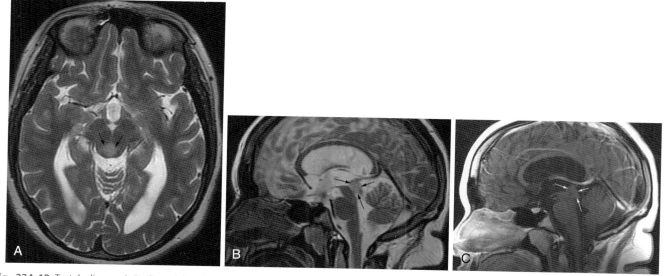

Fig. 33A.18 Tectal glioma. **A-B,** On axial and sagittal T2-weighted images, a faintly hyperintense mass lesion is seen involving the tectum of the midbrain *(arrows)*. There appears to be at least partial obstruction of the aqueduct, resulting in enlargement of the third and lateral ventricles. **C,** Following gadolinium administration, the tumor does not enhance *(arrows)*.

Oligodendroglioma occurs most commonly in young and middle-aged adults, with a median age of onset within the fourth to fifth decades and a male predominance of up to 2:1. Seizure is often the presenting symptom. The most common location is the supratentorial hemispheric white matter, and it also involves the cortical mantle. The tumor often has cystic components and at least microscopically, in 90% of cases also shows calcification. Hemorrhage and necrosis are rare, and the mass effect is not impressive. On MRI (Koeller and Rushing, 2005) the appearance is heterogenous, and the tumor is hypo- and isointense on T1 and hyperintense on T2. With gadolinium, the enhancement is variable, usually patchy, and

the periphery of the lesion tends to enhance more intensely. Oligodendrogliomas are hypercellular and have been noted to appear hyperintense on diffusion-weighted images (**Fig. 33A.19**).

OLIGOASTROCYTOMA

Oligoastrocytomas are tumors consisting of a mixture of neoplastic oligodendroglioma and astrocytoma cell populations that may be separate (in which case the tumor is described as *biphasic*) or intermingled. Oligoastrocytomas cannot be definitively distinguished from oligodendrogliomas on imaging studies, with similar locations, size, and

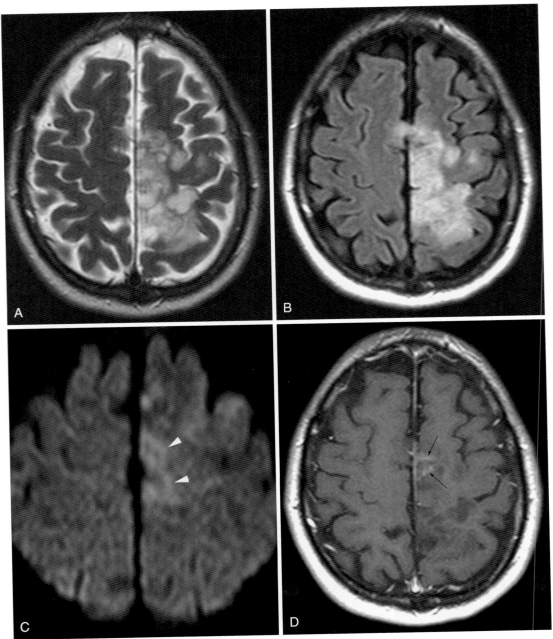

Fig. 33A.19 Oligodendroglioma. A mass lesion is seen in the left medial frontal lobe, involving the cortical mantle and underlying white matter. **A-B,** On T2 and FLAIR images, the tumor is hyperintense. **C,** On diffusion-weighted image, faint hyperintensity due to the hypercellular nature of this tumor is noted *(arrowheads)*. **D,** With contrast, a few areas of enhancement are seen that tend to involve periphery of lesion *(arrows)*.

attenuation/signal characteristics. However, calcification is less common (14%) and enhancement more common (50%) in oligoastrocytomas.

GLIOMATOSIS CEREBRI

Gliomatosis cerebri, a rare glial neoplasm, usually presents in the third decade of life. The glial tumor cells are disseminated throughout the parenchyma and infiltrate large portions of the neuraxis. Macroscopically it appears homogenous and is seen as enlargement/expansion of the parenchyma; the gray/white matter interface may become blurred, but the architecture is otherwise not altered. The hemispheric white matter is involved first, then the pathology spreads to the corpus callosum,

followed by both hemispheres. Later, the deep gray matter (basal ganglia, thalamus, massa intermedia) may be affected as well. Diffuse tumor infiltration often extends into the brainstem, cerebellum, and even the spinal cord. Histologically, most cases of gliomatosis cerebri are WHO grade III.

The MRI appearance is iso- to hypointense on T1 and hyperintense on T2. Hemorrhage is uncommon, and enhancement is also rare, at least in the early stages (**Fig. 33A.20**). Later, multiple foci of enhancement may appear, signaling more malignant transformation. The imaging appearance is similar to that of encephalitis, lymphoma, or subacute sclerosing panencephalitis, but in these disorders, clinical findings are more pronounced.

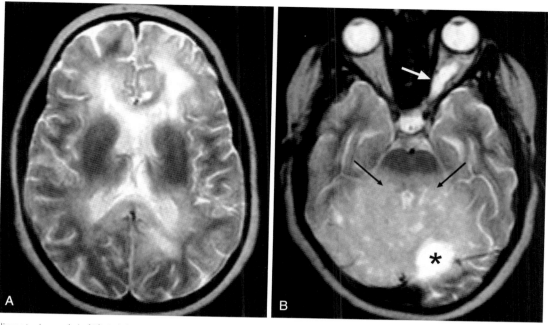

Fig. 33A.20 Gliomatosis cerebri. **(A)** Axial T2-weighted magnetic resonance (MR) image of brain shows bilateral patchy areas of increased signal intensity in periventricular white matter. **(B)** Axial T2-weighted MR image of brain obtained at the level of the upper pons shows diffuse thickening and hyperintensity of left optic nerve *(white arrow)* and increased signal intensity in posterior aspect of pons and in cerebellum *(black arrows)*. A focus of very high signal intensity is present in posterior left cerebellar hemisphere (*). *(From Yip, M., Fisch, C., Lamarche, J.B., 2003. AFIP archives: gliomatosis cerebri affecting the entire neuraxis. Radiographics 23, 247-253.)*

GLIOBLASTOMA MULTIFORME

Glioblastoma multiforme is a highly malignant tumor classified as grade IV by the WHO. It is most common in older adults, usually appearing in the fifth and sixth decades. GBM is the most common primary brain neoplasm, representing 40% to 50% of all primary neoplasms and up to 20% of all intracranial tumors. It forms a heterogenous mass exhibiting cystic and necrotic areas and often a hemorrhagic component as well. The most common locations are the frontal and temporal lobes. The tumor is highly infiltrative and has a tendency to spread along larger pathways such as the corpus callosum and invade the other hemisphere, resulting in a characteristic "butterfly" appearance. GBM has also been described to spread along the ventricular surface in the subarachnoid space and may also invade the meninges. There are reported cases of extracranial glioblastoma metastases.

Structural neuroimaging distinguishes between multifocal and multicentric glioblastomas. The term *multifocal glioblastoma* refers to multiple tumor islands in the brain that arose from a common source via continuous parenchymal spread or meningeal/CSF seeding; therefore, they are all connected, at least microscopically. *Multicentric glioblastoma* refers to multiple tumors that are present independently, and physical connection between them cannot be proven, implying they are separate de novo occurrences. This is less common, having been noted in 6% of cases.

On MRI (**Fig. 33A.21**) glioblastomas usually exhibit mixed signal intensities on T1- and T2-weighted images. Cystic and necrotic areas are present, appearing as markedly decreased signal on T1-weighted and hyperintensity on T2-weighted images. Mixed hypo- and hyperintense signal changes due to hemorrhage are also seen. The hemorrhagic component can also be well demonstrated by gradient echo sequences or by SWI. The core of the lesion is surrounded by prominent edema, which appears hypointense on T1-weighted and hyperintense on T2-weighted images. Besides edema, the signal changes around the core of the tumor reflect the presence of infiltrating tumor cells and, in treated cases, postsurgical reactive gliosis and/or post-irradiation changes. Following administration of gadolinium, intense enhancement is noted, which is inhomogenous and often ringlike, also including multiple nodular areas of enhancement. The surrounding edema and ringlike enhancement at times makes it difficult to distinguish glioblastoma from cerebral abscess. DWI is helpful in these cases; glioblastomas are hypointense with this technique, whereas abscesses exhibit remarkable hyperintensity on diffusion-weighted images.

Owing to its aggressive growth (the tumor size may double every 10 days) and infiltrative nature, the prognosis for patients with glioblastoma is very poor. Despite surgery, irradiation, and chemotherapy the median survival is 1 year.

EPENDYMOMA

Although ependymomas are primarily extraaxial tumors (within the fourth ventricle), intraparenchymal ependymomas arising from ependymal cell remnants of the hemispheric parenchyma are also well known, so this tumor type is discussed here. Ependymomas comprise 5% to 6% of all primary brain tumors; 70% of cases occur in childhood and the first and second decades, and ependymoma is the third most common posterior fossa tumor in children. Ependymomas arise from differentiated ependymal cells, and the most common location (70%) is the fourth ventricle. The tumor is usually well demarcated and is separated from the vermis by a CSF interface. The tumor may be cystic and may contain calcification and hemorrhage, but these features are more

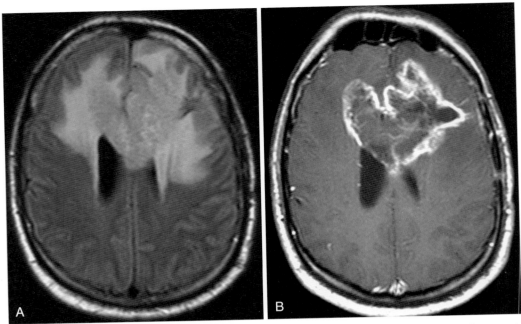

Fig. 33A.21 Glioblastoma multiforme. **A,** Axial FLAIR image demonstrates a mass lesion spreading across the corpus callosum to involve both frontal lobes in a symmetrical fashion ("butterfly" appearance). Tumor is isointense, exerts mass effect on the sulci and the lateral ventricles, and is surrounded by vasogenic edema. **B,** On axial T1 postcontrast imaging, tumor exhibits heterogenous irregular enhancement, most marked at its periphery.

common in supratentorial ependymomas. It may extrude from the cavity of the fourth ventricle through the foramina of Luschka and Magendie. Spreading via CSF to the spinal canal (drop-metastases) may occur, but on spine imaging ependymoma is more commonly noted to arise from the ependymal lining of the central canal, presenting as an intramedullary spinal cord tumor. A subtype, myxopapillary ependymoma, is almost always restricted to the filum terminale.

Ependymomas are hypo- to isointense on T1-weighted, and iso- to hyperintense on T2-weighted images. With gadolinium, intense enhancement is seen, mostly involving the solid components of the tumor, whereas the cystic components tend to exhibit rim enhancement. The differential diagnosis for infratentorial ependymoma includes medulloblastoma, pilocytic astrocytoma, and choroid plexus papilloma.

LYMPHOMA

Primary CNS lymphoma (PCNSL) is a non-Hodgkin lymphoma, which in 98% of cases is a B-cell lymphoma. It once accounted for only 1% to 2% of all primary brain tumors, but this percentage has been increasing, mostly because of the growing acquired immunodeficiency syndrome (AIDS) population. The peak age of onset is 60 in the immunocompetent population and age 30 in immunocompromised patients. Lesions may occur anywhere within the neuraxis, including the cerebral hemispheres, brainstem, cerebellum, and spinal cord, although the most common location (90% of cases) is supratentorial. PCNSL lesions are highly infiltrative and exhibit a predilection for sites that contact subarachnoid and ependymal surfaces as well as the deep gray nuclei.

The imaging appearance of PCNSL depends on the patient's immune status. The tumor is hypo- to isointense on T1-weighted and hypo- to slightly hyperintense on T2-weighted images. Contrast enhancement is usually intense. In

immunocompetent patients (Zhang et al., 2010) the lesion is often single, tends to abut the ventricular border (Costa et al., 2006), and ring enhancement is uncommon (**Fig. 33A.22**). In immunocompromised patients, usually multiple, often ring-enhancing lesions are seen, which are most commonly located in the periventricular white matter and the gray/white junction of the lobes of the hemispheres, but the deep central gray matter structures and the posterior fossa may be involved as well. Overall, the imaging appearance appears more malignant in the immunocompromised cases and may be difficult to differentiate from toxoplasmosis. Other components of the differential diagnosis in patients with multiple PCNSL lesions include demyelination, abscesses, neurosarcoidosis, and metastatic disease.

HEMANGIOBLASTOMA

Hemangioblastomas represent only 1% to 2% of all primary brain tumors, but in adults they are the most common type of primary intraaxial tumor of the posterior fossa (cerebellum and medulla). These tumors are WHO grade I, well circumscribed, and exhibit a vascular nodule with a usually larger cystic cavity. On MRI the solid portion is hypo- to isointense on T1 and hyperintense on T2-weighted images. Sometimes hyperintense foci are noted on T1; this is due to occasional lipid deposition or hemorrhage within the tumor. The cystic component is usually hypointense on T1 (but may be hyperintense relative to CSF due to high protein content) and markedly hyperintense on T2. On FLAIR images, the cyst fluid is not completely nulled, resulting in bright signal, and the nodule is also hyperintense. There is usually mild surrounding edema. With gadolinium, the solid component exhibits intense enhancement. Hemangioblastomas are seen in 50% of patients with von Hippel-Lindau disease, and approximately one-fourth of all hemangioblastomas occur in these patients (Neumann et al., 1989).

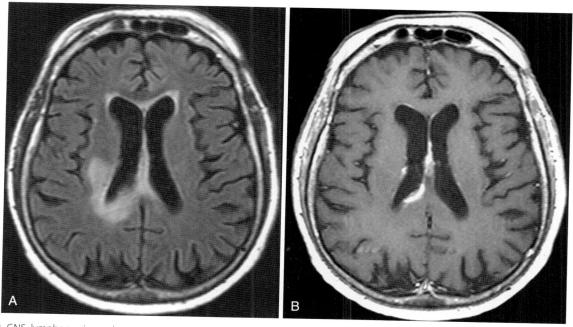

Fig. 33A.22 CNS lymphoma in an immunocompetent individual. **A,** FLAIR sequence depicts a single hyperintense lesion with spread along the ventricular border. **B,** After contrast administration, multiple areas of enhancement are seen within the lesion, without a ringlike enhancement pattern.

Extraaxial Primary Brain Tumors

Descriptions of the rarer extraaxial primary brain tumor types—esthesioneuroblastoma, central neurocytoma, and subependymoma—are available in the online version of this chapter (www.expertconsult.com).

MENINGIOMAS

Meningiomas are the most common primary brain tumors of non-glial origin and make up 15% of all intracranial tumors. The peak age of onset is the fifth decade, and there is a striking female predominance that may be related to the fact that some meningiomas contain estrogen and progesterone receptors. These tumors arise from meningothelial cells. In 1% to 9% of cases, multiple tumors are seen. The most common locations are the falx (25%), convexity (20%), sphenoid wing, petrous ridge (15% to 20%), olfactory groove (5% to 10%), parasellar region (5% to 10%), and the posterior fossa (10%). Rarely an intraventricular location has been reported. Meningiomas often appear as smooth hemispherical or lobular dural-based masses (**Fig. 33A.23**). Calcification is common, seen in at least 20% of these tumors. Meningiomas also often exhibit vascularity. The extraaxial location of the tumor is usually well appreciated owing to a visible CSF interface between tumor and adjacent brain parenchyma. Meningiomas may become malignant, invading the brain and eroding the skull. In such cases, prominent edema may be present in the brain parenchyma, to the extent that the extraaxial nature of the tumor is no longer obvious.

On T1-weighted images, meningiomas are usually iso- to slightly hypointense. The appearance on T2 can be iso-, hypo-, or hyperintense to the gray matter. Although MRI does not reveal the histological subtypes of meningiomas with absolute certainty, there have been observations according to which fibroblastic and transitional meningiomas tend to be iso- to hypointense on T2-weighted images, whereas the meningothelial or angioblastic type is iso- or more hyperintense. Not uncommonly, the skull adjacent to a meningioma will exhibit subtle thickening, a useful diagnostic clue in some cases.

After gadolinium administration, meningiomas typically exhibit intense homogenous enhancement. A quite typical imaging finding on postcontrast images is the *dural tail sign*, which refers to the linear extension of enhancement along the dura, beyond the segment on which the tumor is based. Earlier this had been attributed to en plaque extension of the meningioma along these dural segments and was thought to be specific for this type of tumor. However, recently it has been recognized that this imaging appearance is not specific to this situation and may be seen in other tumors, secondary to increased vascularity/hyperperfusion or congestion of the dural vessels after irradiation and as a postsurgical change.

SCHWANNOMA

Schwannomas arise from the Schwann cells of the nerve sheath, and the most commonly affected nerve is the vestibular portion of the vestibulocochlear nerve. They are typically bilateral in neurofibromatosis (NF) type 2 (see **Fig. 33A.69**). The unilateral form sporadically occurs in non-NF patients, with slight female predominance. Schwannomas typically arise in the intracanalicular segment of the eighth cranial nerve where myelin transitions from central (oligodendroglia) to peripheral (Schwann cell) type. If untreated, the tumor grows toward the internal auditory meatus and eventually bulges into the cerebellopontine angle, where it may deform and displace the brainstem. The intra- and extracanalicular parts of the tumor together result in a mushroom or ice cream cone–like appearance. The tumor is iso- to hypointense on T1-weighted images and iso- to hyperintense on T2-weighted images. This pattern may be modified by the presence of cystic changes or calcification. Gadolinium administration causes homogenous enhancement that,

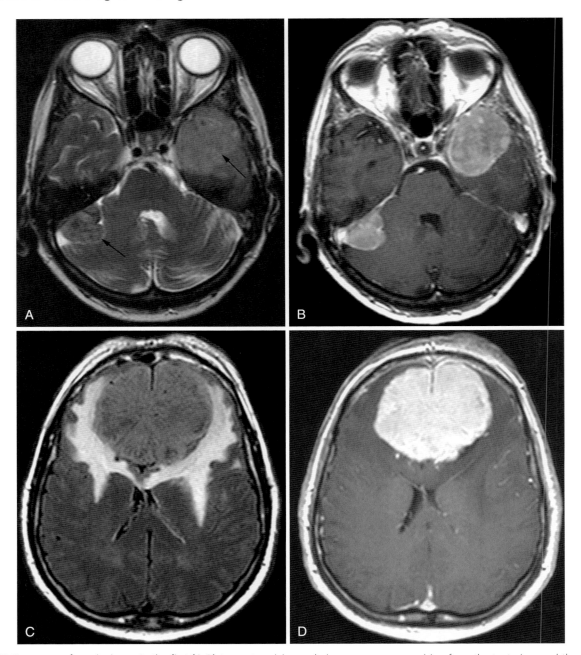

Fig. 33A.23 Two cases of meningioma. In the first **(A-B)** two extraaxial mass lesions are seen, one arising from the tentorium and the other from the sphenoid wing in the left middle cranial fossa *(arrows)*. These compress the right cerebellar hemisphere and the left temporal lobe, respectively. **A,** On T2-weighted image, the masses are mostly isointense with foci of hypointensity. **B,** After gadolinium administration, the masses enhance homogenously. Note the small dural tail along the tentorium. In the second case **(C-D)** a large olfactory groove meningioma is presented that exerts significant mass effect on the frontal lobes, corpus callosum, and lateral ventricles. **C,** On FLAIR image, hyperintense vasogenic edema is seen in the compressed brain parenchyma. **D,** Tumor enhances homogeneously with gadolinium.

together with the performance of axial and coronal thin-slice T2-weighted images, allows for the visualization of even very small intracanalicular schwannomas.

PRIMITIVE NEUROECTODERMAL TUMOR

Primitive neuroectodermal tumor (PNET) is a collective term that includes several tumors arising from cells that are derived from the neuroectoderm and are in an undifferentiated state. The main tumors that belong to the PNET group are medulloblastomas, esthesioneuroblastomas, and pinealoblastomas.

The tumors belonging to the PNET group are fast growing and highly malignant. The most common mode of metastatic spread for PNETs is via CSF pathways, an indication for imaging surveillance of the entire neuraxis when these tumors are suspected.

MEDULLOBLASTOMA

Medulloblastomas arise from the undifferentiated neuroecto-dermal cells of the roof of the fourth ventricle (superior or inferior medullary velum, vermis). They represent 25% of all

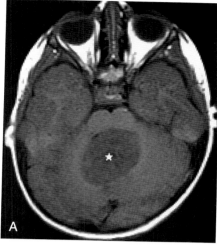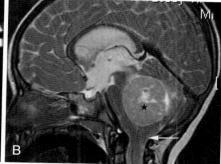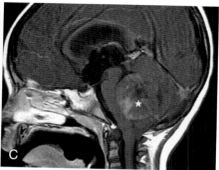

Fig. 33A.24 Medulloblastoma. A large mass lesion is seen (*) filling and expanding the fourth ventricle. **A,** On T1-weighted image, tumor is partially iso- but mostly hypointense. **B,** On T2-weighted image, tumor shows iso- and hyperintense signal change; it compresses/displaces the brainstem and cerebellum. On sagittal images, note the secondary Chiari malformation (caudal displacement of cerebellar tonsils) due to mass effect *(arrow)*. **C,** On T1 postcontrast image, there is a heterogeneous enhancement pattern.

cerebral tumors in children, usually presenting in the first and second decade. The tumor fills the fourth ventricle, extending rostrally toward the aqueduct and caudally to the cisterna magna, frequently resulting in obstructive hydrocephalus. Leptomeningeal and CSF spread may also occur, resulting in spinal drop metastases. Cystic components and necrosis may be present. Calcification is possible. On CT, medulloblastoma typically appears as a heterogeneous, generally hyperdense midline tumor occupying the fourth ventricle, with mass effect and variable contrast enhancement. The MRI signal (Koeller and Rushing, 2003) is heterogenous; the tumor is iso- or hypointense on T1 and hypo-, iso-, or hyperintense on T2. Contrast administration induces heterogenous enhancement (**Fig. 33A.24**). Restricted diffusion may be seen on DWI/ADC (Gauvain et al., 2001). Consistent with its site of origin, indistinct borders between the tumor and the roof of the fourth ventricle may be observed, aiding in the differential diagnosis, which in children includes atypical rhabdoid-teratoid tumor, brainstem glioma, pilocytic astrocytoma, choroid plexus papilloma, and ependymoma. The adult differential diagnosis includes the latter two entities in addition to metastasis and hemangioblastoma. Medulloblastoma does not tend to extrude via the foramina outside of the fourth ventricle, facilitating differentiation from ependymoma. In children, choroid plexus papilloma is more likely to occur within the lateral ventricle.

PINEOBLASTOMA

Pineoblastomas are highly cellular tumors that are similar in MRI appearance to pineocytomas. However, they tend to be larger (>3 cm), more heterogenous, frequently cause hydrocephalus, and also may spread via the CSF. This tumor is isointense to gray matter on T1, with moderate heterogeneous enhancement following administration of gadolinium. Like other PNETs, the hypercellularity of pineoblastoma results in T2-weighted signal that tends to be iso- or hypointense relative to gray matter, and restricted diffusion may also be seen. Cysts within the tumor may appear markedly hyperintense on T2, peripheral edema less so. In cases accompanied by hydrocephalus, FLAIR imaging may reveal uniform

hyperintensity in a planar distribution along the margins of the lateral ventricles due to transependymal flow of CSF. Peripheral calcifications or intratumoral hemorrhage will exhibit markedly hypointense signal with blooming artifact on T2* (pronounced *T2-star*) images. Differential diagnostic considerations include germ cell tumor, pineocytoma, and (uncommonly) metastases.

OTHER PINEAL REGION TUMORS

Besides pineoblastomas, which histologically belong to the group of primitive neuroectodermal tumors, the pineal gland may also develop tumors of pinealocyte origin (pineocytoma) and germ cell tumors.

Pineocytoma

Pineocytomas are homogenous masses containing more solid components, but cysts may also be present. These tumors have a round, well-defined, noninvasive appearance. Calcification is commonly seen, but hemorrhage is uncommon. These tumors may be hypointense on T2 and exhibit a variable (central, nodular) pattern of intense enhancement after gadolinium administration (Fakhran and Escott, 2008).

Germ Cell Tumors (Germinoma)

Masses in the pineal region are most often germ cell tumors, usually germinomas. Less common types include teratoma, choriocarcinoma, and embryonal carcinoma. Germinomas are well-circumscribed round or lobulated lesions. Hemorrhage and calcification are rare. Metastases may spread via CSF, so the entire neuraxis should be imaged if these tumors are suspected. MRI signal characteristics are variable, with iso- to hyperintense signal relative to gray matter on both T1 and T2. With gadolinium, intense contrast enhancement is seen.

Subependymal Giant Cell Astrocytoma

Subependymal giant cell astrocytoma, a WHO grade I tumor, arises from astrocytes in the subependymal zone of the lateral ventricles and develops into an intraventricular tumor in the region of the foramen of Monro. It is seen almost exclusively in patients with tuberous sclerosis. Just like central

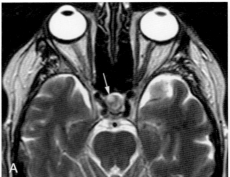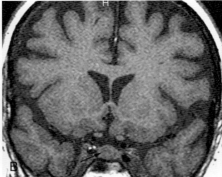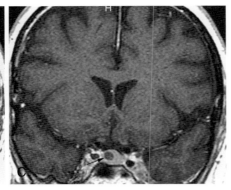

Fig. 33A.25 Pituitary microadenoma. **A,** Axial T2-weighted image demonstrates a round area of hyperintensity on right side of pituitary gland *(arrow)*. **B,** On coronal noncontrast T1-weighted image, the gland has an upward convex morphology, and there is a vague hypointensity in its right side *(arrow)*. **C,** On coronal T1-weighted postcontrast image, the microadenoma is well seen as an area of hypointensity *(arrow)* against the background of the normally enhancing gland parenchyma.

neurocytoma, this tumor is also prone to cause obstructive hydrocephalus. The tumor is heterogeneously hypo- to isointense on T1 and heterogeneously hyperintense on T2-weighted images, with possible foci of hypointensity due to calcification. On FLAIR, an isointense to hyperintense solid tumor background may be punctuated by hyperintense cysts. FLAIR is also useful to assess for the possible presence of hyperintense cortical tubers, which if present aid in the differential diagnosis. With gadolinium, intense enhancement is seen.

Choroid Plexus Papilloma

Choroid plexus papilloma is a well-circumscribed, highly vascular, intraventricular WHO grade I tumor derived from choroid plexus epithelium. In children it is usually seen in the lateral ventricle, while in adults it tends to involve the fourth ventricle. General imaging characteristics include a villiform or bosselated "cauliflower-like" appearance. Hemorrhage and calcification are noted occasionally in the tumor bed. The tumor's location frequently causes obstructive hydrocephalus. On MRI, the appearance is hypo- or isointense to normal brain on T1 and iso- to hyperintense on T2-weighted images. The latter may also show punctate or linear/serpiginous signal flow voids within the tumor. Calcification (25%) or hemorrhage manifest as a markedly hypointense blooming artifact on T2* gradient echo images. With gadolinium, intense enhancement is seen. Choroid plexus carcinomas are malignant tumors that may invade the brain parenchyma and may also spread via CSF.

Tumors in the Sellar and Parasellar Region

The sellar and parasellar group of extraaxial masses include pituitary micro- and macroadenomas and craniopharyngiomas. Meningiomas, arachnoid cysts, dermoid and epidermoid cysts, optic pathway gliomas, hamartomas, metastases, and aneurysms are also encountered in the para- and suprasellar region.

PITUITARY ADENOMAS

The distinction between micro- and macroadenomas is based on their size: tumors less than 10 mm are microadenomas, the larger tumors are macroadenomas. These tumors may arise from hormone-producing cells, such as prolactinomas or growth hormone–producing adenomas, resulting in characteristic clinical syndromes. Pituitary adenomas are typically hypointense on T1-weighted and hyperintense on T2-weighted images, relative to the surrounding parenchyma. This signal change, however, is not always conspicuous, especially in the case of small microadenomas. Gadolinium administration helps in these cases, when the microadenoma is visualized as relative hypointensity against the background of the normally enhancing gland (**Fig. 33A.25**). Following a delay, this difference in enhancement is often no longer apparent, and if the postcontrast images are obtained in a later phase, a reversal of contrast may be noted. The adenoma takes up contrast in a delayed fashion and is seen as hyperintense against the more hypointense gland from where the contrast has washed out. Sometimes when the signal characteristics are not conspicuous, only alteration of the size and shape of the pituitary gland or shifting of the infundibulum may indicate the presence of a microadenoma. Because of this, it is important to be familiar with the normal range of pituitary gland sizes, which depend on age and gender. In adults, a gland height of more than 9 mm is worrisome. In the younger population, however, different normal values have been established. Before puberty, the normal height is 3 to 5 mm. At puberty in girls, the gland height may be 10 to 11 mm and may exhibit an upward convex morphology. In boys at puberty, the height is 6 to 8 mm, and the upward convex morphology can be normal. The size and shape of the gland may also change during pregnancy: convex morphology may appear, and a gland height of 10 mm is considered normal.

While microadenomas are localized to the sellar region, macroadenomas may become invasive and extend to the suprasellar region and displace/compress the optic chiasm or even the hypothalamus. Extension to the cavernous sinus is also possible.

CRANIOPHARYNGIOMA

Craniopharyngiomas are believed to originate from the epithelial remnants of the Rathke pouch. This WHO grade I tumor may be encountered in children, and a second peak incidence is in the fifth decade (Eldevik et al., 1996). The most common location is the suprasellar cistern (**Fig. 33A.26**), but intrasellar tumors are also possible. The tumor may cause expansion of the sella or erosion of the dorsum sellae. In the suprasellar region, displacement of the chiasm, the anterior cerebral arteries, or even the hypothalamus is possible.

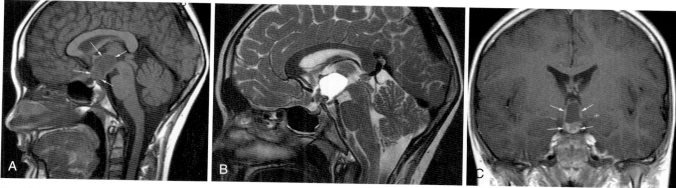

Fig. 33A.26 Craniopharyngioma. **A,** On sagittal T1-weighted image, a suprasellar mass lesion has a prominent T1 hypointense cystic component *(arrows).* **B,** On sagittal T2-weighted image, the cyst is hyperintense. **C,** With gadolinium, both the rim of the cyst and the solid portion of the mass exhibit enhancement *(arrows).*

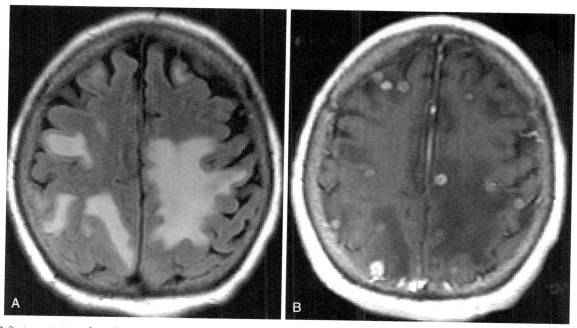

Fig. 33A.27 Brain metastases from breast cancer. **A,** On axial FLAIR image, multiple areas of vasogenic edema extend into subcortical white matter with fingerlike projections. **B,** On axial T1-weighted postcontrast image, numerous small enhancing mass lesions are scattered in both hemispheres at the gray/white junction. Both homogeneous and ringlike enhancement patterns are present.

Craniopharyngiomas have both solid and cystic components. Histologically, the more common adamantinomatous and the less common papillary forms are distinguished. The adamantinomatous type frequently exhibits calcification. The MRI signal is heterogeneous. Solid portions are iso- or hypointense on T1, whereas cystic components exhibit variable signal characteristics depending on the amount of protein or the presence of blood products. On T2, the solid and cystic components are sometimes hard to distinguish, as they are both usually hyperintense. Areas of calcification may appear hypointense on T2. With contrast, the solid portions of the tumor exhibit intense enhancement.

Metastatic Tumors

Intracranial metastases are detected in approximately 25% of patients who die of cancer. Cerebral metastases comprise over half of brain tumors (Vogelbaum and Suh, 2006) and are the most common type of brain tumor in adults (Klos and O'Neill, 2004). Most (80%) metastases involve the cerebral hemispheres, and 20% are seen in the posterior fossa. Pelvic and colon cancer have a tendency to involve the posterior fossa. Intracranial metastases, depending on the type of tumor, may involve the skull and the dura, the brain, and also the meninges in the form of meningeal carcinomatosis. Among all tumors that metastasize to the bone, breast and prostate cancer and multiple myeloma are especially prone to spread to the skull and dura. Most often, carcinomas involve the brain and get there by hematogenous spread. Systemic tumors with the greatest tendency to metastasize to brain are lung (as many as 30% of lung cancers give rise to brain metastases), breast (**Fig. 33A.27**), and melanoma (**Fig. 33A.28**). Cancers of the gastrointestinal tract (especially colon and rectum) and the kidney are the next most common sources. Other possibilities include gallbladder, liver, thyroid gland, pancreas, ovary, and testicles. Tumors of the prostate, esophagus, and

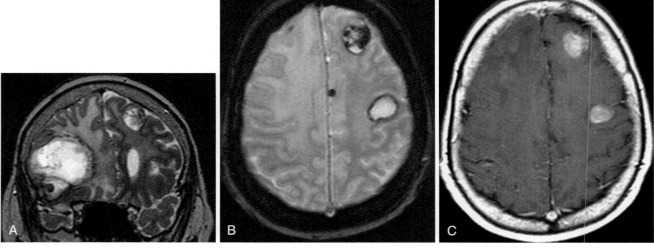

Fig. 33A.28 Hemorrhagic melanoma metastases. **A,** Coronal T2-weighted image demonstrates a large hyperintense mass in the right frontal lobe, with associated hyperintense vasogenic edema and mass effect. A smaller mass lesion with similar signal characteristics is present at the gray/white junction in the left frontal lobe. Note surrounding rim of hypointensity, indicating hemosiderin deposition within these hemorrhagic metastases. **B,** On gradient echo, hypointense blood degradation products are well seen within the metastases. **C,** Following gadolinium administration, intense enhancement is noted.

skin (other than melanoma) hardly ever form brain parenchymal metastases.

It is important to highlight the potential imaging differences between primary and metastatic brain tumors, since a significant percentage of patients found to have brain metastasis have no prior diagnosis of cancer. Cerebral parenchymal metastases can be single (usually with kidney, breast, thyroid, and lung adenocarcinoma) or (more commonly) multiple (in small cell carcinomas and melanoma) and tend to involve the gray/white matter junction. Seeing multiple tumors at the corticomedullary junction favors the diagnosis of metastatic lesions over a primary brain tumor. The size of metastatic lesions is variable, and the mass effect and peritumoral edema is usually prominent and, contrary to that seen with primary brain tumors, frequently out of proportion to the size of the tumor itself. The edema is vasogenic, persistent, and involves the white matter, highlighting the intact cortical sulci as characteristic fingerlike projections. It is hypointense on T1 and hyperintense on T2 and FLAIR. The tumor itself exhibits variable, often heterogenous signal intensity, especially if the metastasis is hemorrhagic (15% of brain metastases). Tumors that tend to cause hemorrhagic metastases include melanoma; choriocarcinoma; and lung, thyroid, and kidney cancer. The tumor signal characteristic can be unique in mucin-producing colon adenocarcinoma metastases, where the mucin and protein content cause a hyperintense signal on T1-weighted images.

Detection of intracerebral metastases is facilitated by administration of gadolinium, and every patient with neurological symptoms and a history of cancer needs to have a gadolinium-enhanced MRI study. The enhancement pattern of metastatic tumors can be solid or ringlike. To improve the diagnostic yield, triple-dose gadolinium or magnetization transfer techniques have been used, which improve detection of smaller metastases that are not so conspicuous with single-dose contrast administration. A triple dose of gadolinium improves metastasis detection by as much as 43% (van Dijk et al., 1997). Meningeal carcinomatosis can also be detected by contrast administration, which can reveal thickening of the meninges and/or meningeal deposits of the metastatic tumor.

Ischemic Stroke
ACUTE ISCHEMIC STROKE

With the introduction of thrombolytic therapy in the treatment of acute ischemic stroke, timely diagnosis of an ischemic lesion, determining its location and extent, and demonstrating the amount of tissue at risk has become essential (see Chapter 51A). CT imaging remains of great value in the evaluation of acute stroke; it is readily available, and newer CT modalities including CT angiography and CT perfusion imaging are coming into greater use. The applicability of CT to acute stroke continues to be enhanced by the ever-increasing rapidity with which scans can be acquired, allowing for greater coverage of tissues with thinner slices. The technological advances allowing for rapid acquisition of data have led to 4D imaging, where complete 3D data sets of the brain are serially obtained over very short time intervals, allowing for higher temporal and spatial resolutions in brain perfusion studies of acute ischemic stroke patients.

CT is very useful in detecting hyperdense hemorrhagic lesions as the cause of stroke. Early ischemic stroke, however, may not cause any change on unenhanced CT, making it difficult to determine the extent of the ischemic lesion and the amount of tissue at risk. CT is especially limited in evaluating ischemia in the posterior fossa, owing to streak artifacts at the skull base. Despite these limitations, early signs of acute ischemia on unenhanced CT may be helpful in the first few hours after stroke. CT signs of acute ischemia include blurring of the gray/white junction and effacement of the sulci due to ischemic swelling of the tissues. Blurring of the contours of the deep gray matter structures is of similar significance. In cases of internal carotid artery occlusion, middle cerebral artery main segment (M1) occlusion, or more distal occlusions, intraluminal clot may be seen as a focal hyperdensity, sometimes referred to as a *hyperdense MCA*, or *hyperdense dot sign* (**Fig. 33A.29**).

Several MRI modalities as well as CT perfusion studies are capable of providing data regarding cerebral ischemia and perfusion to assist in the evaluation for possible thrombolytic therapy very early after symptom onset. DWI with

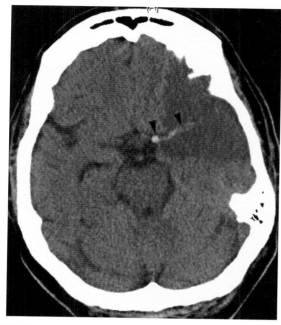

Fig. 33A.29 Evolving ischemic stroke in the territory of the left middle cerebral artery. On this noncontrast CT scan, a hyperdense signal is seen in the distal left internal carotid artery and in the M1 segment of the left middle cerebral artery, indicating presence of a blood clot *(arrowheads)*. There is hypodensity in the corresponding area of the left hemisphere, demonstrating the evolving ischemic infarct.

ADC mapping is considered to be the most sensitive method for imaging acute ischemia (**Figs. 33A.30 to 33A.33** [**Figs. 33A.31, *B*; 33A.32, *B*; and 33A.33** available online only]). In humans, the hyperintense signal indicating restriction of diffusion is detected within minutes after onset (Hossmann and Hoehn-Berlage, 1995).

TEMPORAL EVOLUTION OF ISCHEMIC STROKE ON MAGNETIC RESONANCE IMAGING

Acute Stroke

Initially, the hyperintense signal on DWI is caused by decreased water diffusivity due to swelling of the ischemic nerve cells (for the first 5 to 7 days), then it increasingly results from the abnormal T2 properties of the infarcted tissue (T2 shine-through). For this reason, a reliable estimation of the age of the ischemic lesion is not possible by looking at DWI images alone. Imaging protocols for acute ischemic stroke usually include T1- and T2-weighted fast spin echo images, FLAIR sequences, and DWI with ADC maps. These sequences together confirm the diagnosis of ischemia, determine its extent, and allow for an approximate estimation of the time of onset (Srinivasan et al., 2006). On ADC maps, the values decrease initially after the onset of ischemia (i.e., the signal from the affected area becomes progressively more hypointense). This reaches a nadir at 3 to 5 days but remains significantly low until the seventh day after onset. After this time, the values increase (the signal gets more and more hyperintense) and return to the baseline values in 1 to 4 weeks (usually in 7 to 10 days). Therefore, ADC maps are quite useful for the estimation of the age of the lesion: if the signal of the area is hypointense on an ADC map, the lesion is likely less than 7 to 10 days old. If the area is isointense or hyperintense on the ADC map, the onset was likely more than 7 to 10 days ago. As already noted, although these signal changes take place on ADC maps, the DWI images remain hyperintense, without noticeable changes of intensity by visual inspection.

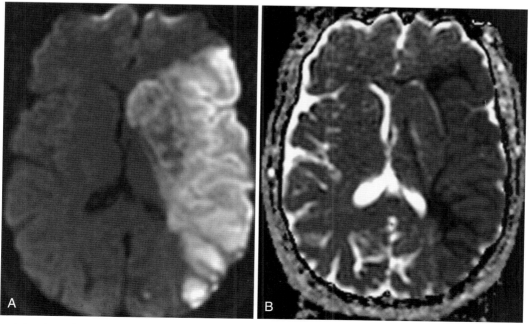

Fig. 33A.30 Acute ischemic stroke in the territory of the middle cerebral artery. **A,** On diffusion-weighted imaging, a hyperintense area of restricted diffusion is seen in the territory of the left middle cerebral artery. Note evolving mass effect on the sulci and left lateral ventricle and the mild midline shift. **B,** On apparent diffusion coefficient map, corresponding hypointensity is seen in the same area.

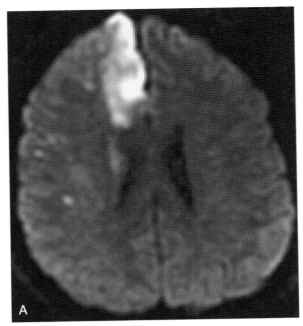

Fig. 33A.31 Acute ischemic stroke in the territory of the anterior cerebral artery. **A,** On diffusion-weighted imaging, a hyperintense area of restricted diffusion is seen in the right medial frontal lobe, involving the territory of the anterior cerebral artery. **B,** On apparent diffusion coefficient map, corresponding hypointensity is seen in the same area (for the image, see online version of this chapter).

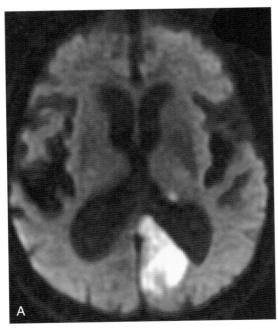

Fig. 33A.32 Acute ischemic stroke in the territory of the posterior cerebral artery. **A,** On diffusion-weighted imaging, a hyperintense area of restricted diffusion is seen in the left medial occipital lobe, involving the territory of the posterior cerebral artery. **B,** On apparent diffusion coefficient map, corresponding hypointensity is seen in the same area (for the image, see online version of this chapter).

On T2-weighted (including FLAIR) images, the signal intensity of the ischemic area is normal in the initial hyperacute stage, increases markedly over the first 4 days, then becomes stable. In a research setting, computing the numerical values of hyperintensity in infarcted tissue on serial T2-weighted scans can demonstrate a consistent sharp signal increase after 36 hours, distinguishing lesions younger or older than 36 hours. This is certainly not possible by visual inspection used in clinical practice.

One purpose of MRI in the evaluation of acute stroke is to determine the extent of irreversible tissue damage and to identify tissue that is at risk but potentially salvageable. The combination of DWI and PWI is frequently used for this purpose (**Fig. 33A.34**). Evaluation is based on the premise that diffusion-weighted images delineate the tissue that suffered permanent damage (although in some cases, restricted diffusion is reversible, corresponding to ischemia without infarction), whereas areas without signal change on DWI but abnormal signal on perfusion-weighted images represent tissue at risk, the so-called ischemic penumbra. If there is a mismatch between the extent of DWI changes and perfusion deficits, the latter being larger, reperfusion treatment with intravenous or intraarterial thrombolysis or other intravascular techniques is justified to salvage the brain tissue at risk. If the extent of diffusion and perfusion abnormalities is similar or the same, the tissue is thought to be irreversibly injured, with no penumbra, and therefore the potential benefit from reperfusion treatment may not be high enough to justify the risk of hemorrhage associated with thrombolytic treatment.

Subacute Ischemic Stroke (1 Day to 1 Week after Onset)

In this stage, there is an ongoing increase of cytotoxic edema due to swelling of the ischemic neurons. Parallel with this, the involved tissue becomes more and more hypointense on T1 and also gradually more hyperintense on T2 and FLAIR sequences. Cytotoxic edema is usually maximal 2 to 3 days after onset, but in the case of malignant middle cerebral artery strokes, it may keep increasing until day 5. Arterial wall enhancement is seen during this stage, whereas parenchymal enhancement usually begins at the end of the first week.

Reperfusion usually occurs at this stage and may be associated with petechial hemorrhages or even frank hemorrhage within the infarcted tissue. Petechial hemorrhages are very common; microbleeds (not always visible with CT or MRI) occur in as much as 65% of ischemic stroke patients (Werring, 2007). Frank hemorrhagic transformation, however, is much less common.

Late Subacute Ischemic Stroke (1 to 3 Weeks after Onset)

In this stage, gradual resolution of the edema is seen. As the infarcted tissue is disintegrating and resorbed, the T1 hypointensity and T2 hyperintensity of the lesion become more marked. Gray matter enhancement (which in the case of infarcted cortex has a gyriform pattern) is intense throughout this stage.

Chronic Ischemic Stroke (3 Weeks and Older)

Areas of complete tissue destruction with death not only of neurons but of glia and necrosis of other supporting tissues as well, will eventually appear as cavitary lesions filled with fluid

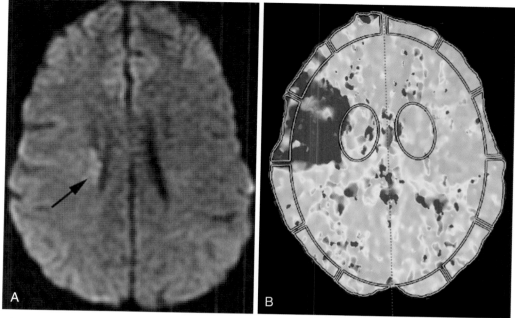

Fig. 33A.34 Ischemic penumbra in acute right middle cerebral artery stroke. **A,** Diffusion-weighted image reveals a small, circumscribed area of restricted diffusion in the paraventricular region of the right centrum semiovale *(arrow).* **B,** Magnetic resonance perfusion-weighted image demonstrates a much larger perfusion deficit, as revealed by increased mean transit time, indicated in red. The perfusion deficit outside the small area of restricted diffusion represents the ischemic penumbra.

that have signal characteristics identical to CSF: hyperintensity on T2-weighted images and marked hypointensity on T1 images and FLAIR sequences. The region of encephalomalacia is bordered by a glial scar (reactive gliosis) that is hyperintense on T2 and FLAIR images (**Fig. 33A.35**; Fig. 33A.35, *B* available online only). Although the initial signal changes on DWI frequently predict the final extent of tissue destruction, changes on DWI can also disappear, and the final size of tissue cavitation can be best determined on T1-weighted images, which should be part of every stroke follow-up imaging protocol. Tissue in the margins of the cavitary lesion, and often in other areas of the brain as well, may have undergone extensive neuronal loss resulting only in atrophy but not in signal intensity changes, even on T2-weighted images (partial infarction).

Besides signal changes, chronic ischemic infarcts lead to secondary changes in the brain. Owing to the loss of tissue, ex vacuo enlargement of the adjacent CSF spaces (sulci and adjacent ventricular segments) occurs. Pathways that originate from or pass through the infarcted area undergo wallerian degeneration, which is seen as T2-hyperintense signal change along the course of these pathways (**Fig. 33A.36**). Later, the hyperintensity may resolve, but the loss of pathways may result in volume loss of the structures they pass through (e.g., cerebral peduncle, pons, medullary pyramid), noted as decreased cross-sectional area.

Stroke Etiology

Structural imaging provides data on the morphology and location of ischemic cerebral lesions, which can be very helpful to determine stroke etiology: lacunar, atherothrombotic, embolic, hypoperfusion-related, or venous. Diagnostic

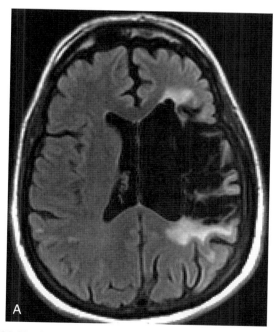

Fig. 33A.35 Chronic ischemic stroke. **A,** On FLAIR image, a large area of encephalomalacia is seen in the territory of the left middle cerebral artery. Hypointense CSF-like cavity is surrounded by hyperintense signal change in adjacent parenchyma, indicating gliosis. Note ex-vacuo enlargement of adjacent segment of left lateral ventricle. **B,** On noncontrast T1-weighted image, the cavity of encephalomalacia appears as CSF-like hypointensity. Areas of gliosis appear as faint zones of hypointensity (for the image, see online version of this chapter).

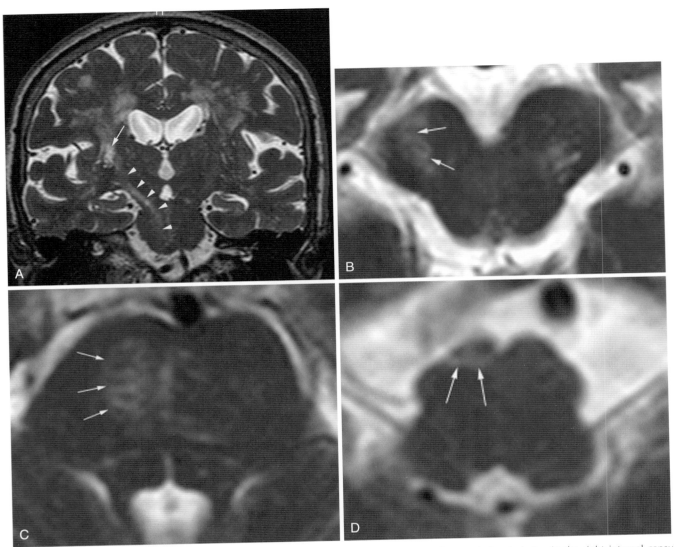

Fig. 33A.36 Wallerian degeneration. **A,** Coronal T2-weighted image demonstrates a chronic lacunar ischemic lesion in the right internal capsule *(arrow).* From here, a linear hyperintense signal change is seen extending caudally along the course of the degenerating corticospinal tract fibers, through the right cerebral peduncle into the pons *(arrowheads).* **B-D,** Serial T2-weighted axial images of the brainstem demonstrate the hyperintense signal of the degenerating fibers *(arrows)* in the right cerebral peduncle **(B),** right pontine tegmentum **(C),** and in the right medullary pyramid **(D).**

evaluation and treatment of a patient with stroke, as well as secondary stroke prevention, is often dependent upon structural imaging. A discussion of the neuroimaging aspects of the various stroke etiologies is in the online-only version of this book, available at www.expertconsult.com.

Other Cerebrovascular Occlusive Disease
MICROVASCULAR ISCHEMIC WHITE MATTER LESIONS, "WHITE MATTER DISEASE," BINSWANGER DISEASE

Diffuse or patchy T2-hyperintense signal changes in the deep hemispheric and subcortical white matter are probably the most common abnormal findings on MRI in the adult and elderly patient population. The terms *microvascular ischemic changes* or *chronic small vessel disease* are frequently used to describe these lesions on imaging studies. Their etiology and clinical significance have been debated extensively.

Certain hyperintense signal changes are considered normal incidental findings, with no clinical relevance. A uniformly thin, linear, T2 hyperintensity that has a smooth outer border along the border of the body of the lateral ventricles is often seen in the elderly population and likely represents fluid or gliotic changes in the subependymal zone. It tends to be more pronounced at the tips of the frontal horns *(ependymitis granularis).* This finding is thought potentially to be due to focal loss of the ependymal lining with gliosis and/or influx of interstitial fluid into these regions.

Patchy signal changes within the white matter of the cerebral hemispheres beyond a relatively low threshold (generally, one white matter hyperintensity per decade of life is felt to fall within the normal range) are pathological and are most commonly of ischemic origin. According to the most accepted hypothesis, these hyperintensities are the result of gradual narrowing or occlusion of the small vessels of the white matter, the diameters of which are less than 200 micrometers (hence the terms *microvascular lesions* or *small vessel disease*). Pathologically, these lesions are composed of focal demyelination and gliosis. The lumen of the involved vessels is narrow or occluded; their walls may exhibit arteriosclerotic changes and commonly amyloid deposits. On imaging studies, they have a chronic appearance, with diffuse borders and no surrounding edema or evidence of mass effect. They are generally associated with some degree of central atrophy, which tends to worsen with higher lesion loads. The distribution of these lesions changes only very gradually on serial scans, often showing minimal to no significant difference on studies spaced several years apart.

While age by itself can cause such changes, and the incidence of these lesions increases with age in people 40 years or older, there are several other risk factors that can make them more numerous. These include hypertension, diabetes, hypercholesterolemia, and smoking. Indeed, patients with these medical problems are more likely to have an elevated number of ischemic white matter lesions.

Chronic ischemic white matter lesions are hypodense on CT, but MRI is much more sensitive and reveals more extensive lesions (**Fig. 33A.38**; **Fig. 33A.38, B-C** available online only). On MRI, the lesions are hyperintense on T2 and FLAIR sequences. They may or not be visible as T1 hypointensities. It is possible that only lesions visible on T1-weighted images may be clinically significant. Common locations are the periventricular (PV) and more commonly, the deep white matter, but subcortical lesions are also common, with sparing of the U-fibers. The lesions can be isolated, scattered, or more confluent, especially in the PV zone. Morphologically, individual lesions generally exhibit indistinct borders with a diffuse "cotton-wool" appearance and range in size from punctate to small. Regions of confluent lesions may appear large and more commonly affect the deep white matter anterior and posterior to the bodies of the lateral ventricles, symmetrically within the parietal and frontal lobes. Deep white matter lesions also often

occur in a distribution parallel to the bodies of the lateral ventricles on axial views, with an irregular band-like or "beads-on-string" appearance often separated from the PV lesions by an intervening band of relatively unaffected white matter. Involvement of the external capsules is also characteristic. These patterns of lesion distribution and morphology are often best seen on FLAIR. Contrary to the lesions of multiple sclerosis (MS), microvascular ischemia tends not to involve the temporal lobes or the corpus callosum. Besides the hemispheric white matter, microvascular ischemic lesions often also involve the basis pontis.

The clinical significance of ischemic white matter lesions depends on their extent and location. The presence of a few small, scattered, ischemic white matter lesions on T2-weighted images is clinically meaningless, and these are usually considered a normal imaging manifestation of aging. Patients may feel more comfortable with descriptions such as "age spots of the brain" to convey their benign nature when verbally discussing results. More extensive lesions also visible on T1-weighted sequences, however, are more likely to be associated with neurological abnormalities such as abnormal gait, dementia, and incontinence. In ischemic arteriolar encephalopathy or Binswanger disease, there is pronounced, widely distributed, and confluent PV and deep white matter signal change. In more severe cases, the confluent hyperintensity also involves the internal and external capsules or subcortical white matter. Besides confluent lesions, coexisting multiple scattered T2 hyperintensities are also very common. Ischemic white matter lesions are often intermixed with lacunar ischemic strokes and generalized cerebral volume loss is also frequently noted.

Scattered small, nonspecific-appearing, seemingly microvascular white matter hyperintensities have a broader differential diagnosis in the younger patient population. Multiple small T2 hyperintense lesions in the hemispheric white matter can be caused by migraine, trauma, inborn errors of metabolism, vasculitis (including Sjögren syndrome, lupus, Behçet disease, and primary CNS vasculitis), Lyme disease, and MS. Since the MRI appearance of these is nonspecific, clinical correlation is always warranted. In many instances, these white matter lesions are idiopathic, and future serial imaging studies are needed for follow-up.

CADASIL

Cerebral autosomal dominant arteriopathy with subcortical infarcts and leukoencephalopathy (CADASIL) is an autosomal dominant inherited vascular disease. Pathologically there is destruction of the smooth muscle cells in the small and medium-sized penetrating arteries, with deposition of osmiophilic material and fibrosis leading to progressive thickening of the arterial wall and narrowing of the lumen. As a result, leukoencephalopathy and multiple ischemic strokes occur. Over 90% of patients have detectable mutations of the NOTCH3 gene, which encodes a transmembrane receptor primarily expressed in arterial smooth muscle cells. On MRI, multiple focal infarcts and T2-hyperintense white matter lesions are seen. The white matter lesions may involve the external capsules and, very characteristically, the anterior temporal lobe white matter in a confluent fashion that includes the subcortical arcuate fibers (**Fig. 33A.39**). This latter finding is helpful for the structural imaging diagnosis and helps distinguish CADASIL from "sporadic" ischemic arteriosclerotic vascular disease.

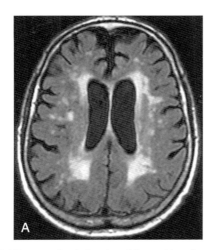

Fig. 33A.38 Microvascular ischemic white matter changes. **A,** Axial FLAIR image reveals extensive hyperintense areas in the hemispheric white matter bilaterally. Some are confluent at the borders of the ventricles, others are scattered in other regions. Note the "band" of hyperintensity in the left hemisphere parallel to the border of the lateral ventricle. **B-C,** On axial FLAIR and T2-weighted images, faint hyperintense signal changes are seen in the pontine tegmentum bilaterally, exhibiting the typical imaging appearance of microvascular ischemia *(arrows)* (for images, see online version of this chapter).

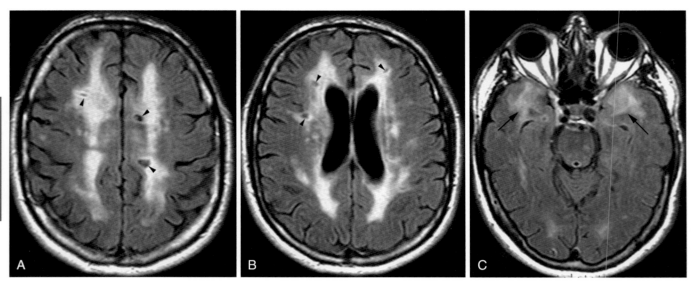

Fig. 33A.39 CADASIL. **A-C,** Axial FLAIR images demonstrate diffuse, confluent hyperintense signal changes in the deep and subcortical white matter. Multiple chronic lacunar infarcts are also seen bilaterally *(arrowheads)*. Note characteristic confluent hyperintensity *(arrows)* in the anterior temporal lobe white matter **(C)**, involving the subcortical fibers as well.

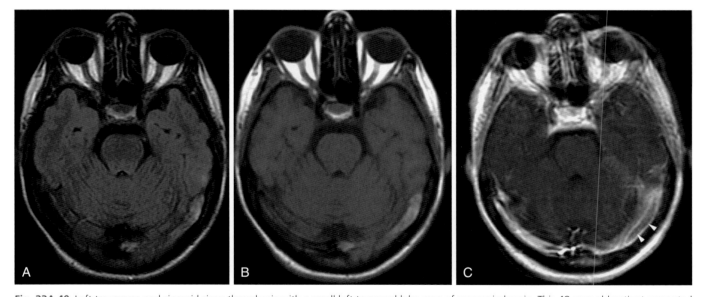

Fig. 33A.40 Left transverse and sigmoid sinus thrombosis with a small left temporal lobe area of venous ischemia. This 48-year-old patient presented with a new-onset seizure and right visual field deficit that resolved later. **A,** Axial FLAIR image reveals abnormal hyperintense signal in the left transverse and sigmoid sinus, indicating thrombosis. Compare to the right transverse sinus, with the normal hypointense flow void. This FLAIR image also shows a small but noticeable area of hyperintensity due to venous ischemia in the left temporal lobe. **B,** Noncontrast T1-weighted image also reveals abnormal hyperintense signal in the involved venous sinuses. Again, compare with the contralateral sinus. **C,** Postcontrast T1-weighted image reveals normal filling in the sinus on the right, but there is no filling along the visualized segment of the left transverse sinus *(arrowheads)*.

CEREBRAL VENOUS SINUS THROMBOSIS

Acute cerebral venous sinus thrombosis results in diminished or absent flow in the involved sinuses. Cerebral venous sinus thrombosis usually causes typical signal changes on MRI (**Fig. 33A.40**) and severely attenuated or absent flow signal on magnetic resonance venography (MRV). MRV techniques include flow-sensitive modalities such as 2D time of flight and phase contrast imaging, as well as postcontrast high-resolution 3D-SPGR, which offers excellent visualization of the sinuses with a very high spatial resolution and contrast-to-noise ratio.

In the appropriate clinical context, a useful sign of venous sinus thrombosis is the absence of a normal hypointense flow void in the involved sinuses on T1- and T2-weighted images and absent flow in the involved sinus on MRV. Nonflowing blood generally results in increased signal intensity on T1 and T2. In the early acute stage, however, the sinuses may still be hypointense. This is followed by signal that is isointense to the gray matter. The typical hyperintense signal on T1- and T2-weighted images appears when methemoglobin is present in the clot. At all stages, therefore, simultaneous review of the MRV or CT angiogram for lack of flow signal and lack of contrast filling in conjunction with conventional MRI may be particularly useful to increase the sensitivity and specificity of detection of sinus thrombosis while also adding information regarding the age of the clot.

Following administration of gadolinium, there may be enhancement of the dural wall of the sinus and along the periphery of the clot, but not within the clot itself, resulting in an "empty delta" appearance. This is classically a CT finding, but the same concept also applies to MRI in the context of the T1-weighted clot signal that varies with clot age. MR demonstrates lack of flow, appearing as absence of contrast-related signal in the involved sinuses. CT angiogram reveals no contrast filling in the thrombosed sinuses. The cortical veins that drain into the involved sinuses may appear engorged on MRV. However, if the thrombosis also involves these draining veins, they too may exhibit lack of signal on MRV, lack of filling on CT angiogram, and lack of flow voids in conjunction with iso- or hyperintense signal on T1- and T2-weighted images.

Variations in the speed of blood flow and anatomical variants of the venous sinuses may change their usual signal characteristics, leading to a false diagnosis of venous sinus thrombosis. Slow flow in a venous sinus may cause increased signal on T1- and T2-weighted images, potentially leading to a false assumption of thrombosis. Gadolinium-enhanced images help in these cases, demonstrating contrast filling/enhancement in the sinuses and confirming the absence of thrombosis. A normal variant of venous sinus hypoplasia/aplasia may result in decreased/absent flow signal on MRV, falsely interpreted as thrombosis. T1- and T2-weighted images, however, are usually able to demonstrate the absence of thrombus in the sinus. These examples highlight the importance of reviewing all necessary image modalities (MRV, T2-weighted images, T1-weighted images with and without contrast) to make or reject a diagnosis of venous sinus thrombosis.

Hemorrhagic Cerebrovascular Disease

Structural neuroimaging is crucial in the evaluation of hemorrhagic cerebrovascular disease. Besides detection of the hematoma itself, its location can provide useful information regarding its etiology. Lobar hematomas, especially along with small, scattered, parenchymal microbleeds, raise the possibility of cerebral amyloid angiopathy, whereas putaminal, thalamic, or cerebellar hemorrhages are more likely to be of hypertensive origin. Other underlying lesions such as brain tumors causing hemorrhages can be detected by structural imaging. This section discusses hemorrhagic cerebrovascular disease and cerebral intraparenchymal hematoma, whereas other causes of hemorrhage such as trauma or malignancy are discussed in other sections. Please also refer to Chapter 51B for a clinical neurological review of intracerebral hemorrhages.

For decades, noncontrast CT scanning has been (and in most emergency settings still is) the essential tool for initial evaluation of intracerebral hemorrhage. In hyperacute (<12 hours after onset) and acute hemorrhage (12 to 48 hours), the patient's hematocrit largely determines the lesion's degree of density on CT. With a normal hematocrit, both retracted and unretracted clots exhibit hyperdensity that contrasts sufficiently with the isodense background of brain parenchyma to be easily detectable. In cases of anemia, however, small hemorrhagic lesions may potentially be overlooked owing to their lower CT density and may even be isodense to brain. The

following sections describing the appearance of hemorrhage on CT and MRI studies all assume a normal hematocrit.

In the acute stage, the hematoma is seen as an area of hyperdensity on CT. The associated mass effect depends on the size and location. Effacement of the ventricles, cortical sulci, or basal cisterns is often seen. Various degrees of midline shift or subtypes of herniation (transtentorial, subfalcine, etc.) may occur. The surrounding edema is seen as hypodensity and tends to appear irregular with varying thickness depending on the degree of involvement of adjacent white matter tracts, which are preferentially affected. The initially distinct border of the hematoma changes within days to a few weeks after onset and becomes irregular and "moth-eaten" due to the phagocytic activity of macrophages. Small hematomas may disappear on CT within 1 week; in the case of larger hematomas, the process may take more than a month. Small hemorrhages may resolve without any residual change, while those that are larger are gradually replaced by an encephalomalacic cavity of decreased density and ex vacuo enlargement of the adjacent CSF spaces.

The appearance of hemorrhagic cerebrovascular disease on MRI is very complex regarding both signal heterogeneity on individual scans and subsequent changes in appearance over successive imaging studies. Signal characteristics of hemorrhage vary widely across different pulse sequences (T1, T2, T2* gradient echo) depending on the age of the hemorrhage; presence of oxyhemoglobin, deoxyhemoglobin, methemoglobin, and hemosiderin; changing water content within the clot; and integrity of erythrocyte membranes. Understanding the typical MRI appearance of each stage in the evolution of a hemorrhage allows one to estimate its age, because biochemical and structural changes characteristic of each stage (macroscopic and microscopic) occur along a predictable time line. In addition to conventional (T1- and T2-weighted) images, the gradient echo technique has been used to detect even small intracerebral hemorrhages, given its sensitivity to the paramagnetic properties (magnetic field distorting effects) of various blood products. More recently introduced into clinical practice, the technique of SWI offers the greatest sensitivity for chronic hemorrhage to date and is particularly useful in evaluating punctate hemorrhages in patients with diffuse shear injury secondary to prior head trauma.

A discussion of the MR imaging features of hemorrhage is best organized according to the stages of hemorrhage evolution as follows.

HYPERACUTE HEMORRHAGE (0 TO 24 HOURS)

In the early (hyperacute) phase of intraparenchymal hemorrhage (<24 hours) the red blood cells are intact, and a mixture of oxy- and deoxyhemoglobin is present (Bakshi et al., 1998). In this stage, the signal on T1-weighted images is isointense to the brain, so even larger hematomas may be missed on this pulse sequence. On T2-weighted images, the oxyhemoglobin portion is hyperintense and deoxyhemoglobin is hypointense, resulting in the gradual appearance of a hypointense rim and gradually increasing hypointense foci within the hematoma as the amount of deoxyhemoglobin increases from the periphery. Such hypointense foci are also seen on FLAIR. Between the clot and the deoxyhemoglobin-containing rim, thin intervening clefts of fluid-like T2 hyperintensity may be seen as an initial manifestation of clot retraction. On gradient echo images, hyperacute hemorrhage will exhibit heterogeneously isointense to markedly hypointense signal,

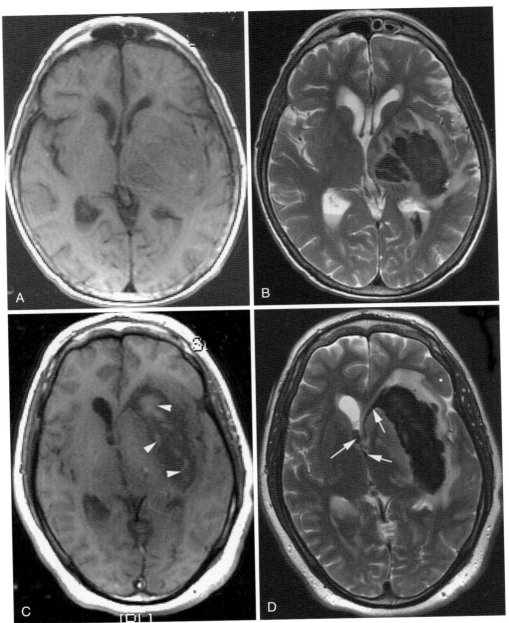

Fig. 33A.41 Two cases of acute parenchymal hemorrhage. **A-B,** Large acute left basal ganglia hemorrhage. On noncontrast T1-weighted image **(A)** only faint hypointensity is noted. On axial T2-weighted image **(B)** the hematoma appears as a striking hypointensity with developing hyperintense edema in surrounding parenchyma. Note associated mass effect. **C-D,** In this case, the basal ganglia hematoma is in a more advanced stage. On T1-weighted image **(C)** the area is still mostly hypointense, but its center is now turning hyperintense because of intracellular methemoglobin *(arrowheads)*. On corresponding T2-weighted image **(D)** the hematoma is still hypointense (as extracellular methemoglobin is also hypointense on T2), but the surrounding hyperintense edema is more prominent, and the mass effect is increased as well. Note that hemorrhage is also present within the ventricle, making the prognosis worse *(arrows)*.

the latter corresponding to deoxyhemoglobin content in more peripheral portions of the clot. The amount of edema is mild in this stage, usually seen as a thin rim that is hyperintense on T2 and FLAIR images and hypointense on T1-weighted images (Atlas and Thulborn, 1998).

ACUTE HEMORRHAGE (1 TO 3 DAYS)

During this stage, hemoglobin is transformed to deoxyhemoglobin, but the membranes of the erythrocytes are still

intact (Bakshi et al., 1998). The hematoma becomes slightly hypointense on T1 and strikingly hypointense on T2-weighted images (**Fig. 33A.41**). On GRE, proton spins in the presence of paramagnetic deoxyhemoglobin dephase rapidly during TE, resulting in signal loss and, therefore, hypointensity of the hematoma on this pulse sequence. The surrounding edema, which is more extensive during this stage, is hypointense on T1 and hyperintense on T2.

EARLY SUBACUTE HEMORRHAGE (3 DAYS TO 1 WEEK)

As blood degradation evolves, deoxyhemoglobin is converted to methemoglobin. At this stage, the blood degradation products are still intracellular (Bakshi et al., 1998). Intracellular methemoglobin is hyperintense on T1 and hypointense on T2-weighted images. T1 shortening is primarily the result of dipole-dipole interactions between heme iron and adjacent water protons, facilitated by a conformational change that occurs when deoxyhemoglobin is converted to methemoglobin.

Signal changes on T2 occur via a different mechanism. Sequestration of methemoglobin within the intact red blood cell membrane results in a locally paramagnetic environment adjacent to the diamagnetic, methemoglobin-free extracellular compartment. These differences in the local magnetic fields, present at a microscopic level, cause rapid dephasing of proton spins and signal loss during TE as water molecules diffuse rapidly through this heterogeneous environment. Therefore, on T2-weighted images the presence of intracellular methemoglobin results in hypointensity of the hemorrhage. These signal changes start from the periphery of the hematoma where the deoxyhemoglobin-to-methemoglobin transformation first occurs. During this stage, the amount of edema starts to decrease.

LATE SUBACUTE HEMORRHAGE (1 TO 4 WEEKS)

In the late subacute phase, the membranes of the red blood cells disintegrate, and methemoglobin becomes extracellular (Bakshi et al., 1998). Extracellular methemoglobin contains Fe^{3+}, which has five unpaired electrons. This leads to a dipole-dipole interaction which, contrary to intracellular methemoglobin, causes hyperintense signal change on both T1- and T2-weighted images (**Fig. 33A.42**).

During this stage (usually 2 weeks after the hemorrhage) hemosiderin deposition begins, typically at the periphery of the hematoma where macrophages reside. A dark peripheral rim appears on GRE and T2-weighted images, initially thin, then progressively thicker. The amount of edema around the hematoma continues to decrease gradually.

CHRONIC HEMORRHAGE (>4 WEEKS)

In the chronic stage (Bakshi et al., 1998), the core of larger hematomas turns into a slitlike or linear cavity with CSF signal characteristics, being hypointense on T1 and FLAIR and hyperintense on T2-weighted images. At the periphery of the lesion, macrophages continue to remove iron from the extracellular methemoglobin; hemosiderin and ferritin are deposited in their lysosomes, resulting in a rim of hypointense signal on T2-weighted and GRE images. This hypointense rim becomes progressively more prominent during the transition from the late subacute to chronic stage (**Fig. 33A.43**).

If the hemorrhage is small, eventually its entire area will be occupied by hemosiderin deposition. Smaller hemorrhages or microbleeds, such as those seen in amyloid angiopathy or after head trauma, are visualized as multiple uniformly hypointense foci on GRE images. Susceptibility-weighted images are even more sensitive to magnetic filed distortion due to blood products and can reveal microbleeds that are missed even by conventional gradient echo images. It is important to keep in mind that because of magnetic field distortion, the area of hypointensity on GRE or susceptibility-weighted images is larger than the actual size of the bleed. GRE or, ideally, SWI should be part of every MRI protocol for brain trauma.

Hemorrhage, like many other lesions to the brain, provokes reactive gliosis. In the chronic stage, surrounding gliosis is seen as mildly hyperintense signal on T2 and FLAIR images.

Superficial siderosis, a chronic sequela of bleeding into the subarachnoid space, and cerebral amyloid angiopathy, a

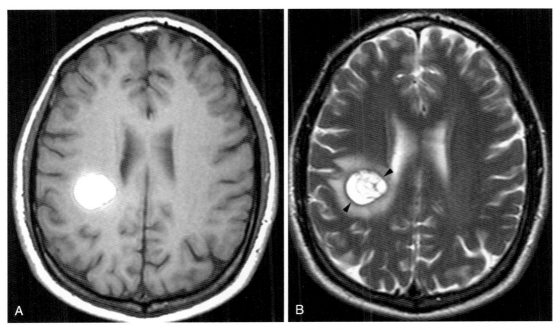

Fig. 33A.42 Late subacute parenchymal hemorrhage. **A,** On noncontrast T1-weighted image, there is a hematoma in the right corona radiata. This exhibits homogeneous hyperintense signal. **B,** On T2-weighted image, the hematoma also appears as homogeneous hyperintensity. Signal characteristics are typical for the presence of extracellular methemoglobin in a late subacute hematoma. Note beginning of hypointense hemosiderin deposition at the rim of the hematoma on T2-weighted image *(arrowheads)*.

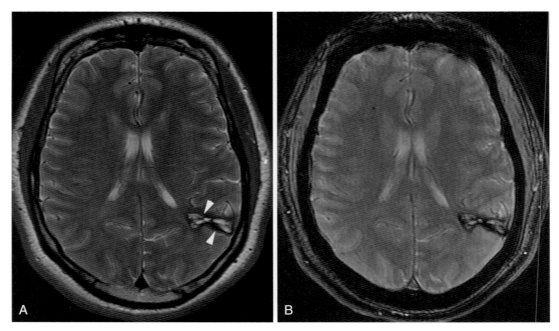

Fig. 33A.43 Chronic parenchymal hemorrhage. **A,** Axial T2-weighted image reveals a slitlike cavitary lesion in the left parietal lobe. Its center has CSF-like hyperintense signal, but there is a rim of hypointensity due to hemosiderin deposition along its border *(arrowheads)*. **B,** Axial gradient echo image reveals markedly hypointense hemosiderin deposition along the border of the chronic hemorrhage.

hemorrhage-prone condition, are discussed in the online version of this book. Please visit www.expertconsult.com for more information.

Infection

Structural neuroimaging can provide useful information for evaluating infectious diseases of the CNS. The imaging modality of choice is MRI, which is able to demonstrate even subtle parenchymal abnormalities and inflammatory involvement of the meninges. For a review of the etiology, clinical presentation, and treatment of infections of the nervous system, see Chapter 53. And in addition to the neuroimaging features of infections discussed in the print version of this text, the online version includes features of CNS tuberculosis, cysticercosis, and cytomegalovirus. Please visit www.expertconsult.com for more information.

BACTERIAL MENINGITIS

In the typical uncomplicated form of bacterial meningitis, no abnormalities are seen in the brain parenchyma, and without contrast administration, the meninges may also appear unremarkable. With gadolinium, however, intense meningeal enhancement is seen, usually over the convexities and along the basal cisterns; this is due to vascular engorgement and increased vascular permeability secondary to the inflammatory process. At times, as a complication, ventriculitis may develop, and then the ependymal lining of the ventricles also exhibits enhancement.

CEREBRITIS, ABSCESS

Cerebritis and abscess can arise as complications of bacterial meningitis, but they may also spread to the brain hematogenously from another source such as endocarditis

or pulmonary abscess. *Cerebritis* and *abscess* refer to different stages of the parenchymal infection. In the cerebritis stage, the lesion has poorly defined hyperintensity on T2 and FLAIR sequences and is iso- to hypointense on T1-weighted images. Foci of necrosis may be present. There is surrounding edema, appearing as hypointensity on T1 and hyperintensity on T2 and FLAIR. With gadolinium, a heterogenous irregular enhancement pattern may or may not be present.

If the process continues to cerebral abscess formation, after an average of 2 weeks, the core appears more demarcated, and fibrotic capsule formation is noted. The center of the abscess contains liquefied, necrotic, and purulent material. This is usually hypointense on T1 (but may appear more hyperintense, depending on the protein content) and hyperintense on T2. The rim is iso- to hypointense on T1 and iso- to hypointense on T2. Often the T2 hypointense rim is well seen, separating the hyperintense core from the usually less hyperintense surrounding edema. With gadolinium, the capsule exhibits ring enhancement, which is typically a smooth, thin, complete ring. Sometimes the deeper segment of the enhancing ring is thinner than the superficial. A characteristic feature that supports the diagnosis of abscess is the so-called daughter abscess, which is seen as a smaller ring-enhancing lesion connected to the parent abscess.

Cerebral abscesses are part of the differential diagnosis when ring-enhancing cerebral lesions are encountered. Besides the described ring morphology and the potential presence of daughter abscesses, cerebral abscesses exhibit restriction of diffusion centrally, appearing as hyperintense signal on diffusion-weighted images and hypointensity on ADC maps, which distinguishes them from metastatic and most primary brain tumors (**Fig. 33A.45**).

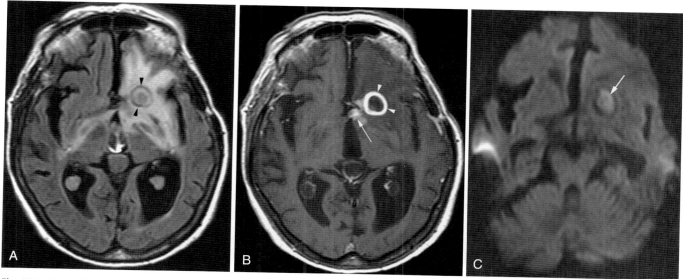

Fig. 33A.45 Cerebral abscess. **A,** Axial FLAIR image shows a round lesion in the deep left frontal lobe, surrounded by a hypointense rim *(arrowheads)*. Hyperintense edema in adjacent parenchyma extends to various white matter regions. **B,** Axial T1-weighted postcontrast image shows complete ring enhancement in the capsule of the abscess *(arrowheads)*. Diffuse parenchymal enhancement is noted in the brain medial to the abscess, likely due to cerebritis *(arrow)*. **C,** Abscess cavity is characteristically hyperintense on diffusion-weighted images *(arrow)*.

LYME DISEASE

In the brain parenchyma, Lyme encephalitis may cause multiple lesions that are slightly hypointense on T1 and hyperintense on T2-weighted images. The most common locations are the subcortical and periventricular white matter, but the thalamus, corpus callosum, and pons may be involved as well. The lesions appear nonspecific, their size ranging from a few millimeters to a centimeter. Vasculitis, demyelinating disease, and microvascular ischemia are frequent differential diagnostic considerations. If present, abnormal enhancement along the meninges and cranial nerve segments may indicate involvement of these structures by Lyme disease.

HERPES SIMPLEX ENCEPHALITIS

In adults, herpes encephalitis is caused by herpes simplex virus type 1. The imaging diagnosis is suggested by the location of the lesions. Herpes encephalitis typically involves the medial temporal and limbic frontal regions, including the basal frontal and cingulate gyri and insula. The cerebral cortex is more affected than the white matter. Herpes simplex encephalitis is usually hyperintense on T2 and FLAIR images and mildly hypointense on T1-weighted images (**Fig. 33A.46**). The encephalitis is frequently hemorrhagic, causing additional signal changes depending on the age of the hemorrhage. Areas of necrosis may be seen as well. Typically, a few days after onset, variable patterns of enhancement may be seen (gyriform, nodular, leptomeningeal, or intravascular). In the chronic stage, varying degrees of encephalomalacia, atrophy, calcification, and gliosis are seen in the affected lobes. Early successful treatment may minimize such sequelae.

HUMAN IMMUNODEFICIENCY VIRUS ENCEPHALITIS

Human immunodeficiency virus (HIV) can affect the brain directly, causing a progressive encephalitis (formerly called *AIDS dementia complex*), or indirectly by making the host susceptible to opportunistic infections (cerebral toxoplasmosis, progressive multifocal leukoencephalopathy (PML), cytomegalovirus) and certain malignancies (lymphoma) that involve the CNS. HIV encephalitis microscopically appears as microglial nodules and multinucleated giant cells, with demyelination and vacuole formation. The demyelination is seen as hyperintense signal change on T2 and FLAIR images, usually starting in the PV white matter and centrum semiovale. Later the lesions become progressively more diffuse and confluent. Eventually, basal ganglionic and thalamic involvement is also seen. Along with these changes, prominent cerebral atrophy develops, with progressive enlargement of the central and superficial CSF spaces (**Fig. 33A.47**).

CEREBRAL TOXOPLASMOSIS

Toxoplasmosis lesions are usually multifocal and may involve the basal ganglia, thalamus, gray/white junction, cerebral cortex, and PV white matter. The lesions are iso- to hypointense on T1 and hyperintense on T2-weighted images. A significant amount of edema surrounds the lesions, appearing as T1 hypointensity and T2 hyperintensity. With gadolinium, the smaller lesions enhance homogenously, and the larger ones exhibit ring or nodular enhancement. After antibiotic treatment, chronic lesions frequently show calcification and hemosiderin deposits.

In an HIV patient with cerebral lesions, the most common differential diagnostic consideration is lymphoma. The imaging appearance of HIV-related lymphoma is different from that seen in an immunocompetent host (see the brain tumor section of this chapter for details). Functional imaging with positron emission tomography (PET) or single-photon emission computed tomography (SPECT) may be used to differentiate between lymphoma and toxoplasmosis or other infectious lesions in HIV-positive patients (Heald et al., 1996).

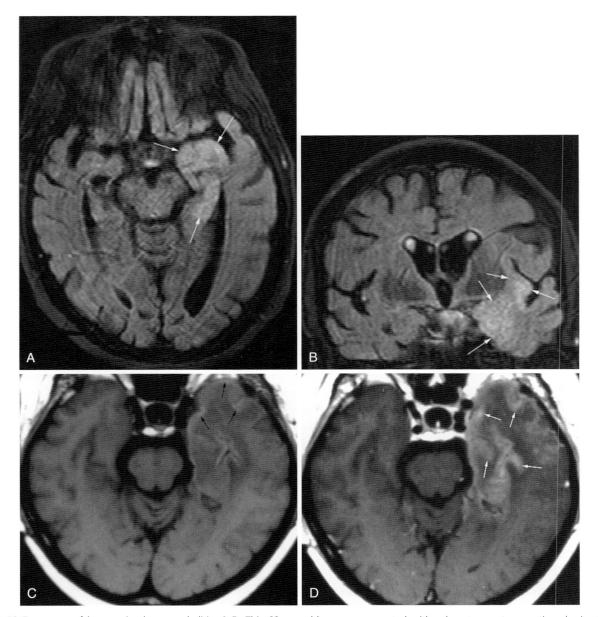

Fig. 33A.46 Two cases of herpes simplex encephalitis. **A-B,** This 68-year-old woman presented with subacute-onset semantic aphasia. Axial and coronal FLAIR images show hyperintense signal involving the left medial temporal lobe and part of the insula *(arrows)*. Involved structures also demonstrate swelling. **C-D,** In a different patient, even more prominent temporal lobe involvement is seen. On a noncontrast T1-weighted image **(C)** the left temporal lobe is swollen, and parts of the cortex show faint hyperintensity, indicating potential hemorrhage *(arrows)*. On the postcontrast T1-weighted image **(D)** gyriform enhancement is seen *(arrows)*.

PROGRESSIVE MULTIFOCAL LEUKOENCEPHALOPATHY

Progressive multifocal leukoencephalopathy is an infectious demyelinating disease caused by the JC polyomavirus. It has been most common in HIV patients, but it is now also a well-known potential complication of natalizumab infusions for MS. The disease initially involves the white matter, most commonly in the frontal, parietal, and occipital lobes. The lesions are hypointense on T1, hyperintense on T2 and FLAIR, usually multifocal, and are initially round or oval then become confluent. They tend to involve the subcortical white matter, including the U-fibers, with later involvement of the deep gray matter, corpus callosum, and posterior fossa. With gadolinium administration, faint enhancement may be present, but usually no enhancement is seen. DWI often reveals restricted diffusion at the spreading outer margins of PML lesions relative to the typically high ADC values within the gliotic and demyelinated central portions, which assists in the differential diagnosis (da Pozzo et al., 2006).

CREUTZFELDT-JAKOB DISEASE

Creutzfeldt-Jakob disease is a rapidly progressing, fatal dementing illness caused by prions—self-replicating, infectious protein particles. In advanced cases, MRI usually reveals prominent atrophy and gray-matter hyperintense signal changes on T2 and FLAIR sequences. The hyperintensity typically involves the cerebral cortex, basal ganglia, and cerebellum. There is no mass effect, and enhancement is rare. In the early stage of the disease, conventional T2-weighted images may be entirely normal, but diffusion-weighted images may show ribbonlike hyperintensity along the cerebral cortex (**Fig. 33A.48**), commonly involving the insula

and cingulate cortex. Hyperintensity may be also seen in the caudate nucleus, lentiform nucleus, and in the thalamus as well, in a nonvascular distribution. Involvement of the pulvinar is characteristic of the mad-cow variant. Cerebellar cortical involvement is also common. The abnormalities may be uni- or bilateral. FLAIR sequences have been known to display these abnormalities earlier than conventional T2-weighted images, but not as conspicuously as DWI (Shiga et al., 2004; Young et al., 2005).

Multiple Sclerosis and Other Inflammatory or White Matter Diseases

Inflammatory and noninflammatory lesions of the corpus callosum, leukodystrophy (Krabbe disease, metachromatic leukodystrophy, adrenoleukodystrophy), radiation leukoencephalopathy, posterior reversible encephalopathy syndrome, and central pontine myelinolysis are discussed only in the online version of this chapter. Please visit www.expertconsult.com for more information.

MULTIPLE SCLEROSIS

Multiple sclerosis is a demyelinating disease with autoimmune inflammatory reaction against the myelin sheath of CNS pathways (see Chapter 54). MRI is essential for the diagnosis of MS by demonstrating the typical inflammatory demyelinating lesions disseminated in time and space (**Fig. 33A.49**). It is also used for disease monitoring and assessment of response to therapy.

MS white matter lesions may occur supratentorially or infratentorially, as well as within the spinal cord (imaging of spinal cord MS lesions is described later). Best evaluated on T2-weighted images, infratentorial lesions may be seen within the medulla, pons, midbrain, or cerebellum. Characteristic locations include the pontine tegmentum, periaqueductal

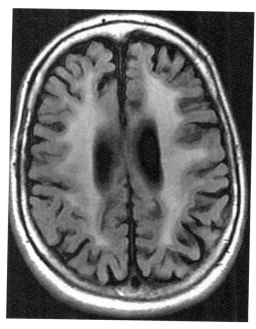

Fig. 33A.47 Human immunodeficiency virus (HIV) encephalopathy. This is a 39-year-old patient with advanced HIV. Axial FLAIR image demonstrates cerebral volume loss and confluent hyperintense demyelination of the white matter in the centrum semiovale and subcortical regions bilaterally.

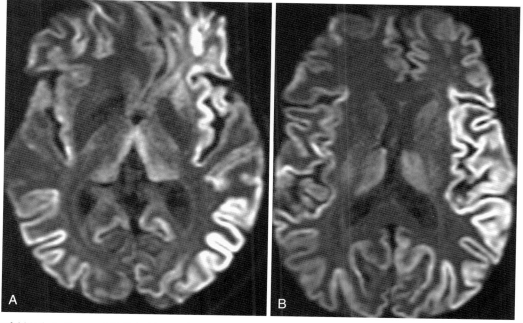

Fig. 33A.48 Creutzfeldt-Jakob disease. **A-B,** This 47-year-old patient presented with rapid cognitive decline, unsteady gait, and myoclonus. Diffusion-weighted images demonstrate hyperintense signal that characteristically involves the cortical ribbon of the frontal and parietal lobes, more so on the left side, and the insula. Hyperintense signal change is also seen in the thalamus bilaterally.

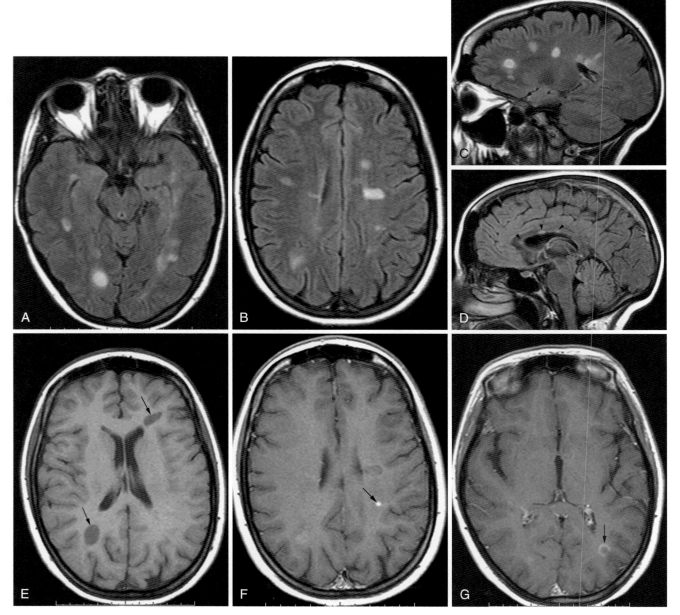

Fig. 33A.49 Multiple sclerosis. **A-C,** Axial and sagittal FLAIR images demonstrate multiple hyperintense lesions in the white matter. The majority of these abut the lateral ventricles, including the temporal horns bilaterally. Several lesions are linear and oriented perpendicular to ventricular borders. On sagittal FLAIR image **(C)** some lesions exhibit characteristic Dawson fingerlike appearance. **D,** On midsagittal FLAIR image, lesions are present in the corpus callosum *(arrowheads)*. **E,** On T1-weighted noncontrast image, two prominently hypointense lesions exhibit a "black hole" appearance *(arrows)*. **F-G,** Axial T1 postcontrast images demonstrate two enhancing lesions. One is a small, homogeneously enhancing lesion in the left centrum semiovale *(arrow)*, the other is seen in the left parietal subcortical area *(arrow)*. This latter lesion exhibits an "open-ring" enhancement pattern which is very typical for active demyelinating lesions.

region, cerebral peduncles, middle and superior cerebellar peduncles, and the white matter of the cerebellar hemispheres. Punctate or small lesions that are present directly adjacent to the fourth ventricle or cisterns are sometimes difficult to detect on T2-weighted images but are not uncommon. Infratentorial lesions are generally smaller than supratentorial lesions and are also less frequently hypointense on conventional T1-weighted images; they commonly appear hypointense on T1-weighted 3D spoiled gradient echo pulse sequences.

Supratentorial white matter lesions are usually best appreciated using the FLAIR pulse sequence, which nulls out CSF signal that may obscure periventricular abnormalities on conventional T2-weighted images. PV and subcortical white matter lesions typically are small in size and morphologically are generally ovoid or round on axial images. On sagittal views, PV lesions often exhibit a thin linear or fingerlike morphology (Dawson fingers), with the long axis of the lesion oriented perpendicularly to the wall of the lateral ventricle in a PV distribution. The PV distribution of many MS lesions is well demonstrated on SWI imaging, which reveals a single tiny, profoundly hypointense dot or thin linearity at the center of a significant proportion of demyelinating lesions. It represents a venule and is visible because of the magnetic susceptibility effects of deoxygenated venous blood, to which SWI is particularly sensitive.

Although the distribution of white matter lesions in MS has a somewhat random appearance, the hemispheres characteristically match each other in terms of lesion load, which typically is highest around the ventricles. On sagittal views, PV lesions are usually most numerous adjacent to the bodies and atria of the lateral ventricles, with less involvement of the white matter adjacent to the occipital and temporal horns. The deep white matter of the frontal and parietal lobes typically also tends to exhibit a greater number of lesions than either the occipital or temporal lobes. However, the presence of lesions adjacent to the temporal horns favors a diagnosis of MS. Juxtacortical demyelination is less commonly seen. Juxtacortical lesions, which involve the U-fibers, often exhibit a crescentic morphology and are usually seen only on FLAIR, proton density, or T2-weighted images. Occasionally they are hypointense on T1 as well. When present, this type of lesion favors the diagnosis of MS. Corpus callosum lesions are also relatively specific for MS. They are best visualized on sagittal FLAIR images, typically as punctate hyperintensities along the septocallosal margin (undersurface of the corpus callosum). Thin hyperintense linearities that are contiguous with and perpendicular to the undersurface may also be present. These findings are often superimposed upon a thin irregular band of T2 hyperintensity running along the undersurface of the corpus callosum rostrocaudally. Isolated lesions within the central fibers of the corpus callosum that are noncontiguous with the septocallosal margin are less typical and should raise the level of suspicion for alternate differential diagnoses, discussed in the following section.

Although it is well known from histopathological studies that MS affects not only the hemispheric white matter but also the cortex and deep gray nuclei, cortical gray matter lesions are uncommonly seen on conventional MRI studies. They may be seen more often with the use of high-field scanners (3.0 T or higher). Of the conventional pulse sequences, high spatial resolution FLAIR images are the most sensitive for cortical gray matter lesions. Detection is limited because the subtle hyperintensity of cortical lesions on FLAIR is only slightly greater than the already relatively hyperintense background of the cortical gray matter. A cortical gray matter lesion may be verified by correlation of the finding on separate FLAIR image stacks acquired in orthogonal planes or by detection of a hypointense lesion of identical morphology and location on T1-weighted 3D spoiled gradient echo pulse sequences. Cortical gray matter lesions generally have a curvilinear contour that conforms to the topology of the cortex but may also overlap with the adjacent white matter. Like deep gray-matter lesions, cortical gray-matter hyperintensities visible on MRI are usually small, in the millimeter range. Deep gray-matter MS lesions tend to be round or oval and are most frequently seen in the thalami.

T1-weighted images are useful for the detection of "black holes," markedly hypointense lesions that have been shown histopathologically to exhibit more extensive demyelination and axonal loss than other lesions. They always exhibit a correlating hyperintensity on T2-weighted images but may

appear centrally hypointense on FLAIR owing to their relatively high free water content. Conversely, not all T2-weighted lesions exhibit T1 hypointensity, and therefore the T1 lesion load is always less extensive than the T2 lesion load. Some MS cases, usually earlier in disease progression, exhibit no T1 hypointense lesions.

T1-weighted postcontrast images are useful for the detection of enhancing lesions in patients with clinical exacerbations. Enhancement may be solid or ringlike. Open-ring configurations are more typical for MS than other disease entities that also exhibit ring enhancement, such as tumors and infections (Masdeu et al., 2000). Five minutes between gadolinium injection and the acquisition of postcontrast images is the minimum acceptable delay for detecting acute demyelinating lesions, but longer delays of up to 30 minutes can significantly increase sensitivity, as can incorporation of magnetization transfer techniques and double or triple doses of gadolinium.

Chronic MS lesions do not exhibit restricted diffusion, appearing on DWI as either isointense to the surrounding brain parenchyma or, less commonly, hyperintense due to T2 shine-through artifact. On the corresponding ADC maps, chronic lesions exhibit normal or high apparent diffusion coefficients. However, as recently described, acute enhancing demyelinating lesions may on rare occasions exhibit high signal on DWI, with corresponding low pixel values (hypointense) on the ADC map, consistent with restricted diffusion (Balashov et al., 2009). Rapid resolution of restricted diffusion in these acute lesions is the rule, and they often evolve to exhibit increased ADC values on follow-up studies.

Nonconventional MRI pulse sequences are commonly used to assess MS in the research environment. SWI is a newer technique that is exquisitely sensitive to the small venules as well as iron deposition, the latter thought to play a pathophysiological role in MS. Magnetization transfer imaging may be used to generate histograms of pixel values within the normal-appearing white matter; such histograms are typically shifted to the left, with lower peak values than in normal individuals. Diffusion tensor imaging is a more advanced application of DWI that is used to measure the directional diffusion of water molecules within white matter tracts. Like magnetization transfer imaging, DTI is useful for the quantification of pathology within normal-appearing white matter.

ACUTE DISSEMINATED ENCEPHALOMYELITIS

Acute disseminated encephalomyelitis (ADEM) is an acute demyelinating disease that, unlike MS, is typically monophasic. It may follow vaccination or a viral infection. On MRI, multiple hyperintense lesions are seen in the hemispheric white matter, cerebellum, and brainstem. The hemispheric lesions are often subcortical. Although MS may also involve the gray matter, this is much more common in ADEM, and basal ganglia or thalamic lesions are seen in 30% to 40% of cases. The lesions may exhibit vasogenic edema, and hemorrhage may also be seen. The lesions may show diffuse faint enhancement with gadolinium.

NEUROSARCOIDOSIS

The prevalence of nervous system involvement in sarcoidosis is approximately 5%. In the brain parenchyma, multiple periventricular T2 hyperintense lesions are frequently noted, which may be due to a vasculitic process and often cannot be distinguished from MS or ischemic microvascular changes. Sarcoidosis may also involve the pituitary infundibulum and hypothalamus (resulting in endocrine symptoms). The granulomatous inflammation may affect the cranial nerves and/or their meningeal coverings as well, resulting in enlargement, hyperintense signal change, and abnormal enhancement. Although sarcoidosis may involve the dura, following gadolinium administration, leptomeningeal enhancement is more commonly noted. It is typically seen along the penetrating blood vessels and the adjacent leptomeninges, and is due to perivascular spread of the granulomatous process (**Fig. 33A.50**). Sometimes larger intraparenchymal or meningeal enhancing lesions are noted which may be mistaken for

primary or metastatic tumors. When involved, the pituitary infundibulum and hypothalamus may also exhibit enhancement. Neurosarcoidosis may also lead to hydrocephalus, either by interfering with CSF absorption through the arachnoid granulations or by obstructing the ventricular system.

Trauma

Both CT and MRI have a pivotal role in the evaluation of craniocerebral trauma (Chapter 50B). In the emergency room setting, the first imaging modality is usually a noncontrast CT scan. CT bone windowing is the best tool for evaluating skull fractures (**Fig. 33A.54**), whereas brain windowing is of great

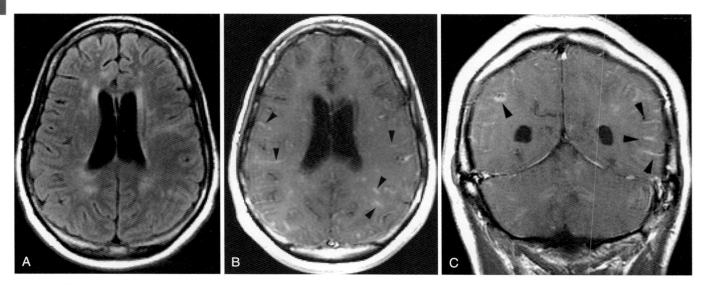

Fig. 33A.50 Neurosarcoidosis. **A,** Axial FLAIR image reveals multiple hyperintense lesions in the deep and subcortical white matter bilaterally. **B-C,** Axial and coronal T1 postcontrast images show multiple linear areas of enhancement in a leptomeningeal and perivascular distribution, a pattern characteristic of neurosarcoidosis *(arrowheads)*.

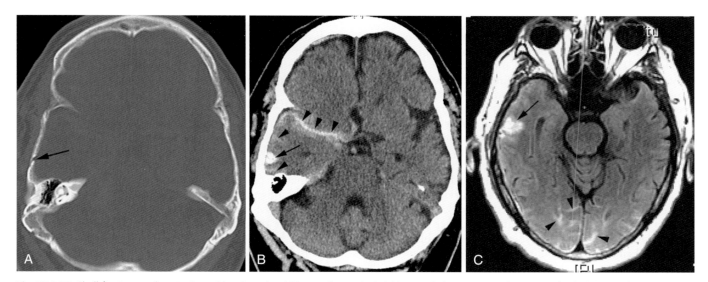

Fig. 33A.54 Skull fracture and contusion with subarachnoid hemorrhage. **A,** Axial bone window computed tomography (CT) image demonstrates a right temporal bone fracture *(arrow)*. **B,** Axial brain window CT scan reveals a hyperdense area at the right temporal lobe surface, consistent with contusion and hemorrhage *(arrow)*. There is hyperdensity in the right temporal lobe sulci and even more so in the right middle cranial fossa of the brain, due to traumatic subarachnoid blood *(arrowheads)*. **C,** Axial FLAIR image demonstrates hyperintense signal change in the right temporal lobe, consistent with contusion *(arrow)*. There is also bilateral hyperintense signal due to the presence of subarachnoid blood in the sulci of the occipital lobes, which settled in these dependent regions because of the prolonged supine position of the patient *(arrowheads)*.

value for visualizing subarachnoid, epidural, subdural, intra-ventricular, or intraparenchymal hemorrhages. MRI is very useful in detecting traumatic lesions of the brain parenchyma, especially when more subtle changes are present, such as small contusions, parenchymal microbleeds, and the small or punctate lesions of diffuse axonal injury. The various consequences of trauma that we will review next seldom occur in isolation but tend to occur in various combinations (e.g., cortical contusion is frequently associated with subarachnoid hemorrhage).

TRAUMATIC SUBARACHNOID HEMORRHAGE

Traditionally, a noncontrast CT scan has been the first-line imaging study to demonstrate traumatic subarachnoid hemorrhage. Acute blood appears hyperdense in the subarachnoid space. The hemorrhage may be seen in the sylvian fissures, interhemispheric fissure, basal cisterns, or in the cortical sulci at the convexities, depending on the site of trauma. Subarachnoid hyperdensity tends to resolve within 5 to 7 days after the hemorrhage, but depending on the amount of subarachnoid blood, this may be a shorter or longer process.

Until FLAIR pulse sequences became available, MRI was inferior to CT in detecting subarachnoid blood, especially in the first few days. Conventional T1- and T2-weighted images may completely miss subarachnoid blood in these early stages. However, subarachnoid blood appears hyperintense on FLAIR images (see **Fig. 33A.54**), and this pulse sequence is considered equal or superior to CT in detecting subarachnoid blood (Woodcock et al., 2001), especially in the posterior fossa and at the skull base, where CT images are often compromised by beam-hardening artifacts. The hyperintense signal change is due to the presence of blood, which changes the zero point of the inversion time of CSF, and therefore signal attenuation in subarachnoid regions containing hemorrhage will not be complete. An important caveat is that subarachnoid hyperintensity on FLAIR may also result from other causes. A common cause is magnetic susceptibility artifact, seen in patients who have braces or other metal devices that distort the magnetic field, which results in a lack of CSF signal suppression and the artifactually hyperintense appearance of CSF adjacent to the anterior frontal lobes.

Besides detection of blood in the acute phase, structural neuroimaging is also very useful to evaluate the potential later complications of subarachnoid hemorrhage. Subarachnoid blood may occlude the arachnoid granulations, leading to impaired CSF absorption, communicating hydrocephalus, and ventriculomegaly. Another late phenomenon that tends to follow repeated episodes of subarachnoid hemorrhage is superficial siderosis. In this condition, hemosiderin is deposited along the leptomeninges and appears as linear areas of hypointensity on T2-weighted images (see **Fig. 33A.44** online at www.expertconsult.com).

SUBDURAL HEMORRHAGE

Subdural hematomas are common sequelae of head trauma and are thought to result from rupture of the bridging veins (veins that drain from the cerebral surface and pierce the dura to enter the adjacent venous sinus). Morphologically they follow the contour of the cerebral surface and can cross the cranial suture lines but not the midline at the falx cerebri and cerebelli. Depending on the size, there is a varying degree of mass effect on the adjacent brain; in the more severe cases,

effacement of the adjacent ventricles, midline shift, and various herniation syndromes may occur.

As subdural hematomas age, their imaging appearance changes both on CT and MRI. On CT, acute subdural hematomas appear hyperdense. If the patient remains in a recumbent position, the cellular elements settle to the lower part of the hematoma, which will appear more hyperdense, whereas the "supernatant" is less so. With time, hemoglobin degradation occurs and the density of the hematoma will decrease, eventually becoming hypodense. During this process there is a transitional stage when the density of the hematoma will be very similar or the same as that of the brain, rendering its detection more difficult. Just as with intraparenchymal hematomas, the density depends on the hematocrit, and in severely anemic patients, even acute subdural hematomas may appear iso- or hypodense, leading to erroneous dating.

On MRI, subdural hematomas exhibit a signal evolution similar to that seen with intraparenchymal hemorrhages, but the pace of evolution is different due to a slower decrease of the oxygen content within the hematoma. Acute subdural hematomas (**Fig. 33A.55**) are initially isointense on T1 and hyperintense on T2, but as deoxyhemoglobin appears, the signal on T2-weighted images becomes hypointense. In the subacute phase, the signal is hyperintense on T1 and hypointense on T2, but in the late subacute stage, the signal will be hyperintense on both T1- and T2-weighted images because of extracellular methemoglobin (**Fig. 33A.56**). It is important to remember that these stages are not separated sharply, and mixed patterns are often seen; this is due to the presence of oxy- and deoxyhemoglobin in the acute stage and intra- and extracellular methemoglobin in the chronic stage. Rebleeding into an existing subdural hematoma may also occur, resulting in the presence of clots of various ages.

Chronic subdural hematomas (**Fig. 33A.57**) are hypointense relative to the brain but, having higher protein content, are mildly hyperintense relative to the CSF on T1-weighted images and hyperintense on T2-weighted images. Hemosiderin deposition is not as prominent as in parenchymal hemorrhages because macrophages tend to be cleared by the meningeal circulation. Chronic subdural hematomas may look similar to hyperacute ones on noncontrast images, but because of their vascular membrane, with gadolinium they exhibit enhancement along their periphery. On CT, chronic subdural hematomas appear as hypodense subdural collections. Mass effect is variable depending on the size of the hematoma and degree of cerebral atrophy. If repeated hemorrhage occurs into the subdural collection, the hyperdense fresh blood is seen within the chronic hypodense collection (**Fig. 33A.58**).

EPIDURAL HEMORRHAGE

Contrary to subdural hematoma, epidural hemorrhage is usually arterial in origin and due to laceration of a meningeal artery, most commonly the middle meningeal artery. Epidural hematomas are often lens shaped, respect cranial suture lines, and sometimes the dura itself is seen as a linear structure pushed toward the brain. The evolution of CT and MRI signal characteristics is similar to that of subdural hematomas.

CORTICAL CONTUSION

Cerebral contusions result from the brain hitting against the inner table of the skull or sliding against the bony ridges of the base of the skull. The most common locations include the

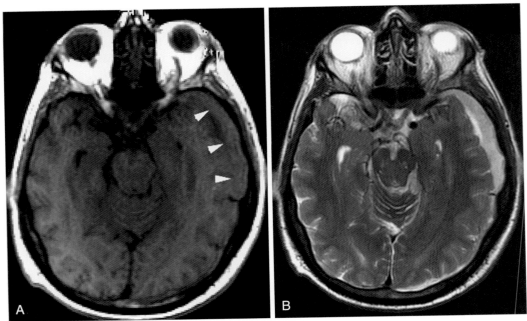

Fig. 33A.55 Acute subdural hematoma. **A,** Axial noncontrast T1-weighted image shows a subdural collection over the left temporal lobe, which is isointense to the brain parenchyma and therefore somewhat difficult to notice *(arrowheads)*. **B,** Axial T2-weighted image helps by revealing a much more obvious hyperintense subdural collection in the same area.

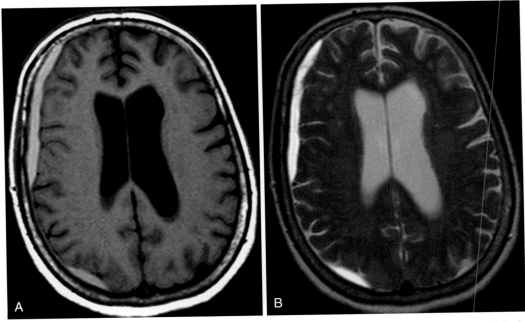

Fig. 33A.56 Subacute subdural hematoma. **A,** On axial T1-weighted image, the subacute subdural hematoma over the right frontal and parietal lobes is hyperintense and easily noticeable. **B,** On axial T2-weighted image, the hematoma is also hyperintense.

poles and inferior surfaces of the frontal, temporal, and occipital lobes. The injured brain parenchyma exhibits foci of hemorrhage and varying degrees of edema, which may progress later to more confluent hematoma and more swelling. On CT, acute contusions appear as foci of hyperdense hemorrhage with or without swelling. The hematomas get reabsorbed later, and the swelling decreases. In the chronic stage, no residual findings or varying degrees of encephalomalacia may be seen. On MRI, with the appearance of deoxyhemoglobin, a hypointense signal is seen on T2; the surrounding edema is hyperintense on T2 and FLAIR sequences (**Fig. 33A.59**). Later, in the subacute stage, extracellular methemoglobin is hyperintense on T1- and T2-weighted images. Gradient echo and susceptibility-weighted images are very useful to show the hemorrhagic component of the lesion. Chronic contusions are associated with encephalomalacic cavities of various sizes, exhibiting CSF signal characteristics and surrounded by a hyperintense rim of reactive gliosis on T2 and FLAIR sequences.

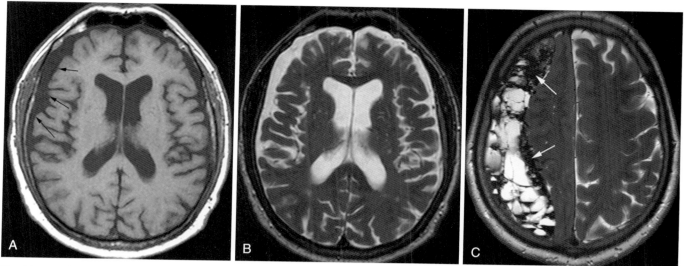

Fig. 33A.57 Chronic subdural hematoma. **A,** Axial T1-weighted image reveals a right frontal chronic subdural hematoma with signal similar to CSF *(arrows)*. **B,** On axial T2-weighted image, the chronic hematoma is hyperintense. **C,** Axial T2-weighted image of a different case. Within the hyperintense subdural collection, multiple hypointense zones are seen; these are due to hemosiderin deposition *(arrows)*. There is prominent mass effect on the hemisphere.

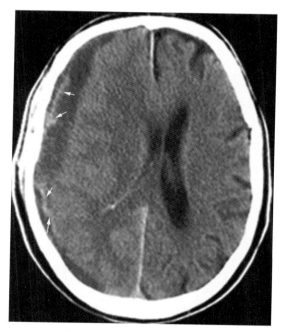

Fig. 33A.58 Chronic subdural hematoma on computed tomography (CT). Axial noncontrast CT scan shows a hypodense subdural collection over the right frontal and parietal lobes. Right hemisphere is compressed, and midline shift is present. Note hyperdense areas within the subdural collection, suggestive of another more recent bleeding episode *(arrows)*.

Variable degrees of hemosiderin deposition appear hypointense on FLAIR, gradient echo, and SWI.

DIFFUSE AXONAL INJURY

The underlying pathomechanism of this entity is shearing injury of the white matter pathways. This may involve the corpus callosum, other fiber tracts of the corona radiata and centrum semiovale, and may also involve the brainstem. The changes on structural neuroimaging can be very subtle, usually in the few-millimeter size range. Such lesions are usually not detected by CT. MRI is the study of choice. On MRI, the lesions appear as foci of hyperintensity seen on T2 and FLAIR sequences. Foci of hemorrhage (usually microbleeds) are also present. For detection of the microbleeds associated with axonal injury, gradient echo or susceptibility-weighted images (**Fig. 33A.60**) are the most sensitive (Li and Feng, 2009).

CEREBRAL PARENCHYMAL HEMATOMA

The imaging appearance of cerebral hematomas is discussed in the section on hemorrhagic cerebrovascular disease. As described there, for detection of smaller hemorrhagic lesions or microbleeds, gradient echo or SWI are the most sensitive techniques and should be part of every trauma imaging protocol.

Metabolic and Toxic Disorders

This section is in the online-only version of this chapter. Please visit www.expertconsult.com for more information, and also refer to Chapters 56 through 58 and 62 for further discussions of these topics.

Genetic and Degenerative Disorders Primarily Causing Ataxia (Cerebellar Disorders)

Structural neuroimaging has a limited role in the evaluation of hereditary and degenerative cerebellar disorders. The neurological examination, family history, and genetic testing are most helpful in finding the specific diagnosis, whereas imaging usually has a supportive role—for instance, by defining the degree of involvement of the pontine nuclei in the differential diagnosis of olivopontocerebellar atrophy. Nevertheless, imaging is almost always obtained in patients who present with progressive ataxia for the purpose of ruling out other potential causes, such as an enlarging posterior fossa neoplasm. Additionally, certain ataxic disorders (multiple system atrophy, spinocerebellar ataxias, Friedrich ataxia, ataxia-telangiectasia, fragile X premutation syndrome)

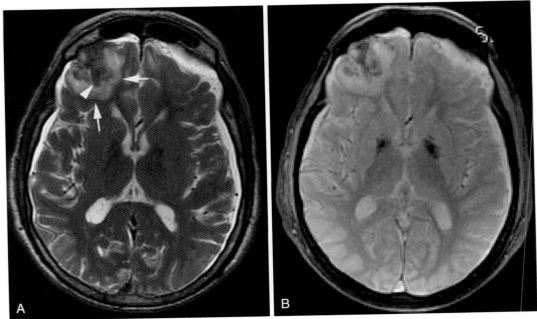

Fig. 33A.59 Contusion with subdural hematoma. **A,** Axial T2-weighted image demonstrates an area of mixed signal change in the right frontal lobe *(arrows).* Its center contains hypointense hemorrhagic changes *(arrowhead)* and is surrounded by hyperintense edema. Note coexisting bilateral traumatic subdural hematomas. **B,** Gradient echo image reveals more clearly a hypointense signal in the center of the contusion, owing to the presence of blood degradation products.

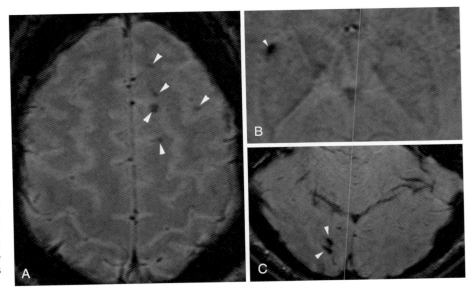

Fig. 33A.60 Diffuse axonal injury. Magnetic resonance image from a 42-year-old assault victim. Susceptibility-weighted images reveal multiple hypointense areas *(arrowheads)* in the left frontal lobe **(A)**, right external capsule **(B)**, and right occipital lobe **(C)**. These are areas of microbleeds associated with axonal injury.

may present with characteristic MRI changes. These are discussed in the online-only version of this chapter (visit www.expertconsult.com). Please also refer to Chapters 20 and 72 for review of ataxic disorders.

Genetic and Degenerative Disorders Primarily Causing Parkinsonism or Other Movement Disorders

Structural neuroimaging has a limited role in the evaluation of parkinsonian syndromes and other movement disorders. Diagnosis of these entities is still largely dependent on a detailed history and thorough neurological examination. In equivocal cases or in the academic/research setting, functional imaging has shown value in the evaluation of various movement disorders. Nevertheless, structural imaging is frequently obtained in patients presenting with movement disorders, and it is therefore necessary to discuss the potential structural imaging findings in the most common parkinsonian syndromes and other common movement disorder syndromes. This discussion is in the online-only version of this chapter (www.expertconsult.com). Please also refer to Chapters 21 and 71 on movement disorders.

Degenerative Disorders Primarily Causing Dementia

AGE-RELATED INVOLUTIONAL CHANGES

The aging brain displays multiple potential changes that usually are of no clinical significance but should be distinguished from pathologic processes (**Fig. 33A.65**). Many of these findings appear on CT, but in general, MRI is more sensitive as to their extent and nature. Cerebral volume loss is commonly seen in the elderly brain (prevalence is 50% in the eighth decade), even in the absence of neurological signs or symptoms. Atrophy involves the hemispheres, mostly the frontal lobes, as revealed by prominence of the sulci, but enlargement of the cisterns, sylvian fissures, and third and lateral ventricles is also frequent.

T2 hyperintense signal changes in the hemispheres is another common finding. A typical pattern is "capping" of the frontal horns, with or without additional signal changes along the borders of the lateral ventricles, seen as a T2 hyperintense lining that has a smooth outer margin. These findings are believed to be related to ependymal cell loss and gliosis. Scattered T2 hyperintense areas of signal change that are of variable size and shape are also commonly found within the cerebral hemispheric white matter in both PV and subcortical locations. These patches of abnormal signal may be due to dilation of periarteriolar spaces or to ischemic demyelination and gliosis and can result from hypertension, narrowing of small vessels, hypoxia, hypoperfusion, or small emboli. In many individuals these are asymptomatic, and their clinical prognostic significance as well as their relation to the more extensive symptomatic microangiopathy, leukoaraiosis, and Binswanger disease has been debated.

Normal aging at times may also be accompanied by iron deposition in the brain. This appears as symmetrical hypointense signal on T2-weighted images, the most commonly affected structures being the globus pallidus, substantia nigra, red nuclei, and dentate nuclei. Iron deposition in the putamen may later occur.

Enlargement of the perivascular spaces may be noted at any age, but it is seen more commonly in the elderly. These enlarged spaces follow CSF signal characteristics and are often seen in the basal ganglia region at the level of the anterior commissure, but also in the hemispheres within the centrum semiovale. They should not be mistaken for chronic lacunar ischemic lesions. For further discussion of the imaging characteristics of perivascular spaces, see the "nonneoplastic cystic lesion" section of this chapter online (www.expertconsult.com).

ALZHEIMER DISEASE

CT and MR imaging may provide helpful findings in Alzheimer disease (AD) (**Fig. 33A.66**), in addition to excluding other pathologies that can also lead to cognitive decline, such as stroke or frontotemporal tumors. Atrophy begins in the entorhinal cortex, eventually involving the rest of the anterior and medial part of the temporal lobes and progressing through the limbic structures to the neocortex. Insular cortex is affected early, while paracentral cortex is resistant to the disease. The temporal horns and sylvian fissures are frequently enlarged. It is important to remember that volume loss occurs in the aging brain; at times patients with marked atrophy are asymptomatic, whereas patients with mild or moderate AD may have little volume loss, at least by visual inspection. Computerized volumetric analysis of the hippocampal formation and other brain regions is the most precise way to measure atrophy. Studies using this technique continue toward the goals of establishing ranges of normal values relative to age, correlating measurements with the degree of cognitive impairment, and differentiating between dementia subtypes (for a review see Chapter 66) with sufficient accuracy and efficiency to allow for its regular clinical use.

FRONTOTEMPORAL LOBAR DEGENERATION, INCLUDING PICK DISEASE

Frontotemporal lobar degeneration (FTLD) is a category of dementing illness with three clinical subtypes: behavioral-type FTLD, primary progressive aphasia (PPA) (also termed *progressive nonfluent aphasia*), and semantic dementia. Formerly, *Pick disease* was a term used for the clinical syndromes now encompassed by FTLD, but it is currently used to refer to only one of the several types of pathology that cause these conditions. FTLD subtypes, just like AD, cannot be diagnosed with structural neuroimaging, but CT and MRI show changes that can assist in differentiating them from each other and other dementias, as well as excluding other etiologies. A characteristic finding in these dementias is atrophy of the frontal and temporal lobes, which may be asymmetrical or symmetrical. When the disease is advanced, gyral atrophy may be so prominent that it has been termed *knife-edge atrophy* (**Fig. 33A.67**).

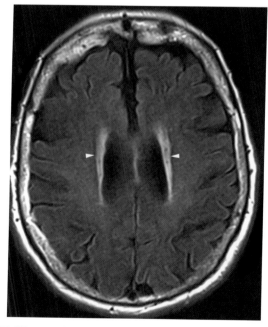

Fig. 33A.65 Normal aging. Magnetic resonance image of a cognitively intact 85-year-old person. There is linear T2 hyperintense signal bordering the bodies of the lateral ventricles. It has a smooth outer margin (*arrowheads*), most likely representing ependymal cell loss and gliosis. Faint ground-glass T2 hyperintensity is seen in the white matter, likely due to microvascular changes. Note the mild frontal lobe atrophy. There is some thickening and fatty marrow transformation of the calvarium.

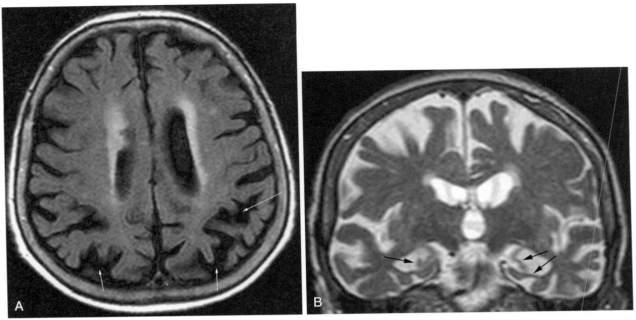

Fig. 33A.66 Alzheimer disease. **A,** Axial FLAIR image close to the vertex demonstrates enlargement of the parietal lobe sulci bilaterally, indicating atrophy *(arrows)*. **B,** Coronal T2-weighted image reveals prominent medial temporal lobe/hippocampal atrophy *(arrows)* and as a result, enlargement of the temporal horns.

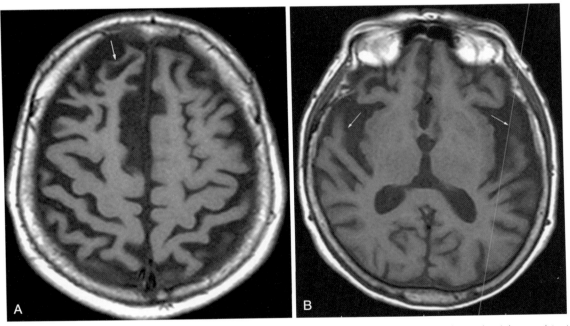

Fig. 33A.67 Frontotemporal dementia. **A,** Axial T1-weighted image reveals enlargement of the frontal lobe sulci on the right, consistent with frontal lobe atrophy. Some gyri fit the description of "knife-edge" atrophy *(arrow)*. **B,** Another axial T1-weighted image shows widening of the sylvian fissures due to temporal lobe atrophy *(arrows)*.

Neurocutaneous Syndromes

Structural neuroimaging features of the neurocutaneous syndromes (neurofibromatosis, hamartoma, neurofibroma, tuberous sclerosis [Bourneville disease], cortical tubers, subependymal nodules, white matter lesions, von Hippel-Lindau disease, Sturge-Weber syndrome) are discussed in the online-only version of this chapter. Please visit www.expertconsult.com and also refer to Chapter 65 for further review of this topic.

Congenital Anomalies of the Brain

This topic is available in the online version of the chapter at www.expertconsult.com.

Nonneoplastic Congenital Cystic Lesions

In addition to the following nonneoplastic congenital cystic lesions, the commonly encountered dilated Virchow-Robin spaces are discussed in the online-only version of this chapter, available at www.expertconsult.com.

EPIDERMOID

These lesions, also known as *squamous epithelial cysts*, congenital keratin cysts, or ectodermal inclusion cysts are formed by epidermal cells. Most epidermoids are congenital and due to the inclusion of epidermal cells of the ectoderm during neural tube closure, but rarely they are acquired secondary to traumatic inoculation of epidermal cells by skin sutures or spinal tap. The most common locations of the congenital type are the basal cisterns, cerebellopontine angle (40% to 50%), parasellar region, third or fourth ventricle, temporal horn, and sometimes within the hemispheres. Epidermoids are generally hypointense to brain on T1-weighted images but in 75% of cases are slightly hyperintense to CSF. Sometimes, triglyceride and fatty acid deposition in the cyst yield a T1 appearance that is hyperintense to brain, referred to as a *white epidermoid*. On T2 they are isointense or slightly hyperintense to CSF. On FLAIR, the signal of the cystic contents is not suppressed completely. Importantly, on diffusion-weighted images, epidermoids appear bright because diffusion is restricted. This may be the only imaging feature that reliably distinguishes them from arachnoid cysts (**Fig. 33A.76**). Epidermoids do not enhance with gadolinium.

DERMOID

Like epidermoids, dermoids are also ectodermal inclusion cysts. However, in addition to epidermal cells, dermoid cysts also contain derivatives of the dermis, such as cells of sebaceous and sweat glands, hair follicles, and adipocytes. The most common locations are in the midline: sellar, parasellar, frontonasal regions, midline vermis, and fourth ventricle. Dermoids are hyperintense on T1 because of their lipid content, and as a result their signal is diminished with fat suppression sequences. On T2-weighted images, they appear heterogeneous, from hypo- to iso- to hyperintense. Hair content may appear as curvilinear hypointensity. Dermoid cysts do not

enhance with gadolinium. At times dermoid cysts rupture, and their hyperintense fat content may be seen scattered in the subarachnoid space on noncontrast T1-weighted images. This may cause chemical meningitis, with associated abnormal enhancement of the meninges.

COLLOID CYST

Colloid cysts originate from the infolding neuroepithelium of the tela choroidea and are located almost exclusively in the anterior third of the third ventricle at the level of the foramen of Monro. Although histologically benign, colloid cysts represent a potential life-threatening emergency owing to their location. Sudden obstruction of the interventricular foramina of Monro by a colloid cyst may even cause acute hydrocephalus, coma, and death due to herniation or neurogenic cardiac dysfunction with subsequent cardiac arrest. The homogeneous signal characteristics of colloid cysts vary depending on the content of the cyst. Most often it is hyperintense on T1 and hypointense on T2-weighted images; this is due to mucus or protein content. If close attention is paid to the anterior third ventricle, the usually hyperintense colloid cyst on T1-weighted images is readily recognizable (**Fig. 33A.77**). A potential problem can arise if the protein content of a colloid cyst is low and results in an isointense rather than hyperintense signal; such a cyst may escape detection. This emphasizes the importance of reviewing all available pulse sequences. Another potential problem is small cyst size. If a colloid cyst is less than 5 mm in diameter, it may be missed if the 5-mm thick slices of a conventional MRI study happen to skip it. The epithelial lining of colloid cysts may appear as a thin rim of enhancement after gadolinium administration.

ARACHNOID CYST

Arachnoid cysts are extraaxial CSF-filled cysts lined by arachnoid membrane. Considering their structure, the term *intraarachnoid cyst* would be more appropriate, as these cysts are formed between the layers of the arachnoid membrane.

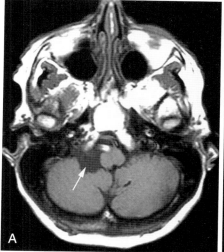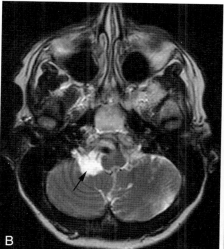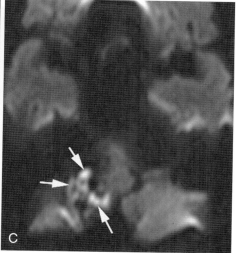

Fig. 33A.76 Epidermoid cyst. **A,** Axial T1-weighted image shows a cystic lesion in the posterior fossa on the right *(arrow)*. It is hypointense, exerts mass effect on the adjacent cerebellar hemisphere, and displaces the medulla. **B,** On an axial T2-weighted image, the same cystic lesion is hyperintense *(arrow)*. **C,** On a diffusion-weighted image, the lesion is bright *(arrows)*, a characteristic finding of an epidermoid cyst as opposed to an arachnoid cyst.

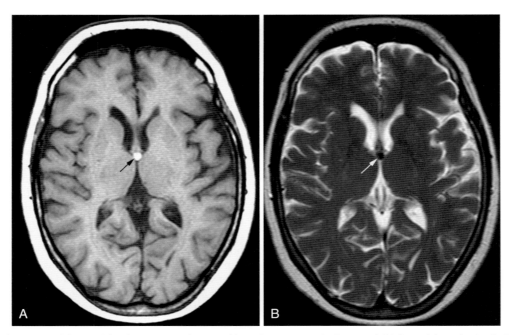

Fig. 33A.77 Colloid cyst. **A,** Axial T1-weighted image reveals a round hyperintense mass in the rostral third ventricle at the level of the interventricular foramen of Monro *(arrow)*. **B,** Axial T2-weighted image shows the cyst in the same location; hypointensity is due to protein or mucus content *(arrow)*.

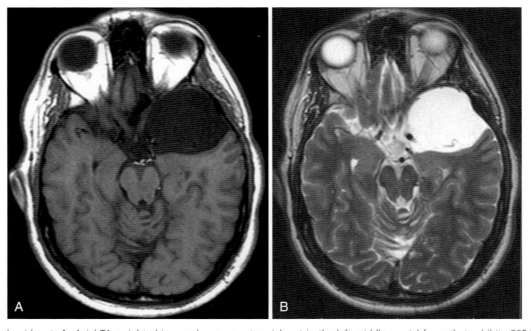

Fig. 33A.78 Arachnoid cyst. **A,** Axial T1-weighted image shows an extraaxial cyst in the left middle cranial fossa that exhibits CSF-like hypointense signal. There is mass effect with resultant compression and posterior displacement of the left temporal lobe. **B,** Axial T2-weighted image demonstrates the same arachnoid cyst with CSF-like hyperintense signal.

Arachnoid cysts are frequent incidental findings on MRI. The most common locations are the middle and posterior fossa, the suprasellar region, and at the vertex. In general, arachnoid cysts exhibit CSF signal characteristics, being hypointense on T1 and FLAIR and hyperintense on T2-weighted images (**Fig. 33A.78**). However, the composition of the fluid inside the arachnoid cyst may be different from that of CSF. The fluid secreted by the cyst wall may have higher protein content and therefore appear slightly more hyperintense on T1-weighted images than the CSF. Pulsation, flow turbulence, or (rarely) intracystic hemorrhage may also result in alteration of the signal within the cyst. When evaluating a suspected arachnoid cyst, the pulse sequences should include DWI to distinguish it from an epidermoid cyst. Epidermoid cysts, unlike arachnoid cysts, are hyperintense on DWI. Arachnoid cysts do not enhance with gadolinium.

Vascular Malformations

The various vascular malformations (arteriovenous malformations, cavernous malformations, developmental venous anomaly, and capillary telangiectasia) are discussed in the online-only version of this chapter. Please visit www.expertconsult.com, and also see Chapters 33B and 51D for review.

Cerebrospinal Fluid Circulation Disorders

Abnormalities in CSF and intraspinal cord flow cause changes in the brain or spinal cord that are readily identifiable by CT or MRI. Hydrocephalus is an abnormal intracranial accumulation of CSF that interferes with normal brain function (see Chapter 59). It should be distinguished from dilation of the ventricles and subarachnoid space due to decreased brain volume, which can be normal or pathological and has been called *hydrocephalus ex vacuo*. We will avoid using this term, because true hydrocephalus often requires treatment by shunting. Hydrocephalus may follow increased CSF production or impaired resorption. Resorption occurs not only via the pacchionian granulations in the venous sinuses but through the brain lymphatic system as well. Traditionally, two main types of hydrocephalus are distinguished: obstructive and nonobstructive. Nonobstructive hydrocephalus is due to increased CSF production, as with choroid plexus papillomas in children. Depending on whether CSF flow from the ventricular system to the subarachnoid space is intact or impeded, we can distinguish between communicating and noncommunicating types of obstructive hydrocephalus. Some processes increase CSF ICP but not the volume of intracranial CSF, causing the syndrome of idiopathic intracranial hypertension (known as *pseudotumor cerebri*). Interruption of CSF circulation can also happen at the craniocervical junction, where pathologies that interfere with the return of CSF from the spinal subarachnoid space to the intracranial compartment, as happens in the Chiari malformations, can arise. Finally, CSF intracranial volume may be abnormally reduced, causing the syndrome of intracranial hypotension.

OBSTRUCTIVE, NONCOMMUNICATING HYDROCEPHALUS

Depending on the site of obstruction, various segments of the ventricular system will enlarge. Obstruction at the foramen of Monro causes unilateral or bilateral enlargement of the lateral ventricles. Aqueductal stenosis, which may be congenital, leads to enlargement of the third and lateral ventricles, but the fourth ventricle is normal in size (**Fig. 33A.79**). Obstruction of the foramina of Luschka and Magendie results in enlargement of the third, fourth, and lateral ventricles. Other possible imaging findings include thinning and upward bowing of the corpus callosum. In third ventricle enlargement, the optic and infundibular recesses are widened. When the evolution of the hydrocephalus is rapid, transependymal CSF flow induces a T2 hyperintense signal (best seen on FLAIR sequences) along the walls of the involved ventricular segments, and in the case of the lateral ventricles, most pronounced at the frontal horns.

NORMAL-PRESSURE HYDROCEPHALUS

In this type of hydrocephalus, there is enlargement of the ventricles, most pronounced for the third and lateral ventricles (**Fig. 33A.80**). The subarachnoid spaces at the top of the convexity are typically compressed, but the larger sulci, such as the interhemispheric sulcus and the sylvian fissure, may be dilated as well as the ventricles (Kitagaki et al., 1998). In this case, the cross-sections of the dilated sulci often have the appearance of a "U" rather than the appearance of a "V" characteristic of atrophy (**Figs. 33A.81 and 33A.82** [online only]; also seen in **Fig. 33A.80**). These morphologic findings are more helpful than flow studies. Increased CSF flow in the

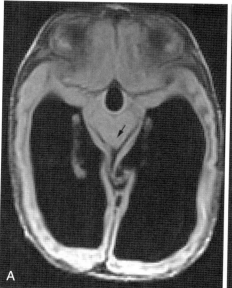
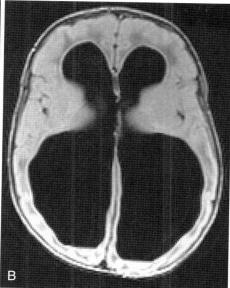
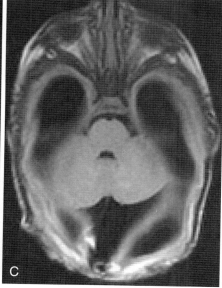

Fig. 33A.79 Obstructive hydrocephalus. **A-C,** In this case of congenital obstructive hydrocephalus, the cerebral aqueduct appears stenotic *(small arrow)*. There is extreme dilatation of the third and lateral ventricles, with the cerebral tissue being extremely thinned. The fourth ventricle is normal in size.

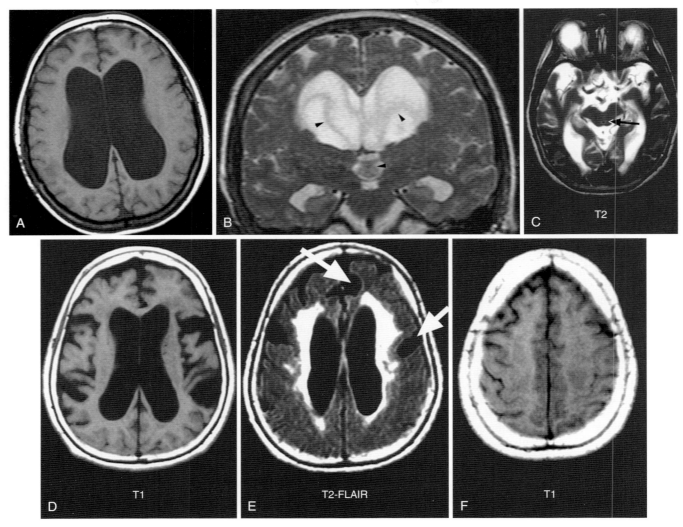

Fig. 33A.80 Two cases of normal-pressure hydrocephalus. In the first case **(A)** axial noncontrast T1-weighted images demonstrate significant enlargement of the ventricles, which is clearly out of proportion to the size of the superficial CSF spaces. The parietal sulci appear somewhat effaced. **B,** Coronal T2-weighted image also exhibits prominent ventricular enlargement. Note intraventricular artifact due to CSF pulsation *(arrowheads)*, indicating hyperdynamic flow. The second case demonstrates communicating hydrocephalus. Images **C-F** are axial sections of the MRI from a 71-year-old woman with progressive gait and cognitive impairment, as well as urinary incontinence. Note the low signal in the sylvian aqueduct, owing to a flow void from high velocity CSF flow through this structure *(C, arrow)*. Although basal cisterns **(C)** and interhemispheric and sylvian fissures **(D-E)** are dilated, sulci in the high convexity **(F)** are compressed. Trans-ependymal reabsorption of CSF, suggested by the homogeneous high signal in the periventricular white matter **(E)**, need not occur in all cases of symptomatic hydrocephalus. In addition to the compressed sulci in the convexity, the U shape of some of the dilated sulci *(E, white arrows)* is helpful to make the diagnosis.

cerebral aqueduct may cause a hypointense "jet-flow" sign on all sequences. Quantitative CSF flow studies (cine phase-contrast MR imaging) are frequently used for evaluation of patients with suspected normal-pressure hydrocephalus. However, the distinction between using MRI to diagnose normal-pressure hydrocephalus versus determining the probability of clinical improvement from shunt placement should be kept in mind, as studies seem to show that MRI may be better at the former than the latter. Although CSF flow studies had been thought to help to predict shunt responsiveness (Bradley et al., 1996), later studies have challenged this view (Dixon et al., 2002; Kahlon et al., 2007). Traditionally it has been hypothesized that in this condition there is a problem with CSF absorption at the level of the arachnoid granulations, since normal-pressure hydrocephalus has been observed

as a late complication after meningitis or subarachnoid hemorrhage that caused meningeal involvement/scarring. But this syndrome, often associated with vascular disease in older people, may also be the result of decreased superficial venous compliance and a reduction in the blood flow returning via the sagittal sinus (Bateman, 2008). The term *normal pressure* is a misnomer because long-term monitoring of ventricular pressure has shown recurrent episodes of transient pressure elevation.

CHIARI MALFORMATION

Depending on associated structural abnormalities, different types of Chiari malformation are distinguished. In the most common, type 1 Chiari, there is caudal displacement of the tip of the cerebellar tonsils 5 mm or more below the level

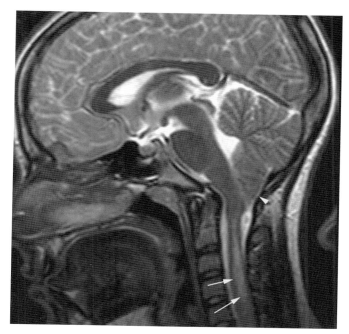

Fig. 33A.81 Chiari type 1 malformation. Sagittal T2-weighted image demonstrates caudal displacement of the cerebellar tonsil through the foramen magnum into the cervical spinal canal *(arrowhead)*. The tonsil is characteristically peg shaped. There is a prominent longitudinal hyperintense cavity in the visualized cervical spinal cord segment, consistent with a syrinx *(arrows)*.

of the foramen magnum. Most often this malformation is accompanied by a congenitally small posterior fossa. However, acquired forms of tonsillar descent also exist, either due to space occupying intracranial pathology or to a low-pressure environment in the spinal canal, such as after lumboperitoneal shunt placement. In typical Chiari 1, the ectopic cerebellar tonsils are frequently peg shaped, but otherwise the cerebellum is of normal morphology. There is usually crowding of the structures at the level of the foramen magnum. The 5-mm diagnostic cutoff value has been selected in adults, as this condition tends to be symptomatic and clinically significant at this or higher measured values. If the tonsils are caudal to the level of the foramen magnum by less then 5 mm, the term *low-lying cerebellar tonsils* is used; this is frequently an asymptomatic incidental finding. When evaluating younger patients or children, it is to be remembered that the considered "normal" position of the cerebellar tonsils is different in the various age groups. In the first decade, 6 mm below the foramen magnum is considered the upper limit of normal, and with increasing age, there is an "ascent" of the tonsils, with a 5-mm cutoff value in the second and third decades, 4 mm up to the eighth decade, and 3 mm in the ninth decade of life (for review see Nash et al., 2002). Tonsillar ectopia and crowding at the foramen magnum interfere with return of CSF from the spinal to the intracranial subarachnoid space. This may lead, by still-disputed mechanisms, to syrinx formation in the spinal cord (see **Fig. 33A.81**). If there is imaging evidence of a Chiari malformation on brain MRI, it is essential to image the cervical and thoracic cord to rule out a syrinx.

In Chiari type 2 malformation, there is a developmental abnormality of the hindbrain and caudal displacement not only of the cerebellar tonsils but also the cerebellum, medulla, and fourth ventricle. The cervical spinal nerve roots are stretched/compressed, and there is often a spinal cord syrinx present. Other abnormalities include lumbar or thoracic myelomeningocele; hydrocephalus is often present as well. Chiari type 3 malformation is an even more severe developmental abnormality, with cervical myelomeningocele or encephalocele.

For a description of idiopathic intracranial hypertension (pseudotumor cerebri) and of the imaging sequelae of intracranial hypotension please see the online-only version of this chapter at www.expertconsult.com.

Orbital Lesions

The structural neuroimaging of orbital lesions is discussed in the online-only version of this chapter. Please visit www.expertconsult.com for more information.

Spinal Diseases
Spinal Tumors

Tumors affecting the spinal region can be classified according to their predominant location, intrinsic to the vertebral column itself or within the spinal canal. Spinal canal tumors may be intramedullary or extramedullary. Intramedullary tumors involve the spinal cord parenchyma, whereas extramedullary tumors are outside the spinal cord but within the spinal canal. Depending on their relation to the dura, extramedullary tumors may be classified as intradural or extradural. As tumors grow, they can spread to other compartments. For example, metastases in the vertebral bodies often extend to the epidural space and cause spinal cord compression. Tumors in pre- and paravertebral locations may also extend to the extradural space, either through the vertebral bodies, as happens with metastatic lung cancer, or through the neural foramina, as in lymphoma.

VERTEBRAL METASTASES, EXTRADURAL TUMORS

In the majority of cases, tumors involving the vertebrae are metastatic in origin. Half of all vertebral metastatic tumors are from lung, breast (**Fig. 33A.86**), and prostate cancer. Kidney and gastrointestinal tumors, melanoma, and those arising from the female reproductive organs are other common sources. Of all structural neuroimaging techniques, MRI is the imaging modality of choice to evaluate vertebral metastases, with sensitivity equal to and specificity better than bone scan (Mechtler and Cohen, 2000). MR imaging protocols for the evaluation of vertebral metastases typically include T1-weighted images with and without gadolinium, T2-weighted images, and STIR sequences. Typically, osteolytic metastases appear as hypointense foci on noncontrast T1-weighted images, hyperintense signal on T2 and STIR sequences, and enhance on postcontrast images. The enhancement may render the previously T1 hypointense metastatic foci isointense, interfering with their detection. Therefore, precontrast T1-weighted images should always be obtained as well. Osteoblastic metastases, such as seen in prostate cancer, are hypointense on T2-weighted images. Besides the vertebral bodies, metastases preferentially involve the pedicles. With marked involvement, the vertebral body may collapse.

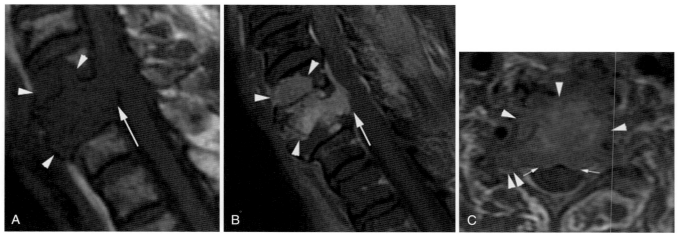

Fig. 33A.86 Spinal metastasis. MRI from a 52-year-old woman with breast cancer. **A,** Sagittal T1-weighted image reveals hypointense signal in two adjacent vertebral bodies *(arrowheads)*. Metastatic mass extends beyond the vertebral bodies into the epidural space *(arrow)*. **B,** Sagittal T1-weighted, fat-suppressed postcontrast image better delineates the extent of the tumor. **C,** Axial postcontrast image demonstrates tumor spread toward the pre- and paravertebral space *(arrowheads)*, into the epidural space *(small arrows)* and into the pedicle *(double arrowheads)*.

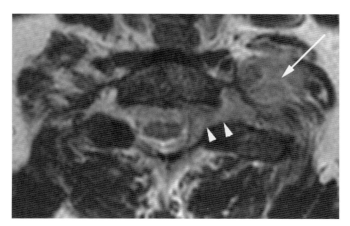

Fig. 33A.87 Lymphoma. A left paravertebral tumor *(arrow)* extends through the left neural foramen into the cervical spinal canal *(arrowheads)*.

Extradural tumors most commonly result from spread of metastatic tumors to the epidural space, directly from the vertebral body or from the prevertebral/paravertebral space. These mass lesions in the epidural space initially indent the thecal sac, and as they grow, they displace and eventually compress the spinal cord or cauda equina. If spinal cord compression is long-standing and severe enough, T2 hyperintense signal change may appear in the involved cord segment as a result of edema and/or ischemia secondary to compromised local circulation. An example of tumor spread from a paravertebral focus is lymphoma, which may extend into the spinal canal through the neural foramen. When intraspinal extension is suspected in a patient with lymphoma, MRI is the study of choice (**Fig. 33A.87**). In cases of epithelial tumors, by the time of presentation, plain radiographs reveal the intraspinal extension with more than 80% sensitivity, but in patients with lymphoma, plain radiographs are still normal in almost 70% of the cases (Mechtler and Cohen, 2000).

In the smaller group of extradural primary spinal tumors, multiple myeloma is the most common in adults. Involvement of the vertebral bone marrow may occur in multiple small foci, but diffuse involvement of an entire vertebral body is also possible. Myelomatous lesions are hypointense on T1, hyperintense on T2-weighted images, and highly hyperintense on STIR sequences. There is marked enhancement after gadolinium administration.

EXTRAMEDULLARY INTRADURAL SPINAL TUMORS

This group of tumors includes leptomeningeal metastases, meningiomas, nerve sheath tumors, embryonal tumors (teratoma), congenital cysts (epidermoid, dermoid), and lipoma.

LEPTOMENINGEAL METASTASES

Leptomeningeal metastases result from tumor cell infiltration of the leptomeningeal layers (pia and arachnoid). Non-Hodgkin lymphoma, leukemia, breast and lung cancer, melanoma, and gastrointestinal cancers are the most common sources of metastases. Leptomeningeal seeding also occurs from primary CNS tumors such as malignant gliomas, ependymoma, and neuroblastomas. The optimal imaging modality to detect leptomeningeal seeding is gadolinium-enhanced MRI, which reveals linear or multifocal nodular enhancing lesions along the surface of the spinal cord or nerve roots. The diagnostic yield can be improved by using higher doses of gadolinium.

SPINAL MENINGIOMAS

Most (90%) spinal meningiomas are intradural, but extradural extension also occurs. The tumors displace/compress the spinal cord or nerve roots. MRI signal characteristics can be variable: they often exhibit isointense signal to the spinal cord on both T1- and T2-weighted images, but T2 hypointensity may also be seen. Similar to intracranial meningiomas, these tumors enhance in an intense homogeneous fashion (**Fig. 33A.88**). In patients with neurofibromatosis type 2, the entire spine should be imaged because multiple meningiomas may be present.

Nerve sheath tumors and embryonal tumors that belong to this group of spinal tumors are described in the online-only version of this chapter. Please visit www.expertconsult.com for more information.

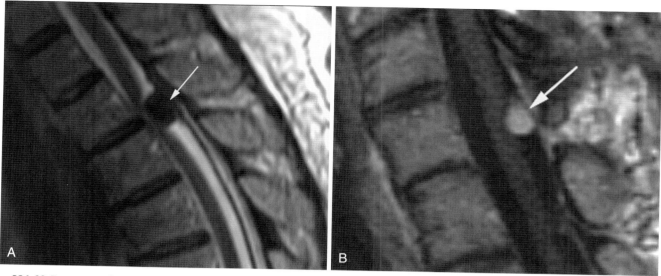

Fig. 33A.88 Two cases of meningioma. **A,** Sagittal T2-weighted image demonstrates a hypointense extramedullary dural-based mass lesion that causes marked spinal cord compression *(arrow).* **B,** Sagittal T1-weighted postcontrast image reveals an extramedullary dural-based mass lesion in a similar location. The mass enhances homogeneously *(arrow).*

INTRAMEDULLARY TUMORS

The most common primary spinal cord tumors are astrocytomas and ependymomas, representing 80% to 90% of all primary malignancies. For best structural assessment of intramedullary tumors (primary and metastatic), MR imaging with and without gadolinium should be obtained.

EPENDYMOMA

Ependymomas are more common in males and in about 50% of cases involve the lower spinal cord in the region of the conus medullaris and cauda equina. The myxopapillary type arises from the ependymal remnants of the filum terminale. Ependymomas are usually well demarcated and may exhibit a T1 and T2 hypointense pseudocapsule. This is important from a surgical standpoint, because these tumors may usually be removed with minimal injury to the surrounding cord parenchyma. The involved cord is expanded. On T1-weighted images, ependymomas are usually isointense to the spinal cord or, rarely, hypointense. On T2-weighted images, they are usually hyperintense relative to the spinal cord. The tumor may have a hemorrhagic component as well, in which case the signal characteristic is usually heterogenous, depending on the stage of the hemorrhage. Ependymomas are often associated with a rostral or caudal cyst, which is hypointense on T1 and hyperintense on T2-weighted images. With gadolinium, intense homogeneous enhancement is seen within the solid portion of the tumor.

ASTROCYTOMA

Astrocytomas occur in both the pediatric and adult populations. Their peak incidence is in the third to fifth decades of life. They have a preference for the thoracic cord segments. Up to three-quarters are low grade. They exhibit T1 hypointensity and appear hyperintense on T2-weighted images. Although the tumor margin is usually poorly defined, subtotal resection is often possible. A cyst or syringomyelic cavity is associated with spinal cord astrocytoma in up to 50% of cases. Contrary to intracranial low-grade gliomas,

spinal astrocytomas typically enhance, often in a heterogeneous fashion (**Fig. 33A.90**).

INTRAMEDULLARY METASTASES

Lung and breast cancer are the most common sources of intramedullary metastases, but lymphoma, colorectal cancer, and renal cell cancer may also metastasize to the cord. Metastases have some preference for the conus medullaris but may be multiple in 10% of cases and involve other cord segments as well. Their signal intensity varies; mucus-containing breast or colon cancer metastases can be hyperintense on noncontrast T1-weighted images. On postcontrast images, intense enhancement is seen, which may be homogeneous or ringlike. Associated edema is frequently seen as surrounding T1 hypointensity and T2 hyperintensity. The cord may be expanded to variable degrees.

Vascular Disease

This section of the chapter is available in the online-only version at www.expertconsult.com. Please also refer to Chapter 51D.

Infection

Infections of the spine may involve the disc spaces as well as the vertebral bodies. Neurological emergency occurs when the infection proceeds to the epidural space, leading to abscess formation that can result in spinal cord compression.

DISCITIS AND OSTEOMYELITIS

The most common pathogen responsible for discitis and osteomyelitis is *Staphylococcus aureus*. The most common route of transmission is hematogenous, and in these cases the lumbar spine is involved most frequently, usually at the L3/4 or L4/5 levels. Contiguous spread of infection may also occur, and postoperative causes (such as after instrumentation) have been documented as well. In adults the discitis/osteomyelitis

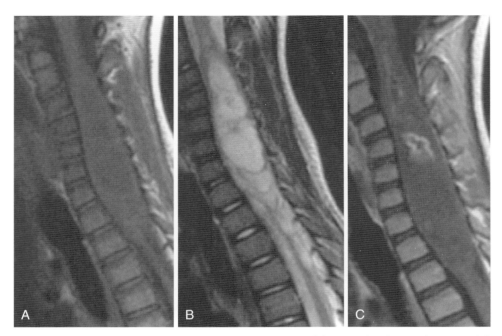

Fig. 33A.90 Astrocytoma. **A,** Sagittal T1-weighted image reveals prominent expansion of the cervical and upper thoracic cord due to a T1-hypointense intramedullary tumor. **B,** Sagittal T2-weighted image demonstrates the hyperintense mass. **C,** Sagittal T1-weighted postcontrast image reveals a patchy heterogeneous pattern of enhancement.

complex generally begins with infection of the subchondral bone marrow inferior to the cartilage endplate. Infection of the subchondral region of a vertebral body results in subsequent perforation of the vertebral endplate, leading to infection of the intervertebral disc, or discitis. The infected disc decreases in height and in conjunction with spread of infection through the disc, the adjacent vertebral body is infected. In children, a direct hematogenous route to the disc can cause discitis to occur before the development of osteomyelitis. Discitis and osteomyelitis are typically hypointense relative to normal discs and vertebrae on T1-weighted images and hyperintense on T2-weighted images, indicating edema. On STIR, markedly hyperintense signal correlates with the signal changes on T1 and T2. There is destruction of the endplates, and therefore the endplate/disc margin is poorly seen. With gadolinium, there is enhancement of the infected marrow and irregular peripheral enhancement at the periphery of the involved disc (**Fig. 33A.92**). Pathological fractures of the infected vertebrae may also be seen.

EPIDURAL ABSCESS, PARAVERTEBRAL PHLEGMON

The pathologies of epidural abscess and paravertebral phlegmon are most commonly seen as complications of discitis and osteomyelitis. Since epidural abscess and resultant spinal cord compression represent a neurological emergency, besides the affected vertebral bodies and discs, it is important to always evaluate the epidural space for abscess and the paraspinal tissues for phlegmon (purulent inflammation and diffuse infiltration of soft or connective tissue) if discitis and/or osteomyelitis are seen. Epidural abscess may be missed on conventional T1 and T2-weighted images because its signal characteristics may blend in with its surroundings. The central portion of the abscess may exhibit hyperintensity similar to CSF on T2-weighted images while exhibiting iso- to hypointense

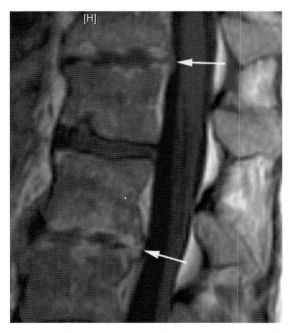

Fig. 33A.92 Discitis and osteomyelitis. Two levels are involved *(arrows)*. Sagittal T1-weighted postcontrast image demonstrates decreased disc height and destruction of the adjacent endplates. With gadolinium, there is irregular enhancement of the infected marrow.

signal relative to the spinal cord on T1-weighted images. With gadolinium administration, however, intense enhancement is noted (**Fig. 33A.93**). Just as may occur with compression due to epidural tumors, the compressed spinal cord segment may exhibit T2 hyperintense signal alteration. Phlegmon in the paravertebral tissues also enhances peripherally with gadolinium. This paravertebral infectious process is also well seen

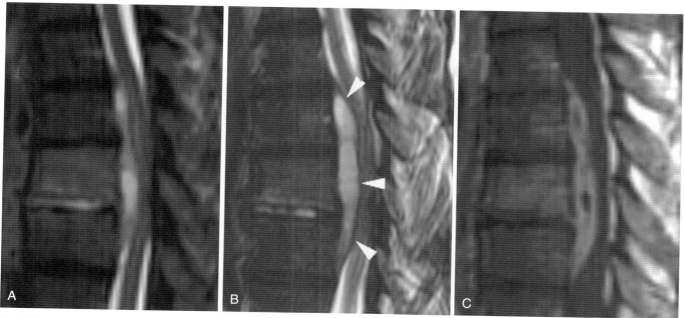

Fig. 33A.93 Discitis, osteomyelitis, and epidural abscess. **A,** Sagittal fat-suppressed image reveals hyperintense signal in the involved disc and hyperintense edema in the vertebral body marrow. Note associated hyperintense epidural collection that displaces the spinal cord. **B,** Sagittal T2-weighted image reveals the discitis and involvement of the inferior endplate of the vertebral body above. The epidural abscess is hyperintense, and the hypointense contour of the dura is well seen *(arrowheads)*. **C,** Sagittal T1-weighted postcontrast image demonstrates intense enhancement of the abscess.

on STIR sequences as hyperintensity against the hypointense signal of the fat-suppressed bone marrow background.

Noninfectious Inflammatory Disorders
MULTIPLE SCLEROSIS

Multiple sclerosis (see Chapter 54) commonly affects the spinal cord. Simultaneous cerebral demyelinating lesions are usually seen in the same patient but less frequently in cases of Devic disease (neuromyelitis optica), which is associated with anti-aquoporin-4 antibodies (Matsushita et al., 2010). On MRI studies of the spinal cord in MS patients, the cervical segments are most commonly involved (**Fig. 33A.94**). The lesions are hyperintense on T2-weighted images and are seen even more conspicuously on sagittal STIR sequences. The lower signal-to-noise ratio of STIR makes this sequence less specific than T2-weighted images for cord lesions, but it is more sensitive. STIR is generally useful only in the sagittal plane, and findings on this sequence should always be correlated with T2 images. Lesional signal changes with either technique are patchy and segmental, often discretely overlapping with the dorsal, anterior, or lateral columns of the spinal cord. The lateral and dorsal columns are affected most frequently. The signal changes are usually in the peripheral regions of the cord, but individual lesions may intersect with the central cord gray matter as well. In MS, the lesions typically do not span more than two vertebral lengths rostrocaudally and tend to involve less than half of the cross-section of the cord. Following administration of gadolinium, active cord lesions may exhibit homogeneous or open-ring enhancement. Large active MS lesions may cause swelling, with local expansion of the cord. In patients with a severe clinical picture or a long-standing history of MS, varying degrees of spinal cord atrophy

may be seen. In less severe cases, volumetric analysis may reveal atrophy not detectable by visual inspection.

ACUTE DISSEMINATED ENCEPHALOMYELITIS

The widespread demyelinating lesions in this condition commonly involve the spinal cord as well. Diffuse or multifocal T2 hyperintense signal changes with variable degrees of cord swelling may be seen (**Fig. 33A.95**). There is a variable amount of enhancement after gadolinium administration.

TRANSVERSE MYELITIS

Transverse myelitis is an inflammatory disorder of the spinal cord that involves the gray as well as the white matter. The inflammation involves one or more (typically 3 to 4) cord segments and usually more than two-thirds of the cross-sectional area of the cord (**Fig. 33A.96**). Transverse myelitis etiologies include viral infection, postviral or post-vaccine autoimmune reactions, vasculitis, mycoplasma infection, syphilis, antiparasitic and antifungal drugs, and even intravenous heroin use (Sahni et al., 2008). The imaging modality of choice is MRI. Acutely, there is T2 hyperintense signal change and cord swelling. In more severe cases, hemorrhage and necrosis may also occur. Following gadolinium administration, diffuse or multifocal patchy enhancement is seen. In the subacute and chronic stages, the swelling and enhancement subside, and the T2 hyperintense signal decreases in extent. In the chronic stage, there may be a variable amount of faint residual T2 hyperintensity. In more severe cases, focal cord atrophy or myelomalacia may be seen.

Spinal sarcoidosis and vacuolar myelopathy are described in the online-only version. Please visit www.expertconsult.com for more information on these noninfectious inflammatory disorders.

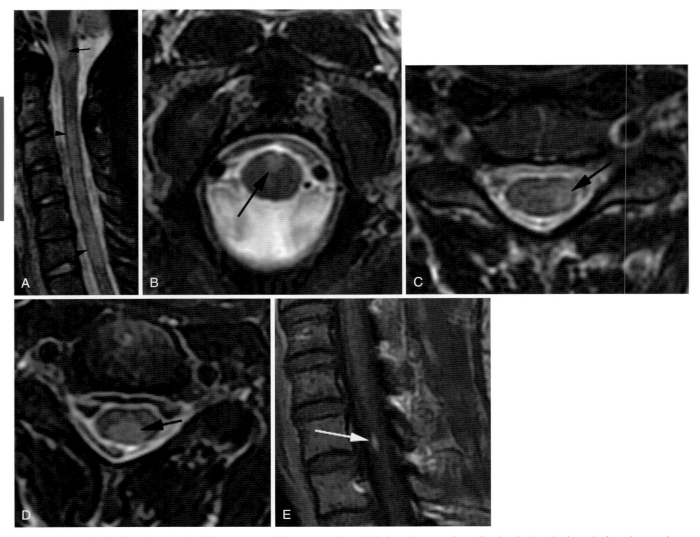

Fig. 33A.94 Multiple sclerosis. **A,** Sagittal fat-suppressed image reveals multiple hyperintense demyelinating lesions in the spinal cord parenchyma *(arrowheads)*, including at the cervicomedullary junction *(arrow)*. On axial T2-weighted images, hyperintense demyelinating lesions are seen in the **(B)** anterior, **(C)** lateral, and **(D)** posterior columns of the cord *(arrows)*. **E,** Sagittal T1-weighted postcontrast image reveals an enhancing lesion in the cord parenchyma *(arrow)*.

Trauma

Structural neuroimaging has an essential role in the emergency evaluation and surgical planning of injured patients. Bone window CT images are an excellent tool for evaluating vertebral column trauma, whereas MRI is more useful in displaying disc trauma, injury involving the spinal cord parenchyma and/or nerve roots, and for the assessment of hemorrhage and soft-tissue damage. Some mechanisms of injury have a predilection for certain spine segments, such as burst fractures due to axial force in the lower thoracic and lumbar spine or axial flexion/extension and resultant distraction injuries at the junctions of mobile and rigid segments of the spine (cervicothoracic and thoracolumbar junctions). Traumatic injuries are typically not isolated but occur in various combinations; for instance, facet joint subluxation may be combined with spondylolisthesis, disc rupture, and spinal cord contusion.

Traumatic lesions to the skeletal elements of the spine (hangman's fracture, odontoid fracture, burst fracture, Jefferson fracture, facet joint disruption) are discussed in the online-only version of this chapter, available at www.expertconsult.com.

SPINAL EPIDURAL HEMATOMA

Epidural hematoma appears as an extradural, usually spindle-shaped collection of blood. It may occur at any segment of the spinal column. Varying degrees of spinal cord or cauda equina compression may be present. In the acute stage, the hematoma is hyperdense on CT. On MRI, the acute hematoma is usually isointense to the cord on T1 and appears hypointense on T2-weighted images. The signal characteristics change as the hematoma undergoes degradation. In subacute and chronic cases, the signal becomes hyperintense (**Fig. 33A.102**). Similar to spinal subdural hematomas, epidural hematomas enhance after gadolinium administration along their periphery; this is due to dural hyperemia. Occasionally, contrast material may also leak into the hematoma.

SPINAL SUBDURAL HEMATOMA

Hemorrhage into the spinal subdural space may occur after trauma or as an iatrogenic phenomenon after lumbar puncture (LP) in patients with coagulopathy. With structural neuroimaging, an intradural collection is seen that exerts a variable degree of mass effect on the spinal cord or cauda equina. The collection is hyperdense on CT and exhibits variable signal intensity on MRI, depending on the stage of the hematoma. A large intradural hypointensity on T2 or gradient echo pulse sequences is a common finding in the acute stage, with hyperintense epidural fat along its periphery. The lower thoracic or lumbar spine is affected most frequently. In posttraumatic cases, the imager should look for other stigmata of trauma

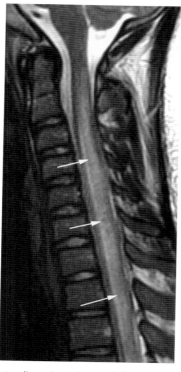

Fig. 33A.95 Acute disseminated encephalomyelitis (ADEM). Sagittal T2-weighted image shows a diffuse hyperintense lesion spanning the length of the cervical cord *(arrows)*. Note the enlarged caliber of the cord, which is due to swelling.

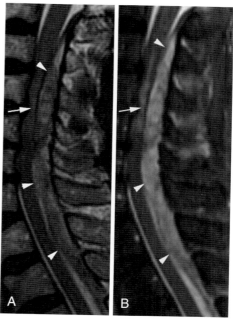

Fig. 33A.102 Spinal epidural hematoma. **A,** Sagittal T2-weighted image demonstrates a prominent mixed but mostly hyperintense epidural collection *(arrowheads)* that displaces the spinal cord. Note the hyperintense signal change in the compressed cord parenchyma *(arrow)*. **B,** Sagittal fat-suppressed image shows the epidural hematoma *(arrowheads)* and demonstrates the cord signal change even more conspicuously *(arrow)*.

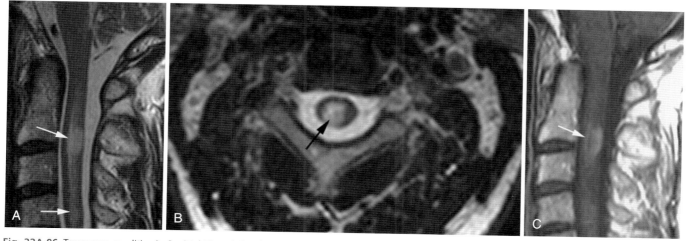

Fig. 33A.96 Transverse myelitis. **A,** Sagittal T2-weighted image demonstrates a longitudinal hyperintense spinal cord lesion spanning three vertebral segments *(arrows)*. **B,** On an axial T2-weighted image, the lesion involves more than two-thirds of the cord's cross-sectional area *(arrow)*. **C,** Sagittal T1-weighted postcontrast image shows an enhancing area within the lesion *(arrow)*.

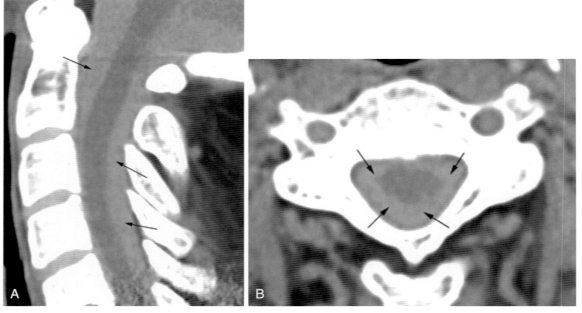

Fig. 33A.103 Spinal subarachnoid hemorrhage. Sagittal **(A)** and axial **(B)** computed tomography images reveal hyperdense blood throughout the spinal and visible intracranial subarachnoid space *(arrows)*.

such as spinal cord contusion/hematoma, vertebral fracture, disc rupture, or changes in vertebral alignment.

SPINAL SUBARACHNOID HEMORRHAGE

Traumatic subarachnoid hemorrhage in the spinal canal may be seen in primary spinal trauma or after an LP but also as a secondary phenomenon in cases of intracranial subarachnoid hemorrhage when the blood reaches the spinal compartment via CSF circulation. In the acute phase, CT scan is a sensitive imaging modality to detect hyperdense subarachnoid blood (**Fig. 33A.103**).

SPINAL CORD TRAUMA

While CT bone window images are best for evaluating traumatic changes of the vertebral column, the imaging modality of choice for spinal cord trauma is MRI. Spinal cord trauma may cause early and delayed changes. Early changes include cord contusion, compression, or varying degrees of transsection due to the traumatic displacement of an intervertebral disc or bony elements. On MRI, they are expressed as variable degrees of cord swelling, with T2 hyperintensity due to edema and complex signal changes due to hemorrhage (see hemorrhage section for a review). In this early phase, gradient echo images are useful for assessment of cord hemorrhage, which appear as hypointense signal change within the parenchyma. A milder form of early traumatic change is in spinal cord concussion, where imaging may reveal some transient swelling and faint T2 hyperintense signal change only. The spinal cord may be damaged without bony compression; in cases of hyperextension, axonal shear injury and cord hemorrhage may develop, typically causing a central cord syndrome. Chronically after severe spinal cord trauma, myelomalacia tends to develop, with microcystic changes and reactive gliosis in the damaged parenchyma, which is hyperintense on T2-weighted images; the involved cord segment is normal in size or atrophic.

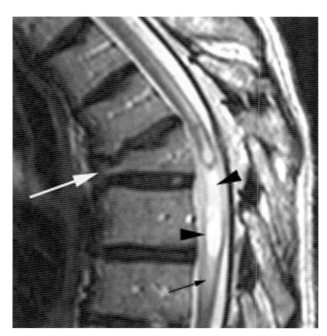

Fig. 33A.104 Posttraumatic syrinx. Sagittal T2-weighted image shows a chronic vertebral body compression fracture *(arrow)*. The formerly traumatized spinal cord reveals a hyperintense posttraumatic syrinx *(arrowheads)*. The surrounding hyperintense signal in the cord parenchyma is reactive gliosis *(small arrow)*.

Besides early traumatic changes, delayed progressive forms of posttraumatic myelopathy may occur. They include spinal cord cysts with CSF signal characteristics (**Fig. 33A.104**). These cysts may enlarge and show CSF pulsation. Cyst shunting may relieve the pressure on the remaining functional cord tissue. Another chronic phenomenon, fibrotic changes in the spinal canal, may result in progressive tethering of the spinal cord to the dura, which can be toward the anterior, lateral, or posterior border of the spinal canal. In addition to deforming the cord and causing neurological symptoms, tethering may also contribute to delayed spinal cord cyst formation.

A special type of spinal cord trauma, SCIWORA (spinal cord injury without radiologic abnormality) is discussed in the online-only version of the chapter (www.expertconsult.com). For a clinical review of spinal cord trauma, see also Chapter 50C.

Metabolic and Hereditary Myelopathies

Here we group metabolic disorders that potentially cause myelopathy, as well as hereditary and degenerative diseases that result in myelopathy by progressive loss of spinal neurons and/or degeneration of spinal cord pathways. Some of the pathologies result in characteristic signal alterations of the spinal cord, such as that seen in subacute combined degeneration due to vitamin B_{12} deficiency. Others (most degenerative diseases) do not alter the signal characteristics but cause cord atrophy, with or without atrophy of other CNS structures.

The most common entities belonging to this group of myelopathies (subacute combined degeneration, adrenomyeloneuropathy, spinocerebellar ataxias, Friedreich ataxia, amyotrophic lateral sclerosis, and hereditary spastic paraplegia) are discussed in the online-only version of this chapter. Please visit www.expertconsult.com for more information.

Degenerative Spine Disease

Degenerative changes are very commonly seen on neuroimaging studies of the spine. These changes may involve the intervertebral discs, the vertebral bodies, and the posterior elements (facet joints, ligamentum flavum) in various combinations.

DEGENERATIVE DISC DISEASE

In young people, the intervertebral discs have a fluid-rich center (nucleus pulposus) that appears hyperintense on T2-weighted images (**Fig. 33A.106**). With aging, the nucleus pulposus loses water, becoming progressively more hypointense, and the disc flattens. This phenomenon is no longer considered to be abnormal but an age-related involutional change. However, the often concurrent weakening of the annulus fibrosus raises the chance of annular tear and resultant disc abnormalities.

The nomenclature of disc abnormalities (Fardon and Milette, 2001) is complex (**Fig. 33A.107**). A *disc bulge* is symmetrical presence of disc tissue "circumferentially" (50% to 100%) beyond the edges of the ring apophyses. On sagittal views, disc bulges have a "flat-tire" appearance. Disc bulges are not categorized as herniations and in the majority of cases do not have any clinical significance.

The term *disc protrusion* refers to extension of a disc past the borders of the vertebral body. A disc protrusion (1) is not classifiable as a bulge, and (2) any one distance between the edges of the disc material beyond the disc space is *less than* the distance between the edges of the base when measured in the same plane. We distinguish between focal and broad-based disc protrusions depending on whether the base of protrusion is less or more than 25% of the entire disc circumference. Disc protrusions may or may not be clinically significant. Whether they affect the neural structures depends

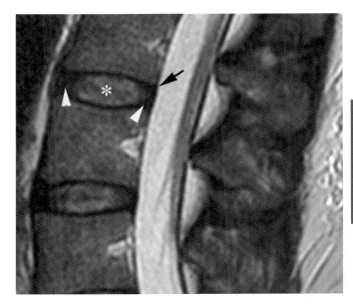

Fig. 33A.106 Normal intervertebral discs. Sagittal T2-weighted image demonstrates normal disc height. Note the T2 hyperintense nucleus pulposus (*) and the hypointense annulus fibrosus *(arrowheads)*. The disc does not extend beyond the borders of the vertebral body *(arrow)*.

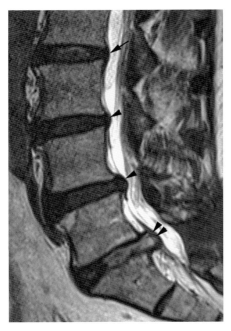

Fig. 33A.107 Disc bulge, protrusion, and herniation. Sagittal T2-weighted image demonstrates examples for all stages of disc pathology. Going from rostral to caudal, a disc bulge *(arrow)*, a small and more prominent protrusion *(arrowheads)*, and a herniation *(double arrowhead)* are seen.

on multiple factors. In a congenitally narrow spinal canal, even a small disc protrusion may result in spinal cord or cauda equina compression. In a normal spinal canal, a central disc protrusion may not do anything other than indent the thecal sac. A protrusion of the same size, however, may cause nerve root compression when situated in the lateral recess (**Fig. 33A.108**) or neural foramen (paracentral or lateral disc protrusion).

Disc extrusion refers to a herniation in which any one distance between the edges of the disc material beyond the disc space is *greater than* the distance between the edges of the base measured in the same plane. It occurs when the inner content of the disc, the nucleus pulposus, herniates through a tear of the outer annulus fibrosus. If the extruded disc material loses its continuity with the disc of origin, it is referred to as a *sequestrated* or *free fragment*. Sometimes it is difficult to determine whether continuity exists or not. The term *migration* is used when there is displacement of disc material away from the site of extrusion, regardless of whether it is sequestrated or not, so it may be applied to displaced disc material irrespective of its continuity with the disc of origin (**Fig. 33A.109**). On T2-weighted images, an annular tear may be appreciated as a dotlike or linear hyperintensity against the hypointense background of the annulus fibrosus. This is sometimes also referred to as a *high intensity zone* (HIZ).

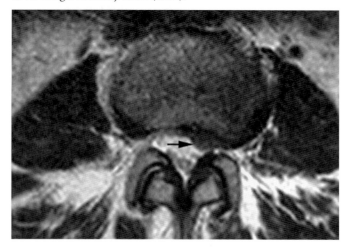

Fig. 33A.108 Disc protrusion. Axial T2-weighted image shows a left paracentral disc protrusion *(arrow)* that indents the thecal sac and narrows the left lateral recess.

Disc herniation frequently reaches considerable size and clinical significance owing to compression of the exiting/descending nerve roots of the spinal cord (**Fig. 33A.110**). Disc protrusions and extrusions/herniations may compromise the spaces to various degrees. As a general guide, spinal canal or neural foraminal stenosis of less than one-third of their original diameter is mild; between one- and two-thirds is moderate; and stenosis involving more than two-thirds of the original caliber is considered severe.

Disc abnormalities are most common in the lumbar spine, particularly at the L4/5 and L5/S1 levels, and second most common at the cervical levels C5/6 and C6/7. These regions represent the more mobile parts of the spinal column.

DEGENERATIVE CHANGES OF THE VERTEBRAL BODIES

The bone marrow of the vertebral bodies undergoes characteristic changes with age that are well demonstrated by MRI. In younger people, it is largely red marrow composed of hemopoietic tissue. In this age group, the only area of fatty conversion, appearing as a linear T1 hyperintensity, is at the center of the vertebral body around the basivertebral vein. In people older than 40 years, additional foci of fatty marrow changes appear T1 hyperintense in other regions of the vertebral body. The size and extent of these fatty deposits increases with advancing age.

In degenerative disc disease, characteristic degenerative changes often occur in the adjacent vertebral body endplates as well, seen as linear areas of signal change in these regions (**Fig. 33A.111**). The process of degenerative endplate changes has been thought to occur in stages which have their characteristic MRI signal change patterns. These patterns were traditionally referred to as *Modic type 1, 2,* and *3 endplate changes* (for review see Rahme and Moussa, 2008). This nomenclature has been largely abandoned. The most common change, formerly Modic type 2, is a linear hyperintensity in the endplate region of variable width on T1- as well as T2-weighted images,

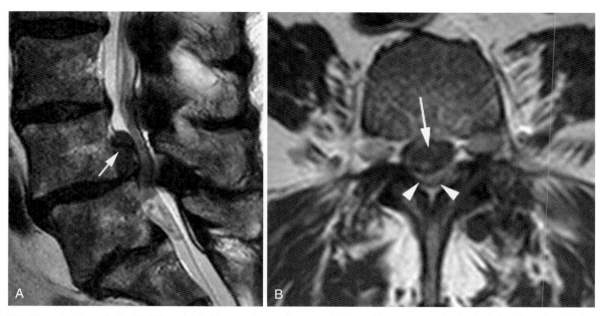

Fig. 33A.109 Disc migration. **A,** Sagittal T2-weighted image shows disc material that did not stay at the level of the disc of origin but migrated cranially *(arrow)*. **B,** Axial T2-weighted image demonstrates the migrated disc material *(arrow)* and the compressed thecal sac *(arrowheads)*.

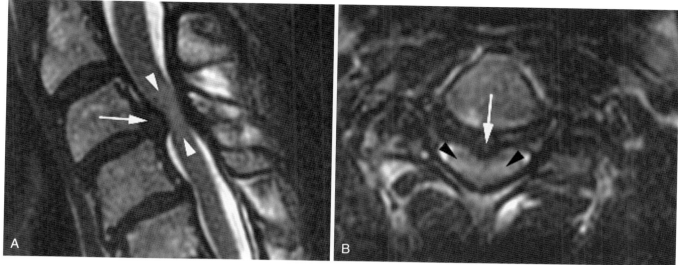

Fig. 33A.110 Disc herniation, spinal cord compression. **A,** Sagittal T2-weighted image demonstrates a disc herniation at the C3-C4 level that compresses the cervical spinal cord *(arrow)*. Note the hyperintense signal abnormality in the compressed cord parenchyma *(arrowheads)*. **B,** Axial T2-weighted image shows the herniation, which has a central component *(arrow)*. The hyperintense signal change in the cord is also well seen *(arrowheads)*.

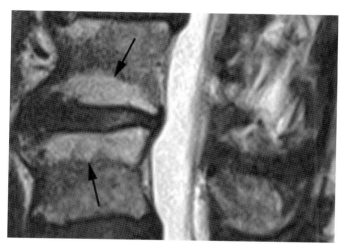

Fig. 33A.111 Degenerative endplate change. Sagittal T2-weighted image reveals hyperintense bands of signal change parallel with the disc space in the endplate region of the adjacent vertebral bodies *(arrows)*.

with corresponding hypointense signal loss on STIR sequences. These changes have been attributed to degenerative fat deposition in these regions.

Besides signal changes, vertebral bodies may also undergo morphological changes. In cases of disc protrusion or extrusion, the bone of the vertebral body may grow along the disc and form osteophytes or spurs. These may contribute to the narrowing of spaces and compromise of the neural elements. Large osteophytes may fuse across vertebral bodies, forming spondylotic bars.

DEGENERATIVE CHANGES OF THE POSTERIOR ELEMENTS

Facet joint arthropathy and ligamentum flavum hypertrophy are common findings in degenerative disease of the spine. In facet arthropathy, the synovial surface of the joint becomes poorly defined, and hyperintense synovial fluid may

accumulate. The joint becomes hypertrophied. Sometimes the synovial fluid accumulation results in outpouching of the synovium, which emerges from the joint, forming a synovial cyst. When prominent enough, this cyst may compromise the diameter of the spinal canal and (rarely) compress the neural elements (**Fig. 33A.112**). Hypertrophy of the T2 hypointense ligamentum flavum is also frequent and may contribute to compromise of the spaces and neural elements.

SPONDYLOLYSIS, SPONDYLOLISTHESIS

Spondylolysis and spondylolisthesis are pathologic changes that often occur together and are most common in the lumbar spine. *Spondylolysis* refers to a defect in the pars interarticularis of the vertebral arch resulting in separation of the articular processes from the vertebral body. A traumatic etiology is common, but it may happen in the setting of advanced degenerative disease as well. A common cause is stress microfractures resulting from episodes of axial loading force on the erect spine, such as when landing after a jump, diving, weight lifting, or due to rotational forces. This abnormality can be visualized with CT or MRI. On sagittal views, the pars defect is well seen; on axial images, the spinal canal may appear slightly elongated at the level of the spondylolysis.

Spondylolisthesis is shifting of one vertebral body relative to its neighbor, either anteriorly (anterolisthesis) or posteriorly (retrolisthesis). It is often associated with spondylolysis (**Fig. 33A.113**). Four grades of spondylolisthesis are distinguished, depending on the degree of shifting. *Grade I spondylolisthesis* refers to shifting over less than one-fourth of a vertebral body's anteroposterior diameter; grade II is shifting over one-fourth to one-half the diameter; grade III is up to three-fourths; and the most severe, grade IV, is shifting over the full vertebral body diameter.

Isolated spondylolysis results in elongation of the spinal canal, whereas spondylolisthesis causes segmental spinal canal narrowing, the extent of which depends on the degree of listhesis. In severe cases, there is compression of the spinal cord

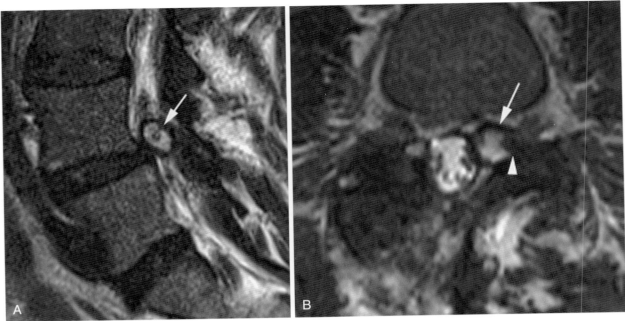

Fig. 33A.112 Synovial cyst. **A,** Sagittal T2-weighted image demonstrates a hyperintense cyst with hypointense rim in the spinal canal *(arrow)*. **B,** Axial T2-weighted image reveals that this cyst *(arrow)* arises from the left facet joint *(arrowhead)*, consistent with a synovial cyst. It narrows the left lateral recess and neural foramen.

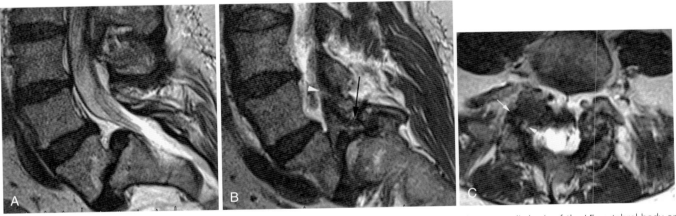

Fig. 33A.113 Spondylolysis, grade 2 anterolisthesis. **A,** Sagittal T2-weighted image demonstrates grade 2 anterolisthesis of the L5 vertebral body on S1. **B,** Sagittal T2-weighted image reveals separation of the L4/L5 facet joint *(arrowhead)* and forward displacement of the L5 articular process *(arrow)*. **C,** Axial T2-weighted image also reveals the spondylolysis *(arrows)*.

or cauda equina, and the changes also frequently cause narrowing of the neural foramina and compromise of the exiting nerve roots at the involved level.

Indications for Computed Tomography or Magnetic Resonance Imaging

Structural neuroimaging studies are probably the most commonly ordered diagnostic tests in both inpatient and outpatient neurological practice. Imaging greatly helps with the diagnosis of various neurological diseases and does so in a relatively quick and noninvasive way. This section summarizes the most common indications for obtaining a neuroimaging study in clinical neurological practice. Selection of the imaging study should be guided by the patient's history and objective findings on neurological examination, as opposed to shooting in the dark and obtaining "all-inclusive" imaging studies of the entire neuraxis. The availability and cost of the various techniques should also be factored into the decision of what tests to obtain in a given clinical situation.

Selecting CT Versus MRI for Neuroimaging in Practice

The decision whether to obtain a CT scan or an MRI is guided by practical factors and the nature of the disorder to be studied. Although MRI often allows for better visualization of anatomy and pathology, availability may limit its more widespread usage. Smaller practices and smaller local or rural hospitals often do not have MRI on site, and the delay in transportation to an MR imaging facility may be a concern. Even larger tertiary-care centers may not have overnight or weekend MRI coverage. In these situations, regardless of the suspected pathology, CT scanning is the first step in the imaging diagnostic process, especially if the patient's condition is urgent. CT scanning has the additional advantage of being less expensive and faster to obtain, minimizing the need for patient cooperation. Patients with pacemakers and other implanted devices cannot have MRI, nor can those with claustrophobia, unless the study is performed in an open unit. Besides these practical issues, CT renders better images of bony structures and calcification. Subarachnoid hemorrhage is better visualized on CT than on MRI, although FLAIR sequences are being found to be of comparable efficacy. CT angiogram, especially when color-coded 3D reconstruction is used, is superior to conventional MR angiogram in evaluating aneurysms.

On the other hand, when neural parenchymal lesions are being investigated, the better resolution of MRI makes it the ideal study. MRI is especially useful in the evaluation of posterior fossa lesions, where CT images are often compromised by artifact. Imaging of acute stroke, staging of hemorrhage, detection of microbleeds, evaluation of brain tumors, or detection of subtle structural or congenital lesions, such as in a seizure patient, are some of the instances when MRI should be used if possible. MRI has the additional advantage of not exposing the patient to harmful irradiation. MRI has no known harmful effects on humans. MRI—without gadolinium administration—is also considered safe in the second and third trimesters of pregnancy and is in fact suitable for examination of the fetus as well.

Neuroimaging in Various Clinical Situations
Sudden Neurological Deficit

Sudden onset and/or rapid evolution of neurological deficits, especially when focal and localized to the CNS, represent an obvious indication for imaging. Ischemic or hemorrhagic strokes, space-occupying lesions in the intracranial or intraspinal region, and lesions due to trauma have to be evaluated on an emergent basis. Unless a subarachnoid hemorrhage is strongly suspected, MRI is the technique of choice; it provides better visualization not only of the compromised tissue but also of the vessels, thus facilitating an etiologic diagnosis. Diffusion- and perfusion-weighted images should be performed in suspected ischemia. If a 64 CT is available, a comparable study may be obtained, although using radiation and contrast is not necessarily innocuous in an acute stroke patient.

Headache

There are several potential features in the presentation of a headache patient which, if present, raise a red flag and require an imaging study. These include new-onset severe headaches in a patient with no significant headache history (such as thunderclap headaches, often associated with aneurysm rupture), progression of the headaches including increasing frequency or severity, worst headache ever experienced, headaches that are always localized to one area, headaches that do not respond to treatment, headaches in a

cancer patient (always with contrast administration), and headaches associated with fever, altered mental status, or a focal neurological deficit. MRI, often followed by gadolinium administration if the nonenhanced study is negative, is the technique of choice.

Visual Impairment

The most common imaging indications that belong to this group include sudden unilateral visual loss, amaurosis fugax that is potentially due to embolism from an ipsilateral carotid stenosis, visual field deficits, such as hemianopia due to temporo-occipital lesions, bitemporal hemianopia due to compression of the optic chiasm, bilateral visual loss/cortical blindness, and double vision that raises the suspicion of pathology in the brainstem or base of the brain. MRI, often followed by gadolinium administration depending on the findings on the non-enhanced study, is the technique of choice.

Vertigo and Hearing Loss

Although there are several neurological signs that help to distinguish between vertigo of central and peripheral origin, new-onset vertigo—especially when associated with headache, impairment of consciousness, or ataxia—or vertigo that does not respond to therapy requires imaging to look for posterior fossa lesions, including cerebellopontine angle pathology. Although vertigo with prominent autonomic symptoms usually signals a peripheral etiology, a cerebellar hematoma or an expanding tumor may present with an identical clinical appearance. Sudden or progressive hearing loss also necessitates evaluation of the cerebellopontine angle, internal acoustic canal, and visible structures of the inner ear. MRI, often followed by gadolinium administration, is the technique of choice.

Progressive Weakness or Numbness of Central or Peripheral Origin

A careful neurological examination is needed to determine whether progressive weakness is of central or peripheral origin, and if central, what level of the neuraxis is involved. Hemiparesis that includes the face implies intracranial pathology. Hemiparesis without facial involvement or quadriparesis calls for imaging of the cervical spine. Paraparesis, central or peripheral-type with sphincter abnormalities, requires imaging of the thoracic and lumbar spine, respectively. Coexisting progressive upper and lower motor neuron signs and weakness in all four extremities, although typical for ALS, requires MRI imaging of the cervical spine, because pathologies there may cause an identical clinical presentation.

Progressive Ataxia, Gait Disorder

A neurological examination is essential to localize the level of dysfunction, and the history will provide the most likely etiology. Cerebellar ataxia warrants MRI imaging to look for cerebellar or spinocerebellar atrophy or an expanding tumor. Unsteadiness may have multiple other intracranial causes as well, including subdural hematomas, hydrocephalus, microvascular disease of the brain, or cerebellar/

brainstem demyelinating lesions. Ataxia due to impaired dorsal column sensory modalities requires MRI imaging of the spinal cord.

Movement Disorders

Diagnosis of the majority of movement disorders remains firmly based on history and neurological examination. Nevertheless, in certain circumstances, structural imaging is also helpful. Examples include Huntington disease, with its typical finding of bilateral caudate atrophy, and cervical dystonia in children, which may result from a posterior fossa tumor. Visualization of the posterior fossa requires MRI.

Cognitive or Behavioral Impairment

Imaging is justified in both slowly and rapidly evolving cognitive deficits. Rapidly evolving cognitive and behavioral impairment requires urgent imaging of the brain to look for acute pathology such as stroke, trauma, or an expanding mass lesion. Structural neuroimaging has a role in evaluation of the slowly progressive cognitive disorders (e.g., degenerative dementias) as well. The purpose of imaging in these cases is to look for changes that are compatible with the disease (e.g., atrophy of the frontal and temporal lobes in frontotemporal lobar degeneration) and also to look for other possible pathologies that may have similar presentations, such as multiple strokes, extensive microvascular changes, or a slowly expanding space-occupying lesion (e.g., olfactory groove meningioma). Structural imaging with CT or MRI is sufficient to rule out nondegenerative dementias and provides some useful data for the diagnosis of degenerative dementia. For instance, predominant medial temporal atrophy is characteristic of AD. However, characteristic changes appear earlier on functional imaging with PET, which can also be used to visualize amyloid deposition in the brain.

Epilepsy

Imaging is essential for the evaluation of patients with seizures. Besides showing pathology that may require immediate attention (trauma, stroke, expanding tumor), MRI is useful for more subtle underlying pathologies including developmental abnormalities (cortical dysplasia, heterotopia, polymicrogyria, etc.) and mesial temporal sclerosis. When epilepsy surgery is planned, MRI is indispensable to delineate the seizure focus in conjunction with electroencephalography (EEG) and functional imaging studies.

Trauma

Serious head or spine trauma may require imaging even in the absence of a neurological deficit. An unstable fracture or an expanding epidural hematoma should be detected before neural tissue is compressed and a deficit ensues. A fracture can sometimes be detected on plain x-ray films, but CT scanning is more sensitive and allows visualization of intracranial or perispinal tissues. It is also superior to MRI for imaging the bony skull and spine. Bone window images should be performed in cranial or spinal trauma, especially when a fracture is suspected. MRI is better than CT for depicting small areas of contusion and white matter injury with edema and microhemorrhages.

Myelopathy

Signs and symptoms of myelopathy on neurological evaluation necessitate imaging, which may be required urgently depending on the nature of the suspected myelopathy. If there is no contraindication (such as a pacemaker), MRI is the study of choice. The neurological examination should guide which level of the neuraxis is imaged. However, in certain cases, for instance in a cancer patient who presents with myelopathy and may have widespread disease, the entire spine has to be evaluated.

Low Back Pain

Besides headaches, low back pain is one of the most common reasons for neurological consultation. While the majority of cases (especially chronic back pain) are due to musculoskeletal causes, and on exam there is no evidence of involvement of the neural elements, there are potential signs and symptoms in a back pain patient that necessitate obtaining an imaging study. These include low back pain patients with objective signs of radiculopathy or a conus lesion (weakness, sensory loss, reflex loss in a radicular distribution, sphincter abnormalities). Other presentations necessitating an imaging study include patients with progressively worsening pain, pain aggravated by Valsalva maneuver, worsening of pain in the recumbent position, low back pain after trauma, pain with fever and/or palpation tenderness, and back pain in a patient with cancer. In these cases, the ideal imaging modality is MRI.

References

The complete reference list is available online at www.expertconsult.com.

Neuroimaging
Vascular Imaging: Computed Tomographic Angiography, Magnetic Resonance Angiography, and Ultrasound

Peter Adamczyk, David S. Liebeskind

Computed Tomographic Angiography

Computed tomographic angiography (CTA) is a relatively rapid, thin-section volumetric spiral (helical) CT technique performed with a time-optimized bolus of contrast medium to enhance visualization of the cerebral circulation. This approach may be tailored to illustrate various segments of the circulation from arterial segments to the venous system. The ongoing development of multidetector CT scanners has advanced CTA, with increasing numbers of detectors used in recent years to further improve image acquisition and visualization.

Methods

Helical CT scanner technology, providing uninterrupted volume data acquisition, can rapidly image the entire cerebral circulation from the neck to vertex of the head within minutes. Typical CT parameters use a slice (collimated) thickness of 1 to 3 mm with a pitch of 1 to 2, which represents the ratio of the table speed per rotation and the total collimation. Data are acquired as a bolus of iodinated contrast medium traverses the vessels of interest. For CTA of the carotid and vertebral arteries in the neck, the helical volume extends from the aortic arch to the skull base. Typical acquisition parameters are 7.5 images per rotation of the x-ray tube, 2.5-mm slice thickness, and a reconstruction interval (distance between the centers of two consecutively reconstructed images) of 1.25 mm. For CTA of the circle of Willis and proximal cerebral arteries, the data acquisition extends from the skull base to the vertex of the

head. Typical acquisition parameters for this higher spatial resolution scan are 3.75 images per rotation, 1.25-mm slice thickness, and an interval of 0.5 mm. A volume of contrast ranging from 100 to 150 mL is injected into a peripheral vein at a rate of 2 to 3 mL/sec and followed by a saline flush of 20 to 50 mL. Adequate enhancement of the arteries in the neck or head is obtained approximately 15 to 20 seconds after injection of the contrast, although this may vary somewhat in each case. Image acquisition uses automated detection of bolus arrival and subsequent triggering of data acquisition. The resulting axial source images are typically post-processed for two-dimensional (2D) and three-dimensional (3D) visualization using one or more of several available techniques including multiplanar reformatting, thin-slab maximum-intensity projection (MIP), and 3D volume rendering. Recently introduced CT with 320 detector rows enables dynamic scanning, providing both high spatial and temporal resolution of the entire cerebrovasculature (4D CTA). The cervical vessels are imaged by acquisition of an additional spiral CT scan analogous to 64-detector row CT. Validated clinical applications of this advanced technique currently remain under investigation (Diekmann et al., 2010).

Limitations
Contrast-Induced Nephropathy

Careful consideration must be made for performing contrast-enhanced CT studies in patients with renal impairment. Exposure to all contrast agents may result in acute renal failure, called *contrast-induced nephropathy* (CIN), which is typically

DOI: 10.1016/B978-1-4377-0434-1.00036-0

reversible but may potentially result in adverse outcomes. The incidence of renal injury appears to be associated with increased osmolality of contrast agents, which have been steadily declining with the newer generations of nonionic agents. Patients with a creatinine level above 1.5 gm/dL or estimated glomerular filtration rate below 60 mL/min/1.73m^2 remain at a higher risk for developing CIN. Treatment for this condition relies on prevention of this disorder, and agents such as *N*-acetylcysteine and intravenous (IV) saline and/or sodium bicarbonate have been demonstrated to reduce the incidence of CIN. Avoidance of volume depletion and discontinuation of nonsteroidal antiinflammatory drugs, which may cause renal vasoconstriction, is recommended for patients prior to the procedure. Patients on hemodialysis are recommended to undergo dialysis as soon as possible afterwards to reduce contrast exposure (Asif and Epstein, 2004; Kim et al., 2010).

Metal Artifacts

Metallic implants such as clips, coils, and stents are generally safe for CT imaging, but it should be noted that they may lead to severe streaking artifacts, limiting evaluation. These artifacts occur because the density of the metal is beyond the normal range of the processing software, resulting in incomplete attenuation profiles. Several processing methods are available to reduce the artifact signal, and operator-dependent techniques such as gantry angulation adjustments and use of thin sections to reduce partial volume artifacts may help decrease this signal distortion. Generally, knowledge of the composition of metallic implants may help in determining the potential severity of artifacts on CT. Cobalt aneurysm clips produce much more artifact than titanium clips. For patients with stents, careful consideration must be made in evaluating stenosis, as these implants may lead to artificial lumen narrowing on CTA. The degree of artificial lumen narrowing decreases with increasing stent diameter. Lettau et al. evaluated patients with various types of stents and found that CTA may be superior to magnetic resonance angiography (MRA) at 1.5T for stainless steel and cobalt alloy carotid stents, whereas MRA at 3T may be superior for nitinol carotid stents (Lettau et al., 2009; van der Schaaf et al., 2006).

Applications
Extracranial Circulation
CAROTID ARTERY STENOSIS

In evaluating occlusive disease of the extracranial carotid artery, CTA complements conventional or digital subtraction angiography (DSA) and serves as an alternative to MRA (**Fig. 33B.1**). In the grading of carotid stenosis using the North American Symptomatic Carotid Endarterectomy Trial (NASCET) criteria, Randoux and colleagues (2001) found that the rate of agreement between 3D CTA and DSA was 95%. Relative to DSA (the reference standard), severe stenosis (70%-99%) was detected with a sensitivity and specificity of 100% and 100%, respectively, for CTA and 93% and 100%, respectively, for contrast-enhanced MRA (CE-MRA). In addition, CTA and CE-MRA were significantly correlated with DSA in depicting the length of the stenotic segment.

Other investigators have reported lower sensitivity (80%-89%) yet comparable specificity (96%-100%) for CTA in detecting severe stenosis (Binaghi et al., 2001; Magarelli et al., 1998). Those investigators found that time-of-flight (TOF) MRA had higher sensitivity (92%-93%) than CTA and similar specificity (98%-100%). Binaghi and colleagues also compared CTA with DSA and showed that the sensitivity was the same (89%), whereas specificity was higher for CTA (100%) than for DSA (81%). In 2006, Wardlaw et al., performed a meta-analysis on studies comparing CTA with DSA for the diagnosis of carotid artery stenosis. For detection of severe (70% to 99%) stenoses, CTA demonstrated a pooled sensitivity and specificity of 77% and 95%, respectively. Data for moderate (50%-69%) stenoses were determined to be sparse and unreliable (Wardlaw et al., 2006). An earlier systematic review found CTA to be a reliable method for detecting severe (70%-99%) stenoses, with a sensitivity and specificity of 85% and 93%, respectively. For detection of a complete occlusion, the sensitivity and specificity were 97% and 99%, respectively (Koelemay et al., 2004). Saba et al. evaluated the use of multidetector CTA and carotid ultrasound in comparison to surgical observation for evaluating ulceration, which is a severe complication of carotid plaques. CTA was found to be

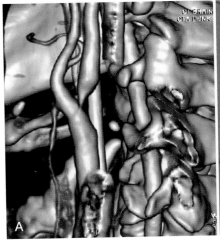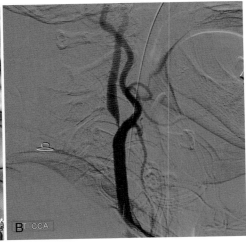

Fig. 33B.1 Computed tomographic angiography (CTA) compared to digital subtraction angiography (DSA) in a patient with proximal internal carotid artery (ICA) stenosis. **A,** Three-dimensional reconstructed CTA image of left ICA reveals severe stenosis distal to the ICA bifurcation. **B,** DSA confirms severe stenosis seen on CTA due to an atherosclerotic plaque.

superior, with 93.75% sensitivity and 98.59% specificity compared to carotid ultrasound, which demonstrated 37.5% sensitivity and 91.5% specificity (Saba et al., 2007).

Fibromuscular dysplasia (FMD), which often involves a unique pattern of stenoses in the cervical vessels, may be detected by CTA, although no large studies have evaluated the sensitivity and specificity for detection. This disorder, which characteristically demonstrates a string-of-beads pattern of vascular irregularity on angiography, has been reliably demonstrated on carotid artery evaluations from case reports. This may potentially reduce the need for more invasive angiographic imaging in the future, although further studies in this area are required (de Monye et al., 2007).

Currently, either CTA or MRA is used to evaluate suspected carotid occlusive disease, with the choice of method determined by clinical conditions (e.g., pacemaker), accessibility of CT and MR scanners, and additional imaging capabilities (CT or MR perfusion brain imaging).

CAROTID AND VERTEBRAL DISSECTION

Dissections of the cervicocephalic arteries, including the carotid and vertebral arteries, account for up to 20% of ischemic strokes in young adults (Leys et al., 1995). CTA findings include demonstration of a narrowed eccentric arterial lumen in the presence of a thickened vessel wall, with occasional detection of a dissecting aneurysm. In subacute and chronic dissection, CTA has been shown to detect a reduction in the thickness of the arterial wall, recanalization of the arterial lumen, and reduction in size or resolution of dissecting aneurysm. CTA or MRA is superior to DSA in depicting the distal portions of the cervical internal carotid artery (ICA), a common site of dissection. CTA is likely superior to MRI alone in evaluating aneurysms at these sites because MRI findings are often complicated by the presence of flow-related artifacts. CTA depiction of dissections at the level of the skull base may be complicated in some cases because of to beam hardening and other artifacts that obscure dissection findings, including similarities in the densities of the temporal and sphenoid bones with the dissected ICA.

A retrospective review compared combined multidetector CT/CTA with MRI/MRA among 18 patients with 25 dissected vessels in both anterior and posterior circulations. CT/CTA was preferred for diagnosis in 13 vessels, whereas MRI/MRA

was preferred in 1 vessel, and the techniques were deemed equal in the remaining 11 vessels. It should be noted that such combinations of noninvasive angiographic study with other CT or MRI components is common and therefore does not reflect the role of CTA or MRA alone. A significant preference for CT/CTA was noted for vertebral artery dissections but not for ICA dissections (Vertinsky et al., 2008). When compared with DSA, a small retrospective review of patients found that multidetector CTA had a sensitivity of 100% and specificity of 95% for detecting vertebral artery dissections (Pugliese et al., 2007). A small study evaluated multislice CTA with cervical axial T1-weighted MRI and MRA among seven patients with carotid artery dissection. The combination of MRI and MRA identified dissection in five of the seven patients that were identified by CTA. Additionally, a dissecting aneurysm was identified by CTA that was missed by MRI and MRA. These findings suggest that CTA may be at the very least a complementary study to provide additional information (Elijovich et al., 2006).

Intracranial Circulation
ACUTE ISCHEMIC STROKE

Computed tomography angiography is a reliable alternative to MRA in evaluating arterial occlusive disease near the circle of Willis in patients with symptoms of acute stroke (Knauth et al., 1997; Shrier et al., 1997) (**Fig. 33B.2**). CTA shows clinically relevant occlusions of major cerebral arteries and enhancement caused by collateral flow distal to the site of occlusion. CTA may be superior to transcranial Doppler (TCD) ultrasound in diagnosing atherothrombotic MCA disease in Asian patients presenting with middle cerebral artery (MCA) stroke (Suwanwela et al., 2002). CTA detected MCA stenosis measuring more than 50% in twice as many patients as TCD. The difference resulted primarily from improved detection by CTA of distal M1 and M2 stenosis. Because half of the patients studied by Suwanwela and colleagues had distal M1 and M2 disease, the authors concluded that TCD should not be used to screen for MCA stenosis.

In the detection of intracranial steno-occlusive disease, Hirai and colleagues (2002) have shown that combined CTA and MRA provide substantially higher sensitivity, specificity, and accuracy than MRA alone. Review of the CTA depiction

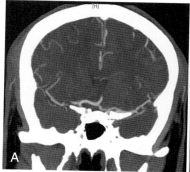
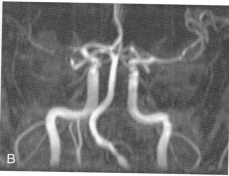
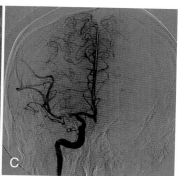

Fig. 33B.2 Right middle cerebral artery (MCA) stenosis in a patient who subsequently received intracranial stent placement. **A,** Coronal image from computed tomographic angiography (CTA) shows focal distal M1 segment stenosis prior to stenting. **B,** 1.5T 3D time-of-flight (TOF) magnetic resonance angiography (MRA) demonstrates a focal flow gap of the right M1. MRA overestimates degree of stenosis when compared to CTA. **C,** Digital subtraction angiography (DSA) image after stent placement reveals right MCA restenosis.

of vessels in conjunction with the 3D time-of-flight (TOF) MRA reduced the frequency of overestimation of stenosis when compared with MRA alone. In the identification of 50% or greater stenosis, the sensitivity, specificity, and accuracy for the combined CTA and MRA evaluation were 100%, 99%, and 99%, respectively, and the values for 3D TOF-MRA alone were 92%, 91%, and 91%, respectively. The grading of stenosis by the combined approach agreed with DSA grading in 98% of cases. In a retrospective review of their cases, the authors found that CTA did not always correctly delineate arterial lumina with circumferential calcification and the cavernous portion of the ICA. Nguyen et al. evaluated 475 vessel segments in 41 patients who received both CTA and DSA studies and found that for arterial occlusions, CTA had demonstrated 100% sensitivity and specificity. For detection of 50% or more stenosis, CTA had 97.1% sensitivity and 99.5% specificity. There was no difference observed in CTA accuracy for vessel segments in the anterior versus posterior circulation (Nguyen-Huynh et al., 2008). In a recent review of published studies, Latchaw et al. found that in comparison to conventional angiography, CTA demonstrated sensitivities ranging from 92% to 100% and specificities of 82% to 100% for the detection of intracranial vessel occlusion. The sensitivities for detection of intracranial stenoses range from 78% to 100%, with specificities of 82% to 100% (Latchaw et al., 2009). CTA is considered to be superior to TCD in detecting intracranial stenoses and occlusions, with a high false-negative rate noted for Doppler ultrasound. Studies also suggest that CTA has a higher sensitivity when directly compared with 3D TOF-MRA. Bash et al. found that CTA had a sensitivity of 98% while MRA had a sensitivity of 70% for detection of intracranial stenosis. The sensitivity for detecting occlusions on CTA was 100% and only 87% on MRA. Additionally, CTA was noted to superior to both MRA and DSA in detecting posterior circulation stenoses when slow or balanced flow states were present, possibly owing to longer scan time, which allows for more contrast to pass through a critical stenosis. Although previous studies noted decreased accuracy with the presence of atheromatous calcifications, the sensitivity and specificity of CTA for stenosis quantification were not compromised by this when appropriate window and level adjustments were made to account for the blooming artifacts that are frequently associated with heavy calcifications (Bash et al., 2005).

Computed tomography angiography source images (CTA-SI) may be used to provide an estimate of perfusion by taking advantage of the contrast enhancement in the brain vasculature that occurs during a CTA, possibly making it unnecessary to perform a separate CT perfusion study with a second contrast bolus. In normal perfused tissue, contrast dye fills the brain microvasculature and appears as increased signal intensity on the CTA-SI. In ischemic brain regions with poor collateral flow, contrast does not readily fill the brain microvasculature. Thus, these regions demonstrate low attenuation (Schramm et al., 2002). The hypoattenuation seen on CTA-SI correlate with abnormality on diffusion-weighted MRI (DWI) and have been found to be more sensitive than noncontrast CT scans for the detection of early brain infarction (Camargo et al., 2007). The sensitivity of CTA-SI and DWI when directly compared has been found to be similar in detecting ischemic regions, but DWI is better at demonstrating smaller infarcts and those in the brainstem and posterior fossa. Such findings

may be useful for patients with symptoms of acute infarction who cannot undergo MRI (Latchaw et al., 2009).

In addition to perfusion status, CTA imaging may potentially be used for prognostication in patients undergoing acute stroke intervention. The 10-point Clot Burden Score (CBS) was devised as a semiquantitative analysis of CTA to help determine prognosis in acute stroke (**Fig. 33B.3**). The CBS subtracts 1 or 2 points each for absent contrast opacification on CTA in the infraclinoid internal carotid artery (ICA) (1), supraclinoid ICA (2), proximal M1 segment (2), distal M1 segment (2), M2 branches (1 each), and A1 segment (1). The CBS applies only to the symptomatic hemisphere. A CBS below 10 was associated with reduced odds of independent functional outcome (odds ratio (OR) 0.09 for a CBS of 5 or less; OR 0.22 for CBS 6 to 7; OR 0.48 for CBS 8 to 9; all versus CBS 10). The quantification of intracranial thrombus extent with the CBS predicts functional outcome, final infarct size, and parenchymal hematoma risk acutely. This scoring system requires external validation and could be useful for patient stratification in stroke trials (Puetz et al., 2008).

The Alberta Stroke Program Early CT Score (ASPECTS) is a 10-point analysis of topographic CT scan score used in patients with MCA stroke (**Fig. 33B.4** and **Box 33B.1**). Segmental assessment of MCA territory is made, and 1 point is removed from the initial score of 10 if there is evidence of infarction in the following regions: putamen, internal capsule, insular cortex, anterior MCA cortex, MCA cortex lateral to insular ribbon, posterior MCA cortex, anterior MCA territory immediately superior to M1, lateral MCA territory immediately superior to M2 and posterior MCA territory immediately

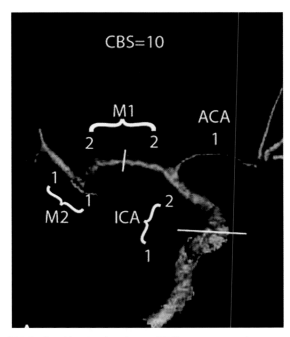

Fig. 33B.3 The Clot Burden Score (CBS) on computed tomographic angiography (CTA). This is a 10-point imaging-based score where two points are subtracted for thrombus found on CTA in the supraclinoid internal carotid artery (ICA) and each of the proximal and distal segments of the middle cerebral artery (MCA) trunk. One point is subtracted for thrombus in the infraclinoid ICA and A1 segment and for each M2 branch.

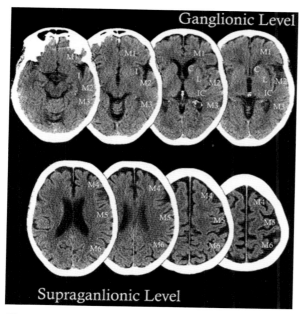

Fig. 33B.4 Axial noncontrast head computed tomography (CT) demonstrating middle cerebral artery (MCA) territory regions defined by the Alberta Stroke Program Early CT Score (ASPECTS). *C,* Caudate, *I,* insular ribbon, *IC,* internal capsule, *L,* lentiform nucleus.

Box 33B.1 Alberta Stroke Program Early CT Score*

Aspects Territories

Caudate
Putamen
Internal capsule
Insular cortex
M1—Anterior MCA cortex
M2—MCA cortex lateral to insular ribbon
M3—Posterior MCA cortex
M4—Anterior MCA territory immediately superior to M1
M5—Lateral MCA territory immediately superior to M2
M6—Posterior MCA territory immediately superior to M3

ASPECTS, Alberta Stroke Program Early CT Score; *CT,* computed tomography; *MCA,* middle cerebral artery.

*Box demonstrates a 10-point quantitative scoring system for patients with acute MCA-territory strokes. Segmental assessment of MCA territory is made, and 1 point is removed from the initial score of 10 if there is evidence of infarction in that region.

---

superior to M3. An ASPECTS score of 7 or less predicts worse functional outcome at 3 months as well as symptomatic hemorrhage. Puetz et al. sought to determine whether the ASPECTS scoring system could be applied to CTA-SI and combined with the CBS system for improved prognostication. A 10-point ASPECTS score based on CTA-SI and the 10-point CBS were combined to form a 20-point score for patients presenting acutely with stroke who received thrombolysis treatment. For patients with a combined score of 10 or less, only 4% were functionally independent, and mortality was 50%. In contrast, 57% of patients with scores of 10 or greater were functionally independent, and mortality was 10%. Additionally, parenchy-

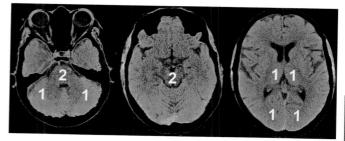

Fig. 33B.5 Cerebral map defining the posterior circulation Acute Stroke Prognosis Early CT score (pc-ASPECTS) territories. From 10 points, 1 or 2 points each (as indicated) are subtracted for early ischemic changes or hypoattenuation on computed tomographic angiography source images (CTA-SI) in left or right thalamus, cerebellum, or posterior cerebral artery (PCA) territory, respectively (1 point); and any part of midbrain or pons (2 points).

mal hematoma rates were 30% versus 8%, respectively (Puetz et al., 2010). A similar semiquantitative scoring system for CTA-SI was devised for patients presenting with acute basilar artery occlusion and termed the posterior circulation (*pc*)-*ASPECTS* (**Fig. 33B.5**). This 10-point scoring system subtracts 1 or 2 points each for areas of hypoattenuation in the left or right thalamus, cerebellum, or posterior cerebral artery (PCA) territory, respectively (1 point), or any part of the midbrain or pons (2 points). Median follow-up pc-ASPECTS was lower in patients with a CTA-SI pc-ASPECTS less than 8 compared with patients with a CTA-SI pc-ASPECTS of 8 or higher, respectively. Hemorrhagic transformation rates were 27.3% versus 9.5%, respectively, for patients who received thrombolysis. The results indicate that such analysis can predict a larger final infarct extent in patients with basilar artery occlusion. Larger prospective trials are required for validation, but the systematic acute evaluation of CTA along with CTA-SI may potentially be used to help guide future stroke treatments (Puetz et al., 2009).

INTRACEREBRAL HEMORRHAGE

Patients presenting acutely with intracerebral hemorrhage (ICH) within the first few hours of symptom onset are known to be at increased risk for hematoma expansion. However, only a fraction of such patients arrive at a hospital within this time frame, so alternative means of identifying potential hemorrhage expansion have been sought because it is an important predictor of 30-day mortality. One such prognostic marker has been identified on CTA: the *spot sign*, defined as a tiny, enhancing foci seen within hematomas, with or without clear contrast extravasation. A prospective study by Wada et al. of 39 consecutive patients with spontaneous ICH within 3 hours of symptom onset identified this sign in 33% of cases. Sensitivity was found to be 91%, and specificity was 89% for predicting hematoma expansion. In patients with the spot sign, mean volume change was greater, extravasation was more common, and median hospital stay was longer (Wada et al., 2007).

A larger retrospective analysis determined that the presence of three or more spot signs, a maximum axial dimension of 5 mm or greater, and maximum attenuation of 180 Hounsfield units or more were independent predictors of significant hematoma expansion (Delgado et al., 2009). In another study,

Delgado et al. noted that the presence of any spot sign increased the risk of in-hospital mortality (OR, 4.0) and poor outcome among survivors at 3-month follow-up (OR, 2.5). This was determined to be an independent predictor of both measures. The spot sign currently requires further validation but remains a promising use of CTA in guiding acute ICH management (Delgado et al., 2010).

BRAIN DEATH

The absence of cerebral circulation is an important confirmatory test for brain death, and CTA is emerging as an important alternative means of testing. A novel 4-point score was devised, with points subtracted based on the lack of opacification of the cortical segments of the MCAs and internal cerebral veins. Frampas et al. used this system to prospectively evaluate 105 patients who were clinically brain dead and found a sensitivity of 85.7% and specificity of 100%. This appears to be a possible alternative means of detecting cerebral circulatory arrest, and given that it is a fast and noninvasive technique, it may become a useful confirmatory test (Frampas et al., 2009; Escudero et al., 2009).

CEREBRAL VENOUS THROMBOSIS

The diagnosis of cerebral venous thrombosis (CVT) was previously often made with conventional angiography and more recently by MRI techniques. Magnetic resonance venography (MRV) is commonly considered the most sensitive noninvasive test in diagnosing CVT. However, given the prolonged imaging time and often limited availability, CTA has been studied as a potential alternate means of detecting CVT. Spiral CT with acquisition during peak venous enhancement has been implemented with single-section systems but remains limited in spatial and temporal resolution. One study directly comparing CTV with MRV demonstrated a sensitivity and a specificity of 75% to 100%, depending on the sinus or venous structure involved (Khandelwal et al., 2006). Multidetector-row CTA (MDCTA) offers higher spatial and temporal resolution, which allows for high-quality multiplanar and 3D reformatting. Two recent small studies found 100% specificity and sensitivity with MDCTA when compared to MRV. The venous sinuses could be identified in 99.2% and the cerebral veins in 87.6% of cases. MDCTA may be equivalent to MRV in visualizing cerebral sinuses, but further studies are needed to evaluate the diagnostic potential of MDCTA in specific types of CVT such as cortical venous thrombosis, thrombosis of the cavernous sinus, and thrombosis of the deep cerebral veins. The advantages of MDCTA include the short exam duration and the possible simultaneous visualization of the cerebral arterial and venous systems with a single bolus of contrast. MDCTA visualizes thrombus via contrast-filling defects and remains less prone to flow artifacts. A potential problem with this technique lies in the fact that in the chronic state of a CVT, older organized thrombus may show enhancement after contrast administration and may not produce a filling defect, leading to a false-negative result. The addition of a noncontrast CT with the MDCTA is sometimes used to remove another potential to obtain false-negative results from the presence of a spontaneously hyperattenuated clot that could be mistaken for an enhanced sinus. This phenomenon is known as the *cord sign* and may be seen in 25% to 56% of acute CVT cases (Gaikwad et al., 2008; Linn et al., 2007).

CEREBRAL ANEURYSMS

Digital subtraction angiography has been the standard imaging method for diagnosis and preoperative evaluation for patients with ruptured and unruptured cerebral aneurysms. However, DSA is invasive and subject to complications resulting from catheter manipulation. Thus, in asymptomatic patients at greater risk for cerebral aneurysms, the use of non-invasive techniques such as MRA and CTA to screen for aneurysms is particularly attractive. These techniques have advantages and disadvantages. The most thoroughly investigated MRA technique is 3D TOF-MRA, and its main disadvantages are long scanning times, difficulty in detecting very small aneurysms, difficulty in establishing the relationship of the aneurysm to adjacent (and surgically important) osseous anatomy, and occasional difficulty in distinguishing between patent lumen, high-grade stenosis, and occlusion.

The main disadvantages of CTA are radiation exposure, the use of iodinated contrast material, and difficulty in detecting very small aneurysms and imaging artifacts from endovascular coils in treated aneurysms. CTA is nondiagnostic for determining the presence of a residual lumen and the size/location of the remnant neck of a treated aneurysm because of the streak artifacts caused by coils.

Although 3D TOF-MRA and dynamic 3D CE-MRA have similar sensitivity and specificity to CTA for detection of intracerebral aneurysms at least 5 mm in diameter, they have lower sensitivity for aneurysms smaller than 5 mm (Villablanca et al., 2002; White et al., 2001) (**Figs. 33B.6 and 33B.7**). The results of the International Study of Unruptured Intracranial Aneurysms (ISUIA) (Wiebers et al., 2003) suggest that MRA, despite its lower sensitivity for smaller aneurysms, would not significantly change management, because incidental aneurysms smaller than 10 mm should not be treated (exceptions may be made for individuals with daughter aneurysm formation, a family history of subarachnoid hemorrhage, and young patients). However, in general, the accuracy of CTA is felt to be at least equal if not superior to that of MRA in most circumstances, and in some cases, its overall accuracy approaches that of DSA (Latchaw et al., 2009).

Using optimized helical CTA acquisition and post-processing protocols that included 3D volume-rendered images, 3D thick-slab and grayscale 2D single-section images, and thick-slab multiplanar reformatted 2D images, Villablanca and colleagues (2002) reported a sensitivity for the detection of small aneurysms (<5 mm diameter) of 98% to 100%, compared with 95% for DSA. The specificity of both CTA and DSA was 100%. CTA image analysis times ranged from 6 to 36 minutes (mean, 16 minutes). The smallest aneurysm detected was $1.9 \times 1.6 \times 1.3 \text{ mm}^3$, and 48% of aneurysms were detected in the presence of subarachnoid hemorrhage. The sensitivity of CTA exceeded that of DSA, primarily because the optimal projection necessary to visualize some aneurysms could be displayed on the post-processed CTA images but was not or could not be displayed by the 2D DSA. Other disadvantages of DSA that have been noted by investigators include superimposition of normal vessels, obscuring a small aneurysm, and the lack of an internal image scale for estimating the aneurysm sac and neck dimensions. Villablanca et al. (2002) showed that CTA can provide quantitative information such as dome-to-neck ratios and aneurysm characterization such as the presence of mural thrombi or calcium, branching

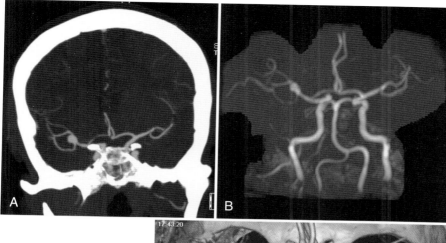

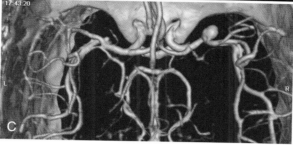

Fig. 33B.6 Right middle cerebral artery aneurysm seen on both computed tomographic angiography (CTA) and magnetic resonance angiography (MRA). **A,** Coronal section on CTA reveals aneurysm in right middle cerebral artery (MCA) bifurcation. **B,** MRA also displays aneurysm with less definition. **C,** Three-dimensional reconstruction of CTA better defines saccular appearance of this aneurysm.

pattern at the neck, and the incorporation of arterial segments in the aneurysm. The 3D images in particular provided a surgically useful display of the aneurysm sac in relation to skull base structures (see **Fig. 33B.7**). The authors concluded that clinically relevant aneurysms can be detected by CTA using published protocols, routine scanners, and commercially available image-processing workstations. Furthermore, CTA can be a reliable source of information for treatment planning.

Cerebral veins show much more anatomical variation than arteries. The presence of an unexpected vein or the lack of collateral drainage from a region drained by a vein that may need to be sacrificed during surgery can alter the approach to resection of an aneurysm. Kaminogo and colleagues (2002) used 3D CTA to demonstrate the venous anatomy accurately. They showed the usefulness of this information in selecting a therapeutic procedure (surgery versus endovascular coiling) and in planning the approach for surgical treatment.

Recent data indicate that CTA is a safe and accurate imaging technique for evaluating most extracranial and intracranial vessels to detect the presence of stenoses or occlusions, as well as for the detection of intracranial aneurysms. The accuracy of CTA appears equal to or superior to MRA imaging in most circumstances, and its accuracy sometimes approaches that of DSA. The development of new advanced CT scanners with more detectors may further enhance the accuracy of this technique (Latchaw et al., 2009).

Magnetic Resonance Angiography

Methods

Numerous techniques are used in the acquisition of MRA images. In general, TOF-MRA and phase-contrast (PC) MRA do not use a contrast bolus and generate contrast between flowing blood in a vessel and surrounding stationary tissues. In 2D TOF-MRA, sequential tissue sections (typically 1.5 mm thick and approximately perpendicular to the vessels) are repeatedly excited, and images are reconstructed from the acquired signal data. This results in high intravascular signal and good sensitivity to slow flow. In 3D TOF-MRA, slabs that are a few centimeters thick are excited and partitioned into thin sections less than 1 mm thick to become reconstructed into a 3D data set. A 3D TOF-MRA has better spatial resolution and is more useful for imaging tortuous and small vessels, but because flowing blood spends more time in the slab than that in a 2D TOF section, a vessel passing through the slab may lose its vascular contrast upon exiting the slab.

In TOF-MRA, stationary material with high signal intensity, such as subacute thrombus, can mimic blood flow. PC-MRA is useful in this situation because the high signal from stationary tissue is eliminated when the two data sets are subtracted to produce the final flow-sensitive images. This technique provides additional information that allows for delineation of flow volumes and direction of flow in various structures from proximal arteries to the dural venous sinuses. In the 2D phase-contrast technique, flow-encoding gradients are applied along two or three axes. A projection image displaying the vessel against a featureless background is produced. Compared with the 2D techniques, 3D PC-MRA provides higher spatial resolution and information on flow directionality along each of three flow-encoding axes. The summed information from all three flow directions is displayed as a speed image, in which the signal intensity is proportional to the magnitude of the flow velocity. The data set in TOF-MRA or PC-MRA may be used to visualize the course of vessels in 3D by mapping the hyperintense signal from the vessel-containing pixels onto a desired viewing plane using a MIP algorithm, producing a projection image. MIP images are generated in several viewing planes and then evaluated

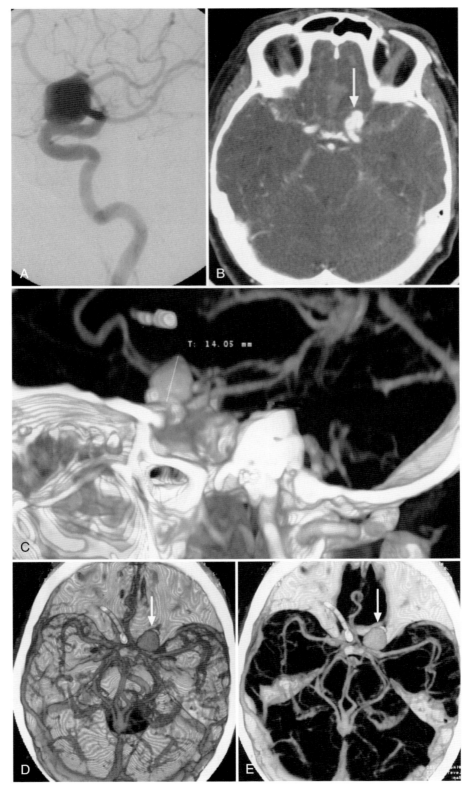

Fig. 33B.7 Left internal carotid artery (ICA) aneurysm. Comparison of computed tomographic angiography (CTA) postprocessed images with catheter angiography. **A,** Catheter angiography lateral view, following left ICA injection, shows aneurysm originating from supraclinoid portion of ICA. **B,** CTA axial source image reveals lobulated aneurysm *(arrow)*. **C-E,** CTA three-dimensional (3D) volume-rendered images with transparency feature for user-selected tissue regions (called *4D angiography*). **C,** Lateral view from left side of patient demonstrates relationship of the aneurysm, measuring 14 mm from neck to dome, to the anterior clinoid process. **D,** View of aneurysm *(arrow)*, skull base, and circle of Willis from above. **E,** Same view as **D** but edited to remove most of skull base densities and improve visibility of vessels.

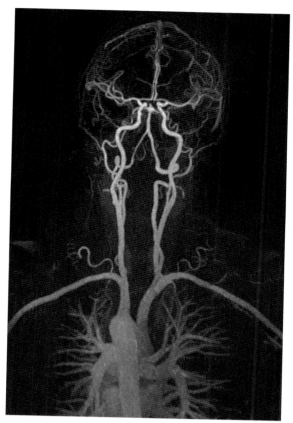

Fig. 33B.8 3T contrast-enhanced magnetic resonance angiography (CE-MRA) of the cerebrovascular system.

together to view the vessel architecture. A presaturation band is applied and represents a zone in which both flowing and stationary nuclei are saturated by a radiofrequency pulse that is added to the gradient recalled echo (GRE) pulse sequence. The downstream signal of a vessel that passes through the presaturation zone is suppressed because of the saturation of the flowing nuclei. Presaturation bands may be fixed or may travel, keeping the same distance from each slab as it is acquired. In general, the placement of presaturation bands can be chosen so as to identify flow directionality and help distinguish arterial from venous flow.

Contrast-enhanced MRA (CE-MRA) uses scan parameters that are typical of 3D TOF-MRA but uses gadolinium to overcome the problem of saturation of the slow-flowing blood in structures that lie within the 3D slab (**Fig. 33B.8**). The scan time per 3D volume is on the order of 5 to 10 minutes, and data are acquired in the first 10 to 15 minutes after the bolus infusion of a gadolinium contrast agent (0.1-0.2 mmol/kg). Presaturation bands usually are ineffective at suppressing the downstream signal from vessels when gadolinium is present. In 3D CE-MRA (called *fast, dynamic,* or *time-resolved CE-MRA*), the total scan time per 3D volume (usually about 30-50 partitions) is reduced to 5 to 50 seconds (Fain et al., 2001; Melhem et al., 1999; Turski et al., 2001). Data are acquired as the bolus of the gadolinium contrast agent

(0.2-0.3 mmol/kg and 2-3 mL/sec infusion rate) passes through the vessels of interest, taking advantage of the marked increase in intravascular signal (first-pass method). Vessel signal is determined primarily by concentration of injected contrast, analogous to conventional angiography. Because 3D CE-MRA entails more rapid data acquisition, and hence higher temporal resolution, than TOF-MRA, spatial resolution may be reduced. The most common approaches to synchronizing the 3D data acquisition with the arrival of the gadolinium bolus in the arteries are measurement of the bolus arrival time for each patient using a small (2 mL) test dose of contrast followed by a separate synchronized manual 3D acquisition (Foo et al., 1997) by the scanner operator (Fain et al., 2001; Foo et al., 1997). Another method rapidly and repeatedly acquires 3D volumes (<10 sec per volume) in the neck, beginning at the time of contrast bolus injection to ensure that at least one 3D volume showing only arteries will be acquired (Turski et al., 2001). Subtraction of preinjection source images from arterial phase images, termed *digital subtraction MRA*, is sometimes used to increase vessel-to-background contrast.

The advent and increasing availability of MRI scanners with 3.0 tesla (T) or even higher field strengths (up to 7T) in selected centers may also be used to improve MRA by capitalizing on higher signal-to-noise ratios and parallel imaging (Nael et al., 2006; Pruessmann et al., 1999). Parallel imaging at 3T or greater can be used to improve spatial resolution, shorten scan time, reduce artifacts, and increase anatomical coverage in first-pass CE-MRA. Recent investigation with 7T TOF-MRA demonstrated that such ultrahigh field strength allows vivid depiction of the large vessels of the circle of Willis with significantly more first- and second-order branches and can even distinguish diseased diminutive vessels in hypertensive patients (Hendrikse et al.; 2008; Kang et al., 2009; Kang et al., 2010). The 4D time-resolved MRA (4D MRA) is a novel contrast-enhanced vascular imaging method under investigation that uses novel processing techniques to achieve subsecond temporal resolution while maintaining high spatial resolution. Dynamic MRA scans may be obtained up to 60 times faster and with higher spatial resolution at 3T. The resulting images may attain the diagnostic performance of conventional DSA, allowing for better characterization of various vascular lesions (Hope et al., 2010; Parmar et al., 2009; Willinek et al., 2008).

Limitations
Nephrogenic Systemic Fibrosis

Clinicians should be aware that a rare but serious complication of contrast-enhanced MRI studies includes the development of nephrogenic systemic fibrosis (NSF). This condition is characterized by widespread thickening and hardening of the skin, with the potential for rapid systemic progression and immobility over several weeks. Although the precise mechanism remains unclear, NSF was first noted in 1997 and occurs exclusively in patients with renal failure. The majority of reported cases involved exposure to a gadolinium chelate within 2 to 3 months prior to disease onset in dialysis-dependent patients. A large percentage of cases has been specifically associated with gadodiamide (Omniscan), with a possible dose-dependent effect, although it should be noted that cases have been reported with all gadolinium agents. Careful consideration must be made for gadolinium administration in patients with renal impairment (glomerular filtration rate <30 mL/min/1.73m^2), especially those on dialysis. The risks and benefits should be carefully discussed prior to any contrast-enhanced procedures, and the dose of gadolinium should be minimized. Additionally, for patients on hemodialysis, prophylactic dialysis is generally recommended as soon as possible, ideally within 3 hours after contrast administration (Kuo et al., 2007).

Metal Implant Contraindications

Limitations due to the presence of metallic materials (clips, stents, coils) remains a common concern in patients undergoing vascular imaging. Aneurysm clips made from martensitic stainless steels remain a contraindication for MRI procedures, because excessive magnetic forces may displace these implants and cause serious injury. However, most clips are now made of metals that are non-ferromagnetic, and all patients with any metallic implants require screening to determine whether they are safe to undergo an MRI study. For the majority of coils and stents that have been tested, it is unlikely that these implants would become moved or displaced as a result of exposure to MRI systems operating at 1.5T or even 3T. Additionally, it is often unnecessary to wait an extended period of time after a procedure to perform an MRI study in a patient with an implant made of non-ferromagnetic material unless there are concerns associated with MRI-related heating. Dental materials including wires and prostheses do not appear to pose a risk, although they may result in artifact on MRI. Artifacts from metal may have varied appearances on MRI related to the type or configuration of the piece of metal. Artifact sizes may increase at 3T compared to 1.5T, depending on the implant type and composition, but these distortions may be substantially reduced by optimizing imaging parameters. Patients who are deemed unsafe for MRI upon screening

may be considered for CT evaluation (Olsrud et al., 2005; Shellock, 2002).

Applications
Extracranial Carotid and Vertebral Circulation
TIME-OF-FLIGHT MRA

Earlier clinical reports outlined the advantages and pitfalls of TOF-MRA for imaging of the extracranial circulation and estimation of degree stenosis at the carotid bifurcation (Norris and Rothwell, 2001). The degree of stenosis tends to be overestimated by the traditional 2D TOF-MRA method. A corollary of this observation is that a 2D TOF study with normal or near-normal findings effectively excludes the possibility of severe (70% to 99%) stenosis. The most accurate results are obtained when short TE and small voxel size are used. Second, a consensus estimate of stenosis derived from a combination of the 2D and 3D TOF methods results in greater specificity than 2D TOF alone. This improvement results primarily from the inclusion of the 3D TOF method, in which stenosis is less likely to be overestimated, particularly if original (**Fig. 33B.9**) or reformatted source images are evaluated rather than the MIP images. In the combined TOF approach, the 2D TOF method is used primarily to distinguish slow flow from occlusion and, in general, the combined TOF approach is considered superior to DSA in differentiating high-grade stenosis from occlusion. A *flow gap*, which is a segmental dropout of signal from the carotid (or other vessels) caused by intravoxel phase dispersion or saturation, is often taken as a sign of stenosis measuring 70% or more. This association should be viewed with caution, however, because in one published series of patients, flow gap was observed with the 2D TOF technique at sites of 50% to 60% stenosis as determined by DSA.

Third, in detecting stenosis appropriate for carotid endarterectomy, TOF-MRA is less sensitive than DSA (75% MRA, 87% DSA) but more specific (88% MRA, 46% DSA); however, when stenosis estimates by TOF-MRA and DSA are

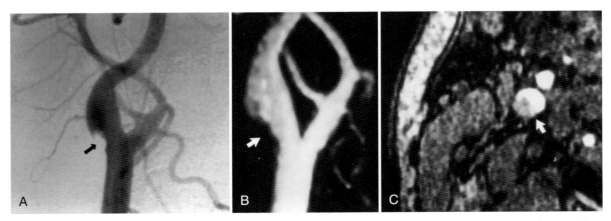

Fig. 33B.9 Carotid stenosis. Comparison of magnetic resonance angiogram and source image to catheter angiogram. **A,** Catheter angiogram of the right carotid system shows narrowing *(arrow)* at the origin of the internal carotid artery. Findings suggest intraluminal thrombus. **B,** Three-dimensional (3D) time-of-flight (TOF) angiogram demonstrates similar narrowing *(arrow)*. **C,** Axial 3D TOF source image at the site of stenosis shows clearly that the lumen is narrowed *(arrow)* by approximately 50%. In this case, there is agreement between the narrowing shown on source image and that detected by the maximum-intensity projection image **(B)**.

concordant and are then taken together, the combined MRA and DSA examination is more sensitive (96%) and specific (85%) than either study alone. Furthermore, when patients are classified as to whether carotid endarterectomy is indicated by the noninvasive examination and then judged against the results of DSA, the misclassification rate for the concordant MRA and DSA results is much lower than that of either test alone (MRA and DSA 7.9%, MRA 18%, DSA 28%) (Johnston and Goldstein, 2001). Therefore, surgical decisions are more likely to be correct when based on concordant TOF-MRA and DSA results.

THREE-DIMENSIONAL CONTRAST-ENHANCED MRA

Compared with 2D and 3D TOF-MRA, 3D CE-MRA delineates carotid arterial stenosis better (Willig et al., 1998) (**Fig. 33B.10**). Surface morphology (e.g., ulcerated plaque) and nearly occluded vessels (e.g., "string sign") are more easily identified, and arterial occlusions are more confidently identified. Severe carotid bifurcation stenosis may be detected by 3D CE-MRA with high sensitivity (93%-100%) and specificity (88%-96%) (Huston et al., 1998; Johnson et al., 2000; Lenhart et al., 2002; Remonda et al., 2002; Wutke et al., 2002) using DSA as the standard method of diagnosis. TOF techniques yield similar results to 3D CE-MRA for mild to moderate stenosis, thus obviating time spent on CE-MRA setup and processing. Advantages of 3D CE-MRA include greater anatomical coverage (**Fig. 33B.11**). For high-grade stenosis, which can cause intravascular flow gaps on TOF MIP images, the addition of CE-MRA to the imaging protocol provides sensitivity and specificity equivalent to CTA in determining the severity of stenosis (relative to DSA as the reference standard).

TOF-MRA and CE-MRA have been found to achieve high accuracy for the detection of high-grade ICA stenoses and occlusions, with CE-MRA having slight benefit over TOF-MRA. A systematic review and meta-analysis of 37 TOF-MRA studies and 21 CE-MRA studies was performed by Debrey et al. and found that for the detection of high-grade (≥70-99%) ICA stenoses, TOF-MRA had an overall sensitivity of 91.2%, with a specificity of 88.3%. The sensitivity of CE-MRA was higher at 94.6%, with a specificity of 91.9%. For the detection of complete ICA occlusions, the sensitivity of TOF-MRA was 94.5%, and the specificity was 99.3%, while CE-MRA demonstrated a sensitivity of 99.4% and specificity of 99.6%. However, for moderately severe ICA stenoses (50%-69%), sensitivity was found to be poor in TOF-MRA and only fair in CE-MRA studies. TOF-MRA had a sensitivity of only 37.9% and a specificity of 92.1%, while CE-MRA had a sensitivity of 65.9% with a specificity of 93.5% (Debrey et al., 2008).

The ability to detect an FMD pattern of stenoses by MRA in the carotid vessels remains uncertain. This disorder may not be as well delineated on TOF-MRA owing to limited resolution, although no large comparative studies with CE-MRA have been performed. In one series evaluating FMD in the renal arteries, Willoteaux found the sensitivity and specificity of CE-MRA to be 97% and 93%, respectively. These findings suggest that using CE-MRA to identify FMD in the cervical vessels may be possible, although further studies are required (Willoteaux et al., 2006).

Atherosclerotic narrowing of the vertebral artery commonly involves the origin or distal intracranial portion. For TOF-MRA evaluation of posterior-circulation cerebrovascular disease, the vertebral origins usually are not evaluated for the same reasons the common carotid origins are not evaluated. Typically, a 3D TOF study covering the vertebrobasilar system from the C2 level to the tip of the basilar artery is done (**Fig. 33B.12**). However, sequential 2D TOF-MRA of the neck is useful in determining whether proximal occlusion is present and in demonstrating flow direction in the vertebral arteries in patients with suspected subclavian steal. A 2D TOF study obtained with no presaturation band shows flow enhancement in both vertebral arteries, whereas a study obtained with a superiorly located walking presaturation band shows flow only in the vertebral artery with normal anterograde flow. The 3D CE-MRA techniques can display both the origins and distal intracranial portions of the vertebral arteries in a single acquisition and are particularly useful in evaluating vertebral artery segments with partial or complete signal loss caused by slow flow and in-plane saturation effects. The accuracy of 3D CE-MRA measurements of stenosis at the vertebral artery origin has yet to be reported, although the accuracy is unlikely

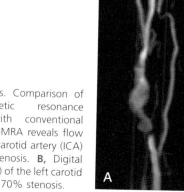
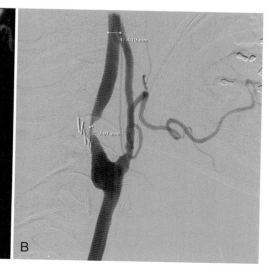

Fig. 33B.10 Carotid stenosis. Comparison of contrast-enhanced magnetic resonance angiography (CE-MRA) with conventional catheter angiography. **A,** CE-MRA reveals flow gap in proximal left internal carotid artery (ICA) suggestive of high-grade stenosis. **B,** Digital subtraction angiography (DSA) of the left carotid system confirms greater than 70% stenosis.

to equal that of carotid bifurcation measurements because of the smaller size of the vertebral origins (Kollias et al., 1999). Nevertheless, an analysis of the elliptical centric encoding technique predicts that it can achieve an isotropic spatial resolution of 1 mm (before zero filling) in a field of view typically used for bilateral carotid and vertebral imaging (Fain et al., 1999). Stenosis or occlusion of the subclavian artery is now routinely evaluated with 3D CE-MRA.

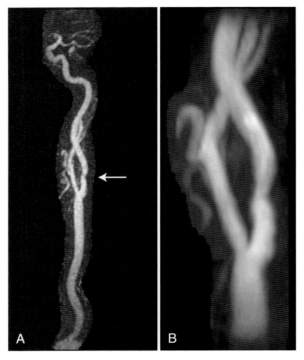

Fig. 33B.11 Similar appearance of mild stenosis *(arrow)* of left internal carotid artery on oblique maximum-intensity projection (MIP) images. **A,** Three-dimensional (3D) contrast-enhanced magnetic resonance angiography (CE-MRA). **B,** 3D time-of-flight (TOF) MRA. Note the greater coverage of the carotids afforded by CE-MRA compared with TOF-MRA. *(From Bowen, B.C., 2007. MR angiography versus CT angiography in the evaluation of neurovascular disease. Radiology 245, 357-361.)*

In patients with carotid or vertebral artery dissection, MRA is complemented by MRI with fat-saturation sequences that aid in detection and characterization of dissecting hematoma, associated dissecting aneurysm, and the length and caliber of the residual patent lumen, especially at the skull base (**Fig. 33B.13**). Subacute hyperintense thrombus is better seen if fat suppression is implemented on thin T1-weighted images to eliminate the high signal intensity from perivascular adipose tissue. When the evaluation includes a 2D or 3D TOF combined study or 3D CE-MRA (Kollias et al., 1999), the detection of stenosis, pseudoaneurysm, or occlusion is improved. Also, the presence of a thrombosed false lumen is more convincingly demonstrated when spin-echo images are supplemented with phase-contrast or TOF images showing absence of flow in the false lumen. The improved recognition of these features afforded by MRA impacts on treatment decisions, such as deployment of stents and other endovascular devices. Serial MRA examinations are required to evaluate for recanalization of the vessel following the dissection (**Fig. 33B.14**) and also to evaluate for dissecting aneurysms that may occasionally develop as the hematoma resolves.

The MRA assessment of vascular stenosis after placement of a metallic stent is limited by turbulence and susceptibility effects. Stent geometry, the relative orientation of the magnetic field, and alloy composition contribute to signal intensity alterations within the stent lumen (Lenhart et al., 2000) (**Fig. 33B.15**). CTA is also limited in determining stenosis of the lumen of a stented vessel. The limitation is primarily due to streak artifacts from the stent, which obscure the residual lumen. Also, widened window settings and volume averaging often result in overestimation of stenosis on CTA (see **Fig. 33B.15**).

Intracranial Circulation

The accuracy of TOF-MRA in detecting stenosis or occlusion of the proximal intracranial arteries, compared with that of DSA, has been studied by several investigators (Furst et al., 1996; Stock et al., 1995). Initially, accuracy was limited by technical shortcomings such as long TE, lower spatial resolution, and single thick-slab acquisition. These resulted in a decrease in vascular signal due to intravoxel phase dispersion,

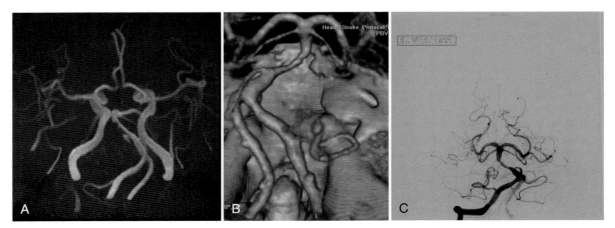

Fig. 33B.12 Basilar artery stenosis seen on both magnetic resonance angiography (MRA) and computed tomographic angiography (CTA). **A,** A 3T time-of-flight (TOF)-MRA reveals moderate luminal narrowing in mid to distal portion of basilar artery. **B,** Three-dimensional reconstruction of CTA images reveals a 1 cm area of irregular narrowing in the basilar artery, with 65% stenosis.

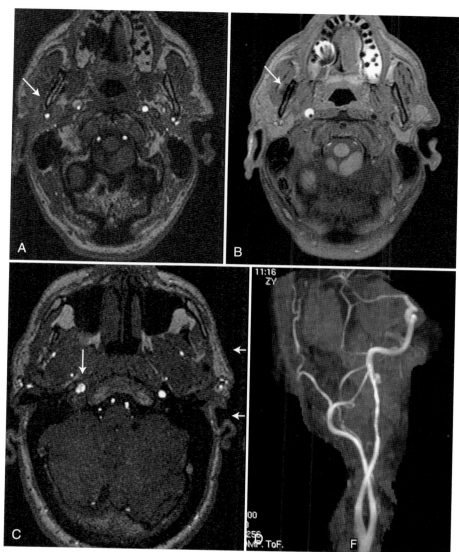

Fig. 33B.13 Right internal carotid artery dissection with intramural hematoma causing severe narrowing of the residual patent lumen as well as pseudoaneurysm at the skull base. **A,** Three-dimensional (3D) time-of-flight (TOF) axial source image. **B,** Fat-suppression T1-weighted axial image at C1-C1 shows the narrowed cervical carotid lumen with flow and the thickened wall with unsuppressed hyperintensity consistent with subacute hematoma *(arrows)*. **C,** 3D TOF axial source image at the level of the carotid canal entrance shows outpouching of pseudoaneurysm *(arrow)*. **D,** Oblique maximum-intensity projection image displays the length of the narrowed lumen *(between arrows)*, ending at the carotid canal and the pseudoaneurysm *(large arrow)*. *(From Bowen, B.C., 2007. MR angiography versus CT angiography in the evaluation of neurovascular disease. Radiology 245, 357-361.)*

susceptibility effects, and saturation effects. Signal loss was typically evident in the petrous, cavernous, and supraclinoid segments of the ICA and in the proximal M1 segment of the MCA. Second- and third-order branches of the cerebral arteries were poorly shown. Later studies reported that normal vessels and completely occluded vessels could be graded correctly when compared with DSA results, but stenotic segments were correctly graded (as either < or > 50% narrowing) only about 60% of the time. Subsequently, technical improvements in the 3D TOF method (variable flip angle, magnetization transfer suppression, multiple thin-slab acquisitions, and higher spatial resolution [512 matrix or greater]) improved the accuracy of stenosis grading, with investigators reporting that 80% of stenoses greater than 70% and 88% of stenoses less than 70% are quantified correctly with MRA.

The current approach to evaluating the intracranial arteries uses a multi-slab 3D TOF acquisition that covers the head from the foramen magnum extending superiorly to the areas of interest. Each slab has a transaxial orientation and may or may not have a superiorly located presaturation band. The axial source images and the reprojected MIP images (**Fig.**

33B.16) are reviewed in conjunction with other MR images. In the setting of acute infarction with the potential for thrombolytic treatment, protocols often include a rapidly acquired 2D PC-MR study of the circle of Willis instead of the more time-consuming 3D TOF study. Other clinical settings in which MRA reportedly complements routine MRI include sickle cell disease, moyamoya syndrome, hemifacial spasm, and trigeminal neuralgia. Flow dynamics (magnitude and direction) in the circle of Willis are more easily determined with the PC method, especially when vessel diameters are 1 mm or more.

The simplest type of 3D CE-MRA technique uses scan parameters typical of 3D TOF-MRA acquisitions with scan times on the order of 5 to 10 minutes per 3D volume. Under these steady-state conditions, visibility of the small intracranial arteries is greater after IV gadolinium administration; however, the intracranial veins also show a much greater increase in visibility. Consequently, the MIP images become cluttered with veins, resulting in greater difficulty in identifying and delineating specific arteries. With dynamic 3D CE-MRA, as used for extracranial carotid imaging, temporal resolution is improved, and visibility of arteries is greater than that of veins. Some investigators have suggested the use of region-of-interest MIP postprocessing to further exclude veins from intracranial artery displays. Despite the limits placed on spatial resolution by the dynamic 3D CE-MRA technique, Parker and colleagues (1998) have shown that in theory, imaging with a TR of 7 to 10 msec (e.g., scan time approximately 1 minute per 3D volume) and a T1 relaxation time of 25 to 50 msec for flowing blood containing gadolinium (first-pass arterial concentration of approximately 5-10 mM) can produce images of the intracranial arteries ($\approx$0.5 mm diameter) with vascular contrast comparable to that produced by the steady-state 3D CE-MRA technique. Dynamic 3D CE-MRA may play a prominent future role in evaluating intracranial arterial steno-occlusive disease, but the accuracy, reproducibility, and reliability of CE-MRA measurements compared with those of DSA and TOF-MRA warrant further delineation.

SUBCLAVIAN STEAL SYNDROME

Subclavian steal syndrome describes the reversal of normal direction of flow in the vertebral artery ipsilateral to a severe stenosis or occlusion occurring between the aortic arch and vertebral artery origin. DSA remains the standard in

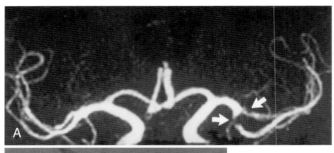

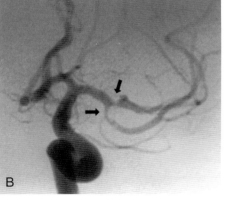

Fig. 33B.16 Proximal middle cerebral artery (MCA) stenosis (same patient as in **Fig. 33B.4**). **A,** Coronal projection magnetic resonance angiogram was produced from the axial source images shown in **Fig. 33B.4**. Coronal view shows better than the axial view (**Fig. 33B.4,** C) that there is stenosis *(arrows)* involving both M2 branches of the MCA. **B,** Catheter angiography confirms the presence of both stenoses *(arrows)*.

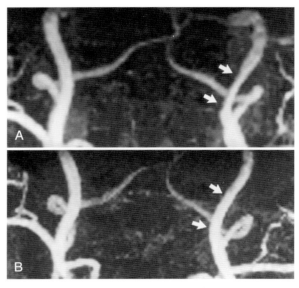

Fig. 33B.14 Resolution of carotid dissection followed with magnetic resonance angiography (MRA). **A,** MRA produced by the three-dimensional time-of-flight technique shows a segmental stenosis *(arrows)* involving the distal cervical portion of the left internal carotid artery. **B,** Repeat study obtained after anticoagulant therapy demonstrates return to normal caliber of the internal carotid artery segment *(arrows)*.

Fig. **33B.15** Stent device in the distal left vertebral artery. **A,** Coronal time-of-flight magnetic resonance image demonstrates loss of enhancement in the distal portion of the stent placement, suggesting a severe stenosis. **B,** Axial images of the neck after contrast administration is unable to accurately determine the degree of residual luminal narrowing. Widening the window settings results in overestimation of stenosis, and a later digital subtraction angiography demonstrated only mild stenosis.

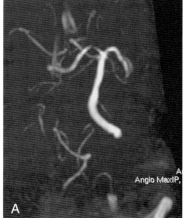

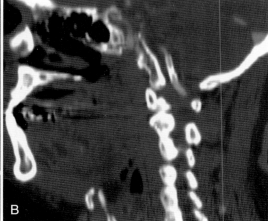

visualizing disease in the great vessels, along with abnormal retrograde filling of the affected vertebral artery. Given the invasive nature of DSA, Doppler sonography is often used, but this study may be limited by lack of visualization of the relevant pathology in the subclavian artery. Therefore, MRA offers a reliable comprehensive means to test patients with suspected subclavian steal syndrome. PC-MRA methods encode direction of flow and can accurately depict subclavian stenosis along with reversal of flow in the vertebral artery. Although TOF-MRA does not possess true flow-encoded information, flow direction can be deduced with suppression of flow from a single direction by a saturation pulse that allows for selective arterial or venous MRI, with reversal of flow presenting as a flow void. This finding may also be seen with severe stenosis or occlusion but may be distinguished by anatomical imaging of vessel patency, such as with 3D CE-MRA. A 3D CE-MRA has a potential disadvantage in the lone evaluation of subclavian steal syndrome, because it does not possess inherent flow-encoded information. However, the low-resolution 2D TOF localizer acquisition that is often performed beforehand has been shown to provide the same information as a formal TOF-MRA sequence (Sheehy et al., 2005).

ACUTE ISCHEMIC STROKE

As advances are made in rapid MRI techniques, a novel application for MRA has been the use of this technique to potentially guide acute stroke intervention. In a study by Marks et al., patients with isolated MCA occlusion and early recanalization at TOF-MRA demonstrated more favorable clinical response than those with tandem ICA/MCA occlusion and early recanalization, among those treated with IV tissue plasminogen activator (tPA) 3 to 6 hours after symptom onset (Marks et al., 2008). The correlation of early angiographic findings with clinical outcomes in stroke has prompted further investigation into utilizing MRA as predictive instrument. The Boston Acute Stroke Imaging Scale (BASIS) was devised as a simple classification instrument to help predict outcomes in acute stroke. In this algorithm, patients are classified as having major stroke if they either demonstrate a proximal cerebral artery occlusion (distal intracranial ICA, proximal [M1 or M2] MCA, and/or basilar artery) or if large parenchymal acute ischemia is found on diffusion MRI or early CT imaging in the event no proximal cerebral artery occlusion is identified. All other circumstances are classified as a minor stroke by imaging. Using this classification, Torres-Mozqueda et al. found that a total of 71.4% of major stroke survivors and 15.4% of minor stroke survivors were discharged to a rehabilitation facility, whereas 14.3% and 79.2%, respectively, were discharged to home. The mean length of hospitalization was 12.3 days for major stroke and 3.3 days for minor stroke. Prospective validation of the BASIS classification instrument, along with future investigations examining dynamic MRA changes, remain promising potential uses of MRA for guidance of stroke treatment (Torres-Mozqueda et al., 2008).

CEREBRAL ANEURYSMS

Three-dimensional TOF-MRA is now readily accepted as a noninvasive screening tool for familial aneurysmal disease. It has also been used as an alternative to DSA for the surgical management of patients with ruptured aneurysms. A review of the relevant literature for 1988 to 1998 found that TOF-MRA

(and CTA) depicted aneurysms with an accuracy of about 90% (White et al., 2000). Sensitivity was much greater for detection of aneurysms larger than 3 mm (94%) than for detection of aneurysms 3 mm or smaller (38%). Diagnostic accuracy was similar for anterior and posterior circulation aneurysms (**Fig. 33B.17**). In general, noninvasive imaging evaluation includes a review of T1- and T2-weighted (fast) spin-echo images and T2*-weighted gradient echo images, in addition to the source images and MIP images from the MRA acquisition.

The role of 3D TOF-MRA in assessing intracranial aneurysms before endovascular treatment is adjunctive to the definitive DSA study (Adams et al., 2000). Based on a composite assessment that included aneurysm detection rate, aneurysm morphology, neck interpretation, and branch vessel relationship to the aneurysm, Adams and colleagues found MRA to be inferior to DSA overall and to have missed aneurysms smaller than 3 mm. Nevertheless, MRA provided complementary information to DSA in anatomically complex areas or in the presence of intramural thrombus. The authors applied the assessment to four different types of image data display: axial source images, multiplanar reconstruction (MPR) of the source image data, MIP images, and 3D isosurface-rendered images. Among these types of images, the MPR and 3D isosurface-rendered images were comparable to the DSA images in all categories of the composite assessment, whereas the MIP images scored poorly in all categories except aneurysm detection. These findings indicate that better noninvasive characterization of aneurysms with TOF-MRA can be achieved by adding MPR or 3D isosurface-rendered images to the source and MIP images that are now routinely reviewed in clinical practice.

Endovascularly coiled intracranial aneurysms are increasingly being followed with MRA imaging to detect aneurysm recurrences, although the data remain mixed regarding its accuracy (**Fig. 33B.18**). One meta-analysis evaluated 16 studies that compared 1.5T TOF-MRA and 1.5T CE-MRA with DSA in the follow-up of coiled intracranial aneurysms. Pooled sensitivity and specificity of TOF-MRA for the detection of residual flow within the aneurysmal neck or body were 83.3% and 90.6%, respectively. Pooled sensitivity and specificity of CE-MRA for the detection of residual flow were 86.8% and 91.9%, respectively, but were not found to be significantly different. The included studies were of moderate methodological quality, and all pooled estimates were subject to heterogeneity (Kwee and Kwee, 2007). A prospective analysis was performed to compare TOF-MRA and CE-MRA at 1.5T and 3T to a reference standard of DSA in the evaluation of previously coiled intracranial aneurysms. For the detection of any aneurysm remnant, the sensitivity was 90%, 85%, 88%, and 90% for 1.5T TOF, 1.5T CE, 3T TOF, and 3T CE-MRA, respectively. These sensitivities dropped to 50%, 67%, 50%, and 67%, respectively, for the detection of only larger (class 3 and 4) aneurysm remnants, because several of these remnants were underclassified as a smaller remnant by MRA. CE-MRA at 1.5T and 3T had a better sensitivity for larger remnants than TOF-MRA, which may be related to greater flow-related artifacts within larger aneurysm remnants on TOF-MRA compared with the luminal contrast-filling characteristics of aneurysms on CE-MRA. Specificities of these four MRA techniques for detecting any aneurysm remnant were 52%, 65%, 52%, and 64%, respectively. Specificities improved to 85%,

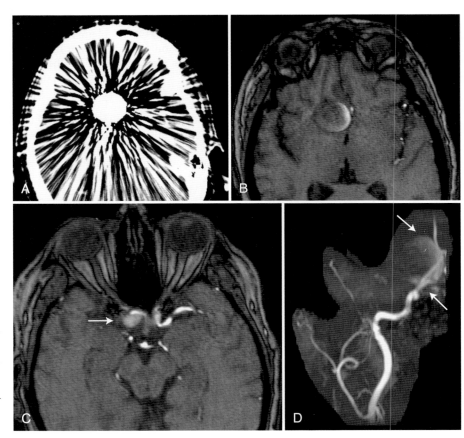

Fig. 33B.17 Anterior communicating artery aneurysm. **A,** A three-dimensional time-of-flight magnetic resonance angiogram (3D TOF-MRA) on 1.5T reveals a lobulated, saccular aneurysm arising from the junction of the A1 and A2 segments. **B,** Digital subtraction angiogram (DSA) prior to coil embolization also demonstrates this anterosuperiorly directed aneurysm.

Fig. 33B.18 Right ophthalmic artery aneurysm following coil embolization. **A,** Computed tomographic angiography source image non-diagnostic for residual lumen due to streak artifacts. **B,** Three-dimensional time-of-flight magnetic resonance angiogram (3D TOF-MRA) axial source image at level of aneurysm dome reveals central and eccentric hypodensity due to packed coils and peripheral hyperintensity due to flow-related enhancement in residual lumen. **C,** 3D TOF-MRA axial source image at level of aneurysm neck also shows evidence of flow through patent neck remnant *(arrow)*. **D,** Coronal maximum-intensity projection image demonstrates continuity of flow into neck and dome remnants of coiled aneurysm *(arrows)*. *(From Bowen, B.C., 2007. MR angiography versus CT angiography in the evaluation of neurovascular disease. Radiology 245, 357-361.)*

84%, 85%, and 87%, respectively, for the detection of larger (class 3 and 4) aneurysm remnants, reflecting the difficulty in detecting smaller remnants with MRA. Regarding the detection of any aneurysm growth since previous comparison angiograms, sensitivities for these MRA techniques were 28%, 28%, 33%, and 39%, respectively, and specificities were 93%, 95%, 98%, and 95%. Although CE-MRA is more likely than TOF-MRA to classify larger aneurysm remnants appropriately, TOF-MRA better identifies the location of coil masses and may be more advantageous if suboptimal CE-MRA contrast bolus is given. Therefore, the advantage of CE-MRA over TOF-MRA remains uncertain and consideration for both

exams may be made in the follow-up of patients with coiled intracranial aneurysms (Kaufmann et al., 2010).

VENOUS DISORDERS

Imaging of the cerebral venous system differs from approaches tailored to the arterial system because of the lower velocity of venous flow and the morphology of the venous sinuses. For suspected dural sinus occlusion resulting from thrombosis or tumor invasion, the primary technique is 2D TOF-MRA in conjunction with spin-echo imaging. To establish the diagnosis of venous thrombosis, lack of visualization of a vein or sinus on the source images and angiogram must be

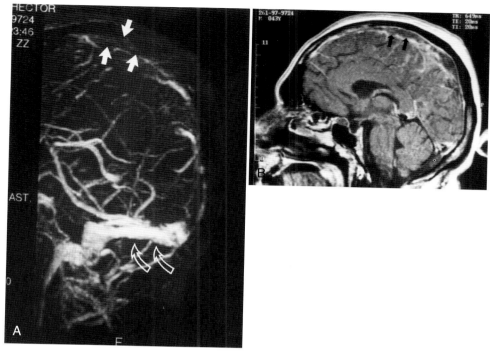

Fig. 33B.19 Acute superior sagittal sinus thrombosis. **A,** Magnetic resonance angiogram (lateral view) produced from 80 sequential two-dimensional time-of-flight coronal sections covering posterior half of the head. Flow-related signal is observed in transverse *(open arrows)* and sigmoid sinuses but not in superior sagittal sinus *(closed arrows)* or straight sinus. Short segments of vessels projecting over posterior course of superior sagittal sinus represent patent superficial cerebral veins lateral to the sinus. **B,** Postgadolinium midsagittal T1-weighted image shows hypointense signal in superior sagittal sinus and enhancing margins. Combined with the results in **A,** findings are consistent with the presence of intraluminal thrombus.

accompanied by identification of the clot on the spin-echo images at the location of the suspected occlusion (**Fig. 33B.19**). With the 2D TOF technique, optimal flow enhancement in a section is achieved when it is perpendicular to the flow direction. This condition is best approximated using coronal sections to image the sagittal, straight, and transverse sinuses (as well as the internal cerebral veins, basal veins of Rosenthal, and to a lesser degree, the vein of Galen). The acquisition of coronal sections can be augmented by the acquisition of oblique sagittal sections to allow better flow enhancement in the posterior portions of the transverse sinuses and the cortical veins draining into the superior sagittal sinus. With the 2D TOF-MR venography technique, arterial signal is reduced or eliminated by an axial presaturation band placed across the upper neck below the skull base. A common diagnostic pitfall of the technique is the presence of flow gaps in the transverse sinus. Ayanzen and colleagues (2000) observed these gaps in 31% of patients with normal MRI findings. Flow gaps were not observed in the superior sagittal, straight, or dominant transverse sinuses, so gaps occurring in these locations should raise suspicion of venous obstruction. The authors found that the nondominant transverse sinuses (90% of gaps) or codominant transverse sinuses (10%) that demonstrated the flow gaps were hypoplastic yet patent by DSA.

Alternative techniques for demonstrating cerebral veins and dural venous sinuses lack the robustness of the 2D TOF technique. The 3D TOF technique suffers from saturation effects and hence frequent signal loss in the veins and dural sinuses. The 2D phase-contrast technique is limited by gradient heterogeneity, eddy currents, aliasing artifacts, and lower

spatial resolution. Although the phase-contrast technique can be useful in differentiating very slow flow in the dural sinuses from thrombosis, it was recently found to be inferior to the 2D TOF technique and a contrast-enhanced 3D FLASH (fast low-angle shot) MRA technique in displaying the normal septal veins, internal cerebral veins, and the basal veins (Kirchhof et al., 2002). Both the 3D FLASH technique and a 3D magnetization-prepared, rapid-acquisition gradient echo MRI technique (Liang et al., 2001) are contrast-enhanced methods and reportedly are superior to the 2D TOF technique in depicting normal venous structures, especially in overcoming the flow gap artifact. These contrast-enhanced techniques, though, have two potential limitations: (1) both techniques involve rapid acquisition (1-2 minutes per 3D volume), so the intensity of the intravascular signal depends on the timing of the contrast infusion relative to data acquisition, and (2) chronic thrombus may enhance with gadolinium and mimic a patent lumen. Consequently, these two contrast-enhanced techniques should be viewed as adjuncts to the 2D TOF technique.

VASCULAR MALFORMATIONS

Traditional MRA methods (2D and 3D TOF and PC-MRA) have played a secondary role to DSA in evaluating intracranial arteriovenous malformations (AVMs) because of a lack of consistent and complete demonstration of all components of an AVM: feeding arteries, nidus, and draining veins. For this reason, and because of the general impression that TOF-MRA adds little to the spin-echo MRI findings useful for preliminary staging of an AVM (nidus size and location and central versus

Table 33B.1 **Spetzler-Martin Grading System***					
Lesion Size		**Location**		**Venous Drainage**	
Small (<3 cm)	1	Non-eloquent site	0	Superficial only	0
Medium (3-6 cm)	2	Eloquent site[†]	1	Any deep	1
Large (>6 cm)	3				

*Assigns cumulative points based on arteriovenous malformation characteristics, with higher scores indicating increased surgical risk.
[†]Eloquent areas include sensorimotor, language, visual, thalamus, hypothalamus, internal capsule, brainstem, cerebellar peduncles, and deep cerebellar nuclei.

peripheral pattern of venous drainage in the Spetzler-Martin Grading Scale) before definitive DSA, many investigators have considered TOF-MRA of AVMs superfluous (**Table 33B.1**). Phase-contrast techniques have been used by some investigators to estimate blood flow velocities and volume flow rates in the largest arteries supplying the AVM. A high-resolution 3D gradient echo technique based on the paramagnetic property of deoxyhemoglobin has been used to detect cerebral veins with submillimeter resolution, resulting in greater sensitivity in identifying the presence of small AVMs. But compared with TOF-MRA, the technique provides poorer detection of feeding arteries and is markedly limited in its delineation of nidus size and shape when there are susceptibility artifacts from nearby bone, air, or blood products (hemosiderin) (Essig et al., 1999). High-resolution, real-time, auto-triggered, elliptic, centric-ordered 3D CE-MRA (Farb et al., 2001) and lower-resolution time-resolved 2D CE-MRA (Klisch et al., 2000) have also been applied to the evaluation of AVMs and the results compared with those of TOF-MRA and intraarterial DSA. In an initial investigation, Farb and colleagues found that their 3D CE-MRA technique was superior to 3D TOF-MRA, particularly in depicting nidus and draining veins. The 3D CE-MRA technique consistently showed AVM components and their spatial relationships on MIP images and was equivalent to DSA in depicting AVM components in 70% to 90% of cases (total patients = 10), based on blinded independent assessments by two experienced neuroradiologists. Several small studies prospectively examined 4D CE-MRA at 3T for evaluating AVM and found that 4D CE-MRA yielded 100% accuracy in classifying Spetzler-Martin classification (nidus size, venous drainage, eloquence) of cerebral AVMs when compared to DSA. One study demonstrated a 93% rate of detection of feeding arteries using 4D MRA alone. However, the combined use of selective ASL provided additional functional or anatomical information in 4 of 16 cases (25%), enabling the detection of a cross-filling feeding artery that was not identified by 4D MRA without selective arterial spin labeling (ASL) technique, and improved sensitivity to 96% (Kukuk et al., 2010). These novel techniques may prove to be a noninvasive alternative to DSA in the assessment of patients with cerebral AVMs (Hadizadeh et al., 2008).

Dural arteriovenous fistulas (AVFs) most commonly involve the cavernous, transverse, and sigmoid sinuses along the skull base. Arterial feeders not seen on spin-echo MR sometimes are detected on 3D TOF-MRA but much less often than on catheter angiography. Transverse and sigmoid sinus occlusion and dilated cortical veins are detected better by MRA than spin-echo imaging, yet neither technique achieves the accuracy of catheter angiography. Traditional 3D TOF-MRA is useful in detecting cavernous sinus fistulas, because flow enhancement

in the cavernous sinus and contiguous veins can provide evidence of the fistula (**Fig. 33B.20**). This finding must be regarded with caution because venous flow signal has been observed in the cavernous sinus and inferior petrosal sinus in a variable percentage (from 4% to 36%, depending on unspecified technical differences between MR scanners) of patients without clinical evidence of carotid-cavernous fistula (Ouanounou et al., 1999). Farb et al. compared the use of 3T time-resolved MRA for the diagnosis and classification of a cranial dural AVF with DSA. Patients underwent a commercially available contrast-enhanced time-resolved imaging of contrast kinetics (TRICKS) MRA (trMRA) technique that combines k-space segmentation into central, mid, and peripheral zones with superimposed elliptic centric-view ordering. High temporal resolution is obtained by sampling the central zones of the k-space at a more frequent rate than peripheral zones. The high spatial and temporal resolution allows for identification of dural AVFs by identifying both early opacification of a dural sinus and reflux into the connecting cortical veins if present. In 93% (39/42) of dural AVF cases, investigators had unanimously correct interpretations of the trMRA to correctly identify or exclude all fistulas and accurately classify them when found. The small series suggests that trMRA may be a reliable technique in the screening and surveillance of DAVFs in certain clinical situations, but further validation studies are required (Farb et al., 2009).

The diagnostic imaging features of venous malformations (angiomas, developmental venous anomalies) are well shown on postgadolinium T1-weighted spin-echo images. These features include the radially oriented collection of small vessels (medullary veins) that produce a caput medusa or spoke-wheel configuration. This is contiguous with a large trunk vein that drains into either subependymal or superficial cerebral veins or a dural sinus. The 2D TOF technique and the phase-contrast method with low anticipated maximum blood flow velocity often display these slow-flow malformations without the use of gadolinium and allow determination of flow direction. However, the 3D TOF technique, which provides greater spatial resolution, requires gadolinium to avoid saturation effects. Cavernous malformations and capillary telangiectasias do not show flow enhancement on MRA studies, and the former usually are identified on spin-echo and gradient echo images by the heterogeneous signal intensity caused by blood products from prior hemorrhage.

Spine Disorders

Spinal MRA is used as an adjunct to MRI to improve the visibility of the millimeter-sized intradural vessels and to help differentiate abnormal from normal ones. The combined MR

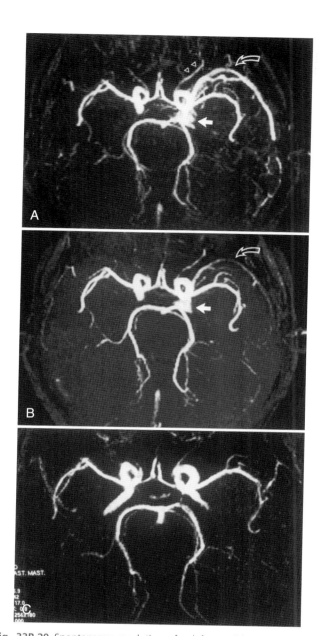

Fig. 33B.20 Spontaneous resolution of a left carotid-cavernous dural arteriovenous fistula (AVF). Magnetic resonance angiograms (axial maximum-intensity projection images) of sellar region and circle of Willis were acquired with three-dimensional time-of-flight technique (no gadolinium enhancement). The studies, performed at the time of clinical presentation **(A)**, 3 months later **(B)**, and 3 years later **(C)**, show progressive resolution of venous drainage from the AVF. Flow-related signal in left cavernous sinus *(closed arrow)*, sphenoparietal sinus *(open arrow)*, and cerebral veins results from shunting of high-flow-rate arterial blood through fistula. Note progressive decrease in signal in the sphenoparietal sinus. Flow-related signal in the left orbit is caused by the ophthalmic artery *(arrowheads)*, not the superior ophthalmic vein, which was found by catheter angiography to be thrombosed at the time of presentation.

examination provides better characterization of spinal vessels and thus more effective noninvasive screening for vascular lesions (e.g., dural AVFs) than MRI alone (Saraf-Lavi et al., 2002). The improved screening facilitates decisions regarding invasive catheter angiography for definitive diagnosis and

endovascular treatment. The combined MR examination also allows the largest normal vessels to be localized noninvasively before surgical or endovascular procedures that carry a risk of cord injury (Yamada et al., 2000).

Enhancement of the intradural vessels with gadolinium contrast agents has been found necessary for optimal detection on MRA. The 3D CE-MRA technique with steady-state conditions (i.e., TOF pulse sequence parameters) detects the largest intradural veins in healthy volunteers: the posterior and anterior median veins and the great medullary veins draining from the surface of the cord to the epidural space. This technique, and to a lesser extent the 3D phase-contrast technique, also detects the abnormally enlarged and tortuous veins draining dural AVFs (**Fig. 33B.21**) and intramedullary AVMs. In detecting the presence of dural AVFs, the steady-state 3D CE-MRA technique combined with spin-echo MRI had a sensitivity ranging from 80% to 100%, specificity of 82%, and accuracy of 81% to 94% in a randomized blinded review by 3 neuroradiologists of 11 control subjects and 20 patients with proven dural AVFs (Saraf-Lavi et al., 2002). More importantly, in determining the vertebral level of the fistula, the correct level was predicted in 73% of cases by combined MRA and MRI, representing a significant improvement over MRI alone. Improved noninvasive localization of the fistula level potentially expedites the subsequent invasive catheter angiography study. Preliminary studies of spinal vascular malformations using time-resolved or fast 3D CE-MRA indicate that such first-pass studies may provide better depiction of the dural AVF in the neural foramen because of diminished extradural venous enhancement and improved visibility of the feeding arteries of AVMs (Binkert et al., 1999). Studies have also shown that patients undergoing catheter angiography following MRA require half the fluoroscopy time and half the volume of iodinated contrast if the level and side of the fistula have been identified on screening MRA (Luetmer et al., 2005). MRA and CTA are reported to have similar sensitivities in screening for the level of the artery of Adamkiewicz (Yoshioka et al., 2003).

The use of 3T time-resolved spine MRA has been recently investigated for presurgical localization of the artery of Adamkiewicz prior to reimplantation of the feeding intercostal artery, lumbar artery, or both during aortic aneurysm repair. Bley et al. identified the artery of Adamkiewicz and the location of the feeding intercostal and/or lumbar artery with high confidence in 88% of cases (68 patients). The artery of Adamkiewicz and the anterior spinal artery were identified and differentiated from the great anterior radiculomedullary vein, even in patients with substantially altered hemodynamics from aortic disease (Bley et al., 2010).

Ultrasound

Methods

The physics and underlying methodology of ultrasound techniques used in clinical practice is an extensive topic that has been explained in detail elsewhere. Ultrasound studies are often reported in the relatively simplistic terms of flow-velocity measurements and associated diagnoses of steno-occlusive lesions in the cerebral circulation. Comprehending the physical basis of such findings may provide the clinician with an even greater appreciation for subtle findings and

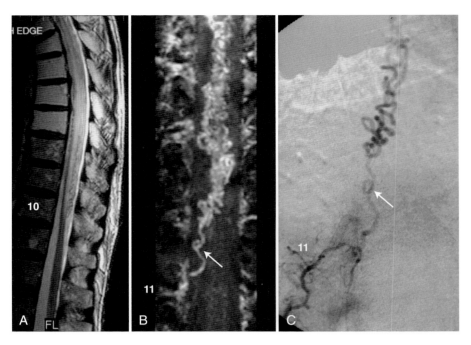

Fig. 33B.21 Spinal dural arteriovenous fistula (AVF). **A,** Sagittal T2-weighted fast-spin-echo image of thoracic spine shows hyperintensity of spinal cord and vertebra above T8, as well as serpentine "intradural flow voids" in a patient with a history of radiation therapy for lung carcinoma and progressive myelopathy. **B,** Coronal maximum-intensity projection image from three-dimensional steady-state contrast-enhanced magnetic resonance angiography of the same thoracic region reveals an enlarged, tortuous vessel *(arrow)* extending from approximately the right T11 foramen to abnormal vessels on the cord surface. Findings are typical for a dural AVF and are confirmed by subsequent catheter angiography **(C)**. Anteroposterior view **C** shows the enlarged vessel *(arrow)* to be the medullar vein draining from the fistula in the T11 foramen to the coronal venous plexus on the cord surface. *(From Bowen, B.C., 2007. MR angiography versus CT angiography in the evaluation of neurovascular disease. Radiology 245, 357-361.)*

insight on the strengths and limitations of these ultrasound techniques (Kremkau, 2006; Tegeler and Ratanakorn, 1999).

Most diagnostic ultrasound devices operate at frequencies of 2 to 10 MHz and evaluate acoustic properties of blood and tissue to obtain both hemodynamic and anatomical information for vessels. Transducers for Doppler ultrasonography, using a single element, may continuously transmit and receive (continuous-wave Doppler) acoustic information to accurately identify flow velocities or intermittently emit and receive a series of short pulses of sound (pulsed-wave Doppler) to sample a specific depth or a time window for recording. Many hemodynamic parameters are obtained, such as flow direction, peak systolic velocity, and end-diastolic flow velocity, as well as several indirect or derived parameters such as width or spread of the spectral band of velocities, flow acceleration time (systolic acceleration slope), pulsatility, and resistivity index. An embolic particle passing through the Doppler sample volume has acoustic impedance that can be distinguished from surrounding blood, resulting in transient high-intensity signals called *microembolic signals* (MES). Individual vessels also have characteristic spectral appearances primarily caused by distal peripheral resistance and specific spectral patterns, particularly very high- or low-resistance signals, and provide indirect clues about hemodynamics and potential pathological conditions both proximally and distally.

In brightness-mode (B-mode) imaging, the transducer is swept in a single plane to produce a 2D structural and anatomical display of a slice of tissue based on its acoustic properties (Tegeler et al., 2005). These are static images, but the image can be updated 15 to 30 times per second so that it appears to be moving in real time. Duplex ultrasonography makes use of both pulsed-wave Doppler ultrasound and B-mode imaging to obtain both hemodynamic and anatomical information (**Fig. 33B.22**). Color-flow imaging (CFI) uses Doppler flow-velocity information obtained from multiple sample volumes within the image, which is then color-coded based on the speed and direction of flow and overlaid onto

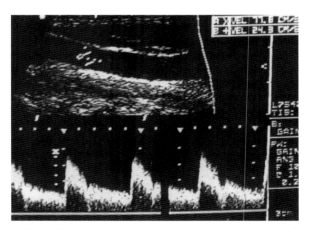

Fig. 33B.22 Duplex ultrasonography. Combined Doppler velocity spectral display and brightness-mode image-guided placement of the sample volume.

the appropriate anatomical site in the grayscale B-mode image (**Fig. 33B.23**) (Tegeler et al., 2005). Modern transducers for extracranial high-resolution B-mode carotid imaging operate at frequencies of 7.5 to 10.0 MHz, whereas those used for transcranial CFI operate at 2 to 3 MHz. Power Doppler imaging (PDI) is a variation of CFI that uses the integrated intensity or amplitude of power in the Doppler spectrum to provide information regarding the amount of blood flow detected at each point, rather than the mean velocity (Bluth et al., 2000; Griewing et al., 1996).

Techniques
Carotid Ultrasonography

Duplex examination of the carotid arteries must include Doppler flow-velocity sampling of the proximal, mid, and distal common carotid arteries (CCAs), proximal and distal

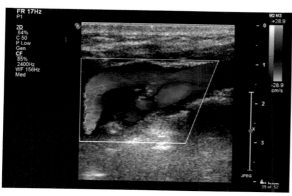

Fig. 33B.23 Color-flow imaging. Duplex color-flow imaging superimposes the color-coded velocity information onto the brightness-mode image of the carotid bifurcation, internal carotid artery, and external carotid artery.

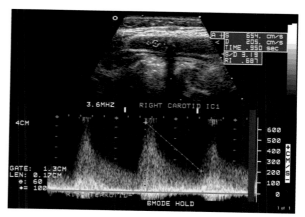

Fig. 33B.24 Doppler ultrasound with tight stenosis. Spectral display of duplex Doppler flow velocities suggesting 75% to 90% internal carotid artery stenosis, with high systolic (654 cm/sec) and diastolic velocities (205 cm/sec) and spectral broadening.

ICAs, and the ECAs bilaterally. The proximal great vessels (innominate and subclavian arteries) are also studied if they can be visualized. If disease is detected, additional Doppler sampling of the vessel proximal to, at the point of, and distal to the stenosis should be included. Sampling should be across the entire vessel diameter to avoid missing a high-velocity jet along the vessel wall. Sampling should be done using a standard angle of insonation, or at least within a standard range of angles. Most sonographers try to sample at a 60-degree angle, but any angle between 45 and 60 degrees is acceptable. Enough of the study should be videotaped to allow review of both the spectral display and the audible signals from all target vessels or regions of abnormality. Transducer frequencies for Doppler interrogation usually are between 4.0 and 7.5 MHz.

Because of predictable hemodynamic changes as stenosis develops, duplex Doppler ultrasound can be used to estimate the severity of stenosis. Very mild degrees of stenosis have little hemodynamic effect and cause little change in flow velocity or in the Doppler spectral waveform. Progressive stenosis first causes increased peak-systolic velocity across the narrowed segment. Additional narrowing causes further increase in the peak-systolic velocity and a disturbed flow pattern, or *turbulence*, emerges (**Fig. 33B.24**). Severe stenosis prevents adequate blood-flow volume across the lesion, even though the peak-systolic and end-diastolic velocity values are both increased. In very tight carotid stenosis approaching occlusion, peak-systolic and end-diastolic velocity values may increase even further or may begin to decrease as critical narrowing is reached.

These changes in velocity and pattern of flow are used to estimate the severity of stenosis. Most criteria used for interpretation are based primarily on the peak-systolic velocity, end-diastolic velocity, and ratios of velocities in the ICA and CCA. The ratio of velocities is helpful because the velocity in the stenotic segment remains high when compared to the velocity proximal or distal to the stenosis, even when cardiac dysfunction exists. Any set of criteria should serve as a guideline for interpretation of velocity data and should not be considered as hard inflexible rules. Interpreters also must consider the overall clinical picture in every patient and exercise judgment and flexibility in reaching conclusions. Current ultrasound laboratories should strive for an accuracy of approximately 90% for identification of tight carotid

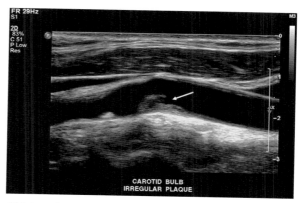

Fig. 33B.25 Atherosclerotic plaque. Longitudinal B-mode image of an atherosclerotic plaque in the region of the carotid bifurcation and proximal internal carotid artery, with possible crater formation (arrow).

stenosis, as documented by a program of ongoing quality assurance.

High-resolution carotid B-mode real-time imaging should be done with transducers having frequencies greater than 5 MHz and preferably exceeding 7 MHz. Imaging should include visualization of the CCA, CCA bifurcation, ICA, ECA (including anterior, lateral, posterior, and transverse views), or a circumferential scan at each level to include all of these views. Real-time recording of these images allows study of pulsation patterns and movement of intimal flaps or complex plaques. Measurements of the plaque thickness and residual lumen are performed frequently. Plaque severity can be classified by thickness, with minimal (1.1-2.0 mm), moderate (2.1-4.0 mm), and severe (>4.0 mm) categories. The posterolateral approach is usually optimal for measurements of plaque formation and residual lumen because plaques most often occur on the posterior wall of the carotid bifurcation and ICA, and B-mode imaging is most accurate when the sound beam is at 90 degrees to the interface being imaged.

High-resolution B-mode imaging also has a unique ability to evaluate the specific features of atherosclerotic plaques (**Fig. 33B.25**) (Tegeler et al., 2005). Identifiable characteristics include the distribution of plaque (concentric, eccentric, length), surface features (smooth, irregular, crater), echodensity and presence of any calcification producing acoustic shadowing, and texture (homogeneous, heterogeneous, or intraplaque hemorrhage). The presence of hypoechoic plaques and the presence of plaques that are quite heterogeneous with prominent hypoechoic regions (complex plaque) identify an increased risk of stroke (Polak et al., 1998). High-resolution B-mode imaging is more accurate than Doppler ultrasound testing for defining atherosclerosis of the vessel wall early in the course of the disease. Measurement of the intima-media thickness, which increases in the early stages of plaque formation, has been correlated with risk of cardiovascular disease and is used as a surrogate endpoint for clinical trials assessing whether lipid-lowering medications might slow or reverse atherosclerosis (Polak, 2005). The sensitivity of B-mode imaging for detection of surface ulceration is approximately 77% in plaques causing less than 50% linear stenosis and 41% for plaques causing more than 50% linear stenosis, with no significant differences between B-mode carotid imaging and arteriography. Although associated with a somewhat worse outcome, surface irregularity or crater formation appears to be a less important morphological risk factor than echodensity and heterogeneity.

Advantages of CFI include rapid determination of the presence and direction of blood flow, with more accurate placement of the Doppler sample volume and determination of the angle of insonation. Absence of color filling in what appears to be the vessel lumen provides clues about the presence of a hypoechoic plaque, and the contour of the color column can provide information about surface features. If a crater or ulcer is open to the lumen, color further details the surface architecture. Newer instruments with sensitive CFI designed to detect very low flow velocities are able to accurately differentiate critical stenosis from total occlusion (87%-100% sensitivity, 84% specificity versus angiography), negating the need for conventional angiography (Sitzer et al., 1996). The addition of CFI improves understanding of many unusual anatomical configurations such as kinks or coils. Although difficult to quantify accurately, CFI probably adds approximately 5% to the overall diagnostic accuracy of carotid duplex ultrasound.

The addition of PDI offers more potential to improve accuracy in some difficult situations. In the setting of high-grade stenosis, PDI improves identification of stenosis and measurement of residual lumen and may improve visualization of plaque surface features, even in the presence of calcification.

Conventional criteria for reporting carotid stenosis use flow velocity to estimate the linear percent stenosis. However, increased flow velocity may be seen in other conditions such as a hyperperfusion state seen in anemia that might be misconstrued as stenosis. To avoid such mistakes, various methods have been devised to evaluate volume flow rate in the extracranial cerebral vessels. Processing techniques such as color velocity imaging quantification (CVI-Q) may be implemented, and normal volume flow rate values (330 mL/minute for women and 375 mL/minute for men) have been defined. Use of the CCA volume flow rate in patients with carotid stenosis reveals characteristic decreases in the rate with progressive stenosis. In some laboratories, measurement of CCA volume flow rate is a standard part of the carotid evaluation for patients whose flow velocity suggests 75% or greater carotid stenosis (**Fig. 33B.26**); this technique may better delineate hemodynamic changes (Knappertz et al., 1996; Tan et al.,

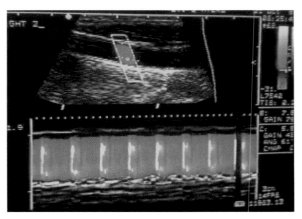

Fig. 33B.26 Volume flow rate. Measurement of volume flow rate using color velocity imaging quantification with a color M-mode display of the flow velocities across the common carotid artery and tracking of the vessel diameter. Flow volume is in milliliters per minute.

2002). There appears to be an acceptable correlation between results of CVI-Q and Doppler-based methods (Likittanasombut et al., 2006), and diminished extracranial cerebral volume flow rate may identify increased risk for recurrent stroke (Han et al., 2006).

The optimal noninvasive imaging method for determining severity of carotid artery stenosis remains uncertain. MRA and CTA are being used with rapidly increasing frequency to determine the degree of stenosis. Although duplex carotid ultrasound should not be used as the sole method for definitive diagnosis of carotid disease, this inexpensive imaging technique remains a valid screening tool. A systematic review of published studies comparing carotid ultrasound with DSA showed that for distinguishing severe stenosis (70%-99%), duplex carotid ultrasound had a pooled sensitivity of 86% and a pooled specificity of 87%. For recognizing occlusion, duplex carotid ultrasound had a sensitivity of 96% and a specificity of 100% (Nederkorn, van der Graaf, Hunink, 2003). Another study found high concordance rates among CTA, contrast-enhanced MRA, and ultrasound for patients with asymptomatic carotid stenosis (Nonent et al., 2004). However, a study comparing ultrasound and MRA to DSA determined that ultrasound alone would have misassigned 28% of patients to receive carotid endarterectomy, whereas ultrasound combined with CE-MRA reduced this misassignment rate to 17% (Johnston et al., 2000).

Vertebral Ultrasonography

Because posterior circulation cerebrovascular disease is quite common, study of the vertebral arteries is considered part of the routine extracranial duplex ultrasound examination. The same techniques described for use in the carotid arteries can be used to study the vertebral arteries and the proximal subclavian or innominate arteries. As such, there should be duplex Doppler and B-mode imaging of these arterial segments. CFI is also helpful for identification and interrogation of the vertebral arteries. The vertebral artery can virtually always be evaluated in the pretransverse and intertransverse cervical segment of C5-C6, whereas the origin can be studied only on the right in 81% and on the left in 65% of cases. Because there is mostly a low-resistance distal vascular bed, the vertebral artery usually shows a low-resistance Doppler spectral pattern similar to that seen with the ICA. Unlike the carotid arteries, there are no widely accepted criteria for stenosis in the extracranial vertebral artery. As with the carotid system, spectral analysis provides insight into proximal and distal disease. Another confounding factor is contralateral occlusive disease, associated with increased carotid volume flow which may result in an overestimation of the severity of stenosis. Given the variable factors associated with carotid duplex sonography, it has been recommended that each laboratory validate its own Doppler criteria for clinically relevant stenosis and undergo certification by an independent organization such as the Intersocietal Commission for Accreditation of Vascular Laboratories Essentials and Standards for Accreditation in Noninvasive Vascular Testing. Studies have shown that the accuracy of duplex ultrasound examination is much better from accredited versus nonaccredited laboratories (Latchaw et al., 2009).

Transcranial Doppler Ultrasonography

Most commercially available TCD ultrasonography instruments use a low-frequency 2-MHz probe to allow insonation through the cranium. These pulsed-wave Doppler instruments have an effective insonation depth range of 3.0 to 12.0 cm or more that can be evaluated by increments of 2 or 5 mm. At an insonation depth of 50 mm, the sample volume is usually 8 to 10 mm axially and 5 mm laterally. TCD probes also differ from the 4- to 10-MHz transducers used to monitor the progress of intraoperative neurosurgical procedures (Unsgaard et al., 2002). Advantages of TCD include the maneuverability of the relatively small probes, the Doppler sensitivity, and—compared to transcranial color-coded duplex and MRA—the relatively low price of instruments.

Routine TCD testing relies on three natural acoustic windows to study the basal segments of the main cerebral arteries. Insonation through the temporal bone window allows detection of flow through the MCA M1 segment and the anterior cerebral artery A1 segment. Normal blood flow direction is toward the probe in the MCA and away from it in the anterior cerebral artery. The supraclinoid ICA is also detected but may occasionally be difficult to distinguish from the MCA. Depending on the position of the window, the probe usually has to be tilted frontally to detect these vessels. A posterior (or occipital) tilt of the probe enables insonation of the PCAs. The occipital window takes advantage of the foramen magnum's opening into the skull. Flow in the distal vertebral artery and proximal to mid-portions of the basilar artery can be detected; its direction is away from the probe in these arterial segments. A considerable degree of natural variation occurs in the position and caliber of these arteries, making insonation occasionally difficult. The ophthalmic artery and carotid siphon can be studied through the orbital window. Flow in the ophthalmic artery is toward the probe and has a high resistance pattern. Flow in the ICA siphon can be either toward or away from the probe, depending on the insonated segment. The power output of the instrument must be decreased when insonating through the orbital window, because prolonged exposure to high-intensity ultrasound has been associated with cataract formation.

Flow velocities change with age and differ among men and women. Normal values are available. Repeated measurements of flow velocities are highly reproducible. Thus, based on the general knowledge of the location of intracranial arteries and flow direction, a comprehensive map of the basal arteries can be generated. This map is clinically useful because common pathological conditions affecting the intracranial arteries (e.g., atherosclerosis, sickle cell disease, vasospasm associated with aneurysmal subarachnoid hemorrhage) often affect arterial segments that can be insonated. Convexity branches of the cerebral arteries are beyond the reach of TCD.

Transcranial Color-Coded Duplex Ultrasonography

Examinations performed with 2.25-MHz phased array and 2.5-MHz 90-degree sector transducers enable color-coded imaging of intracranial arterial blood flow in red and blue, respectively, indicating flow toward and away from the probe. The main advantages of transcranial color-coded duplex (TCCD) ultrasonography are the ability to visualize and positively identify the insonated vessel, thus increasing the ultrasonographer's confidence and the ability to correct for the angle of insonation. In addition, TCCD provides a limited B-mode image of intracranial structures.

Applications
Acute Ischemic Stroke

Transcranial Doppler studies obtained within hours from the onset of symptoms of stroke in the carotid territory may reveal stenosis or occlusion of the distal intracranial ICA or proximal MCA in 70% of patients. When compared with DSA, TCD is more than 85% sensitive and specific in detecting supraclinoid ICA or MCA M1 segment lesions. The use of contrast-enhanced color-coded duplex sonography can be especially useful in this context. The use of TCD in the early hours of stroke may also provide important prognostic information. Patency of the MCA by TCD testing within 6 hours of the onset of stroke symptoms is an independent predictor of better outcome (Allendoerfer et al., 2006).

Transcranial Doppler can also help in monitoring the effect of thrombolytic agents. Testing before and after the administration of streptokinase or tPA can assess the agent's efficacy in obtaining arterial patency and ascertain continued patency during the days after treatment (Yasaka et al., 1998). In addition, investigators have adjusted the dosage and duration of IV thrombolytic agent administration based on information provided by continuous TCD monitoring. Rapid arterial recanalization is associated with better short-term improvement (Alexandrov et al., 2001). Continuous TCD insonation during IV thrombolysis and for 1 hour thereafter significantly increases the rate of recanalization or improvement in the stroke severity score (Alexandrov et al., 2004). The addition of microbubbles during this period of monitoring may further improve the results. Ultrasound energy has been observed to accelerate enzymatic fibrinolysis, possibly by allowing increased transport of drug molecules into the clot and promoting the motion of fluid throughout the thrombus. This observation has led to studies that allow for real-time monitoring of vessel recanalization while potentially providing additional therapeutic benefit from the ultrasound energy. Studies have demonstrated that IV tPA combined with continuous TCD safely increased recanalization rates and produced a trend toward better functional outcomes compared with IV tPA alone. Other small trials demonstrated an improvement in clot lysis when TCCD was combined with IV tPA. In one small study of patients with acute M1 MCA occlusions, 1.8-MHz pulsed-wave ultrasound combined with IV tPA demonstrated higher recanalization rates than patients who received IV tPA alone (58% versus 22%). However, 16% developed a symptomatic intracranial hemorrhage compared to 6% in the non-ultrasound group (Eggers et al., 2008). Another study using ultrasound-mediated thrombolysis found a 36% rate of symptomatic ICH when IV tPA was administered with a 300-kHz therapeutic ultrasound. These studies highlight the need to determine minimum and safe amounts of ultrasound energy necessary to enhance thrombolysis (Rubiera and Alexandrov, 2010). One meta-analysis looking at various ultrasound technologies found that the rate of symptomatic ICH was 3.8% in the IV tPA plus TCD group, 11.1% in the IV tPA plus TCCD group, 35.7% in the IV tPA plus low-frequency ultrasound group, and 2.9% in the IV tPA–alone group. Complete recanalization rates were higher in patients receiving a combination of TCD with IV tPA compared to patients treated with IV tPA alone (37.2% versus 17.2%) (Tsivgoulis et al., 2010). Administration of microbubbles using Perflutren lipid microspheres remains under investigation and may transmit energy momentum from an ultrasound wave to residual flow to promote further recanalization, thereby enhancing the effect of ultrasound on thrombolysis (Alexandrov et al., 2008; Molina et al., 2009). Additional operator-independent devices, different microbubble-related techniques, and other means of improving sonothrombolysis are currently being studied in clinical trials.

Transcranial power motion–mode Doppler (PMD-TCD) is a technique that along with spectral information simultaneously displays real-time flow signal intensity and direction over 6 cm of intracranial space. One study compared PMD-TCD with CTA and found a sensitivity of 81.8% and specificity of 94% for detecting an acute arterial occlusion. The sensitivity for detecting MCA occlusions was 95.6%, and the specificity was 96.2%. For the anterior circulation, PMD-TCD demonstrated a sensitivity of 100% and specificity of 94.5%. For the posterior circulation, sensitivity was 57.1%, and specificity was 100% (Brunser et al., 2009).

Recent Transient Ischemic Attack or Stroke

Compared to other available methods, ultrasound testing offers a safe, accurate, noninvasive, and less expensive method to evaluate for extracranial cerebrovascular disease. It is considered the initial test of choice for identifying significant carotid stenosis in patients with recent transient ischemic attack (TIA) or stroke (Tegeler and Ratanakorn, 1998). For the carotid territory, this should include duplex ultrasonography, with or without CFI. Reports should address the severity of stenosis based on Doppler flow-velocity measurements. There also must be information provided about the presence of any plaque, as well as the morphology, based on high-resolution B-mode imaging. Additional helpful ultrasound tools include PDI and volume flow rate measurement. Results of carotid ultrasound testing must then be integrated with

other available testing modalities if additional information is needed. At present, this often means a combination of ultrasound and MRA or CTA, with DSA reserved for those in whom results of the preceding tests are technically inadequate, equivocal, or contradictory. The combination of ultrasound and MRA is more cost-effective than the use of routine DSA in this setting. However, the best algorithm for evaluation may vary depending on the services and expertise available at each medical center.

MCA or basilar artery occlusion is associated with an absence or severe reduction of Doppler signal at the appropriate depth of insonation at a time when signals from the other ipsilateral basal cerebral arteries are detectable. Follow-up studies often show spontaneous recanalization of previously occluded segments. The latter can be detected within hours from the onset of symptoms, the majority of symptomatic occlusions being recanalized within 2 days and followed by a period of hyperperfusion.

Collateral flow patterns associated with severe cervical carotid stenosis or occlusion can also be detected by TCD. They include retrograde flow of the ophthalmic artery and anterior or posterior communicating artery flow toward the hemisphere distal to the stenosed or occluded ICA. Among patients with symptomatic carotid occlusions, one study found that compared with DSA, TCD detection of collateral flow via the major intracerebral collateral branches had a sensitivity of 82% and a specificity of 79% in the anterior portion of the circle of Willis. In the posterior communicating artery, TCD demonstrated a sensitivity of 76% and a specificity of 47% (Hendrikse et al., 2008). Lesions causing stenosis of the V4 segment of the vertebral artery and the proximal basilar artery can be imaged by TCD. Focal increases of the peak-systolic and mean velocities to 120 cm/sec and 80 cm/sec or more, respectively, at depths of insonation corresponding to these arterial segments are considered significant. Velocities often exceed 200 cm/sec with lesions causing more than 50% stenosis. Compared to DSA, the sensitivity of TCD is approximately 75% in detecting vertebrobasilar stenotic lesions, and its specificity exceeds 85%. Frequent variation in the size and course of the vertebrobasilar trunk and its contribution of collateral flow to the anterior cerebral circulation are the main reasons for these relatively low figures. Contrast media and TCCD imaging can be particularly helpful in this setting (Stolz et al., 2002).

Microembolic signals detected by TCD correspond to gaseous microbubbles or emboli composed of platelets, fibrinogen, or cholesterol moving in intracranial arteries. Such MES can be detected spontaneously or with provocative stimuli such as the Valsalva maneuver.

In patients with extracranial carotid disease, these signals are associated with a history of recent TIAs or cerebral infarction in the distribution of the insonated artery, and they correlate with the presence of ipsilateral severe stenosis and plaque ulceration. They are detected mainly during the week following symptoms of cerebral ischemia and resolve afterward. MES also can be detected in subjects with cardiac prosthetic valves but often correspond to gaseous microbubbles in that setting. They are less common in adequately anticoagulated patients with atrial fibrillation. The clinical impact of microembolus detection studies remains limited at this time. The presence of these signals in an arterial territory is useful in identifying proximal "active" lesions. This is especially relevant when a symptomatic patient has more than one potential lesion, such as cervical carotid stenosis and atrial fibrillation, or a suboptimal history. In this situation, laboratory data can help identify the specific cause of cerebral infarction. In addition, because the presence of MES is predictive of future cerebral ischemic events in the insonated artery's territory (Markus et al., 2005), detecting these signals may affect therapeutic decisions. In the future, microembolus detection studies may be useful in monitoring the effect of antithrombotic agents (Junghans and Siebler, 2003). Microemboli monitoring is also of interest in the context of CEA and coronary artery bypass graft surgery. MES have been reported in 43% of patients with symptomatic carotid stenosis and 10% of patients with asymptomatic carotid stenosis. MES were reported in 25% of symptomatic versus 0% of patients with asymptomatic intracranial stenosis. In patients with cervical artery dissection presenting with TIA or stroke, 50% had MES, compared to 13% with local symptoms. Among patients with aortic embolism, patients with plaques 4 mm or larger demonstrated MES more frequently than patients with smaller plaques. MES has been shown to be useful for risk stratification in patients with carotid stenosis, but data from published studies remain insufficient to reliably predict future events in patients with intracranial stenosis, cervical artery dissection, and aortic embolism (Ritter et al., 2008).

Extracranial Stenotic Lesions

Ultrasound remains a safe and noninvasive method to monitor patients with carotid or vertebral artery disorders. Periodic evaluation can be helpful for assessing the progression or regression of existing plaques or the development of new lesions, whether symptomatic or asymptomatic. The timing of follow-up carotid testing must be individualized depending on the severity and type of lesions, as well as the onset of new or recurrent symptoms. The identification of asymptomatic carotid stenosis has become an important clinical mandate since the Asymptomatic Carotid Atherosclerosis Study (ACAS) showed the benefit of CEA in asymptomatic patients with 60% to 99% stenosis, when compared with treatment with 325 mg of aspirin daily (Executive Committee for the Asymptomatic Carotid Atherosclerosis Study, 1995). Yet, it is not cost-effective to screen the entire population, even with ultrasound. Asymptomatic individuals with cervical bruits should be studied, even though bruits are often due to another cause. Patients with multiple risk factors probably warrant study, but the clinical utility of this has not yet been confirmed. Practice guidelines are being developed for carotid screening in high-risk individuals to identify stenosis that may need clinical treatment or intervention (Qureshi et al., 2007). If vessel disease is identified, stenosis of less than 50% might be initially restudied in 12 to 24 months, whereas lesions with 50% to 75% stenosis and uncomplicated plaques might wait 6 to 12 months. For 50% to 75% stenosis with complicated plaque features, or for more than 75% stenosis, initial restudy at 3 to 6 months is appropriate. Lack of progression for several years allows lengthened intervals before restudy. When evidence of asymptomatic progression is present, a shorter interval is recommended. Development of new symptoms should prompt urgent reevaluation. After CEA, repeat ultrasound is often done at approximately 1 month after surgery and then yearly to identify potential restenosis.

Large population studies such as the Atherosclerosis Risk in Communities and the Cardiovascular Health Study have documented the association between risk factors and intima-media thickening in the wall of the carotid artery on B-mode imaging (Polak, 2005; Polak et al., 1998). This may represent an early stage in the development of atherosclerosis; the presence of significant thickening correlates with risk of heart attack as well as abnormalities on MRI of the brain. Further investigations remain ongoing regarding the clinical utility of identifying increased intima-media thickness values, but it has been suggested that B-mode imaging for evaluation of intima-media thickness should be used clinically to identify patients at high risk for coronary or cerebrovascular events or to assess responses to risk factor modification (AHA Prevention Conference V Writing Group III, 2000; Polak, 2005). The hope is that such early identification of atherosclerotic changes will allow intervention to prevent later development of clinical events.

Intracranial Stenotic Lesions

Intracranial atherosclerotic plaques are dynamic lesions that may increase in degrees of stenosis or regress over relatively short periods of time. TCD enables noninvasive monitoring of these lesions. It is often obtained at baseline in conjunction with DSA, CTA, or MRA and is subsequently repeated during the follow-up period (**Fig. 33B.27**). Monitoring also enables detection of new atherosclerotic plaques. However, clinical experience is limited, and further prospective investigations are needed to make recommendations regarding the frequency and timing of follow-up studies.

Aneurysmal Subarachnoid Hemorrhage

Vasoconstriction of intracerebral arteries is the leading cause of delayed cerebral infarction and mortality after aneurysmal subarachnoid hemorrhage. Vasospasm is clinically detected 3 or 4 days after the hemorrhage and usually resolves after day 12. Although the exact cause of vasospasm remains unknown, its presence correlates with the volume and duration of exposure of an intracranial artery to the blood clot. Laboratory and animal models indicate that blood breakdown products can lead to vasoconstriction. The detection of vasospasm is important because it may potentially be treated with medications, hemodynamic management, and endovascular interventions. These treatments are not innocuous, so the ability to noninvasively detect and monitor vasospasm has considerable clinical importance. Although vasospasm can be angiographically detected in 30% to 70% of patients with aneurysmal subarachnoid hemorrhage, only 20% to 40% develop clinical signs of cerebral ischemia. Thus, the presence of vasospasm is not a sufficient condition for development of a clinical focal ischemic deficit. Several factors including the severity of spasm, presence of collateral flow, condition of the patient's intravascular volume, and cerebral perfusion pressure are considered mitigating factors. TCD studies show an increase in the flow velocities of basal cerebral arteries, usually starting on day 4 after subarachnoid hemorrhage and peaking by days 7 to 14 (**Fig. 33B.28**). Although a diffuse increase in velocities is often detected in patients with severe hemorrhage, arterial segments in close proximity to the subarachnoid blood clot usually have the highest velocities.

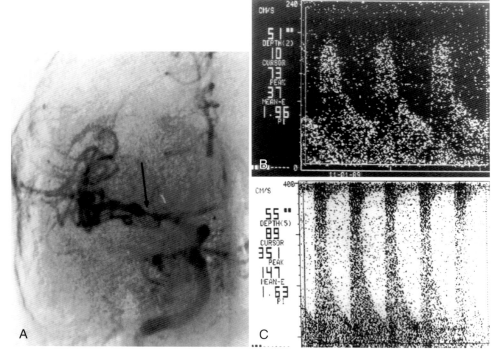

Fig. 33B.27 Monitoring of intracranial atherosclerotic lesions. **A,** Cerebral angiogram shows an area of stenosis *(arrow)* in the M1 segment of the right middle cerebral artery. **B,** The first transcranial Doppler study obtained within 48 hours of angiography shows a corresponding peak-systolic velocity of 188 cm/sec. **C,** Repeat transcranial Doppler study 34 months later shows a further increase of the peak-systolic velocity to approximately 350 cm/sec. *(Reprinted with permission from Schwarze, J.J., Babikian, V., DeWitt, L.D., et al., 1994. Longitudinal monitoring of intracranial arterial stenoses with transcranial Doppler ultrasonography. J Neuroimaging 4, 182-187).*

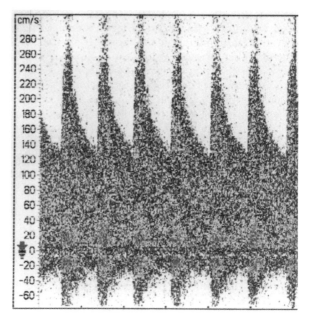

Fig. 33B.28 Subarachnoid hemorrhage. Temporal bone window; depth of insonation of 56 mm. Increased flow velocities indicating moderate to severe vasospasm in the middle cerebral artery M1 segment.

Severe vasospasm in an arterial segment can be associated with reduced regional cerebral blood flow in the artery's distal territory. There is a linear inverse relationship between the severity of vasospasm and the amplitude of flow-velocity increase in an arterial segment. It is valid until the vasoconstriction is so severe that the flow volume is reduced, flow velocities drop, and the TCD signal becomes difficult to detect. The linear relationship can also be affected by several factors, including the presence of hyperperfusion. Angiographic studies confirm the presence of at least some degree of MCA vasospasm when the mean flow velocities are higher than 100 cm/sec, but values below 120 cm/sec are not usually considered clinically significant. Mean velocities in the 120 to 200 cm/sec range correspond to 25% to 50% angiographically determined diameter reduction; values exceeding 200 cm/sec correspond to more than 50% luminal narrowing (Sloan et al., 1999). The 200 cm/sec threshold and rapid flow-velocity increases exceeding 50 cm/sec on consecutive days are associated with subsequent infarction. TCD is used also to monitor the effects of endovascular treatment of vasospasm. Flow velocities decrease after successful angioplasty or papaverine infusion. Persistent increases after treatment indicate either extension of vasospasm to new arterial segments or hyperemia in the treated arterial segment and may constitute a valid reason for repeat cerebral angiography.

The accuracy of TCD in detecting vasospasm depends to some degree on the location of the involved arterial segment. Although TCD criteria are more than 90% specific in detecting MCA and ACA vasospasm, they are respectively

80% and less than 50% sensitive in detecting disease in these arterial segments (Sloan et al., 1999). Basilar artery vasospasm is detected with an approximate sensitivity of 75% and specificity of 80%. Several factors including the effects of hyperemia, increased intracranial pressure (ICP) and blood pressure changes, the presence of vasospasm in convexity branches not accessible by TCD, and difficulties in assessing vasospasm by angiography contribute to these findings. Because of these limitations in accuracy, the combined use of TCD and SPECT or xenon-enhanced CT has been advocated, with the expectation that it will provide a more comprehensive and accurate assessment of the clinical condition. Overall, however, TCD is considered to have acceptable accuracy for the evaluation of vasospasm in aneurysmal subarachnoid hemorrhage. It is a useful tool with limitations that must be taken into consideration in the clinical setting.

Brain Death

A characteristic pattern of changes can be detected by TCD in patients with increased ICP. Early findings consist of a mild decrease in the diastolic flow velocity and an increase in the difference between peak-systolic and end-diastolic velocities. When ICP increases further and reaches the diastolic blood pressure level, flow stops during diastole, and the corresponding flow velocity drops to zero; flow continues during systole, and spiky systolic peaks are observed. A further increase in ICP is associated with a reverberating flow pattern, with forward flow in systole and retrograde flow in diastole (see **Fig. 33B.28**). The net volume of flow decreases and can reach zero. At cerebral perfusion pressure values close to zero, either small systolic spikes are observed (**Fig. 33B.29**), or no signal at all is detected. This corresponds to a complete arrest of flow as demonstrated by cerebral angiography. The pattern of TCD changes is not specific to a particular neurological disease and can occur in a variety of conditions associated with increased ICP.

These changes are also observed in patients clinically diagnosed as brain dead. Experience remains variable among different institutions, and one retrospective study found that TCD evaluation was able to confirm brain death in 57% of patients but remained inconclusive in 43% (Sharma et al., 2010). Another recent study found that the specificity of TCD testing was 100%, with a sensitivity of 82.1%. When the evaluation was augmented by insonation of the extracranial ICA, the sensitivity was increased to 88% by allowing the detection of cerebral circulatory arrest in patients lacking temporal windows. The addition of serial examinations further increased sensitivity to 95.6% (Alexandrov et al., 2010). Thus, although TCD is useful in detecting cerebral circulatory arrest, it cannot be recommended as the sole diagnostic test for the diagnosis of brain death. The latter has to be established based on the clinical presentation and neurological examination findings. TCD and other laboratory tests can help confirm the clinical impression.

Cerebrovascular Reactivity

Cerebrovascular reactivity testing evaluates the presence of abnormal cerebral hemodynamic changes to potentially identify patients at an increased risk of recurrent stroke. Both IV

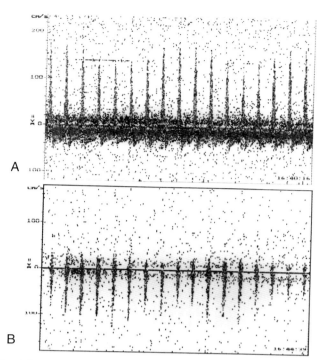

Fig. 33B.29 Raised intracranial pressure. Reverberating flow pattern **(A)** and small systolic spikes **(B)** seen in a patient with markedly increased intracranial pressure.

acetazolamide administration and carbon dioxide inhalation are used to assess cerebrovascular reactivity. In patients with exhausted cerebrovascular reactivity reserves, flow velocities fail to adequately increase after the IV administration of acetazolamide or have a decreased response to hypercapnia and hypocapnia. In patients with ICA occlusion and impaired cerebrovascular reactivity determined by TCD or by xenon-enhanced CT, the annual rate of distal cerebral ischemic events is approximately 10%. Further investigation remains to determine whether such testing can reliably identify patients who might benefit from a revascularization procedure.

Sickle Cell Disease

An occlusive vasculopathy characterized by a fibrous proliferation of the intima often involves the basal cerebral arteries of patients with sickle cell disease. Cerebral infarction is a common complication of this vasculopathy and has a frequency of approximately 5% to 15%. As in all patients with anemia, flow velocities are diffusely increased in individuals with sickle cell anemia. Additional focal velocity increases in the basal cerebral arteries can be detected in some subjects. A time-averaged mean of the maximum velocity of 200 cm/sec or greater in the distal ICA and proximal MCA identifies neurologically asymptomatic children at an increased risk for first-time stroke (Adams et al., 1998). In addition to standard insonation techniques with the TCD probe, a recent study determined that extending the submandibular approach to include infrasiphon portions of the ICA increased the sensitivity to better identify sickle cell patients with potential sources of cerebral infarction (Gorman et al., 2009). Periodic red blood cell transfusion is associated with a 90% reduction in the rate of stroke. A Clinical Alert from the National Heart, Lung and Blood Institute recommended that children with sickle cell disease between ages 2 and 16 receive baseline TCD testing and that those with normal study results be restudied every 6 months (National Heart, Lung and Blood Institute, 1997). Discontinuation of transfusion therapy can result in a reversal of abnormal blood-flow velocities and stroke (STOP 2 Trial, 2005).

Periprocedural Monitoring

Carotid endarterectomy (CEA) and carotid artery stenting (CAS) remain important interventions for certain cases of asymptomatic and symptomatic carotid stenosis. Monitoring is often performed to identify and correct periprocedural events that can lead to cerebrovascular complications. Monitoring tests currently in use for CEA include electroencephalography. These tests are useful in detecting cerebral hypoperfusion or its consequence, cerebral ischemia, and investigations remain ongoing to determine their effectiveness in reducing the perioperative stroke rate. TCD monitoring during CEA shows a consistent pattern of flow-velocity changes. The most significant changes occur at the time of carotid clamping, with persistent and severe flow-velocity decreases to less than 15% of pre-clamp values in up to 10% of patients (**Fig. 33B.30**). Patients with velocities decreasing to this level usually are considered candidates for shunting. Although definitive TCD criteria for shunting have not yet been established, a post-clamp peak-systolic or mean flow-velocity decrease to less than 30% of the pre-clamp value is often considered an acceptable criterion.

TCD monitoring also has the unique capability of detecting microembolism as it occurs. This provides a considerable edge to TCD when compared with other monitoring techniques, because the majority of perioperative infarcts are thought to be secondary to cerebral embolism. Microemboli are detected at specific stages of surgery; dissection, clamp insertion and release, and the immediate postoperative period are the high-risk periods (**Fig. 33B.31**). The presence of solid and gaseous microemboli in patients undergoing CEA and/or carotid stenting have been associated with procedure-related acute ipsilateral ischemic strokes on MRI as well as postoperative cognitive decline (Skjelland et al., 2009). One study evaluating patients who underwent carotid endarterectomy under TCD monitoring found that low MCA mean blood-flow velocity (≤28 cm/sec) during carotid dissection was significantly associated with new postoperative neurological deficits in patients with 10 or greater MES during carotid dissection. This combined evaluation resulted in improved specificity and positive predictive value when compared with either criterion used

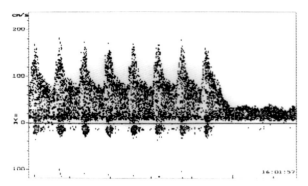

Fig. 33B.30 Carotid endarterectomy. At clamp insertion, the peak-systolic flow velocity decreases from approximately 175 to 35 cm/sec.

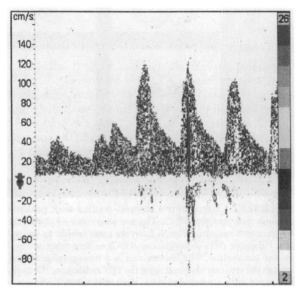

Fig. 33B.31 Carotid endarterectomy. At clamp release, flow velocities are restored, and microembolic signals are seen.

alone (Ogasawara et al., 2008). TCD remains a relative newcomer to the field of periprocedural monitoring and provides useful information to potentially avert cerebrovascular complications.

References

The complete reference list is available online at www. expertconsult.com.

Neuroimaging
Functional Neuroimaging: Functional Magnetic Resonance Imaging, Positron Emission Tomography, and Single-Photon Emission Computed Tomography

Philipp T. Meyer, Michel Rijntjes, Cornelius Weiller

Structural imaging modalities such as computed tomography (CT) and magnetic resonance imaging (MRI) are essential techniques for evaluating various central nervous system (CNS) disorders, providing superb structural resolution and tissue contrast. On the other hand, functional imaging modalities like functional MRI (fMRI), positron emission tomography (PET), and single-photon emission computed tomography (SPECT) visualize brain functions that are not necessarily related to brain structure, most notably cerebral blood flow and metabolism, receptor binding, and enzyme activity. Functional neuroimaging is particularly valuable for mapping brain functions or depicting disease-related molecular changes that occur independently of or before structural changes. The principles of fMRI, PET, and SPECT and their applications in clinical neurosciences will be discussed in this chapter. Regarding applications of PET and SPECT, the focus will be on investigations of cerebral blood flow (CBF) and glucose metabolism in dementia, parkinsonism, brain tumors, and epilepsy. These applications are particularly well established and important in clinical practice. Localization of brain function may be the main focus of fMRI research at present and is increasingly utilized in presurgical mapping. Furthermore, one of the oldest questions in clinical neurology is how brain function is lost and can be regained. Numerous fMRI studies in stroke patients have demonstrated relevant plasticity in the human brain and that cerebral reorganization is related to improvement of function, which can be reinforced by training. Studies using fMRI suggest links in the clinical manifestations underlying apparently unrelated diseases like stroke and multiple sclerosis (MS); such knowledge could be vital to the development of treatment strategies.

Functional Neuroimaging Modalities

Functional Magnetic Resonance Imaging

Today, fMRI is the most widespread technique in neuroscience brain imaging. It mainly relates to the blood oxygen level–dependent (BOLD) effect, which is due to a local hyperoxygenation of the venous blood, resulting in a relative increase of signal. The BOLD effect is related to changes in regional CBF as well as to neuronal activity. Experimental trials are presented either in a block design (about 20-25 seconds stimulus followed by 20-25 seconds rest, repeated, e.g., 3-4 times per condition) or event related ($\approx$30-40 stimuli of each type are presented in a counterbalanced order, each followed by some baseline period). Experiments are often conducted with multiple subjects, which requires stereotactic normalization into a standard space. Time series are analyzed in a *general linear model* (GLM), allowing inferences on effect sizes. Resulting maps illustrate regions with a task-specific statistically significant difference in brain activation. Time series of fMRI studies are used to detect functional dependencies between brain regions ("functional" or "effective" connectivity) with mathematical approaches such as dynamic causal modeling, directed partial correlations using Granger causality, Bayesian learning networks, graph theory, and others.

In addition to fMRI, structural imaging has recently gained more attention. Voxel-based morphometry (VBM) allows voxel-by-voxel comparison of the relative contribution of white or gray matter to the signal between groups. A well-known application to learning was the increase of parietal regions used for visuospatial integration in people who learned to juggle (Draganski et al., 2004). Integrity of tracts may be determined through diffusion tensor imaging (DTI). DTI measures the diffusion vector in each voxel. It is feasible to detect the direction of diffusion across longer distances by analyzing and relating the values in several neighboring voxels. As diffusion is facilitated along axes, in contrast, probabilistic fiber tracking identifies the most likely course of fiber tracts (Kreher et al., 2008). Comparison of diffusivity (i.e., fractional anisotropy) voxel by voxel across the entire brain allows the differentiation of tracts between groups, analogous to VBM. For instance, stutterers have a less smooth connection below a region responsible for preparation of articulation (Sommer et al., 2002).

Positron Emission Tomography

Although the first attempts to use positron emitters for medical imaging were made as early as the 1950s, the concept of modern PET was developed during the 1970s (Phelps et al., 1975). The underlying principle of PET, and also of SPECT, is to image and quantify a physiological function or molecular target of interest (e.g., blood flow, metabolism, receptor binding) in vivo by noninvasively assessing the spatial and temporal distribution of the radiation emitted by an intravenously injected target-specific probe (radiotracer). Importantly, PET and SPECT tracers are administered in a non-pharmacological dose (micrograms or less), so they neither disturb the underlying system nor cause pharmacological or behavioral effects. Because of their ability to visualize molecular targets and functions on a macroscopic level with unsurpassed sensitivity, down to picomolar concentration, PET and SPECT are also called *molecular imaging techniques*. (See Cherry et al., 2003, for an excellent textbook on PET and SPECT physics.)

In the case of PET, a positron-emitting radiotracer is injected. The emitted positron travels a short distance in tissue (effective range < 1 mm for common PET nuclides) before it encounters an electron, yielding a pair of two 511-keV annihilation photons emitted in opposite directions. This photon pair leaving the body is detected quasi-simultaneously (within a few nanoseconds) by scintillation detectors of the PET detector rings that surround the patient's head. Assuming that the annihilation site is located on the line connecting both detectors (known as the *line of response* [LOR]), three-dimensional (3D) PET image data sets of the distribution of the PET tracer and its target in tissue are generated by standard image reconstruction algorithms using the LOR data. To actually gain quantitative PET images (i.e., radioactivity/tracer concentration per unit tissue), the acquired data are corrected for scatter and random coincidences and photon attenuation by tissue absorption (e.g., using a measured CT or $^{68}Ge/^{68}Ga$ transmission scan). The spatial resolution of modern PET or combined PET/CT systems is about 3 to

5 mm. Thus, PET is susceptible to partial volume effects if the object or lesion size is below two times the scanner resolution (as a rule of thumb).

Commonly used radionuclides in neurological PET studies are oxygen-15 (^{15}O, physical half-life = 2.03 minutes), carbon-11 (^{11}C, half-life = 20.4 minutes), and fluorine-18 (^{18}F, half-life = 109.7 minutes), which are all cyclotron products. Whereas the relatively long half-life of ^{18}F allows shipping ^{18}F-labelled tracers from a cyclotron site to a distant PET site, this is not possible in the case of ^{15}O and ^{11}C. This clearly limits the clinical use of ^{15}O-labelled water, molecular oxygen, and carbon dioxide for quantification of CBF, cerebral metabolic rate of oxygen, and oxygen extraction fraction. This also applies to clinically very interesting ^{11}C-labelled tracers like [^{11}C]raclopride (dopamine D_2/D_3 receptor), [^{11}C]flumazenil (GABA$_A$ receptor), [^{11}C]methionine (amino acid transport), and [^{11}C]PIB (amyloid beta [Aβ]). Thus, ^{18}F-labelled substitutes have been proposed and are currently under investigation.

In this chapter on perfusion and metabolism, we will focus on PET studies using the glucose analog, 2-deoxy-2-(^{18}F) fluoro-D-glucose ([^{18}F]FDG), to assess cerebral glucose metabolism. With the rate of glucose metabolism being closely related to maintenance of ion gradients and transmitter turnover (in particular, glutamate), [^{18}F]FDG represents an ideal tracer for assessment of neuronal function and its changes (Sokoloff, 1977). After uptake in cerebral tissue by specific glucose transporters, [^{18}F]FDG is phosphorylated by hexokinase. Since [^{18}F]FDG-6-P is neither a substrate for transport back out of the cell nor can it be metabolized further, it is virtually irreversible trapped in cells. Therefore, the distribution of [^{18}F]FDG in tissue imaged by PET (started 30-60 minutes after injection to allow for sufficient uptake; 5-20 minute scan duration) closely reflects the regional distribution of cerebral glucose metabolism. By use of appropriate pharmacokinetic models and a plasma input function (i.e., [^{18}F]FDG concentration in arterial or arterialized venous plasma), the absolute cerebral metabolic rate of glucose (CMRglc in μmol/min/100 g tissue) can be estimated. In the case of [^{18}F]FDG, absolute quantification is usually not necessary for routine clinical studies, since the diagnostic information can often be obtained from the cerebral pattern of [^{18}F]FDG uptake or relative estimates of regional glucose metabolism gained by normalizing regional [^{18}F]FDG uptake to the uptake of a suitable reference region unaffected by disease.

Single-Photon Emission Computed Tomography

The first SPECT measurements were performed in the 1960s (Kuhl and Edwards, 1964). As explained earlier, SPECT relies on the same radiotracer principle as PET. Unlike PET, SPECT employs gamma-emitting radionuclides that decay by emitting a single gamma ray. Typical radionuclides employed for neurological SPECT are technetium-99m (^{99m}Tc; half-life = 6.02 hours) and iodine-123 (^{123}I; half-life = 13.2 hours). Gamma cameras are used for SPECT acquisition, whereby usually two or three detector heads rotate around the patient's head to acquire two-dimensional planar images (projections) of the head from multiple angles (e.g., in 3-degree steps). Whereas radiation collimation is achieved by coincidence detection in PET, hardware collimators with lead septa are placed in front of the detector heads in the case of SPECT scanners. Finally, 3D image data reconstruction is done by conventional reconstruction algorithms. With combined SPECT/CT systems, a CT transmission scan can replace the less accurate calculated attenuation correction.

The different acquisition principles outlined above imply that SPECT possesses a considerably lower sensitivity than PET. Thus, rapid temporal sampling (image frames of seconds to minutes) as a prerequisite for pharmacokinetic analyses is the strength of PET, whereas a single SPECT acquisition usually takes 20 to 30 minutes. Furthermore, the spatial resolution of modern SPECT is only about 7 to 10 mm, deteriorating with increasing distance between object and collimator (i.e., higher resolution for cortical than subcortical structures; distance between patient and collimator should be minimized for optimal resolution). SPECT is considerably more susceptible to partial volume effects than PET, which can be a particular drawback when it comes to imaging small structures or lesions (e.g., brain tumors). Nevertheless, brain-dedicated SPECT instruments have been proposed that allow for optimized spatial and temporal sampling and pharmacokinetic data quantification (Meyer et al., 2008), and further technical developments are underway (Jansen and Vanderheyden, 2007). The important advantages of SPECT over PET are the lower costs, the broad availability of SPECT systems, and the availability of SPECT radionuclides in smaller community hospitals and private practices. While [123I]-labelled tracers (e.g., [123I]FP-CIT and [123I]IBZM for dopamine transporter and receptor imaging, respectively) can easily be shipped over long distances, technetium-99m can be eluted onsite from molybdenum-99 ([99Mo]/[99mTc] generators and used for labeling commercially available radiopharmaceutical kits. Although [99mTc] is an almost ideal radionuclide from the perspective of imaging physics, chemical incorporation of [99mTc] into tracers is much more demanding than in case of the aforementioned PET radionuclides, limiting the diversity of [99mTc]-labelled tracers.

We will focus on the two most widely used CBF tracers, hexamethylpropyleneamine oxime ([99mTc]HMPAO) and ethylcysteinate dimer ([99mTc]ECD). Owing to their lipophilic nature and thus high first-pass extraction, both radiotracers are rapidly taken up by the brain. They are quasi-irreversibly retained after conversion into hydrophilic compounds (enzymatic de-esterification of [99mTc]ECD; instability, and possibly interaction with glutathione in the case of [99mTc]HMPAO). Differences in uptake mechanisms may explain slight differences in biological behavior (e.g., in stroke), with [99mTc]HMPAO being more closely correlated to perfusion, while [99mTc]ECD uptake is also influenced by metabolic activity. Despite the fact that cerebral radiotracer uptake is virtually complete within just 1 to 2 minutes after injection, SPECT acquisition is usually started after 30 to 60 minutes to allow for sufficient background clearance.

Given the fact that the CBF is closely coupled to cerebral glucose metabolism, and thus to neuronal function (with a few rare exceptions), [99mTc]HMPAO and [99mTc]ECD are used to assess neuronal activity. However, since cerebral autoregulation is also affected by many other factors (e.g., carbon dioxide level) and possibly diseases, cerebral glucose metabolism represents a more direct and probably less variable marker of neuronal activity. Given the technical limitations mentioned earlier, [18F]FDG PET is generally preferred to CBF SPECT. One important exception, however, is the use of ictal CBF SPECT in the assessment of patients with epilepsy.

Clinical Applications

Dementia

Early and accurate diagnosis of dementia is of crucial importance for appropriate treatment (including possible enrollment into investigational trials on novel therapies and avoidance of possible side effects of treatments), for prognosis, and for adequate counseling of patients and caregivers. The diagnostic power of [18F]FDG PET in this situation is well established (Herholz, 2003). In clinical practice, [18F]FDG PET studies are interpreted by qualitative visual readings. These readings are commonly assisted by voxel-based statistical analyses in comparison to aged-matched normal controls (Herholz et al., 2002; Minoshima et al., 1995), which have become state of the art in recent years. PET studies should always be interpreted with parallel inspection of a recent CT or MRI scan to detect structural defects (e.g., ischemia, atrophy, subdural hematoma) that cause regional hypometabolism.

The typical finding in Alzheimer disease (AD), the most frequent neurodegenerative dementia, is bilateral hypometabolism of the temporal and parietal association cortices, with the temporoparietal junction being the center of impairment. As the disease progress, frontal association cortices also get involved (**Figs. 33C.1 and 33C.2**). The magnitude and

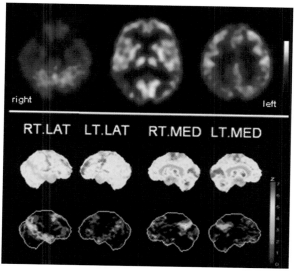

Fig. 33C.1 [18F]FDG PET in early Alzheimer disease. Early disease stage is characterized by mild to moderate hypometabolism of temporal and parietal cortices and posterior cingulate gyrus and precuneus. As in this case, distinct asymmetry is often noticed. As disease progresses, frontal cortices also become involved. *Upper panel,* Transaxial PET images of [18F] FDG uptake (color coded, see color scale on right; orientation in radiological convention as indicated). *Lower panel,* Results of voxel-based statistical analysis using Neurostat/3D-SSP. Three-dimensional stereotactic surface projections of [18F]FDG uptake (*upper row*) and statistical deviation of the individual's examination (as z score) from age-matched healthy controls. Data are color coded in rainbow scale (see lower right for z scale). Given are right and left lateral and mesial views. *(Neurostat/3D-SSP analysis based on Minoshima, S., Frey, K.A., Koeppe, R.A., et al., 1995. A diagnostic approach in Alzheimer's disease using three-dimensional stereotactic surface projections of fluorine-18-FDG PET. J Nucl Med 36, 1238-1248.)*

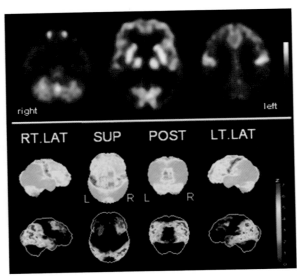

right
left

RT.LAT SUP POST LT.LAT

L R L R

z

Fig. 33C.2 [¹⁸F]FDG PET in advanced Alzheimer disease. Advanced disease stage is characterized by severe hypometabolism of temporal and parietal cortices and posterior cingulate gyrus and precuneus. Frontal cortex is also involved, while sensorimotor and occipital cortex, basal ganglia, thalamus, and cerebellum are spared. Mesiotemporal hypometabolism is also apparent. *Upper panel*, Transaxial PET images of [¹⁸F]FDG uptake. *Lower panel*, Results of voxel-based statistical analysis using Neurostat/3D-SSP. Given are right and left lateral, superior, and posterior views (see **Fig. 33C.1** for additional details). *(Neurostat/3D-SSP analysis based on Minoshima, S., Frey, K.A., Koeppe, R.A., et al., 1995. A diagnostic approach in Alzheimer's disease using three-dimensional stereotactic surface projections of fluorine-18-FDG PET. J Nucl Med 36, 1238-1248.)*

extent of the hypometabolism increases with progressing disease, with relative sparing of the primary motor and visual cortices, the basal ganglia, and the cerebellum (often used as reference regions). The degree of hypometabolism is usually well correlated with the dementia severity (Herholz et al., 2002; Minoshima et al., 1997; Salmon et al., 2005). Furthermore, cortical hypometabolism is often asymmetrical, corresponding to predominant clinical symptoms (language impairment if dominant or visuospatial impairment if nondominant hemisphere is affected, respectively). Voxel-based statistical analyses consistently show that the posterior cingulate gyrus and precuneus are also affected even in the earliest AD stages (Minoshima et al., 1997). It is unclear whether the hypometabolism in this rather circumscribed area is in fact particularly pronounced in early AD or more narrowly and consistently localized (compared to other regions) and thus preferentially detected by statistical methods (Herholz et al., 2002). In any case, it is an important diagnostic clue in early AD that should not be missed. The hippocampus is particularly affected by AD pathology and, consequently, neurodegeneration. However, studies on hippocampal metabolism in AD yielded conflicting results, mostly showing no significant hypometabolism. This may be due to the relatively low-normal [¹⁸F]FDG uptake, small size, and AD-related atrophy of this structure, which render visual and voxel-based statistical analyses insensitive. Region-based analyses like a recently proposed automated hippocampal masking technique can help overcome these limitations and provide valuable incremental diagnostic information (Mosconi et al., 2005).

In [¹⁸F]FDG PET studies on autopsy-confirmed AD patients with memory complaints, the pattern of temporoparietal hypometabolism as assessed by visual readings alone showed a high sensitivity of 84% to 94% for detecting pathologically confirmed AD, with a specificity of 63% to 74% (Hoffman et al., 2000; Jagust et al., 2007; Silverman et al., 2001). As a diagnostic tool, visual inspection of [¹⁸F]FDG PET was found to be of similar accuracy as a clinical follow-up examination performed 4 years after PET (Jagust et al., 2007). In two recent large multicenter trials, voxel-based statistical analyses of cortical [¹⁸F]FDG uptake provided a sensitivity of 93% to 99% and a specificity of 93% to 98% for the distinction between mild to moderate AD (clinical diagnosis) and normal controls (Herholz et al., 2002; Mosconi et al., 2008). The specificity of the differentiation between AD and dementia with Lewy bodies (DLB) and frontotemporal dementia (FTD) was lower (71% and 65%, respectively) if done by voxel-based cortical analyses alone. However, the use of an additional hippocampal analysis greatly improved specificity (100% and 94%, respectively), yielding an overall classification accuracy of 96% for the aforementioned patient groups and controls (Mosconi et al., 2008). Patterns of hypoperfusion observed with CBF SPECT in AD are very similar, but according to a SPECT meta-analysis (Dougall et al., 2004) and direct comparisons (Herholz et al., 2002), [¹⁸F]FDG PET provides higher diagnostic accuracy (also see recommendation in Dubois et al., 2007).

The syndrome of mild cognitive impairment (MCI) (Petersen et al., 1999) represents a risk state for dementia. More than half of subjects progress to manifest dementia within 5 years, with AD being the most frequent underlying cause, particularly in the group with amnestic MCI (Gauthier et al., 2006). Several studies demonstrated that an AD-like [¹⁸F]FDG PET pattern can be observed in high frequency among MCI patients (e.g., 79% and 31% of multidomain and amnestic MCI patients, respectively; Mosconi et al., 2008), and that this pattern is highly predictive of subsequent progression to manifest dementia, with a sensitivity of 92% to 93% and a specificity of 82% to 89% in two recent studies in which overall accuracy of [¹⁸F]FDG PET for prediction of progression was higher than of ApoE genotype or in-depth memory assessment (Anchisi et al., 2005; Drzezga et al., 2005). In addition, a recent meta-analysis showed that [¹⁸F]FDG PET performs better on prediction of rapid progression to AD than CBF SPECT and MRI (Yuan et al., 2009). Finally, it has been demonstrated that cognitively normal healthy controls at risk for AD owing to being an ApoE ε4 carrier and/or having a positive family history (maternal in particular) exhibited significantly reduced glucose metabolism in those cortical areas typically affected by AD (Mosconi et al., 2007; Reiman et al., 1996; Small et al., 1995). This was also found in young ApoE ε4 carriers (mean age of 30 years) and thus decades before the possible onset of AD (Reiman et al., 2004). Follow-up studies in subjects at risk for AD also demonstrated that the subsequent decline in cerebral glucose metabolism in AD-typical regions was significantly greater compared to non-at-risk subjects (Mosconi et al., 2009; Reiman et al., 2001; Small et al., 2000). Taken together, these results emphasize that [¹⁸F]FDG PET is not only a very powerful method for accurate diagnosis of manifest AD and prediction of progression in possibly prodromal AD (MCI) but may also be useful to investigate preclinical stages of AD (e.g., in prevention and treatment trials).

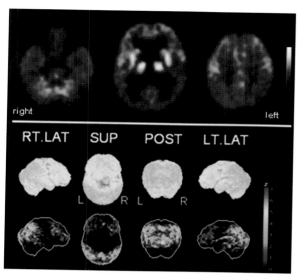

Fig. 33C.3 [¹⁸F]FDG PET in dementia with Lewy bodies (DLB). This disorder affects similar areas as those affected by Alzheimer disease (AD). Occipital cortex is also involved, which may distinguish DLB from AD; mesiotemporal lobe is relatively spared in DLB. A very similar, if not identical, pattern is observed in Parkinson disease with dementia (PDD). *Upper panel,* Transaxial PET images of [¹⁸F]FDG uptake. *Lower panel,* Results of voxel-based statistical analysis using Neurostat/3D-SSP. Given are right and left lateral, superior, and posterior views (see **Fig. 33C.1** for additional details). *(Neurostat/3D-SSP analysis based on Minoshima, S., Frey, K.A., Koeppe, R.A., et al., 1995. A diagnostic approach in Alzheimer's disease using three-dimensional stereotactic surface projections of fluorine-18-FDG PET. J Nucl Med 36, 1238-1248.)*

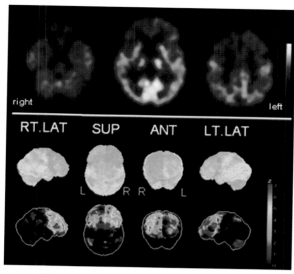

Fig. 33C.4 [¹⁸F]FDG PET in frontotemporal dementia (FTD). Bifrontal hypometabolism is usually found in FTD, sometimes in a somewhat asymmetrical distribution, as in this case. At early stages, frontomesial and frontopolar involvement is most pronounced, while parietal cortices are affected later in disease course. *Upper panel,* Transaxial PET images of [¹⁸F]FDG uptake. *Lower panel,* Results of voxel-based statistical analysis using Neurostat/3D-SSP. Given are right and left lateral, superior, and posterior views (see **Fig. 33C.1** for additional details). *(Neurostat/3D-SSP analysis based on Minoshima, S., Frey, K.A., Koeppe, R.A., et al., 1995. A diagnostic approach in Alzheimer's disease using three-dimensional stereotactic surface projections of fluorine-18-FDG PET. J Nucl Med 36, 1238-1248.)*

Dementia with Lewy bodies is considered the second most frequent cause of dementia. The typical [¹⁸F]FDG PET pattern observed in DLB resembles the pattern observed in AD, with the exception of additional hypometabolism of the primary visual cortex and the occipital association cortex (Albin et al., 1996) (**Fig. 33C.3**). The latter has been linked to the occurrence of typical visual hallucinations in DLB patients (particularly in those with relatively preserved posterior temporal and parietal metabolism) (Imamura et al., 1999). Occipital hypometabolism was found to be a valuable diagnostic feature to separate clinically diagnosed patients with AD and DLB (sensitivity 86%-92%, specificity 91%-92%) (Higuchi et al., 2000; Ishii et al., 1998a). This was confirmed in a study with autopsy confirmation (sensitivity 90%, specificity 80%) (Minoshima et al., 2001). Recent studies have demonstrated that hippocampal metabolism is preserved in DLB but reduced in AD (Ishii et al., 2007; Mosconi et al., 2008). The aforementioned multicenter study (Mosconi et al., 2008) found considerably enhanced accuracy of [¹⁸F]FDG PET for differentiating DLB from AD, FTD, and controls if an additional hippocampal analyses were included (92%). It has to be mentioned that differences may be hard to appreciate in routine clinical examination of individual patients. In this situation, PET or SPECT examinations of nigrostriatal integrity (e.g., using [¹⁸F]FDOPA or a dopamine transporter ligand like [¹²³I]FP-CIT) can be very helpful in differentiating between AD and DLB (McKeith et al., 2007). One has to bear in mind that nigrostriatal projections may also be damaged in FTD (Rinne et al., 2002) and atypical parkinsonian syndromes with dementia (e.g., PSP

and CBD; see below). DLB is clinically distinguished from Parkinson disease with dementia (PDD) by the so-called 1-year rule, referring to the duration of parkinsonism prior to dementia. Although the separation between DLB and PDD is controversial, it is still recommended for several reasons (Lippa et al., 2007; McKeith, 2007). In line with the notion that both diseases most likely represent manifestations of the same disease process (Lewy body disease), [¹⁸F]FDG PET studies in PDD (Peppard et al., 1992; Vander Borght et al., 1997) found very similar results to those in DLB. In a recent direct comparison, there were only minor differences between both groups (barely significant lower metabolism in DLB compared to PDD in the anterior cingulate cortex) (Yong et al., 2007). Of note, however, in a recent [¹¹C]PIB PET study, the majority of DLB patients (11/13) showed increased Aβ binding, while the majority of PDD patients (10/12) did not (Edison et al., 2008).

Frontotemporal lobar degeneration (FTLD) probably represents the third most common cause of dementia. It comprises the three prototypical syndromes: frontotemporal dementia (FTD), semantic dementia (SD), and progressive nonfluent aphasia (PA) (Neary et al., 1998). FTLD is caused by a spectrum of underlying, possibly related, pathologies (also including corticobasal degeneration [CBD] and progressive supranuclear palsy [PSP]) which lead to a variety of overlapping clinical presentations that hinder predicting the underlying pathology by the clinical phenotype (so-called Pick complex) (Kertesz et al., 2005). FTD is usually associated with a bilateral, sometimes asymmetrical, frontal hypometabolism which is most pronounced in the mesial (polar) frontal cortex (**Fig. 33C.4**) (Garraux et al., 1999; Salmon et al.,

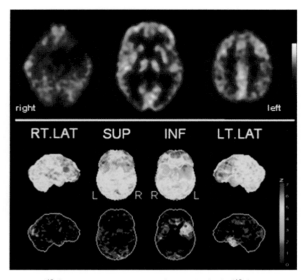

Fig. 33C.5 [¹⁸F]FDG PET in semantic dementia (SD). [¹⁸F]FDG PET scans in SD may initially appear normal because SD leads to hypometabolism of temporal poles, sometimes hard to recognize by visual inspection alone. Voxel-based statistical analyses can be particularly helpful. Usually, both temporal poles are affected (left greater than right), but sometimes degeneration is very asymmetrical, as in this case. *Upper panel*, Transaxial PET images of [¹⁸F]FDG uptake. *Lower panel*, Results of voxel-based statistical analysis using Neurostat/3D-SSP. Given are right and left lateral, superior, and inferior views (see **Fig. 33C.1** for additional details). *(Neurostat/3D-SSP analysis based on Minoshima, S., Frey, K.A., Koeppe, R.A., et al., 1995. A diagnostic approach in Alzheimer's disease using three-dimensional stereotactic surface projections of fluorine-18-FDG PET. J Nucl Med 36, 1238-1248.)*

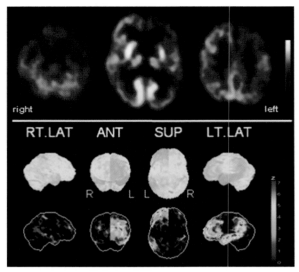

Fig. 33C.6 [¹⁸F]FDG PET in progressive aphasia (PA). [¹⁸F]FDG PET finding in PA is a very asymmetrical hypometabolism of left (speech dominant) hemisphere, which is usually already fairly pronounced when PA is first diagnosed. Both more frontal and more temporoparietal involvements have been described. In this case, there is also a pronounced striatal involvement. *Upper panel*, Transaxial PET images of [¹⁸F]FDG uptake. *Lower panel*, Results of voxel-based statistical analysis using Neurostat/3D-SSP. Given are right and left lateral, superior, and posterior views (see **Fig. 33C.1** for additional details). *(Neurostat/3D-SSP analysis based on Minoshima, S., Frey, K.A., Koeppe, R.A., et al., 1995. A diagnostic approach in Alzheimer's disease using three-dimensional stereotactic surface projections of fluorine-18-FDG PET. J Nucl Med 36, 1238-1248.)*

2003). The putamen, thalamus, and temporal and parietal cortices are also affected, although to a lesser extent (Garraux et al., 1999; Ishii et al., 1998). Despite the fact that FTD and AD affect overlapping cortical areas, the predominance of frontal and temporoparietal deficits, respectively, is usually very apparent and allows a clear distinction between FTD and AD. In line with this, a voxel-based statistical analysis provided a diagnostic accuracy of 90% (sensitivity 98%, specificity 86%) for separating FTD and AD in an autopsy-confirmed study, which was clearly superior to clinical diagnosis alone (Foster et al., 2007). As mentioned, additional hippocampal analyses may enable an even higher diagnostic accuracy (94%) for distinguishing FTD from AD, DLB, and control subjects (Mosconi et al., 2008). SD and PA are rather rare disorders, and PET studies are less abundant. Unlike FTD patients, SD patients usually show a predominant hypometabolism of the temporal lobes, most pronounced for the temporal poles, which is usually leftward asymmetrical (**Fig. 33C.5**) (Diehl et al., 2004; Rabinovici et al., 2008). In contrast, a strikingly greater left than right perisylvian hypometabolism of frontal, temporal, and parietal cortices is found in PA (**Fig. 33C.6**), with left insular/frontal opercular involvement being particularly associated with nonfluent aphasic features (Josephs et al., 2010; Nestor et al., 2003; Panegyres et al., 2008; Rabinovici et al., 2008). Given the relatively rare incidence of these syndromes and the controversy regarding their classification (Knibb et al., 2006), studies are missing that address the diagnostic value of [¹⁸F]FDG PET to distinguish between FTLD

subgroups (including additional entities not discussed here) and to separate these from other dementias.

Finally, pure vascular dementia (VD) seems to be rather rare in North America and Europe and more prevalent in Japan; [¹⁸F]FDG PET adds little to the diagnosis of VD. In agreement with CT and MRI, PET may show defects of [¹⁸F]FDG uptake corresponding to ischemic infarcts in all cerebral regions, including primary cortices, striatum/thalamus, and cerebellum. Since the latter are usually well preserved in AD, defects in these regions can be an important diagnostic clue. Deficits due to vascular lesions can be considerably larger or cause remote deficits of [¹⁸F]FDG uptake due to diaschisis. Furthermore, cerebral glucose metabolism was reported to be globally reduced (Mielke et al., 1992), but without absolute quantification this finding cannot be reliably assessed.

Parkinsonism

The current application of [¹⁸F]FDG PET and CBF SPECT in movement disorders focuses mostly on the diagnostic workup of parkinsonism, whereas their use for investigations of other movement disorders like Huntington or Wilson diseases is of little practical clinical importance in the era of gene analyses. Similar conclusions can also be drawn from CBF SPECT, but as noted earlier, the diagnostic accuracy is expected to be lower.

Most studies using quantitative [¹⁸F]FDG PET in idiopathic Parkinson disease (PD) reported a global decrease of

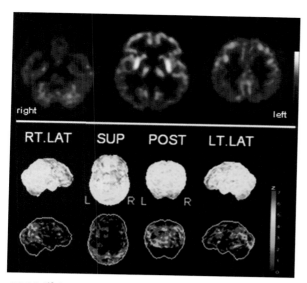

Fig. 33C.7 [^{18}F]FDG PET in Parkinson disease (PD). PD is typically characterized by (relative) striatal hypermetabolism. Temporoparietal hypometabolism can be observed in a significant fraction of PD patients without apparent cognitive impairment. As shown here, hypometabolism can be fairly pronounced, strongly resembling the typical finding in dementia with Lewy bodies/PD with dementia. However, it still unclear whether this represents preclinical dementia. *Upper panel,* Transaxial PET images of [^{18}F]FDG uptake. *Lower panel,* Results of voxel-based statistical analysis using Neurostat/3D-SSP. Given are right and left lateral, superior, and posterior views (see **Fig. 33C.1** for additional details). *(Neurostat/3D-SSP analysis based on Minoshima, S., Frey, K.A., Koeppe, R.A., et al., 1995. A diagnostic approach in Alzheimer's disease using three-dimensional stereotactic surface projections of fluorine-18-FDG PET. J Nucl Med 36, 1238-1248.)*

gray-matter CMRglc in nondemented PD patients compared to controls (Hu et al., 2000; Kuhl et al., 1984; Peppard et al., 1992). This global hypometabolism was more pronounced in demented PD patients, with accentuation in temporo-parieto-occipital cortices (Kuhl et al., 1984; Peppard et al., 1992; Vander Borght et al., 1997). Cerebral hypometabolism correlated with dementia severity (Piert et al., 1996). Interestingly, temporo-parieto-occipital hypometabolism may also been seen in nondemented PD patients (Hu et al., 2000), raising the important and so far unresolved question of whether this finding indicates an increased risk of subsequent dementia.

In addition, several studies investigated abnormalities in relative regional glucose metabolism (regional [^{18}F]FDG uptake normalized to global [^{18}F]FDG uptake), either by direct comparison between PD patients and controls or by more sophisticated methods like spatial covariance analyses. Both approaches yielded very similar findings in terms of affected regions and local effects (Eckert et al., 2005; Eidelberg et al., 1994; Tang et al., 2010a): relatively increased activity is usually observed in putamen, globus pallidus, thalamus, pons, cerebellum, and primary motor cortex, whereas decreased activity is detected in bilateral parietal, occipital, and frontal cortices (dorsolateral prefrontal, premotor, and supplementary motor areas) (**Fig. 33C.7**). Of note, however, since global normalization is performed, the aforementioned relative changes do not necessarily imply corresponding changes in absolute glucose metabolism (Borghammer et al., 2009).

Spatial covariance analyses can be powerful methods to identify abnormal cerebral networks as biomarkers for assessment of disease severity, progression, treatment efficacy, and differential diagnosis (Hirano et al., 2009). The expression of two distinctive spatial covariance patterns characterize PD: one related to motor manifestations and one related to cognitive manifestations. Alteration of metabolic brain network activity has been found to correlate with the cardinal motor symptoms of PD (PDRP), and a PD-related cognitive pattern (PDCP) has been described that correlates with cognitive impairment and affective disorder. A recent study showed that abnormal PDRP activity may precede motor symptom onset by 2 years (Tang et al., 2010b). Such analyses can also be useful for early diagnosis of suspected PD (separating PD from controls) (Eckert et al., 2005; Eidelberg et al., 1994, 1995), but it is unlikely that they will be superior to PET and SPECT examinations using molecular probes to investigate integrity of nigrostriatal dopaminergic projections like [^{18}F]FDOPA or [^{123}I]FP-CIT (Brooks, 2010; Piccini and Whone, 2004). The strength of [^{18}F]FDG PET in parkinsonism lies in the differential diagnosis of PD and atypical parkinsonian syndromes (APS) like multiple system atrophy (MSA), PSP, and CBD, that cannot be reliably differentiated on an individual patient basis by the aforementioned studies of nigrostriatal integrity, but present with distinct metabolic patterns on [^{18}F] FDG PET.

In a very recent large clinicopathological study (Ling et al., 2010) with extensive review of all medical records available, the sensitivity the clinical diagnosis was report to be 92.8% for PD, while the sensitivity was only 70.1% for MSA, 73.1% for PSP, and 26.3% for CBD. Specificity was 85.8% for PD and better than 95% for MSA, PSP, and CBD (Ling et al., 2010). In line with the fact that decisive diagnostic features tend to develop over time (often years) and that a considerable fraction of APS patients show some initial response to L-dopa, the sensitivity of the initial clinical diagnosis was reported to be lower: 73.5% for PD (Litvan et al., 1998), approximately 60% for MSA (Litvan et al., 1997, Osaki et al., 2002), and less than 50% for PSP (Osaki et al., 2004). Consequently, for appropriate therapy selection (including therapy trials), prognosis, and counseling of patients and caregivers, improving early differential diagnosis is essential, and [^{18}F] FDG PET can significantly contribute to this endeavor by providing disease-specific patterns of cerebral glucose metabolism. In MSA, decreased glucose metabolism is commonly found in striatum, brainstem, and cerebellum (**Fig. 33C.8**), which can be used as a reliable discriminator from PD (Antonini et al., 1997; Eidelberg et al., 1993; Ghaemi et al., 2002; Otsuka et al., 1997; Taniwaki et al., 2002). While patients with olivopontocerebellar atrophy have predominant cerebellar hypometabolism, predominant striatal hypometabolism is found in striatonigral degeneration (Perani et al., 1995). In addition, there is a reduction of cerebral glucose metabolism in the frontal cortices, which appears to spread to temporal and parietal cortices during the disease course, with subsequent cognitive decline (Lyoo et al., 2008; Otsuka et al., 1996). In PSP, glucose metabolism was consistently reported to be reduced in caudate nucleus and putamen, thalamus, pons/midbrain, and the mesial and dorsal frontal cortex (most notably in anterior cingulate cortex, precentral, dorso- and ventrolateral premotor and prefrontal areas) (Foster et al., 1988; Garraux et al., 1999; Hosaka et al., 2002; Juh et al., 2005;

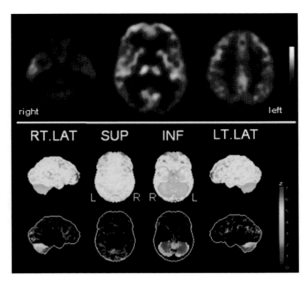

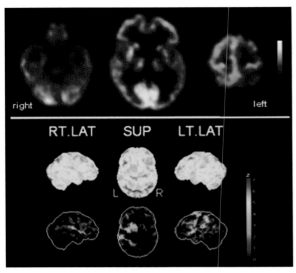

Fig. 33C.8 [¹⁸F]FDG PET in multiple system atrophy (MSA). In contrast to Parkinson disease, striatal hypometabolism is commonly found in MSA, particularly in those patients with striatonigral degeneration (SND, or MSA-P). In patients with olivopontocerebellar degeneration (OPCA, or MSA-C), cerebellar hypometabolism particularly evident, as shown here. *Upper panel,* Transaxial PET images of [¹⁸F]FDG uptake. *Lower panel,* Results of voxel-based statistical analysis using Neurostat/3D-SSP. Given are right and left lateral, superior, and inferior views (see **Fig. 33C.1** for additional details). *(Neurostat/3D-SSP analysis based on Minoshima, S., Frey, K.A., Koeppe, R.A., et al., 1995. A diagnostic approach in Alzheimer's disease using three-dimensional stereotactic surface projections of fluorine-18-FDG PET. J Nucl Med 36, 1238-1248.)*

Fig. 33C.10 [¹⁸F]FDG PET in corticobasal degeneration (CBD). In line with the clinical presentation, CBD is characterized by a strongly asymmetrical hypometabolism of frontal and parietal areas, striatum, and thalamus. Most pronounced hypometabolism is often found in parietal lobe, but patients with the clinical syndrome of CBD may also show a one-sided PSP-like pattern on [¹⁸F]FDG PET. *Upper panel,* Transaxial PET images of [¹⁸F]FDG uptake. *Lower panel,* Results of voxel-based statistical analysis using Neurostat/3D-SSP. Given are right and left lateral and superior views (see **Fig. 33C.1** for additional details). *(Neurostat/3D-SSP analysis based on Minoshima, S., Frey, K.A., Koeppe, R.A., et al., 1995. A diagnostic approach in Alzheimer's disease using three-dimensional stereotactic surface projections of fluorine-18-FDG PET. J Nucl Med 36, 1238-1248.)*

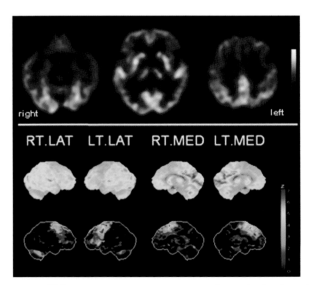

Fig. 33C.9 [¹⁸F]FDG PET in progressive supranuclear palsy (PSP). Typical finding in PSP is bilateral hypometabolism of mesial frontal and premotor/prefrontal areas. Thalamic and midbrain hypometabolism is usually also present. In line with overlapping pathologies in FTD and PSP, patients with clinical FTD can show a very PSP-like pattern, and vice versa. *Upper panel,* Transaxial PET images of [¹⁸F]FDG uptake. *Lower panel,* Results of voxel-based statistical analysis using Neurostat/3D-SSP. Given are right and left lateral and mesial views (see **Fig. 33C.1** for additional details). *(Neurostat/3D-SSP analysis based on Minoshima, S., Frey, K.A., Koeppe, R.A., et al., 1995. A diagnostic approach in Alzheimer's disease using three-dimensional stereotactic surface projections of fluorine-18-FDG PET. J Nucl Med 36, 1238-1248.)*

Karbe et al., 1992) (**Fig. 33C.9**). Comparing FTD and PSP, which both show frontal lobe involvement, striatofrontal metabolic impairment is greater in FTD, whereas mesencephalothalamic impairment was only observed in PSP (Garraux et al., 1999). Finally, the hallmark [¹⁸F]FDG PET of clinically diagnosed CBD is a highly asymmetrical cerebral hypometabolism in the thalamus, striatum, and predominantly parietal cortex but also frontal cortex (including cingulate cortex, precentral, premotor, and prefrontal areas) of the hemisphere contralateral to the side most clinically affected (Eidelberg et al., 1991; Garraux et al., 2000; Hosaka et al., 2002; Juh et al., 2005; Nagahama et al., 1997) (**Fig. 33C.10**). In a direct comparison of PSP and CBD, midbrain, thalamus, and cingulate cortex hypometabolism is greater in PSP, whereas asymmetry of the parietal lobes, sensorimotor area, and striatal involvement was more pronounced in clinical CBD (Garraux et al., 2000; Hosaka et al., 2002; Juh et al., 2005; Nagahama et al., 1997).

Few large-scale studies have explored the diagnostic value of [¹⁸F]FDG PET for differential diagnosis of uncertain parkinsonism. In one study, qualitative readings assisted by voxel-based statistical analyses were used to differentiate between PD, MSA, PSP, CBD, and healthy controls, using clinical diagnosis after a 2-year follow-up as reference. Disease-characteristic templates were used for data interpretation, which were generated by direct comparison of subsets of patients and controls (diagnostically most relevant features: PD, hypermetabolism in putamen; MSA, hypometabolism in putamen and cerebellum; PSP, hypometabolism in brainstem and midline frontal cortex; CBD, cortex and basal ganglia hypometabolism contralateral to the most affected body side) (Eckert et al., 2005). The following diagnostic accuracies were achieved in the individual groups: 97.7% in early PD, 91.6% in late PD, 96.0% in MSA, 85.0% in PSP, 90.1% in CBD, and 86.5% in controls. Except for the sensitivity in classifying PSP (85%) and controls (86%), sensitivity and specificity exceeded 90% in all other groups (Eckert et al., 2005). In a subsequent very recent study by the same group (Tang et al., 2010a), an automated image-based classification procedure relying on spatial covariance analyses was used to classify a large cohort of clinically diagnosed patients with PD, MSA, and PSP (follow-up > 6 months; on average, 2.6 years). The authors used a two-level analysis (first level: APS versus PD; second level: MSA versus PSP) to automatically classify patients according to disease-related metabolic patterns (see earlier discussion). Again, a high diagnostic accuracy was achieved in classifying PD (sensitivity/specificity 84%/97%), MSA (85%/96%), and PSP (88%/94%) (Tang et al., 2010a). However, it has to be acknowledged that this does not necessarily reflect the clinical situation. A typical clinical population also includes patients with CBD and possibly also patients with DLB, AD, and FTD, and finally, a relevant fraction of subjects without neurodegenerative parkinsonism (if not excluded beforehand by a preceding [123I]FP-CIT SPECT or [18F]FDOPA PET). Thus, an automated classification approach will probably result in a less optimal outcome in a typical clinical population. The overall classification accuracy in a four-class categorization (76%-84%; PD, MSA, PSP, and controls) was inferior to a three-class categorization (92%-94%; PD, MSA, and PSP only) using an automated classification based on principal component analysis (Spetsieris et al., 2009). On the other hand, an experienced observer will probably correctly recognize the majority of "unexpected" cases as such (e.g., AD and non-neurodegenerative patients).

As mentioned, an important caveat exists regarding the use of the clinical diagnosis of MSA, PSP, and even more so, CBD (Ling et al., 2010) as gold standards in diagnostic trials. In particular, the clinical distinction of CBD from PSP is questionable, since PSP is a common clinical misdiagnosis of pathologically verified CBD and a common pathological substrate of clinical CBD (Ling et al., 2010; Wadia and Lang, 2007). This issue gets even more complex if one considers that FTLD is often caused by PSP and CBD pathology (Kertesz et al., 2005). Thus, autopsy-confirmed imaging studies are ultimately needed to unravel this uncertainty and validate the use of [18F]FDG PET in parkinsonism.

Brain Tumors

Imaging with [18F]FDG PET or PET/CT is a well-established and often indispensable modality for diagnosis, staging, treatment monitoring, and follow-up of oncological patients with various malignancies of virtually all organs. Imaging of brain tumors was actually the first oncological application of [18F]FDG PET (Chen, 2007; Di Chiro et al., 1982; Herholz et al., 2007; Patronas et al., 1982). The degree of [18F]FDG uptake in brain tumors correlates with the grade of malignancy. The basis of this observation is not fully understood. As with other malignancies, both increased hexokinase activity and an increased glucose transport into the cell have been proposed. The use of [18F]FDG PET in brain tumors was recently

reviewed by a National Comprehensive Cancer Network (NCCN) panel. Based on current lower-level evidence (lack of randomized studies) and panel consensus (corresponding to category 2A), a role for [18F]FDG PET in managing brain tumors was proposed for diagnosis/staging, restaging/recurrence, prognosis, and possibly also for treatment planning/response monitoring (Podoloff et al., 2009).

The use of [18F]FDG PET in brain tumor imaging is complicated by the high physiological uptake of [18F]FDG in gray matter. Thus, unlike tumors of other organs that are usually visualized as areas of intense [18F]FDG uptake compared to the surrounding tissue, brain tumors with little [18F]FDG uptake present as uptake deficits in cortex or are hardly discernable when localized in white matter. In turn, tumors with high [18F]FDG uptake may be masked by physiological [18F]FDG uptake of the cortex. Thus, co-registration of the [18F]FDG PET scan to a recent MRI scan is mandatory for sufficient [18F]FDG PET interpretation to accurately delineate the area of interest (Borgwardt et al., 2005; Chao et al., 2001; Wong et al., 2004). This is of particular importance in tumors with low and heterogenous uptake as is often the case after therapy. Other PET radiotracers like 3'-deoxy-3'-18F-fluorothymidine ([18F]FLT; a marker of cell proliferation/DNA synthesis) or [11C]methionine and O-(2-[18F]fluoroethyl)-L-tyrosine ([18F]FET; markers of amino acid transport into the cell) offer the advantage of very low physiological brain uptake. The radiotracers [11C]methionine and O-(2-[18F]fluoroethyl)-L-tyrosine ([18F]FET) have been particularly well evaluated and represent very promising alternatives to [18F]FDG. They enable a very high lesion–to–normal brain contrast, particularly in high-grade gliomas but also in the majority of low-grade gliomas without contrast enhancement on MRI. Thus, they are particularly well suited for tumor delineation for treatment planning (surgery and radiation therapy) and biopsy guidance, comparing favorably with [18F]FDG (Goldman et al., 1997; Kaschten et al., 1998; Pauleit et al., 2009; Pirotte et al., 2004). Although some studies suggests that [18F]FET may also be a suitable tracer of brain tumor grading and therefore of prognostic relevance, this is still a matter of debate, particularly in comparison to [18F]FDG. Finally, the aforementioned tracers appear to be very suitable for the detection of persistent or recurrent brain tumors after therapy. However, given the limited availability of these tracers in routine clinical practice, we direct the interested reader to recent reviews (Chen, 2007; Herholz et al., 2007; Langen et al., 2006).

From the very early days of [18F]FDG PET scanning, it was known that high-grade gliomas (World Health Organization [WHO] grade III-IV) show a significantly higher [18F]FDG uptake than low-grade gliomas (WHO grade I-II) (Di Chiro et al., 1982). Low-grade gliomas usually have an [18F]FDG uptake that is below or roughly comparable to white matter (**Fig. 33C.11**), while high-grade gliomas commonly exhibit an [18F]FDG uptake that is distinctly higher than white matter. In fact, glioblastomas (WHO grade IV) commonly show areas of increased [18F]FDG uptake similar to or above that of gray matter, while uptake of anaplastic gliomas (WHO grade III) often falls below gray matter but noticeably above white matter (**Fig. 33C.12**). Several studies reported a high accuracy of [18F]FDG PET in differentiating low- and high-grade brain tumors, with a diagnostic sensitivity and specificity ranging from 84% to 94% and 77% to 95%, respectively (Delbeke

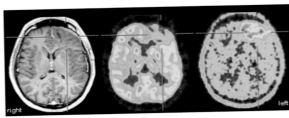

Fig. 33C.11 [^{18}F]FDG and [^{18}F]FET PET in a left frontal low-grade oligodendroglioma (WHO grade II). [^{18}F]FDG uptake *(middle)* of low-grade gliomas is usually comparable to white-matter uptake, prohibiting a clear demarcation of tumor borders. In contrast, the majority of low-grade gliomas (particularly oligodendroglioma) show intense and well-defined uptake of radioactive amino acids like [^{18}F]FET *(right)* even without contrast enhancement on MRI *(left)*. *(Courtesy Karl-Josef Langen, MD, Institute of Neuroscience and Medicine, Research Center Juelich, Germany.)*

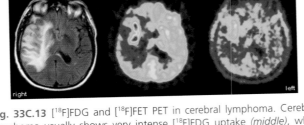

Fig. 33C.13 [^{18}F]FDG and [^{18}F]FET PET in cerebral lymphoma. Cerebral lymphoma usually shows very intense [^{18}F]FDG uptake *(middle)*, while metabolism of surrounding brain tissue is suppressed by extensive tumor edema (see MRI, *left*). [^{18}F]FET uptake *(right)* of cerebral lymphoma can also be high. *(Courtesy Karl-Josef Langen, MD, Institute of Neuroscience and Medicine, Research Center Juelich, Germany.)*

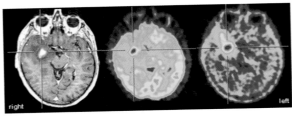

Fig. 33C.12 [^{18}F]FDG and [^{18}F]FET PET in a right mesial temporal high-grade astrocytoma (WHO grade III). In contrast to low-grade gliomas, high-grade tumors usually have [^{18}F]FDG uptake *(middle)* that is distinctly higher than white matter and sometimes even above gray matter, as in this case. Nevertheless, the [^{18}F]FET scan *(right)* clearly depicts a rostral tumor extension that cannot be identified by [^{18}F]FDG, owing to high physiological [^{18}F]FDG uptake by adjacent gray matter. Tumor delineation is clearer on [^{18}F]FET PET than on MRI *(left)*. *(Courtesy Karl-Josef Langen, MD, Institute of Neuroscience and Medicine, Research Center Juelich, Germany.)*

et al., 1995; Meyer et al., 2001; Padma et al., 2003). Qualitative readings were found to be at least as accurate as semiquantitative region-of-interest analyses (Meyer et al., 2001), and such differentiation is also possible in gliomatous and nongliomatous tumors (e.g., meningioma, angioma, etc.) (Delbeke et al., 1995; Meyer et al., 2001). Common causes of false-positive [^{18}F]FDG PET scans mimicking malignancy include brain abscesses, pituitary adenomas, juvenile pilocytic astrocytomas, choroid plexus papillomas, and gangliogliomas. High [^{18}F]FDG uptake in benign brain tumors is particularly often found in children, but [^{18}F]FDG PET has nevertheless been demonstrated to be a powerful method for tumor grading of childhood CNS tumors (Borgwardt et al., 2005). Finally, cerebral lymphomas usually possess extraordinary high [^{18}F]FDG uptake, making [^{18}F]FDG PET a powerful method to detect cerebral lymphoma (**Fig. 33C.13**). This can be particularly useful in differentiating nonmalignant CNS lesions in patients with acquired immunodeficiency syndrome (AIDS) (Hoffman et al., 1993).

It has been shown that the degree of [^{18}F]FDG uptake strongly predicts overall survival of patients with gliomas. Patients with increased tumor [^{18}F]FDG uptake had a significantly shorter survival (Alavi et al., 1988; Kim et al., 1991; Patronas et al., 1985). Importantly, this was also true within histological groups of high-grade tumors (in particular

glioblastoma multiforme), indicating that [^{18}F]FDG PET provides prognostic information beyond histological grading and may represent a more accurate marker of tumor aggressiveness (De Witte et al., 2000; Hölzer et al., 1993; Kim et al., 1991; Patronas et al., 1985). In a more recent large retrospective analysis, 94% of patients with low uptake (less or equal to white matter) survived for more than 1 year (median survival 28 months), while only 29% of patients with higher uptake (more than white matter) survived for more than 1 year (median survival 11 months) (Padma et al., 2003). Patients with primary brain tumors that exhibited persistent low [^{18}F]FDG uptake on follow-up studies had a significantly longer survival than those with increased [^{18}F]FDG uptake (Schifter et al., 1993). This is of particular relevance for follow-up and management of patients with low-grade gliomas that commonly show a malignant transformation during follow-up. Earlier studies demonstrated that malignant transformation of low-grade glioma is accompanied by focal hypermetabolism (Francavilla et al., 1989), which is associated with a considerably worse prognosis (De Witte et al., 1996). Thus, the diagnostic and prognostic information gained from [^{18}F]FDG PET can be of high therapeutic relevance (e.g., by selecting a more aggressive treatment).

Based on the observation that tumor areas with the highest [^{18}F]FDG uptake represent the most aggressive portions of the tumor, [^{18}F]FDG PET can also be used to direct stereotactic biopsies and tumor resections. It was demonstrated that incorporation of [^{18}F]FDG PET in biopsy planning considerably increased the diagnostic yield of biopsies, particularly in high-grade tumors with heterogenic tissue composition (Goldman et al., 1997; Pirotte et al., 1994). Furthermore, [^{18}F]FDG and [^{11}C]methionine PET was found to be helpful in targeting the resection to hypermetabolic/anaplastic tumor areas in high-grade gliomas (Pirotte et al., 2006). Complete removal of hypermetabolic tissue was associated with an increased survival in anaplastic gliomas and glioblastomas, whereas a total resection of MRI contrast-enhancing areas was not (Pirotte et al., 2009). With the same rationale, information on active tumor tissue from [^{18}F]FDG PET was also incorporated into radiation treatment planning (Douglas et al., 2006; Gross et al., 1998; Solberg et al., 2004; Tralins et al., 2002). Based on the few available studies, however, neither tumor volume definition nor targeting dose escalation by [^{18}F]FDG PET had a noticeable impact on survival of patients with high-grade gliomas, compared to literature data and historical

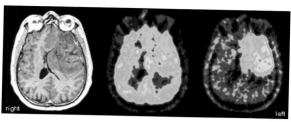

Fig. 33C.14 [^18^F]FDG and [^18^F]FET PET in a recurrent high-grade astrocytoma (WHO grade III). [^18^F]FDG uptake *(middle)* is clearly increased above expected background in several areas of suspected tumor recurrence on MRI *(left)*, confirming viable tumor tissue. In comparison to [^18^F]FDG PET, [^18^F]FET PET *(right)* more clearly depicts area of active tumor. *(Courtesy Karl-Josef Langen, MD, Institute of Neuroscience and Medicine, Research Center Juelich, Germany.)*

controls (Douglas et al., 2006; Gross et al., 1998). However, volumes of abnormal [^18^F]FDG uptake were of higher predictive value regarding time to progression and survival than MRI (Tralins et al., 2002).

Another important, albeit controversial, use of [^18^F]FDG PET imaging in brain tumors is the evaluation of persistent or recurrent disease—in particular, differentiation from radiation necrosis. In earlier studies, the sensitivity and specificity of differentiating recurrent brain tumors (including gliomas and metastases of various origins) from radiation necrosis was 80% to 100% and 40% to 100%, respectively (Langleben und Segall, 2000). False-negative findings may result from very recent radiation therapy, pretreatment low FDG uptake (e.g. in low-grade gliomas or metastases with low FDG avidity), and small tumor volumes (due to partial volume effects). Conversely, intense inflammatory reaction after (stereotactic) radiation therapy and seizure activity (possibly unnoticed) may result in false-positive PET findings. Earlier studies were done without PET/MRI co-registration, which can be a relevant source of error. Since [^18^F]FDG uptake in recurrent brain tumors and neighboring tissue is often lower than the uptake before radiation therapy, it is crucial to evaluate tumor uptake with reference to the expected background uptake in adjacent brain tissue (Chen, 2007). This is hardly possible without accurate anatomical information from MRI. In more recent reports, the sensitivity and specificity for detecting recurrent brain tumors was reported to be 76% to 78% and 95% to 96%, respectively, for gliomas (low and high grade) (Gómez-Río et al., 2008; Wang et al., 2006) and 82% to 86% and 80% to 97%, respectively, for brain metastases (Chao et al., 2001; Wang et al., 2006). Despite these fairly good results, the use of [^18^F]FDG PET for the purpose of detecting recurrent brain tumors remains controversial, and PET studies with amino acid tracers are probably superior (**Fig. 33C.14**).

Magnetic resonance spectroscopy (MRS) has been suggested in addition to MRI to help in the characterization of brain tumors by detecting metabolic alterations that may be indicative of the tumor class (Callot et al., 2008). MRS emerged as a clinical research tool in the 1990s, but it has not yet entered clinical practice. Of the principal metabolites that can be analyzed, *N*-acetylaspartate (NAA) is present in almost all neurons. Its decrease corresponds to neuronal death or injury or the replacement of healthy neurons by other cells (e.g., tumor). Choline-containing compounds increase whenever

there is cellular proliferation. Creatine is a marker of overall cellular density. Myoinositol is a sugar only present in glia. Lactate concentrations reflect hypoxic conditions as well as hypermetabolic glucose consumption. The most frequently studied chemical ratios to distinguish tumors from other brain lesions with MRS are choline/creatine, choline/NAA and lactate/creatine. Specifically, a choline/NAA ratio greater than 1 is considered to be indicative of neoplasm. The differentiation between astrocytoma WHO grade II and III is especially difficult. MRS in conjunction with structural MRI has been used to differentiate cystic tumor versus brain abscess (Chang et al., 1998), low-grade glioma versus gliomatosis cerebri, and edema versus infiltration (Nelson et al., 2002). Recent studies have shown that positive responses to radiotherapy or chemotherapy may be associated with a decrease of choline (Lichy et al., 2005; Murphy et al., 2004).

Epilepsy

In drug-refractory focal epilepsy, surgical resection of an epileptogenic focus offers patients the opportunity for a seizure-free outcome or greatly reduced seizure frequency, making epilepsy surgery the treatment method of choice in these patients. Accurate focus localization as a prerequisite for successful surgery is commonly accomplished by a comprehensive presurgical evaluation including neurological history and examination, neuropsychological testing, interictal and ictal electroencephalogram (EEG) depth recordings, high-resolution MRI, and video-EEG monitoring. To circumvent the necessity or, if necessary, to target invasive EEG recordings, [^18^F]FDG PET and CBF SPECT are often used to gain valuable information about the location of seizure onset. In contrast to the aforementioned PET and SPECT indications in which PET is superior to SPECT, both modalities are equally essential and often complementary in presurgical assessment of patients with drug-refractory focal epilepsy (Goffin et al., 2008). In general, PET and SPECT are of particular diagnostic value if surface EEG and MRI yield inconclusive or normal results (Casse et al., 2002; Knowlton et al., 2008; Willmann et al., 2007). Several neurotransmitter receptor ligands (most notably [^11^C]/[^18^F]flumazenil) have been proposed for diagnostic imaging in epilepsy. However, their use is still rather experimental, and their superiority compared to [^18^F]FDG PET and ictal SPECT have not been validated (Goffin et al., 2008).

Because of their rapid and virtually irreversible tissue uptake and their long physical half-lives, CBF SPECT tracers like [^99m^Tc]ECD and [^99m^Tc]HMPAO (in its stabilized form) can be used in combination with video-EEG monitoring to image the actual zone of seizure onset. To do so, the patient is monitored by video-EEG, and the tracer is administered as fast as possible after the onset of seizure or EEG discharges to capture the associated CBF increase. For rapid tracer administration and radiation safety reasons, the radiotracers should be stored in a shielded syringe pump (e.g., conventional contrast agent pump) and injected via remote control from the surveillance room. Actual SPECT acquisition can then be done at a later time point (preferably within 4 hours after injection) when the patient has recovered and is cooperative.

Although ictal SPECT alone may show a well-defined region of hyperperfusion corresponding to the seizure onset zone, it is generally recommended to acquire an additional

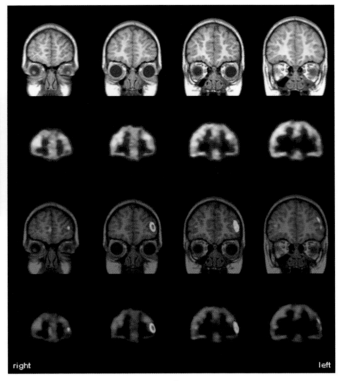

Fig. 33C.15 [¹⁸F]FDG PET and ictal [⁹⁹ᵐTc]ECD SPECT in left frontal lobe epilepsy. In this patient, MRI scan *(top row)* was normal, whereas [¹⁸F]FDG PET showed extensive left frontal hypometabolism *(second row)*. Additional ictal and interictal ⁹⁹ᵐTc]ECD SPECT scans were performed for accurate localization of seizure onset. Result of a SPECT subtraction analysis (ictal – interictal; blood flow increases above a threshold of 15%, maximum 40%) was overlaid onto MRI and [¹⁸F]FDG PET scan *(third and forth rows, respectively)*, clearly depicting the zone of seizure onset within the functional deficit zone given by [¹⁸F]FDG PET.

interictal SPECT scan (also under EEG monitoring to exclude seizure activity). By comparison of both scans, even areas with low ictal CBF increases or CBF increases from an interictally hypoperfused state to an apparent "normal" perfused ictal state can be reliably defined. In addition to visual inspection, quantitative analysis of both scans (e.g., SPECT image subtraction with statistical thresholding after accurate co-registration, global count rate normalization, and filtering for noise reduction) and overlay of areas of significant CBF changes onto a corresponding MRI are optimal for focus localization. Such analyses (e.g., subtraction ictal SPECT co-registered to MRI [SISCOM]) have been demonstrated to improve the accuracy and inter-rater agreement of seizure focus localization with ictal SPECT, particularly in frontoparietal neocortical epilepsy (Lee et al., 2006; O'Brien et al., 1998; Spanaki et al., 1999) (**Fig. 33C.15**). The area with the most intense and extensive ictal CBF increase is commonly assumed to represent the seizure onset zone. However, depending on the time gap between seizure onset and cerebral tracer fixation, ictal SPECT not only depicts the onset zone but also the propagation zone. Therefore, accurate knowledge about the time of tracer injection relative to seizure onset is crucial for ictal SPECT interpretation. CBF increases may propagate to various cortical areas during seizure progression, including the contralateral temporal lobe, insula, basal ganglia, and

frontal lobe in patients with temporal lobe epilepsy (TLE), reflecting seizure semiology (Shin et al., 2002). In patients with focal dysplastic lesions, four distinct ictal SPECT perfusion patterns have been observed depending on seizure propagation, during which the area of most intense CBF increase may actually migrate away from the seizure onset zone (Dupont et al., 2006). This underlines the need for rapid tracer injection after seizure onset to localize the onset zone most clearly. An injection delay of 20 to 45 seconds enables optimal localization results (O'Brien et al., 1998; Lee et al., 2006). At later time points and after seizure termination, a so-called postictal switch occurs, leading to hypoperfusion of the onset zone. Thus, within 100 seconds from seizure onset, about two-thirds of ictal SPECT studies can be expected to show hyperperfusion; after that (>100 seconds postictally), hypoperfusion will be observed (Avery et al., 1999).

The diagnostic sensitivity of ictal SPECT to correctly localize the seizure focus (usually with reference to surgical outcome) has been described to be 84% to 97% in TLE and 66% to 92% in extratemporal lobe epilepsy (ETLE) (Devous et al., 1998; Newton et al., 1995; Weil et al., 2001; Zaknun et al., 2008). Focus localization can also be successful by postictal tracer injection, capturing postictal hypoperfusion. However, localization accuracy will be lower (about 70%-75% in TLE and 50% in ETLE) (Devous et al., 1998; Newton et al., 1995). In contrast, interictal SPECT to detect (possibly mild) interictal hypoperfusion is insufficient for focus localization (sensitivity about 50% in TLE; of no diagnostic value in ETLE) (Newton et al., 1995; Spanaki et al., 1999; Zakun et al., 2008).

In contrast to ictal SPECT, [¹⁸F]FDG PET studies are regularly performed in the interictal state to image the functional deficit zone, which shows abnormal metabolism between seizures and is generally assumed to contain also the seizure onset zone. The etiology of this hypometabolism is not fully understood and probably relates to functional (e.g., surround inhibition of areas of seizure onset and propagation as a defense mechanism) and structural changes (e.g., neuronal or synaptic loss due to repeated seizures). Therefore, the hypometabolism found on interictal [¹⁸F]FDG PET usually extends considerably beyond the actual seizure onset zone. A direct comparison of ictal perfusion abnormalities detected by SISCOM and interictal [¹⁸F]FDG PET hypometabolism in TLE patients demonstrated high concordance, suggesting that seizures are generated and spread in metabolically abnormal regions (Bouilleret et al., 2002). To ensure an interictal state, the patient should ideally be seizure free for at least 24 hours before PET and be monitored by EEG after [¹⁸F]FDG injection to rule out possible subclinical epileptic activity. The use of a voxel-wise statistical analysis to supplement visual analysis is recommended. Visual analysis by an experienced observer is at least as accurate in TLE patients (**Fig. 33C.16**), but accuracy and interobserver agreement of focus localization is considerably improved by additional voxel-wise statistical analyses in ETLE (Drzezga et al., 1999) (**Fig. 33C.17**). Since PET imaging in epilepsy patients relies on hypometabolic areas, its diagnostic value can be severely compromised if a hypometabolic structural abnormality or lesion is present (e.g., low-grade tumor, infarct, contusion). In such cases, ictal SPECT should be preferred to directly image the area of seizure onset.

In recent meta-analyses, the sensitivity of [¹⁸F]FDG PET for focus lateralization (rather than localization given the extent of hypometabolism) in TLE was reported to be around 86%,

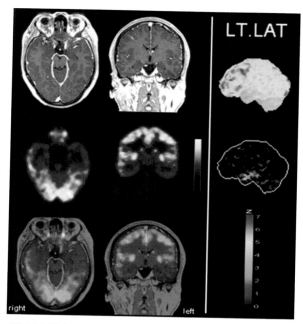

Fig. 33C.16 [^{18}F]FDG PET in left temporal lobe epilepsy. Diagnostic benefit of [^{18}F]FDG PET is greatest in patients with normal MRI *(left panel, top row)* in which [^{18}F]FDG PET still detects well-lateralized temporal lobe hypometabolism *(second row:* left temporal lobe hypometabolism). As in this patient with left mesial temporal lobe epilepsy, the area of hypometabolism often extends to the lateral cortex (functional deficit zone; *third row:* PET/MRI fusion). *Right panel,* Results of voxel-based statistical analysis of [^{18}F]FDG PET scan using Neurostat/3D-SSP. Given are left lateral views *(top image:* [^{18}F]FDG uptake; *bottom image:* statistical deviation of uptake from healthy controls, color-coded as z score; see **Fig. 33C.1** for additional details). *(Neurostat/3D-SSP analysis based on Minoshima, S., Frey, K.A., Koeppe, R.A., et al., 1995. A diagnostic approach in Alzheimer's disease using three-dimensional stereotactic surface projections of fluorine-18-FDG PET. J Nucl Med 36, 1238-1248.)*

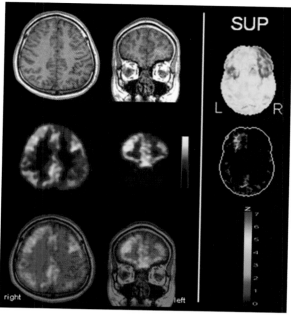

Fig. 33C.17 [^{18}F]FDG PET in left frontal lobe epilepsy. Despite normal MRI scan *(left panel, top row)*, [^{18}F]FDG PET *(second row)* depicts a circumscribed area of left frontal hypometabolism (i.e., functional deficit zone; *third row:* PET/MRI fusion). Additional voxel-based statistical analysis of [^{18}F]FDG PET scan is strongly recommended in extratemporal lobe epilepsy to improve sensitivity and reliability *(right panel:* results of a Neurostat/3D-SSP analysis. Given are views from superior of [^{18}F]FDG uptake *(top)* and of statistical deviation of uptake from healthy controls, color-coded as z score *(bottom)*; see **Fig. 33C.1** for additional details. *(Neurostat/3D-SSP analysis based on Minoshima, S., Frey, K.A., Koeppe, R.A., et al., 1995. A diagnostic approach in Alzheimer's disease using three-dimensional stereotactic surface projections of fluorine-18-FDG PET. J Nucl Med 36, 1238-1248.)*

whereas false lateralizations to the contralateral side of the epileptogenic focus rarely occur (<5%) (Casse et al., 2002; Willmann et al., 2007). Consequently, presurgical unilateral temporal hypometabolism predicts a good surgical outcome (Engel Class I-II) in 82% to 86% of total TLE cases and even 80% and 72% in TLE patients with normal MRI and nonlocalized ictal scalp EEG, respectively (Casse et al., 2002; Willmann et al., 2007). In contrast, asymmetrical thalamic metabolism (particularly in reverse direction to temporal lobe asymmetry) and extratemporal cortical hypometabolism (in particular of the contralateral hemisphere) are associated with poor postoperative seizure control (Choi et al., 2003; Newberg et al., 2000). In ETLE, the sensitivity of [^{18}F]FDG PET is lower, providing a seizure focus localization in about 67% of ETLE patients (Casse et al., 2002; Drzezga et al., 1999). Again, correct localization by [^{18}F]FDG PET was demonstrated to be a significant predictor of a good surgical outcome in a recent large study in patients with neocortical epilepsy (Yun et al., 2006).

Few large-scale studies directly compared ictal SPECT and interictal [^{18}F]FDG PET. Comparing rates of correct lateralizations provided by [^{18}F]FDG PET and [^{99m}Tc]HMPAO SPECT in patients with good surgical outcome revealed that the overall performance of [^{18}F]FDG PET was slightly better (86%, compared to 78% for SPECT), mainly because of higher accuracy in TLE cases (90% versus 83%; 64% versus 62% in

ETLE) (Won et al., 1999). In patients with focal cortical dysplasia (FCD), [^{18}F]FDG PET showed a corresponding focal hypometabolism in 71% and SPECT an ictal hyperperfusion in 60% of cases. However, unlike the extent of lesion resection and pathological features, neither PET nor SPECT findings predicted good surgical outcome in FCD (Kim et al., 2009a). A prospective study was recently performed in patients who had ETLE in the majority of cases and in which seizure onsets could not be localized by scalp EEG and MRI. In this challenging patient population, the sensitivity/specificity (with respect to surgical outcome) of PET and SPECT were 59%/79% and 50%/72%, respectively (Knowlton et al., 2008). Finally, in pediatric patients, [^{18}F]FDG PET was found particularly valuable in TLE (correct lateralization/localization 96%/73%), whereas ictal CBF SPECT with SISCOM was more accurate in ETLE (correct lateralization/localization 92%/85%) (Kim et al., 2009).

Presurgical Brain Mapping

The use of BOLD-based fMRI for presurgical mapping has been one of the first clinical applications for fMRI. Despite multiple efforts to develop standardized and reproducible paradigms for routine use, there has been a certain reluctance to use fMRI as a presurgical tool. There is uncertainty about the origin and basis for the BOLD signal and about the physiological meaning of "activation" foci measured with fMRI. In a scientific research environment, in which the pros and cons of fMRI can be carefully weighed, information from fMRI has been extremely helpful. But is the technique foolproof enough for widespread use in clinical diagnostic and therapeutic decision making? An absolute requirement on the part of the treating physician is a profound and detailed understanding of the potentials and pitfalls of this technique. As brain function is organized in networks, sparing a "focus of activation" during operation does not necessarily mean preservation of function, and vice versa. The reason for this is the "the trouble with cognitive subtraction" (Friston et al., 1996). Subtracting an "easy" control task from a more difficult one does not reflect the way the brain works, as interaction analyses have shown. In addition, fMRI data are usually thresholded to dissociate true activations from spurious "activations," thus minimizing type I errors. Unfortunately, this is not absolute, since statistical thresholding can only reduce the errors but not completely avoid them. Using fMRI for presurgical planning poses a different problem, namely that of sensitivity minimizing type II error (false negative results). This is a difficult task because when using very low thresholds in fMRI analyses, many areas of the brain are seen as activated. Furthermore, the BOLD signal differs significantly between individuals, and therefore absolute thresholds set for a whole population are unreliable (Klöppel and Büchel, 2005). Nevertheless, the potential use seems very attractive for clinicians, and every effort should be made to improve the quality and interpretation of these measurements. Paradigms involving verbal fluency, semantic decisions, or verb generation activate frontal language areas. The combination with auditory comprehension tasks can increase the validity of lateralization testing (Carpentier et al., 2001). Lehéricy et al. (2000) found no significant correlation between Wada test lateralization and fMRI activation patterns in temporal areas but did find correlations in frontal areas and the anterior insula for semantic fluency and story-listening tasks. Prediction of postsurgical naming ability is more reliable with fMRI than with Wada testing (Sabsevitz et al., 2003). Verbal memory is reduced on the side of the seizure focus in mesial temporal lobe epilepsy (Jokeit et al., 2001). On a single subject level, Janszky et al. (2005) found a high correlation between lateralization in fMRI and memory outcome. Standard procedures for presurgical mapping with fMRI (e.g., in epilepsy surgery) have been developed (Fernández et al., 2001) that include fiber tracking as well as BOLD-based fMRI. Robust fiber tracking with definite-endpoint tools should significantly facilitate this application (Kreher et al., 2007, 2008). Moreover, maps of fiber connections in the human brain may be used as a priori knowledge for the interpretation of functional neuroimaging data. These approaches are expected to contribute significantly to the development of models of brain function but have not really been used thus far.

Imaging with [18F]FDG PET has also been employed for preoperative functional mapping of eloquent cortices using language or motor activation tasks. By contrasting an activation scan with a rest scan, a sensitivity of 94% and a specificity of 95% for identification of motor-associated brain areas have been reported in comparison to direct cortical electrostimulation (DCES) (Schreckenberger et al., 2001). Of note, the rest scan can also be used for diagnostic brain tumor workup. Despite the fact that such studies yield strong and robust

activation signals (e.g., 21% and 17% metabolism increases for hand and foot movement, respectively) (Schreckenberger et al., 2001), presurgical PET activation studies assessing CBF changes with [15O]water offer the advantage of allowing multiple studies covering several eloquent areas in shorter time because of the short half-life of oxygen-15. In conjunction with statistical parametric mapping (SPM), such [15O]water PET activation studies were demonstrated to be a suitable method for mapping of motor and language functions and possible detection of functional reorganization processes in brain tumor patients (Meyer et al., 2003a, 2003b). Functional MRI offers the advantage of being widely available (in contrast to [15O]water PET, which is dependent on an onsite cyclotron) and easily implemented in clinical practice. Presurgical fMRI has been validated against [18F]FDG and [15O]water activation PET and DCES (Krings et al., 2001; Reinges et al., 2004). Functional MRI provides comparable results in motor activation tasks, but in speech activation tasks, PET offers the advantages of greater activation signals (higher sensitivity), lower susceptibility to motion artifacts (e.g., during overt articulation, important to verify adequate task performance), and considerably lower ambient noise.

Recovery from Stroke

During the last 20 years, the application of functional brain imaging to stroke patients has brought new insights into the field of rehabilitation (Rijntjes and Weiller, 2002). We understand better what happens in the brain after stroke. For example, we "see an active ipsilateral motor cortex" when we notice mirror movements of the healthy hand during ward rounds, or we assume the resolution of diaschisis when language performance improves abruptly from one day to the next within the first week after a stroke.

Imaging the acute phase of stroke (i.e., the first days after stroke onset) offers the opportunity for unique insights into the function and dysfunction of the brain. Various effects may be differentiated, resulting in the observed clinical deficit (**Fig. 33C.18**, *A*).

Ischemia directly affects functionally relevant gray- or white-matter structures, resulting in either complete or incomplete infarction (Weiller et al., 1993b). In the acute phase, symptoms often fluctuate owing to the instability of the lesion. This is mainly caused by changes in cerebral perfusion and the extension of the peri-infarct edema. For example, reperfusion of the left posterior middle temporal and frontal areas may be associated with early improvement in picture naming (Hillis et al., 2006).

The structural lesion itself may cause a dysfunction in remote noninfarcted but connected areas. The concept of "diaschisis" was introduced by von Monakow (1906). *Diaschisis* is seen as a temporary disturbance of function through disconnection. Von Monakow thereby integrated localist ideas with holistic views. Taken together, the lesion of a critical network component may result in an acute global network breakdown. In this situation, we typically observe a more severe functional deficit.

Reversal of diaschisis may explain acute functional improvements. Von Monakow related this phenomenon predominantly to higher cortical functions such as language. **Fig. 33C.19** shows an example of early fMRI activation in a patient with acute global aphasia due to a left temporal middle

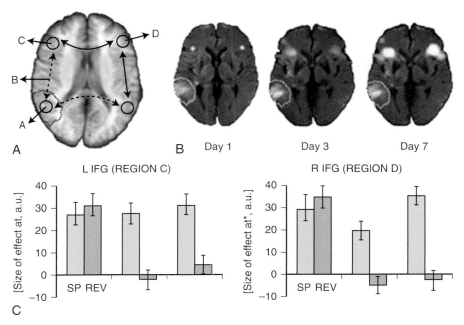

Fig. 33C.18 A, Schematic diagram of direct and indirect consequences of focal ischemia on language network. Dotted lines indicate ischemic areas in left temporal cortex; black circles indicate candidate language areas in both hemispheres. Ischemia may cause direct damage of language-relevant gray (A) and white (B) matter *(dashed lines)*, resulting in a functional and anatomical disconnection of remote areas C and D due to missing functional input (diaschisis). **B,** Demonstration of fMRI activation for a patient with a left (dominant) temporal infarction performing two auditory language comprehension tasks, one being listening to speech and the other being listening to speech presented in reverse. The fMRI analysis that contrasts speech with reversed speech is displayed ($P < 0.05$, corrected for multiple comparisons). Infarct is outlined with a dashed line. At day 1, no language-specific activation was detectable (i.e., no significant difference in language-area activation when language task (speech) was contrasted with non-language task [reversed speech]). At this time, patient presented with acute global aphasia. Follow-up examinations at days 3 and 7 revealed increased language-specific activation in language areas (bilateral inferior frontal gyrus [IFG]) in parallel with improvement of behavioral language function. **C-D,** Effect sizes for fMRI activation, extracted from left (region C) and right (region D) IFG. Notably, at day 1, there is a strong effect for both language task (speech [SP]) and non-language task (reversed speech [REV]). However, left and right IFG did not distinguish between these two conditions, indicating an acute dysfunction of preserved remote areas in terms of diaschisis. This ability to distinguish between speech and reversed speech is recovered at days 3 and 7, indicating a resolution of diaschisis in parallel with language behavioral gains.

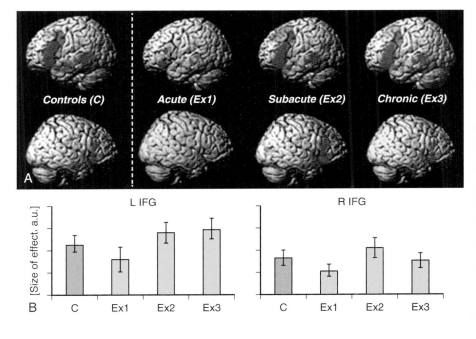

Fig. 33C.19 A, Dynamics of language-specific (speech [SP] contrasted with reversed speech [REV]) fMRI activation in healthy control subjects (first column, a single fMRI exam) and in 14 patients with acute aphasia (columns 2-4, representing the three exams). Activation is shown for left hemisphere in top row and for right hemisphere in bottom row. Note that there is little or no left hemisphere activation in acute stage. This is followed by a bilateral increase in activation in the subacute stage, peaking in right hemisphere homolog of the Broca area. In chronic phase, consolidation and gradual normalization emerged, with a "re-shift" to left hemisphere. **B,** Parameter estimates extracted in left and right inferior frontal gyrus (IFG), indicating a continuous increase of activation in left IFG over time but a biphasic course in right IFG. *(Modified from Saur, D., Lange, R., Baumgaetner, A., et al., 2006. Dynamics of language reorganization after stroke. Brain 129, 1371-1384.)*

cerebral artery (MCA) infarction. In an auditory language comprehension task, the patient listened to three sentences of intelligible speech (SP) and also listened to sentences of reversed speech (REV). Extraction of condition-wise effect sizes (see **Fig. 33C.19, *B***) showed that in the hyperacute phase about 10 hours after onset, remote left and right inferior frontal gyrus (IFG) were dysfunctional. Although a strong effect for both the SP and REV conditions was observed, neither area distinguished between intelligible SP and unintelligible REV, inasmuch as activation was the same for both tasks. However, 3 and 7 days later, in parallel with improvements in language behavior, a clear differentiation between conditions returned to both brain areas, indicating functional recovery of these remote areas, which most likely might be explained by a resolution of diaschisis. That is, injury to the left temporal language areas produced diaschisis in bilateral IFG, which produced dysfunction and inability to distinguish SP from REV. With resolution of diaschisis, bilateral IFG function returned, and these language network areas were able to function and thereby contribute to effective language behavior and thus compensate for the deficit (Saur et al., 2006b).

Imaging the acute state in patients with aphasia may offer another lesson related to our understanding of subcortical aphasia. Aphasia in striatocapsular infarction was related to the cortical hypoperfusion caused by an occlusion of the proximal segment of the MCA, rather than the subcortical infarction itself. This cortical hypoperfusion led to a subsequent cortical atrophy 1 year later (Weiller et al., 1990), interpreted as selective neuronal loss (Weiller et al., 1993), which is typically invisible on conventional MRI but detectable with [^{123}I]iomazenil SPECT (Saur et al., 2006a). This observation was later confirmed by a perfusion imaging study by Hillis et al. (2002), who demonstrated that aphasia due to acute subcortical infarction can be largely explained by concurrent cortical hypoperfusion. These findings underline the importance of accurately characterizing acute ischemia, including registration of hypoperfused tissue by performing multiparametric MRI sequences.

A note of caution is warranted here. Obviously fMRI is only associated with relative changes in cerebral perfusion performed with the BOLD technique. This may and will produce misleading results in patients with altered global blood flow, as in the acute or subacute state of stroke (e.g., hypoperfusion, hyperemia). The BOLD response is affected by internal carotid artery occlusion (Altamura et al., 2009; Hamzei et al., 2003). In these situations, currently the only reliable approach is to use absolute measurements performed with PET. In the future, arterial spin labeling may be used for fMRI studies as a means to ultimately obtain absolute quantification for perfusion studies (Hernandez-Garcia et al., 2010; Kelly et al., 2010). The infarct does affect the normalization procedure, BOLD responses vary with age, making the use of age-matched controls mandatory, and finally, the relation of function (e.g., force) to rCBF may be different in stroke patients from normals requiring different approaches in data analysis (Dettmers et al., 1997).

Neural reorganization of language functions may be better understood by imaging the recovery process throughout all phases after stroke, which allows one to relate changes in language performance to changes in language-related brain activation. Saur et al. (2006) performed the same auditory comprehension task as described earlier for the single subject study on a heterogeneous group of 14 aphasic patients suffering from a left MCA stroke affecting temporal, frontal, and subcortical brain regions. The fMRI data were collected in the acute (<4 days after stroke, Exam 1), subacute (about 2 weeks after stroke, Exam 2), and chronic (4-12 months after stroke, Exam 3) phases of recovery. Across these three fMRI exams, patients recovered from aphasia. Group analysis of the fMRI data (see **Fig. 33C.19, *A***) revealed little or no left hemisphere (see **Fig. 33C.19, *A, top row***) activation in the acute stage, followed by a strong bilateral increase in activation in the subacute stage, peaking in the right hemisphere (see **Fig. 33C.19, *A, bottom row***), the homolog of the Broca area. In the chronic phase, a consolidation and gradual normalization emerged, with a "re-shift" to the left hemisphere. Language-specific effect sizes (see **Fig. 33C.19, *B***; SP contrasted with REV) showed a continuous increase throughout all phases in left inferior frontal gyrus, while in the right hemisphere homologue, a more biphasic course with a temporary increase in the subacute stage was observed. The early increase of activation in right hemisphere homolog of the Broca area correlated with early improvement of language function. Since in this study, an overall pattern of reorganization was derived from a heterogeneous group of stroke patients, relating of the group activation to the lesion site was not possible. Consequently, Saur et al. (2009) investigated a homogeneous group of eight patients who all suffered from a left temporal infarction. The greatest lesion overlap in this group was found in the anterior temporal lobe. The longitudinal study design was the same as described earlier. Again, in the acute phase, reduced activation in the entire language network was found, including the uninfarcted left frontal cortex. Since in all patients, left inferior frontal cortex was intact, we interpreted the reduced activation in this area as a demonstration of diaschisis due to disconnection of left temporal cortex and left frontal cortex. In the subacute phase, an increase in bilateral frontal region was observed. Finally, in the chronic phase, perilesional activation in posterior temporal areas emerged. This perilesional activation was found in areas also activated in healthy subjects, indicating a reactivation of temporarily dysfunctional tissue rather than a true recruitment of novel brain areas. From these studies, a longitudinal three-phase model of brain reorganization during recovery from aphasia was derived (Rijntjes and Weiller, 2002; Saur et al., 2006). In the acute phase, nearly complete abolishment of language function is reflected by little if any activation in brain regions which later can be activated by language tasks. In this acute phase, there is a global network breakdown in which "diaschisis" or ischemic stunning (Alexandrov et al., 2004) is the key factor. A second "hyperactive" stage of brain activation follows in which the altered function recovers at a rapid pace. It is characterized by a sudden return of activation in the left hemisphere and often a hyperactivation of homolog right hemisphere areas and may include reversal from diaschisis. In the third stage, a consolidation of activation resembling the patterns in healthy controls follows. It is unclear whether similar patterns occur in the motor system following infarction.

The majority of imaging studies on language recovery were performed in the chronic phase after stroke. In these studies, patients who recovered to various degrees were examined one or more times with PET or fMRI to identify the pattern of the activation in the lesioned brain. These studies with very heterogeneous designs, methods, and patients have shown that brain reorganization after stroke comprises areas that are also activated under normal conditions during language tasks, involve both the lesioned and the contralesional hemisphere, and often require compensatory mechanisms (Heiss et al., 1999; Leff et al., 2002; Musso et al., 1999; Rosen et al., 2000; Sharp et al., 2004; Warburton et al., 1999; Weiller et al., 1995; Zahn et al., 2006). More specific conclusions can be drawn by correlating the proficiency of a particular function with task-related activation in a cross-sectional design. For instance, Crinion and Price, (2005) demonstrated in a group of 17 patients with left temporal lobe stroke that performance in auditory sentence comprehension was positively correlated with activation in the right lateral superior temporal gyrus. These results demonstrate that in the chronic phase, too, right hemisphere activation might be beneficial. Additional evidence comes from a dynamic challenge in which repetitive behavioral studies are performed. Musso et al. (1999) showed that after repeated 8-minute sessions of language comprehension training, subsequent behavioral improvement correlated with an increase of activation in the right temporal cortex, supporting a role for right hemisphere language homolog areas in language function after stroke.

Several studies have shown task-related activation changes from pre- to posttreatment scans. Even short-term treatment may influence the neural basis of language processing. Studies by Musso et al. (1999) and Blasi et al. (2002) demonstrated increased activity in the right frontal cortex associated with learning a word retrieval task. Studies performing long-term training found left (Cornelissen et al., 2003; Leger et al., 2002; Meinzer et al., 2008; Vitali et al., 2007), right (Crosson et al., 2005; Raboyeau et al., 2008), or bilateral activation to be associated with treatment-induced improvement (Fridriksson et al., 2006, 2007; Meinzer et al., 2007). In contrast, Richter et al. (2008) found no significant changes of fMRI activation at all after 2 weeks of "constraint-induced aphasia therapy." This heterogeneity of results is best explained by differences in treatment strategies and language impairments, as well as differences in lesion sites and sizes. In post-stroke brain reorganization, as with many aspects of stroke recovery, many factors can contribute to differences between patients. However, these studies do demonstrate clearly that remodeling of cortical functions is possible even years after stroke and typically occurs in both the left and right hemispheres as well as perilesional language zones, similar to what has been described in the motor system (Liepert et al., 2000).

Most brain functions are organized in distributed, segregated, and interconnected networks, and brain reorganization due to lesions or interventions mainly takes place within the framework of these networks (Rijntjes and Weiller, 2002; Weiller and Rijntjes, 1999). Language is a brain function especially suited to assessing a network approach during recovery after injury, as it is represented in a widespread bilateral fashion. Recent combinations of fMRI with probabilistic fiber tracking, integrating pairwise point-to-point anatomical connections along with measurements of functional connectivity, resulted in a relatively complete network description of language processing around the sylvian fissure (Saur et al., 2008, 2010). In contrast to classical diagrams that suppose speech comprehension to be localized in the temporal lobe, speech production in the inferior frontal lobe, and both regions connected through the arcuate fascicle, the modern anatomical view proposes that the left temporal lobe connects to most of

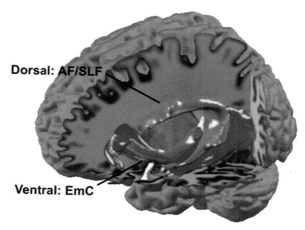

Fig. 33C.20 Diffusion tensor imaging tracking results for ventral and dorsal language pathways projecting to the prefrontal and premotor cortex. *AF,* Arcuate fasciculus; *EmC,* extreme capsule; *SLF,* superior longitudinal fasciculus. *(Modified from Saur, D., Kreher, B.W., Schnell, S., et al., 2008. Ventral and dorsal pathways for language. Proc Natl Acad Sci USA 105, 18035-18040.)*

the frontal lobe along two segregated and integrating large association tracts (Anwander et al., 2007; Frey et al., 2009; Makris et al., 2008; Saur et al., 2008) (**Fig. 33C.20**). A dorsal route along the arcuate fasciculus/superior longitudinal fasciculus mainly projects to premotor cortices for automated sensory-motor mapping, while several aspects of language comprehension utilize a ventral route via the extreme capsule mainly projecting to the prefrontal cortex. These new findings not only require a new description of anatomical correlation of language functions and dysfunctions but also imply various routes of compensation after stroke.

The network view addresses another frequent misconception, namely the assumption of functional independence of brain "centers." As an example, *conduction aphasia*, which is often defined as an isolated repetition failure with preserved comprehension and spontaneous speech, is supposed to result from a destruction of the pathway (i.e., the arcuate fascicle) connecting the sensory and the motor speech centers, which themselves are intact. Such a conclusion assumes that the temporal lobe suffices for comprehension, and the inferior frontal cortex for language production, and that a disruption of the connecting pathway does not affect the function of either area. We know from imaging experiments that this is not true. Semantic tasks activate the Broca area and propositional speech as well as the temporal lobe (Vigneau et al., 2006). The various constituents of language circuitry are not independent from each other; interruptions in the network have an impact on the remaining parts of the network. In other words, the functions of the Broca or Wernicke areas with an intact arcuate fascicle may not be the same as after that fascicle's destruction. The network view takes this into account when interpreting symptoms and activations in patients with aphasia.

If the individual nodes of the network influence each other through their connections, the importance of a network node might be determined by the number of its connections used for a certain task. This leads directly to the concept of critical lesions. The more important a network node is to a behavior, the more behavioral effects its lesioning will have. Using a combination of functional and anatomical connectivity to identify networks subserving auditory language comprehension within a temporofrontal network, the posterior part of the middle temporal gyrus and the inferior frontal gyrus in the left hemisphere were identified as having the most functionally relevant connections (Saur et al., 2008). Therefore, both regions are especially important in comprehension. One question posed was how much of the left hemisphere network had to be spared to prevent right hemisphere recruitment (Rijntjes and Weiller, 2002). The network approach described previously would focus this question to critical lesions of the left hemisphere (i.e., those that affect the regions with most connections). For example, in patients with temporal lesions sparing the posterior temporal region, it is exactly this posterior region which shows the best correlation with language performance over time (Sauer et al., 2010). In contrast, if this posterior region is spared, the contralateral hemisphere comes into play (Weiller et al., 1995). However, there is also a clear hierarchy between the nodes of a network such as the Broca area, which is indispensable for grammar (Musso et al., 2003).

Combining functional and structural network identification procedures is a promising approach to improve our understanding of loss and recovery of brain functions. However, beyond this more theoretical interest, we suggest that a precise description of the lesioned network might be useful to guide the application of focal brain stimulation techniques such as transcranial direct current stimulation, or rTMS (e.g. Naeser et al., 2005; see also Chapter 32C). In future settings, patients will be investigated with fMRI and diffusion tensor imaging prior to brain stimulation. Processing of the impaired language function will be analyzed with the earlier-mentioned network identification procedures. Subsequent brain stimulation and adjuvant therapies might then be applied to the identified central processing nodes to support behavioral training.

Although our understanding about what changes take place during stroke recovery has increased immensely, functional imaging still has not found a firm place in clinical rehabilitation, primarily because there are still many unanswered questions about what these reorganization processes mean in terms of therapeutic interventions.

Three phases of reorganization after stroke with aphasia or hemiparesis can now be described in some detail, and it is probable that therapies should be adjusted depending on the phase the patient is in. For example, to stimulate the second phase in motor stroke, characterized by bilateral activations, it might be opportune to offer therapies that also involve the ipsilateral contralesional hemisphere (Winhuisen et al., 2005). However, there is still a complete lack of relating the phase of recovery with overt performance. At the moment, no clinical correlate is known for determining, for example, whether a patient is in the second phase or third phase of recovery.

The clinical relevance of different activations in different patients is still unclear. If after motor stroke, patients show a strong activation in the ipsilateral motor cortex, should this mean that a therapy with emphasis on bilateral movements is warranted, or would it be better to counter this activation pattern and concentrate on stimulating the contralateral lesioned hemisphere using constraint-induced movement therapy (CIMT)? Many studies on reorganization use small groups of patients and do not investigate the long-tem benefit of therapies, which limits the informative value of these findings.

Functional imaging has shown that improvement can be associated with different patterns of reorganization (Feydy et al., 2002; Weiller et al., 1993). For example, in motor stroke, improvement after CIMT can be associated either with an increase or a decrease of activation in the primary motor cortex, depending on the size of the pyramidal tract lesion (Hamzei et al., 2006, 2008). However, it is unclear whether one pattern is more beneficial than the other in the long term, or if patients with one pattern need more or different therapy.

In rehabilitation from stroke, information about the relationship between the amount of therapy and the amount of improvement is scarce. Similar to pharmacological studies, dose-response curves should be developed (Dobkin, 2005). Functional imaging could point to the appropriate time for the application of certain therapies and might be helpful to see whether a plateau of activation is reached, which could indicate that a change of strategy is required.

The relationship between changes in motor or language scores and BOLD signal is not fully understood. Scores are not continuous and were developed for interobserver reliability, consistency over time, or for comparisons between patients, not for comparison with brain activity. If one patient on a clinical scale improves from grade 2 to grade 4 and another one from grade 4 to grade 6, should they show similar increases in activation? Already, early studies have shown that the relationship between performance and activation is not necessarily a linear one (Dettmers et al., 1995).

In summary, it is probable that therapies should be tailored to the anatomical lesion, clinical deficit, and maybe even the activation patterns of individual patients. Currently, many new therapies are being investigated with the intention of stimulating the remaining network after stroke (Liepert, 2008). Functional imaging is very well suited to assess which therapies might be appropriate for which patient, and when an increase or a change of therapy is indicated. However, to achieve this, the clinical correlate of activation patterns should be better known, and therapies should be verified in randomized controlled studies.

Multiple Sclerosis

In recent years, there have been a number of functional imaging studies in patients with MS that have shown cortical reorganization similar to that observed in stroke patients. It is worthwhile to compare data from these two diseases, because the process can lead to new ideas about symptoms and therapies in each of them. The present comparison is limited to the motor system, which has been studied most extensively. Two recent reviews summarize the principal findings of patterns of brain reorganization in patients with MS (Pantano et al., 2006; Rocca and Filippi, 2007). Like in ischemic stroke (Ward et al., 2003), the first reaction of the sensorimotor system to an MS lesion that leads to paresis is an up-regulation of the whole network, with a subsequent gradual decrease toward normal levels as the paresis improves (Reddy et al., 2000).

In cross-sectional studies in relapsing-remitting (Pantano et al., 2002; Saini et al., 2004), primary progressive (Rocca et al., 2002), and secondary progressive MS patients (Rocca et al., 2003), the patients activate the sensorimotor network more than healthy controls. In all three variants of the disease, there is a strong association with the lesion burden, measured by standard T2-weighted imaging, by fractional anisotropy in diffusion tensor MRI data, or by spectroscopic assessment of NAA levels using MRS. Prominent examples of up-regulation have been found in the premotor cortex, SMA, ipsilateral or contralateral sensorimotor cortex, and cerebellum (Lee et al., 2000; Pantano et al., 2006; Rocca and Filippi, 2007). There has been some variability in these observations, although this seems to be more related to the activation magnitude than to the overall pattern, while increased recruitment of the bilateral motor system correlates with lesion load (Giorgio et al., 2010; Rocca et al., 2002, 2003). Variations probably depend more on the lesion localization than on the type of MS, which is also well documented in stroke patients (Rijntjes, 2006).

As in stroke (Foltys et al., 2003), simple movements elicit activation patterns in patients that are normally associated with the performance of difficult movements in healthy controls (Filippi et al., 2004). Whether MS patients regain complete function after hemiparesis seems to depend on the ability to involve motor areas of the affected hemisphere (Mezzapesa et al., 2008), a finding also reported in stroke patients (Rijntjes, 2006).

One interesting recent finding is that in patients with MS in which reorganization of the motor system has taken place, learning a new task is not accompanied by training-dependent reductions in activation, as is known from healthy subjects (Morgen et al., 2004). This question has not yet been investigated in stroke patients.

The adaptive changes in the brain probably limit the symptoms of MS, but the eventual exhaustion of these plastic capabilities may lead to clinical manifestations of the respective deficit (Pantano et al., 2006; Rocca and Filippi, 2007). It is tempting to suggest that fatigue, which is a common symptom in MS patients, occurs when this capacity for recruitment of additional parts of the network is exhausted. Two studies in MS patients found a clear-cut correlation between the degree of fatigue and the amount of activation in the sensorimotor system (Filippi et al., 2002; Tartaglia et al., 2004).

The issue of what mechanisms play a role in this plasticity on a neuronal level cannot be determined with functional imaging, but so far, there are no indications that fundamentally different mechanisms are involved in the cortical reorganization processes in patients with stroke and MS. The reorganization patterns in MS and stroke have thus far mainly been investigated in parallel, but the similarities lead to the following clinical hypotheses.

Lessons from Stroke Relevant to Multiple Sclerosis

Several centrally acting drugs have been successfully employed in stroke patients, inducing reorganizational changes in the motor system and correlating with clinical improvement (Liepert, 2008). It might be worthwhile to consider whether one or more of them might also be beneficial for MS patients.

Physical therapy is a basic strategy for treating the motor deficits in both diseases. In stroke patients, CIMT (Taub et al., 2002) has been proven to induce cortical reorganization, and there is probably no reason not to try this form of therapy in MS patients with hemiparesis.

Studies that investigate reorganization in stroke usually include patients with a single lesion, but the size and extent of the lesion generally correlates poorly with the functional disability (Binkofski et al., 2001). However, if precise anatomical information on the posterior limb of the internal capsule is available (Wenzelburger et al., 2005), a rough prognosis can be made. In MS studies, a different approach is usually taken, where the complete lesion load in the brain is correlated with motor performance. Although a correlation is commonly found in these studies, a more precise anatomical delineation of lesions would perhaps lead to an even better correlation with clinical deficits. Of course, the possibility of spinal cord lesions in MS patients should be taken into account using this approach.

Lessons from Multiple Sclerosis Relevant to Stroke

Fatigue is a well-known problem in MS patients but not commonly diagnosed in stroke patients, maybe because therapists tend to focus on the focal deficit. However, older anecdotal (Brodal, 1973) and recent multisubject reports indicate that fatigue might also be common in stroke patients (Carlsson et al., 2003, 2004; Choi-Kwon et al., 2005). It would be interesting to investigate whether the same principles apply as have been shown in MS.

So-called silent reorganization—changes in the organization of the sensorimotor system that possibly prevent clinical deficits in MS—might also prevent patients with microangiopathy from developing symptoms in the early stage. In one study in patients with cerebral autosomal-dominant arteriopathy with subcortical infarcts and leukoencephalopathy (CADASIL), a similar pattern of silent reorganization has been demonstrated (Reddy et al., 2002).

Reorganization of the motor system in MS patients interferes with the normal activation changes seen in healthy subjects during learning a new task (Morgen et al., 2004). It should be investigated whether this phenomenon is also present in stroke patients and whether it correlates with the ability to maintain performance.

Lessons for Both

Disabilities in stroke and MS patients are usually measured on different disease-specific scales. Functional imaging does not provide a physiological basis for this. For comparison of therapy effects, it might be more practical to apply the same motor scores in both groups.

It is through functional imaging that the similarities on a functional level of these two disparate CNS diseases is recognized, and this method is also eminently well suited to investigate these questions.

Conscious and Unconscious Processes

If the wish to grab a pencil leads to an appropriate motion of the hand, brain activations occurring before and during this time will be interpreted as responsible for this goal-directed movement. However, several recent experiments have highlighted the difference between conscious and unconscious processes and that both are not necessarily always congruent.

Sleeping subjects show enhanced activity in those parts of the brain that were active while the individual was awake

(Maquet et al., 2000). Patients with apallic syndromes (vegetative states) do not show meaningful responses to outside stimuli, which is usually interpreted to mean that they are not capable of conscious thought. However, surprisingly, some of them still seem to understand at least some tasks: when lying in a scanner and instructed to image walking around at home, they sometimes show activations in areas that are similar to healthy subjects doing the same task (Owen et al., 2006). It should be asked, therefore, to what extent is consciousness preserved in these patients. In conscious persons, unconscious processes can be visualized with functional imaging. For example, in patients with chronic pain, the so-called placebo-effect leads to activations in regions in the brainstem and spinal cord that correlate with the pain-relieving impact of the placebo (Eippert et al., 2009a, 2009b).

Functional imaging has also been used to investigate moral questions. It is possible to correlate activation patterns with deliberate lying (Langleben et al., 2005) or with psychopathic traits (Fullam et al., 2009). Some investigators call this *forensic imaging*. In certain experimental settings, an investigator can recognize from the pattern of activation whether a promise will subsequently be broken, even if subjects report that they had not yet reached a decision at that time point (Baumgartner et al., 2009).

Experiments like these again raise the philosophical question as to whether humans have a free will, or that what we are aware of is just the surface of a pool of unconscious processes that we can only partly influence. Such experiments have also led to a public discussion about responsibility; if a suspect shows "pathological" activations, is his culpability reduced? In these discussions, care should be taken to realize that arguments concern three levels of representation: the brain level, the personal level, and the societal level. The conclusions about such experiments should be drawn at each separate level: the relevance for society should be judged by society itself and cannot be in the realm of neurology or psychiatry.

At the moment, there is hardly a state of mind in disease and health that is not investigated with functional imaging. Even religious feelings have been "captured" in the scanner. It has long been known that some patients with temporal epilepsy report strong religious experiences, and it is possible to evoke such feelings with magnetic fields in healthy subjects (Booth et al., 2005). Using functional imaging, it appears that brain areas active during a religious experience in believers (Azari et al., 2001; Beauregard and Paquette, 2006; Kapogiannis et al., 2009) are also involved in ethical decisions, empathy for the feelings of other persons ("theory of mind"), and strong emotions (Greene et al., 2004; Hein and Singer, 2008; Young et al., 2007). Again, very divergent conclusions from these findings are possible. For some, they point to the possibility that religion evolved from processes that developed during evolution and that have to be applied in daily life for a person functioning properly as a member of society (Boyer, 2008). In this interpretation, religion could be a product of evolution. However, for those who believe in divine revelation, the information that religious feelings are processed by brain areas that are competent for them will be wholly unspectacular.

In general, caution should prevail in interpretating experiments about psychopathology and "unconscious" contributions to behavior. As with most other ethical questions, the appraisal of psychological and psychopathological findings will surely depend on the mood of the time.

References

The complete reference list is available online at www.expertconsult.com.

Neuroimaging
Chemical Imaging: Ligands and Pathology Seeking Agents

A. Jon Stoessl

Functional imaging is of particular benefit for providing insight into neurochemical pathology and the normal functions of neurotransmitters, particularly in situations where structural changes may be minimal. By labeling the chemical of interest with a radioactive tag, its function can be studied in a quantitative fashion. This is of particular benefit in neurodegenerative and behavioral disorders. More recently, radiolabeled agents have been developed to permit the assessment of pathological processes such as inflammation or abnormal protein deposition.

Principles of Positron Emission Tomography

Positron emission tomography (PET) is based on the detection of radiation when a molecule of interest is labeled with an unstable isotope that emits positrons (positively charged electrons). Positrons travel a short distance before colliding with electrons, resulting in an annihilation reaction from which two photons (511 keV) arise, traveling in opposite directions. By accepting only those events that simultaneously activate photosensitive crystals at 180 degrees (coincident events), fairly good anatomical specificity can be achieved. Single-photon emission computed tomography (SPECT) is also dependent on the detection of γ-rays, but in this case only single photon events rather than coincident events are detected. In both cases, it is important to remember that one is simply measuring radioactivity, and the biological interpretation of the images depends on knowledge and/or assumptions about how the radiolabeled molecule is handled after injection and arrival in the brain. This typically requires the application of a variety of mathematical models of varying complexity, as well as dynamic scanning (i.e., the collection of data at multiple time points) and determination of the input function, derived either from arterial plasma or from a tissue reference region.

Most positron-emitting isotopes are highly unstable, with half-lives ranging from 2 minutes (oxygen-15 [^{15}O]) to 2 hours (fluorine-18 [^{18}F]). Many studies of biological compounds are performed using carbon-11 (^{11}C), which has a half-life of 20 minutes. The advantage of the longer half-life of F-18 is not only the more leisurely pace at which the study can be performed (most PET studies have to be performed in close proximity to the cyclotron at which the isotopes are produced) but also the ability to scan for longer times. This may be particularly helpful for molecules that require longer times to undergo the biological process of interest (e.g., enzymatic conversion, trapping in synaptic vesicles, equilibrium state for receptor binding). On the other hand, fluorine chemistry can be difficult, and the labeling process may change the biological activity of the compound. Radioisotopes with short half-lives can be administered repeatedly over the course of a day, and this may be useful for assessing the effects of an intervention (e.g., cerebral blood flow [CBF] responses to a behavioral task, changes in receptor occupancy following administration of a pharmacological agent).

Positron Emission Tomography versus Single-Photon Emission Computed Tomography

Both PET and SPECT can provide useful information on neurochemistry and neuroreceptor function. Traditionally, PET

DOI: 10.1016/B978-1-4377-0434-1.00038-4

has been regarded as having superior resolution, but with newer generations of SPECT cameras, this is not necessarily the case. For studies requiring dynamic data acquisition, PET is preferable. Attenuation of the emitted radioactivity by brain and skull can be measured directly with PET, whereas this must be estimated for SPECT. Both techniques are expensive, but for PET this is particularly true because a significant infrastructure is required, as is reasonable proximity to a cyclotron. Thus, PET is performed at specialized centers, often for research rather than diagnostic purposes, whereas most centers have a nuclear medicine department with SPECT capability, and the longer isotope half-lives mean that tracers can be shipped from elsewhere rather than produced on site. The majority of the discussion in this chapter will be based on PET studies, but in many cases, similar studies can be performed with SPECT.

Neurochemical Targets of Interest

General studies of cerebral glucose metabolism or regional CBF can be found in Chapter 33C. Neurochemical systems of interest that have been well studied using PET—monoamines (particularly dopamine and serotonin), cholinergic systems, opioid and non-opioid peptides, and amino acids—will be addressed in this chapter (**Table 33D.1**).

Monoamines

Dopaminergic function (**Fig. 33D.1**) can be assessed using 6-[^{18}F]fluoro-L-dopa (FD), an analog of levodopa that is decarboxylated to [^{18}F]fluorodopamine and trapped in synaptic vesicles, or by its false neurotransmitter analog 6-[^{18}F] fluoro-meta-tyrosine (FMT). The membrane dopamine transporter (DAT) can be assessed using either PET or SPECT using a variety of tropane (cocaine-like) analogs labeled with C-11, F-18, iodine-123 (^{123}I), or technetium-99m (^{99m}Tc), or with the non-tropane [^{11}C]d-threo-methylphenidate. FD uptake/decarboxylation and expression are subject to changes that may arise as a compensatory mechanism or in response to pharmacological manipulations. In contrast, [^{11}C]dihydrotetrabenazine (DTBZ), which labels the vesicular monoamine transporter type 2 (VMAT2) responsible for packaging monoamines into synaptic vesicles, is theoretically less subject to

such influences. VMAT2 is, however, expressed by all monoaminergic neurons and is therefore not specific for dopamine (although dopaminergic nerve terminals represent the majority of VMAT2 binding in the striatum).

Dopamine receptors can be studied using a variety of C-11- or F-18-labeled ligands for the D_2 receptor (some ^{123}I-labeled ligands are available for SPECT as well), with fewer options available for the D_1 receptor. Some D_2 receptor ligands are susceptible to competition from endogenous dopamine or by pharmacological agents that bind to dopamine receptors. On the one hand, this can lead to problems of interpretation because differences in binding could potentially reflect alterations in receptor occupancy by endogenous neurotransmitter rather than changes in receptor expression. However, this property may also be extremely useful for estimating changes in dopamine release in response to a variety of behavioral (Monchi et al., 2006), pharmacological (Piccini et al., 2003; Tedroff et al., 1996), or physical (Strafella et al., 2003) interventions.

Serotonin (5-hydroxytryptamine [5HT]) nerve terminal function can be studied by the radiolabeled precursor α-[^{11}C] methyl-L-tryptophan (analogous to FD uptake as a measure of dopaminergic integrity) or by agents that bind to the membrane 5HT transporter, of which the most widely accepted example is [^{11}C]DASB. The 5HT$_2$ receptor can be labeled with [^{11}C]MDL 100,907 or [^{18}F]setoperone, but these tracers have suboptimal kinetics (MDL) or selectivity (setoperone). Another option is [^{18}F]altanserin, whose binding characteristics are very similar to those of [^{3}H]MDL 100,907 in vitro (Kristiansen et al., 2005). Binding is relatively insensitive to endogenous 5HT, and interpretation could theoretically be affected by the presence of radiolabeled metabolites that cross the blood-brain barrier (BBB) (Price et al., 2001), but standard graphical analysis appears to be adequate, and changes are seen in Alzheimer disease (AD; decreased) (Marner et al., 2010) and Tourette syndrome (TS; increased) (Haugbol et al., 2007). Binding of [^{18}F]altanserin correlates with response to tonic heat pain (Kupers et al., 2009), and 5HT$_{1A}$ receptors can be labeled with [^{11}C]WAY 100,635. In the raphe, the latter agent binds to presynaptic somatodendritic autoreceptors, and its binding accordingly gives an indirect measure of serotonergic integrity, whereas binding in other regions is predominantly postsynaptic. Unlike the situation with dopamine receptor binding, changes in the binding of serotonergic ligands cannot routinely be used to assess alterations in the availability of endogenous 5HT.

Cholinergic Systems

Presynaptic cholinergic function can be assessed using agents that bind to the vesicular cholinergic transporter, such as [^{123}I] iodo-benzovesamicol or substrates for acetylcholinesterase such as [^{11}C]PMP or [^{11}C]MP4A. The latter are hydrolyzed and cleared, and it is the clearance that is measured as an indicator of neuronal activity.

A number of ligands have been developed for both muscarinic (Asahina et al., 1998; Eckelman, 2006) and nicotinic (Ding et al., 2006; Horti et al., 2010) cholinergic receptors.

Neuropeptides

Opioid peptide receptors have been most widely studied using PET with [^{11}C]diprenorphine (nonselective) or [^{11}C]

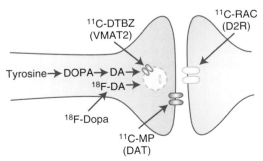

DOPAMINERGIC NERVE TERMINAL

Fig. 33D.1 Schematic of a dopaminergic nerve terminal with examples of positron emitting labels. *^{11}C-DTBZ*, [11C]dihydrotetrabenazine; *^{11}C-MP*, [11C]d-threo-methylphenidate; *^{11}C-RAC*, [11C]raclopride; *DAT*, plasmalemmal dopamine transporter; *D_2R*, dopamine D2 receptor; *^{18}F-dopa*, 6-[18F]fluoro-l-dopa; *^{18}F-DA*, 6-[18F]fluorodopamine; *VMAT2*, type 2 vesicular monoamine transporter.

Table 33D.1 Neurochemical Tracers and Pathology-Seeking Agents

MONOAMINES

Dopamine

Vesicular monoamine transporter type 2	[^{11}C]dihydrotetrabenazine
Dopamine transporter	[^{11}C]*d-threo*-methylphenidate [^{11}C]- and [^{18}F]-fluoropropyl-CIT [^{123}I]β-CIT [^{99m}Tc]TRODAT Numerous other tropanes (cocaine analogs)
Dopa decarboxylase	6-[^{18}F]fluoro-L-dopa
D$_1$ receptors	[^{11}C]SCH 23390
D$_2$ receptors	[^{11}C]raclopride (also dopamine release) [^{11}]N-methylspiperone [^{18}F]benperidol [^{11}C]FLB 457 (extrastriatal sites) [^{11}C] or [^{18}F]fallypride (extrastriatal)

Serotonin

Tryptophan hydroxylase/kynurenin	α-[^{11}C]-L-methyltryptophan
5HT transporter	[^{11}C]DASB
5HT1A receptors	[^{11}C]WAY 100635 [^{18}F]MPPF [^{18}F]FCWAY
5HT2 receptors	[^{11}C]MDL 100907 [^{18}F]setoperone [^{18}F]altanserin

CHOLINERGIC

Acetylcholinesterase	[^{11}C]MP4A [^{11}C]PMP
Cholinergic vesicular transporter	[^{123}I]iodobenzovesamicol
Muscarinic receptors	[^{11}C]N-methyl-piperidyl benzylate [^{123}I]quinuclidinyl benzylate
Nicotinic receptors	[^{11}C]N-methyl-iodo-epibatidine

OPIOID RECEPTORS

μ-Opioid receptor	[^{11}C]carfentanil
Non-selective opioid receptor	[^{11}C]diprenorphine

AMINO ACID RECEPTORS

GABA$_A$/benzodiazepine receptor	[^{11}C]flumazenil
Excitatory amino acid receptors:	
NMDA receptors	[^{18}F]fluoroethyl-diarylguanidine [^{11}C]GMOM
mGluR5 receptors	[^{11}C]MPEP [^{11}C]ABP688 [^{18}F]FE-DABP688 [^{18}F]SP203 [^{18}F]FP-ECMO [^{18}F]PEB

NEUROINFLAMMATION

Peripheral benzodiazepine receptor (microglia)	[^{11}C]PK 11195

BLOOD-BRAIN BARRIER FUNCTION

P-glycoprotein	[^{11}C]verapamil
Amyloid and other protein deposition	[^{11}C]Pittsburgh compound B [^{18}F]AV-45 [^{18}F]BAY94-9172 [^{18}F]FDDNP

carfentanil (selective for μ-opioid receptors). Both agents are thought to be susceptible to competition from endogenous opioids. In the case of [^{11}C]carfentanil, this property has been used to demonstrate opioid release in response to pain (Zubieta et al., 2001) and to placebo analgesia (Zubieta et al., 2005). In vivo imaging of opioid receptors has been extensively reviewed in a recent paper (Henriksen and Willoch, 2008).

Amino Acids

The agent [^{11}C]flumazenil is a benzodiazepine receptor inverse agonist and can be used to assess γ-aminobutyric acid (GABA)$_A$ receptors. It is not clear, however, whether its binding is susceptible to competition from endogenous GABA. The peripheral benzodiazepine receptor is used as a marker of microglial activation and will be discussed later under pathology-seeking agents.

There has been relatively limited use of agents to study excitatory amino acid receptors, but recently agents for the mGluR5 (Honer et al., 2007; Kimura et al., 2010; Lucatelli et al., 2009; Mu et al., 2010; Patel et al., 2007; Sanchez-Pernaute et al., 2008; Treyer et al., 2007; Yu, 2007), as well as the N-methyl-D-aspartate (NMDA) (Robins et al., 2010; Waterhouse, 2003) and glycine-binding site of the NMDA receptor (Fuchigami et al., 2009) have been developed.

Assessment of Pathology

Functional imaging can give insights into the pathological processes underlying neurological disease. This may be of particular benefit in early disease, since the changes that occur later may be secondary and nonspecific. From this perspective, a number of agents are of particular interest.

Inflammation

The peripheral benzodiazepine receptor (PBR) ligand, [^{11}C] PK 11195, has been used as a marker of microglial activation; [^{11}C]PK 11195 binding is increased in disorders with known inflammatory response such as multiple sclerosis (MS) (Banati et al., 2000), encephalitis (Banati et al., 1999; Cagnin et al., 2001b), and stroke (Gerhard et al., 2000), but changes can also be seen in neurodegenerative disorders, lending support to an inflammatory contribution to these conditions. More recently, other agents with higher affinity for the PBR have been developed. These may presumably have a higher sensitivity for detecting inflammatory changes.

Blood-Brain Barrier Function

The P-glycoprotein (P-gp) is responsible for extrusion of potential toxins across the BBB; [^{11}C]verapamil is a putative substrate for P-gp. Thus, increased [^{11}C]verapamil binding may be seen as evidence of impaired P-gp function. A number of studies have been conducted in Parkinson disease (PD) and related disorders, with somewhat unclear findings (see Clinical Studies).

Abnormal Protein Deposition

A number of agents have been developed for imaging amyloid deposition. [^{18}F]FDDNP appears to bind to aggregated protein and is therefore not specific for β-amyloid deposition. This may be an advantage if one is interested in assessing the deposition of other aberrant proteins. In contrast, the thioflavin Pittsburgh Compound B (PiB) labeled with C-11 (and more recent congeners labeled with F-18) appears to be specific for β-amyloid; its deposition in disorders other than AD is still likely to reflect deposition of this protein (see later discussion).

Clinical Studies

Parkinson Disease

In PD, FD uptake, DAT binding, and VMAT2 binding are all reduced in a similar pattern, with a rostral-caudal gradient in which the posterior striatum is maximally affected and the caudate nucleus is relatively spared (**Fig. 33D.2**). The degree of abnormality is typically asymmetrical, in keeping with clinical findings, but even patients with clinically unilateral disease have evidence of bilateral striatal dopamine denervation on PET or SPECT (Marek et al., 1996). With disease progression, uptake of all tracers declines according to an exponential function. The rostral-caudal gradient of involvement is maintained throughout the course of the illness, but the asymmetry between sides lessens over time (Nandhagopal et al., 2009). Because the symptoms of PD do not become manifest until loss of approximately 50% of nigral neurons or 80% of striatal dopamine, imaging may be used to detect preclinical abnormalities in individuals at high risk of developing parkinsonism, including persons exposed to the selective nigral toxin, N-methyl-4-phenyl-1,2,3,6-tetrahydropridine (MPTP) (Calne et al., 1985); twins of persons with PD (Piccini et al., 1999); family members from pedigrees with dominantly inherited PD (Adams et al., 2005; Nandhagopal et al., 2008); and individuals with REM sleep behavior disorder (Albin et al. 2000). Interestingly, family members from kindreds with recessively inherited PD who carry heterozygous mutations also demonstrate imaging evidence of dopamine denervation (Hilker et al., 2001; Khan et al., 2002; Khan et al., 2005). The significance of the latter observation is unclear. While imaging can be used to assess disease progression, there have been numerous examples of discordance between PET or SPECT findings and clinical observations, particularly in studies designed to assess the effects of potential disease-modifying or cell-based therapies (Fahn et al., 2004; Marek et al., 2002; Olanow et al., 2003; Whone et al., 2003). This has led to caution with respect to the use of imaging as a surrogate marker in such studies (Brooks et al., 2003; Ravina et al., 2005).

By using displacement of [^{11}C]raclopride as a measure of dopamine release, it can be shown that PD patients who go on to develop fluctuations in response to levodopa therapy have a relatively large but poorly sustained increase in synaptic dopamine following levodopa, compared to those who have a stable response to medication, in whom dopamine release is lower in magnitude but more sustained. These differences are evident even at a time when both groups still have a stable response to medication (de la Fuente-Fernandez et al., 2001a). Levodopa-induced dopamine release increases with disease progression and is also increased in patients with medication-induced dyskinesias (de la Fuente-Fernandez et al., 2004). A similar approach has been used to demonstrate increased levodopa-derived dopamine release in the ventral (but not

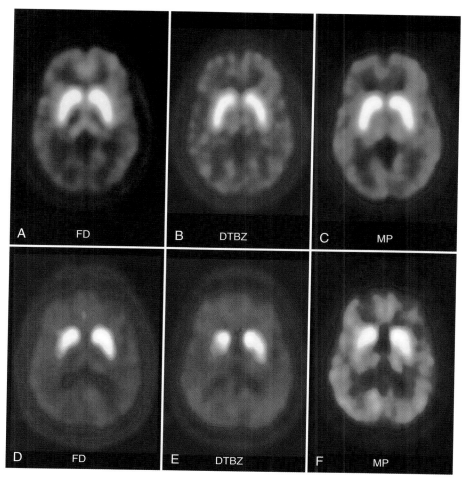

Fig. 33D.2 FD uptake, VMAT2 (DTBZ) and DAT (MP) binding in a healthy control *(upper panel)* and an individual with early Parkinson disease (PD) *(lower panel)*. Note the asymmetrical reduction of uptake in the patient with PD, maximally affecting the posterior putamen, with relative sparing of the caudate nucleus.

dorsal) striatum of patients with the dopamine dysequilibrium syndrome (Evans et al., 2006). In this situation, dopamine release correlates with how much subjects want the drug as opposed to how much they enjoy the effects. Dopamine release is also increased during performance of a gambling task with monetary reward, and this effect is enhanced in PD patients with pathological gambling (Steeves et al., 2009).

The same technique has been used to demonstrate dopamine release underlying the placebo effect in PD (de la Fuente-Fernandez et al., 2001b). This finding, initially demonstrated using placebo medication, has been confirmed with sham repetitive transcranial magnetic stimulation, which also induces ventral striatal dopamine release (Strafella et al., 2006).

PET has been used to investigate depression in PD, and the results are somewhat surprising. Using the selective 5HT transporter ligand, [¹¹C]DASB, Guttman and colleagues demonstrated widespread reductions in 5HT transporter binding in PD compared to healthy controls, in keeping with loss of serotonergic fibers (Guttman et al., 2007). In PD patients with depression, however, 5HT transporter binding was increased, particularly in dorsolateral and prefrontal cortex (Boileau et al., 2008); 5HT transporter binding correlated with clinical ratings of depression. Although somewhat surprising, this finding is reminiscent of those in major depression, where 5HT transporter binding is increased in those subjects with negativistic dysfunctional attitude (Meyer et al., 2004).

Dementia in PD (PDD) is associated with marked reductions in cholinergic activity (Bohnen et al., 2003; Hilker et al., 2005) greater than those seen in AD (see later discussion). The pathology of PDD is mixed but will often include cortical Lewy body deposition (with or without evidence of AD pathology), so there has been considerable interest in whether agents that bind to aberrantly folded protein can be used to image dementia with Lewy bodies (DLB) or PDD. Most studies to date have suggested that [¹¹C]PiB binding is increased in DLB but not in PDD. This may be seen as somewhat surprising, as many investigators consider these to represent variations of the same disorder. It is possible that patients with PDD who demonstrate [¹¹C]PiB uptake in fact have concurrent AD pathology, as suggested by a relationship to ApoE4 allele and CSF $A\beta_{42}$ levels (Maetzler et al., 2009), as well as recent postmortem (Burack et al., 2010) and in vitro (Fodero-Tavoletti et al., 2007) studies.

As is the case for other neurodegenerative disorders, there has been great interest in the possibility of an inflammatory component to the pathogenesis and progression of PD. Using the peripheral benzodiazepine ligand, [¹¹C]PK 11195, as a marker of microglial activation, Ouchi et al. demonstrated increased binding in the substantia nigra of PD patients that correlated with dopaminergic nerve loss and with clinical measures of disease severity (Ouchi et al., 2005). In contrast, Gerhard et al. found more widespread increases in [¹¹C]PK 11195 binding that did not correlate with either FD uptake or

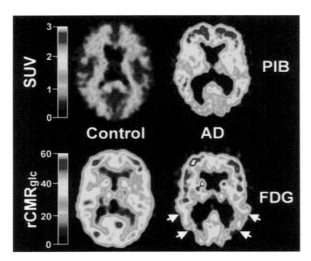

Fig. 33D.3 Amyloid binding (PIB = Pittsburgh Compound B; *upper panel*) and glucose (2-deoxy-2-(18F)fluoro-d-glucose [FDG]) metabolism *(lower panel)* in a healthy control subject *(left)* and a patient with Alzheimer disease *(right)*. Note the diffuse increase in amyloid deposition in the patient, combined with reduced glucose metabolism in parietotemporal cortex. *SUV*, Standardized uptake value; *rCMRglc*, regional cerebral metabolic rate for glucose. *(From Klunk, W.E., Engler, H., Nordberg, A., et al., 2004. Imaging brain amyloid in Alzheimer's disease with Pittsburgh Compound-B. Ann Neurol 55, 306-319.)*

clinical measures of disease progression (Gerhard et al., 2006). Quantitation with this tracer is difficult, and results vary according to the analytical model employed; furthermore, binding is apparently not reduced in response to treatment with celecoxib (Bartels et al., 2010).

Another tantalizing possibility for pathogenic mechanisms in PD was raised by the observation that [11C]verapamil binding was increased in the midbrain of patients with PD (Kortekaas et al., 2005). In the initial report, this was interpreted by the authors as reflecting impairment of BBB P-gp function, resulting in reduced extrusion of toxins. Similar abnormalities have been reported in the basal ganglia of patients with multiple system atrophy (MSA) and progressive supranuclear palsy (PSP) (Bartels et al., 2008b). However, the pathogenic significance of this finding in PD is questionable, as it is not seen in patients with early PD (Bartels et al., 2008a).

Alzheimer Disease

Both [11C]PiB and [18F]FDDNP bind to β-amyloid, and their uptake is increased in cortical and subcortical regions in AD (Klunk et al., 2004; Shoghi-Jadid et al., 2002) (**Fig. 33D.3**). Since [18F]FDDNP binds to neurofibrillary tangles as well as amyloid plaques, one might anticipate some differences between the uptake of the two ligands. This does appear to be the case, with voxel-based analysis revealing preferential uptake of [18F]FDDNP in the hippocampus (Shin et al., 2010). Similarly, global [11C]PiB uptake is inversely associated with CSF Aβ$_{1-42}$ levels, while [18F]FDDNP binding correlates with CSF τ (Tolboom et al., 2009a). Increased [18F]FDDNP binding seems to correlate better with impairment of episodic memory, while [11C]PiB binding may be associated with more widespread cognitive deficits (Tolboom et al., 2009b). Binding of

[11C]PiB does not necessarily correlate with the Mini-Mental State Examination, even where glucose metabolism does (Jagust et al., 2009). Both agents reveal increased uptake in subjects with minimal cognitive impairment (MCI) (Small et al., 2006), although there is some variability reported in the ability of [18F]FDDNP to differentiate between control, MCI, and AD (Tolboom et al., 2009c). In healthy aging, [11C]PiB binding is increased, particularly in carriers of the ApoE-ε4 allele (Rowe et al., 2010). Perhaps not surprisingly, binding is also increased in healthy adults with a family history of late-onset AD (Mosconi et al., 2010). Increased binding in subjects with minimal cognitive impairment (Okello et al., 2009) or indeed in apparently healthy controls (Morris et al., 2009) is associated with a significant risk of progression to dementia. While [11C]PiB binding appears to be sensitive to the effects of therapeutic interventions such as monoclonal anti-amyloid antibodies, placebo-treated patients showed ongoing accumulation (Rinne et al., 2010).

Clearly these agents may be helpful in differentiating AD from other disorders resulting in dementia. Thus [11C]PiB binding may distinguish between AD and frontotemporal lobar dementia (FTLD). A significant proportion of patients with clinical evidence of FTLD may display increased [11C]PiB binding, and it is as yet unclear whether this represents false positivity, misdiagnosis, or concurrent AD (Rabinovici et al., 2007). Binding of [18F]FDDNP is increased in the cerebellum, neocortex, and subcortical structures of patients with the prion amyloid disorder, Gerstmann-Sträussler-Scheinker disease and in caudate and thalamus of some asymptomatic mutation carriers (Kepe et al., 2010).

One obvious disadvantage of [11C]-labeled agents is their requirement for proximity to a cyclotron. When an [18F]-labeled agent is used, the longer half-life permits a somewhat greater degree of flexibility. Other β-amyloid–selective agents with favorable kinetic properties are [18F]AV-45 (flobetapir) (Wong et al., 2010) and [18F]BAY94-9172 (Rowe et al., 2008); like [11C]PiB, these agents demonstrate widespread increased binding in patients with AD compared to healthy controls.

Binding of [11C]PK 11195 suggests increased microglial activation in entorhinal, temporoparietal, and cingulate cortex of patients with AD (Cagnin et al., 2001a).

Epilepsy

Studies of CBF and/or glucose metabolism have a long-established indication in the assessment of epilepsy and will not be discussed further in this chapter, whose focus is neurochemical and pathology-seeking ligands.

There is abundant evidence for altered opioid transmission in experimental models of seizures. Combined PET studies using both the δ-opioid antagonist, [11C]N-methylnaltrindole, and the μ-opioid agonist, [11C]carfentanil, in patients with temporal lobe epilepsy (TLE) revealed increases in the binding of both ligands (associated with reduced glucose metabolism), although with somewhat different distributions (Madar et al., 1997). In contrast, binding of the nonselective opioid ligand, [11C]diprenorphine, was reduced during reading-induced seizures, compared to the baseline state, suggestive of opioid release in patients with reading epilepsy (Koepp et al., 1998), although [11C]diprenorphine binding increased in the fusiform gyrus and temporal pole following seizures in patients with TLE (Hammers et al., 2007).

The GABA$_A$/benzodiazepine receptor has been studied using [^{11}C]flumazenil. In patients with mesial temporal epilepsy and hippocampal sclerosis, binding is reduced in the affected hippocampus (with or without concurrent reductions in binding in the amygdala), but variable increases or decreases may be seen in neocortical regions (Hammers et al., 2001). Focal abnormalities (increases, decreases, or both concurrently) may be seen in many patients with cortical epilepsy. In some patients, these abnormalities are seen in periventricular regions, possibly representing neuronal migration abnormalities (Hammers et al., 2003).

Multiple lines of evidence suggest dysfunction in serotonergic mechanisms in patients with epilepsy. Uptake of the 5HT precursor, α-[^{11}C]-methyl-L-tryptophan (AMT), is increased in the hippocampus of patients with TLE and preserved hippocampal volume (Natsume et al., 2003), and focal cortical increases of this tracer in children with intractable epilepsy are often associated with epileptogenic cortical developmental abnormalities (Juhasz et al., 2003). Increases in AMT uptake are smaller in extent and have a lower sensitivity but greater specificity compared with areas of altered glucose metabolism. Decreases in 5HT$_{1A}$ binding have been demonstrated in epileptogenic regions of TLE patients using the antagonist ligands, [^{18}F]MPPF (Merlet et al., 2004) and [^{18}F]FCWAY (Liew et al., 2009).

More recent studies also suggest abnormalities in dopamine transmission. Uptake of 6-[^{18}F]-fluoro-L-dopa was reduced in patients with multiple types of epilepsy (Bouilleret et al., 2005). Striatal and thalamic binding of [^{11}C]raclopride is increased in patients with Unverricht-Lundborg myoclonic epilepsy (Korja et al., 2007), also in keeping with a striatal dopaminergic deficit. This is further supported by reduced dopamine transporter binding, which is restricted to the midbrain in juvenile myoclonic epilepsy but found in the putamen in patients with generalized tonic-clonic epilepsy (Ciumas et al., 2010). In patients with mesial TLE, dopamine D$_2$/D$_3$ receptor binding (as measured by [^{18}F]fallypride) is reduced at the pole and in lateral aspects of the epileptogenic temporal lobe, possibly corresponding to the "irritative zone" (Werhahn et al., 2006).

Concluding Comments

For many years, the chief diagnostic applications of brain PET have been in the fields of oncology (not discussed here) and epilepsy (traditionally using fluorodeoxyglucose, but more recently with other neurochemically specific agents, as discussed earlier). Studies with specific ligands have largely been used for research purposes and have provided significant insights into the pathophysiology of neurodegenerative disorders and their complications. This situation may be changing, however. In the case of AD, imaging with amyloid agents may become an integral part of the diagnostic workup, particularly for participation in clinical trials, where it is increasingly being used as an outcome measure. Caution must be used, however; in PD, there have been many examples of discordance between the effects of disease interventions on imaging biomarkers and clinically relevant outcomes. Functional imaging studies are increasingly useful for preclinical identification of disease, particularly in individuals who carry an increased risk. By reassigning phenotype, such studies may assist in the identification of new disease-causing mutations, and by identifying people at the earliest stages of disease, they may also permit testing of novel neuroprotective strategies.

References

The complete reference list is available online at www.expertconsult.com.

Chapter **33E**

Neuroimaging
Interventional Neuroradiology: Neurological Endovascular Therapy in Hemorrhagic and Ischemic Strokes

Marco Zenteno, Fernando Vinuela

Historical Background

Neurological endovascular therapy is a relatively new subspecialty dealing with a wide range of pathologies linked to central nervous system (CNS) hemorrhagic (Jabbour et al., 2009; Pearl et al., 2010) or ischemic (Santos-Franco et al., 2009; Thorisson and Johnson, 2009; Zenteno-Castellanos et al., 2009) disorders of arteries and veins (Caso et al., 2008) and of the head and neck (Gandhi et al., 2008; Sekhar et al., 2009; Turowski and Zanella, 2003). Working closely with different disciplines—stroke neurology, diagnostic and interventional neuroradiology, neurosurgery, neurointensive care, and neurorehabilitation (Connors et al., 2005; Qureshi et al., 2008)—endovascular therapy plays a key role in patient management.

Endovascular therapy has evolved in the last 25 years. Thanks to rapid technological developments, better knowledge of applied neuroanatomy, and greater understanding of the pathological processes, many procedures that were previously risky and often ineffective now produce excellent clinical results with low morbidity and mortality (Naggara et al., 2010). The implementation of neurointerventional procedures requires a multidisciplinary team including neuroanesthesiologists (Brekenfeld et al., 2010; Varma et al., 2007; Young, 2007), neurosurgeons, radiologists, critical care specialists (Bruder et al., 2008; Connolly et al., 2005), and neurologists, along with a well-trained staff of nurses (Galimany-Masclans et al., 2009; Wright, 2007) and technologists. Additionally, some studies comparing the length of stay and total hospital charges have recently favored interventional treatment over surgical procedures in selected cases (Hoh et al., 2010).

Since the first in vivo angiography performed by Edgas Moniz in 1927, this technique has evolved significantly from direct puncture of cervical vessels to transfemoral or transradial approaches to the neurovascular structures (Jo et al., 2010). In the late 1970s, most of the procedures were limited to the extracranial vasculature. In 1976, Kerber described a balloon catheter with a calibrated leak as a new system for super-selective angiography and occlusive catheter therapy. Flow-guided catheters were soon replaced by more soft, trackable devices. The use of latex/silicone detachable balloons and mechanically driven coils were also soon complemented by the addition of particles, liquid embolic agents, and electrically detachable coils.

The diagnostic and technical excellence brought by digital subtraction angiography was also improved with the development of new guide wires and hydrophilic microcatheters. New angiography techniques were incorporated, such as high-speed serial imaging, road mapping (Rossitti and Pfister, 2009), contrast injectors, and the availability of biplanar rotational (Dorfler et al., 2008) three-dimensional (3D) flat-panel angiography and C-arm flat-detector computed tomography (CT) (Kamran et al., 2010). Noninvasive imaging techniques such as computed tomography angiography (CTA) and magnetic resonance angiography (MRA) complement the use of digital 3D subtraction angiography, though the latter remains the diagnostic gold standard owing to its more accurate assessment of intracranial and spinal vascular anatomical and dynamic information (Mo et al., 2010). Interventional neuroradiology is a discipline that brings together

DOI: 10.1016/B978-1-4377-0434-1.00039-6

three major branches of the neurosciences: observation through neuroradiology, technical mastery of neurosurgery, and clinical skills of neurology. Combining these three skill sets allows endovascular therapy to be both comprehensive and effective in the diagnosis and management of patients with vascular disorders of the CNS.

Intracranial Vascular Malformations

Brain Arteriovenous Malformations

As seen in **Table 33E.1**, arteriovenous malformations (AVMs) can be divided into two different groups (Chaloupka and Huddle, 1998). The group in the left column is suitable for neurointerventional management.

Epidemiology and Pathology

Brain AVMs are the more frequent type of vascular malformations and those which cause the most morbidity and mortality. The true incidence is difficult to estimate, but some retrospective population-based studies have shown that the incidence of symptomatic intracranial hemorrhage (ICH) due to any type of intracranial vascular malformations was 0.8 per 100,000 (Brown et al., 1996a). The New York Island Arteriovenous Malformation Study was the first ongoing prospective population-based survey to determine the incidence of AVM hemorrhage and associated morbidity and mortality rates in New York City. Initial results calculated an AVM detection rate of 1.34 per 100,000 person-years and an acute AVM hemorrhage rate of 0.51 per 100,000 person-years (Stapf et al., 2003).

Some 90% of brain AVMs are supratentorial, and 10% are infratentorial. An AVM is a complex tangled bundle of abnormal arteries and veins linked by one or more fistulas (Choi and Mohr, 2005). An important anatomical feature of this vascular conglomerate, also known as a *nidus*, is the lack of a capillary bed (Choi and Mohr, 2005). The nidus is surrounded by gliotic tissue with traces of hemosiderin and calcifications due to previous bleeds. Most AVMs harbor intracranial aneurysms, which can be intranidal, related to the AVM (distal or proximal arising from the feeder vessels), or located in different parts of the arterial circulation.

Natural History

The clinical presentation generally occurs between the second and fourth decades of life. The natural history of unruptured AVMs is unclear. A Randomized Trial of Unruptured Brain

Arteriovenous Malformations (ARUBA) is underway to address this issue (Stapf et al., 2006). About 50% of patients harboring a brain AVM present with hemorrhage (intraparenchymal, subarachnoid, or intraventricular) (Brown et al., 1996b). In the Cooperative Study of Intracranial Aneurysms and Subarachnoid Hemorrhage, symptomatic AVMs were found in 8.6% of all patients with nontraumatic subarachnoid hemorrhages. Seizures are the second most common presentation, followed by headache and progressive focal neurological deficit. The risk of hemorrhage is 1.3% to 3.9% yearly after diagnosis of an AVM in patients who present without ICH. For patients with a previous hemorrhage, the risk of rebleeding is between 6% and 17% in the first year (Fleetwood and Steinberg, 2002), diminishing thereafter.

Various angiographic and clinical factors predictive of bleeding have been identified in retrospective studies and include (Fleetwood and Steinberg, 2002): previous hemorrhage, deep venous drainage, unique venous drainage, venous stenosis or aneurysms, intranidal aneurysms, venous reflux into a venous sinus, small nidus size, high-feeding artery pressure, slow arterial filling, and deep/periventricular location.

Imaging and Classification

Several imaging findings in brain AVMs influence the patient's therapeutic and clinical management decisions. The most important ones are those known to be associated with hemorrhage or risk of future hemorrhage (evidence of previous hemorrhage, intranidal aneurysms, venous stenosis, deep venous drainage, and deep location of the nidus) (Geibprasert et al., 2010). Magnetic resonance imaging (MRI) is more sensitive than CT in the diagnosis of an AVM and is useful in accurately identifying its location and relationship to functional regions. The most significant features are flow-void signal and hemosiderin deposits in T1- and T2-weighted images. Functional MRI plays an important role in interventional management because it facilitates the localization of functionally important brain areas adjacent to the AVM nidus (Schlosser et al., 1997). Although MRA provides useful information on AVM feeder arteries and draining veins, digital 3D cerebral angiography is the gold standard (Strozyk et al., 2009) for the acquisition of accurate anatomical and dynamic information. The addition of superselective catheterization and angiography of AVM arterial feeders adds key information on AVM angioarchitecture (identification of high-flow arteriovenous fistulas [AVFs], intranidal aneurysms, and selective stenosis of AVM-draining veins).

AVMs can be superficial (sulcal/gyral) or deep (deep parenchymal/choroid plexus). In the sulcal type, the nidus is located in the subpial space and has a conical or wedge-shaped morphology. In the gyral type, AVMs tend to be spherical, since they are covered with cortex. These AVMs have feeding arteries that continue beyond the lesion to supply healthy brain tissue (arteries "en passage") (Choi and Mohr, 2005).

Mixed malformations are larger and have sulcal and gyral features. The location of the AVM nidus is important because it can predict its pattern of venous drainage. Cortical AVMs typically drain through cortical veins into a dural sinus. When they have a subcortical or ventricular extension, they have superficial and deep venous drainage. Angiography should provide information on: (1) the nidus (single or multiple

Table 33E.1 Types of Arteriovenous Malformations with and without Shunts	
ARTERIOVENOUS SHUNT	
Present	**Absent**
Arteriovenous malformation	Capillary vessel malformations (telangiectasias)
Pial arteriovenous fistulas	Developmental venous anomalies (venous angiomas)
Dural arteriovenous fistulas	Cavernous angiomas

compartments, plexiform, fistulous), (2) the number and origin of feeding arteries (pial, dural, leptomeningeal, choroidal, or perforating), (3) type of venous drainage, and (4) presence of intranidal aneurysms.

Morphological characteristics (size and location) and drainage patterns of the AVM are used to classify patients for the risk of persistent neurological deficits from surgery (Choi and Mohr, 2005).

The classification used in clinical practice for surgical management is the Spetzler-Martin grading scale based on three criteria: (1) size of the AVM, (2) venous drainage, and (3) location (eloquent parenchyma corresponds to sensorimotor cortex, areas of language, visual cortex, hypothalamus, thalamus, internal capsule, brainstem, cerebellar peduncles, and deep cerebellar nuclei). However, one of the original authors has redesigned the grading system into a three-tiered classification of cerebral AVMs (class A combines grades I and II, class B are grade III, and class C combines grades IV and V), offering simplification of the previous placement of patients into five categories, which is intended to provide a guide to treatment and be predictive of outcome (Spetzler and Ponce, 2010). Spetzler-Martin grades were specifically designed to classify surgical patients and do not apply when the patient is managed endovascularly. Risk assessment and outcome determination in brain AVM patients treated by endovascular techniques seem adequate and clinically feasible using other scales (Feliciano et al., 2010).

Treatment

Multimodality treatment is the best approach in patients with complex AVMs (Yuki et al., 2010). The present therapeutic approaches include radiosurgery (with latency to obliteration of 1 to 3 years) (Yen et al., 2010), surgery (Rubin et al., 2010), and embolization (Valle et al., 2008; Vinuela et al., 2005; Xu et al., 2010). Medium and large AVMs (Valle et al., 2008) or AVMs with large AVFs or intranidal aneurysms also require a multidisciplinary strategy. The endovascular occlusion of large AVFs or intranidal aneurysms associated with an AVM nidus decreases endovascular or surgical complications, mostly related to local and regional high venous pressure and intraoperative bleeding.

Embolization focuses on occlusion of surgically difficult-to-reach arteries (deep arteries), intranidal aneurysms, and AVFs (Yuki et al., 2010). A 48- to 72-hour interval is advised between AVM embolization and final surgical removal. If embolization is performed before radiosurgery (Shtraus et al., 2010), its primary goal is to reduce the size of the AVM, close fistulas, and treat intranidal aneurysms (see **Fig. 33E.2**). If an AVM is small and has few afferent pedicles, endovascular treatment can be complete and permanent (Oran et al., 2005) (**Fig. 33E.1**). Embolic materials include:

- Polyvinyl alcohol particles (PVAs): ranging from 14 to 1000 μm. PVAs cause a foreign body inflammatory reaction. Disadvantages are their adhesivity to the

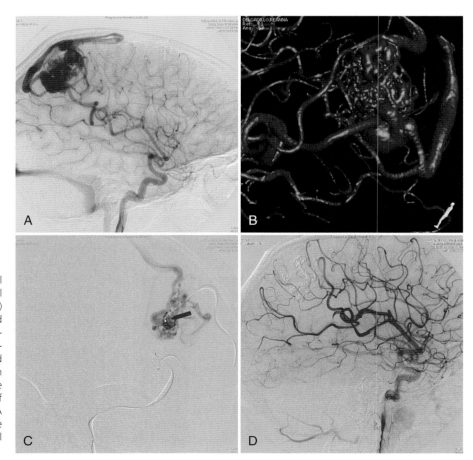

Fig. 33E.1 Embolization of a right parietal arteriovenous malformation (AVM). **A,** Lateral view of right internal carotid artery (ICA) angiogram shows a right parietal AVM supplied by middle cerebral artery feeders. **B,** Three-dimensional subtraction angiography demonstrates the AVM nidus, arterial feeders, and draining veins. **C,** Superselective angiogram performed with a microcatheter identifies the area to be embolized; arrow identifies tip of microcatheter. **D,** Postembolization right ICA angiogram shows complete occlusion of the AVM nidus and preservation of normal arterial circulation.

microcatheter and high recanalization rates (Sorimachi et al., 1999).

- *N*-2-butyl-cyanoacrylate (NBCA) (Starke et al., 2009; Yu et al., 2004) causes an inflammatory reaction in arteries and surrounding tissue, leading to necrosis/fibrosis of the vessel. NBCA polymerizes in contact with ionic solutions. An iodized oil-based contrast agent (Lipiodol) is added to the NBCA to control its polymerization rate as well as to opacify the mixture for angiographic visualization (Calvo et al., 2001). The microcatheter must be flushed with 10% dextrose to prevent NBCA polymerization within it. Occlusion of cerebral AVMs with NBCA is generally permanent (Wikholm, 1995). It is essential to deliver the acrylic into the AVM nidus and not in the parent artery alone. Proximal arterial occlusion elicits early AVM recanalization by local collateral circulation, making the postembolization surgical AVM resection more difficult.

- Onyx (Hauck et al., 2009; Xu et al., 2010) is a copolymer of ethylene vinyl alcohol (EVOH) solved in dimethyl sulfoxide (DMSO). When the compound comes in contact with a liquid, it precipitates and forms a sponge-like material. The precipitation progresses centripetally, and the center remains fluid and continues its anterograde flow. Use of Onyx requires DMSO-compatible microcatheters, which are stiffer and often require guide wires for navigation (Weber et al., 2007). The injection of Onyx is slower and more controllable than the NBCA injection. In experienced hands, the percentage of complete AVM occlusion with Onyx reaches 50% (Maimon et al., 2010). NBCA is preferred in fistulous arteriovenous shunts, perforating arteries, leptomeningeal collaterals, and catheter positions distal from the nidus.

- Microcoils are used to occlude high-flow AVFs in combination with AVM nidus. Their main role is to decrease untoward embolization of liquid embolic agents into the AVM venous drainage, dural venous sinus, and pulmonary circulation.

Dural Arteriovenous Fistulas

Dural arteriovenous fistulas (DAVFs) are characterized by discrete AVFs involving the intracranial meninges covering the venous sinuses. Although their etiology remains unknown, in most cases there is evidence that the fistula formation is preceded in some instances by trauma resulting in skull fracture, sinus thromboses, or venous outlet stenoses (Berenstein et al., 2004). They are often located in the cavernous sinus, transverse sigmoid sinus, superior sagittal sinus, foramen ovale, tentorium, and anterior or middle cranial fossae.

The clinical features associated with DAVFs depend on location of the lesion, extent of AV shunting, and associated recruitment pial veins. Symptoms may be benign (asymptomatic, tinnitus, ocular symptoms, cranial nerve palsies) or serious (ICH, focal neurological deficits, dementia, papilledema, and even death). These symptoms are associated with cortical venous reflux and/or development of intracranial hypertension. The risk of bleeding is 2% per year and depends on location and hemodynamics. Bleeding is always of venous origin. Several classifications have been proposed and compared (Davies et al., 1996). The most widely accepted ones are from Cognard et al. (1995) and Borden et al. (1995).

Therapeutic Approach to Cavernous Dural Arteriovenous Fistulas

Intermittent manual compression of the carotid artery may be effective in occluding the cavernous sinus. The ipsilateral carotid artery is compressed using the contralateral hand for approximately 5 minutes every waking hour for 1 to 3 days. If this is tolerated, the compression time is increased to 10 to 15 minutes of compression per waking hour. The compression produces concomitant partial obstruction of the ipsilateral carotid artery and jugular vein. This results in the transient reduction of arteriovenous shunting by decreasing arterial flow while simultaneously increasing the outlet venous pressure, thereby promoting spontaneous thrombosis within the cavernous sinus (Katsaridis, 2009).

Treatment of DAVF may be endovascular (Kathleen et al., 2009; Katsaridis, 2009), radio-surgical, or surgical. The endovascular approach can be performed with detachable coils, cyanoacrylate, or Onyx (Cognard et al., 2008; Jiang et al., 2010) or via the venous route, packing the sinus with coils or Onyx (Lv et al., 2009) (**Fig. 33E.2**). The objective of the arterial approach is to close the fistula at the origin of the main draining vein. Occlusion of a meningeal fistula proximal to its draining vein elicits rapid development of arterial collaterals and fistula recanalization ("medusa head" angiographic appearance).

Carotid-Cavernous Fistulas

Carotid-cavernous DAVF should be differentiated from direct AVFs involving the cavernous sinus. A well-accepted classification divides them into:

- Direct carotid cavernous fistula (CCF) (Barrow type A): related to trauma or a ruptured aneurysm of the intracavernous internal carotid artery. These are high-flow fistulas.

- Indirect CCF (Barrow types B, C, and D): with abnormal arterial flow into the cavernous sinus from meningeal arteries arising from the internal and external carotid arteries. They are often spontaneous and occur more frequently in menopausal women.

Symptoms and signs tend to be mild, and parenchymal hemorrhage is rare. Orbital pain, proptosis, chemosis, ophthalmoplegia, pulsating noise, increased intraocular pressure, and decrease in visual acuity are usually seen (Jabbour et al., 2009; Zenteno et al., 2010). The treatment of a CCF depends on the severity of clinical symptoms, its angiographic characteristics, and the risk it presents for ICH. In most instances, endovascular treatment is preferred.

Treatment of the CCF can be:

- Intraarterial: detachable balloons (latex/silicone) (Teng et al., 2000), platinum coils, or stent-assisted coiling (Moron et al., 2005). Self-expandable covered stents look very promising but are still under investigation (Gomez et al., 2007). Cyanoacrylate embolization has a high rate of complete closure but can be associated with serious complications. Onyx injection into the cavernous sinus has also been used, with excellent clinical and angiographic results.

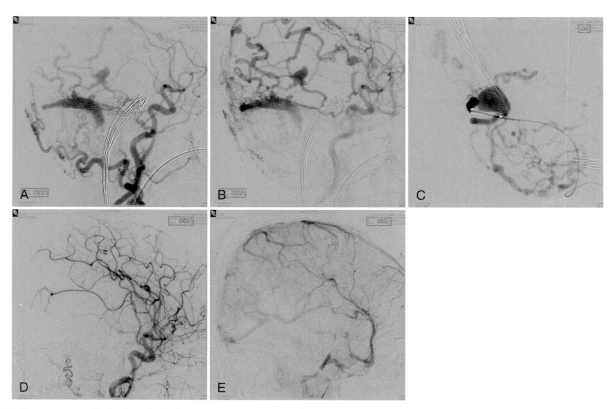

Fig. 33E.2 Transvenous embolization of dural transverse arteriovenous fistula. **A,** Lateral view of left common carotid angiogram shows a partially thrombosed dural transverse sinus with extensive recruitment of cortical pial veins. **B,** Late venous phase shows severe recruitment of cortical veins throughout left brain hemisphere. **C,** Superselective contrast injection through microcatheter shows enhancement of the residual sinus and recruited cortical veins. Occlusion of the sinus was performed with a combination of detachable coils and Onyx. Arterial **(D)** and venous **(E)** phases of left common carotid angiogram show complete occlusion of the dural arteriovenous fistula.

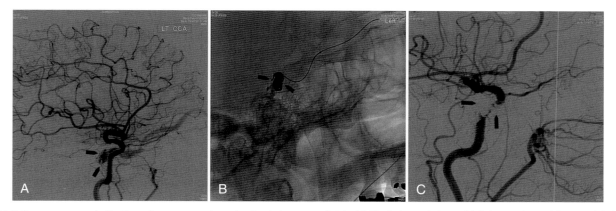

Fig. 33E.3 Transvenous embolization of cavernous sinus dural arteriovenous fistula (AVF). **A,** Lateral view of left internal carotid artery (ICA) shows a dural cavernous AVF draining into a large superior ophthalmic vein. The arrows show early opacification of the cavernous sinus. **B,** Lateral skull view shows microcatheter located in cavernous sinus through superior ophthalmic vein, and Onyx has been delivered into cavernous sinus. Arrows show cavernous sinus filled with Onyx. **C,** Lateral view of left ICA angiogram shows complete obliteration of the dural cavernous sinus fistula. Arrows identify occluded cavernous sinus.

■ Intravenous: embolization with coils or Onyx (Saraf et al., 2010) is the treatment of choice in indirect fistulas (**Fig. 33E.3**).
■ Parent vessel sacrifice: a last resort (Gemmete et al., 2009a, 2009b).

Brain High-Flow Arteriovenous Fistulas

Intracranial pial high-flow AVFs may be classified as:

■ Pial AVF (subependymal).
■ Vein of Galen aneurysmal malformations (VGAM).

Intracranial Pial Arteriovenous Fistula

An intracranial pial AVF is a rare cerebrovascular lesion that has only recently been recognized as a distinct pathological entity. According to a series reported by Halbach et al. (1989), pial AVFs account for 1.6% of all intracranial vascular malformations. Intracranial pial AVFs have a single or multiple arterial connections to a single venous channel. They differ from brain AVMs in that they lack a true nidus and differ from dural AVFs in that they derive their arterial supply from pial or cortical arteries and are not located within the dura mater (Hoh et al., 2001).

Pial AVFs can be congenital or may result from a traumatic injury (Lee et al., 2008). Little is known about their pathophysiological mechanisms. The clinical suspicion of pial AVFs should be followed by prompt appropriate treatment because of their natural history. They are associated with congestive heart failure, intracranial varices, increased intracranial pressure due to venous hypertension, and rarely with ICH.

Direct surgical exposure and occlusion of these vascular lesions is associated with high morbidity and mortality (Passacantilli et al., 2006). Today, most intracranial high-flow pediatric and adult AVFs are treated endovascularly. Accurate identification of the arteriovenous shunt and its precise occlusion with embolic materials make the neurointerventional approach the gold standard for this kind of cerebrovascular lesion.

Vein of Galen Aneurysmal Malformation

Vein of Galen aneurysmal malformations (VGAM) are rare intracranial AVFs that present almost exclusively in children. They are disproportionately represented in pediatric neurovascular disorders, accounting for up to 30% of intracranial vascular abnormalities (Gupta et al., 2006; Kumar et al., 2006). A VGAM consists of multiple AVFs draining into a dilated median prosencephalic vein of Markowski (Hoang et al., 2009). This embryonic vein does not drain normal tissue and does not communicate with normal cerebral veins. In many cases, the straight sinus is absent, and the vein drains directly into the superior sagittal sinus through the falcine sinus. VGAMs can be categorized into choroidal or mural, depending upon their arterial supply.

Clinical manifestations vary according to age:

- Infants: loud intracranial bruit, severe cyanosis, and cardiac failure.
- Early childhood: hydrocephalus with or without congestive heart failure.
- Older toddlers: macrocephaly, seizures, mental retardation.

The primary indication for treating neonates with VAGMs is congestive heart failure refractory to medical treatment (Horowitz et al., 2005). Elective embolization is performed to close the arteriovenous shunt by the arterial route (Bhattacharya and Thammaroj, 2003). Endovascular techniques include transarterial embolization with cyanoacrylate or Onyx, transvenous embolization with use of coils and Onyx, and combined techniques (Pearl et al., 2010) (**Fig. 33E.4**). Endovascular embolization has considerably improved outcomes in patients with VGAM. More recently, with the continued development and improvement of endovascular techniques, many patients are found to be neurologically normal on clinical follow-up, and mortality rates have dropped substantially when compared with microsurgical treatment (Khullar et al., 2010).

Intracranial Aneurysms
Epidemiology

Intracranial aneurysms are the most frequent cause of nontraumatic subarachnoid hemorrhage (SAH). Their prevalence in adults ranges from 0.4% to 6%, depending on whether data are collected retrospectively (e.g., from autopsy series) or prospectively (from angiographic series). The incidence of intracranial aneurysms is associated with age, gender, race, tobacco and alcohol consumption, hypertension, family history, and some hereditary disorders (polycystic kidney disease, Ehlers-Danlos syndrome, neurofibromatosis type 1, and Marfan syndrome). Global mortality of SAH can be as high as 25%, and morbidity among survivors is 50% (Locksley, 1966).

The main complications of aneurysmal SAH are:

- Vasospasm: from day 3 to 5 after bleeding. The main predictive factor is the amount of blood in the subarachnoid space (Fisher scale).
- Rebleeding: particularly in the first 24 hours after hemorrhage.
- Hydrocephalus.
- Medical complications (neurological, cardiac, pulmonary, digestive, electrolytic).

The most important predictive factor of the patient's prognosis is the patient's clinical status at admission: Glasgow Coma Scale, Hunt and Hess Scale, and the classification of the World Federation of Neurologic Surgeons (WFNS) (Teasdale et al., 1988). Comparing the high prevalence of brain aneurysms with the relatively low incidence of SAH, it seems that only a small number of aneurysms actually do rupture. However, neurological sequelae after aneurysmal rupture may justify treatment of asymptomatic aneurysms in selected cases (Locksley, 1966).

Diagnosis

The first diagnostic modality for patients with possible SAH should be unenhanced CT. If the head CT is negative and clinical suspicion is high, a lumbar puncture is mandatory. Noninvasive imaging techniques such as CTA and MRA may show an intracranial aneurysm, but their resolution and sensitivity are inferior to 2D or 3D digital subtraction angiography (Anxionnat et al., 2001). Both carotid and both vertebral arteries must be angiographically explored because more than 20% of patients have multiple aneurysms. If cerebral angiography is negative, it should be repeated 2 weeks later. Sometimes an intra-aneurysmal clot or local arterial vasospasm may hide a small ruptured saccular or dissecting aneurysm. External carotid angiography should also be performed, looking for a DAVF with intracranial pial venous drainage.

Treatment

Ruptured intracranial aneurysms must be treated endovascularly or surgically as soon as possible to avoid aneurysm rebleeding (Heros, 2006). In asymptomatic aneurysm found

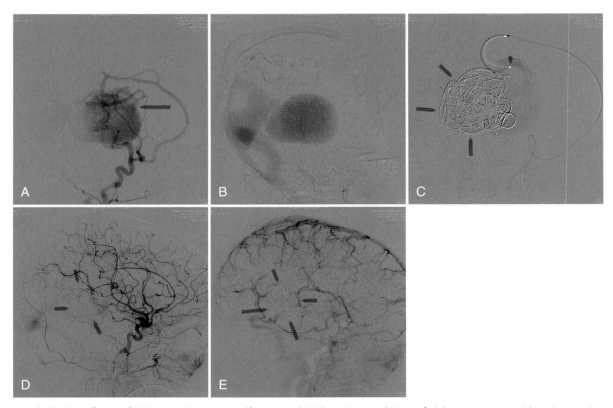

Fig. 33E.4 Embolization of vein of Galen arteriovenous malformation (AVM). **A-B,** Lateral view of right common carotid angiogram in a neonate shows a vein of Galen AVM. Arrow shows entrance of arterial feeders into dilated vein of Galen. **C,** Microcatheter was positioned in vein of Galen using a transarterial approach. Multiple coils are seen in the vein of Galen *(long arrows)*. Short arrow shows tip of microcatheter in main arterial feeder. Coil embolization was followed by injection of Onyx. **D-E,** Postembolization lateral view of right common carotid angiogram shows almost complete occlusion of the vascular malformation. Arrows show coils in vein of Galen. Patient tolerated the procedure well and has only minimal neurological dysfunction after 5 years.

incidentally, the conservative versus active decision should be based on the benefit/risk ratio associated with treatment and the natural history of the aneurysm.

The International Study of Unruptured Intracranial Aneurysms (ISUIA) investigated the natural history of intracranial aneurysms according to the characteristics of the patient, aneurysm size, and morbidity and mortality of the treatment (Wiebers et al., 2003). In the subgroup of small aneurysms (up to 7 mm in diameter) diagnosed and managed conservatively, some of them remained stable and others grew, increasing their risk of rupturing. Some neurointerventional centers perform anatomical follow-up imaging studies (CTA or MRA) with aneurysm fluid dynamic evaluations using computer flow analysis (CFA). The goal of this new evaluation is to depict hemodynamic characteristics in aneurysms related to a higher incidence of aneurysm growth and/or rupture (Chien et al., 2009; Ford et al., 2008).

Intracranial aneurysms can be treated by endovascular embolization or surgical clipping. In the comparative ISAT (International Subarachnoid Aneurysm Trial) study, embolization yielded better results in terms of short-term morbidity and mortality when compared to open surgery (Molyneux et al., 2002). However, the mid-term follow-up showed that surgery had better anatomical results and a lower incidence of aneurysm rebleeding and recanalization (Molyneux et al., 2009).

A turning point in the history of interventional neuroradiology occurred in the early 1990s with the advent of the Guglielmi Detachable Coils (GDC, Target). This device is a platinum coil released by electrolytic detachment when properly placed within the aneurysm. If necessary, it can be removed or placed in another position before detachment (**Fig. 33E.5**). Today more than 100 types of detachable coils are being manufactured. They differ in shape (spiral, 2D, 3D), stiffness, and coating (bioabsorbable polymer or hydrogel).

After embolization, poor packing of the coils may lead to aneurysm regrowth or recanalization (Nguyen et al., 2007). Alternative techniques have been developed to reduce aneurysm recanalization in small aneurysms with wide necks (>4 mm), large (>10 mm in diameter) and giant (>25 mm in diameter) aneurysms.

BALLOON REMODELING TECHNIQUE

In the balloon remodeling technique, a small nondetachable balloon is inflated intermittently within the parent artery at the neck of the aneurysm to provide a transient support for coil placement, reducing untoward coil herniation into the parent artery and distal intracranial coil migration (Moret et al., 1997) (**Fig. 33E.6**).

STENT-ASSISTED EMBOLIZATION

The placement of a stent across the neck of an aneurysms leads to:

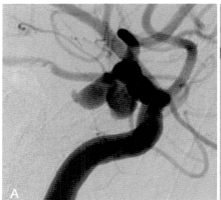
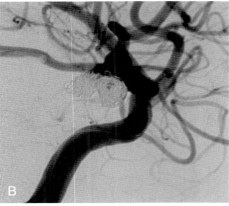

Fig. **33E.5** Endovascular coil embolization of ruptured aneurysm. **A,** Lateral view of left internal carotid artery angiogram shows a posterior communicating bi-lobulated aneurysm. **B,** Postembolization angiogram shows complete filing of the aneurysm with detachable coils.

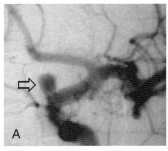
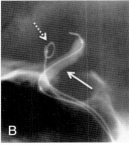
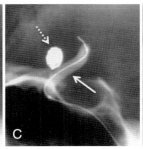
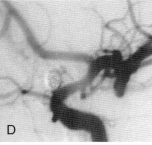

Fig. **33E.6** Balloon-assisted technology in embolization of a wide-neck aneurysm. **A,** Oblique view of left internal carotid artery (ICA) shows a small carotid-ophthalmic aneurysm *(arrow)*. **B,** Detachable coil *(broken arrow)* being delivered into the aneurysm while an inflated balloon *(solid arrow)* closed the neck of the aneurysm. **C,** Complete aneurysm occlusion was obtained *(broken arrow)*. Balloon through neck of aneurysm remains inflated *(solid arrow)*. **D,** Postembolization oblique view of left ICA shows complete aneurysm embolization and preservation of lumen of parent artery.

1. Redistribution and decrease of blood flow into the aneurysm.
2. Later neo-intimal formation and endothelialization of the stent into the wall of the parent vessel, with permanent blockade of the aneurysm from the arterial circulation.
3. A permanent scaffold at the neck of the aneurysm to prevent late herniation of coils (Lubicz et al., 2009).

This technique is associated with an increased risk of thromboembolic events and acute stent thrombosis if antiplatelet drugs are not administered before the procedure. Antiplatelet medication must continue for several months after the procedure as well. Stents may be used alone or in combination with coils. They may be overlapped across the aneurysmal neck, or they can be deployed with a Y-configuration in terminal aneurysms (Doerfler et al., 2004). More recently, stent flow diverters have been developed. These special stents do not require coil embolization, because they elicit hemodynamic changes that produce aneurysm thrombosis between 3 and 10 days (Merlin, Silk, Pipeline embolization devices) (Lylyk et al., 2009) (**Fig. 33E.7**). As noted earlier, Onyx is a novel liquid embolic material (EVOH, DMSO, and micronized tantalum), and when it comes in contact with water or blood, the copolymer precipitates because of rapid diffusion of the DMSO solvent. This liquid embolizing agent may be used alone or in association with other devices (stents, coils, etc.). A temporary balloon occlusion is performed at the neck of the aneurysm while injecting Onyx through a microcatheter to decrease the chances of untoward Onyx migration into the parent artery. Onyx has been mostly used to embolize large and giant aneurysms. In experienced hands, it has shown satisfactory anatomical and clinical outcomes, but it requires a more complex technique than the aneurysm coil or stent embolizations (Molyneux et al., 2004).

Extracranial Carotid Atherosclerosis

About 25% of ischemic strokes are secondary to arteriosclerotic stenotic or occlusive pathology of the internal carotid artery (ICA) at its cervical bifurcation. Carotid endarterectomy (CEA) remains the gold standard for carotid revascularization. It is supported by solid class IA evidence from NASCET (North American Symptomatic Carotid Endarterectomy Trial), ECST (European Carotid Surgery Trial), ACAS (Asymptomatic Carotid Atherosclerosis Study) and ACST (Asymptomatic Carotid Surgery Trial). The surgical target rates for perioperative stroke and death are 6% in symptomatic patients and 3% in asymptomatic patients. A 5-year 17% stroke reduction was demonstrated in symptomatic patients and a 5.9% in asymptomatic patients.

Carotid angioplasty and stenting (CAS) is a valid alternative to surgery in selected patients. The first carotid angioplasty was published by Bockenheimer and Mathias in 1983. The first carotid angioplasty and stenting with distal embolic protective device (EPD) was published by Jacques Theron in 1996 (Theron et al., 1996). A review of the present literature on CAS finds numerous single-center studies with conflicting

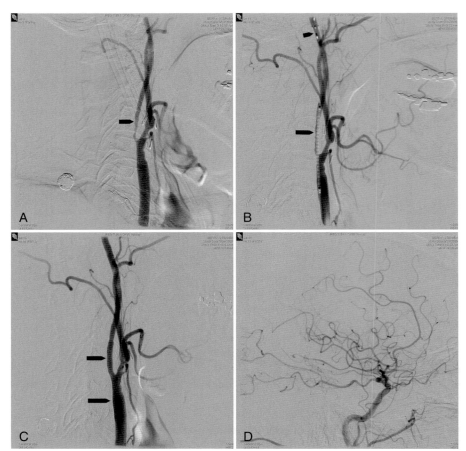

Fig. 33E.7 Carotid balloon angioplasty/stenting with embolic protection device (EPD). **A,** Lateral view of right internal carotid artery (ICA) shows severe post-endarterectomy ICA stenosis *(arrow)*. **B,** Lateral view shows a distal embolic protection device *(short arrow)* and a non-deployed stent in the area of ICA stenosis *(long arrow)*. **C,** Postangioplasty and stenting of right ICA shows reestablishment of normal ICA lumen after stent deployment *(arrows)*. **D,** Postangioplasty intracranial view of right ICA angiogram shows no signs of distal embolization of cerebral circulation.

results, industry-sponsored registries, and randomized trials comparing CEA to CAS.

The SAPPHIRE trial (Stenting and Angioplasty with EPD in Patients at High Risk for Endarterectomy) was a prospective noninferiority design trial (a clinical trial that shows that a new treatment is equivalent to standard treatment) with randomization of high-risk asymptomatic and symptomatic patients to CAS or CEA (Yadav et al., 2004). Its primary endpoint was stroke/death/myocardial infarction (MI) at 30 days plus ipsilateral stroke or death at 1 year. This was the pivotal study leading to Centers for Medicare and Medicaid Services (CMS) approval for reimbursement of CAS with EPD in high-risk symptomatic octogenarian patients with angiographic evidence of greater than 70% ICA stenosis. Clinical follow-up at 3 years showed no significant differences between patients who underwent carotid stenting with an EPD and those who underwent carotid endarterectomy (Gurm et al., 2008).

The CREST trial (Carotid Revascularization Endarterectomy versus Stenting Trial) has being the largest prospective randomized carotid revascularization trial ever conducted (2502 symptomatic and asymptomatic patients) (Brott et al., 2010). Its primary endpoint was periprocedural stroke/death/MI and ipsilateral stroke at 4 years. Brott et al. reported that in the 30-day period following the procedure, the rate of stroke was 2.3% in the surgical patients and 4.1% in the stenting group. However, the heart attack rate was higher in the surgical group: 2.3% compared to 1.1% of the stenting group. The difference in heart attack and stroke between the groups was statistically significant.

CAS is now approved by the U.S. Food and Drug Administration (FDA) for use in patients with high anatomical/clinical risk for surgery (symptomatic ≥50% stenosis and asymptomatic ≥80% stenosis). CAS is CMS approved (reasonable and necessary) for high-risk symptomatic patients with 70% or greater stenosis. This approval is based upon category B investigational device exemption (IDE) studies such as the SAPPHIRE WW. The advantages of CAS over CEA are that it does not require general anesthesia, the patient's neurological status can be assessed during the procedure, recovery time is shorter, and there is no need for a neck incision (risks of cervical hematoma and cranial nerve injuries).

Angioplasty with a balloon and placement of a stent create an intimal lesion favoring thrombosis, so patients must be on an appropriate postprocedural antiplatelet regime. During the procedure, the risk of stroke due to intracranial migration of fresh thrombus or a friable atheromatous plaque exists and may cause neurological deficits. To minimize this risk, several devices are available, distal protection filters being the most commonly used (see **Fig. 33E.7**). Carotid stents should be self-expandable; balloon-expandable stents have a higher collapse rate. The morphology can be straight or conical (corresponding to the differences in diameter between internal and common carotid arteries). The use of bioactive or drug-eluting stents is under current assessment for the prevention of restenosis.

All these techniques should be performed by trained neurointerventionalists to avoid serious complications: embolism, dissection, vasospasm, intracranial bleeding, acute stent thrombosis, or death. Neurological evaluation should guide patient selection, management of comorbidities, lesion criteria, and operator experience to clarify the place of CAS in the management of carotid artery atherosclerosis.

Intracranial Arterial Atherosclerosis

Some 8% of all ischemic strokes are caused by arteriosclerotic intracranial stenosis (ICS). ICS becomes symptomatic by producing distal embolization, compromising cerebral perfusion or developing an in situ atherothrombosis.

The Warfarin-Aspirin Symptomatic Intracranial Disease (WASID) study of arterial stenosis showed the potentially severe prognosis of ICS (Chimowitz et al., 2005). In patients entering the study with a stroke and 70% or greater arterial stenosis, the ipsilateral stroke rate was 23% per year. Patient enrollment was stopped after 569 patients because of concerns about the safety of patients assigned to warfarin (death, 4.3% versus 9.7%; hemorrhage, 2.9% versus 7.3%). The 2-year rate for ischemic stroke in this trial was 19.7% in the aspirin group and 17.2% in the warfarin group. These data indicated that intracranial stenosis is a high-risk disease for which alternative therapies are needed (e.g., aggressive management of risk factors, alternative antiplatelet regimens, intracranial angioplasty and stenting).

Intracranial angioplasty and stenting was first performed using coronary devices. The first stent manufactured for intracranial stenosis was the Wingspan intracranial stent. The Wingspan intracranial stent was manufactured by Boston Scientific Corporation for use in ICS (**Fig. 33E.8**). The first Wingspan Humanitarian Device Exemption (HDE) study was performed in 17 centers outside the United States and was a prospective single-arm study that incorporated 45 patients presenting with recurrent stroke attributable to atherosclerotic disease refractory to medical therapy and ICS of 50% or more. A U.S. multicenter study of Wingspan stents in 78 patients with 82 intracranial atheromatous lesions, 54 of which had 70% or greater stenosis, was published in 2007 (Fiorella et al., 2007). Of the 78 patients, 48 presented with a stroke ipsilateral to the ICS, 28 had a transient ischemic attack (TIA), and 59 failed antiplatelet therapy. Of the 82 lesions treated, there were 5 (6.1%) major periprocedural neurological complications, 4 of which ultimately led to patient death

within 30 days of the procedure. The National Institutes of Health Registry on use of the Wingspan stent enrolled 129 patients with symptomatic 70% to 99% ICS. Its primary endpoint was stroke/death up to 30 days or any ipsilateral stroke beyond 30 days. These events occurred at 5% at 24 hours, 9.2% at 30 days, and 13.9% at 6 months (Zaidat et al., 2008). The technical success rate was 96.7%. The frequency of > or 50% restenosis on follow-up angiography was 13/52 (25%). Fiorella et al. (2009) noted a 27% restenosis rate (36/129 patients) after Wingspan stenting; 29 of those 36 cases required retreatment, and 9 required multiple endovascular angioplasties.

The SAMMPRIS trial (Stenting versus Aggressive Medical Management for Preventing Recurrent Stroke in Intracranial Stenosis) was up and running in the United States starting in November 2008 (Registry, 2010). This was an investigator-initiated, phase III, multicenter, randomized, blindly adjudicated, clinical trial of angioplasty and stenting with aggressive medical management versus medical management alone. This trial's main objective was to determine whether intracranial stenting (using the Wingspan self-expanding nitinol stent [Boston Scientific, Natick, Massachusetts]) and intensive medical therapy were superior to intensive medical therapy alone for preventing the primary endpoint (any stroke or death within 30 days after enrollment, any stroke or death after revascularization of the qualifying artery, any stroke or death within 30 days of re-angioplasty of symptomatic restenosis of the qualifying lesion, or stroke in the territory of the symptomatic intracranial artery beyond 30 days) during a mean follow-up of 2 years in high-risk patients with symptomatic stenosis of a major intracranial artery (middle cerebral, carotid, vertebral, basilar). Patients in the medical arm who underwent angioplasty for recurrent TIAs (i.e., crossovers) and who had a stroke or death within 30 days also met this endpoint. In April 2011, NINDS decided that enrollment in the study should be stopped and that the trial currently available indicates that aggressive medical management alone is superior to angioplasty combined with stenting in patients with recent symptoms and high grade intracranial arterial stenosis. At the time of the most recent data safety board review, 14% of patients treated with angioplasty combined with stenting experienced a stroke or died within the first 30 days after enrollment compared with 5.8% of patients

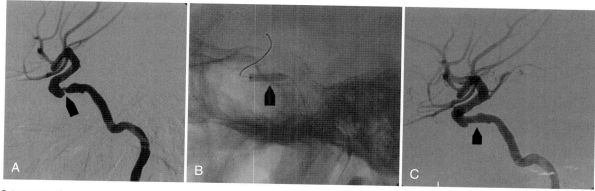

Fig. 33E.8 Intracranial angioplasty and stenting of severe intracavernous internal carotid artery (ICA) stenosis in symptomatic patient. **A,** Lateral view of left ICA shows severe stenosis involving its intracavernous portion *(arrow)*. **B,** Balloon dilatation of the ICA intracavernous stenosis. Arrow shows inflated balloon through stenosis. **C,** Left ICA angiogram after stent deployment shows complete restoration of arterial lumen *(arrows)*.

treated with medical therapy alone, a highly significant difference.

Neurointerventional Management of Acute Stroke

Stroke can be defined as an acute vascular injury of the CNS. Acute ischemia accounts for approximately 80% of all strokes. It is the third leading cause of death in the United States, and every year about 600,000 individuals will experience a stroke. It causes 150,000 deaths per year, and is also a major cause of disability in adults. The estimated direct and indirect costs related to stroke in the United States amounted to $45.4 billion in 2001.

Before effective therapies for acute ischemic stroke were introduced, the primary role of imaging consisted in excluding hemorrhage and other stroke mimics such as infection and neoplasm.

New therapeutic alternatives became available, such as intravenous (IV) or intraarterial thrombolysis, and their use was established in some cases during the past decade. Fibrinolytic therapy offers substantial benefits in selected patients with acute brain ischemia.

Imaging of Stroke
Computed Tomography

The sensitivity for detection of acute ischemia within the first 6 hours after onset is below 50% for CT. Unenhanced CT is fast, readily and widely available, and may contribute not only to ruling out hemorrhage (a contraindication to thrombolytic therapy) but also to detection of early acute ischemia (**Box 33E.1**).

The *hyperdense vessel sign* also may be seen in the presence of high hematocrit levels or middle cerebral artery (MCA) calcification, but in such cases hyperattenuation is usually bilateral.

The Alberta Stroke Program Early CT Score (ASPECTS) was developed to offer the reliability and utility of a standard CT examination with a reproducible grading system to assess early ischemic changes (<3 hours from symptom onset) on pretreatment CT studies in patients with acute ischemic stroke of the anterior circulation (Pexman et al., 2001). It is a 10-point quantitative topographic CT scan score using a segmental assessment of MCA territory. One point is removed from the initial score of 10 if there is evidence of infarction in each of the 10 regions (M1, M2, M3, M4, M5, M6, caudate nucleus, lentiform nucleus, internal capsule, and insular cortex). The baseline ASPECTS correlates inversely with the National Institutes of Health Stroke Score (NIHSS), and as the ASPECTS score decreases, the likelihood of dependence, death, and symptomatic hemorrhage is increased.

Computed Tomographic Angiography

Computed tomographic angiography is best performed on a late-generation multislice CT scanner on which a fast thin-section volumetric spiral examination is performed during a time-optimized bolus of IV contrast material injection with opacification of blood vessels (Tomandl et al., 2003). Complete imaging of the craniocervical circulation from the aortic arch through the circle of Willis region can be performed in as little as 20 seconds. High-resolution 2D (multiplanar reformatted [MPR]) or 3D reconstructed images presented as maximum intensity projection (MIP) or shaded surface display (SSD) images (see **Fig. 33E.7**) can be obtained. CTA can be performed at the same time that a dedicated cranial CT examination is performed, as CTA requires relatively little patient cooperation, is a quick examination, and can identify sites of intracranial or extracranial vessel stenosis or occlusion as possible underlying causes of a patient's acute symptoms. It can therefore potentially identify the source of an ischemic process to aid in the planning of (sometimes emergent) definitive therapy.

Computed Tomographic Perfusion Imaging

Computed tomography perfusion imaging is 75.7% to 86% accurate for detecting stroke and 94.4% accurate in determining the extent of stroke (Shetty and Lev, 2005). **Table 33E.2** lists perfusion imaging parameters, and **Table 33E.3** describes typical perfusion imaging findings with this technique.

Magnetic Resonance Imaging in Acute Stroke Evaluation

Conventional spin-echo MRI is more sensitive and more specific than CT for the detection of acute cerebral ischemia within the first few hours after the onset of stroke. It has the additional benefit of depicting the pathological entity (stroke and its mimics) in multiple planes. The MR sequences

---

Box 33E.1 Early Computed Tomography Signs of Acute Ischemia

Computed tomography features in acute ischemia:
- Hyperdense vessel sign
- Thrombus in intracranial vessel
- Insular ribbon sign
- Obscuration of the lentiform nucleus
- Loss of contrast between gray matter/white matter due to cytotoxic edema

---

Table 33E.2	Perfusion Imaging Parameters
Cerebral blood volume	The volume of blood per unit of brain tissue; normal range = 4-5 mL/100 g
Cerebral blood flow	The volume of blood flow per unit of brain tissue per minute; normal range in gray matter = 50-60 mL/100 g/min
Mean transit time	Time difference between the arterial inflow and venous outflow
Time to peak enhancement	Time from the beginning of contrast material injection to the maximum concentration of contrast material within a region of interest (ROI)

Table 33E.3 **Computed Tomography Perfusion Imaging Findings in Acute Stroke**

Computed tomography perfusion imaging findings in acute stroke:

	Penumbra with autoregulatory mechanisms	Penumbra without autoregulatory mechanisms	Infarcted tissue
Mean transit time (MTT)	Moderately increased	Increased	Increased
Cerebral blood volume (CBV)	Normal or increased CBV (80%-100% or higher)	Moderately reduced CBV (<60%)	Severely decreased CBV (<30%)
Cerebral blood flow (CBF)	Moderately decreased (<60%)	Markedly reduced (<30%)	(<40%)

Box 33E.2 Magnetic Resonance Imaging Results in Acute Stroke

MRI findings:

  Hyperintense signal in white matter
  Loss of gray matter/white matter differentiation
  Sulcal effacement
  Mass effect
  Loss of the arterial flow voids seen on T2-weighted images
  Stasis of contrast material within vessels in the affected territories
  Low-signal-intensity or high-signal-intensity vessel sign due to intravascular thrombus on MR T2*-weighted gradient echo or FLAIR respectively

typically used in the evaluation of acute stroke include T1-weighted spin-echo, T2-weighted fast spin-echo, fluid-attenuated inversion recovery, T2*-weighted gradient echo, and gadolinium-enhanced T1-weighted spin-echo sequences (Schellinger et al., 2001). Common MRI results in acute stroke can be found in **Box 33E.2**.

Conventional MRI is less sensitive than diffusion-weighted MRI in the first few hours after a stroke (hyperacute phase). Diffusion-weighted MRI must be included in any MRI protocol for evaluation of acute stroke.

Statistically significant correlations have been demonstrated repeatedly between the acute infarct volume on diffusion-weighted images and various neurological scales for the assessment of acute and chronic stroke, including the NIHSS, Canadian Neurologic Scale, Barthel Index, and Rankin Scale. It also has been shown that patients who have lesions with a larger volume on perfusion-weighted MRI than on diffusion-weighted MRI have worse outcomes and larger final infarct volumes. Thus, the evaluation of images for a diffusion/perfusion mismatch at a very early stage of stroke may help predict the clinical outcome.

Perfusion-weighted MRI is used to identify areas of reversible ischemia.

Intravenous Thrombolysis

Intravenous thrombolysis is an IV therapeutic modality that was FDA approved in 1996 for patients arriving before 3 hours of onset of symptoms. This decision was based upon results published by the National Institute of Neurological Disorders and Stroke rtPA Stroke Study Group (1995).

For every 100 patients treated with tPA, 32 benefit and 3 deteriorate. It is necessary to treat 8.3 patients to see a patient completely recovered, and 3.1 patients to observe clinical improvement (Saver 2004).

Del Zoppo reported in 1992 that IV recombinant tissue plasminogen activator (rtPA) is more efficient in smaller arteries such as the M2 and M3 portions of the MCA and less so in the ICA and M1 portion of the MCA (Saver, 2004). He reports an 8% recanalization rate in the ICA, 26% in MCA M1, 35% in M2, and 40% in M3.

Intraarterial Thrombolysis

The technique of intraarterial thrombosis requires intracranial navigation with a microcatheter and guide wire and location of the tip of the microcatheter distal to the clot (**Fig. 33E.9**). The contrast injection must be delivered gently, avoiding arterial perforators and distal emboli. A dose of 2 mg of rtPA is delivered distal to the clot before introducing the microcatheter tip into the middle of the clot. Then 10 to 20 mg of rtPA is delivered in situ over 60 to 120 minutes, checking with contrast injections every 15 to 20 minutes. A gentle mechanical manipulation of the clot with the guide wire can also be done.

Two prospective trials of intraarterial thrombolysis were reported. The PROACT I reported arterial recanalization in 57% of recombinant pro-urokinase (rpro-UK) patients and 14% of placebo patients ($P = .017$). Hemorrhages with clinical deterioration occurred in 15% of rpro-UK patients and 7% of placebo patients (ns). Heparin dose influenced hemorrhage frequency and deterioration. Overall, 6 angiographic responders (35.3%) had a modified Rankin score of 0 or 1 at 90-day follow-up compared with 5 nonresponders (21.7%) ($P = .48$).

In the primary analysis, the PROACT II reported 40% of rpro-UK patients and 25% of control patients had a modified Rankin score of 2 or less ($P = .04$). Mortality was 25% for the rpro-UK group and 27% for the control group. The recanalization rate was 66% for the rpro-UK group and 18% for the control group ($P < .001$). ICH with neurological deterioration within 24 hours occurred in 10% of rpro-UK patients and 2% of control patients ($P = .06$).

The authors concluded that despite an increased frequency of early symptomatic ICH, treatment with intraarterial rpro-UK within 6 hours of the onset of acute ischemic stroke caused by MCA occlusion significantly improved clinical outcome at 90 days (Furlan et al., 1999).

Mechanical Thrombectomy

The increased rate of cerebral hemorrhagic complications observed with the use of intraarterial rtPA in PROACT I and PROACT II directed the neurointerventionist to explore

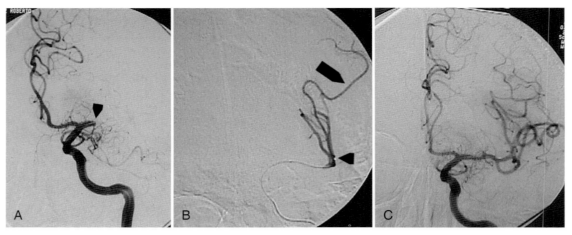

Fig. 33E.9 Intraarterial thrombolysis of an intracranial clot with the injection of recombinant tissue plasminogen activator (rtPA). **A,** Anteroposterior (AP) view of left internal carotid artery (ICA) angiogram shows embolic occlusion of M1 portion of left middle cerebral artery (MCA) *(arrow).* **B,** Angiogram of left MCA with a microcatheter located distal to clot. Small arrow shows tip of microcatheter; long arrow identifies left MCA branches. **C,** AP view of left ICA angiogram showing complete MCA recanalization after intraclot injection of 12 mg of rtPA.

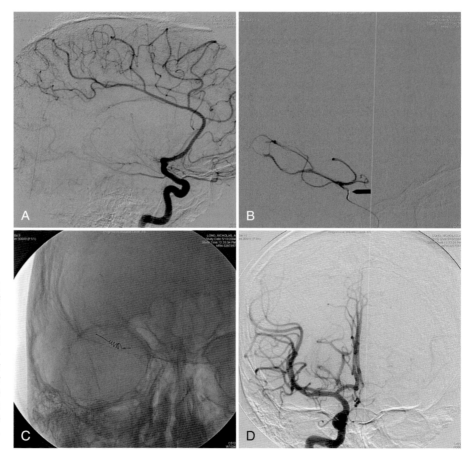

Fig. 33E.10 Mechanical retrieval of intracranial clot using a MERCI device. **A,** Lateral view of right internal carotid artery (ICA) shows complete occlusion of middle cerebral artery (MCA) in a patient known to have septic endocarditis and presenting with a right MCA syndrome. **B,** Selective right MCA angiogram by a microcatheter positioned distal to clot *(arrow).* **C,** Anteroposterior view of skull shows position of MERCI device before clot retrieval. **D,** Right ICA angiogram performed post MERCI retrieval shows complete recanalization of right cerebral arterial circulation. Patient was discharged neurologically intact.

the possibility of using mechanical instead of pharmacological thrombolysis. The potential advantages of this endovascular technology includes a faster recanalization, a potential for lower rates of intracranial bleeding, the possibility of decreasing therapeutic time, and thrombus retrieval for clot analysis.

The mechanical thrombectomy may be performed by clot retrieval devices (Merci Retriever, Neuronet Basket, microsnare), suction thrombectomy (Syringe suction, Angiojet/

Neurojet, and the Penumbra System), and primary angioplasty/stenting.

MERCI Retriever

The MERCI Retriever is an FDA-approved device intended to restore blood flow by removing intracranial thrombus in patients experiencing an ischemic stroke (**Fig. 33E.10**). It may be used alone or in combination with intraarterial rtPA.

The Multi-MERCI Trial involved 14 sites in the United States and Canada and recruited 111 patients up to 8 hours after onset of symptoms. It included anterior and posterior circulation arteries, intraarterial thrombolysis was permitted, and its primary endpoint was arterial recanalization. The study reported an overall Thrombolysis in Myocardial Infarction grading system (TIMI) 2+3 recanalization rate, 2.4% device-related complications, and 5.5% procedure-related complications. Total ICH at 24 hours was 40.2% (30.5% asymptomatic and 9.8% symptomatic). Some 36% of patients had a 90-day good outcome (modified Rankin Scale <2); mortality was 34% at 90 days. In the cases of successful arterial recanalization, good outcome was observed in 49% of patients and in 10% of patients with poor arterial recanalization (Smith et al., 2008).

Penumbra System

The Penumbra intracranial aspiration device is also FDA approved for acute stroke management. It has a reperfusion catheter with a special design for efficient navigation and aspiration, a separator guide wire (it clears the reperfusion catheter enabling continuous aspiration), and a Penumbra aspiration pump and aspiration tube.

The Penumbra Pivotal Stroke Trial reported its results in the journal *Stroke* in 2009. A total of 125 target vessels in 125 patients were treated by the Penumbra system. Post procedure, 81.6% of the treated vessels were successfully revascularized to TIMI 2 to 3. There were 18 procedural events reported in 16 patients (12.8%); 3 patients (2.4%) had events that were considered serious. A total of 35 patients (28%) were found to have ICH on 24-hour CT, of which 14 (11.2%) were symptomatic. All-cause mortality was 32.8% at 90 days, with 25% of the patients achieving a modified Rankin Scale score of 2 or below. The authors concluded that their results suggest the Penumbra system allows safe and effective revascularization in patients experiencing ischemic stroke secondary to large-vessel occlusive disease who present within 8 hours from symptom onset.

References

The complete reference list is available online at www.expertconsult.com.

Chapter **34**

Neuropsychology

Justin J.F. O'Rourke, Leigh Beglinger, Jane S. Paulsen

Neuropsychology is the scientific study of neural correlates for cognition and behavior, with a specific clinical interest in patients presenting a range of medical, neurological, and psychiatric illnesses. Neuropsychologists are specialized clinicians who receive extended fellowship training (with available board certification) in functional neuroanatomy, neurobiology, psychopharmacology, neurological illness or injury, neuroimaging, personality and mood testing, clinical psychology, and neuropsychological assessment. Neuropsychological evaluation refines neuroimaging and neurological examinations by determining the extent to which cognition is affected by brain dysfunction and by assisting the neurologist in objectively quantifying cognition and behavior. A complete clinical neurological examination would be lacking if it did not consider the patient's decision-making ability, judgment, attention, memory, language, and the effect changes in these domains can have on functional capacity. Detailed cognitive evaluation can contribute to diagnosis and prognosis, treatment planning, and the ability to monitor changes over time.

In this chapter, we begin by explaining the utility of neuropsychology and describing the neuropsychological evaluation. Guidelines are then suggested for brief cognitive screening in clinical settings. Finally, the typical patterns of cognitive impairments associated with major neurological disorders are discussed.

Goals of Neuropsychology

When neural damage is present or cognitive changes are observed or reported during clinical evaluation, an extended neuropsychological evaluation is appropriate. The prominent neuropsychologist, Arthur Benton (1975), best described neuropsychology as "a refinement of clinical neurological observation [that] serves the function of enhancing clinical observation [and] is closely allied to clinical neurological evaluation and in fact can be considered to be a special form of it." (p. 68) In clinical settings, neuropsychological assessment aims to extend the clinical neurological exam by: (1) providing important diagnostic information and predictions, even in conditions not detected via other procedures (e.g., anoxia), (2) attributing cognitive strengths and weaknesses to their appropriate factors (e.g., psychiatric symptoms, neurological disease, demographic factors), (3) predicting functional ability to enhance treatment planning, and (4) monitoring cognitive changes and treatment effectiveness across time (Lezak et al., 2004). Neuropsychological assessment is also used in forensic settings and for research in neuroscience, but discussion on these topics is beyond the clinical focus of this chapter.

Before the advent of neuroimaging in the 1970s and 1980s, one of the main goals of neuropsychology was lesion localization. Since current structural imaging techniques are capable of localizing lesions with remarkable accuracy, the focus of neuropsychology has shifted toward characterizing patients' cognitive and behavioral profiles. Such profiles can be used to make differential diagnosis decisions, especially when lesions may not be evident. For example, some types of dementias present with a *cortical profile* (i.e., impairments of memory and language), whereas others present with a characteristic *subcortical profile* (i.e., impairments of processing speed, executive functioning, and mood) (**Table 34.1**). Repeated neuropsychological evaluations can also be a sensitive method for monitoring the progression of neurodegenerative diseases over time (e.g., Huntington disease [HD], Alzheimer disease

Table 34.1 Neuropsychological Characteristics of Cortical versus Subcortical Dementia Using Alzheimer Disease and Huntington Disease as Examples

	Alzheimer Disease (Cortical Dementia)	Huntington Disease (Subcortical Dementia)
LEARNING AND MEMORY		
Episodic memory	Impaired encoding/consolidation Poor delayed recall and recognition memory	Impaired information retrieval Recognition memory is better than delayed recall
Retrograde amnesia	Severe, temporally graded, retrograde amnesia	Mild, non-graded, retrograde amnesia
Priming	Impaired	Preserved
Implicit procedural/motor learning	Preserved	Impaired
Implicit cognitive skill learning	Preserved	Impaired
ATTENTION/CONCENTRATION	Relatively preserved	Poor auditory and visual attention
PROCESSING SPEED	Relatively intact	Very slow
EXECUTIVE FUNCTIONING		
Set shifting	Better able to shift focus	Difficulty with perseveration
Working memory	Mild deficits in ability to manipulate information, but preserved phonological loop and visuospatial sketchpad	Early notable deficits in phonological loop, visuospatial sketchpad, and ability to manipulate information
LANGUAGE AND SEMANTIC KNOWLEDGE		
Speech	Preserved	Dysarthric and slow
Fluency	More impaired semantic fluency than phonemic fluency	Severe and equal impairment in phonemic and semantic fluency
Naming	Impaired; more semantic errors (e.g., calling a lion "an animal")	Relatively preserved; more perceptual errors (e.g., calling a bucket "a cup")
Structure of semantic knowledge	Tend to focus on concrete perceptual information	Able to focus on abstract conceptual knowledge

Adapted from Salmon, D.P., Filoteo, J.V., 2007. Neuropsychology of cortical versus subcortical dementia syndromes. Semin Neurol 27, 7-21.

[AD]), recovery after an acute injury (e.g., stroke or traumatic brain injury [TBI]), or postoperative recovery following neurosurgery (e.g., temporal lobectomy). Evaluating the effectiveness of medical procedures also entails repeated assessment of cognitive abilities with pre- and post-treatment testing.

Another goal of neuropsychology is to attribute cognitive strengths or deficits to their appropriate causes. Whereas neurological disease might account for some cognitive deficits, so can demographic factors (e.g., age, education, race, cultural background), psychiatric symptoms (e.g., depression, anxiety), and other medical conditions (e.g., chronic obstructive pulmonary disease [COPD], alcoholism, hypoglycemia). Therefore, the neuropsychologist weighs the differential impact of all of these confounding factors in the test performances.

In addition to offering information regarding diagnosis and clinical significance of neuroanatomical dysfunction, the neuropsychological assessment is unique in its ability to address patients' functional abilities. Clinicians of all disciplines are often called on to assess patients' abilities to make financial and healthcare decisions, provide supervision, drive a car, and live independently, and neuropsychologists can bring vital information to these decisions. Neuropsychological evaluation can help determine patients' occupational capacity or when they are able to return to work after an injury. Cognitive assessments may also be used to determine appropriate adjustments to patients' treatment plans.

Neuropsychological Evaluation

The neuropsychological evaluation is primarily focused on answering the referral question and typically involves a review of patient records, clinical interview, test selection, administration and scoring, test interpretation, diagnosis, and treatment and rehabilitation recommendations. Evaluations may vary in length, given the presenting concerns of the patient. A complete interview covers the onset and course of the patient's cognitive problems, developmental background, medical and psychiatric history, family medical history, academic performance, vocational achievements, psychosocial functioning, and current functional capacity. Information obtained from collateral sources such as caregivers or spouses about the patient's medical and psychosocial history can also be critical because some patients lack insight. Besides gathering data, the interview serves two additional goals. One is to develop rapport and educate the patient about his or her role in the evaluation. Oftentimes, patients arrive for appointments expecting to be passive participants, as with a neuroimaging procedure. They need to be educated that their involvement is crucial in collecting valid data that will better inform their healthcare providers. A second goal of the interview is to develop hypotheses about the patient's cognitive status. Behavioral observations of the patient during the interview and testing are an important source of information that can influence test selection and interpretation.

Test Administration

Two major approaches to neuropsychological evaluation currently dominate the field: the fixed battery approach and the flexible battery approach (Barr, 2008). The fixed battery approach requires that the same tests are administered to every patient in a standardized manner. One example of a

---

Box 34.1 Heaton Adaptation of Halstead-Reitan Neuropsychological Test Battery

Tactual Performance Test
Finger Oscillation Test
Category Test
Seashore Rhythm Test
Speech Sounds Perception Test
Aphasia Screening Test
Sensory-Perceptual Examination
Grip Strength Test
Tactile Form Recognition Test
Wechsler Adult Intelligence Scale–Revised
Wechsler Memory Scale–Revised

Adapted from Heaton, R.K., Grant, I., Matthews, C.G., 1991. Comprehensive Norms for Expanded Halstead-Reitan Battery: Demographic Corrections, Research Findings, and Clinical Applications. Psychological Assessment Resources, Odessa, Florida.

---

fixed battery is the Halstead-Reitan battery (**Box 34.1**), for which comprehensive norms have been published by Heaton and colleagues (Heaton et al., 1991). An advantage to the fixed battery approach is that the information gathered is comprehensive and systematically assesses multiple domains of cognitive functioning. Additionally, if repeated assessments are available, test scores can be directly compared with baseline information, and tests are well validated and normed. Drawbacks of the fixed battery approach include its length (up to 8 hours), because it may be too long for some patients to tolerate and is difficult to afford with the limited reimbursement schedules in managed care. Furthermore, an extended assessment may not be necessary to address the referral question.

In contrast to the fixed battery approach, the flexible battery (or hypothesis-driven) approach allows neuropsychologists to develop a test battery based on the referral question, the patient's history, and the clinical interview. In the flexible battery approach, a brief set of basic tests is initially administered, and additional tests of more specific abilities are used to conduct in-depth follow-up assessments based on each particular patient's needs. For example, clinicians using the Iowa-Benton method (Tranel, 2008) specifically tailor testing to each patient based on their presenting concern by administering the appropriate portions of a core battery, which are then followed up with tests that assess suspected impairments in more detail (**Fig. 34.1**). Considerations when selecting tests include age, primary language, level of education, ethnicity/cultural factors, reading level, expected level of global cognitive impairment (to avoid ceiling or floor effects in testing), and physical disabilities (Smith et al., 2008). Although this approach is more tailored to the individual needs of the patient (and is therefore briefer), it can be less comprehensive than the fixed battery approach. Most neuropsychologists' approaches fall somewhere between the use of a set battery and a completely individualized examination.

Regardless of clinicians' preferences, all tests are administered according to standardized instructions by neuropsychologists or trained psychometricians. The testing environment requires adequate light, appropriate seating and equipment, and a private office where distractions are controlled so patient performance is optimized. Patients are to bring any assistive

devices (e.g., hearing aid, glasses) to the testing session. Specifics on test administration and scoring are beyond the scope of this chapter; the interested reader is referred to the test manuals that accompany most published assessment instruments.

Test Interpretation

Test interpretation requires the integration of neuropsychological test scores with findings from the clinical interview, the patient's history, the neurological examination, neurophysiology and neuroimaging data, and the relevant literature. Before proper interpretation can be accomplished, however, the raw test scores must be compared to an appropriate reference standard. Several approaches are used in interpreting neuropsychological test scores, including the use of normative data, cut scores, and comparisons with an individual's own prior testing results.

Neuropsychological test scores are interpreted most often by using group statistics to make inferences about individual patients through the use of normative data, which are typically collected by test developers as a standardization sample. Normative data aid in test interpretation by accounting for variables that are likely to influence test performance (e.g., demographic factors) so that accurate and appropriate conclusions are drawn. Confounding variables are accounted for by stratifying test scores according to gender, age, and/or level of education. An individual's raw score is compared with the distribution of scores from his or her peer group to determine where it falls within the range of expected performances. **Fig. 34.2** and **Table 34.2** show a normal distribution and interpretive guidelines for use in neuropsychological interpretation. The usefulness of normative data depends strongly on the size and representativeness of the standardization sample. Clinical interpretation can also be greatly affected by the goodness-of-fit between the individual patient and the standardization sample. For example, it would not be appropriate to make determinations about the test performance of an 82-year-old man with 8 years of education by comparing his test score with those of a group of 40-year-olds with an average of 12 years of education. Furthermore, it is important to use the most recent norms available, because cohort effects may lead to differences between current patients and those from whom data were collected years ago. When appropriate norms are not available, there is a danger of overdiagnosis or underdiagnosis of cognitive impairment. Accurate interpretation of neuropsychological test performance necessarily incorporates information about the sample from which the test norms were developed.

Another approach to test interpretation is through the use of cut scores. Tests that rely on cut scores often measure performances with low base rates or deficits very few healthy people demonstrate. Some tests are fairly straightforward in their capability to measure abilities that are largely intact in normal subjects but impaired in disordered patients. For example, most people are able to bisect a line without difficulty, but patients with left-sided visuospatial neglect typically identify the midpoint of the line to be to the right of center. Other tests, however, are more complex and require more sophisticated analyses to develop valid cut scores. Smith et al. (2008) provide an excellent explanation for how cut scores are useful individual statistics (i.e., test scores) that allow inferences about which diagnostic group a patient is

CORE BATTERY   FOLLOW-UP TESTS

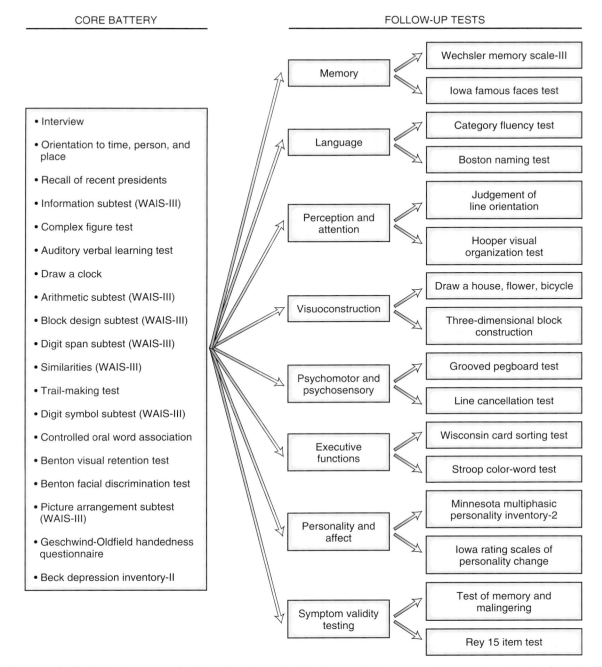

Fig. 34.1 Example of a flexible battery approach. *(Adapted from Tranel, D., 2008. Theories of clinical neuropsychology and brain-behavior relationships, in: Morgan, J.E., Ricker, J.H. (Eds), Textbook of Clinical Neuropsychology. Taylor & Francis, New York, pp. 25-37.)*

likely to belong to (e.g., AD versus mild cognitive impairment versus healthy). Test validation studies commonly use sensitivity and specificity data and base rate information to calculate likelihood ratios and positive predictive values for individual tests. Likelihood ratios and positive predictive values are differing expressions of the probability that a patient has a particular condition given his or her test score. Smith et al. (2008) put these concepts another way by saying, "the positive predictive value allows for statements such as: 'Based on the patient having earned a score of *y* on test *z*, the probability that this patient has the condition of interest is *x*.'" (p. 47). A common example of the application of cut scores can be found in the use of screening instruments to quickly identify

potential impairments. For example, a cut score of 23 on the Mini-Mental State Examination (MMSE) has frequently been used as an indicator of cognitive impairment for dementia. Although cut scores can save time and provide useful heuristics, these scores may miss "true hits" and identify "false positives."

The comparison of current performance with past test scores is another important component of test interpretation, especially if cognitive decline is suspected. Rarely, however, do individuals have previous test data available for these comparisons. When no previous test scores are available, evidence of the patient's premorbid intellectual functioning is estimated. Several techniques are available for estimating premorbid

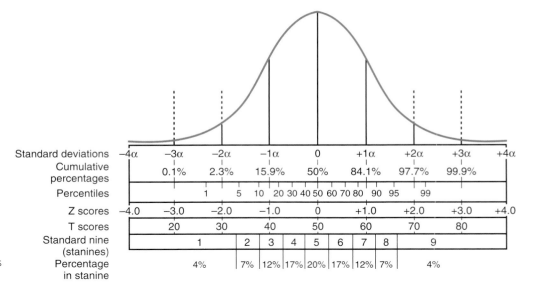

Fig. 34.2 The normal curve and its relationship to derived scores.

Table 34.2 Descriptive Terms Associated with Performance within Various Ranges of the Normal Distribution

Qualitative Terms	Standard Deviation Score	Percentile Rank	T Score
Severely impaired	<3.0	<1	<20
Moderately to severely impaired	2.6 to 3.0	<1	20-24
Moderately impaired	2.07 to 2.53	1-2	25-29
Mildly to moderately impaired	1.6 to 2.0	2-5	30-34
Mildly impaired	1.07 to 1.53	6-14	35-39
Below average	0.6 to 1.0	16-27	40-44
Average	0.53 to +0.53	30-70	45-55
Above average	+0.60 to +1.0	73-84	56-60
High average	+1.07 to +1.53	86-94	61-65
Superior	+1.6 to +2.0	95-98	66-70
Very superior	+2.07 to +2.53	98-99	71-75
Upper extreme	>+2.53	>99	>75

NOTE: The patient's educational history and premorbid level of functioning should be taken into consideration in applying any qualitative label.

Box 34.2 Barona Regression-Based Premorbid IQ Estimation Formula

Barona premorbid IQ estimation formula: VIQ = 54.23 + 0.49 (age) + 1.92 (sex) + 4.24 (race) + 5.25 (education) + 1.89 (occupation) + 1.24 (region)

Age: 16 to 17 years = 1; 18 to 19 years = 2; 20 to 24 years = 3; 25 to 34 years = 4; 35 to 44 years = 5; 45 to 54 years = 6; 55 to 64 years = 7; 65 to 69 years = 8; and 70 to 74 years = 9

Sex: female = 1; male = 2

Race: black = 1; other ethnicity = 2; white = 3

Education in years: 0 to 7 years of school = 1; 8 years = 2; 9 to 11 years = 3; 12 years = 4; 13 to 15 years = 5; and 16 or more years of school = 6

Occupation: farm laborers, farm foremen, and laborers (unskilled workers) = 1; operatives, service workers, farmers, and farm managers (semiskilled) = 2; not in the labor force = 3; craftsmen and foremen (skilled workers) = 4; managers, officials, proprietors, clerical, and sales workers = 5; professional and technical = 6

Region: Southern region = 1; North Central region = 2; Western region = 3; Northeast region = 4

Adapted from Barona, A., Reynolds, C., Chastain, R., 1984. A demographically based index of premorbid intelligence for the WAIS-R. J Clin Consult Psychol 52, 885-887.

intellect. Measures known as *hold tests* (i.e., cognitive tests that are resistant to neurological insult), such as reading ability measures, are frequently used because they are more resistant to many processes that cause decline in cognitive functioning (Smith-Seemiller et al., 1997). Some common measures of reading ability are the National Adult Reading Test (Nelson, 1982), Wide Range Achievement Test Revision 4 (Wilkinson and Robertson, 2006), and Wechsler Test of Adult Reading (Psychological Corporation, 2001), all of which assess the ability to read irregularly spelled words aloud. In some cases, reading ability measures may not be appropriate estimates, because they are affected by the progression of disease (e.g., dementia) (Cockburn et al., 2000; Taylor, 1999). In such conditions, estimates that use demographic variables (e.g., age, education level, primary occupation) in regression-based formulas to predict premorbid IQ may be more useful (e.g., the Barona formula; see **Box 34.2**). Similarly, academic records (e.g., college grade point average, achievement tests from middle school) can provide estimates of functioning prior to illness or injury. Most contemporary neuropsychologists use a combination of these strategies, either formally (e.g.,

Oklahoma Premorbid Intelligence Estimate-3) (Schoenberg et al., 2002) or informally, to arrive at the best estimate of premorbid ability.

Ultimately, feedback about the results of the neuropsychological evaluation, along with diagnostic impressions and treatment recommendations, are communicated to the referring physician. Some form of written report is typical in neuropsychological evaluations, and these tend to vary in length and level of detail (e.g., <1 to 8 pages). Additionally, feedback to the patient can also occur through a brief follow-up appointment or copy of the written report.

Brief Mental Status Examination

Before referring a patient for a neuropsychological evaluation, the neurologist typically has either clinical or historical evidence of cognitive concerns. This might come from patient or collateral report, an informal mental status examination, or a brief objective screening measure of mental status. Although many mental status examinations are conducted in a nonstandard manner, neurologists are encouraged to develop a standardized method of mental status examination so interpretations across time and patients can be reliably made. A few suggested objective screening measures of cognitive functioning that are useful for neurologists to administer are briefly described in this section.

Mini-Mental State Examination

One of the most widely used mental status examinations is the MMSE (Folstein et al., 1975), a 30-point standardized screening tool for assessing orientation, attention, short-term recall, naming, repetition, simple verbal and written commands, writing, and construction (**Fig. 34.3**). The MMSE has been used in a variety of settings (e.g., community,

1. "What is the year? ____
 season? ____
 date? ____
 day of week? ____
 month? ____
 ____/5

2. "Where are we? state? ____
 county? ____
 town? ____
 hospital? ____
 floor? ____
 ____/5

3. Repeat 3 words: ____
 (use list) ____
 ____

"Here are three words I want you to remember." Repeat up to 6 times.
 # words on 1st trial ____
 # repetitions ____
 ____/3

4. Serial 7's: 93 ____
 86 ____
 79 ____
 72 ____
 65 ____
 ____/5

"Start with 100 and count backward by 7. For example: What is 100–7? Keep subtracting 7. Stop after five responses."

Spell "world" backward:
 D ____
 L ____
 R ____
 O ____
 W ____
 ____/5

5. Recall 3 words: ____
 (Set used in #3) ____
 ____
 ____/3

6. Name a: Pencil ____
 Watch ____
 ____/2

7. Read and obey ____/1

CLOSE YOUR EYES

8. Copy design ____/1

(Must have 10 angles and intersect)

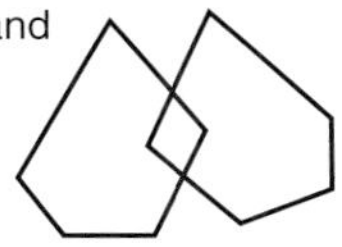

9. Write a sentence: ____/1

(Must have subject and verb make sense)

10. Repeat the following:
 "no ifs, ands, or buts" ____/1

11. Follow a 3-stage command:
 a. take a paper in your right hand ____
 b. fold it in half ____
 c. put it on the floor ____
 ____/3

"Now I will give you some directions to follow. Please listen carefully and do as I say. Take this paper in your right hand, fold it in half, and put it on the floor."

____ TOTAL
MAX = 30

Fig. 34.3 Mini-Mental State Examination. *(Reprinted with permission from Folstein, M.F., Folstein, S.E., McHugh, P.R., 1975. Mini-Mental State: a practical method for grading the cognitive state of patients for the clinician. J Psychiatr Res 12, 189-198.)*

institutions, general hospital, specialty clinics), with many different neurological and psychiatric conditions (e.g., dementia, stroke, depression), across age ranges, and with different cultural and ethnic subgroups. Demographic variables such as age and education have been shown to systematically influence MMSE scores, so normative data or cut scores should account for these variables. One example of appropriate norms comes from the Epidemiologic Catchment Area study (Crum et al., 1993); these are presented in **Table 34.3**. Whereas many intact individuals achieve total scores near 30, a cut score of 23 on the MMSE has been shown to have adequate sensitivity and specificity (86% and 91%, respectively) for detecting dementia in community samples (Cullen et al., 2005). However, when working with highly educated patients (i.e., ≥16 years of formal education) a cut score of 27 is recommended. A cut score of 27 has correct classification rate of 90.1% and a likelihood ratio of 9.6, which means that highly educated individuals with cognitive complaints and MMSE scores below 27 are almost 10 times more likely to have dementia than those with scores greater than 27 (O'Bryant et al., 2008). MMSE scores can also track changes across time. Longitudinal studies have found patients with AD show an average annual rate of change of 2.81 points, although change rates are not uniform across illness stages or gender (Chatfield et al., 2007).

Despite its widespread use, the MMSE has some drawbacks. One potential threat to the test's internal validity is the nonstandardized administration of some of the items. Examples of these frequent adaptations of the MMSE include the use of nonorthogonal (i.e., semantically related) word stimuli for registration and recall, nonstandard scoring of serial 7s, and nonstandard inclusion of spelling *world* backwards. Standard scoring instructions can alleviate some of these problems. Another drawback of the MMSE is that it has "ceiling effects" that can miss cognitive impairments in high-functioning individuals. The MMSE also has difficulty differentiating individuals with mild cognitive impairment (MCI) from controls and those with dementia (Mitchell, 2009). Finally, because this test relies on a single total score, partial administration of the measure (e.g., due to sensory impairments of the patient) provides no information about cognitive status.

Modified Mini-Mental State Examination

Some of the criticisms of the MMSE led to the development of the Modified Mini-Mental State Examination (3MS) (Teng and Chui, 1987), a 15-item extension of the MMSE that assesses orientation (self, time, place), attention (simple and complex), memory (recall and recognition), language (naming, verbal fluency, repetition, following commands, writing), construction, and executive functioning (similarities). It remains relatively brief to administer (10 minutes), and age- and education-corrected normative data are available (Tschanz et al., 2002). Regression-based prediction formulas for the 3MS allow for more accurate assessments of change across time (Tombaugh, 2005). The broader scoring range (0 to 100) has been shown to be more sensitive than that of the MMSE in identifying dementia (McDowell et al., 1997; Tschanz et al., 2002) and other cognitive disorders (Bland and Newman, 2001) in large community samples. A cut score for cognitive impairment is typically 77 (Bland and Newman, 2001; McDowell et al., 1997), and a change of 5 points over the

course of 5 to 10 years indicates the presence of clinically meaningful decline (Andrew and Rockwood, 2008).

Montreal Cognitive Assessment

The Montreal Cognitive Assessment (MoCA) was originally developed as a screening tool to correct the MMSE's insensitivity to MCI (Nasreddine et al., 2005). Executive functioning, immediate and delayed memory, visuospatial abilities, attention, working memory, language, and orientation to time and place are all assessed in this one-page measure (**Fig. 34.4**). The total score ranges from 0 to 30 points, and a cut score of 26 has demonstrated very good specificity (by correctly identifying 87% of healthy participants) and excellent sensitivity when differentiating MCI (90%) and AD (100%) from healthy comparisons (**Table 34.4**). More importantly, the positive predictive value of the MoCA was 89% for both MCI and AD. The psychometric properties of the MoCA contrast with the MMSE's sensitivity of 18% for MCI and 78% for AD (although the MMSE had a specificity of 100% in the same study, meaning it correctly ruled out dementia in all cases) (**Fig. 34.5**). Studies in Parkinson disease (PD) (Hoops et al., 2009; Nazem et al., 2009) and HD (Videnovic et al., 2010) populations have also shown that the MoCA has promise as a measure sensitive to early stages of different types of dementia. The MoCA has the advantage of assessing more cognitive domains, therefore reducing the likelihood that impairments or disorders would be overlooked (e.g., executive dysfunction, a hallmark symptoms of vascular dementia). Another advantage is that the test is free to clinicians (http://www.mocatest.org) and has been translated into 31 different languages and dialects.

Telephone Interview for Cognitive Status—Modified

The Telephone Interview for Cognitive Status—Modified (mTICS) is a relatively brief screening instrument that was designed to quickly and accurately assess cognition over the telephone, although it can also be used in face-to-face settings. This 13-item measure is heavily weighted toward immediate and delayed free recall, which might make it particularly useful in detecting mild impairments (Duff et al., 2009; Lines et al., 2003) such as amnestic MCI (**Fig. 34.6**). Age-, education-, gender-, and race-corrected normative data are available (Hogervorst et al., 2004).

As with many screening instruments, these instruments are gross measures of cognitive functioning that are relatively insensitive to the various domains of cognitive dysfunction. Results from these instruments are also likely to be confounded by individual characteristics of the patients (e.g., age, education, anxiety, visual impairment, paralysis), including brain dysfunction. Overall, these instruments should be used to complement behavioral observations from the neurological examination to suggest whether further testing is necessary.

Neuropsychological Characteristics of Neurological Disease

In this section we briefly address the neurocognitive sequelae of some of the major neurological disorders. Although many

Table 34.3 Mini-Mental State Examination Score by Age and Educational Level, Number of Participants, Mean, Standard Deviation, and Selected Percentiles

AGE (YEARS)	18-24	25-29	30-34	35-39	40-44	45-49	50-54	55-59	60-64	65-69	70-74	75-79	80-84	≥85	Total
EDUCATIONAL LEVEL															
0-4 yr	17	23	41	33	36	28	34	49	88	126	139	112	105	61	892
Mean	22	25	25	23	23	23	23	22	23	22	22	21	20	19	22
SD	2.9	2.0	2.4	2.5	2.6	3.7	2.6	2.7	1.9	1.9	1.7	2.0	2.2	2.9	2.3
5-8 yr	94	83	74	101	100	121	154	208	310	633	533	437	241	134	3223
Mean	27	27	26	26	27	26	27	26	26	26	26	25	25	23	26
SD	2.7	2.5	1.8	2.8	1.8	2.5	2.4	2.9	2.3	1.7	1.8	2.1	1.9	3.3	2.2
9-12 yr or H.S. diploma	1326	958	822	668	489	423	462	525	626	814	550	315	163	99	8240
Mean	29	29	29	28	28	28	28	28	28	28	27	27	25	26	28
SD	2.2	1.3	1.3	1.8	1.9	2.4	2.2	2.2	1.7	1.4	1.6	1.5	2.3	2.0	2.8
College experience	783	1012	989	641	354+	259	220	231	270	358	255	181	96	52	5701
Mean	29	29	29	29	29	29	29	29	29	29	28	28	27	27	29
SD	1.3	0.9	1.0	1.0	1.7	1.6	1.9	1.5	1.3	1.0	1.6	1.6	0.9	1.3	1.3
Total	2220	2076	1926	1443	979	831	870	1013	1294	1931	1477	1045	605	346	18,056
Mean	29	29	29	29	28	28	28	28	28	27	27	26	25	24	28
SD	2.0	1.3	1.3	1.8	2.0	2.5	2.4	2.5	2.0	1.6	1.8	2.1	2.2	2.9	2.0

Data from the Epidemiologic Catchment Area household surveys in New Haven, Connecticut; Baltimore, Maryland; St Louis, Missouri; Durham, North Carolina; and Los Angeles, California, between 1980 and 1984. The data are weighted based on the 1980 U.S. population census by age, sex, and race. Adapted from Crum, R.M., Anthony, J.C., Bassett, S.S., et al., 1993. JAMA 269, 2386-2391.

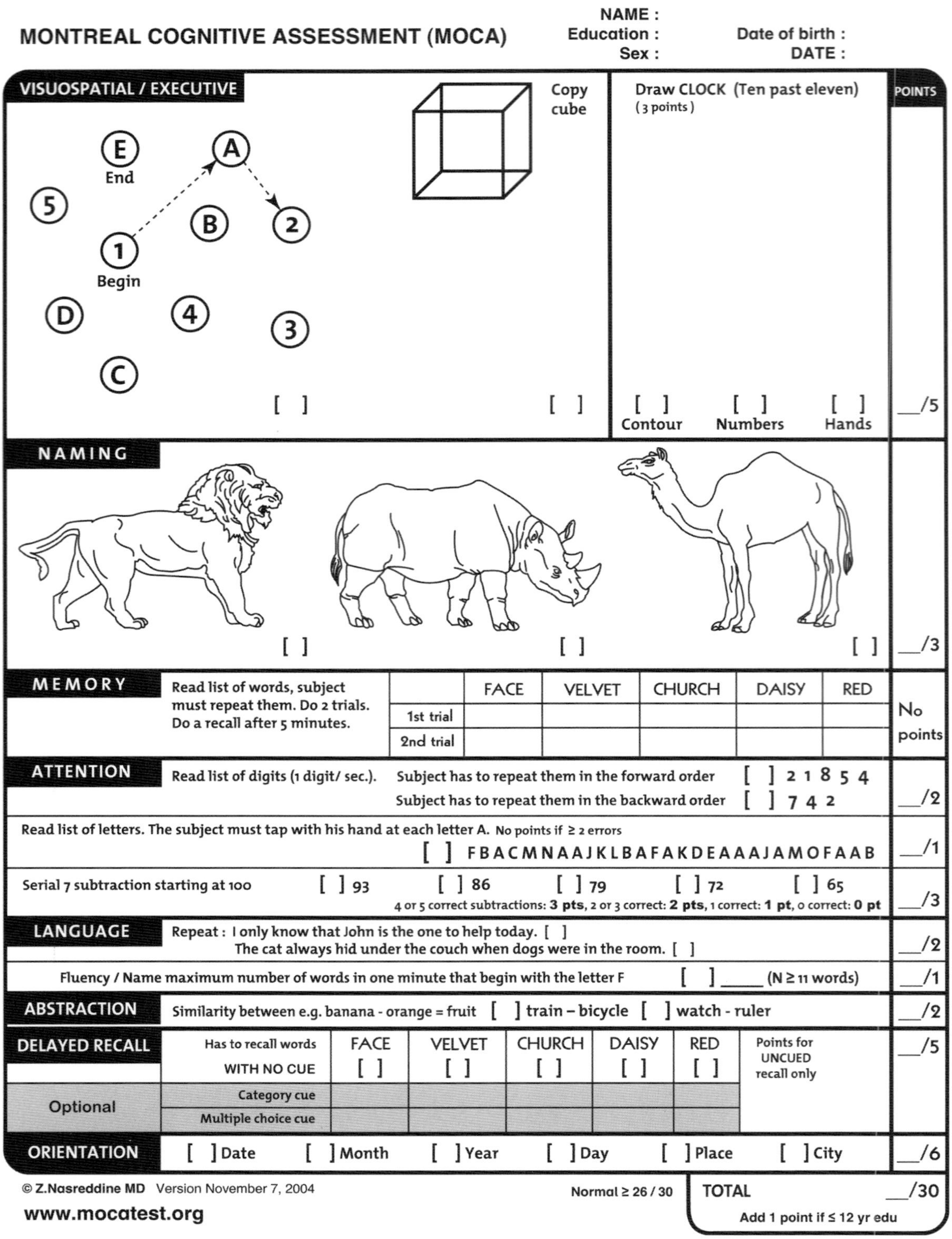

MONTREAL COGNITIVE ASSESSMENT (MOCA)

NAME :
Education :
Sex :
Date of birth :
DATE :

VISUOSPATIAL / EXECUTIVE		Copy cube	Draw CLOCK (Ten past eleven) (3 points)	POINTS

(E) End   (A)
(5)   (B)   (2)
(1) Begin
(D)   (4)   (3)
(C)

[ ]   [ ]   [ ] Contour   [ ] Numbers   [ ] Hands   __/5

NAMING

[ ]   [ ]   [ ]   __/3

MEMORY	Read list of words, subject must repeat them. Do 2 trials. Do a recall after 5 minutes.		FACE	VELVET	CHURCH	DAISY	RED	No points
		1st trial						
		2nd trial						

ATTENTION	Read list of digits (1 digit/ sec.).	Subject has to repeat them in the forward order	[ ] 2 1 8 5 4	__/2
		Subject has to repeat them in the backward order	[ ] 7 4 2	

Read list of letters. The subject must tap with his hand at each letter A. No points if ≥ 2 errors

[ ] F B A C M N A A J K L B A F A K D E A A A J A M O F A A B   __/1

Serial 7 subtraction starting at 100   [ ] 93   [ ] 86   [ ] 79   [ ] 72   [ ] 65   __/3
4 or 5 correct subtractions: **3 pts**, 2 or 3 correct: **2 pts**, 1 correct: **1 pt**, 0 correct: **0 pt**

LANGUAGE	Repeat : I only know that John is the one to help today. [ ] The cat always hid under the couch when dogs were in the room. [ ]	__/2

Fluency / Name maximum number of words in one minute that begin with the letter F   [ ] _____ (N ≥ 11 words)   __/1

ABSTRACTION	Similarity between e.g. banana - orange = fruit [ ] train – bicycle [ ] watch - ruler	__/2

DELAYED RECALL	Has to recall words WITH NO CUE	FACE [ ]	VELVET [ ]	CHURCH [ ]	DAISY [ ]	RED [ ]	Points for UNCUED recall only	__/5
Optional	Category cue							
	Multiple choice cue							

ORIENTATION	[ ] Date [ ] Month [ ] Year [ ] Day [ ] Place [ ] City	__/6

© Z.Nasreddine MD   Version November 7, 2004
www.mocatest.org

Normal ≥ 26 / 30   **TOTAL** __/30   Add 1 point if ≤ 12 yr edu

Fig. 34.4 Montreal Cognitive Assessment. *(Reprinted with permission from Nasreddine, Z.S., Phillips, N.A., Bedirian, V., et al., 2005. The Montreal Cognitive Assessment, MoCA: a brief screening tool for mild cognitive impairment. J Am Geriatr Soc 53, 695-699.)*

of these disorders have psychiatric characteristics as well, these will only be briefly discussed. Please see Chapter 8, Behavior and Personality Disturbances, for a more comprehensive discussion on the psychiatric aspects of neurological disorders.

Mild Cognitive Impairment

Research into aging and dementia is increasingly focused on characterizing the earliest period of cognitive impairment before the development of dementia, and evidence points to

Table 34.4 Normative Data for the Montreal Cognitive Assessment

	Normal Controls (NC)	Mild Cognitive Impairment (MCI)	Alzheimer Disease (AD)
Number of subjects	90	94	93
MoCA average score	27.4	22.1	16.2
MoCA standard deviation	2.2	3.1	4.8
MoCA score range	25.2-29.6	19.0-25.2	21.0-11.4
Suggested cutoff score	≥26	<26	<26*

MoCA, Montreal Cognitive Assessment.

*Although the average MoCA score for the AD group is much lower than the MCI group, there is overlap between them. The suggested MoCA cutoff score is thus the same for both. The distinction between AD and MCI is mostly dependent on the presence of associated functional impairment, not on a specific score on the MoCA test.

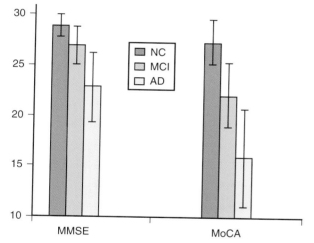

Fig. 34.5 Means and standard deviations for the Mini-Mental State Examination and Montreal Cognitive Assessment for individuals with mild cognitive impairment, Alzheimer disease, and healthy comparisons. *(Reprinted with permission from Nasreddine, Z.S., Phillips, N.A., Bedirian, V., et al., 2005. The Montreal Cognitive Assessment, MoCA: a brief screening tool for mild cognitive impairment. J Am Geriatr Soc 53, 695-699.)*

Initially, MCI was defined as a purely amnestic condition, with a focus on deficits in immediate and delayed recall of verbal and nonverbal information. Isolated difficulties in other cognitive abilities were not fully considered in diagnosis. More recently, however, the criteria have been broadened to include other cognitive domains beyond memory. Several different subtypes of MCI have been proposed, including single-domain impairment (either memory or non-memory) and multiple-domain impairments (with or without memory impairment) (Petersen et al., 2009). To illustrate, Duff et al. (2010c) applied criteria for amnestic and non-amnestic MCI to individuals in the prodromal phase of Huntington disease and found that nearly 40% of these individuals met criteria for some type of MCI. Unlike single-domain amnestic MCI, which tends to progress into Alzheimer dementia, the most common deficit in prodromal HD was slow processing speed, not poor memory. Furthermore, the prevalence of MCI increased as patients' motor symptoms worsened and they approached clinical diagnosis. Other MCI subtypes are hypothesized to progress to their own dementia outcomes. For example, single, non-memory, executive dysfunction domain subtype might reflect a prodromal stage of frontotemporal dementia or, if either executive dysfunction or visuospatial deficits are present, Lewy body disease (Molano et al., 2010). Multiple domain MCI (e.g., deficits in memory and processing speed) might be indicative of eventual vascular dementia. Neuropsychological testing is essential for obtaining the necessary information to differentiate MCI subtypes and track their progression into the various forms of dementia.

MCI has attracted so much attention because of its prognostic value, with a 10-fold increase in the rate of dementia for individuals with MCI (Petersen et al., 1999). Patients of memory disorders clinics with MCI progress to dementia at a rate of 10% to 15% per year (Farias et al., 2009) and community dwelling adults at an annual rate of 6% to 10% per year (Petersen et al., 2009). Individuals with MCI also experience global cognitive decline at over twice the rate of what is observed in nonimpaired individuals (Wilson et al., 2010). Since not everyone with MCI progresses to dementia, several predictors of the progression from MCI have been identified. On neuropsychological testing, more severe memory deficits have been associated with transition from MCI to dementia, as has mild executive dysfunction (Griffith et al., 2006), visuospatial dysfunction (Molano et al., 2010), and processing speed (Duff et al., 2010c). An absence of expected practice effects has also been linked to continued cognitive decline (Duff et al., 2007). Despite this growing research, no standard has yet been established for predicting the MCI-to-dementia conversion.

Alzheimer Disease

Alzheimer disease-related dementia is the most common type, with prevalence rates as high as 10% in community-based samples (Fitzpatrick et al., 2004) and 68% in memory disorder clinics (Paulino Ramirez Diaz et al., 2005). Definitive diagnosis requires postmortem neuropathological examination of brain tissue for the hallmark signs of plaques and neurofibrillary tangles in the hippocampal and entorhinal regions (Braak and Braak, 1991); however, premortem diagnostic criteria are widely employed in clinical and research settings. Currently, the diagnosis of dementia in AD can be made with evidence of a gradually progressive episodic memory impairment plus

a long prodromal period. This transitional stage between normal aging and dementia has been referred to as *mild cognitive impairment* (Petersen, 2004). The initial diagnostic criteria for MCI, defined by Petersen and colleagues at the Mayo Clinic, are subjective memory complaints, an objective memory deficit approximately 1.5 standard deviations below peers, otherwise intact cognition, no functional impairments, and the absence of dementia. By definition, objective cognitive testing is required to diagnose MCI. Objective deficits must be observed across multiple memory tests to accurately classify persons with amnestic MCI (Brooks et al., 2008).

impairment in at least one other cognitive ability (aphasia, apraxia, agnosia, or executive dysfunction) alongside functional decline (American Psychiatric Association, 2000). For research purposes, the National Institute of Neurological and Communicative Disorders and Stroke Alzheimer's Disease and Related Disorders Association (NINCDS-ADRDA) criteria for probable AD are the most commonly used. Recently, workgroups convened by the National Institutes of Aging and the Alzheimer's Association have proposed revised criteria for MCI, preclinical AD, and AD dementia to improve upon the 25-year-old NINCDS-ADRDA standards (Alzheimer's Association, 2010). The aim of the revisions is to differentiate the various stages of AD pathology and to differentiate AD dementia from other acknowledged dementia etiologies (e.g., FTD, vascular dementia [VaD]). Advantages of the new revisions include the incorporation of biomarkers, neuroimaging, and genetic findings into the diagnostic criteria. The proposed criteria particularly emphasize the importance of measurable cognitive decline, especially for MCI and preclinical AD. Formal neuropsychological assessment is needed to measure

AD related declines, using the most sensitive and accurate tools available. The bedside exams mentioned earlier in this chapter also have some degree of utility in detecting cognitive changes, but their comparatively limited scope and sensitivity and their susceptibility to ceiling effects make them better suited for screening purposes.

Complaints about "memory problems" are what often lead to a clinical evaluation of possible AD (Godbolt et al., 2005; Lehrner et al., 2005). Consistent with patient report and behavioral observations, performances across a comprehensive battery of neuropsychological assessment measures is likely to identify stark memory deficits for both verbally (e.g., lists, stories, paired associates) and visually (e.g., concrete or abstract figures) mediated information (Harciarek and Jodzio, 2005). An inability to recall more than 50% of previously learned information is not unusual (Au et al., 2003). Deficits in delayed recall are also notable in AD (Moulin et al., 2004), and intrusion errors are common (e.g., adding extra words to delayed recall trials on word-list memory tasks). Furthermore, performance on recognition trials with memory

Modified Telephone Interview for Cognitive Status (mTICS)

1. What is your name?_____   /2

2. What is your telephone number?_____   /2

3. What is today's date (month, date, year, season, day)? (5 points maximum, 1 point per correct response)

    Month: _____   /1
    Date: _____   /1
    Year: _____   /1
    Season: _____   /1
    Day: _____   /1   /5

4. I'm going to read you a list of 10 words. Please listen carefully and try to remember them. When I am done, tell me as many as you can in any order. Ready? (10 points maximum, 1 point per correctly recalled word)

Cabin	
Pipe	
Elephant	
Chest	
Silk	
Theatre	
Watch	
Whip	
Pillow	
Giant	
TOTAL	

/10

5. Please count backwards from 20 to 1.   /2

    20 19 18 17 16 15 14 13 12 11 10 9 8 7 6 5 4 3 2 1

Fig. 34.6 Modified Telephone Interview for Cognitive Status. (*Data from Welsh, K.A., Breitner, J.C.S., Magruder-Habib, K.M., 1993. Detection of dementia in the elderly using telephone screening of cognitive status. Neuropsychiatry Neuropsychol Behav Neurol 6, 103-110.*)

6. Please take 7 away from 100. Now continue to take away 7 from what you have left over until I ask you to stop. (5 points maximum, 1 point per correct response)

        93: _____ /1

        86: _____ /1

        79: _____ /1

        72: _____ /1

        65: _____ /1   /5

7. What do people usually use to cut paper?_____ /2

8. What is the prickly green plant found in the desert?_____ /2

9. Who is president of the United States now?_____ /2

10. Who is the vice president of the United States now? _____ /2

11. What word is opposite of east?_____ /2

12. Please say this: "Methodist Episcopal"   /2
       Correct response (circle one): YES NO

13. Please tap your finger 5 times on the part of the phone you speak into.
      (2 points if they tap 5 times, 1 point if they tap more or less than 5 times)   /2

14. Please repeat the list of 10 words I read earlier.

Cabin	
Pipe	
Elephant	
Chest	
Silk	
Theatre	
Watch	
Whip	
Pillow	
Giant	
TOTAL	

             /10

             TOTAL: /50

Fig. 34.6, cont'd For legend see facing page.

cues is as impaired as free recall trials (Delis et al., 2005), with few correct "hits" and relatively high numbers of false-positive errors. Other cognitive deficits are seen in a number of other domains including language functions (e.g., paraphasias, naming), semantic knowledge, visuospatial abilities, executive functioning, and motor planning (Smith and Bondi, 2008). Indeed, according to the newly proposed AD diagnostic criteria, a non-memory cognitive deficit may be the primary cognitive presentation of AD if it is present alongside a known AD biomarker or genetic risk factor. Global cognitive functioning in AD declines at a rate nearly four times faster than what is observed in cognitively intact individuals of the same age (Wilson et al., 2010). Given the pattern of deficits in AD, it is not surprising that measures of semantic fluency, delayed free recall, and global cognitive status demonstrate the highest levels of sensitivity and specificity for detecting patients with early AD (Salmon et al., 2002), even over other measures commonly used in the diagnosis of AD (e.g., confrontation naming) (Testa, et al., 2004). Many patients with AD are also anosognosic, which means they are unaware of the extent of their cognitive deficits, if at all (Smith and Bondi, 2008).

Although memory deficits are usually glaring compared to other deficits in AD, some studies suggest that older AD patients (i.e., older than 80) do not have the same disproportionate performances as their younger counterparts (Bondi et al., 2003). As dementia progresses to moderate stages, learning and memory performances are likely to produce floor effects on many standardized neuropsychological measures, and more profound deficits are apparent in other cognitive domains. Deficits in praxis also begin to develop. These pervasive declines in late AD often make formal neuropsychological testing unnecessary or impossible.

Vascular Dementia

Cerebrovascular disease frequently leads to cognitive impairment, which is to be expected given the high prevalence of vascular pathology in both demented and non-demented individuals (Matthews et al., 2009). Extracerebellar lacunar, large vessel, or strategically placed infarcts and hemorrhage lead to varying types and degrees of cognitive impairment. Small vessel disease is the most frequently observed vascular pathology that leads to cognitive declines. Cognitive changes can occur abruptly and in a stepwise pattern with coinciding cerebrovascular accidents (CVAs), or they may fluctuate or remain static. Neuroimaging is likely to detect lesions that are a result of a CVA and enhance diagnostic certainty, but imaging is not required to accurately identify dementia with a vascular etiology. Neurological evidence (e.g., history of strokes, sensorimotor changes consistent with stroke) in combination with cognitive changes can also signify vascular dementia (VaD) (American Psychiatric Association, http://www.dsm5.org).

The clinical presentation of VaD varies depending on the number of infarcts, severity of neural damage following stroke, and location of the CVA. Although many VaD patients may acknowledge "memory problems," which may lead to suspicions of AD, further questioning reveals that these complaints are quite different from those typically seen in AD. Since many patients do not experience a notable stroke preceding the onset of VaD, they may not present to memory disorder clinics because their primary symptoms are an inability to solve simple problems, slowed cognitive processing, apathy, and/or depression (Roman, 2005). Classic dementia symptoms might be reported (e.g., difficulty remembering names, appointments, medications) but changes in instrumental activities of daily living that require complex organizational and problem-solving skills (e.g., managing finances, following directions, "figuring things out") are likely more prominent in a patient with VaD compared to one with AD. Depression, emotional lability, and delusions are also reported, and apathy is a hallmark symptom (McKeith and Cummings, 2005). Upon first inspection, VaD may initially be cognitively indistinguishable from other dementias in many ways; VaD and AD patients have similarly poor orientation to time, person, and place, for example (Mathias and Burke, 2009). Yet, during a detailed neuropsychological examination, behavioral observations and formal tests are likely to reveal a unique pattern of deficits in VaD. VaD patients tend to have better long-term verbal memory than their AD counterparts but worse frontal-executive functioning (Looi and Sachdev, 1999). Declines in speeded processing and complex attention are also prominent in VaD, and they tend to have a rapid initial onset (Boyle et al., 2004). Free recall might occasionally appear similar in VaD and AD, but patients with VaD significantly outperform their AD counterparts on tests of recognition memory (Tierney et al., 2001). Better recognition memory suggests that encoding processes are relatively intact in VaD compared to AD patients, but information retrieval is deficient. This retrieval deficit appears to be quite common in subcortical dementias, with which VaD appears to have several components in common. Patients with VaD also perform more poorly on phonemic fluency tasks relative to semantic fluency tasks, which suggests greater executive dysfunction due to disruption of the frontal subcortical circuitry rather than degeneration in the temporal lobes. Lastly, VaD patients often perform worse than AD patients on emotion recognition tasks (Mathias and Burke, 2009).

Mixed Dementia

More common than AD and VaD in their pure forms is mixed dementia, which involves the coexistence of AD and VaD pathology or a combination of AD and VaD with another pathological process (e.g., Lewy bodies). Across several studies, from 25% to 50% of patients with AD also have sufficient vascular pathology to be deemed VaD (Langa et al., 2004; Zekry et al., 2002), and in autopsy studies the prevalence of mixed dementia ranges from 2% to 56% (Jellinger and Attems, 2007). Persons with multiple pathologies are three times more likely to develop dementia than others with only one identifiable diagnosis (Schneider and Arvanitakis et al., 2007). Neuropsychological and neuroimaging comparisons between AD, VaD, and mixed dementia tend to show that the latter two conditions are most similar (Zekry et al., 2002). Multiple types of dementia pathology can co-occur, with each leading to its own pattern of deficits and impairments.

Frontotemporal Dementia

Frontotemporal dementia is another common type of dementia and is in fact the second most common in those younger than age 65 (Arvanitakis, 2010). Current estimates suggest that 4% of dementia patients will be diagnosed with FTD (Brunnstrom et al., 2009), and it is frequently misdiagnosed as AD. The term *frontotemporal lobar degeneration* (FTLD) is also frequently used in connection with FTD, but usually when referring to the pathological aspects of FTD, not the clinical entity (McKhann et al., 2001). As the newly proposed criteria for FTD in the DSM-V suggests (American Psychiatric Association, http://www.dsm5.org), FTD has multiple clinical manifestations that include behavioral and language variants. Behavioral observations, neuropsychological testing, and neuroimaging (e.g., frontal or temporal lobe atrophy on computed tomography [CT] or magnetic resonance imaging [MRI], hypoperfusion or hypometabolism on single-photon emission tomography [SPECT] or positron emission tomography [PET]) are used in combination to establish a clinically probable diagnosis of FTD. A definitive diagnosis can be made with histopathological evidence through biopsy or postmortem examination.

Although cognitive deficits are clearly evident on formal testing, the earliest and most common complaints for the behavioral variant of FTD are related to changes in personality and behavior (Arvanitakis, 2010). Increases in impulsive actions and disinhibition, poor judgment, compulsive and stereotypic behaviors, lack of hygiene, hyperorality, and loss of social graces are all prominent. A formerly mild-mannered and conscientious patient who develops the behavioral variant of FTD may present as overly frank, crass, and uncaring. The patient is usually indifferent to their behavior, but spouses and adult children are usually embarrassed by his or her conduct. Many of these behavioral issues may have underlying cognitive components. Patients' indifference to their behavior ultimately reflect an inability to cognitively recognize emotions or perspectives in others (Gregory et al., 2002). Deficits on cognitive testing typically involve impaired mental flexibility, planning deficits, slowed word/design generation, multiple response errors, and impairments in reversal learning. The Wisconsin Card Sorting Test, Trail Making Test-Part B, and the Stroop Color-Word Test are all common tests of executive functioning that capture decline in the behavioral variant of FTD. Phonemic fluency also tends to be more impaired than semantic fluency. As the disease progresses, even simple go/no go tasks are difficult. Despite the array of cognitive deficits in FTD, visuospatial functioning tends to be well preserved, and some suggest that a lack of deficits in this domain might be one of the best ways to differentiate FTD from other diseases such as PD (Arvanitakis, 2010).

The language variants of FTD are different clinical entities than the behavioral variant, and they develop if there is disproportionate atrophy, hypometabolism, or hypoperfusion in the temporal lobes (Arvanitakis, 2010). Confrontation naming, word finding, speech production, comprehension, and/or syntax all gradually worsen over the course of disease. Memory functioning and visuospatial skills are relatively spared. The proposed DSM-V diagnostic criteria suggest that the language variant of FTD be divided into four subtypes: primary progressive aphasia (PPA), semantic variant, nonfluent/agrammatic variant, and logopenic/phonologic variant (American Psychiatric Association, http://www.dsm5.org). All of these variants involve impaired confrontation naming (e.g., poor Boston Naming Test scores) but have otherwise unique neuropsychological profiles. Primary progressive aphasia is characterized by the insidious and gradual decomposition of nearly all language functions such as word finding, object naming, grammar, speech production, and comprehension. The semantic variant of FTD involves impaired single-word comprehension, object and/or person knowledge, and dyslexia in the presence of spared single-word repetition, motor speech production, and syntax. Non-fluent/agrammatic FTD results in impaired motor speech production, grammatical errors, and comprehension of complex sentences, with intact single-word comprehension and object knowledge. Lastly, the logopenic/phonologic variant presents with deficits in spontaneous word retrieval and repetition of sentences and phrases, while single-word comprehension, object knowledge, and motor speech and grammar production are spared. Needless to say, neuropsychological testing may be the ideal exam for parsing out the complexity of FTD variants, given the details of their cognitive profiles.

Parkinson Disease with Dementia and Dementia with Lewy Bodies

Parkinson disease with dementia (PDD) and dementia with Lewy bodies (DLB) have been collectively classified as *Lewy body dementias* given their shared α-synuclein pathology (Lippa et al., 2007). The neuropsychological findings in the two disorders are largely similar, so they are often distinguished by differences in the onset of signs and symptoms (Metzler-Baddeley, 2007). The cognitive symptoms of PDD often develop after the onset of motor signs (e.g., bradykinesia, gait instability, tremor, rigidity), while the cognitive symptoms in DLB tend to precede motor features or occur within 1 year of the manifestation of motor signs. Furthermore, cognition fluctuates more drastically, and motor signs develop more quickly in DLB when compared to the insidious onset of PDD signs and symptoms (McKeith et al., 2005). Although the time course of cognitive symptoms and motor signs in DLB and PDD may serve as a helpful heuristic, caution should be used when differentiating these dementias from one another based on onset alone, since subtle cognitive declines can be detected early in the course of PDD (Tröster, 2008).

The neuropsychological profiles of PDD and DLB are similar (Tröster and Fields, 2008). Up to 40% of PD patients progress to dementia at some point during their illness (Padovani et al., 2006). There is considerable heterogeneity in the presentation and progression of cognitive deficits, with some patients displaying only minor cognitive slowing. Overall, the neuropsychological profile of PDD includes bradyphrenia, memory impairment, visuospatial deficits, and executive dysfunction (Troster and Fields, 2008). Of these cognitive difficulties, executive dysfunction—including impairments in decision making, planning, set shifting, and monitoring of goal-directed behaviors—may be among the earliest signs of cognitive decline in PDD. Language problems (e.g., decreased verbal fluency, poor comprehension, difficulty producing syntactically complex sentences) can occur frequently. Memory problems in PDD reflect the subcortical dementia profile, with poor initial learning and delayed recall but relatively intact recognition (Beatty et al., 2003). Psychiatric manifestations are also common in PD, including mood disturbances, anxiety, apathy, and psychosis (Richard, 2005; Weintraub and Stern, 2005; Williams-Gray et al., 2006). Similar psychiatric problems are also observed in patients with DLB; however, the most striking symptom in these patients is the development of well-formed visual hallucinations (Metzler-Baddeley, 2007). These hallucinations are typically not frightening to the patient, and they can be any visual object; however, they often take human form.

In addition to characterizing the cognitive sequelae of PD and the effects of pharmacological treatment, neuropsychologists are often called upon to evaluate candidates for deep brain stimulation (DBS) of the subthalamic nucleus. If patients with PD are severely cognitively impaired, DBS may be contraindicated, since significant declines in executive function, learning and memory, and verbal fluency can occur following surgery (Parsons et al., 2006). Furthermore, older PD patients with MCI prior to DBS may be at greater risk for postoperative declines (Halpern et al., 2009).

Huntington Disease

Huntington disease is a genetically transmitted neurodegenerative condition that primarily affects the basal ganglia and is characterized by a triad of clinical symptoms: choreoathetosis, cognitive decline, and psychiatric dysfunction. The diagnosis of HD is based on a neurological evaluation (e.g., Unified Huntington's Disease Rating Scale [UHDRS]) (Huntington Study Group, 1996) with the manifestation of an unequivocal extrapyramidal movement disorder, although the cognitive and behavioral alterations can be the most debilitating aspect of the disease and place the greatest burden on HD families (Nehl and Paulsen, 2004).

Slowed processing speed, followed by declines in episodic memory and visuospatial processing, may be some of the earliest cognitive changes in people with the HD gene expansion (Duff et al., 2010c; Solomon et al., 2007). The perception of time and timing precision are also affected in HD (Paulsen et al., 2004), and differences in this ability are particularly sensitive to approaching diagnosis in the prodromal phase of the disease (Paulsen et al., 2004; Rowe et al., 2010). Executive dysfunction (e.g., strategies in planning and problem solving, self-monitoring, cognitive flexibility) and "frontal" neurobehavioral symptoms such as apathy and disinhibition are also prominent, even in prodromal HD (Duff et al., 2010a, 2010b). Patients with HD are impaired on cognitive tests that require executive functions, such as the Wisconsin Card Sorting Test, the Stroop Color-Word Test (Beglinger et al., 2005; Montoya et al., 2006), and clinical rating scales of executive control (Paulsen et al., 1996). Even extremely face-valid tests of judgment and decision making have detected impairments in HD (Stout et al., 2001). Another cognitive deficit observed in HD and prodromal HD is poor attention and concentration, affecting such processes as resource allocation, response flexibility, and vigilance (Montoya et al., 2006; Nehl et al., 2001). Recent research has suggested that poor attention in HD may be due to an inability to automatize task performance, which results in the diversion of cognitive resources to tasks that are normally automatic in healthy people (Thompson et al., 2010). Memory problems are also frequently reported by patients with HD and their families. Objective deficits in learning and memory have been widely reported, with these patients displaying a typical subcortical profile (Duff et al., 2010a; Paulsen et al., 1995). Additionally, emotion recognition declines regardless of modality (i.e., facial expression, verbal intonation), especially for fear, anger, and disgust (Johnson et al., 2007; Snowden et al., 2008).

Language deficits may initially appear present in HD; however, communication deficits are likely due to dysarthria—one of the more prominent motor features of HD—and not cognitive decline per se. Dysarthria-related changes include insufficient breath support, varying prosody, increased response latencies, and mild misarticulations (Rohrer et al., 1999). As HD progresses, phrase length decreases, and pauses in speech output are extended. Dysarthria likely accounts for the deficits observed on tasks of letter and category fluency early in the disease (Henry et al., 2005). These deficits are best described as a "paucity of speed" as opposed to dysfluency. Regardless of impairments in speech production, other language functions remain intact, including syntactic structure, content, and the integrity of word associations. Speech output continues to worsen as the disease progresses, typically resulting in a profound communication deficit.

Multiple Sclerosis

Estimates of the prevalence of cognitive disability in multiple sclerosis (MS) range between 40% and 50% in community-based samples (Amato et al., 2006; Jonsson et al., 2006) to more than 55% in clinical settings (Feinstein, 2004). Slowed processing speed is perhaps the most prominent neuropsychological deficit in MS (Parmenter et al., 2007; Rao et al., 1991). A variety of other cognitive declines observed in MS include working memory, cognitive flexibility, inhibition, problem solving, attention, verbal fluency, and spatial reasoning. Confrontation naming and verbal comprehension are generally not affected in MS, and dementia is uncommon (Rao et al., 1991). Consistent correlations between brain lesion magnitude and severity of cognitive dysfunction have also been reported (Benedict et al., 2002).

A distinct cognitive profile is difficult to establish in MS, since individual differences in the microscopic and macroscopic pathology of the disease lead to tremendous variability

depending on the location of sclerotic plaques (e.g., subcortical white matter versus spinal cord). Furthermore, the cognitive sequelae of MS are complicated by the fact that deficits vary across the different subtypes of MS, with progressive subtypes performing worse over time (Huijbregts et al., 2006). Although deficits vary, the typical cognitive profile of MS has been described as a subcortical one, similar to PD or HD, given the deficits outlined above. Depression and other disturbances of emotional functioning occur in nearly half of these patients (Siegert and Abernethy, 2005). Psychiatric disturbances have also been linked with additional cognitive disability (Feinstein, 2004). Depression in MS has also been found to be related to cognitive deficits, particularly speeded attention and executive functioning (Arnett et al., 2002).

Epilepsy

The cognitive effects of epilepsy are unique for each patient, because there is no single cognitive profile associated with any epilepsy subtype (e.g., partial seizures, complex partial, primary generalized). Cognitive deficits also vary according to the location of the seizure foci, frequency of seizures, duration of seizure disorder, age of onset, and antiepileptic drug effects (Jokeit and Schacher, 2004; Lee and Clason, 2008). Regardless of whether a seizure is part of a single idiopathic event or a chronic epileptic disorder, the abnormal electrical activity produced during the ictal period is usually associated with cognitive and psychiatric changes. In chronic conditions, residual interictal alterations in cognition and mood also occur. Given the heterogeneity of cognitive deficits in epilepsy, neuropsychological testing is particularly indicated to provide an accurate characterization of patients' unique cognitive deficits.

Memory deficits are one of the most common clinical manifestations of cognitive impairment in epilepsy, likely due to the high incidence of seizures originating in the medial temporal lobes (MTL) (Bornstein et al., 1988). Research has suggested that patients with focal seizure onset in the right MTL may experience greater nonverbal and visual memory loss, whereas those with onset in the left MTL have a reduced capacity for verbal information (Davis et al., 2006; Glosser and Donofrio, 2001; Kim et al., 2003). However, these findings must be interpreted with caution, since other studies have had contrasting results (Giovagnoli et al., 2005; Raspall et al., 2005). Although visual memory deficits have been observed in right MTL epilepsy, general visuospatial functioning and perception are not usually impaired in these patients (Lee and Clason, 2008). In addition to memory, Lee and Clason (2008) note in their review of the literature that general intellectual functioning can be impaired. In general, those with left MTL seizures and less cognitive reserve (i.e., protective factors, such as education, that generate resilience against the behavioral effects of neuropathology) tend to demonstrate broader cognitive deficits (Oyegbile et al., 2004). Narrative discourse (i.e., the ability to formulate and tell a story) is also affected in epilepsy. Bell and colleagues (2003) found that temporal lobe epilepsy (TLE) patients used non-communicative language, produced less story content, and spoke slower than healthy controls when asked to tell a story. Interestingly, there were no differences between controls and epilepsy patients in procedural discourse (i.e., explaining how to do a task). Confrontation naming is also impaired in some epilepsy patients (Raspall et al., 2005). Language deficits are usually more pronounced if the focus of seizure activity is in the language dominant hemisphere. Postictal language recovery is also affected by seizure origin and generalization in frontal lobe epilepsy patients. Patients with seizures originating in the left frontal lobe and spreading to the language dominant temporal lobe have a slower recovery when compared to their counterparts with either right frontal lobe seizures or seizures confined to the frontal lobe only (Goldberg-Stern et al., 2004). Executive functioning is primarily affected in frontal lobe epilepsy, especially if seizures originate in left frontal lobe, but less so in TLE. Dysfunction is usually characterized by poor cognitive flexibility, response inhibition, and perseveration (McDonald et al., 2005; Milner, 1963).

Neuropsychological evaluation is an integral part of neurosurgical treatments for pharmaco-resistant epilepsy (Helmstaedter, 2004). Preoperative evaluations and Wada testing provide useful information about the localization and lateralization of seizure-induced cognitive impairment. Assessment of patients' cognitive reserve can be useful for predicting postoperative outcomes (e.g., better memory performance at baseline usually means greater memory loss after resection). Postoperative testing is also useful for treatment planning and quality control following resection, and ultimately refines the effectiveness of surgical procedures. Neuropsychological test batteries for surgery candidates are usually very extensive. Given the frequency of temporal lobectomy surgery relative to other procedures, most batteries are heavily focused on assessing memory and language functioning; however, executive functioning, attention, cognitive efficiency, and visuoperception are also examined thoroughly. Although fMRI has potential as a noninvasive method for lateralizing function, Wada testing is still well suited for determining how the nonepileptic hemisphere will function in isolation. Helmstaedter (2004) suggests that the Wada procedure is indicated when neuropsychological testing suggests that seizures are originating from cortex directly involved in language functioning, or if there is an atypical lateralization of language functioning. Other indications include early seizure onset (due to the increased potential for cortical reorganization) and left-handedness. Ultimately, neuropsychological assessment in Wada testing can help reduce the potential for post-surgical disconnection syndromes, aphasia, and functional loss due to unexpectedly poor contralateral compensation.

In addition to the cognitive aspects of epilepsy, psychiatric and behavioral disorders are prevalent (McCagh et al., 2009). Depression is the most common mood disorder, with 40% to 60% of epilepsy patients reporting symptoms, particularly persons with TLE in the dominant hemisphere (Grabowska-Grzyb et al., 2006). Symptoms of depression also appear to be associated with the future onset of focal seizures in some patients. One study found that depression can increase the likelihood of unprovoked seizures by six times (Hesdorffer et al., 2000). Increased anxiety is also present in about 1 in 5 epilepsy patients and does not appear to be directly associated with the neuropathology of epilepsy, but rather the unpredictability of seizures, social consequences of epilepsy, and societal stigmatization (Mensah et al., 2007).

A complicating issue in identifying cognitive and behavioral deficits associated with epilepsy is the independent effect antiepileptic drugs (AEDs) commonly have on neuropsychological functioning (Carreno et al., 2008). Episodic memory, concentration, and psychomotor functioning are the most frequently affected by both classic and new AEDs, although only modestly in most cases (Meador, 2002). The varying effects these medications have on cognition must be weighed against the benefits of minimizing the frequency and severity of seizures.

Traumatic Brain Injury

Traumatic brain injury is one of the most common forms of neurological damage in the United States, particularly in young adults (National Center for Injury Prevention and Control, 2003). In cases of moderate to severe injury, impairments in several cognitive domains can occur, depending on what caused the injury (i.e., blunt force versus projectile), the severity of the injury, site of the lesion, premorbid cognitive and personality factors, and treatment received after the injury. Advances in knowledge regarding the various cognitive sequelae of TBI has allowed for better diagnostic clarity. Beyond the established methods for staging the severity of TBI (e.g., length of loss of consciousness or posttraumatic amnesia, Glasgow Coma Scale [GCS]), neuropsychological

Table 34.5 Common Neurocognitive Sequelae of Moderate to Severe Traumatic Brain Injury

Cognitive Domain	Clinical Manifestation of Impairment
Attention	Difficulty with sustained attention Poor concentration Psychomotor impersistence
Memory	Problems with acquiring and retaining new verbal or nonverbal information Problems in retrieving verbal and nonverbal memories
Speed of information processing	Slowed sensorimotor skills and information processing
Executive functioning	Problems in convergent and divergent reasoning Poor judgment Difficulty planning Problems in self-monitoring and self-correcting behavior
Awareness of symptoms	Difficulty recognizing deficits Unrealistic expectations concerning the recovery of functions Problems related to poor treatment compliance
Language and communication	Problems in word comprehension Impaired reading, spelling, and writing ability Tendency to become fragmented in free speech
Integrative functions	Problems in adequate or time efficient execution of various perceptual-motor-spatial-sequential tasks

testing can be used to increase diagnostic accuracy by measuring the classic cognitive deficits that result from head injury.

Neuropsychological testing is frequently indicated in TBI, because the range of deficits following parenchymal damage can vary significantly. For example, a circumscribed TBI involving the ventromedial prefrontal cortex can produce changes in moral reasoning and social judgment that result in impulse control problems, utilitarian moral reasoning, marked misinterpretation of social cues, or lowered frustration tolerance (Koenigs et al., 2007; Young et al., 2010). Yet, a milder TBI elsewhere might only lead to subtle deficits in attention and processing speed. Despite individual clinical variability, several common neurobehavioral sequelae of moderate to severe TBI can be identified (**Table 34.5**). Cognitive recovery is protracted for moderate to severe TBIs, with improvements still occurring 2 years after the injury; however, even after this length of time, individuals do not necessarily return to preinjury levels.

In addition to moderate and severe TBI, the cognitive sequelae of mild TBI (mTBI) have become an increasing concern, since estimates suggest that 80% of all 2 million TBIs in the United States fall under this classification (National Center for Injury Prevention and Control, 2003; Kraus et al., 1996). In their review of the literature, Mittenberg and Roberts (2008) identified reduced memory, processing speed, and attention span as the most common deficits in mTBI. Global cognitive functioning is also affected in mTBI, but much less so than what is observed in moderate to severe TBI. Furthermore, cognition appears to recover for 95% of patients within 1 to 3 months following the injury (Schretlen and Shapiro, 2003). Other symptoms following mTBI may linger. For instance, a potential concern following mTBI is postconcussion syndrome (PCS), which is characterized by headaches, fatigue, irritability, depression, and poor concentration. Approximately 28% of mTBI patients exhibit symptoms of PCS 6 months following their injury, well past the point of neuropsychological recovery, indicating that PCS may be more related to anxiety surrounding the injury and not underlying neuropsychological impairment, although this is controversial (Mittenberg and Strauman, 2000; Panayiotou et al., 2010; Ryan and Warden, 2003). Treatment for patients with persisting PCS frequently involves education about what they can reasonably expect from their injury and prognosis.

References

The complete reference list is available online at www.expertconsult.com.

Neuro-ophthalmology: Ocular Motor System

Patrick J.M. Lavin

I do not know of any kind of work better fitted for correcting loose habits of observation and careless thinking than a study of the ocular motor nerves.

John Hughlings Jackson, 1877

This chapter discusses diplopia, strabismus, nystagmus, saccadic intrusions such as ocular flutter, opsoclonus, and other ocular oscillations. A brief outline of the anatomy, physiology, and innervation of the extraocular muscles is followed by a discussion of the mechanisms, types, treatment of nystagmus, the development and supranuclear control of the ocular motor system, supranuclear gaze disorders, and oculographic recording techniques.

Neuro-ophthalmology bridges the disciplines of ophthalmology and neurology. Despite sophisticated technological advances in neuroimaging, competence in neuro-ophthalmological diagnosis still requires basic clinical skills that include attentive listening, use of empathetic and timely probing questions, knowledge of neuroanatomy and disorders that affect the afferent and efferent visual pathways, skill in examination of the visual system and cranial nerves, and experience and expertise in evaluating supplementary investigations including perimetry, fluorescein angiography, optical coherence tomography, and neuroimaging. Often a thorough clinical examination and careful thought preempt uncomfortable, invasive, and expensive procedures.

DOI: 10.1016/B978-1-4377-0434-1.00045-1

The human fovea is a highly sensitive part of the retina capable of resolving angles of less than 20 arc seconds. The ocular motor system places images of objects of regard on the fovea and maintains fixation (foveation) if the object or head moves. Each eye has six extraocular muscles (**Table 35.1**) yoked in pairs (**Table 35.2**) that move the eyes conjugately (versions) to maintain alignment of the visual axes (**Fig. 35.1**). The actions of the medial and lateral recti are essentially confined to the horizontal plane. The actions of the superior and inferior recti are solely vertical when the eye is abducted 23 degrees. The oblique muscles, the main cyclotortors, also act as pure vertical movers when the eye is adducted 51 degrees (**Fig. 35.2**). For practical purposes, the vertical actions may be tested at 30 degrees of adduction and abduction. According to the Hering law of dual innervation, yoked muscles receive equal and simultaneous innervation while their antagonists are inhibited (the Sherrington law of reciprocal inhibition), thereby allowing the eyes to move conjugately and with great precision. The pulling actions of the extraocular muscles evolved to move the eyes in the planes of the semicircular canals, which are not strictly horizontal or vertical. These pulling actions are influenced by both the conventional insertions of the global layer of each extraocular muscle directly into the eyeball and by the insertion of the orbital layer into the fibromuscular connective tissue sheath that envelopes each rectus muscle (**Fig. 35.3**). This arrangement forms a pulley system that is actively innervated (Demer, 2002), stabilizes rotation of the globes in three-dimensional space during complex eye movements (e.g., when a horizontal muscle contracts during upgaze), and prevents excessive retraction of the globe within the orbit during extraocular muscle contraction.

Images of the same object must fall on corresponding points of each retina to maintain binocular single vision (fusion) and stereopsis (**Fig. 35.4**). If the visual axes are not aligned, the object is seen by noncorresponding (disparate) points of each retina, and diplopia results (**Fig. 35.5**). In patients with paralytic strabismus, the image from the nonfixating paretic eye is the false image and is displaced in the direction of action of the weak muscle. Thus, a patient with esotropia has uncrossed diplopia (see **Fig. 35.5, A**), and a

Table 35.1	**Actions of Extraocular Muscles**		
Muscle	**Primary**	**Secondary**	**Tertiary**
Medial rectus	Adduction		
Lateral rectus	Abduction		
Superior rectus	Elevation	Intorsion	Adduction
Inferior rectus	Depression	Extorsion	Adduction
Superior oblique	Intorsion	Depression	Abduction
Inferior oblique	Extorsion	Elevation	Abduction

Table 35.2	**Yoked Muscle Pairs**
Ipsilateral	**Contralateral**
Medial rectus	Lateral rectus
Superior rectus	Inferior oblique
Inferior rectus	Superior oblique

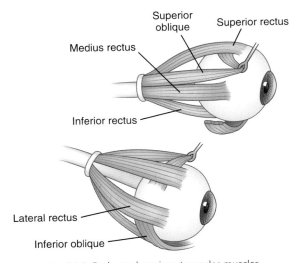

Fig. 35.1 Each eye has six extraocular muscles.

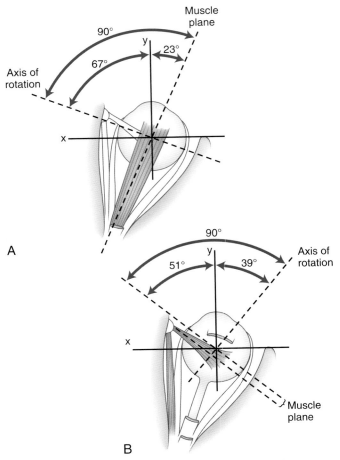

A

B

Fig. 35.2 A, Relationship of muscle plane of vertical rectus muscles to x- and y-axes. **B,** Relationship of muscle plane of oblique muscles to x- and y-axes. *(Reprinted with permission from Von Noorden, G.K., 1985. Burian-Von Noorden's Binocular Vision and Ocular Motility, third ed. Mosby, St. Louis.)*

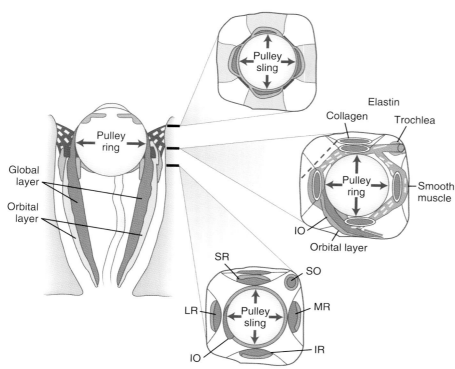

Fig. 35.3 Diagrammatic representation of the structure of orbital connective tissues and their relationship to the fiber layers of the rectus extraocular muscles. Coronal views are represented at levels indicated by the arrows in horizontal section. *IR,* Inferior rectus; *LR,* lateral rectus; *MR,* medial rectus; *SO,* superior rectus. *(Redrawn from Demer, J.L., 2002. The orbital pulley system: a revolution in concepts of orbital anatomy. Ann N Y Acad Sci 956, 17-32.)*

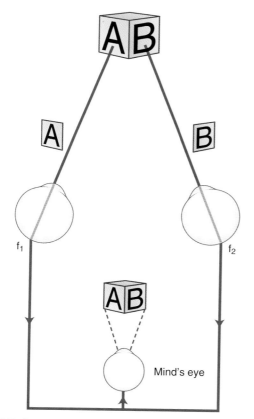

Fig. 35.4 Each eye views the target, AB, from a different angle. The fovea of the left eye (f_1) views the "A" side of the target; the fovea of the right eye (f_2) views the "B" side of the target. The occipital cortex—the cyclopean (mind's) eye—integrates the disparate images so that a three-dimensional image (AB) of the target is perceived. This phenomenon is called *sensory fusion*.

patient with exotropia has crossed diplopia (see **Fig. 35.5,** *B*). After a variable period, the patient person learns to ignore or suppress the false image. If suppression occurs before visual maturity (approximately 6 years of age) and persists, central connections in the afferent visual system fail to develop fully, leading to permanent visual impairment in that eye (developmental amblyopia). Amblyopia is more likely to develop with esotropia than with exotropia, because exotropia is commonly intermittent. After visual maturity, suppression and amblyopia do not occur; instead, the patient learns to avoid diplopia by ignoring the false image.

Heterophorias and Heterotropias

When the degree of misalignment—that is, the angle of deviation of the visual axes—is constant, the patient has a comitant strabismus (heterotropia). When it varies with gaze direction, the patient has a noncomitant (paralytic or restrictive) strabismus. In general, comitant strabismus is ophthalmological in origin, whereas noncomitant strabismus is neurological. Some form of ocular misalignment is present in 2% to 3% of preschool children and some form of amblyopia in 3% to 4%.

Most people have a latent tendency for ocular misalignment, *heterophoria*, which may become manifest (*heterotropia*) under conditions of stress such as fatigue, exposure to bright sunlight, or ingestion of alcohol, anticonvulsants, or sedatives. In nonparalytic (comitant) strabismus, the image is projected in the direction opposite the deviation. When such a latent tendency for the visual axes to deviate is unmasked, the diplopia usually is present in most directions of gaze (relatively comitant).

Divergent eyes are designated *exotropic* and convergent eyes are *esotropic*. Vertical misalignment of the visual axes is less common: When the nonfixating eye is higher, the patient is

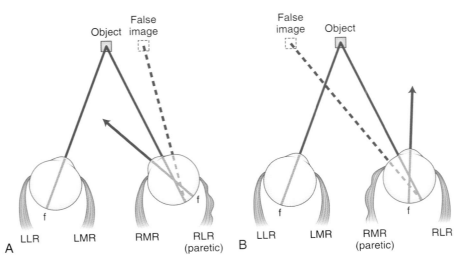

Fig. 35.5 Misalignment of the visual axes. **A,** Esotropia caused by a right lateral rectus (RLR) palsy results in the right eye turning inward so that the image falls on the retina, nasal to the fovea (f), and is projected by the mind's eye to the temporal field. That is, the false image is projected in the direction of action of the paretic muscle, causing uncrossed (homonymous) diplopia. **B,** Exotropia caused by a paretic right medial rectus muscle (RMR) results in the image falling on the retina temporal to the fovea, with projection to the nasal field in the direction of the action of the paretic RMR, causing crossed (heteronymous) diplopia. *LLR,* left lateral rectus; *LMR,* left medial rectus.

said to have a *hypertropia,* and when it is lower, a *hypotonia* (Donahue, 2007), irrespective of which eye is abnormal; for example, with a right hypertropia, the right eye is higher. Asymptomatic hypertropia on lateral gaze often is a congenital condition or "physiological hyperdeviation."

Comitant Strabismus

New-onset strabismus at school age (after age 6 years) is unusual and warrants evaluation for a neurological disorder. Comitant strabismus occurs early in life; the magnitude of misalignment (deviation) is similar in all directions of gaze, and each eye has a full range of movement (i.e., full ductions). Probably, it occurs because of failure of central mechanisms in the brain that keep the eyes aligned. Infantile (congenital) esotropia may be associated with maldevelopment of the afferent visual system, including the visual cortex, and presents within the first 6 months of life; those with comitant esotropia of more than 40 prism diopters (20 degrees) do not "grow out of it" and require surgical correction (Donahue, 2007). Evidence using cortical motion visual evoked potentials indicates that early correction of strabismus (before 11 months of age) improves visual cortical development (Gerth et al., 2008). Cases of comitant esotropia that manifest between the ages of 7 months and 7 years (average 2½ years) are caused by hyperopia (farsightedness) resulting in *accommodative esotropia*: children with excessive farsightedness must accommodate to have clear vision; the constant accommodation causes excessive convergence and leads to persistent esotropia. Accommodative esotropia responds well to spectacle correction alone. Evidence indicates that high-level stereopsis is restored in these children (unlike those with uncorrected infantile esotropia) if treatment is initiated within 3 months of the onset of constant esotropia (Fawcett et al., 2005).

Occasionally, children with Chiari malformations or posterior fossa tumors present with isolated esotropia before the appearance of other symptoms or signs. Features that suggest a structural cause for the esotropia include presentation after age 6, complaints such as diplopia or headache, incomitance in horizontal gaze, esotropia greater at distance than near, and neurological findings such as abduction deficits, ataxia, optic disc edema, pathological nystagmus, and saccadic pursuit. Adults in whom isolated esotropia develops, particularly when

they become presbyopic in their early 40s, should have a cycloplegic refraction to *detect latent hyperopia.* Other causes of adult-onset esotropia include Chiari malformations and acute thalamic hemorrhage (**Box 35.1**).

Esotropia after the age of 3 months is abnormal and, if constant, is usually associated with development delay, cranial facial syndromes, or structural abnormalities of the eye. It should be corrected early unless contraindicated by one of the above underlying conditions. Intermittent exotropia is common and can be treated with exercises, minus-lens spectacles to stimulate accommodation, or surgery.

Box 35.1 Causes of Esotropia

- Congenital esotropia (also acquired, cyclic)
- Duane syndrome
- Accommodative esotropia
- Abducens palsy (unilateral or bilateral)
- Spasm of the near reflex
- Tonic convergence spasm (part of dorsal midbrain syndrome)
- Pseudo–sixth cranial nerve palsy of Fisher
- Acute thalamic esotropia
- Posterior internuclear ophthalmoplegia of Lutz (pseudo-sixth)
- Ocular neuromyotonia
- Divergence insufficiency
- Divergence paralysis
- Cyclical oculomotor palsy (spastic phase)
- Nystagmus blockage syndrome (in congenital and latent nystagmus)
- Abducens palsy with contracture of antagonist (ipsilateral medial rectus) during recovery
- Myasthenia
- Medial rectus entrapment (blowout fracture)
- Thyroid myopathy (rare at presentation)
- Orbital disorders (orbital varix, infiltrative lesions)
- Stiff person syndrome (associated with abduction deficits, hypometric saccades) (Economides and Horton, 2005)
- Wernicke encephalopathy (bilateral abducens palsies)
- Chiari malformation
- Rippling muscle disease

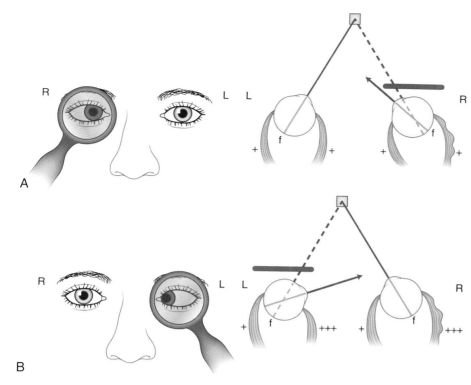

Fig. 35.6 Primary and secondary deviation with palsy of the right lateral rectus muscle. **A,** Right eye is covered with an occluder while left eye fixates on the object. A small right esotropia (primary deviation) is demonstrated. (The opaque occluder is shown here to be partly transparent so the reader can observe the position of the covered eye.) **B,** Left eye is covered while paretic right eye fixates on the object. The right eye can fixate on the object despite the weak right lateral rectus muscle, because that muscle is overdriven by the central nervous system. The normal left medial rectus muscle also is overdriven (the Hering law of dual innervation), resulting in a large esotropia (secondary deviation). *f,* Fovea.

Noncomitant (Incomitant) Strabismus

Noncomitant strabismus occurs when the degree of misalignment of the visual axes varies with the direction of gaze as a result of weakness or restriction of one or more extraocular muscles. When a patient with a noncomitant strabismus fixates on an object with the nonparetic eye, the angle of misalignment is referred to as the *primary deviation*. When the patient fixates with the paretic eye, the angle of misalignment is referred to as the *secondary deviation*. Secondary deviation is always greater than primary deviation in noncomitant strabismus because of the Hering law of dual innervation; it may mislead the examiner to believe that the eye with the greater deviation is the weak one (**Fig. 35.6**).

Diplopia

Theoretically, the onset of double vision should be abrupt. However, in practice the history of onset may be vague for various reasons. The patient may interpret subtle diplopia as blurring unless one eye is covered, or the onset may be uncertain because the diplopia is intermittent initially, of small amplitude, or compensated for by head position, as may be the case in disorders such as congenital superior oblique palsy, ocular myasthenia, and thyroid eye disease. Guidelines for evaluation for diplopia are presented in **Box 35.2**.

Most adult patients with acquired heterotropia complain of frank double vision, but if the images are close together, the patient may not be aware of frank diplopia but merely perceive blurring, overlapping images (ghosting), or strain. Occasionally, visual confusion occurs because each fovea fixates a different object simultaneously, causing the perception of two objects in the same place at the same time (**Fig. 35.7**).

Anxious or histrionic patients may misinterpret physiological diplopia, a normal phenomenon, as a pathological

Box 35.2 Rules for Evaluation for Diplopia

1. *Head tilt*: When the weak extraocular muscle is unable to move the eye, the head moves the eye. Therefore, the head tilts or turns (or both) in the direction of action of the weak muscle (see **Fig. 35.9**).
2. *Image from the nonfixating eye is the false image* and is displaced in the direction opposite the deviation; when the patient fixates with the nonparetic eye, the false image is displaced in the direction of action of the paretic muscle (see **Fig. 35.5**).
3. *False image is the most peripheral image* and is displaced in the direction of action of the weak muscle, except when the patient fixes with the paretic eye. When the lateral rectus is paralyzed, the eyes are *esotropic* (crossed), but the images are uncrossed (see **Fig. 35.5A**). Diplopia is worse at a distance and on looking to the side of the weak muscle. When the medial rectus is paralyzed, the eyes are *exotropic* (wall-eyed), but the images are crossed (see **Fig. 35.5B**). Diplopia is worse at near and on looking to the opposite side.
4. *Images are most widely separated when an attempt is made to look in the direction of the paretic muscle.*
5. *Secondary deviation* (angle of ocular misalignment when paretic eye is fixating) is always greater than primary deviation (when normal eye is fixating; see **Fig. 35.6**). Patients who fixate with the paretic eye may appear to have intracranial disease.
6. *Comitance*: With a comitant strabismus, the angle of ocular misalignment is relatively constant in all directions of gaze. With a *noncomitant (paralytic) strabismus*, the angle of misalignment varies with the direction of gaze.

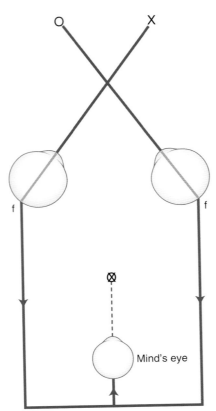

Fig. 35.7 Visual confusion (a rare occurrence). Each fovea (f) views a different object, which is projected to the visual cortex by the cyclopean (mind's) eye and perceived in the same place at the same time.

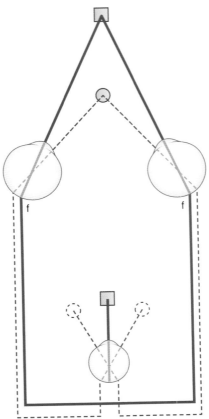

Fig. 35.8 Physiological diplopia. The cyclopean eye views the object *(the square)* as a single object because each fovea (f) fixates it. The images of a nonfixated target *(the circle)* fall on noncorresponding points of each retina, so the object appears double.

symptom. Physiological diplopia occurs when a subject fixates an object in the foreground and then becomes aware of another object farther away but in the direction of gaze. The nonfixated object is seen by noncorresponding parts of each retina and is perceived by the mind's (cyclopean) eye as double (**Fig. 35.8**). Conversely, when the subject fixates a distant object, a near object may appear double.

Isolated vertical diplopia (**Box 35.3**) most commonly is caused by superior oblique muscle palsy. If the palsy is acquired, one image is virtually always tilted—an infrequent finding when the palsy is congenital. If recently acquired diplopia is worse in downgaze, the weak muscle is a depressor. If the diplopia is worse in upgaze, it is an elevator. If one image is tilted, the weak muscle is more likely an oblique rather than a vertically acting rectus.

Spread of comitance—that is, the tendency for the ocular deviation to "spread" to all fields of gaze—occurs in longstanding cases; then the diplopia no longer obeys the usual rules.

If double vision persists when one eye is covered, the patient has *monocular diplopia*, which may be bilateral. The most common cause of monocular diplopia is an optical aberration (refractive error) and warrants appropriate correction (**Box 35.4**). Less commonly, monocular diplopia is psychogenic, but occasionally it can be attributed to dysfunction of the retina or cerebral cortex. The *pinhole test* quickly settles the matter. The patient is asked to look through a pinhole; if the cause is refractive, the diplopia abates because optical distortion is eliminated as the light rays entering the eye through the pinhole are aligned along the visual axis and thus not deflected.

Oscillopsia (see later discussion) may be misinterpreted as diplopia.

Occasionally, disorders that displace the fovea, such as a subretinal neovascular membrane, can cause binocular diplopia by disrupting the alignment of the photoreceptors *(foveal displacement syndrome)*. The diplopia probably results from rivalry between central and peripheral fusional mechanisms (Brazis and Lee, 1998). *Central disruption of fusion* (see later) and *horror fusionis* (in patients with asymmetrical retinal disease) causes intractible diplopia.

Anisoiconia (aniseikonia), defined as a difference of 20% or more between the image size from each eye and usually due to an optical aberration caused by anisometropia or cataract surgery, can cause diplopia that may resolve with complex optical correction. Small differences in image size, even less than 3%, can cause visual discomfort or asthenopia without frank diplopia.

Clinical Assessment

History

Box 35.5 shows the procedure for assessing patients with diplopia. The following points should be clarified if the patient has not volunteered the information: Is the diplopia relieved by covering either eye? (If not, it is monocular diplopia; see **Box 35.4**.) Is it worse in the morning or in the evening? Is it affected by fatigue? Are the images separated horizontally, vertically, or obliquely? If obliquely, is the horizontal or vertical

Box 35.3 **Causes of Vertical Diplopia**

Common Causes

- Superior oblique palsy
- Dysthyroid orbitopathy (muscle infiltration)
- Myasthenia
- Skew deviation (brainstem, cerebellar, hydrocephalus)

Less Common Causes

- Orbital inflammation (myositis, idiopathic orbital inflammatory syndrome [previously designated "pseudotumor"])
- Orbital infiltration (lymphoma, metastases, amyloid)
- Primary orbital tumor
- Entrapment of the inferior rectus (blowout fracture)
- Third nerve palsy
- Superior division third nerve palsy
- Atypical third nerve (partial nuclear lesion)
- Aberrant third nerve reinnervation
- Brown syndrome (congenital, acquired)
- Congenital extraocular muscle fibrosis or muscle absence
- Double elevator palsy (monocular elevator deficiency); controversial in origin

Other Causes

- Chronic progressive external ophthalmoplegia
- Fisher syndrome
- Botulism
- Monocular supranuclear gaze palsy
- Vertical nystagmus (oscillopsia)
- Stiff person syndrome (associated with hypometric saccades, abduction deficits) (Economides and Horton, 2005)
- Superior oblique myokymia
- Dissociated vertical deviation (divergence)
- Wernicke encephalopathy
- Vertical one-and-a-half syndrome
- Monocular vertical diplopia (see **Box 35.4**)

Box 35.4 **Causes of Monocular Diplopia**

- After surgery for long-standing tropia (eccentric fixation)
- Corneal disease (e.g., astigmatism, dry eye, keratoconus)
- Corrected long-standing tropia (eccentric fixation)
- Equipment failure (defective contact lens, ill-fitting bifocals in patients with dementia)
- Foreign body in aqueous or vitreous media
- Iris abnormalities (polycoria, trauma)
- Lens: multirefractile (combined cortical and nuclear) cataracts, subluxation
- Monocular oscillopsia (nystagmus, superior oblique myokymia, eyelid twitching)
- Occipital cortex: migraine, epilepsy, stroke, tumor, trauma (palinopsia, polyopia)
- Psychogenic
- Retinal disease (rarely)

Box 35.5 **Assessment of the Patient with Diplopia**

History

- Define symptoms.
- Effect of covering either eye?
- Horizontal or vertical separation of the images?
- Monocular?
- Effect of distance of target (worse at near or far)?
- Effect of gaze direction?
- Tilting of one image?

Observation

- Head tilt or turn? ("FAT scan")
- Ptosis (fatigue)?
- Pupil size?
- Proptosis?
- Spontaneous eye movements?

Eye Examination

- Visual acuity (each eye separately, and binocularly if primary position nystagmus present)
- Versions (pursuit, saccades, and muscle overaction)
- Convergence (does miosis occur?)
- Ductions
- Ocular alignment (muscle balance) in the "forced primary position"
- Pupils
- Lids (examine palpebral fissures, levator function, fatigue)
- Vestibulo-ocular reflexes (doll's eye reflex)
- Bell phenomenon
- Prism measurements
- Stereopsis (Titmus stereo test)
- Optokinetic nystagmus

General Neurological Examination

Other Tests Where Indicated

- Listen for bruits
- Forced ductions
- Edrophonium (Tensilon) test
- Ice-pack test for ptosis

FAT, Family album tomography—that is, review of old photographs for head tilt, pupil size, lids, ocular alignment, and so on. For magnification, use ophthalmoscope or magnifying glass.

deteriorated? Are there any general health problems? Are there associated symptoms such as headache, dizziness, vertigo, or weakness? What medications are taken? Is there a family history of ocular, neurological, autoimmune, or endocrine disease? Has the patient had a "lazy" eye, worn a patch, or had strabismus surgery?

For example, lateral rectus muscle weakness causes diplopia that is worse at distance and worse on looking to the side of the weak muscle. Acutely, superior oblique weakness causes diplopia that is worse on looking downward to the side opposite the weak muscle and causes difficulty with tasks such as reading, watching television in bed, descending a staircase, and walking on uneven ground. Medial rectus muscle weakness causes diplopia that is worse for near than for distance vision and is worse to the contralateral side.

component more obvious? Is the distance between images constant despite the direction of gaze, or does it vary? Is the diplopia worse for near vision or for distance? Is one image tilted? Do the eyelids droop? Is the diplopia influenced by head posture? Has this condition remained stable, improved, or

General Inspection

Ptosis that fatigues suggests myasthenia gravis (MG). Ptosis associated with a dilated pupil suggests an oculomotor nerve palsy. Lid lag suggests thyroid eye disease or myotonia. Lid retraction suggests thyroid eye disease, aberrant reinnervation after a third nerve palsy, a cyclical third nerve palsy, a dorsal midbrain lesion, hypokalemic periodic paralysis, or chronic corticosteroid use. Proptosis suggests an orbital lesion or, if associated with conjunctival injection and periorbital swelling, an inflammatory disorder such as orbital pseudotumor, orbital lymphoma, dural shunt fistula, or infection. Facial asymmetry suggests a superior oblique palsy that is congenital contralateral to the hemiatrophic side.

Head Posture

Because the weak extraocular muscle cannot move the eye fully, patients compensate by tilting or turning the head in the direction of action of the weak muscle (**Fig. 35.9**). For example, with right lateral rectus palsy, the head is slightly turned to the right; then on attempted right gaze, the patient turns the head farther to the right (see **Fig. 35.9, A**). With a right superior oblique palsy, the head tilts forward and to the left (see **Fig. 35.9, B**). The rule is as follows: The head turns or tilts in the direction of action of the weak muscle.

Sensory Visual Function

Visual acuity, stereopsis, color vision, and confrontation visual fields should be carefully and separately checked in each eye. Patients with nystagmus should have visual acuity checked binocularly as well, because it often is better than with either eye alone.

Stability of Fixation

Fixation and stability of the gaze-holding mechanism should be checked. This is done by having the patient look at a target and then observing for spontaneous eye movements such as drift, microtremor, nystagmus, opsoclonus, ocular myokymia, ocular myoclonus, or saccadic intrusions.

Versions (Pursuit, Saccades, and Ocular Muscle Overaction)

Pursuit movements are tested by asking the patient to fixate and follow (track) a moving target in all directions (**Fig. 35.10, A**). This test determines the range of eye movement and provides an opportunity to observe for gaze-evoked nystagmus. If spontaneous primary-position nystagmus is present, the effects of the direction of gaze and convergence on the nystagmus may be determined. Pursuit movements should be smooth and full. Cogwheel (saccadic) pursuit is a nonspecific finding and is normal in infants. When present in only one direction, however, it suggests a defect of the ipsilateral pursuit system.

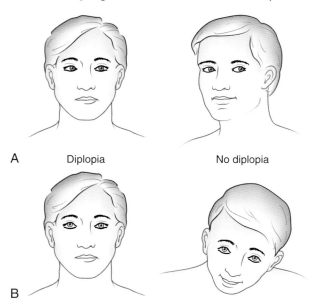

Fig. 35.9 A, Right lateral rectus palsy. A right esotropia is present in primary gaze; however, by turning the head to the right (in the direction of action of the weak right lateral rectus muscle), the patient can maintain both eyes on target (orthotropia), thereby achieving binocular single vision. **B,** Acute right superior oblique muscle palsy. Right eye extorts (excycloduction) because of the unopposed action of the right inferior oblique muscle. When the patient tilts the head to the left and forward (in the direction of action of the weak muscle), the right eye is passively intorted, while the left eye actively intorts to compensate and maintain binocular single vision. The head also tilts forward to compensate for the depressor action of the weak right superior oblique.

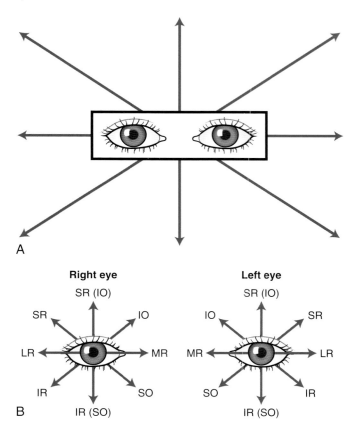

Fig. 35.10 A, The nine diagnostic positions of gaze, used for testing versions (saccades and pursuit). **B,** Ductions are used to test the isolated action of each of the six muscles of each eye (the other five muscles are assumed to be functioning normally). Pure elevation (supraduction) and depression (infraduction) of the eyes are predominantly functions of the superior (SR) and inferior (IR) rectus muscles, respectively, with some help from the oblique muscles. That is, the eyes are rotated directly upward primarily by the SR, with some help from the inferior oblique (IO). The eyes are rotated directly downward primarily by the IR, with some help from the superior oblique (SO). *LR,* Lateral rectus; *MR,* medial rectus.

Saccades (fast eye movements) are tested by asking the patient to look rapidly from one target to another (e.g., from the examiner's nose to a pen) while observing for a delay in initiating the movement (latency) as well as the movement's speed, accuracy, and conjugacy. An internuclear ophthalmoplegia is best detected by this method (Video 35.1, available at www.expertconsult.com). If a specific muscle (particularly an oblique) underacts or overacts, this can be observed in eccentric gaze before testing ductions in each eye separately, as shown in **Fig. 35.10, B**. Assessment of disorders of conjugate (supranuclear) gaze is discussed later.

Convergence

Convergence is tested by asking patients to fixate on a target moving toward the nasion while observing the alignment of the eyes and constriction of the pupils. Miosis confirms an appropriate effort, whereas its absence suggests less than optimal effort.

Ductions

Ductions are tested monocularly by having the patient cover one eye and checking the range of movements of the other eye (see **Fig. 35.10, B**). If ductions are not full, the physician should check for restrictive limitation by moving the eye forcibly (see Forced Ductions, later).

Ocular Alignment and Muscle Balance

Before determining ocular alignment, first the examiner must neutralize a head tilt or turn by placing the patient in the "controlled (or forced) primary position"; otherwise, the misalignment may go undetected because of the compensating head posture. Subjective tests of ocular alignment include the red glass, Maddox rod, Lancaster red-green, and Hess screen tests.

With the *red glass test*, the patient views a penlight while a red filter or glass is placed, by convention, over the right eye. This allows easier identification of each image; the right eye views a red light and the left a white light. The addition of a green filter over the left eye, using red-green glasses, further simplifies the test for younger or less reliable patients. The target light is shown to the patient in the nine diagnostic positions of gaze (see **Fig. 35.10, A**). As the light moves into the field of action of a paretic muscle, the images separate. The patient is asked to signify where the images are most widely separated and to describe their relative positions. Interpretation of the results is summarized in **Fig. 35.11**.

The *Maddox rod test* uses the same principle as for the red glass test, but the images are completely dissociated by changing the point of light seen through the rod, which is a series of half cylinders, to a straight line perpendicular to the cylinders (**Fig. 35.12**). This dissociation of images (a point of light and a line) breaks fusion, allowing detection of heterophorias as well as heterotropias. Cyclotorsion may be detected by asking if the image of the line is tilted (see **Fig. 35.15, B**). The Maddox rod can be positioned to produce a horizontal, vertical, or oblique line.

A further extension of these tests includes the *Lancaster red-green test* and the *Hess screen test*, which use similar principles. Each eye views a different target (a red light through the red filter and a green light through the green filter). The

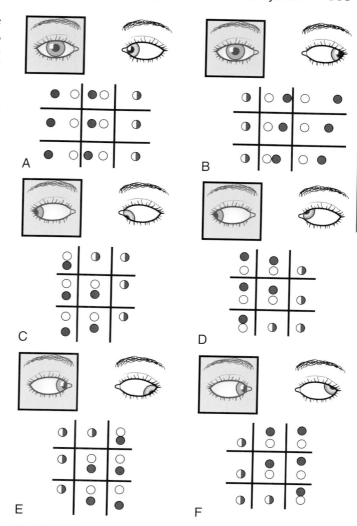

Fig. 35.11 The red glass test. Diplopia fields for each muscle paralysis are shown. By convention, the red glass is placed over the right eye. The charts below each case are displayed as the subject, facing the examiner, indicates the position of the red *(dark circle)* and the white *(white circle)* images in the nine diagnostic positions of gaze. **A,** Right lateral rectus palsy. **B,** Right medial rectus palsy. **C,** Right inferior rectus palsy. **D,** Right superior rectus palsy. **E,** Right superior oblique palsy. **F,** Right inferior oblique palsy. *(Reprinted with permission from Cogan, D.G., 1956. Neurology of the Ocular Muscles, second edition. Charles C Thomas, Springfield, IL. Courtesy Charles C Thomas, Publisher, 1956.)*

relative positions of the targets are plotted on a grid screen and analyzed to determine the paretic muscle. These haploscopic tests are used mainly by ophthalmologists when quantitatively following patients with motility disorders.

The *Hirschberg test*, an objective method of determining ocular deviation in young or uncooperative patients, is performed by observing the point of reflection of a penlight held approximately 30 cm from the patient's eyes (**Fig. 35.13**); 1 mm of decentration is equal to 7 degrees of ocular deviation. One degree is equal to approximately 2 prism diopters. One prism diopter is the power required to deviate (diffract) a ray of light by 1 cm at a distance of 1 m (**Fig. 35.14**).

The *cover-uncover test* is determined for both distance (6 m) and near (33 cm) vision. The patient is asked to fixate an object held at the appropriate distance. The left eye is covered

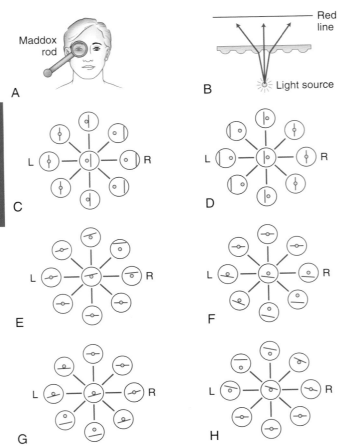

Fig. 35.12 The Maddox rod test. (Unlike in **Fig. 35.11**, the images are displayed as the patient perceives them.) **A,** By convention, the right eye is covered by the Maddox rod, which may be adjusted so the patient sees a red line, at right angles to the cylinders, in the horizontal or vertical plane, as desired (red image seen by the right eye; light source seen by the left eye). **B,** The Maddox rod is composed of a series of cylinders that diffract a point of light to form a line. **C,** Right lateral rectus palsy. **D,** Right medial rectus palsy. **E,** Right superior rectus palsy. **F,** Right inferior rectus palsy. **G,** Right superior oblique palsy. **H,** Right inferior oblique palsy.

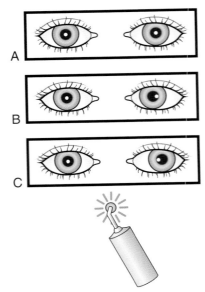

Fig. 35.13 The Hirschberg method for estimating amount of ocular deviation. Displacement of the corneal light reflex of the deviating eye varies with the amount of ocular misalignment. One millimeter is equivalent to approximately 7 degrees of ocular deviation, and 1 degree equals approximately 2 prism diopters. **A,** No deviation (orthotropic). **B,** Left esotropia. **C,** Left exotropia.

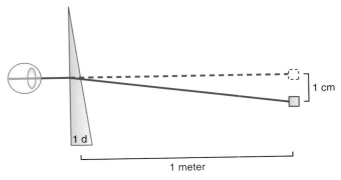

Fig. 35.14 A prism with the power of 1 prism diopter (D) can diffract a ray of light 1 cm at 1 meter.

while the patient maintains fixation on the object. If the right eye is fixating, it remains on target, but if the left eye alone is fixating, the right eye moves onto the object. If the uncovered right eye moves in (adducts), the patient has a right exotropia; if it moves out (abducts), the patient has an esotropia; if it moves down, a right hypertropia; if it moves up, a right hypotropia. The physician should *always* observe the uncovered eye. The test should be repeated by covering the other eye. If the patient has a tropia, the physician must determine whether it is comitant or noncomitant by checking the degree of deviation in the nine diagnostic cardinal positions of gaze (see **Fig. 35.10, A**). With a lateral rectus palsy, the esotropia increases on looking to the side of the weak muscle and disappears on looking to the opposite side (see **Fig. 35.11, A**). Similarly, with a medial rectus weakness, the patient has an exotropia that increases on looking in the direction of action of that muscle (see **Fig. 35.11, B**). Prisms are used mainly by ophthalmologists to measure the degree of ocular deviation (see **Fig. 35.14**). If the diplopia is due to breakdown of a long-standing (congenital) deviation, prism measurement can detect supranormal fusional amplitudes (large fusional reserve). If no manifest deviation of the visual axes is found using

the cover-uncover test, the patient is orthotropic. Then the physician may perform the cross-cover test.

During the *cross-cover test* (alternate-cover test), the patient is asked to fixate an object, then one eye is covered for at least 4 seconds. The examiner should observe the uncovered eye. If the patient is orthotropic, the uncovered eye does not move, but the covered eye loses fixation and assumes its position of rest—latent deviation (heterophoria or phoria). In that case, when the covered eye is uncovered, it refixates by moving back; the uncovered eye is immediately covered and loses fixation. The cross-cover test prevents binocular viewing, and thus foveal fusion, by always keeping one eye covered. Unlike the cover-uncover test, the cross-cover test detects heterophoria. Most normal persons are exophoric because of the natural alignment of the orbits.

Fixation switch diplopia occurs in patients with long-standing strabismus who partially lose visual acuity in the fixating eye, usually as a result of a cataract or refractive error. Such patients normally avoid double vision by ignoring the false image from the nonfixating eye, but a significant decrease in acuity in the "good" eye forces them to fixate with the weak eye. This causes misalignment of the previously good eye and results in diplopia. Fixation switch diplopia usually can be treated successfully with appropriate optical management.

Dissociated vertical deviation (divergence) is an asymptomatic congenital anomaly that usually is discovered during the cover test. While the patient fixates an object, one eye is covered. The covered eye loses fixation and rises; the uncovered eye maintains fixation but may turn inward. This congenital ocular motility phenomenon usually is bilateral but frequently is asymmetrical and often associated with amblyopia, esotropia, and latent nystagmus (LN). Whether the number of axons decussating in the chiasm is excessive, as suggested by evoked potential studies, remains controversial. Dissociated vertical deviation has no other clinical significance.

Three-Step Test for Vertical Diplopia

Eight muscles are involved in vertical eye movements: four elevators and four depressors. The three-step test endeavors to determine whether one particular paretic muscle is responsible for vertical diplopia (**Fig. 35.15**). Using the cover-uncover test, which is objective, or one of the subjective tests such as the red glass test, the physician can perform the three-step test for vertical diplopia. When using one of the subjective tests, it is important to remember that the hypertropic eye views the lower image.

- *Step 1* determines which eye is higher (hypertropic) in primary position. The patient's head may have to be repositioned (controlled primary position) because of a compensatory tilt. If the right eye is higher, the weak muscle is either one of the two depressors of the right eye (inferior rectus or superior oblique) or one of the two elevators of the left eye (superior rectus or inferior oblique).
- *Step 2* determines whether the hypertropia increases on left or right gaze. If it increases on left gaze, the weak muscle is either the depressor in the right eye, which acts best in adduction (i.e., the superior oblique), or the elevator in the left eye, which acts best in abduction (i.e., the superior rectus), and vice versa.
- *Step 3* determines whether the hypertropia changes when the head tilts to the left or the right. If it increases on head tilt left, the weak muscle must be an intortor of the left eye (superior rectus). If it increases on head tilt right, the weak muscle must be an intortor of the right eye (superior oblique).

Two more optional steps:

- *Step 4* uses one of a number of techniques (e.g., double Maddox rod, visual field blind spots, indirect ophthalmoscopy, fundus photography) to determine whether ocular torsion is present. Establishing the degree and direction of ocular torsion, if any, can differentiate a skew deviation from a superior oblique palsy. Because the primary action of the superior oblique muscle is intorsion (see **Table 35.1**), an acute palsy typically results in approximately 5 degrees of extorsion of the affected eye due to unopposed action of the ipsilateral inferior oblique muscle. If either eye is intorted, a superior oblique palsy is not responsible, and the patient may have a skew deviation (Donahue et al., 1999).

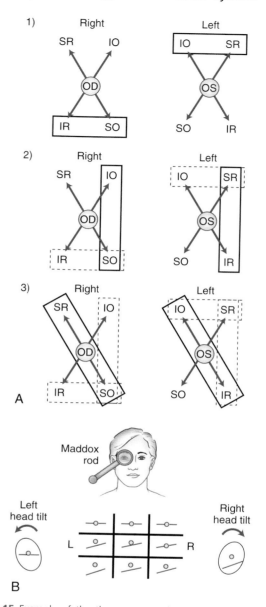

Fig. 35.15 Example of the three-step test in a patient with an acute right superior oblique palsy. **A,** In a patient with hypertropia, one of eight muscles may be responsible for vertical ocular deviation. Identifying the higher eye eliminates four muscles. Step 1: With a right hypertropia, the weak muscle is either one of the two depressors of the right eye (IR or SO) or one of the two elevators of the left eye (IO or SR) *(enclosed by solid line)*. Step 2: If the deviation (or displacement of images) is greater on left gaze, one of the muscles acting in left gaze *(enclosed by solid line)* must be responsible, in this case either the depressor in the right eye (SO) or the elevator in the left eye (SR). Step 3: If the deviation is greater on right head tilt, the incyclotortors of the right eye (SR and SO) or the excyclotortors of the left eye (IR and IO) *(enclosed)* must be responsible, in this case, the right SO—that is, the muscle enclosed three times. If the deviation is greater on left head tilt, the left SR would be responsible. *IO,* Inferior oblique; *IR,* inferior rectus; *SO,* superior oblique; *SR,* superior rectus. **B,** The Maddox rod test (displayed as in **Fig. 35.12,** as the subject perceives the images) in a patient with a right SO palsy shows vertical separation of the images that is worse in the direction of action of the weak muscle and demonstrates subjective tilting of the image from the right eye. When the head is tilted toward the left shoulder, the separation disappears, but when the head is tilted to the right shoulder, to the side of the weak muscle, the separation is exacerbated (Bielschowsky's third step).

Box 35.6 Causes of Positive (Restrictive) Findings on Testing Forced Ductions

- Acquired: superior oblique tendinitis, myositis, or injury
- Brown syndrome
- Carotid-cavernous or dural shunt fistula
- Congenital: superior oblique tendon sheath syndrome
- Duane syndrome
- Entrapment (blowout fracture)
- Extraocular muscle fibrosis (congenital, postoperative)
- Long-standing muscle weakness
- Orbital infiltration: myositis, lymphoma, metastasis, amyloidosis, cysticercosis, trichinosis
- Thyroid ophthalmopathy

- *Step 5* is helpful in the acute phase. If the deviation is greater on downgaze, the weak muscle is a depressor; if it is worse on upgaze, the weak muscle is likely to be an elevator. This fifth step is helpful only in the acute stage, because with time the deviation becomes more comitant.

The examiner should be aware of the pitfalls of the three-step test—namely, the conditions in which the rules break down. These include restrictive ocular myopathies (**Box 35.6**), long-standing strabismus, skew deviation, and disorders involving more than one muscle.

The four fundamental features of the fourth cranial nerve are: (1) it has the longest intracranial course and is the thinnest of all the cranial nerves and thus very susceptible to injury; (2) it is the only cranial nerve that exits the neuraxis dorsally; (3) its nucleus of origin is on the contralateral side of the neuraxis (the oculomotor subnucleus for the superior rectus is on the opposite side also); and (4) the most common cause of isolated vertical diplopia is a fourth nerve (superior oblique) palsy.

Fatigability

Once the weak muscle is identified, the physician should determine whether it fatigues by testing its rapid (saccadic) action repetitively and its ability to sustain eccentric eye position without drift.

Forced Ductions

 If the weak muscle does not fatigue, the physician should determine whether it is restricted by performing forced ductions (Video 35.2, available at www.expertconsult.com). The use of phenylephrine hydrochloride eye drops beforehand reduces the risk of subconjunctival hemorrhage. Although this test is in the realm of the ophthalmologist, it may be performed in the office using topical anesthesia and a cotton-tipped applicator, but great care must be taken to avoid injuring the cornea. The causes of restrictive myopathy are listed in **Box 35.6**; however, any cause of prolonged extraocular muscle paresis can result in contracture of its antagonist.

Signs Associated with Diplopia

When evaluating a patient with diplopia, the examiner should determine whether any of the signs outlined in **Box 35.7** are present.

Box 35.7 Signs Associated with Diplopia

- Extraocular muscle or lid fatigue suggests MG.
- Cogan lid twitch sign suggests MG.
- Weakness of other muscles (e.g., orbicularis oculi, other facial muscles, neck flexors, bulbar muscles) suggests oculopharyngeal dystrophy or MG (see Chapters 25, 78, and 79).
- Narrowing of palpebral fissure and retraction of globe on adduction, associated with an abduction deficit, suggests Duane retraction syndrome (Gutowski, 2000).
- Paradoxical elevation of upper lid on attempted adduction or downgaze, and pupil constriction on attempted adduction or downgaze, occurs with aberrant reinnervation of the third cranial nerve, which is virtually always a result of trauma or compression caused by tumor or aneurysm (see Chapter 70).
- Miosis accompanying apparent bilateral sixth nerve palsy occurs with spasm of the near reflex.
- Horner syndrome, ophthalmoplegia, and impaired sensation in the distribution of the first division of the trigeminal nerve occur with superior orbital fissure and anterior cavernous sinus lesions.
- A third nerve palsy with pupillary involvement most often is due to a compressive lesion; with acute onset, a posterior communicating aneurysm usually is responsible.
- Proptosis suggests an orbital lesion such as thyroid eye disease, inflammatory or infiltrative orbital disease (tumor, pseudotumor, or amyloidosis), or a carotid-cavernous sinus fistula, in which case it may be pulsatile.
- Ocular bruits, often heard by both patient and doctor, occur with carotid-cavernous or dural shunt fistulas.
- Entrapment (blowout fracture) is a sign of periorbital and ocular injury.
- Nystagmus is seen with INO.
- Ophthalmoplegia, ataxia, nystagmus, and confusion suggest Wernicke encephalopathy.
- Pyramidal and spinothalamic signs with crossed hemiparesis suggest brainstem syndromes (Chapter 19).
- Facial pain, hearing loss, and ipsilateral lateral rectus weakness indicate the Gradenigo syndrome.
- Myotonia and RP suggest more widespread disorders.

INO, Internuclear ophthalmoplegia; *MG,* myasthenia gravis; *RP,* retinitis pigmentosa.

Edrophonium (Tensilon) Test

The edrophonium test is discussed in detail in Chapter 78, but a few points are emphasized here. The test must have an objective endpoint (e.g., ptosis, a tropia, limited ductions), and the physician must observe an objective change. When forced ductions are positive, indicating a restrictive myopathy, the edrophonium test will be negative and therefore is not indicated. Myasthenic ptosis may be reversed temporarily with application of an ice pack over the affected lid.

Acute Bilateral Ophthalmoplegia

The causes of acute bilateral ophthalmoplegia are outlined in **Box 35.8**.

Chronic Bilateral Ophthalmoplegia

The causes of chronic bilateral ophthalmoplegia are outlined in **Box 35.9**.

Box 35.8 Causes of Acute Bilateral Ophthalmoplegia*

- AIDS encephalopathy
- Basilar meningitis, hypertrophic cranial pachymeningitis, or neoplastic infiltration[†]
- Botulism
- Brainstem encephalitis[†]
- Brainstem stroke[†]
- Carotid-cavernous or dural shunt fistula[†]
- Cavernous sinus thrombosis (febrile, ill)[†]
- Central herniation syndrome
- Ciguatera poisoning
- Diphtheria
- HMG-CoA reductase inhibitors* (may be transient, may be associated with anti-AChR antibodies) (Negvesky et al., 2000; personal observation, 2002)
- Intoxication (sedatives, tricyclics, organophosphates, anticonvulsants—consciousness impaired)
- Leigh disease (subacute necrotizing encephalomyelitis)
- Fisher syndrome (Miller Fisher syndrome) with or without ataxia (Lee et al., 2008)
- MS
- Myasthenia
- Neuroleptic malignant syndrome (personal observation)
- Orbital pseudotumor[†]
- Paraneoplastic encephalomyelitis
- Pituitary apoplexy[†]
- Polyradiculopathy (associated with)
- PERM, a variant of stiff person syndrome (Hutchinson et al., 2008)
- Psychogenic
- Stiff person syndrome
- Thallium poisoning
- Tick paralysis
- Tolosa-Hunt syndrome[†]
- Trauma (impaired consciousness, signs of injury)[†]
- Wernicke encephalopathy

AChR, Acetylcholine receptor; *AIDS,* acquired immunodeficiency syndrome; *MS,* multiple sclerosis; *PERM,* progressive encephalomyelitis with rigidity and myoclonus.

*All may be unilateral.

[†]Pain may be present. Painful ophthalmoplegia is discussed in Chapter 70.

Box 35.9 Causes of Chronic Ophthalmoplegia

- Brainstem neoplasm
- Chronic basal meningitis (infection, sarcoid, or carcinoma)
- Chronic ophthalmoplegia with anti-GQ1b antibody*
- Congenital extraocular muscle fibrosis
- Dysthyroidism
- Leigh disease
- MS
- MG
- Myopathies (e.g., mitochondrial, fiber-type disproportion [see **Table 35.6**])
- Nuclear, paranuclear, and supranuclear gaze palsies (see **Table 35.6**)
- Vitamin E deficiency

---

*From Reddell, S.W., Barnett, M.H., Yan, W.X., et al., 2000. Chronic ophthalmoplegia with anti-GQ1b antibody. Neurology 54, 1000-1002.
MG, myasthenia gravis; *MS,* multiple sclerosis.

Botulinum toxin is used with mixed success in patients with both comitant and noncomitant strabismus. It may be helpful in patients with acute abducens palsies, particularly if bilateral and traumatic in origin. Extraocular muscle surgery can correct long-standing strabismus (comitant or noncomitant). Finally, orthoptic exercises are of use in patients with convergence insufficiency.

Related Disorders

Asthenopia (the visual equivalent of neurasthenia) is characterized by symptoms and signs such as episodic blurring, watering, itching, diplopia, eyestrain, tiredness of the eyes or lids (especially after reading), sleepiness, and photophobia. Patients with this condition often manifest exaggerated reactions to normal phenomena such as physiological diplopia, floaters, persistence of afterimages, and difficulty reading fine print. Their symptoms may be associated with accommodative insufficiency, headache, and other asthenic complaints. Care must be taken to exclude true refractive errors, anisometropia, defective accommodation, convergence insufficiency, medication effects, dry eye syndrome, diabetes mellitus, and incorrectly made spectacles. Although asthenopia usually is psychogenic, a cause for isolated accommodative insufficiency (e.g., parieto-occipital stroke) may be found. Management includes a thorough examination, recognition of real abnormalities, and confident and authoritative reassurance.

Occasionally after extremely prolonged monotonous visual and vestibular stimulation, as in interstate or highway driving, *"interstate illusions" (highway hallucinosis)* may occur; the environment may appear to be sloping downward when in fact it is flat. This perception is somewhat similar to the prolonged sensation of movement after a long sea voyage (*mal de débarquement*).

Micropsia, defined as the reduction in apparent size of an object of a given retinal angle, is the illusion of objects appearing smaller than normal. It can occur with optical aberrations such as overcorrection of myopia with minus spherical lenses, retinal disorders (e.g., macular edema), and disorders of the parietal region such as stroke or, more commonly, migraine (the so-called "Alice in Wonderland" syndrome). Convergence

Treatment

Patching (occlusive) therapy is used mainly to eliminate one image during the acute phase of diplopia. In children younger than age 6, each eye should be patched alternately to prevent developmental amblyopia. Such young patients should be under the care of an experienced ophthalmologist, with regular follow-up evaluations. Adult patients may wear the patch over whichever eye is more comfortable with patching, although some clinicians feel that alternating the patch reduces the incidence of contractures.

Prisms are helpful in eliminating double vision if the deviation is not too great. A reasonable range of binocular single vision may be achieved with prisms, provided the patient's expectations are not too high and there is no significant cyclodeviation.

and accommodation are associated with micropsia to avoid a sense of enlargement as an object gets closer to the eye. Occasionally a disturbance of convergence or accommodation, or both, can induce micropsia.

Monocular elevator deficiency (double elevator palsy) is discussed later.

Oscillopsia, an illusion of movement or oscillation of the environment, occurs with acquired nystagmus, superior oblique myokymia, other ocular oscillations, and disorders of the vestibulo-ocular reflex.

Triplopia, or triple vision, is rare and anatomically so unlikely that it generally is presumed to be psychogenic. However, in a review of findings in 13 patients who described triplopia, 11 had ocular motor abnormalities, including third nerve palsies in 5, sixth nerve palsies in 2, and internuclear ophthalmoplegia in 4 (Keane, 2006). Generally, the patients reported triplopia when looking in the direction of maximal nystagmus or ocular dissociation, probably as a result of oscillopsia. Psychogenic triplopia was uncommon but recognized by persistence in all directions of gaze and failure to resolve with the pinhole test.

Polyopia, the perception of multiple images, frequently is optical and can be determined by the pinhole test, discussed earlier under Diplopia. Polyopia also may be caused by cortical lesions (see **Box 35.4**).

Palinopsia (or palinopia), the pathological persistence or recurrence of visual images after the stimulus has been removed, may cause cerebral diplopia or polyopia. The images become more apparent and numerous when the target moves relative to the retina, because it provokes multiple persistent afterimages (**Fig. 35.16**). Sometimes patients describe the visual disturbance as trailing, vibrating, echoing, smearing, or ghosting of images. This visual perseveration occurs more frequently in patients with mild left homonymous visual field defects caused by right parieto-occipital lesions; it may be ictal and respond to anticonvulsant medication. Palinopsia can occur with migraine, metabolic disorders, carbon monoxide poisoning, and a variety of drugs including clomiphene, interleukin 2, lysergic acid diethylamide, mescaline, nefazodone, topiramate, trazodone, and 3,4-methylenedioxymethamphetamine ("Ecstasy"). Palinopsia can occur in patients with ocular or optic nerve disease and in apparently healthy people.

Occasionally it may be associated with auditory perseveration (*palinacusis*) (Pomeranz and Lessell, 2000).

Superior oblique myokymia is a small, rapid, monocular torsional-vertical oscillation (discussed later under Superior Oblique Myokymia).

Tortopia, the illusion of tilting or even inversion of the visual environment for a period of seconds to minutes, may occur in patients with posterior fossa disease, most commonly vertebrobasilar ischemia. Tortopia may be associated with headache, dizziness, vertigo, and double vision and is presumed to be due to dysfunction of the vestibulo-otolithic system or its central connections.

Nystagmus

Nystagmus, which interrupts steady fixation, is an involuntary biphasic rhythmic ocular oscillation in which one or both phases are slow (**Fig. 35.17**). The slow phase of jerk nystagmus is responsible for the initiation and generation of the nystagmus, whereas the fast (saccadic) phase is a corrective movement bringing the fovea back on target. Nystagmus often interferes with vision by blurring the object of regard (poor foveation), or making the environment appear to oscillate (oscillopsia), or both.

For clinical purposes, nystagmus may be divided into pendular and jerk forms. Either form may be horizontal or, less commonly, vertical. Jerk nystagmus is labeled conventionally by the direction of the fast phase and is divided into three types on the basis of the shape of the slow phase tracing on oculographic recordings (see **Fig. 35.17**).

Mechanisms

Nystagmus may result from dysfunction of the vestibular end-organ, vestibular nerve, brainstem, cerebellum, or cerebral centers for ocular pursuit. *Pendular nystagmus* (see **Fig. 35.17, A**) is central (brainstem or cerebellum) in origin, whereas *jerk nystagmus* may be either central or peripheral. Jerk nystagmus with a linear (constant velocity) slow phase (see **Fig. 35.17, B**) is caused by peripheral vestibular dysfunction resulting in an imbalance in vestibular input to the brainstem gaze centers.

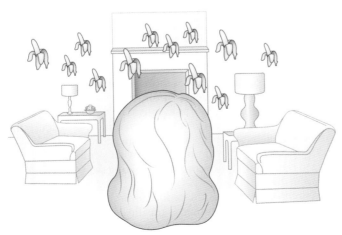

Fig. 35.16 Palinopsia (cerebral polyopia). Visual images experienced by a patient moments after peeling a banana. *(Reprinted with permission from Michel, E.N., Troost, B.T., 1980. Palinopsia: cerebral localization with computed tomography. Neurology 30, 887-889.)*

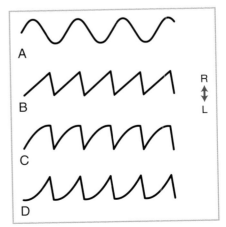

Fig. 35.17 Oculographic diagrams of nystagmus waveforms. **A,** Pendular (sinusoidal) nystagmus. **B,** Left-beating jerk nystagmus with a constant (linear) velocity slow phase. **C,** Left-beating jerk nystagmus with a decreasing (exponential) velocity slow phase. **D,** Left-beating jerk nystagmus with an increasing (exponential) velocity slow phase.

When the slow phase has a decreasing velocity exponential (see **Fig. 35.17, C**), the brainstem neural integrator (NI) is at fault and is said to be "leaky." The integrator is unable to maintain a constant output to the gaze center to hold the eyes in an eccentric position, resulting in gaze-paretic nystagmus. An increasing velocity exponential slow phase (see **Fig. 35.17, D**) in the horizontal plane is central in origin and is the usual form of congenital nystagmus (now termed *infantile nystagmus syndrome*).

Clinical Evaluation

Congenital nystagmus usually is asymptomatic and rarely bothers the patient or causes oscillopsia. The physician should determine whether the nystagmus was present since birth or is acquired and whether there is a family history, a history of amblyopia or lazy eye, and what medications the patient takes. Symptoms such as headache, diplopia, impaired vision, oscillopsia, vertigo, or other neurological abnormalities must be taken into account. Examination should include assessment of visual acuity, confrontation visual fields, ocular motility, pupil reflexes, observing for ocular albinism, and ophthalmoscopy. Ophthalmoscopy may be used to detect subtle nystagmus not apparent to the naked eye. Clinical features that must be determined are listed in **Box 35.10**.

Nystagmus Syndromes

Table 35.3 summarizes the localizing value of nystagmus syndromes and non-nystagmus ocular oscillations.

Box 35.10 Clinical Features to Look for in Patients with Nystagmus

- Are there signs of ocular albinism?
- Is there a spontaneous head tilt or turn?
- Is the nystagmus present in primary position or only with eccentric gaze (gaze-evoked)?
- Is the nystagmus binocular and conjugate, or is it dissociated?
- Is the waveform pendular or jerk? If jerk, what is the direction of the fast phase?
- Is there a latent component (i.e., an increase in nystagmus intensity when one eye is covered)?
- Is there a torsional component?
- Is there spontaneous alteration of direction, as with periodic alternating nystagmus? This entity must be distinguished from rebound nystagmus, for which recognition requires observation over time.
- Is there a null zone (a direction of gaze in which the nystagmus is minimal or absent)?
- Determine whether convergence damps the nystagmus or changes its direction.
- Is the nystagmus altered (accentuated or suppressed) by head positioning or posture or by head shaking (as in spasmus nutans)?
- What is the effect of optokinetic stimulation? In infantile nystagmus syndrome (INS), the response is paradoxical—that is, the fast phase is in the direction of the slow-moving target.
- Are there associated rhythmic movements of other muscle groups (e.g., face, tongue, ears, neck, palate [as in oculopalatal myoclonus/tremor], limbs)?

Congenital Forms of Nystagmus

The three distinct nystagmus syndromes seen in infancy were renamed by the Classification of Eye Movement Abnormalities and Strabismus (CEMAS) Working Group (2003), sponsored by the National Eye Institute. The first of these syndromes, previously known as *congenital nystagmus*, is now called *infantile nystagmus syndrome* (INS); the second, *fusion maldevelopment nystagmus syndrome* (FMNS), includes the latent form and manifest latent nystagmus; and the third, *spasmus nutans syndrome* (SNS), remains virtually unchanged from past classifications.

Infantile nystagmus syndrome usually is present from birth but may not be noticed for the first few weeks, or occasionally even years, of life. It may be accompanied by severe visual impairment but is not the result of poor vision. Disorders that, through genetic association, are responsible for poor vision in patients with INS include those designated by the mnemonic of A's—*a*chiasma (Jansonius et al., 2001), *a*chromatopsia, *a*lbinism (both ocular and oculocutaneous forms), *a*maurotic idiocy of Leber (Leber's congenital amaurosis), *a*niridia, *a*plasia (usually hypoplasia) of the fovea, and *a*plasia (usually hypoplasia) of the optic nerve—and also congenital cataracts and congenital stationary night blindness. Paradoxical pupil constriction in darkness, particularly in patients with poor vision, suggests an associated retinal or optic nerve disorder. High myopia (uncommon early in life) in infants with INS suggests congenital stationary night blindness, and high hyperopia suggests Leber congenital amaurosis; such retinal disorders can be confirmed by electroretinography. INS sometimes is associated with head titubation (head nodding). INS may be familial and is inherited in an autosomal recessive, X-linked dominant or recessive pattern. Genetic defects identified in some families include a dominant form of INS linked to chromosomal region 6p12 (Kerrison et al., 1998), an X-linked form of INS with incomplete penetrance among female carriers associated with a defect on the long arm of the X chromosome (Kerrison et al., 2001), a deletion in the OA1 gene (ocular albinism) in a family with X-linked INS associated with macular hypoplasia and ocular albinism (Preising et al., 2001), and three mutations in the OA1 gene in families with hereditary nystagmus and ocular albinism (Faugere et al., 2003). Self and Lotery (2007) recently reviewed the molecular genetics of INS.

INS appears horizontal in most patients and may be either pendular or jerk in primary position. Pendular nystagmus often becomes jerk on lateral gaze. The horizontal oscillations may be accentuated during vertical tracking. Oculography with three-dimensional scleral search coils demonstrates that many patients with INS have a torsional component phase-locked with the horizontal component (Averbuch-Heller et al., 2002).

Patients with INS often have good vision unless an associated afferent defect is present (see earlier discussion). In INS, the nystagmus damps with convergence; latent superimposition (an increase in nystagmus amplitude occurring when one eye is covered) may be present. A null zone wherein the nystagmus intensity is minimal may be found; if this zone is to one side, the affected person turns the head to improve vision. The head often "oscillates" as well. Both features—damping of nystagmus with convergence and a null zone—can be used in therapy by changing the direction of gaze with prisms or extraocular muscle surgery to improve head posture and visual acuity. Oculographic recordings usually demonstrate

Table 35.3 Localizing Value of Nystagmus Syndromes and Non-Nystagmus Ocular Oscillations

Nystagmus Syndrome	Localization
Downbeat nystagmus	Bilateral cervicomedullary junction (flocculus) Floor of the fourth ventricle
PAN	Cervicomedullary junction (nodulus)
Upbeat nystagmus	Bilateral pontomesencephalic junction Bilateral pontomedullary junction Cerebellar vermis
Pendular nystagmus	Paramedian pons Deep cerebellar (fastigial) nuclei
SSN: Hemi-jerk SSN	Mesodiencephalic junction, chiasm, disorders that disrupt central vision Unilateral mesodiencephalic lesions: upper poles of the eyes jerk toward side of the lesion, and vertical component is always disjunctive (eyes oscillate in opposite directions, with the intorting eye rising and the extorting eye falling) Lateral medullary lesions: upper poles of the eyes jerk away from the side of lesion; but the vertical component may be either conjugate, usually upward, or disjunctive
Alternating hemi-SSN with direction	Middle cerebellar peduncle of vertical pursuit
Rebound nystagmus	Cerebellum
Brun nystagmus	Cerebellopontine angle, AICA territory stroke
Torsional nystagmus, jerk	Central vestibular system
Torsional nystagmus, pendular	Medulla

Atypical INS:
  Asymmetrical horizontal
  Vertical (pendular, downbeat, or upbeat)
	Ocular albinism
	Retina: congenital cone dysfunction, congenital stationary night blindness

Non-nystagmus Ocular Oscillations	**Localization**
Convergence-retraction "nystagmus"	Dorsal midbrain
Opsoclonus	Cerebellar fastigial nuclei or brainstem
Ocular flutter	Deep cerebellum nuclei or brainstem
Ocular dysmetria	Cerebellum (dorsal vermis and fastigial nuclei)
Ocular myoclonus (oculopalatal)	Guillain-Mollaret triangle (central tegmental tract in the pons)
Ocular bobbing	See **Table 35.4**
Square-wave jerks	See **Table 35.7**
Square-wave pulses	Cerebellar outflow tracts (may be associated with rubral tremor)

AICA, Anterior inferior cerebellar artery; *INS*, infantile nystagmus syndrome; *PAN*, periodic alternating nystagmus; *SSN*, seesaw nystagmus.

either a sinusoidal (see **Fig. 35.17, A**) or a slow phase with an increasing exponential waveform (see **Fig. 35.17, D**). However, in the first few months of life, the waveform of INS may be more variable, evolving into the more classic pattern as the child gets older.

Outside the null zone, the nystagmus follows the Alexander law and increases in intensity (amplitude × frequency) on lateral gaze. Thus patients with INS or FMNS may induce an esotropia intentionally to suppress the nystagmus in the adducting eye. This strategy is called the *nystagmus blockage syndrome.*

Patients with INS do not experience oscillopsia (an illusory oscillation of the environment) unless a head injury, decompensated strabismus, or retinal degeneration causes a decline in vision, ocular motor function, or both. Prisms or strabismus surgery may correct such late-onset oscillopsia (Hertle et al., 2001a). Approximately 30% of patients with INS have strabismus (Leigh and Zee, 2006).

Rarely in INS, the nystagmus may be in the vertical plane or circumductory, in which the eyes move conjugately in a circular or cycloid pattern. In patients with retinal disorders

such as achromatopsia, congenital cone dysfunction, or congenital stationary night blindness, INS can have an asymmetrical horizontal (albinism) or vertical waveform that varies among pendular, downbeat, and upbeat (Shawkat et al., 2000). Occasionally INS may be unilateral, occur later in the teens or adult life, or become symptomatic if changes in the internal or external environment alter foveation stability and duration, causing oscillopsia. Less common patterns of INS such as periodic alternating, upbeat, downbeat, and seesaw nystagmus (SSN) are discussed later.

Fusion maldevelopment nystagmus syndrome, as noted earlier, includes both LN and manifest latent nystagmus (MLN). LN occurs with monocular fixation, that is, when one eye is covered. The slow phase is directed toward the covered eye. The amplitude of the oscillations increases on abduction of the fixating eye. With MLN, the oscillations are present with both eyes open, but only one eye is fixating, vision in the other is ignored or suppressed as a result of strabismus or amblyopia. The nystagmus waveform has a linear (decreasing velocity) slow phase (see **Fig. 35.17**), which differs from that of true INS. Some patients with LN can suppress it at will.

The pathogenesis of LN may be related to impaired development of binocular vision mechanisms. Under monocular viewing conditions, rhesus monkeys deprived of binocular vision early in life have poor nasal-to-temporal optokinetic responses. The pretectal nucleus of the optic tract (NOT) is necessary for generation of slow-phase eye movements in response to horizontal full-field visual motion. In normal monkeys, the NOT on each side is driven binocularly and responds well to visual stimuli presented to either eye. In monkeys with LN, each NOT is driven mainly by the contralateral eye. Thus in the altered monkeys, when only one eye is viewing, one optic tract nucleus is stimulated, causing an imbalance between each NOT. This imbalance is believed to be responsible for LN (Kaminski and Leigh, 1997). Of interest, under monocular viewing conditions, patients with congenital esotropia have poor temporal-to-nasal pursuit, and some have LN or MLN. Indeed, in esotropic patients, LN may be unmasked in dim light or by shining a bright light at the dominant eye, as when testing pupil reflexes.

Spasmus nutans syndrome is a transient, high-frequency, low-amplitude pendular nystagmus with onset between the ages of 6 and 12 months that lasts approximately 2 years but occasionally can be as long as 5 years. The direction of the oscillations may be horizontal, vertical, or torsional; the oscillations often are dysconjugate, asymmetrical, even monocular, and variable. SNS may be associated with torticollis and head titubation, and these three features constitute the *spasmus nutans triad*. The titubation has a lower frequency than that of the nystagmus and thus is not compensatory. Patients can improve vision by vigorously shaking the head, presumably to stimulate the vestibulo-ocular reflex and suppress or override the ocular oscillations. Some patients may have esotropia. Clinically, spasmus nutans is distinguished from INS and FMNS by its intermittency, high frequency, vertical component, and dysconjugacy (Leigh and Zee, 2006).

Although spasmus nutans is a benign and transient disorder, it must be distinguished from acquired nystagmus caused by structural lesions involving the anterior visual pathways in approximately 2% of patients. In the latter situation, a careful ophthalmological examination reveals clinical evidence such as impaired vision, a relative afferent pupillary defect, or optic atrophy. Also, retinal disorders may masquerade as spasmus nutans; paradoxical pupil constriction in darkness is suggestive, but an electroretinogram is confirmatory. Kim and associates (2003) reported spasmus nutans in a patient with congenital ocular motor apraxia and cerebellar vermian hypoplasia.

Nystagmus Blockage Syndrome

The nystagmus blockage syndrome is a poorly understood condition in which some patients with INS, or the latent form of FMNS "purposely" induce an esotropia to suppress the nystagmus; this results in a head turn in the direction of the fixating (adducted) eye. An abducting jerk nystagmus reappears with attempted abduction of either eye. In some patients it is believed excessive convergence blocks the nystagmus, in others the waveform of INS converts to MLN (Dell'Osso and Daroff, 1999a). The differential diagnosis includes crossed fixation (the Ciancia syndrome), bilateral sixth nerve paralysis, and Duane's syndrome. The treatment is corrective extraocular muscle surgery.

Pendular Nystagmus

Pendular nystagmus (see **Fig. 35.17, A**) has a sinusoidal waveform and usually is horizontal. It may be either congenital or acquired. Large-amplitude ("searching") pendular nystagmus usually is associated with poor vision as a result of afferent disorders such as optic neuropathy, which can be unilateral, and retinal disorders (see INS). Acquired pendular nystagmus (APN) typically has horizontal, vertical, and torsional components, although one may be dominant. The oscillations of each eye may be so different that the nystagmus may appear monocular clinically (Leigh and Zee, 2006). The most common cause of APN is multiple sclerosis (MS), followed by brainstem vascular disease; MS patients frequently have optic neuropathy that usually is worse in the eye with the larger oscillations. Other disorders of myelin, including Cockayne syndrome, Pelizaeus-Merzbacher disease, peroxisomal disorders, disorders associated with toluene abuse, as well as spinocerebellar disease, hypoxic encephalopathy, and Whipple disease, can cause pendular nystagmus.

Pendular nystagmus probably results from disruption of normal feedback from cerebellar nuclei to the NI (Das et al., 2000). This is in keeping with the predominance of paramedian pontine lesions on magnetic resonance imaging (MRI) in patients with horizontal pendular nystagmus (Lopez et al., 1995, 1996) and with the predominance of medullary lesions in those with torsional pendular nystagmus. The rhythmic pendular oscillations may be the result of deafferentation of the inferior olive by lesions involving the central tegmental tracts, medial vestibular nuclei, or paramedian tracts, causing instability in the system. Disruption of prenuclear ocular motor pathways necessary for orthotropia (and conjugacy) may be a factor as well. A similar mechanism may be responsible for oculopalatal myoclonus (discussed later in this section).

Pendular vergence nystagmus, previously called *convergent-divergent nystagmus*, a rare variant of acquired pendular nystagmus, is dysconjugate and occurs in patients with MS, brainstem stroke, Chiari malformations, cerebral Whipple disease (see Oculomasticatory Myorhythmia), occasionally palated myoclonus, and progressive ataxia (Averbuch-Heller et al., 1995). The eyes oscillate, mainly horizontally, in opposite directions simultaneously, although they sometimes form circular, elliptical, or oblique trajectories, depending on the phase relationship of the horizontal, vertical, and torsional vectors responsible for the oscillations.

Cyclovergent nystagmus (i.e., dysconjugate torsional nystagmus in which the upper poles of the eyes oscillate in opposite directions) was detected by scleral search coil oculography in a patient with progressive ataxia and palatal myoclonus (Averbuch-Heller et al., 1995). On rare occasions, cyclovergent nystagmus may be observed clinically.

Vertical pendular nystagmus closely resembles the vertical ocular oscillation associated with palatal myoclonus (the oculopalatal syndrome) (Dell'Osso and Daroff, 1999a) and may be a form of the same disorder, which also results from lesions of the deep cerebellar nuclei and their connections.

Elliptical pendular nystagmus, with a larger vertical component and superimposed or interposed upbeat nystagmus, is characteristic of Pelizaeus-Merzbacher disease. This nystagmus can be difficult to discern with the naked eye. It is seen more easily with an ophthalmoscope, but oculography using scleral search coils may be necessary to detect it (Dell'Osso and Daroff, 1999b).

Oculomasticatory Myorhythmia

Oculomasticatory myorhythmia, described in patients with Whipple disease and, to date, pathognomonic of that disorder, consists of continuous rhythmic jaw contractions synchronous with dissociated pendular vergence oscillations. It may be associated with supranuclear vertical gaze palsy, altered mentation, somnolence, mild uveitis, or retinopathy (Knox et al., 1995). Myorhythmia of the face and arms is described in Hashimoto encephalopathy (Erickson et al., 2002).

Gaze-Paretic Nystagmus

Gaze-paretic nystagmus, the most common type of nystagmus, usually is symmetrical and evoked by eccentric gaze to either side but is absent in the primary position. Frequently it is present on eccentric vertical gaze, with upward-beating nystagmus on upgaze and downward-beating nystagmus on downgaze. It may be asymmetrical with asymmetrical central nervous system (CNS) disease or with disorders such as myasthenia. It has a jerk waveform, with the fast phase in the direction of gaze. Oculographic recordings show a decreasing exponential slow phase (see **Fig. 35.17, C**). Gaze-paretic nystagmus results from dysfunction of the NI and commonly is caused by alcohol or drug intoxication (by anticonvulsants and tranquilizers). When it is caused by structural disease, it tends to be asymmetrical.

Vestibular Nystagmus

Vestibular nystagmus results from damage to the labyrinth, vestibular nerve, vestibular nuclei, or their connections in the brainstem or cerebellum. Vestibular nystagmus may be divided into central and peripheral forms on the basis of the associated features outlined in Chapter 37. Peripheral vestibular nystagmus, caused by dysfunction of the vestibular end organ or nerve, has a linear slow phase (see **Fig. 35.17, B**), whereas with central lesions, the slow phase may be variable. Usually, peripheral vestibular nystagmus is associated with severe vegetative symptoms and signs including nausea, vomiting, perspiration, and diarrhea; it also may be associated with hearing loss and tinnitus. With central vestibular nystagmus, vegetative symptoms are less severe, but other neurological features may be present, such as headache, ataxia, dysconjugate gaze, and pyramidal tract signs (see Chapter 19).

Caloric-Induced Nystagmus

Caloric-induced nystagmus is discussed in Chapter 37.

Physiological Nystagmus

Physiological (endpoint) nystagmus is a jerk nystagmus observed on extreme lateral or upward gaze. If the bridge of the nose obstructs the view of the adducting eye, physiological nystagmus may be dysconjugate because the amplitude is greater in the abducting eye. A torsional component is sometimes seen. Physiological nystagmus is distinguished from pathological nystagmus by its symmetry on right and left gaze and by the absence of other neurological features. It is not present when the angle of gaze is less than 30 degrees from primary position. Oculographic recordings primarily demonstrate a linear slow phase (see **Fig. 35.17, B**) and may detect transient small-amplitude rebound nystagmus.

Box 35.11 **Causes of Monocular Nystagmus**

- Acquired monocular blindness (nystagmus in blind eye)
- Alternating hemiplegia of childhood
- Amblyopia
- Brainstem infarction (thalamus and upper midbrain)
- Ictal nystagmus
- Internuclear and pseudointernuclear ophthalmoplegia
- Multiple sclerosis
- Nystagmus with monocular ophthalmoplegia
- Nystagmus with one eye absent
- Pseudonystagmus (lid fasciculations)
- Spasmus nutans
- Superior oblique myokymia

Dysconjugate Nystagmus

Dysconjugate (dissociated) nystagmus occurs when the ocular oscillations are out of phase (in different directions). It is seen with internuclear ophthalmoplegia, other brainstem lesions (see earlier discussion of pendular vergence nystagmus under Pendular Nystagmus), and spasmus nutans. Monocular nystagmus also is dysconjugate and may be associated with amblyopia and other forms of vision loss (**Box 35.11**).

Monocular Nystagmus

Monocular nystagmus may be pendular or jerk and also may be horizontal, vertical, or oblique. Oculographic recordings may reveal small-amplitude oscillations in the fellow eye. Monocular nystagmus may occur in patients with *alternating hemiplegia of childhood* (Egan, 2002), amblyopia, strabismus, monocular blindness, spasmus nutans, internuclear ophthalmoplegia, MS, or (rarely) seizures (Grant et al., 2002), and of course when the other eye is completely ophthalmoplegic or absent.

The *Heimann-Bielschowsky phenomenon* is a rare form of monocular vertical pendular oscillation, with a frequency of 1 to 5 Hz, that occurs in an amblyopic eye or after acquired monocular vision loss, such as with cataract. In the latter situation, it may be reversible after successful treatment of the underlying condition or with gabapentin (Rahman et al., 2006).

Superior oblique myokymia may be mistaken for a monocular torsional or vertical nystagmus (see **Box 35.11**).

Upbeat Nystagmus

Upbeat nystagmus is a spontaneous jerk nystagmus with the fast phase upward while the eyes are in primary position (Hirose et al., 1998). It is attributed to interruption of the anterior semicircular canal projections, which are responsible for the upward vestibulo-ocular reflex, causing downward drift of the eyes with corrective upward saccades. The amplitude and intensity of the nystagmus usually increase on upgaze. This finding strongly suggests bilateral paramedian lesions of the brainstem, usually at the pontomedullary or pontomesencephalic junction, the paramedian tract neurons in the lower medulla, or midline cerebellum (vermis). Rarely, upbeat nystagmus may be congenital, or it may result from Wernicke encephalopathy or intoxication with

Table 35.4   Treatment of Nystagmus and Non-Nystagmus Oscillations*

Nystagmus Syndrome	Treatment

Infantile nystagmus syndrome	Prisms
	Contact lenses
	Extraocular muscle surgery
	  Kestenbaum-Anderson procedure
	  Tenotomy (experimental)
	Acetazolamide (Thurtell et al., 2010)
	  Gabapentin (Shery et al., 2006)
	  Gene therapy (experimental) when the nystagmus is associated with retinal disorders
	  (Leigh and Zee, 2006)

APN	Trihexyphenidyl, benztropine, clonazepam, gabapentin, isoniazid, memantine[†] (Leigh and Zee, 2006), valproate, diethylpropion hydrochloride, tenotomy followed by memantine (Tomsak et al., 2006)
Convergence-evoked horizontal	Base-in prisms nystagmus
Downbeat nystagmus	Base-out prisms (if nystagmus damps with convergence) Base-down prisms over both eyes if intensity of nystagmus diminishes in upgaze Baclofen, clonazepam, gabapentin, scopolamine, 4-aminopyridine, 3,4-diaminopyridine

PAN:
  Congenital
  Acquired
	
	Dextroamphetamine, baclofen (occasionally), 5-HT
	Baclofen, phenytoin, memantine

Upbeat nystagmus	Base-up prisms over both eyes if intensity of nystagmus diminishes in downgaze Baclofen gabapentin, 4-aminopyridine, memantine (Thurtell et al., 2010), thiamine
Ocular myoclonus	Chronically patch one eye Baclofen, carbamazepine, cerulein, clonazepam, memantine, gabapentin, scopolamine, trihexyphenidyl, valproate
SSN	Baclofen, clonazepam, gabapentin or memantine (Huppert et al., 2011), base-out prisms
Hemi-SSN	Memantine (Thurtell et al., 2010)
Ictal nystagmus	AEDs

Episodic nystagmus:
  Episodic ataxia-1
  Episodic ataxia-2
	
	Acetazolamide
	Acetazolamide, 4-aminopyridine (Strupp et al., 2011)

Oculomasticatory myorhythmia	Antibiotics for Whipple disease; consider gabapentin or memantine
Torsional nystagmus	Memantine (Thurtell et al., 2010)

Non-Nystagmus Ocular Oscillations	Treatment
Opsoclonus	Treat underlying condition when possible, ACTH, vitamin B1, clonazepam, gabapentin, ondansetron, steroids; if paraneoplastic, protein A immunoabsorption
Superior oblique myokymia	Carbamazepine, gabapentin, oxcarbazepine, other AEDs, topical beta-blockers, memantine, base-down prism over the affected eye, muscle/tendon surgery, microvascular decompression
Ocular neuromyotonia	Carbamazepine
Microflutter	Propranolol, verapamil
Saccadic intrusions	Memantine (Serra et al., 2008)
Square-wave jerks	Valproate (Traccis et al., 1997), amphetamines, barbiturates, diazepam, clonazepam, memantine (Leigh and Zee, 2006)
Square-wave oscillations	Valproate (Traccis et al., 1997)

ACTH, Adrenocorticotropic hormone; *AEDs*, antiepileptic drugs; *5-HT*, 5-hydroxytryptamine; *APN*, acquired pendular nystagmus; *PAN*, periodic alternating nystagmus; *SSN*, seesaw nystagmus.

*Treat underlying cause when possible.

[†]Memantine is reported to exacerbate MS (Villoslada el al., 2009).

anticonvulsants, organophosphates, lithium, nicotine, or thallium (author's personal observation). In infants, upbeat nystagmus may be a sign of anterior visual pathway disease, such as Leber congenital amaurosis (see Chapter 36), optic nerve hypoplasia, aniridia, or cataracts. Small-amplitude upbeat nystagmus may be seen in persons who are carriers of blue-cone monochromatism, whereas affected patients may have intermittent pendular oblique nystagmus. If the intensity of upbeat nystagmus diminishes in downgaze, base-up prisms over both eyes may improve the oscillopsia; gabapentin also may be helpful (**Table 35.4**). For an extensive list of causes of upbeat nystagmus, see Leigh and Zee's textbook (2006).

Downbeat Nystagmus

Downbeat nystagmus is a spontaneous downward-beating jerk nystagmus present in primary position and is attributed to either (1) interruption of the posterior semicircular canal projections, which are responsible for the downward vestibulo-ocular reflex (VOR), causing upward drift of the eyes with corrective downward saccades, or (2) impaired cerebellar inhibition of the vestibular circuits for upward eye movements, resulting in uninhibited upward drifting of the eyes, with corrective downward saccades. The amplitude of the oscillations increases when the eyes are deviated laterally and slightly downward (the Daroff sign).

Downbeat nystagmus may be apparent only with changes in posture (positional downbeat nystagmus), particularly the head-hanging position. Downbeat nystagmus results from either damage to the commissural fibers between the vestibular nuclei in the floor of the fourth ventricle or bilateral damage to the flocculus that disinhibits the VOR in pitch; frequently it occurs with structural lesions at the craniocervical junction (**Box 35.12**). A thorough investigation for such should be made. MRI of the foramen magnum region (in the sagittal plane) is the investigation of choice. Olson and Jacobson suggested that in some cases of unexplained downbeat nystagmus, the cause is a radiographically occult infarction (2001); however, lesions that cause downbeat nystagmus are bilateral (Brandt and Dietrich, 1995). Causes of downbeat nystagmus are listed in **Box 35.12**.

The treatment of downbeat nystagmus involves correction of the underlying cause when possible. When downbeat nystagmus damps on convergence, it may be treated successfully with base-out prisms, reducing the oscillopsia and improving the visual acuity. Baclofen, clonazepam, or 4-aminopyridine may also help (see **Table 35.4**); 4-aminopyridine is more effective in downbeat nystagmus associated with cerebellar atrophy rather than structural lesions (Huppert et al., 2011).

Both upbeat and downbeat nystagmus may be altered in amplitude and direction by a variety of maneuvers (e.g., convergence, head tilting, changes in posture) and by 3,4-diaminopyridine (Leigh and Zee, 2006).

Periodic Alternating Nystagmus

Periodic alternating nystagmus (PAN) is a horizontal jerk nystagmus in which the fast phase beats in one direction and then damps or stops for a few seconds before changing direction to the opposite side every 30 to 180 seconds. During the short transition period, vertical nystagmus or square wave jerks may occur. PAN has the same clinical significance as downbeat nystagmus, and the two entities sometimes coexist. Attention should be focused at the craniocervical junction. PAN also may occur in Creutzfeldt-Jakob disease.

When PAN is congenital, it may be associated with albinism. In one series of patients with congenital PAN, none had pure vertical oscillations, even during the transition period (Gradstein et al., 1997). Although not all patients with acquired PAN have vertical nystagmus during the transition period, its presence may distinguish acquired from congenital PAN (personal observation); this finding does not obviate further evaluation when appropriate. Transient episodes of PAN were provoked by attacks of Ménière disease in a patient with a hypoplastic cerebellum and an enlarged cisterna magna (Chiu

Box 35.12 Causes of Downbeat Nystagmus

- Congenital (rare)
- Transiently in normal neonates
- Craniocervical junction abnormalities:
  - Basilar invagination (e.g., Paget disease)
  - Chiari malformations
  - Dolichoectasia of the vertebrobasilar arterial system
  - Foramen magnum tumors
  - Syringobulbia
- Cerebellar disorders:
  - Alcoholic cerebellar degeneration (chronic usage)
  - Anoxic cerebellar degeneration
  - Anti–glutamic acid decarboxylase antibodies (anti-GAD65 antibodies)
  - Familial spinocerebellar degeneration, particularly SCA-6, and with multiple system atrophy (Leigh and Zee, 2006)
  - Episodic ataxia
  - Cerebellar degeneration following human T-lymphotropic virus types I and II (Castillo et al., 2000)
  - Paraneoplastic cerebellar degeneration
  - Heat stroke–induced cerebellar degeneration
- Metabolic disorders (drugs, toxins, and deficiencies):
  - Alcohol intoxication
  - Amiodarone
  - Anticonvulsants
  - Lithium
  - Opioids (Rottach et al., 2002)
  - Toluene abuse
  - Magnesium depletion
  - Wernicke encephalopathy
  - Vitamin B_{12} deficiency
- Other:
  - Benign paroxysmal positional vertigo: positional downbeat nystagmus with anterior canal lesion
  - Brainstem encephalitis
  - Cardiogenic vertigo (Choi et al., 2011)
  - Carriers of blue-cone monochromatism may have small-amplitude downbeat nystagmus.
  - Cephalic tetanus (Orwitz et al., 1997)
  - Hydrocephalus
  - Leukodystrophy
  - Multiple sclerosis
  - Syncope
  - Vertebrobasilar ischemia

and Hain, 2002). Episodic PAN can be a manifestation of a seizure (see later discussion of ictal nystagmus). An atypical form of paroxysmal alternating skew deviation and nystagmus has followed partial destruction of the inferior uvula and adjacent pyramis during biopsy of a suspected brainstem glioma (Radtke et al., 2001).

Lesions of the cerebellar nodulus cause loss of γ-aminobutyric acid (GABA)-mediated inhibition from the Purkinje cells to the vestibular nuclei, impairing the velocity storage mechanism. It is likely that overcompensation in feedback loops causes cyclical firing between reciprocally connected inhibitory neurons and generates the unusual oscillations of acquired PAN. Affected patients have hyperactive vestibular responses and poor vestibular fixation suppression, attributed to involvement of the nodulus and uvula (Leigh and Zee, 2006).

Treatment of PAN should be directed at correcting the cause, such as a Chiari malformation, when possible. Baclofen, a GABA-b agonist, replaces the missing inhibition and usually is effective in the acquired form of the disease and occasionally in the congenital form. Dextroamphetamine resulted in clinical improvement in a patient with PAN who also had rod-cone dystrophy and strabismus (Hertle et al., 2001b).

Rebound Nystagmus

Rebound nystagmus is a horizontal gaze–evoked nystagmus in which the direction of the fast phase reverses with sustained lateral gaze or beats transiently in the opposite direction when the eyes return to primary position (Video 35.3, available at www.expertconsult.com). The latter is occasionally a physiological finding and caused by dysfunction of the cerebellum or the perihypoglossal nuclei in the medulla. Occasionally, rebound nystagmus may be torsional.

Centripetal Nystagmus

Cerebellar dysfunction can cause a form of gaze-evoked nystagmus in which the fast phase beats toward primary position (i.e., centripetally) and the slow phase drifts peripherally toward an eccentric target. Centripetal nystagmus is similar to rebound nystagmus and may result from overcompensation by the cerebellar nodulus and uvula to adjust for a directional bias by temporarily moving the null zone during eccentric gaze. Centripetal nystagmus in both the horizontal and vertical planes may be associated with Creutzfeldt-Jakob disease.

Convergence-Evoked Nystagmus

Convergence-evoked nystagmus is an unusual ocular oscillation, usually pendular, induced by voluntary convergence (see earlier discussion of pendular vergence nystagmus under Pendular Nystagmus). The movements may be conjugate or dissociated. This condition may be congenital or acquired, such as in patients with MS. A jerk form occurs with Chiari type I malformations. Convergence-evoked vertical nystagmus (upbeat more common than downbeat) also occurs. Convergence-evoked nystagmus should be distinguished from voluntary nystagmus and from convergence retraction nystagmus (see Saccadic Intrusions and Other Non-Nystagmus Ocular Oscillations, later).

Seesaw Nystagmus

Seesaw nystagmus is a spectacular ocular oscillation in which one eye rises and intorts as the other eye falls and extorts. The waveform appears pendular. The oscillations usually become faster and smaller on upgaze but slower and larger on downgaze; they may cease in darkness. Disordered control of the normal ocular counter-rolling reflex may be responsible. Bitemporal hemianopia, caused by acquired chiasmal defects or impaired central vision, plays a significant role in generating SSN. Disruption of retinal error signals necessary for VOR adaptation, which normally are conveyed to the inferior olive by the chiasmal crossing fibers, results in an unstable visuovestibular environment. Fixation and pursuit feedback accentuate

this instability, causing synchronous oscillations of floccular Purkinje cells, which relay to the nodulus, resulting in SSN. This mechanism also may be the basis for the ocular oscillations of oculopalatal myoclonus. The observations of SSN and INS in achiasmatic humans and achiasmatic Belgian sheepdogs support this hypothesis (Dell'Osso and Daroff, 1998). Significantly, the onset of both SSN and oculopalatal myoclonus may be delayed after CNS lesions.

SSN occurs with lesions in the region of the mesodiencephalic junction, particularly the zona incerta and the interstitial nucleus of Cajal. Congenital SSN may be associated with a superimposed horizontal pendular nystagmus; some patients with congenital SSN may be achiasmatic or have septo-optic dysplasia. Acquired SSN may be associated with suprasellar tumors, Joubert syndrome, and Leigh disease, particularly the jerk form described later. Acquired pendular SSN may be accompanied by a bitemporal hemianopia from trauma or an expanding lesion in the third ventricular region, or by severe loss of central vision due to disorders such as choroiditis, cone-rod dystrophy, whole-brain radiation and intrathecal methotrexate, and vitreous hemorrhage (Dell'Osso and Daroff, 1998). Transient (latent) SSN may occur for a few seconds after a blink, perhaps because of loss of fixation, in patients with chiasmal region lesions. If SSN damps with convergence, base-out prisms may be helpful. Baclofen also may be beneficial in SSN.

Reverse congenital seesaw nystagmus is a rare condition in which the rising eye extorts as the falling eye intorts.

A jerk waveform hemi-SSN occurs with unilateral mesodiencephalic lesions, presumably as a result of selective unilateral inactivation of the torsional eye-velocity integrator in the interstitial nucleus of Cajal. During the fast (jerk) phases, the upper poles of the eyes rotate toward the side of the lesion. In hemi-jerk SSN caused by lateral medullary lesions, the fast phases jerk away from the side of the lesion. In both situations, the torsional component is always conjugate. With mesodiencephalic lesions, the vertical component is always disjunctive (the eyes oscillate in opposite directions, with the intorting eye rising and the extorting eye falling), but with medullary lesions it may be either conjugate (usually upward) or disjunctive. Other features of brainstem dysfunction may be necessary to localize the lesion.

Torsional (Rotary) Nystagmus

In torsional nystagmus (TN), the eye oscillates in a pure rotary or plane. TN may be present in primary position or with either head positioning or gaze deviation. Usually it results from lesions in the central vestibular pathways. Pure TN occurs only with central vestibular dysfunction, whereas mixed torsional-linear nystagmus may occur with peripheral vestibular disease. When the waveform of TN is pendular (i.e., torsional pendular nystagmus), the lesion usually is in the medulla (Lopez et al., 1995). Skew deviation frequently coexists with TN.

In patients with lesions of the middle cerebellar peduncle, TN with a jerk waveform—similar to jerk SSN—may be evoked by vertical pursuit eye movement and during fixation suppression of the vertical VOR. The direction of the fast phase changes with pursuit direction; it usually is toward the side of the lesion on downward pursuit and away from the side of the lesion on upward pursuit (FitzGibbon et al., 1996).

Ictal Nystagmus

Ictal nystagmus often accompanies adversive seizures and beats to the side opposite the focus. Ictal nystagmus may be associated with transient pupillary dilation of either the abducting or adducting eye (Masjuan et al., 1997). Pupillary oscillations synchronous with the nystagmus may occur rarely. Ictal nystagmus associated with unformed visual hallucinations, homonymous hemianopia, and unusual MRI findings occurs in patients with non-ketotic hyperglycemia (Lavin 2005). Nystagmus as the only motor manifestation of a seizure is rare; however, there are reports of isolated ictal nystagmus, such as occurs in patients with vivid ictal visual hallucinations. Monocular nystagmus associated with ipsilateral hemianopic visual hallucinations in a binocular patient can occur as the only manifestation of a partial seizure caused by a focal discharge in the contralateral medial occipital lobe (Grant et al., 2002). It is difficult to draw any conclusion clinically regarding the location of the seizure discharge in these patients, because seizure foci were found in occipital, parietal, temporal, and frontal areas. Usually the nystagmus is horizontal, but vertical nystagmus, mainly in comatose patients, was reported on occasion. In comatose patients, periodic eye movements should alert the physician to the possibility of status epilepticus; indeed, PAN associated with periodic alternating gaze deviation and periodic alternating head rotation may be a manifestation of a seizure (Moster and Schnayder, 1998). The monocular abducting nystagmus seen in alternating hemiplegia of childhood is likely ictal in origin.

Brun Nystagmus

Brun nystagmus occurs in patients with large cerebellopontine angle tumors. The nystagmus is bilateral but asymmetrical, with a jerk waveform. It is characterized by large-amplitude, low-frequency fast phases on gaze toward the side of the lesion but small-amplitude, high-frequency fast phases on gaze to the other side. The ipsilateral large-amplitude (coarse) nystagmus has an exponentially decreasing velocity slow phase attributed to compression of the brainstem NI, which includes the ipsilateral medial vestibular nucleus. The contralateral small-amplitude, high-frequency nystagmus has a linear slow phase attributed to ipsilateral vestibular dysfunction (see **Fig. 35.17**). Occasionally an anterior inferior cerebellar artery territory stroke can cause Brun nystagmus (personal observation).

Episodic Nystagmus (Periodic Nystagmus)

Episodic nystagmus is associated with disorders in which the patient has paroxysmal episodes of vertigo, ataxia, and nystagmus lasting up to 24 hours. The nystagmus may be torsional, vertical, or dissociated. The frequency of attacks varies, ranging from once a day to only a few times per year. Such periodic ataxias occur in patients with hereditary inborn errors of metabolism, in an autosomal dominant form without any detectable metabolic defect (channelopathy), in some forms of spinocerebellar degeneration, in basilar migraine, and in MS. Acetazolamide or 4-aminopyridine may alleviate or prevent attacks in the familial form (see Chapter 72).

Perverted Nystagmus

Perverted vestibular nystagmus occurs in a plane different from that of the applied vestibular stimulus and is caused by lesions involving central vestibular connections. For example, horizontal head shaking in a patient with MS caused transient downbeat nystagmus (Minagar et al., 2001).

Lid Nystagmus

Lid nystagmus, characterized by rhythmic jerking movements of the upper eyelids, occurs in the following situations: (1) synchronous with vertical ocular nystagmus, (2) synchronous with the fast phase of gaze-evoked horizontal nystagmus in some patients with the lateral medullary syndrome, (3) evoked by horizontal gaze in some patients with midbrain tumors that injure the M-group of neurons adjacent to the riMLF, and (4) during voluntary convergence (the Pick sign) in some patients with medullary or cerebellar disease (Dell'Osso and Daroff, 1999a; Leigh and Zee, 2006).

Optokinetic Nystagmus

True optokinetic nystagmus (OKN) is a rhythmic involuntary conjugate ocular oscillation provoked by a compelling full visual field stimulus, such as that produced by rotating an image of the environment around the patient or by turning the patient in a revolving chair. The oscillations are biphasic, and the nystagmus consists of initial slow phases provoked by and in the direction of the stimulus, followed by corrective fast phases. Elicitation of OKN in response to a pocket tape is a useful bedside test but only evaluates foveal pursuit and refixation saccades, which is helpful in several circumstances including: (1) detection of a subtle internuclear ophthalmoplegia; (2) provocation of convergence-retraction nystagmus, wherein the tape is moved downward in an attempt to induce upward saccades; (3) congenital nystagmus, wherein the direction of the fast phase may be paradoxical—that is, in the direction of the slowly moving tape or drum; (4) psychogenic blindness or ophthalmoplegia; (5) homonymous hemianopia caused by a large, deep-seated parietotemporo-occipital lesion, in which the OKN response is depressed or absent as the tape moves toward the side of the lesion.

A large mirror may be used to induce true optokinetic movements in patients with psychogenic ophthalmoplegia or psychogenic blindness. The examiner holds the mirror in front of the patient, whose eyes are open. The mirror is gently rocked so that the reflected environment (full visual fields) move. This compelling optokinetic stimulus forces reflex slow eye movements. The patient may close the eyes, look away, or exhibit convergence in an attempt to avoid the reflex response. Care must be taken in diagnosing psychogenic disorders with this test in patients with supranuclear gaze palsies, ocular motor apraxia, or poor vision; even those with "count-fingers" vision may still have an OKN response.

Treatment

Treatments used for the different types of nystagmus are summarized in **Table 35.15**. Underlying causes should be rectified where possible, and visual acuity should be corrected when necessary. With the exception of INS, in which prisms, surgery, and contact lenses are helpful, results of treatment of other forms of nystagmus are less effective; Occasionally, prisms are helpful in acquired nystagmus. Various pharmacological agents are used. For extensive reviews, see the works of Leigh and Zee (2006), Stahl et al. (2002), and Thurtell et al. (2010).

Saccadic Intrusions and Other Non-Nystagmus Ocular Oscillations

Voluntary Nystagmus

Voluntary nystagmus is not true nystagmus but ocular flutter under voluntary control. It consists of a series of fast (saccadic) back-to-back eye movements, without any interval or slow phase (**Fig. 35.18, A**). The oscillations usually are horizontal but may be vertical, torsional, or (rarely) cycloid—a phenomenon reported as "volitional opsoclonus" or multiplanar flutter (Espinosa and Berger, 2005). The ability to induce flutter voluntarily tends to be familial. Usually, persons with this ability must converge their eyes to initiate the oscillation but are unable to sustain it for longer than 30 seconds. Occasionally, patients use this ability to feign illness, but the phenomenon should be recognized easily.

Ocular Flutter

Ocular flutter (see **Fig. 35.18, A**) occurs with brainstem or cerebellar disease and consists of horizontal conjugate back-to-back saccades that occur spontaneously in intermittent bursts. It is aggravated by attempts at fixation. Occasionally it is triggered by a change in posture. Ocular flutter results from loss of

pause cell inhibition of the burst neurons in the paramedian pontine reticular formation (PPRF), caused by injury either to the PPRF (Schon et al., 2001) or to the cerebellar neurons that influence the pause cells, or both. Flutter often is associated with ocular dysmetria and may progress to opsoclonus.

Opsoclonus

Opsoclonus is a spontaneous, chaotic, multivector saccadic eye movement disorder in which the abnormal movements are virtually always conjugate. Opsoclonus is aggravated by attempts at fixation and may be associated with myoclonic jerks of the limbs and cerebellar ataxia (dancing eyes–dancing feet syndrome). Dysfunction of the pause cells in the pons due to cerebellar or brainstem disease is the cause. In two patients with opsoclonus, functional MRI demonstrated activation in the deep cerebellar nuclei that decreased or stopped with the eyes closed (Helmchen et al., 2003). This finding supports the hypothesis that disinhibition of the fastigial nuclei inhibits the omnipause neurons and is responsible for opsoclonus and perhaps other saccadic intrusions. The most common causes (**Box 35.13** and **Table 35.5**) include viral or postviral encephalitis and toxic, metabolic, and paraneoplastic disorders. The paraneoplastic opsoclonus-myoclonus-cerebellar syndrome that is a manifestation of neuroblastoma (2%–3%), found in children, may be responsive to adrenocorticotropic hormone. In adults, opsoclonus may accompany paraneoplastic parenchymal cerebellar degeneration resulting from a remote carcinoma or lymphoma. Opsoclonus also may occur in hyperosmolar states, Wernicke encephalopathy, and with toxic levels of many drugs. The efficacy of immunotherapy in adults with paraneoplastic syndromes is difficult to assess

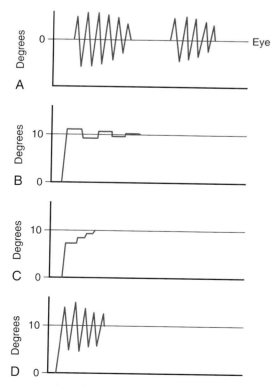

Fig. 35.18 Oculographic diagrams of waveforms in various non-nystagmus oscillations. **A,** Spontaneous ocular flutter in primary position. **B,** Overshoot dysmetria (hypermetria). **C,** Undershoot dysmetria (hypometria). **D,** Flutter dysmetria exacerbated by refixation of 1 to 10 degrees.

Box 35.13 Causes of Opsoclonus

- AIDS-related brainstem encephalitis or lymphoma
- Adults: carcinoma (thiamine-responsive)
- Biotin-responsive multiple carboxylase deficiency
- Celiac disease
- Children: neuroblastoma (corticotropin-responsive)
- Drugs (amitriptyline, chlordecone, cocaine, dichlorodiphenyl-trichloroethane, haloperidol, phencyclidine, phenytoin, diazepam, thallium, toluene, strychnine, vidarabine)
- Encephalitis (viral, pyogenic)
- Hashimoto encephalopathy
- Hydrocephalus
- Hyperosmolar coma
- Lipidoses
- MS
- Paraneoplastic
- Pontine hemorrhage
- Postencephalitic
- Pregnancy (Koide et al., 2004)
- Sarcoid
- Thalamic glioma
- Thalamic hemorrhage
- Transient phenomenon in healthy neonates
- Viral hepatitis (Wong, 2007)
- Wernicke encephalopathy

AIDS, Acquired immunodeficiency syndrome; *MS,* multiple sclerosis.

Table 35.5	Age-Related Likely Causes and Features of Opsoclonus
Neonates	Parainfectious Paraneoplastic (neuroblastoma in chest or abdomen)
Older infants: 8 months to 3 years Older than 3 years	Neural crest tumor or regressed neural crest tumor Regressed neural crest tumor
Children with opsoclonus	Good prognosis for tumor Poor prognosis for ocular movements (Respond to ACTH)
Adults	Paraneoplastic (breast, ovary); may respond to protein A immunoabsorption)

because of spontaneous fluctuations and remissions. In addition to treatment of the underlying neoplasm, however, early and aggressive immunotherapy, including the use of immunoadsorption therapy with plasma exchange through a protein A column (Cher et al., 1995), may be effective in opsoclonus. Responsiveness probably depends on the degree of the inflammatory component rather than on the neuronal loss. Opsoclonus occasionally may respond to thiamine, clonazepam, and antiepileptic agents, specifically gabapentin when associated with the locked-in syndrome (Pistoia et al., 2010).

Ocular Microflutter

Ocular microflutter, previously called *microsaccadic ocular flutter* (a redundant term), is a rare symptomatic ocular oscillation requiring magnification for detection (Dell'Osso and Daroff, 1999b). It may be a form of opsoclonus but in some patients is a variant of voluntary nystagmus. Patients complain of episodes of "shimmering" vision. It is reported with cerebellar degeneration and MS. When it is persistent, patients should be evaluated for occult neoplasms and have long-term follow-up (Leigh and Zee, 2006). Microflutter may respond to propranolol or verapamil (Leigh and Zee, 2006).

Ocular Dysmetria

Ocular dysmetria occurs with refixation saccades that overshoot the target (see **Fig. 35.18, B**) and often oscillate with an intersaccadic latency of approximately 200 milliseconds (Leigh and Zee, 2006) before coming to rest (see **Fig. 35.18, C**). It results from dysfunction of dorsal vermis and fastigial nuclei in the cerebellum.

Flutter Dysmetria

Flutter dysmetria occurs immediately after the patient refixates on a target; the eye then briefly oscillates without intersaccadic intervals across the line of the target for a few cycles (see **Fig. 35.18, D**). Both flutter and opsoclonus result from dysfunction of the pause cells in the PPRF, which tonically suppresses the burst cells. The pause cells have input from the cerebellum; thus, cerebellar or brainstem dysfunction may result in flutter or opsoclonus.

Convergence Retraction Nystagmus

Convergence retraction nystagmus is not a true nystagmus but a rapid dysmetric horizontal eye movement induced by attempted upward saccades. It occurs as part of the dorsal midbrain (Parinaud) syndrome. Clinically, rapid convergence with synchronous retraction of both globes caused by simultaneous co-contraction of the extraocular muscles is followed by a slow divergent movement. Less commonly, if lateral rectus innervation is dominant, a rapid divergent movement occurs initially.

Ocular Bobbing

Ocular bobbing is a rapid downward movement of both eyes followed by a slow drift back to primary position. The oscillation recurs between 2 and 15 times per minute and is found in patients (usually comatose) with severe central pontine destruction and horizontal gaze palsies (**Table 35.6**). In atypical bobbing, horizontal eye movements are spared.

With *reverse bobbing*, the initial fast phase is upward, followed by a slow downward drift, whereas with *inverse bobbing* (dipping), the initial deviation is a slow downward movement followed by a rapid return to primary position. The latter two phenomena occur in patients with severe metabolic disorders or structural damage involving the mesodiencephalic region. *Reverse dipping*, a slow upward movement followed by a fast downward movement, was described in an obtunded patient with a seizure disorder and chronic meningitis. Bobbing may be dysconjugate (see **Table 35.6**).

V-pattern pretectal pseudobobbing, a higher-frequency, more rapid downward convergent movement with a slower than normal return toward primary position, occurs with acute obstructive hydrocephalus and is an indication for urgent decompression. Some patients may exhibit more than one type of bobbing.

Ocular Myoclonus (Oculopalatal Tremor)

Ocular myoclonus is a vertical pendular oscillation with a frequency of approximately 160 Hz, usually associated with similar oscillations of the soft palate (palatal tremor) and sometimes other muscles of branchial origin (Leigh and Zee, 2006). The palatal tremor, referred to as the *oculopalatal syndrome*, occurs after brainstem infarction, particularly of the pons, involving the central tegmental tract. Following a latency of months, hypertrophic degeneration of the inferior olives ensues and the myoclonus begins. The association of a facial nerve palsy and the one-and-a-half syndrome may predict the development of oculopalatal myoclonus, probably because of the proximity of the central tegmental tract to the facial nerve (Wolin et al., 1996). Also, oculopalatal myoclonus can occur spontaneously in association with progressive ataxia, a fourth ventricular tumor, or hydrocephalus following subarachnoid hemorrhage (Eggenberger et al., 2001). Dysfunction of the

Table 35.6 Ocular Bobbing

Type	Movement	Cause
Ocular bobbing (atypical bobbing, horizontal eye movements preserved)	Fast down, slow upward return to primary position	Severe central pontine destruction, central pontine myelinolysis, encephalitis, extra-axial pontine compression (usually a cerebellar hematoma), organophosphate poisoning
Reverse bobbing	Fast up, slow downward return to primary position	Usually nonlocalizing encephalopathy: anoxia, metabolic encephalopathy, head injury, post status epilepticus
Dipping (inverse bobbing)	Slow down, fast upward return to primary position	Anoxic, metabolic, and toxic position encephalopathies, post status epilepticus
Reverse dipping	Slow up, fast downward return to primary position	Cryptococcal meningitis or obtundation (in a patient with acquired immunodeficiency syndrome), pontine stroke
V-pattern pretectal pseudobobbing	Fast downward convergent movements at higher frequency than typical bobbing; slower-than-normal return to primary position	Acute obstructive hydrocephalus

cerebellar nuclei or their connections (Guillain-Mollaret triangle) and disruption of retinal error signals relayed to the inferior olive may be responsible for oculopalatal myoclonus, which is confined to the muscles of branchial origin. Patients may get some relief from anticonvulsants such as carbamazepine, clonazepam, gabapentin, memantine (Thurtell et al., 2010), valproic acid, and agents such as trihexyphenidyl hydrochloride and cerulein, or by chronically patching one eye. Palatal tremor may respond to botulinum injections. In patients with aortic regurgitation, it should be distinguished from pulsations of the uvula that are synchronous with the systolic pulse (Muller sign) (Williams and Steinberg, 2006).

Superior Oblique Myokymia

Superior oblique myokymia is a paroxysmal, rapid, small-amplitude, monocular torsional-vertical oscillation caused by contraction of the superior oblique muscle, predominantly on the right side (Yousry et al., 2002). Patients may complain of monocular blurring, torsional or vertical oscillopsia, torsional or vertical diplopia, or twitching of the eye. Oculography using magnetic search coils has demonstrated both phasic and tonic contractions of intorsion, depression, and to a much lesser extent, abduction of the superior oblique muscle (Leigh and Zee, 2006). MRI demonstrated that the affected superior oblique muscle was smaller in some patients, suggesting antecedent injury to the fourth nerve; this hypothesis is supported by an MRI finding of neurovascular compression of the fourth nerve at its root exit zone (Hashimoto et al., 2001; Yousry et al., 2002).

Superior oblique myokymia may be difficult to detect with the unaided eye and is more easily detected with a direct ophthalmoscope. It may be precipitated by activating the superior oblique muscle when the patient looks down in the direction of action of that muscle or tilts the head toward the affected eye. Superior oblique myokymia has a relapsing-remitting course in otherwise normal, healthy adults. It is reported with adrenoleukodystrophy, lead poisoning, cerebellar astrocytoma, dural arteriovenous fistula, and microvascular compression (Hashimoto et al., 2001; Samii et al., 1998; Yousry et al., 2002).

Superior oblique myokymia may respond dramatically to carbamazepine or gabapentin (Tomsak et al., 2002). Propranolol in low dosage, amitriptyline, baclofen, phenytoin, benzodi-

Box 35.14 Saccadic Oscillations

- Flutter (voluntary, involuntary)
- Flutter dysmetria
- Microsaccadic flutter (variant of voluntary flutter?)
- Opsoclonus
- Macro–square wave jerks (now designated *square-wave pulses*)
- Ocular bobbing, reverse and inverse bobbing, dipping, and reverse dipping
- Superior oblique myokymia
- Convergence-retraction nystagmus
- Abduction nystagmus with internuclear ophthalmoplegia
- Tic-like ocular myoclonic jerks (eye tics)

azepines, or topical beta-blockers (used for glaucoma) also may be helpful. A base-down prism in front of the affected eye may alleviate the patient's symptoms, avoid potential side effects of long-term medication, and obviate superior oblique muscle or tendon surgery, which some clinicians advocate when the disorder is prolonged. Disabling superior oblique myokymia may respond to microvascular decompression of the trochlear nerve at its root exit (Samii et al., 1998; Scharwey et al., 2000).

Saccadic Intrusions and Oscillations

Saccadic intrusions such as square wave jerks are brief, unwanted, nonrepetitive saccadic interruptions of fixation (**Box 35.14**). Other intrusions are saccadic pulses (stepless saccades) that interrupt fixation and are followed by a slow drift back on target (glissade), double saccadic pulses (fragment of flutter), and dynamic overshoots (see **Fig. 35.29**). Macrosaccadic oscillations—macro square wave jerks (Dell'Osso and Daroff, 1999b)—are discussed later.

Generation and Control of Eye Movements

Reasonable understanding and interpretation of gaze disorders require an appreciation of the anatomy and physiology of eye movement control. In the words of J. Hughlings Jackson,

"The study of the cause of things must be preceded by study of things caused."

Normal visual behavior is accomplished by a continuous cycle of visual fixation and visual analysis interrupted by saccades (Schall and Thompson, 1999). Individuals with intact sensory visual systems (optical and afferent) are capable of discerning small details comparable to Snellen acuity of 20/13, provided the image of the target is maintained within 0.5 degree of the center of the fovea. However, 10 degrees from fixation, the resolving power of the retina drops to 20/200. Although the peripheral retina has poor spatial resolution capabilities, it is exquisitely sensitive to movement (temporal resolution). The image of an object entering the peripheral visual field stimulates the retina to signal the ocular motor system to make a rapid eye movement (saccade) and fixate it on the fovea. In the words of American psychologist William James, "The peripheral retina is like a sentinel and when an object of regard falls upon it, it shouts 'hark, who goes there' and calls the fovea to the spot." Visual information concerning spatial resolution (fine detail) and color travels

via retinal ganglion (P) cells to the parvocellular layers of the lateral geniculate nucleus (LGN), whereas information concerning temporal resolution (movement) travels via retinal ganglion (M) cells to the magnocellular layer of the LGN. In turn, neurons in the LGN project via the optic radiations to the primary visual area (V1), the striate cortex (area 17).

Visual processing in the cortex begins in the primary visual area from which issues two processing streams (**Fig. 35.19, A**). The ventral stream, responsible for form and object recognition and emphasizing foveal representation, projects to the temporal lobe via occipital areas V2 and V4. The dorsal stream, responsible for movement recognition, guiding actions in space, and emphasizing peripheral visual field representation, projects to the prestriate cortex; then it relays to the superior temporal sulcus region, which contains cortical areas MT (middle temporal) and MST (middle superior temporal) in monkeys, roughly equivalent to the parietotemporo-occipital junction (PTO) in humans, and encodes for location, direction, and velocity of objects. Both streams converge on the FEF

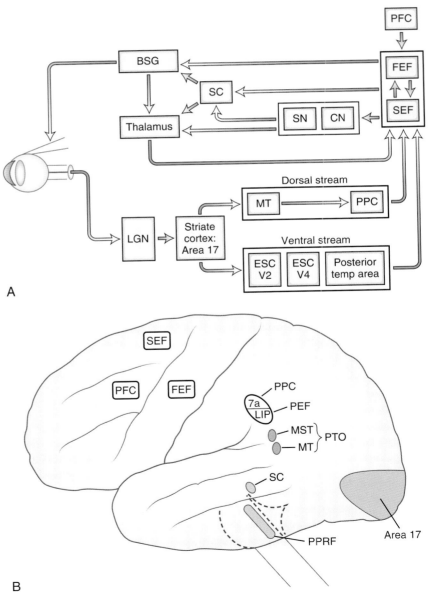

Fig. 35.19 **A,** Overview of the combined afferent and efferent visual system. **B,** Areas in the human brain that are believed to be important in generating saccades and pursuit. *BSG,* Brainstem saccadic generator; *CN,* caudate nucleus; *ESC,* extrastriate cortex; *FEF,* frontal eye field; *LGN,* lateral geniculate nucleus; *LIP,* lateral intraparietal area; *MST,* medial superior temporovisual area; *MT,* middle temporovisual area; *PEF,* parietal eye field; *PFC,* prefrontal cortex; *PPC,* posterior parietal cortex area; *PPRF,* paramedian pontine reticular formation; *PTO,* parietotemporo-occipital junction; *SC,* superior colliculus; *SEF,* supplementary eye fields in the supplementary motor area; *7a,* area 7a; *SN,* substantia nigra. (**A** Redrawn from Stuphorn, V., Schall, J.D., 2002. Neuronal control and monitoring of the initiation of movements. Muscle Nerve 26, 326-339.)

(frontal eye field) and are involved in controlling saccades (see later discussion).

The premotor substrates for conjugate gaze and vergence eye movements are in the brainstem. The substrates specific for vertical gaze, vergence, and ocular counter-rolling are in the mesodiencephalic region, whereas those for horizontal eye movements are mainly in the pons. Our understanding of the mechanisms for eye movements is based on clinicopathological and radiological correlation as well as animal and bioengineering experiments. With the exception of reflexive movements such as the VOR and fast phases of nystagmus, cerebral structures determine *when* and *where* the eyes move, whereas brainstem mechanisms determine *how* they move. In other words, voluntary eye movements are generated in the brainstem but are triggered by the cerebral cortex.

Ocular Motor Subsystems

Eye movements are of two main types: those that redirect gaze to different objects of interest and those that stabilize the image of the target on each retina and maintain binocular foveation during head or target movement, or both. The saccadic system moves the eyes rapidly (up to 800 degrees per second) to fixate new targets (**Fig. 35.20, A**). Saccades may be generated voluntarily or in response to verbal commands in the absence of a visible target. Reflex saccades may occur in

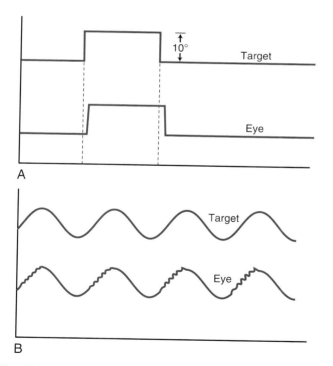

A

B

Fig. 35.20 Simulated eye movement recordings. By convention for horizontal movements, upward deflections represent rightward eye movements, and downward deflections represent leftward eye movements. **A,** Saccades. A target moves rapidly 10 degrees to the right. After a latency of about 200 msec, the eye follows. When the target returns to the center, the sequence is repeated in the opposite direction. **B,** Pursuit. The target moves in a sinusoidal pattern in front of the patient. The eye follows the target after a latency of about 120 msec, but pursuit movements to the right are defective, resulting in the rightward "cogwheel" (saccadic) pursuit. Pursuit to the left is normal.

response to peripheral retinal stimuli such as visual threat or retinal error signals, or to sound. Saccades also are the fast components of nystagmus.

The pursuit system enables the eyes to track slowly moving targets (up to 70 degrees per second) to maintain the image stable on the fovea. Specially trained subjects are capable of smooth-pursuit eye movements as fast as 100 degrees per second. Pursuit eye movements are limited more by the target's acceleration than by its velocity. If the target moves too quickly or changes direction abruptly, or if the pursuit system is impaired, the eyes are unable to maintain pace with the target and fall behind. Consequently, the image moves off the fovea, producing a retinal error signal that provokes a corrective (catch-up) saccade and refixates the target. The cycle then repeats itself, resulting in saccadic ("cogwheel") pursuit (see **Fig. 35.20, B**).

Bidirectionally defective pursuit eye movements, a normal finding in infants, are nonspecific and occur under conditions of stress or fatigue or with sedative medication. However, impaired tracking in one direction suggests a structural lesion of the ipsilateral pursuit system (see **Fig. 35.20, B**).

Fixation allows the eyes to maintain an image of a stationary target on each fovea at rest. The fixation subsystem shares neural circuitry with the optokinetic and pursuit systems (Leigh and Zee, 2006).

The vestibular eye movement subsystem maintains a stable image on the retina during head movements. The semicircular canals respond to rotational acceleration of the head by driving the VOR to maintain the eyes in the same direction in space during head movements. The otoliths (utricle and saccule) are gravity receptors that respond to linear acceleration and static head tilt (gravity)—that is, with ocular counter-rolling. The vestibular system is discussed further in Chapter 37.

The optokinetic system uses visual reference points in the environment to maintain orientation. It complements the vestibulo-ocular system, which becomes less responsive during slow or sustained head movements, to stabilize images on the retina in situations such as large turns or spinning. When the eyes reach their limit of movement in the orbits, a reflex saccade allows refixation to a point further forward in the direction of head rotation. The sequence repeats itself, resulting in OKN.

In humans, the optokinetic system responds predominantly to fixation and pursuit of a moving target (immediate component) and to a lesser extent velocity storage (delayed component), which involves neural circuitry in the vestibular system. (*Velocity storage* is a mechanism by which the CNS, predominantly the vestibular system including the vestibulo-cerebellum, prolongs or perseverates short signals generated by the vestibular end-organ to enhance orientation in space. Velocity storage is largely involuntary.) The optokinetic system probably evolved to supplement the vestibular system during sustained rotations.

The vergence system enables the eyes to move disconjugately (converge and diverge) in the horizontal plane to maintain binocular fixation on a target moving toward or away from the subject. Vergence movements are essential for binocular single vision and stereoscopic depth perception.

The different types of eye movements are listed in (**Box 35.15**).

Box 35.15 Types of Eye Movements

Saccades (Move Eyes from One Target to Another)

- Intentional saccades (internally triggered, with a goal):
  - Visually guided saccades
  - Memory-guided saccades (with visual/vestibular input)
  - Predictive saccades
  - Target-searching saccades
  - Antisaccades*
- Reflexive saccades (externally triggered):
  - Visually guided saccades
  - Auditory saccades
- Spontaneous saccades (internally triggered, without a goal):
  - During another motor activity
  - At rest
  - When sleeping
- Quick phases of nystagmus:
  - Physiological nystagmus:
    - Vestibular nystagmus
    - Optokinetic nystagmus
  - End-point nystagmus
  - Pathologic nystagmus

Eye Movements Stabilizing the Image of the Target on the Fovea

- Smooth pursuit:
  - Foveal pursuit
  - Full-field pursuit (slow phase of optokinetic nystagmus)
- Vestibulo-ocular reflex (horizontal, vertical, torsional)
- Convergence

Ocular Oscillations That May Interfere with Vision

- Double saccadic pulses
- Macrosaccadic oscillations
- Nystagmus (pathological)
- Ocular bobbing
- Ocular dysmetria:
  - Ocular hypometria
  - Ocular hypermetria
  - Ocular lateropulsion
  - Ocular torsipulsion
  - Ocular flutter
- Ocular neuromyotonia
- Ocular tics (myoclonic jerks)
- Oculogyric crisis
- Opsoclonus
- Saccadic pulses
- Square-wave pulses (previously designated *macro–square wave jerks*)
- Square-wave jerks
- Superior oblique myokymia
- Torsional saccades (blips)

*Antisaccades are fast eye movements deliberately made away from a new target. It is a laboratory procedure used to investigate frontal lobe or cognitive function.

Horizontal Eye Movements

When gaze is redirected from one point to another, a saccade moves the eyes conjugately. To enable the small, straplike extraocular muscles to move the relatively large globes and

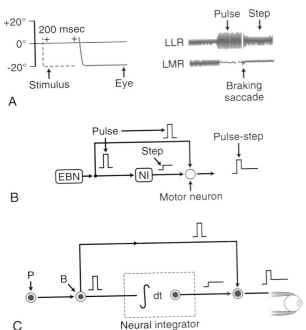

Fig. 35.21 Ocular motor events on gaze left. **A,** After the appearance of a stimulus 20 degrees to the left of fixation (−20 degrees), the eyes move to the target with a saccade after a latency of 200 msec. Idealized electromyography of the left extraocular muscles shows the activity of the agonist (the left lateral rectus [LLR]) and the antagonist (the left medial rectus [LMR]) muscles. **B,** The pulse originates in the excitatory burst neurons (EBNs) and is mathematically integrated by the neural integrator (NI); both signals are added to produce the pulse-step of the innervation to the ocular motor neurons. **C,** The pause cells (P) discharge continuously, suppressing the burst cells (B), except during a saccade, when they "pause," allowing the burst cells to discharge and generate a pulse. *(Reprinted with permission from Lavin, P.J.M., 1985. Conjugate and disconjugate eye movements, in: Walsh, T.J. [Ed.], Neuro-ophthalmology: clinical signs and symptoms. Lea & Febiger, Philadelphia.)*

overcome inertia and the elastic recoil of the viscous orbital contents, the yoked agonist muscles require a surge or *burst* of innervation (pulse) at the same time their yoked antagonists are reciprocally inhibited (**Fig. 35.21, A**). For a leftward saccade, the left lateral rectus and the right medial rectus muscles each receive a pulse of innervation while their antagonists, the left medial and right lateral rectus muscles, are reciprocally inhibited. Excitatory burst neurons (EBNs) contained in the ipsilateral paramedian pontine reticular formation (PPRF) just rostral to the abducens nucleus generate the pulse to initiate the saccade. The EBNs are medium-lead burst cells that discharge about 10 msec before and during all horizontal saccadic eye movements; they preferentially discharge for ipsilateral saccades and create the immediate premotor command, generating pulse activity for saccades.

About half the neurons in the abducens nucleus are interneurons (with different morphological and pharmacological features than the neurons of the abducens nerve) that relay, via the medial longitudinal fasciculus (MLF), to the contralateral medial rectus neurons in the oculomotor nuclear complex (**Fig. 35.22**). Except just before and during a saccade, the EBNs are tonically suppressed by omnipause neurons located in the nucleus raphe interpositus rostral to the abducens nucleus. The trigger that initiates a saccade also inhibits the omnipause

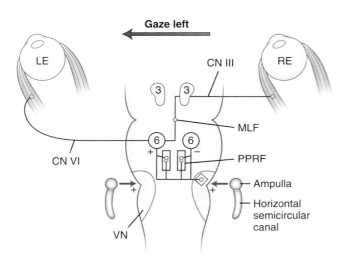

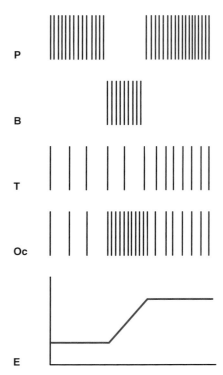

Fig. 35.22 A lateral head turn induces movement of the endolymph in the ipsilateral horizontal semicircular canal toward the ampulla (as would warm water caloric stimulation of an ear), and thus excites the contralateral abducens nucleus and inhibits the ipsilateral abducens nucleus via the vestibular nuclei (VN). Each abducens nucleus innervates the ipsilateral lateral rectus muscle via the abducens nerve and the contralateral medial rectus muscle via the abducens nucleus interneurons, the medial longitudinal fasciculus (MLF), and the neurons for the medial rectus (part of cranial nerve [CN] III nucleus). Neurons in each paramedian pontine reticular formation (PPRF) also have an excitatory input to the ipsilateral abducens nucleus and an inhibitory input to the contralateral abducens nucleus, for saccades and quick phases of nystagmus. *LE*, Left eye; *RE*, right eye. *(Adapted from Lavin, P.J.M., 1985. Conjugate and disconjugate eye movements, in: Walsh, T.J. [Ed.], Neuro-ophthalmology: clinical signs and symptoms. Lea & Febiger, Philadelphia.)*

Fig. 35.23 Electrophysiological events during an eye movement. P represents an intraneuronal recording from a pause cell and demonstrates a constant discharge, which ceases, allowing an excitatory burst neuron (B) to discharge during pulse. T represents the discharge in a tonic neuron, which increases after the pulse as a result of integration of the pulse to a step. Both the pulse (P) and the tonic output (T) of burst-tonic neurons innervate the oculomotor neurons (Oc). The result is a rapid contraction of the extraocular muscle, which moves the eye from primary position and holds it in an eccentric position (E).

neurons. Subsequently, hypothetical latch neurons in the reticular formation, which receive input from the EBNs, inhibit omnipause neurons until the saccade is complete (Leigh and Zee, 2006). Latch neurons are active during pursuit also. Disorders of latch neurons may result in prematurely terminated saccades and very hypometric saccades in disorders such as Parkinson disease. Thus the omnipause neurons, which receive input from the cerebrum, cerebellum, and superior colliculus (SC), mediate the command for a saccade when they cease discharging and allow the burst cells to fire (**Fig. 35.23**). While the EBNs discharge, a group of inhibitory cell-burst neurons that lie caudal to the abducens nucleus in the medial rostral medulla and project across the midline to the contralateral abducens nucleus discharge during the saccade to reciprocally inhibit the yoked antagonist muscles (Leigh and Zee, 2006).

To maintain the eyes on target in an eccentric position at the end of a saccade, the agonist muscles for a leftward movement (left lateral and right medial recti) now require a new level of tonic innervation—a position command—achieved by a group of neurons referred to as the *neural integrator*. (An integrator mathematically converts phasic input to tonic output by using reverberating collateral circuits to reexcite neurons. The efficiency of an integrator depends on its time constant [i.e., the duration it can prolong the activity of the input]. The effective time constant is the period necessary for

the output to decay to 37% of its initial value after the input signal stops.)

The NI for horizontal gaze, thought to be partly in the rostral perihypoglossal nuclear complex and the adjacent rostral medial vestibular nucleus (Leigh and Zee, 2006), receives the velocity command signal (pulse) from the EBNs. The NI then mathematically integrates the pulse to a "tonic" position command (step) before relaying it to the ipsilateral abducens nucleus (see **Figs. 35.21, *B*, and 35.22**).

The cerebellum and the PPRF maintain the output of this NI by controlling the gain, via a positive feedback loop, to keep the eyes on target (**Fig. 35.24**). The *gain* of a system is the ratio of its output to its input. In this case, the output is the innervation required to maintain eccentric fixation, and the input is the pulse signal (see **Fig. 35.21, *C***). If the NI is unable to maintain the gain at unity (output/input = 1), the output falls, causing the eyes to drift off target toward primary position. A corrective saccade then refixates the target, resulting in gaze-evoked (gaze-paretic) nystagmus. Current evidence suggests that all conjugate eye movement commands, including saccades, pursuit, the slow phases of OKN, and the VOR, are initiated as velocity commands and mediated by a final common integrator (**Fig. 35.25**).

Although its anatomical borders are unclear, the PPRF is defined functionally with the medial aspects of the nuclei gigantocellularis, or pontis centralis oralis and caudalis, and is

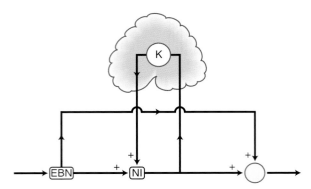

Fig. 35.24 The time constant of the brainstem neural integrator (NI), and therefore the fidelity of its output (innervation for gaze holding), is controlled predominantly by the cerebellum. Dysfunction of the gain control (K) may cause the integrator output to fall (a shortened time constant causes the signal to decay), allowing the eyes to drift back toward primary position. Conversely, an increase in K may result in an unstable integrator and cause the eye to drift eccentrically with an increasing velocity waveform. *EBN*, Excitatory burst neuron. *(Adapted from Lavin, P.J.M., 1985. Conjugate and disconjugate eye movements, in: Walsh, T.J. [Ed.], Neuro-ophthalmology: clinical signs and symptoms. Lea & Febiger, Philadelphia. Reprinted by permission of the author and the publisher.)*

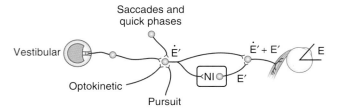

Fig. 35.25 The final common integrator hypothesis. All conjugate eye movements (E) are initiated as eye velocity commands (E′) that are converted to eye position (Ė′) by the neural integrator (NI). Both eye velocity and eye position commands are relayed to the motor neurons. *(Adapted from Cannon, S.C., Zee, D.S., 1988. The neural integrator of the oculomotor system, in: Lessell, S., Van Dalen, J.T.W. [Eds.], Current Neuro-ophthalmology. Chicago, Year Book.)*

located just ventral and lateral to the MLF, extending from the level of the abducens nucleus almost to the trochlear nucleus. The PPRF innervates the ipsilateral abducens nucleus, the rostral medulla (part of the NI), and the midbrain reticular formation (MRF) to coordinate horizontal and vertical eye movements. The PPRF receives direct input from each medial vestibular nucleus, the contralateral FEFs, the ipsilateral posterior parietal region, the SC, and the cerebellum.

A lesion of the abducens nucleus produces paralysis of all ipsilateral versional eye movements. Pontine lesions outside the abducens nucleus may selectively involve certain classes of eye movements while sparing others, demonstrating that the neural signals encoding subclasses of eye movements (e.g., saccades, pursuit, VOR, tonic position) project independently to the abducens nucleus. The PPRF also plays a role in generating vertical eye movements; acute bilateral injury may cause a transient vertical and horizontal gaze palsy. Bilateral injury may cause a persistent horizontal and vertical selective saccadic palsy. A unilateral lesion, in addition to impairing ipsilateral horizontal saccades, may also cause slowing and oblique misdirection of vertical saccades away from the side of injury.

With rare exceptions (Miller et al., 2002), lesions of the abducens nucleus that cause an acquired ipsilateral gaze palsy almost always involve the facial nerve fasciculus as it loops around the abducens nucleus and result in an associated facial nerve palsy.

The vestibular system stabilizes the direction of gaze during head movements by virtue of changes in its tonic input to the ocular motor nuclei. This is most clearly illustrated by the horizontal VOR (see **Fig. 35.22**). Each horizontal semicircular canal innervates the ipsilateral medial vestibular nucleus to inhibit the ipsilateral and excite the contralateral abducens nucleus. The ampulla of the right horizontal semicircular canal is stimulated by turning the head to the right (or warm caloric stimulation). This mechanical information is transduced by the vestibular end-organ to electrical signals and transmitted to the ipsilateral vestibular nucleus. Excitatory information is then relayed to the contralateral abducens nucleus, and inhibitory information to the ipsilateral abducens nucleus, causing the eyes to deviate in the direction opposite to head rotation, thus maintaining the direction of gaze.

Saccades (see **Box 35.15**), or fast eye movements, are initiated mainly in the contralateral frontal lobe and may be classified into four broad groups:

1. Internally triggered saccades, which are voluntary (intentional) and include target-searching, memory-guided, predictive (where the appearance of the target is anticipated), intentional visually guided saccades to an existing target in the peripheral visual field, and antisaccades.
2. Externally triggered saccades are reflexively activated by the appearance of a new target or a sound.
3. Spontaneous saccades, which occur in the absence of a target and are triggered internally by both the FEF and the SC to repetitively scan the environment; they occur at rest, during other motor activities, and during rapid-eye-movement sleep.
4. The quick phases of nystagmus.

A number of specialized areas in the cerebral cortex, identified by both experimental and pathological lesions, by neurophysiological studies (particularly in monkeys), and by transcranial magnetic stimulation, play a major role in controlling saccades (see **Fig. 35.19, B**):

1. The FEF in the precentral gyrus and sulcus (Brodmann area 6 in humans and area 8 in monkeys).
2. The supplementary eye field (SEF) on the dorsomedial aspect of the superior frontal gyrus is anterior to the supplementary motor area.
3. The parietal eye field (PEF) in the lateral intraparietal (LIP) area in monkeys is equivalent to an area in the intraparietal sulcus near the angular gyrus region (Brodmann areas 39 and 40) in humans.

Other cortical areas that have a role in controlling saccades include the posterior parietal cortex (PPC), located in Brodmann area 39 in the upper angular gyrus in humans (equivalent to 7a in monkeys); the dorsolateral prefrontal cortex (PFC), area 46; the vestibular cortex in the posterior aspect of the superior temporal gyrus; and the hippocampus in the medial temporal lobe (Pierrot-Deseilligny et al., 1995). These cortical areas and the superior colliculus are parts of a network that collectively produce saccades and determine when different types of saccades occur and where they go; that is, they calculate their direction and amplitude (accuracy). In summary, this network determines where potential targets for orienting are located; where, whether, and when gaze will shift; and coordinates saccades with visually guided reaching and head movements.

Topographically, the FEF is heavily interconnected with areas in both the dorsal and ventral streams of the extrastriate visual cortex (see **Fig. 35.19, A**) and participates in the transformation of visual signals into saccadic motor commands (Schall et al., 1995). Being extensively connected with extrastriate visual cortical areas, many neurons in the FEF respond to visual stimuli. The FEF and SC are both activated in the same way at the same time in response to visual stimuli before and during saccades.

Also, the FEF plays a direct role in producing saccades. A subpopulation of neurons in the FEF that discharge specifically before and during saccades innervate the deeper layers of the SC and neural circuits in the brainstem that generate saccades.

The FEF projects to the SC mainly by three pathways: a direct pathway through the posterior aspect of the anterior limb of the internal capsule near the genu, an indirect pathway via the thalamus, and another indirect pathway via the caudate nucleus to neurons in the substantia nigra pars reticulata (SNr). These neurons in the SNr project, in turn, to the SC and tonically suppress saccades by a GABA-ergic mechanism. Controlled disinhibition of this basal ganglia system is important for normal visually and auditory-guided saccades and is probably essential for saccades to remembered targets. Saccades of different amplitudes and directions are encoded in neurons in the FEF and SC in a retinotopic fashion (i.e., the size and direction of a saccade is determined by which neurons are stimulated). The SC also has some role in reflexive and orienting saccades. The basal ganglia are involved in sequencing complex memory-guided saccades and perhaps predictive saccades (Pierrot-Deseilligny et al., 1995).

Neurons in the dorsolateral PFC project to the superior colliculus via the anterior limb, genu, and anterior half of the posterior limb of the internal capsule to suppress unwanted saccades to distracting stimuli when attention is directed at an existing target. Clinically, this system may be evaluated with the antisaccade test (Zee and Lasker, 2004).

The SEF parallels the FEF in several respects and also innervates ocular motor centers in the SC and brainstem. However, the SEF seems to play a less essential or less potent role in saccade production, as ablation of SEF causes only minimal and short-lasting gaze impairment.

The role of the PEF (area LIP in monkeys) is uncertain. Although neural activity in the PEF precedes saccades, the PEF does not directly control the initiation of saccades, but signals areas such as the FEF and SC with the location of potential targets for orienting (Colby and Goldberg, 1999; Snyder et al., 2000).

The SC has seven alternating fibrous and cellular layers that are broadly divided into a superficial sensory (dorsal) and a deep, predominantly motor (ventral) division. The superficial sensory division receives a direct orderly input from the retina via the accessory optic tract, bypassing the lateral geniculate body, such that the visual field may be mapped on the surface of the SC (retinotopic). Only about 10% of the retinal ganglion cells project to the SC; the remainder project to the lateral geniculate body to subserve conscious vision. The deep motor division receives visual input from the striate cortex (area 17) and projects to motor areas in the subthalamic region and brainstem. The deeper division also receives input directly from the FEF and PPC and indirectly via the basal ganglia, as well as somatosensory and auditory input. Stimulation of the SC drives the eyes contralaterally to a point in the visual field corresponding to the retinal projection to that site. Thus the SC is essentially a sensory map overlying a corresponding motor map and represents the visual fields (Leigh and Zee, 2006). The SC may also play a role in relaying excitatory information from part of the inferior parietal lobule (IPL), which has some influence in initiating saccades. Isolated lesions of the SC produce minimal but specific defects of saccades. However, when combined with experimental lesions of the FEFs, significant contralateral saccadic defects result. Purely vertical saccades require bilateral simultaneous stimulation of corresponding points of the SC or of the FEFs.

Control of smooth-pursuit eye movements is also complex (see **Fig. 35.19**) but essentially consists of three components: sensory, motor, and attentional-spatial. The stimulus for pursuit is movement of an image across the fovea at velocities greater than 3 to 5 degrees per second. The sensory component includes the striate cortex (area 17), which receives information from the retinal ganglion (M) cells via the magnocellular layer of the lateral geniculate body (nucleus) and the optic radiations. The striate cortex projects to the prestriate cortex (parieto-occipital areas 18 and 19) and then to the superior temporal sulcus region, which contains cortical areas MT and MST in monkeys, equivalent to the PTO junction in humans (Barton et al., 1995). This sensory subsystem encodes for location, direction, and velocity of objects moving in the contralateral visual field and is the major afferent input driving smooth pursuit. It projects bilaterally to the pursuit motor subsystem, which is also located in the PTO region, as well as to the FEF and SEF. This pursuit pathway is indirect and focuses attention on small moving targets. A direct pathway bypassing the attentional-spatial subsystem enables large moving objects, such as full-field OKN stimuli, to generate smooth pursuit contralaterally even when the subject is inattentive. The SC also contributes to pursuit drive. The PTO projects via the internal sagittal stratum and the posterior limb of the internal capsule to the ipsilateral dorsolateral and lateral pontine nuclei. The pursuit pathways control ipsilateral tracking and so must either remain on the same side or undergo a double decussation at least once. In 1992, Johnston and co-workers suggested the pursuit pathways project from the pontine nuclei to the contralateral flocculus and medial vestibular nucleus and then back to the ipsilateral abducens nucleus (**Fig. 35.26**).

Pursuit defects fall into four categories:

1. Retinotopic defects: Lesions of the geniculostriate pathway cause impaired pursuit in both directions in the contralateral visual field defect. Defects also occur with lesions of areas MST or MT; these patients have apparently normal visual fields but selective "blindness" for movement.

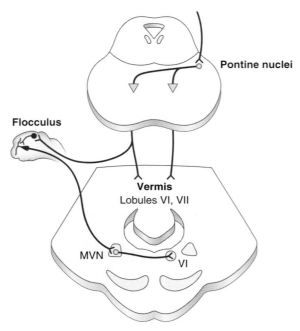

Fig. 35.26 Postulated double decussation of pursuit pathways in the brainstem and cerebellum. The first decussation consists of excitatory mossy fiber projections from the pontine nuclei to granule cells, which excite basket cells and stellate cells in the contralateral cerebellar flocculus. The basket and stellate cells inhibit Purkinje cells, which in turn inhibit neurons in the medial vestibular nucleus (MVN). The second decussation consists of excitatory projections from the MVN to the opposite abducens nucleus (VI). *(Reprinted with permission from Johnston, J.L., Sharpe, J.A., Morrow, M.J., 1992. Paresis of contralateral smooth pursuit and normal vestibular smooth eye movements after unilateral brainstem lesions. Ann Neurol 31, 495-502.)*

2. Impaired pursuit, worse in the ipsilateral direction in both hemifields, occurs with lesions in the lateral aspect of area MST and the foveal representation of area MT in monkeys, similar to a focal PTO lesion in humans. Lesions in the FEFs, posterior thalamus, midbrain, ipsilateral pons, contralateral cerebellum, contralateral pontomedullary junction, and the ipsilateral abducens nucleus also can impair pursuit in both hemifields, worse in the ipsilateral direction.
3. Symmetrically impaired pursuit in both horizontal directions occurs with focal lesions in the parieto-occipital region (area 39). Medication (e.g., anticonvulsants, sedatives, and psychotropic agents), alcohol, fatigue, inattention, schizophrenia, encephalopathy, a variety of neurodegenerative disorders, and age (infants and the elderly) also cause symmetrically impaired pursuit.
4. An acute nondominant (e.g., parietal, frontal) hemisphere lesion associated with a hemispatial neglect syndrome causes transient loss of pursuit beyond the midline into contralateral hemispace.

The cerebellum coordinates the ocular motor system to drive the eyes smoothly and accurately and is richly supplied by afferent fibers conveying ocular information (e.g., velocity, position, neural integration) from the vestibular system, the afferent visual system, the PPRF, and the MRF. The dorsal vermis and fastigial nuclei determine the accuracy of saccades by modulating saccadic amplitude; also, they adjust the innervation to each eye selectively to ensure precise conjugate movements. Lesions of the dorsal vermis and fastigial nuclei result in saccadic dysmetria (often, overshoot dysmetria that is greater centripetally), macrosaccadic oscillations, and disorders of vergence (see following section).

Selective cerebellar lesions have differential effects on eye movements. Bilateral lesions of the fastigial and globose (interpositus) nuclei cause hypermetria of externally triggered saccades but do not affect internally triggered saccades (Straube et al., 1995). Bilateral lesions of the posterior vermis (lobules VI and VII) cause hypometric horizontal and vertical saccades and impaired pursuit. Unilateral lesions of the posterior vermis cause hypometric ipsilateral and hypermetric contralateral saccades, whereas unilateral lesions of the caudal fastigial nucleus cause hypermetric ipsilateral and hypometric contralateral saccades (Büttner and Straube, 1995; Vahedi et al., 1995).

The flocculus, part of the vestibulocerebellum, is responsible for matching the saccadic pulse and step appropriately and for stabilizing images on the fovea. It adjusts the output of the NI and participates in long-term adaptive processing to ensure that eye movements remain appropriate to the stimulus. For example, the amplitude (gain) and even the direction of the slow phases of the VOR are adjusted by the flocculus. Lesions of the flocculus result in gaze-holding deficits such as gaze-evoked, rebound, and downbeat nystagmus. Floccular lesions also impair smooth pursuit, cancellation (suppression) of the VOR by the pursuit system during combined head and eye tracking, and the ability to suppress nystagmus (and vertigo) by fixation. The nodulus, also part of the vestibulocerebellum, influences vestibular eye movements and vestibular optokinetic interaction. Lesions of the nodulus in monkeys and humans produce PAN.

Vergence Eye Movements

In humans and other animals capable of binocular fusional vision, dysconjugate (vergence) eye movements are necessary to maintain ocular alignment on an approaching or retreating object (convergence and divergence, respectively). Electromyography demonstrates that divergence is an active movement, although not as dynamic or as much under voluntary control as convergence. The principal driving stimuli for vergence movements, relayed from the occipital cortex, are accommodative retinal blur (unfocused) and fusional disparity (diplopia). Each of these stimuli can operate independently. Also, during convergence, each eye extorts (more so in downgaze) to facilitate stereoscopic perception (Brodsky, 2002). In addition, the pupils change size synkinetically as part of the near reflex to increase the depth of field and sharpen the focus of the optical system.

Although the precise locations of the convergence and divergence centers are unknown, important areas include the paramedian thalamus, the midbrain pretectum, the nucleus reticularis tegmenti pontis (NRTP), and the dorsal vermis. A group of neurons just lateral to the third cranial nerve nuclear complex fire in relation to the angle of convergence. Lesions to the pretectal region cause accommodative and vergence abnormalities (Ohtsuka et al., 2002). Lesions to the dorsal cerebellar vermis cause small-angle esodeviations in primates (Takagi et al., 2003). The NRTP is contiguous with the PPRF and forms part of a feedback loop by relaying visual information to the cerebellum via a cerebropontocerebellar pathway; the NRTP may also function as a vergence integrator. Experimental lesions of the NRTP in monkeys can cause sustained convergence or pendular convergence-divergence oscillations.

Unilateral stimulation of areas 19 and 22 of the preoccipital cortex caused bilateral convergence, accommodation, and miosis in macaque monkeys. The occipitomesencephalic pathway, involved in vergence, travels more ventrally in the diencephalon and midbrain than does the light reflex pathway and is less susceptible to compression by extrinsic lesions (dorsal midbrain syndrome) (see Chapter 19).

Vertical Eye Movements

The pathways involved in controlling vertical gaze are not fully known, and some of the neural connections discussed here are speculative. The third and fourth cranial nerves innervate the extraocular muscles responsible for both vertical and torsional eye movements. The premotor substrate for vertical and torsional eye movements lies in the midbrain reticular formation (MRF), but some vertical saccades are programmed in the PPRF and relayed to the MRF via a juxta-MLF pathway, presumably to coordinate horizontal, vertical, and oblique trajectories as well as head movement. Lesions of the PPRF can impair both horizontal and vertical saccades and cause a pseudo-PSP syndrome (see Supranuclear Gaze Disturbances). The rostral interstitial nucleus of the medial longitudinal fasciculus (riMLF) on each side contains EBNs for both upward and downward saccades but only for ipsilateral torsional saccades. The EBNs for upward saccades are probably caudal, ventral, and medial in the riMLF and project to the elevator muscles (superior rectus and inferior oblique) bilaterally, with axons crossing within the oculomotor nucleus (**Fig. 35.27, *A***) and not in the posterior commissure (PC) as previously thought (Bhidayasiri et al., 2000). The EBNs for downward saccades are more rostral, dorsal, and lateral in the riMLF and

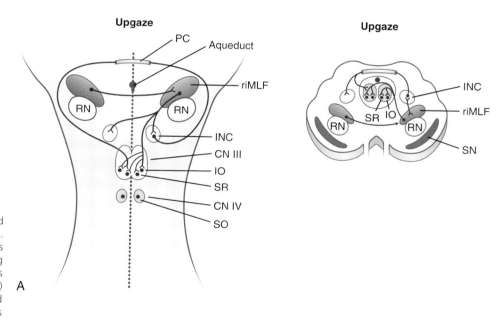

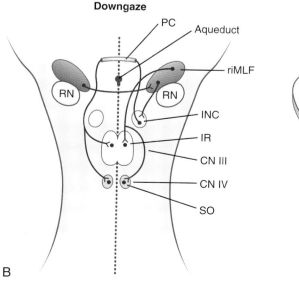

Fig. 35.27 Hypothetical pathways involved in controlling vertical eye movements. **A,** Upward eye movements. Burst neurons for upward saccades are shown projecting from the medial rostral interstitial nucleus of the medial longitudinal fasciculus (riMLF) to the elevator muscles, superior recti and inferior obliques bilaterally, with axons crossing within the oculomotor nucleus. **B,** Burst neurons for downward saccades are shown projecting only to the ipsilateral depressor muscles, the inferior rectus and superior oblique. The axons of the burst neurons for upward saccades also project to the interstitial nucleus of Cajal (INC), which plays a role in neural integration for vertical and torsional gaze. From the INC, the axons project dorsally and laterally to cross in the posterior commissure before turning ventrally to the oculomotor and trochlear nerve nuclei. *CN III,* Third nerve nuclear complex; *CN IV,* fourth nerve nucleus; *IO,* inferior oblique subnucleus; *IR,* inferior rectus subnucleus; *PC,* posterior commissure; *RN,* red nucleus; *SN,* substantia nigra; *SO,* superior oblique nucleus; *SR,* superior rectus subnucleus. *(Redrawn from Bhidayasiri, R., Plant, G.T., Leigh, R.J., 2000. A hypothetical scheme for the brainstem control of vertical gaze. Neurology 54, 1985-1993.)*

project only to the ipsilateral depressor muscles (inferior rectus and superior oblique) (see **Fig. 35.27, B**). The EBNs for vertical saccades also project to the interstitial nucleus of Cajal (INC), which plays a major role in neural integration for vertical and torsional gaze (Bhidayasiri et al., 2000). From the INC, the pathways project dorsally and laterally to cross in the PC before turning ventrally to the oculomotor and trochlear nerve nuclei (see **Fig. 35.27**). The axons to the elevator muscles travel more dorsally and thus are more susceptible to extrinsic compression, such as from a pinealoma.

Although the riMLF is key for vertical saccades, the MRF also has a role because of its reciprocal connections with the SC. Each riMLF also receives input from the nucleus of the posterior commissure, the FEF, the SC, the fastigial nucleus of the cerebellum, and the contralateral riMLF; the latter fibers cross in a commissure ventral to the aqueduct (see **Fig. 35.27**). Each riMLF is supplied by a branch of the proximal posterior cerebral artery, the posterior thalamosubthalamic paramedian artery; sometimes a single anomalous posterior thalamosubthalamic paramedian artery, called the *artery of Percheron*, supplies both riMLFs. Vertical saccades require bilateral supranuclear innervation from the FEF or SC, or both.

The NI for vertical and torsional eye movements (Leigh and Zee, 2006) is located in the INC. Burst-tonic and tonic neurons in the region of the INC discharge in relation to vertical eye position and play a role in vertical pursuit and eye position. These neurons project to the contralateral INC and the ocular motor nuclei via the PC, which plays a critical role in vertical gaze (**Fig. 35.28**). Injury to the PC limits all types of vertical

eye movements, particularly upward movements, although the vertical VORs and Bell phenomenon may be relatively spared.

Retinal slip, the sensory stimulus for vertical pursuit, is encoded by the dorsolateral pontine nuclei and relayed to the flocculus and posterior vermis before converging, via the INC, on the midbrain (see **Figs. 35.26 and 35.27**). The commands for vertical pursuit pass through the pons and cerebellum before turning rostrally to reach the relevant ocular motor neurons in the midbrain.

Development of the Ocular Motor System

At birth, the vestibular system is the most developed of the ocular motor subsystems and is easily tested by rotating the infant, held at arm's length, with the head tilted 30 degrees forward. In normal neonates, the eyes tonically deviate in the same direction as head movement; reflex saccades develop by 2 to 3 weeks after birth. Smooth-pursuit movements may be detected in neonates but only with large targets (such as a human face) at low velocities. These findings, although not well quantified, are consistent with histological maturation of the fovea after at least 8 weeks of age. Also, neonates can generate the smooth-pursuit component of OKN with full-field stimulation.

Fixation is not well developed until about 2 months, although some infants younger than 1 month of age can fixate targets, provided the stimuli are engaging and the infant is alert. By 9 weeks, 90% of full-term infants can fixate and follow the human face. Full-field OKN and larger targets stimulate the parafoveal retina, which matures earlier than the fovea. Stimulation of the saccadic system, also immature in the neonate, is influenced by the infant's attention as well as by the size and appropriateness of the target. Vertical saccades mature more slowly than horizontal saccades and may not be detected for the first month after birth. Vergence movements are also slow to mature but are seen after about the first month.

Ocular alignment in the newborn is usually poor, with transient shifts from esotropia to exotropia during the first few weeks. Ocular alignment depends on both visual input and the maturity of the vergence system. In most infants, ocular alignment is established by 3 to 4 weeks of age but may be delayed as late as 5 months. Small-angle esotropia and intermittent esotropia may spontaneously resolve in infants younger than 20 weeks of age; constant esotropia greater than 40 prism diopters is unlikely to resolve spontaneously. Esotropia after 3 months and exotropia after 5 months are considered abnormal and require appropriate evaluation. Large-angle exotropia may be associated with craniofacial, genetic, or other neurological abnormalities.

Paroxysmal phenomena are common in infancy and may occur in as many as one in four (Reerink et al., 1995). Ocular motor anomalies may occur in the neonate without any pathological significance. About 2% of newborns have a tendency for tonic downward deviation of the eyes in the waking state; during sleep, however, the eyes assume the normal position, and the VORs are intact. Other uncommon abnormalities seen in newborns include opsoclonus, which may regress through a phase of ocular flutter, skew deviation,

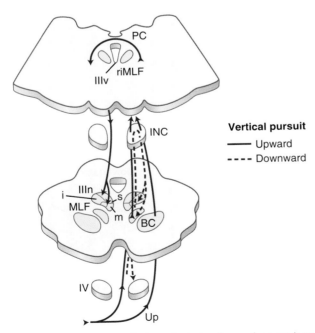

Fig. 35.28 Vertical pursuit. The hypothetical pathways for pursuit reach the midbrain via the dorsal lateral pontine nuclei and travel upward in the brachium conjunctivum (BC) and the medial longitudinal fasciculus (MLF). The interstitial nucleus of Cajal (INC) is involved in pursuit and may also be the neural integrator for vertical position commands. *(Reprinted with permission from Ranalli, P.J., Sharpe, J.A., Fletcher, W.A., 1998. Palsy of upward and downward saccadic, pursuit, and vestibular movements with a unilateral midbrain lesion: pathophysiological correlations. Neurology 38, 114-123.)*

apparent bilateral internuclear ophthalmoplegia, transient downbeat nystagmus, and tonic upward deviation. These findings likely represent delayed maturity of the ocular motor system in neonates.

Supranuclear Gaze Disturbances

Interruption of the saccadic and pursuit pathways before they reach the eye-movement generators in the MRF and PPRF results in a loss of voluntary eye movements but relatively spares reflex movements such as the VOR, optokinetic response, and the Bell phenomenon. This constellation of findings is referred to as a *supranuclear gaze palsy* and occurs classically in progressive supranuclear palsy (PSP) as well as a variety of disorders listed in **Table 35.7**.

A *pseudo-PSP syndrome*, characterized by a selective saccadic palsy (sometimes associated with ataxia, dysarthria, and dysphagia) that progresses over several months can follow aortic or cardiac surgery under hypothermic circulatory arrest. It has the appearance of a supranuclear gaze palsy caused by hemispheric infarction, but injury to the EBNs in the PPRF is more likely (Bernat et al., 2004; Leigh and Tomsak 2004; Mokri et al., 2004). The delayed progression of this syndrome remains unexplained but may represent a form of decelerated apoptosis. Also, a partially treatable PSP-like syndrome can occur in the *stiff person syndrome* (Oskarsson et al., 2008).

Technically, skew deviation and the ocular tilt reaction (OTR), which spare the final common efferent pathway for eye movements, are also supranuclear, but because they are dysconjugate, they are referred to here as *prenuclear*.

Bilateral lesions of the frontomesencephalic pathways cause loss of horizontal saccades in both directions and impair vertical saccades (particularly upward) but spare pursuit, VORs, and the slow phases of OKN. Also, focal lesions in the PPRF can cause selective saccadic defects (see Horizontal Eye Movements).

To evaluate disorders of gaze, first determine the range of versions (conjugate eye movements) to a slowly moving target, and then test saccades as described earlier. If a dysconjugate defect is observed, check ductions, ocular alignment, and comitance. If a conjugate defect (i.e., a gaze palsy) is present, determine whether the eyes move reflexively by testing for the oculocephalic reflex (doll's eye maneuver) or VOR (calorics) and the Bell phenomenon (ocular deviation, usually upward, on forced eyelid closure); their presence indicates supranuclear dysfunction. With supranuclear gaze disorders, saccades may be impaired first, then pursuit, followed by loss of VORs. Causes of gaze palsies and ophthalmoplegias are outlined in **Table 35.21**.

Ocular Motor Apraxia

Ocular motor apraxia is the inability to perform voluntary saccades while spontaneous saccades and reflex eye movements (vestibular and OKN slow phases) are preserved. Sometimes the term is used loosely and incorrectly (see later discussion).

Congenital ocular motor apraxia (COMA) is more common in boys than in girls and is characterized by impaired voluntary horizontal pursuit and saccadic movements but preservation of vertical eye movements (Leigh and Zee, 2006); reflex saccades may be partly retained. Because random eye movements also are absent in many of these children, the term *apraxia* is strictly incorrect; *congenital saccadic palsy* or *congenital gaze palsy* is more accurate (Leigh et al., 1997), but the term *COMA* is now established in the literature. By 4 to 8 months of age, the child develops a thrusting head movement strategy, often with prominent blinking, to overcome the eye movement deficit. Because the VOR prevents a change in direction of gaze on head turning, the child closes the eyes to reduce the degree of reflex eye movement (the gain of the VOR falls with the eyes closed) while thrusting the head beyond the range of the VOR arc to bring the eyes in line with the target. Then, with the eyes open, the child slowly straightens the head while the contralateral VOR maintains fixation. Some patients may use the dynamic head thrust to facilitate saccadic eye movements or reflexively to induce fast phases of vestibular nystagmus.

Because children with COMA cannot easily refixate or pursue new targets, particularly in the first 6 months of life, before they develop the head thrusting strategy, they are sometimes misdiagnosed as being blind. After 6 months of age, children with COMA present because of the head thrusts. The diagnosis of COMA can be confirmed by demonstrating the inability to make saccades; this is most easily done by spinning the infant, as described in Development of the Ocular Motor System. In normal infants, the eyes tonically deviate in the same direction as head movement; persistent absence of reflex saccades (fast phases in the opposite direction) after 2 to 3 weeks of age is abnormal and indicates saccadic palsy.

As children with COMA reach school age, pursuit and voluntary saccades variably improve. However, the condition does not completely resolve and can be detected in adulthood. COMA may be associated with structural abnormalities (**Box 35.16**) and occasionally strabismus, psychomotor developmental delay (particularly reading and expressive language ability), clumsiness, and gait disturbances. COMA may be familial.

Similar ocular motor findings, better described as intermittent saccade failure rather than true apraxia, are found in a variety of disorders listed in **Box 35.16**. In most patients (about 75%), saccadic failure indicates CNS involvement rather than specific diagnoses. Saccadic failure is a constant feature of COMA, whereas head thrusts are detected only in about half the patients (Harris et al., 1996).

Congenital vertical ocular motor apraxia is rare and must be differentiated from metabolic and degenerative disorders that cause progressive neurological dysfunction (e.g., neurovisceral lipidosis) and from stable disorders such as birth injury, perinatal hypoxia, and Leber congenital amaurosis.

Acquired ocular motor apraxia occurs in patients with bilateral parietal damage and with diffuse bilateral cerebral disease (see **Table 35.21**); the head thrusts are not as conspicuous as in the congenital variety.

Early-Onset Ataxia with Ocular Motor Apraxia and Hypoalbuminemia

Early-onset ataxia with ocular motor apraxia and hypoalbuminemia (EAOH), an autosomal recessive disorder described in Japanese families, presents in childhood and is associated

Table 35.7   **Causes of Ophthalmoplegias and Gaze Palsies***

Site	Disorder

Muscle	Ocular myopathies:
	  Congenital myopathy:
	    Central core
	    Centronuclear (myotubular)
	    Fiber-type disproportion
	    Multicore (ptosis, spares EOM)
	    Nemaline
	    Neurocristopathy (EOM fibrosis)
	    Oculopharyngodistal myopathy (Satoyoshi myopathy) (Mastaglias and Laing, 1999)
	    Autosomal dominant
	    Autosomal recessive
	    Reducing body myopathy (ptosis, spares EOM)
	  Dystrophy:
	    Myotonic dystrophy (ptosis, usually spares EOM)
	    Oculopharyngeal dystrophy
	  Inflammatory:
	    Dermatomyositis
	    GCA
	    Idiopathic orbital inflammatory syndrome (orbital pseudotumor)
	  Metabolic and toxic (act at multiple sites, e.g., anticonvulsants)
	  Mitochondrial cytopathy:
	    Kearn-Sayre syndrome
	    CPEO
	    CPEO-like syndrome: mitochondrial toxicity in long-standing AIDS and long exposure to HAART (Pfeffer et al., 2009)
	    Pearson syndrome
	    POLIP syndrome (*p*olyneuropathy, *o*phthalmoplegia, *l*eukoencephalopathy, *i*ntestinal *p*seudo-obstruction)
	    High myopia (large globes cause mechanical restriction)
	    Infiltrative disorders (thyroid, amyloid, metastases, congenital familial fibrosis, cystinosis)
	    Trauma (orbital entrapment)
	    Vitamin E deficiency (associated with malabsorption)

Neuromuscular junction	MG Toxins (e.g., botulism, cosmetic botulinum toxin, organophosphates) Lambert-Eaton syndrome (rarely affects EOM, mainly causes ptosis)
Ocular motor nerves	See Chapter 70

Gaze palsies	Nuclear and paranuclear:
	  Brainstem injury (vascular, MS, encephalitis, paraneoplastic, toxins, tumor)
	  Familial congenital gaze palsy
	  Glycine encephalopathy (nonketotic hyperglycinemia: hiccups, seizures, apneic spells)
	  Machado-Joseph disease (SCA3)
	  Leigh disease
	  Maple syrup urine disease
	  Möbius and Duane syndromes (agenesis of cranial nerve nuclei)
	  PERM, a variant of the stiff person syndrome (Hutchinson et al., 2008)
	  Raised ICP (pseudotumor cerebri, idiopathic ICP hypertension, cerebral venous sinus thrombosis); the precise location is unknown (Friedman et al., 1998)
	  Spinocerebellar degeneration
	  Tangier disease
	  Vitamin E deficiency
	  INO
	  One-and-a-half syndrome:
	Prenuclear:
	  Monocular "supranuclear" elevator palsy
	  OTR
	  Skew deviation
	  Vertical one-and-a-half syndrome
	Supranuclear (predominantly horizontal):
	  Congenital ocular motor apraxia or congenital saccadic palsy
	  Acutely, after hemispheric stroke:
	    Ipsiversive
	    Contraversive (wrong-way eyes)
	  Gaucher disease (types 2 and 3):
	  Ictal (transient, adversive)
	  Juvenile-onset GM_2 gangliosidosis (mimics juvenile SMA)
	  Postictal (transient, ipsiversive)
	  Paraneoplastic (prostatic adenocarcinoma)

Table 35.7	Causes of Ophthalmoplegias and Gaze Palsies—cont'd
Site	**Disorder**

Site	Disorder
	Supranuclear (predominantly vertical):
	Adult-onset GM$_2$ gangliosidosis (mimics MSA or spinocerebellar degeneration) (V>H)
	Congenital vertical ocular motor apraxia (rare)
	ALS (rare, V>H)
	Autosomal dominant parkinsonian-dementia complex with pallidopontonigral degeneration (dementia, dystonia, frontal and pyramidal signs, urinary incontinence)
	Vitamin B$_{12}$ deficiency (U>D)
	Cerebral amyloid angiopathy with leukoencephalopathy
	Dentatorubral-pallidoluysian atrophy (autosomal dominant, dementia, ataxia, myoclonus, choreoathetosis)
	Diffuse Lewy body disease (ophthalmoplegia may be global)
	Dorsal midbrain syndrome
	Familial Creutzfeldt-Jakob disease (U>D)
	Familial paralysis of vertical gaze
	Fisher syndrome
	Gerstmann-Sträussler-Scheinker disease (U>D, dysmetria, nystagmus)
	Guamanian Parkinson disease-dementia complex (Lytico-Bodig disease)
	HARP syndrome (*h*ypoprebetalipoproteinemia, *a*canthocytosis, *r*etinitis pigmentosa, *p*allidal degeneration)
	Hydrocephalus (untreated, decompensated shunt)
	Joseph disease
	Kernicterus (U>D)
	Late-onset cerebellopontomesencephalic degeneration (D>U)
	Neurovisceral lipidosis; synonyms: DAF syndrome (*d*owngaze palsy-*a*taxia-*f*oamy macrophages); dystonic lipidosis; Niemann-Pick disease type C (initially loss of downgaze, may become global)
	Pallidoluysian atrophy (dysarthria, dystonia, bradykinesia)
	Paraneoplastic disorders
	PSP (D>U)
	Stiff person syndrome (Oskarsson et al., 2008)
	Subcortical gliosis (U>D)
	Variant Creutzfeld-Jakob disease (U>D)
	WD (also slow horizontal saccades) (U>D)
	Supranuclear (global):
	Abetalipoproteinemia
	AIDS encephalopathy
	AD (pursuit)
	Cerebral adrenoleukodystrophy
	Corticobasal ganglionic degeneration
	Fahr disease (idiopathic striatopallidodentate calcification)
	Gaucher disease
	Hexosaminidase A deficiency
	HD
	Joubert syndrome
	Leigh disease (infantile striatonigral degeneration)
	Methylmalonohomocystinuria
	Malignant neuroleptic syndrome (personal observation)
	Neurosyphilis
	Opportunistic infections
	Paraneoplastic disorders
	PD (transient gaze palsy with intercurrent infection)
	Pelizaeus-Merzbacher disease (H>V)
	Pick disease (impaired saccades)
	Progressive multifocal leukoencephalopathy
	Pseudo-PSP, a selective saccadic palsy, associated with progressive ataxia, dysarthria, and dysphagia over several months following aortic/cardiac surgery under hypothermic circulatory arrest
	Stiff person syndrome-late (Oskarsson et al., 2008)
	Tay-Sachs disease (infantile GM$_2$ gangliosidosis) (V>H)
	Wernicke encephalopathy
	Whipple disease (V>H)
	X-linked dystonia-parkinsonism (Lubag disease)

AD, Alzheimer disease; *AIDS,* acquired immunodeficiency syndrome; *ALS,* amyotrophic lateral sclerosis; *CPED,* chronic progressive external ophthalmoplegia; *D,* loss of downgaze; *EOM,* extraocular muscles; *GCA,* giant cell arteritis; *global,* loss of horizontal and vertical gaze; *H,* loss of horizontal gaze; *HAART,* highly active antiretroviral therapy; *HD,* Huntington disease; *ICP,* intracranial pressure; *INO,* internuclear ophthalmoplegia; *MG,* myasthenia gravis; *MS,* multiple sclerosis; *MSA,* multiple system atrophy; *OTR,* occular tilt reaction; *PD,* Parkinson disease; *PERM,* progressive encephalomyelitis with rigidity and myoclonus; *PSP,* progressive supranuclear palsy; *SMA,* spinal muscular atrophy; *U,* loss of upgaze; *V,* loss of vertical gaze; *WD,* Wilson disease.

*See also Boxes 35.8 and 35.9.

Box 35.16 Disorders Associated with Ocular Motor Apraxia or Saccadic Palsy

- Aplasia or hypoplasia of the corpus callosum
- Aplasia or hypoplasia of the cerebellar vermis (up to 53% of patients) (Sargent et al., 1997)
- Ataxia with "ocular motor" apraxia type I syndrome
- Aicardi syndrome
- Ataxia telangiectasia
- Autosomal recessive AOA associated with axonal peripheral neuropathy, areflexia, and pes cavus (Barbot et al., 2001) (may be the same as EOAH)
- Bardet-Biedl syndrome
- Bilateral cortical lesions
- Birth injuries (see perinatal/postnatal disorders)
- Carbohydrate-deficient glycoprotein syndrome type Ia (Stark et al., 2000)
- Carotid fibromuscular hypoplasia
- COMA (occasionally may be familial)
- Congenital vertical ocular motor apraxia (rare)
- Cornelia de Lange syndrome
- Cockayne syndrome
- Dandy-Walker malformation
- EOAH (Shimazaki et al., 2002) may be the same disorder as AOA
- GM1 gangliosidosis
- Infantile Gaucher disease
- Infantile Refsum disease
- Hydrocephalus
- Joubert syndrome
- Krabbe leukodystrophy
- Leber congenital amaurosis
- Microcephaly
- Megalocephaly
- Microphthalmos
- Neurovisceral lipidosis
- Occipital porencephalic cysts
- Pelizaeus-Merzbacher disease
- Perinatal and postnatal disorders (hypoxia, meningitis, PV leukomalacia, athetoid cerebral palsy, perinatal septicemia and anemia, herpes encephalitis, epilepsy)
- Propionic acidemia
- Succinic semialdehyde dehydrogenase deficiency
- Wieacker syndrome

From Harris, C.M., Shawkat, F., Russell-Eggitt, I., et al., 1996. Intermittent horizontal saccade failure ('ocular motor apraxia') in children. Br J Ophthalmol 80, 151-158.
AOA, Ataxia with ocular motor apraxia; COMA, congenital ocular motor apraxia; EOAH, early-onset ataxia with ocular motor apraxia hypoalbuminemia; PV, periventricular.

with progressive ataxia with marked cerebellar atrophy on imaging, horizontal and vertical ocular motor apraxia, a peripheral neuropathy with early areflexia and late distal wasting and weakness, and hypoalbuminemia. Some patients have foot deformities, kyphoscoliosis, choreiform movements, facial grimacing, and exaggerated blinking (perhaps in an attempt to initiate saccades). When the condition is advanced, external ophthalmoplegia can mask the saccadic failure. This

disorder is associated with hypercholesterolemia and mimics Friedreich ataxia; patients with EAOH have ocular motor apraxia, chorea, and intention tremor (Shimazaki et al., 2002) but not extensor plantar responses or cardiomyopathy. Leg edema correlates with the degree of albumen; the *pseudo*hypercholesterolemia resolves with replacement of albumen. EAOH is likely a variant of autosomal recessive ataxia with ocular motor apraxia (AOA), described next. Both disorders have missense mutations in the aprataxin (APTX) gene.

Autosomal Recessive Ataxia with Ocular Motor Apraxia

Ataxia with ocular motor apraxia, an autosomal recessive disorder described in Portuguese families, presents in early childhood and is associated with cerebellar ataxia, horizontal and vertical ocular motor apraxia, and very early areflexia that later progresses to a full-blown axonal neuropathy (Barbot et al., 2001). Some patients have pes cavus, scoliosis, dystonia, and optic atrophy. In advanced cases, external ophthalmoplegia can mask the saccadic failure, as in EAOH. AOA resembles ataxia telangiectasia but without the telangiectasia, developmental delay, and immune dysfunction. It is very similar to ataxia with ocular motor apraxia type 1 (AOA1) syndrome.

Ataxia with Ocular Motor Apraxia Type 1 Syndrome

Ataxia with ocular motor apraxia type 1, a late-onset autosomal recessive neurodegenerative form with progressive ataxia and peripheral neuropathy, can mimic ataxia telangiectasia, without the extraneurological features (Criscuolo et al., 2004; Gascon et al., 1995). It is associated with mutations of the APTX gene. Also, ocular motor apraxia was reported in a patient with spasmus nutans and cerebellar vermian hypoplasia (Kim et al., 2003).

Ataxia with Ocular Apraxia Type 2

Ataxia with ocular apraxia type 2 (AOA2), a juvenile-onset autosomal recessive disorder, is a slowly progressive cerebellar ataxia characterized by cerebellar atrophy and a sensory-motor neuropathy. Almost all patients have elevated serum alpha-fetoprotein levels, but ocular motor apraxia is observed in only 47% of patients (Asaka et al., 2006). Thus the disease name, AOA2, could be misleading. The responsible gene (SETX) maps to chromosome 9q34.

Spasm of Fixation

Spasm of fixation, a term introduced by Gordon Holmes in 1930, describes patients who have difficulty shifting visual attention because of impaired initiation of voluntary saccades when looking at a fixation target, but normal initiation of saccades in the absence of such a target or when it is removed. Their saccades have a prolonged latency and may be hypometric in the presence of a central visual target; however, blinks or combined eye and head movements may sometimes facilitate normal saccades. Holmes stressed that fixation was an active process and attributed spasm of fixation to "exaggerated" fixation; evidence from other studies supports this concept.

The lesions that cause spasm of fixation may be bihemispheric and interrupt indirect FEF projections via the caudate nucleus and SNr to the SC. Normally, during saccades to auditory, visual, and remembered targets, neurons in the FEFs discharge via these pathways and disinhibit the SC to allow the saccades and disengage fixation. Interruption of these and perhaps other pathways might contribute to spasm of fixation by maintaining tonic inhibitory suppression of saccades by the SC (Leigh and Zee, 2006).

Familial Horizontal Gaze Palsy

Familial horizontal gaze palsy with scoliosis (HGPS) is an autosomal recessive disorder characterized by paralysis of horizontal gaze from birth and impaired OKN and VORs but intact convergence, vertical eye movements, and progressive scoliosis (Leigh and Zee, 2006). HGPS maps to chromosome 11q23-25 in some kindreds (Jen et al., 2002). Types of nystagmus described in HGPS include a fine pendular horizontal nystagmus, upbeat nystagmus, and see-saw nystagmus (Pieh et al., 2002). Individuals in some families may have facial myokymia, facial twitching, hemifacial atrophy, and situs inversus of the optic disks. Neuroimaging may demonstrate brainstem dysplasia, particularly pontine hypoplasia (Pieh et al., 2002). HGPS is one of a spectrum of disorders of maldevelopment of cranial nerve nuclei that include Duane syndrome, Möbius syndrome (Verzijl et al., 2003), the congenital syndromes of fibrosis of the extraocular muscles, and congenital ptosis (Engle and Leigh, 2002).

Acquired Horizontal Gaze Palsy

Transient gaze deviation, usually of the head and eyes, occurs in about 20% of patients with acute hemisphere stroke and other insults. Because of gaze paresis to the hemiplegic side (i.e., paralyses of gaze and limbs are on the same side) the eyes are deviated towards the side of the lesion (ipsiversive gaze deviation) and may be seen on imaging studies performed at presentation (Simon et al., 2003). In stroke patients, right-sided lesions are more common but smaller; consequently, patients with left-sided lesions (gaze deviation to the left) have a worse prognosis. Ipsiversive gaze deviation occurs more often when the inferior parietal lobule (IPL) or circuits between the FEFs and the IPL or their projections to the brainstem (SC or PPRF) are involved; the FEFs are usually spared. After about 5 days, the intact hemisphere, which contains neurons for bilateral gaze, takes over. Thereafter, subtle abnormalities such as prolonged saccadic latencies and impaired saccadic suppression can be detected only by quantitative oculography.

Because the premotor neural network for voluntary horizontal eye movements in the PPRF is composed of subclasses of neurons with different functions, selective lesions may affect some types of eye movement while sparing others (see Horizontal Eye Movements).

A lesion affecting the ipsilateral abducens nucleus or PPRF causes ipsilateral gaze palsy; a rostral PPRF lesion spares the VOR, whereas a caudal lesion does not.

Horizontal gaze palsies can occur with a variant of the stiff person syndrome, progressive encephalomyelitis with rigidity and myoclonus (PERM), that is responsive to immunotherapy

(Hutchinson et al., 2008) and is similar to paraneoplastic brainstem disorders.

Paraneoplastic brainstem encephalitis can cause supranuclear, internuclear, or nuclear damage, resulting in selective loss of voluntary horizontal and vertical saccades (Crino et al., 1996). Patients with prostatic adenocarcinoma may, after an interval of 3 to 4 years, develop paraneoplastic gaze palsies followed by severe facial and bulbar muscle spasms (probable sustained myoclonus), diplopia, and respiratory insufficiency. Other neurological features that may be associated with such paraneoplastic disorders include ataxia, hyperacusis, muscle spasms, myoclonus, periodic alternating gaze deviation (PAGD), and vertigo. MRI is often unrevealing, particularly in the early stages, but auditory evoked potentials and cerebrospinal fluid analysis may be abnormal. Clonazepam, valproic acid, and botulinum may help the myoclonus and muscle spasms.

Other causes of horizontal gaze palsies are listed in **Table 35.7**.

Wrong-Way Eyes

Conjugate eye deviation to the "wrong" side—that is, away from the lesion and toward the hemiplegia (contraversive gaze deviation)—may occur with supratentorial lesions, particularly thalamic hemorrhage and (rarely) large perisylvian or lobar hemorrhage. The mechanism is unclear, but possibilities include the following:

1. An irritative or seizure focus causing "contraversive ocular deviation" is unlikely, because neither clinical nor electrical seizure activity has been reported in these patients.
2. Because eye movements are represented bilaterally in each frontal lobe, it is conceivable that the center for ipsilateral gaze alone may be damaged, resulting in contraversive ocular deviation.
3. An irritative lesion of the intralaminar thalamic neurons, which discharge for contralateral saccades, could theoretically cause contraversive ocular deviation.
4. Damage to the contralateral inhibitory center could also be responsible.

Postictal "paralytic" conjugate ocular deviation occurs after adversive seizures as part of Todd paresis.

Spasticity of conjugate gaze (lateral deviation of both eyes away from the lesion) during forced eyelid closure, a variant of the Bell phenomenon, can occur in patients with large, deep parietotemporal lesions; eye movements are otherwise normal except for ipsilateral saccadic pursuit.

Psychogenic ocular deviation can occur in patients feigning unconsciousness; the eyes are directed toward the ground irrespective of which way the patient is turned.

Periodic Alternating Gaze Deviation

Periodic alternating gaze deviation (PAGD) is a rare cyclical ocular motor disorder in which the direction of gaze alternates every few minutes. Lateral deviation can be sustained for up to 15 minutes; gaze then returns to the midline for 10 to 20 seconds before changing to the other side. Occasionally, PAGD is associated with structural lesions such as pontine vascular disorders; Chiari malformations; congenital absence or abnormalities of the inferior cerebellar vermis, the uvula, and nodulus; Creutzfeldt-Jakob disease involving the flocculonodular lobe; spinocerebellar degeneration; occipital encephaloceles; and paraneoplastic brainstem encephalitis. A reversible form of PAGD occurs with hepatic encephalopathy and is attributed to derangement of GABA metabolism (Averbuch-Heller and Meiner, 1995).

Periodic alternating nystagmus (PAN) has a similar time cycle to PAGD and also results from lesions of the uvular and nodular regions. Indeed, PAGD may be PAN with loss of corrective saccades because of concomitant saccadic palsy or immaturity of the saccadic system in infants.

Other cyclical ocular motor phenomena, including cyclical esotropia, cyclical ocular motor palsy, springing pupil, alternating skew deviation, and PAN, are discussed in the appropriate sections.

Ping-Pong Gaze

Ping-pong gaze is a slow conjugate horizontal rhythmic oscillation that cycles every 4 to 8 seconds (short-cycle PAGD) and occurs in comatose patients as a result of bilateral cerebral or upper brainstem lesions or metabolic dysfunction; one patient had a vermian hemorrhage. The oscillations can be saccadic. Ping-pong gaze implies that the horizontal gaze centers in the pons are intact. Generally, the prognosis for recovery is poor except in patients with a toxic or metabolic cause (Johkura et al., 1998); occasionally, patients with structural lesions recover (Diesing and Wijdicks, 2004).

Saccadic Lateropulsion

Saccadic lateropulsion is characterized by hypermetric (overshoot) saccades (see **Fig. 35.18, B**) to the side of the lesion (ipsipulsion) and hypometric (undershoot) saccades (see **Fig. 35.18, C**) to the opposite side. In darkness or with the eyelids closed, the patient may have conjugate deviation toward the side of the lesion. Saccadic lateropulsion occurs with lesions of the lateral medulla (most commonly ischemic) involving cerebellar inflow (inferior cerebellar peduncle).

Saccadic lateropulsion with a bias away from the side of the lesion (contrapulsion) may occur with lesions involving the region of the superior cerebellar peduncle (outflow tract) and adjacent cerebellum (superior cerebellar artery territory).

Pulsion of vertical saccades with a parabolic trajectory occurs in patients with lateral medullary injury: both upward and downward saccades deviate toward the side of the lesion with corrective oblique saccades; whereas in those with lesions involving cerebellar outflow, vertical saccades deviate away from the side of the injury.

Torsional Saccades

Pathological rapid torsional eye deviation during voluntary saccades may occur with large lesions involving the midline cerebellum, deep cerebellar nuclei, and dorsolateral medulla. The amplitudes of these torsional saccades ("blips") are larger for ipsilesional (hypermetric) than for contralesional (hypometric) horizontal saccades. Eye movement recordings using a scleral search coil (see Eye Movement Recording Techniques)

demonstrated that the blips are followed by an exponentially slow torsional drift toward the initial torsional eye position. These blips may be a form of torsional saccadic dysmetria (Helmchen et al., 1997).

Slow Saccades

Saccades of low velocity result from pontine disease, presumably because of burst cell dysfunction. They occur in patients with olivopontocerebellar degeneration and other disorders listed in **Box 35.17**. Some patients with hypometric saccades (see **Fig. 35.18, C**) composed of multiple small-amplitude steps (as in myasthenia, Huntington disease, brainstem encephalitis, and striatonigral degeneration) appear to have slow saccades clinically (pseudoslow saccades), but each small saccade has a normal velocity-amplitude relationship.

Prolonged Saccadic Latency

Disorders of saccadic initiation, resulting in prolonged latencies for voluntary saccades, occur in patients with inattention, acquired immunodeficiency syndrome (AIDS)-dementia complex, and a variety of encephalopathies and degenerative disorders of the nervous system, such as Alzheimer disease, the frontotemporal dementias, HD, and PD.

Box 35.17 **Slow Saccades**

- AIDS dementia complex
- ALS
- Anticonvulsant toxicity (consciousness usually impaired)
- Ataxia-telangiectasia
- Brainstem encephalitis
- Hexosaminidase A deficiency
- HD
- INO (slow abduction)
- Joseph disease
- Kennedy disease (X-linked recessive progressive spinomuscular atrophy) (Thurtell et al., 2009)
- Lesions of the paramedian pontine reticular formation
- Lipid storage diseases
- Long-standing cholestasis (probable vitamin E deficiency)
- Lytico-Bodig disease (Guamanian ALS-PD-dementia complex)
- Myasthenia
- Myotonic dystrophy
- Nephropathic cystinosis
- Ocular motor apraxia
- Ocular motor nerve or muscle weakness
- Olivopontocerebellar degeneration (ADCA type I)
- PSP
- Pseudo-PSP
- Striatonigral degeneration
- Wernicke encephalopathy
- Whipple disease
- WD

ADCA, Autosomal dominant cerebellar ataxia; *AIDS,* acquired immunodeficiency syndrome; *ALS,* amyotrophic lateral sclerosis; *ALS-PD,* amyotrophic lateral sclerosis–Parkinson disease; *HD,* Huntington disease; *INO,* internuclear ophthalmoplegia; *PSP,* progressive supranuclear palsy; *WD,* Wilson disease.

Square-Wave Jerks

Square-wave jerks (SWJs) (**Box 35.18**) are spontaneous, small-amplitude, paired saccades with an intersaccadic latency of 150 to 200 msec that briefly interrupt fixation (**Fig. 35.29**). They may occur physiologically in normal subjects (particularly in darkness) without fixation and are usually about 2 degrees in amplitude. They are more common in the elderly and in carriers of blue-cone monochromatism. SWJs are prominent in PSP, multiple system atrophy (MSA), and cerebellar disease; the increased frequency of SWJs in these less dopamine-responsive parkinsonian syndromes (e.g., olivopontocerebellar atrophy [autosomal dominant cerebellar atrophy], PSP, Lewy body disease, MSA) may distinguish them from PD.

Because of the intersaccadic interval (latency), SWJs are thought to be triggered supratentorially, whereas other saccadic intrusions (e.g., saccadic pulses) and oscillations (e.g., flutter and opsoclonus) are caused by dysfunction of the pause cells in the brainstem.

Square-wave pulses (SWPs), previously termed *macrosquare-wave jerks*, also interrupt fixation but differ from SWJs having larger amplitudes (10 to 40 degrees) and shorter latencies (about 80 msec) before the eyes return to the target; they occur in patients with MS and olivopontocerebellar degeneration and may accompany rubral tremor. SWJs and SWPs should be distinguished from macrosaccadic oscillations, which wax and wane across fixation (see **Fig. 35.29**), are not present in darkness, and occur with midline cerebellar lesions.

Box 35.18 Square-Wave Jerks

- Normal subjects (<2 degrees)
- Excitement in normals
- Catecholamine depletion in normals
- Aging
- Carriers of blue-cone monochromatism
- Strabismus
- Congenital nystagmus
- Latent nystagmus
- Dyslexia (suppressed by methylphenidate)
- PSP
- Schizophrenia
- Cerebral hemisphere tumors and stroke
- PD; small SWJs may develop or increase after pallidotomy (Leigh and Zee, 2006)
- Wernicke encephalopathy
- Friedreich ataxia
- Joseph disease
- Gerstmann-Sträussler-Scheinker disease
- Lithium
- Tobacco
- AIDS-dementia complex (HIV encephalitis)
- Square-wave pulses (macro–square wave jerks)
- OPCA
- MS (cerebellar dysfunction)

AIDS, Acquired immunodeficiency syndrome; *HIV,* human immunodeficiency virus; *MS,* multiple sclerosis; *OPCA,* olivopontocerebellar astrophy; *PD,* Parkinson disease; *PSP,* progressive supranuclear palsy.

These and other saccadic oscillations are discussed in detail elsewhere (Dell'Osso and Daroff, 1999a, Chapter 11; Leigh and Zee, 2006, Chapter 10).

Internuclear Ophthalmoplegia

Damage to the MLF between the third and sixth cranial nerve nuclei impairs transmission of neural impulses to the ipsilateral medial rectus muscle (see **Fig. 35.22**). Adducting saccades of the ipsilateral eye are impaired (either slow or absent), depending on the severity of the lesion. Typically nystagmus-like movement of the abduction gives the appearance of dissociated nystagmus but is in fact overshoot dysmetria. Usually upward-beating and torsional nystagmus are present. Convergence may be preserved with an internuclear ophthalmoplegia (INO), but because the patient's attention and effort are necessary for its evaluation, it is not a particularly helpful sign. Patients with bilateral INO may be exotropic, designated the *wall-eyed bilateral INO* (WEBINO) *syndrome* (Komiyama et al., 1998), and have slow-abducting saccades because of impaired inhibition of tone in the medial recti. Other clinical features associated with unilateral INO include a partial contralateral OTR, manifest by skew deviation with ipsilateral hypertropia (Zwergal et al., 2008), and defective vertical smooth pursuit, OKN, and vertical VORs.

A subtle INO may be demonstrated by having the patient make repetitive horizontal saccades, which often discloses slow adduction of the ipsilateral eye. Alternatively, an optokinetic tape may be used to induce repetitive saccades in the direction of action of the suspected weak medial rectus muscle, by moving the tape in the opposite direction and observing for slower and smaller amplitude adducting saccades.

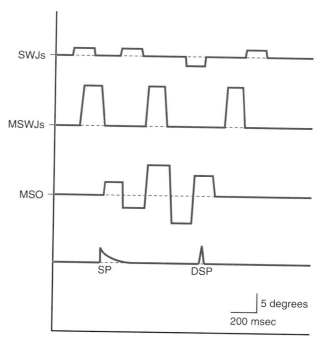

Fig. 35.29 Simulated eye movement recordings of square-wave jerks (SWJs), macrosquare-wave jerks, or square-wave pulses (MSWJs), macrosaccadic oscillations (MSOs), a saccadic pulse (SP), and a double saccadic pulse (DSP).

- Brainstem (pontine) stroke—unilateral
- MS—unilateral or bilateral
- Intrinsic tumor—primary or metastatic
- Meningitis (especially tuberculosis, also AIDS, brucellosis, cystercosis, syphilis) (Keane, 2005)
- Brainstem encephalitis (infective, inflammatory, lupus, paraneoplastic, sarcoid)
- Chemotherapy with radiation therapy
- Drug intoxication:
  Comatose—anticonvulsants, phenothiazines, tricyclics
  Awake—lithium
- Spinocerebellar degeneration
- Fabry disease (vascular)
- Herniation (epidural and acute and chronic subdural hemorrhage, cerebral hematoma) (Keane, 2005)
- Vascular malformations
- Vasculitis
- Wernicke encephalopathy
- PSP
- Syringobulbia associated with a Chiari malformation
- Trauma (closed head injury, neck/vertebral artery injury)
- Hexosaminidase A deficiency
- Kennedy disease (X-linked recessive progressive spinomuscular atrophy) (Thurtell et al., 2009)
- Maple syrup urine disease
- Cerebral air embolism
- Vitamin B_{12} deficiency
- Pseudointernuclear ophthalmoplegia
  - Long-standing exotropia
  - Myasthenia
  - Myotonic dystrophy
  - Neuromyotonia of the lateral rectus muscle
  - Partial palsy of cranial nerve III
  - Previous extraocular muscle surgery
  - Thyroid orbitopathy (lateral rectus restriction)
  - Orbital pseudotumor
  - Other infiltrative disorders of extraocular muscle (neoplasm, amyloid, etc.)
  - Miller-Fisher syndrome (sometimes may be a true ION)

AIDS, Acquired immunodeficiency syndrome; *ION,* internuclear ophthalmoplegia; *MS,* multiple sclerosis; *PSP,* progressive supranuclear palsy.

INO may occur with a variety of disorders (**Box 35.19**) affecting the brainstem (Keane, 2005; Leigh and Zee, 2006) and must be distinguished from the many (primarily peripheral) causes of pseudo-INO (see **Box 35.19**).

Rarely, patients with small lesions in the rostral pons or midbrain, remote from the abducens nerve and nucleus, may have a Lutz posterior INO. In this condition, abduction is impaired, but the adducting eye has nystagmus. The mechanism is due to impaired inhibition of the antagonist medial rectus muscle secondary to damage to uncrossed fibers from the PPRF to the oculomotor nucleus, running close to but separate from the MLF. Patients with type I Duane syndrome may have a similar appearance (pseudo-Lutz posterior INO),

with adducting "nystagmus" (really dysmetria) on attempted lateral gaze (personal observation).

One-and-a-Half Syndrome

The one-and-a-half syndrome is characterized by an ipsilateral gaze palsy with an ipsilateral INO due to a lesion in the caudal dorsal pontine tegmentum involving the ipsilateral PPRF or the abducens nucleus and the ipsilateral MLF (see **Fig. 35.22**) (Komiyama et al., 1998). Abduction of the contralateral eye is the only intact horizontal movement. Some patients have a contralateral OTR (Zwergal et al., 2008); those with facial nerve palsy may develop oculopalatal myoclonus later, probably because of the proximity of the central tegmental tract to the facial nerve fascicle (Wolin et al., 1996). Ocular myasthenia can cause a pseudo-one-and-a-half syndrome.

Disorders of Vertical Gaze

A variety of disorders of conjugate vertical gaze result from discretely placed lesions in the midbrain pretectal region (see **Fig. 35.27**). However, selective deficits of vertical gaze may be overlooked unless the examiner specifically tests for different types of eye movements, particularly saccades.

Paralysis of vertical saccades usually involves loss of downward saccades or combined upward and downward saccades and is often caused by bilateral ischemia of the riMLF. Selective paralysis of downward saccades may occur because the depressor muscles are innervated just unilaterally, whereas the elevator muscles are innervated bilaterally; thus partial riMLF lesions affect the depressor muscles disproportionately (Bhidayasiri et al., 2000).

A unilateral lesion in the midbrain tegmentum involving the riMLF can cause impairment of both upward and downward saccades by injuring ipsilateral burst cells, crossing fibers from the contralateral burst cells, and probably neighboring inhibitory pathways. Experimentally, a unilateral lesion confined to the riMLF should cause only a minimal defect in vertical saccades (mainly downward) unless it extends to involve adjacent structures such as the INC. However, such an isolated lesion causes loss of ipsilateral torsional saccades, detected by tilting the patient's head to the shoulder—that is, in the roll plane (Leigh and Zee, 2006). A lesion of the PC limits all types of vertical eye movements, particularly upgaze.

Upgaze paralysis occurs with lesions at or near the posterior commissure or with bilateral lesions in the pretectal area (see **Fig. 35.27, *A***).

Downgaze paralysis occurs with bilateral lesions of the riMLF or its projections, which course caudally and dorsally (see **Fig. 35.27, *B***). In humans, with the exception of occlusion of an anomalous posterior thalamosubthalamic paramedian artery of Percheron, such isolated lesions are rare (see Vertical Eye Movements). More commonly, bilateral involvement of the pathways for downgaze (as well as upgaze) occurs as a part of diffuse disorders such as PSP, Whipple disease, neurovisceral lipid storage disorders, and complications of AIDS (see **Table 35.7**).

Patients with impaired vertical gaze due to extrinsic compression of the posterior commissure or pretectal region are more likely to have pupillary light-near dissociation (loss of the pupillary light reflex but preservation of the near reflex), because the light reflex pathways are more superficial.

Intrinsic midbrain lesions cause impairment of convergence and accommodation (the near reflex) while sparing the light reflex. With supranuclear disorders of vertical gaze, saccades are impaired initially, followed by pursuit, and then by loss of vertical VORs. Paralysis of upgaze, light-near dissociation of the pupils, impaired convergence, lid retraction, and convergence-retraction nystagmus are features of the dorsal midbrain (Parinaud) pretectal syndrome (see Chapter 19), which occurs with injury to the PC or both INCs.

Disorders of vertical gaze (see **Table 35.7**), particularly downgaze and combined upgaze and downgaze paresis, may be overlooked in patients with brainstem vascular disease because of impaired consciousness as a result of concomitant damage to the reticular activating system.

Two forms of the vertical one-and-a-half syndrome occur with discrete lesions in the upper midbrain. One, which consists of bilateral upgaze palsy associated with monocular paresis of downward movement, can occur with either ipsilateral or contralateral thalamomesencephalic infarctions. The other consists of a downgaze palsy associated with monocular elevator paresis that can occur with bilateral mesodiencephalic lesions.

A crossed vertical gaze paresis, with supranuclear weakness of elevation of the contralateral eye and weakness of depression of the ipsilateral eye, may occur with a lesion involving the mesodiencephalic junction and medial thalamus (West et al., 1995).

Monocular elevator deficiency, also termed *monocular elevator palsy* or *double elevator palsy*, is characterized by limitation of elevation of one eye. The limitation is the same in both adduction and abduction, unlike Brown superior oblique tendon sheath syndrome, in which the limitation is predominantly in adduction. Monocular elevator deficiency can result from paretic or restrictive disorders of the extraocular muscles, such as muscle fibrosis, myositis, myasthenia, infiltrative disease (thyroid orbitopathy, neoplasia), orbital floor fractures, and fascicular lesions of the oculomotor nerve (Gauntt et al., 1995). Some cases may be supranuclear, particularly those with normal ocular alignment in primary position (see later discussion).

When monocular elevator deficiency is congenital or occurs early in life, it may be associated with abnormalities of convergence, amblyopia, a chin-up head position, and ptosis or pseudoptosis. (Pseudoptosis occurs when a patient with a hypotropic eye fixates with the other eye; the upper lid follows the hypotropic eye and appears ptotic. When the patient fixates with the hypotropic eye, the apparent ptosis disappears. Some patients may have both a true ptosis and a superimposed pseudoptosis.) Some congenital cases are supranuclear as a result of congenital unilateral midbrain lesions; when they are long-standing, inferior rectus restriction and fibrosis prevent reflex elevation of the eye (the Bell phenomenon). In those cases, primary orbital disorders such as myositis, thyroid orbitopathy, orbital floor fractures, and infiltrative disease must be excluded. Corrective surgery is sometimes helpful.

Acquired supranuclear monocular elevator palsy results in limitation of elevation of one eye on attempted upgaze, despite intact downgaze and orthotropia in primary position (unlike patients with monocular elevator deficiency, who have an abnormal head posture). This rare condition occurs with unilateral vascular or neoplastic lesions involving either the ipsilateral or contralateral midbrain. Usually the affected eye can

be elevated in response to vestibular stimulation or the Bell phenomenon, and ptosis is usually absent.

Tonic upward deviation of gaze (forced upgaze), a rare sign, is seen in unconscious patients and must be distinguished from oculogyric crises, petit mal seizures, and psychogenic coma. Comatose patients with sustained upgaze after diffuse brain injury (e.g., hypotension, cardiac arrest, heatstroke) usually have cerebral and cerebellar hypoxic damage, with relative sparing of the brainstem; generally, it appears within the first few hours of the insult (Johkura et al., 2004). Those patients who develop myoclonic jerks and large-amplitude downbeat nystagmus later have a very poor prognosis. Rarely, tonic upward gaze deviation may be psychogenic but can be overcome, indeed cured, by cold caloric stimulation of the eardrums.

"Benign" paroxysmal tonic upward (PTU) gaze may occur in association with ataxia in young children who have downbeat nystagmus on attempted downgaze. The duration of the deviation is variable (seconds to hours), but it is usually short and occurs frequently throughout the day. PTU gaze usually starts in the first year of life and lasts about 2 years; the onset may be during or shortly after an infection or vaccination. PTU gaze may be exacerbated by fatigue, relieved by sleep, and sometimes provoked by car travel; there is no evidence that the episodes are seizures or oculogyric crises. The cause of PTU gaze is unknown, but at follow-up, a significant number of patients have developmental delay, intellectual disability, language delay, or ocular motility disorders; these findings imply that PTU gaze is a marker for underlying neurological or developmental abnormalities (Hayman et al.,1998). The condition is reminiscent of the intermittent or periodic ataxias, which may respond to drugs such as acetazolamide (see Chapter 64).

Tonic downward deviation of gaze (forced downgaze) is associated with impaired consciousness in patients with medial thalamic hemorrhage, acute obstructive hydrocephalus, severe metabolic or hypoxic encephalopathy, or massive SAH. Also, the eyes may converge, as if looking at the nose. When tonic downward gaze deviation is the result of hypoxic encephalopathy, it appears later (1 to 7 days) than upward tonic gaze deviation (hours) and almost always predicts a persistent vegetative state (Johkura et al., 2004). Tonic downward gaze deviation may also occur in psychogenic illness, especially feigned coma, but also can be overcome by caloric stimulation. In young children with acute hydrocephalus, tonic downward deviation may be associated with upper lid retraction; because of its appearance, this is called the *setting sun sign*.

In otherwise healthy neonates, downward deviation of the eyes or tonic upgaze while awake may occur as a transient phenomenon caused by uneven delayed development in the vertical otolithic-ocular pathways (Brodsky and Donahue, 2001). Tonic vertical deviation due to ictal activity is rare. A form of paroxysmal ocular downward deviation that lasts seconds and occurs in neurologically impaired infants with poor vision may also be seen in preterm infants with bronchopulmonary dysplasia but subsequent normal development.

Torsional nystagmus with a jerk waveform may be evoked during vertical-pursuit eye movements in patients with lesions of the middle cerebellar peduncle (see section on nystagmus). The direction of the fast phase is usually toward the side of

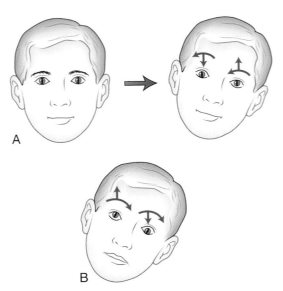

Fig. 35.30 **A,** Normal ocular counter-rolling phenomenon during head tilt. **B,** Ocular tilt reaction consists of spontaneous skew deviation, cyclotorsion of both eyes (upper poles rotated towards lower eye), paradoxical head tilting, and displacement of the subjective visual vertical toward the side of the lower eye.

the lesion on downward pursuit and away from the side of the lesion on upward pursuit (FitzGibbon et al., 1996).

In normal circumstances, a synkinetic movement, ocular counter-rolling, allows people to maintain horizontal orientation of the environment while tilting the head to either side (**Fig. 35.30, A**). When the head is tilted to the left, the left eye rises and intorts as the right eye falls and extorts within the range of the ocular tilt reflex (approximately 10 degrees from the vertical). The initial transient dynamic (phasic) counter-rolling response results from stimulation of the semicircular canals, whereas the sustained (tonic) response is mediated by the otolith organs and holds the eyes in their new position. Lesions of these pathways result in skew deviation.

Skew deviation is a vertical divergence of the ocular axes caused by a "prenuclear" lesion in the brainstem or cerebellum involving the vertical vestibulo-ocular pathways or, occasionally, the vestibular nerve or end-organ. In about 12% of patients, the skew alternates on lateral gaze or spontaneously. A skew deviation is usually, but not always, comitant; when noncomitant, it may mimic a partial third cranial nerve or a fourth cranial nerve palsy. Skew deviation occurs most commonly with vascular lesions of the pons or lateral medulla (Wallenberg syndrome). Brandt and Dieterich (1998) demonstrated ocular torsion of one or both eyes associated with subjective tilting of the visual vertical toward the lower eye in most patients with skew deviations. With lesions caudal to the lower pons, the ipsilateral eye was lower (ipsiversive skew), but with lesions rostral to the midpontine level, the contralateral eye was lower (contraversive skew). Ocular torsion may be present without a vertical deviation and, in either situation, can be detected by blind spot mapping, indirect ophthalmoscopy, fundus photography, double Maddox rod test, or settings of the visual vertical (Mossman and Halmagyi, 1997).

Alternating skew deviation, in which the hypertropia changes sides, results from vascular or demyelinating lesions

at the pretectal-mesodiencephalic junction, usually involving the INC. This phenomenon, also referred to as *paroxysmal skew deviation* and *periodic alternating skew*, may change spontaneously or with the direction of gaze in a regular or irregular manner over periods of seconds to minutes. Disorders affecting the cerebellar pathways or cervicomedullary junction cause alternating skew deviation on lateral gaze, in which the abducting eye is hypertropic. This is probably the result of asymmetrical vestibular input to the yoked superior oblique and contralateral inferior rectus muscles (see **Table 35.2**) as a result of increased central otolithic tone for downgaze (Brodsky and Donahue, 2001). Skew deviation that alternates between up- and downgaze can occur with spinocerebellar degeneration. Congenital superior oblique overaction causes an A-pattern exotropia (eyes diverge on downgaze) and an abducting hypertropia on lateral gaze; often it is associated with disorders of the posterior fossa, such as hydrocephalus and meningomyelocele, and Chiari II malformations. Congenital inferior oblique overaction causes a V-pattern esotropia (eyes converge or cross on downgaze) and is otherwise benign (Brodsky and Donahue, 2001).

Bilateral fourth cranial nerve palsies may mimic gaze-dependent alternating skew, in which the adducting eye is hypertropic; however, diplopia is worse on downgaze, with significant excyclotorsion and a V-pattern esotropia.

The OTR consists of spontaneous skew deviation, cyclotorsion of both eyes (the upper poles rotated towards the lower eye), paradoxical head tilting (**Fig. 35.30, B**), and displacement of the subjective visual vertical, all toward the side of the lower eye. A tonic (sustained) OTR occurs with a prenuclear lesion causing imbalance in the otolithic (gravireceptive) pathways to the ocular motor system, anywhere from the ipsilateral utricle, vestibular nerve, nuclei, or the contralateral MLF, contralateral INC, and medial thalamus. A phasic (paroxysmal) OTR occurs with a lesion in the region of the INC, and it may respond to baclofen or carbamazepine (Rodriguez et al., 2009). An OTR can be induced by sound in patients with perilymph fistulas of the vestibular end-organ (the Tullio phenomenon). A partial OTR in which there is no head tilt, or there is merely ocular torsion, can occur with lesions of the cerebellar nodulus and uvula. This is attributed to an increase in the tonic resting activity of secondary otolithic neurons in the ipsilesional vestibular nucleus as a result of loss of inhibition from the injured nodulus (Mossman and Halmagyi, 1997). A contralateral OTR occurs in patients with INO, and with the one-and-a-half syndrome (Zwergal et al., 2008).

Oculogyric crises are spasmodic conjugate ocular deviations, usually in an upward direction. They occurred in the late stages of postencephalitic PD after the 1918 influenza epidemic, but now most often are caused by neuroleptic medication, particularly haloperidol. They may also occur in patients with head injury, neurosyphilis, herpetic brainstem encephalitis, bilateral paramedian midbrain inflammation (Della Marca et al., 2011), and carbamazepine or lithium carbonate toxicity. Oculogyric crises can occur also in the early stages of autosomal dominant "rapid-onset dystonia-parkinsonism." A typical attack or crisis lasts about 2 hours, during which the eyes are tonically deviated upward, repetitively, for periods of seconds to minutes. The spasms may be preceded or accompanied by disturbing emotional symptoms, including anxiety, restlessness, compulsive thinking, and sensations of increased brightness or distortions of visual background (similar to occipital lobe seizures). The patient may be able to force the eyes back to the primary position temporarily by using voluntary saccades, optokinetic tracking, head rotation, or blinking. Electroencephalograph recordings during the attacks show no epileptiform activity. The eyelids are usually open, although they may rhythmically jerk at times from twitching of the orbicularis oculi. The pupils are not usually involved. Attacks may be precipitated by excitement. They should be differentiated from benign paroxysmal tonic upward gaze (see Disorders of Vertical Gaze). Treatment for oculogyric crises includes diphenhydramine, L-dopa, and high-dose trihexyphenidyl; anticholinergic agents terminate the thought disorders as well (Leigh and Zee, 2006).

Disorders of Convergence

Usually, convergence paralysis is associated with other features of the dorsal midbrain syndrome (see Chapter 19). Patients with psychogenic convergence paralysis may be distinguished from those with organic disease by the absence of pupillary constriction during attempted convergence and preservation of upgaze. Lack of effort is the most common cause of poor convergence, which becomes more difficult with age. Degenerative disorders such as PD and PSP are often associated with poor convergence and can be helped with prisms.

Convergence insufficiency, an idiopathic condition that may be partly psychogenic, occurs most commonly in women between the ages of 15 and 45 years. Symptoms include words running together when reading, occasionally frank diplopia at near, and vague symptoms such as eyestrain, headache, and burning eyes that are often associated with asthenopia. Convergence insufficiency may be seen after head injury. Because the mechanism of convergence insufficiency is an imbalance between accommodation and convergence, orthoptic exercises (pencil push-ups), less commonly prisms, and myopic correction are useful in management.

Spasm of the near reflex, a disorder characterized by intermittent episodes of convergence, miosis, and accommodation, may mimic bilateral (and occasionally unilateral) abducens paresis. The patient may complain of double or blurred vision and is esotropic, particularly at distance; however, prominent miosis is the clue. Occasionally, spasm of the near reflex may occur in patients with organic disorders (Goldstein and Schneekloth, 1996) but is more commonly psychogenic, either in patients with conversion reactions or in anxious patients in whom the "spasm" is a manifestation of misdirected effort. The differential diagnosis is that of esotropia (see **Box 35.1**). Miosis on gaze testing generally establishes the diagnosis but can be difficult to discern. Accommodative esotropia and latent hyperopia must be excluded by obtaining a cycloplegic refraction. Patients with psychogenic spasm of the near reflex have associated somatic complaints and behavioral abnormalities. Blepharoclonus on lateral gaze and poor cooperation in performing motor tasks such as smiling, opening the mouth, protruding the tongue, and the like (features of neurasthenia and asthenopia) often are found during examination (**Box 35.20**). Management should focus on identifying the source of the psychopathology and may require psychiatric evaluation. Strategies such as the use of cycloplegia (homatropine eye drops) to prevent accommodative spasm, thus inhibiting the near triad, are helpful.

> ### Box 35.20 **Features of Spasm of the Near Reflex (Psychogenic)**
>
> - Near tetrad:
>   - Convergence
>   - Miosis
>   - Accommodation (blur at distance, myopia by retinoscopy)
>   - Extorsion (excyclotorsion)
> - Neurasthenic symptoms
> - Blepharoclonus (frequent blink rate)
> - Poor cooperation in other motor tasks
> - Other behavioral changes (e.g., tunnel vision)
> - May disappear with rapid saccades
> - Full range of eye movement:
>   - With pursuit of own hand
>   - With one eye covered
>   - Doll's eyes with fixation
> - Ice-cold calorics:
>   - Normal response
>   - Bizarre behavioral response
> - Normal optokinetic nystagmus if patient encouraged or distracted (e.g., count stripes)
> - Demeanor:
>   - Affective disorder
>   - Tinted glasses or sunglasses
>   - Excessive makeup

Disorders of Divergence

Divergence insufficiency is characterized by sudden-onset esotropia and uncrossed horizontal diplopia at distance, in the absence of other neurological symptoms or signs. The esotropia may be intermittent or constant, but the patients can fuse at near. The esodeviation is greater at distance than near but is comitant in all directions. Versions and ductions are full, and saccadic velocities, if measured quantitatively, appear normal. Fusional divergence is reduced. The origin of divergence insufficiency is unclear, but it may result from a break in fusion in a patient with a congenital esophoria, usually coming on later in life; also, it occurs in patients with midline cerebellar disease particularly hereditary spinocerebellar ataxia (Morrison et al., 2008). The condition is easily treated with base-out prisms for the distance correction and rarely requires extraocular muscle surgery.

Divergence paralysis, a controversial entity that may be difficult to distinguish from divergence insufficiency, usually occurs in the context of a severe head injury or other cause of raised ICP. Such patients also have horizontal diplopia at distance, but quantitatively, abducting saccades are slow. Patients with bilateral palsies of the sixth cranial nerve who recover gradually may go through a phase in which the esotropia becomes comitant with full ductions, mimicking divergence paralysis. Divergence paralysis can also occur with Fisher syndrome, Chiari malformations, pontine tumors, and excessive sedation from drugs.

Central disruption of fusion, or posttraumatic fusion deficiency, can occur after moderate head injury and causes intractable diplopia despite the patient's ability to fuse intermittently and, even briefly, achieve stereopsis. The diplopia fluctuates and varies among crossed, uncrossed, and vertical. Versions and ductions may be full, but vergence amplitudes are reduced greatly. Prism therapy or surgery is ineffective, but an eye patch or centrally frosted lens may provide symptomatic relief. The location of injury is presumed to be in the midbrain. Central disruption of fusion is also reported with brainstem tumors, stroke, removal of long-standing cataracts, uncorrected aphakia, and neurosurgical procedures. This condition must be distinguished from bilateral fourth cranial nerve palsies, when diplopia is constant and associated with cyclodiplopia and excyclotropia (>12 degrees), and also from psychogenic disorders of vergence (see Disorders of Convergence).

A congenital inability to fuse is associated with amblyopia or congenital esotropia.

The hemislide (hemifield slip) phenomenon causes diplopia in patients with large visual field defects, particularly dense bitemporal hemianopias or, occasionally, heteronymous altitudinal defects (Borchert et al., 1996). Because of loss of overlapping areas of visual field, patients have difficulty maintaining fusion and can no longer suppress any latent ocular deviation.

Cyclical esotropia, also called *circadian*, *alternate-day*, or *clock-mechanism esotropia*, usually begins in childhood, although it can occur at any age and can also follow surgery for intermittent esotropia. The cycles of orthotropia and esotropia may run 24 to 96 hours, similar to many other cyclical or periodic biological phenomena of obscure mechanisms. Patients with cyclical esotropia can decompensate into a constant esotropia that can be corrected surgically.

Ocular neuromyotonia is a brief episodic myotonic contraction of one or more muscles supplied by the ocular motor nerves, most commonly the oculomotor nerve (Yee and Purvin, 1998). It may occur spontaneously or be provoked by prolonged gaze in a particular direction. It usually results in esotropia of the affected eye accompanied by failure of elevation and depression of the globe. When the oculomotor nerve is affected, there may be associated signs of aberrant reinnervation (see Chapter 70). The pupil may be fixed to both light and near stimuli or become myotonic (Abulla and Eustace, 1999). Ocular neuromyotonia occurs most often after radiation therapy for sellar region tumors. Less often it is associated with compressive lesions such as pituitary adenomas, cavernous sinus meningiomas or aneurysms, or thyroid orbitopathy, and occasionally it occurs following myelography with thorium dioxide (Yee and Purvin, 1998), with Paget disease of the skull base, or with neurovascular compression by a dolichoectatic basilar artery (Tilikete et al., 2000). Demyelinating lesions in the region of the third cranial nerve fascicle can also cause "paroxysmal spasm" of the muscles innervated by the oculomotor nerve (Ezra and Plant, 1996) but are usually accompanied by other findings such as eyelid retraction or paroxysmal limb dystonia. Occasionally, no cause can be found. Ocular neuromyotonia may respond to carbamazepine or other antiepileptic drugs. It should be distinguished from superior oblique myokymia and the spasms of cyclical oculomotor palsy.

Cyclical oculomotor palsy is characterized by paresis alternating with "cyclic" spasms of both the extra- and intraocular muscles supplied by the oculomotor nerve. It is a rare condition usually noted in the first 2 years of life, although the majority of cases are believed to be congenital and are often associated with other features of birth trauma. During the spasms, which last 10 to 30 seconds, the upper eyelid elevates, the globe adducts, and the pupil and ciliary muscle constrict, causing miosis and increased accommodation (Loewenfeld, 1999); the paretic phase usually lasts longer. Signs of aberrant oculomotor reinnervation (see Chapter 70) are usually present. Spasms, often heralded by twitching of the upper lid, may be precipitated by intentional accommodation or adduction. Cycles occur irregularly, vary from 1.5 to 3 minutes in duration, persist during sleep, may be suppressed by topical cholinergic agents (eserine, pilocarpine), and are abolished by topical anticholinergic agents (atropine, homatropine) or general anesthesia. The cycles usually persist throughout life, but the spasms of the extraocular muscles may abate, leaving only intermittent miosis.

Symptomatic cyclical oculomotor palsy may occur in later life in patients with underlying lesions involving the third cranial nerve, but the features and cycles are atypical. The

---

Box 35.21 Gaze-Evoked Phenomena

Physiological Phenomena

- Blinks
- End-point nystagmus
- Flaring of the nostrils during vertical saccades
- Mentalis contraction during horizontal saccades (personal observation)
- Oculoauricular phenomenon: retraction of ear during lateral gaze (or convergence)
- Orbicularis oculi myokymia
- Phosphenes (more intense in patients with optic neuritis, retinal/vitreous detachment: Moore lightning streaks)

Pathological Sensory Phenomena

- Gaze-evoked amaurosis in the eye ipsilateral to an orbital apex tumor
- Gaze-evoked tinnitus with cerebellopontine angle tumors or following posterior fossa surgery
- Reverse-Tullio phenomenon (gaze-evoked swooshing sound) caused by end-organ damage in a patient with Tullio phenomenon (sound-evoked nystagmus and vertigo) (personal observation)
- SUNCT (sudden unilateral conjunctival injection and tearing) syndrome with saccades
- Tinnitus with periodic saccadic oscillations
- Vertigo

Pathological Motor Phenomena

- Convergence retraction nystagmus on attempted upgaze (dorsal midbrain syndrome)
- Facial twitching, clonic limb movements, blepharoclonus, lid nystagmus, involuntary laughter and seizures
- Gaze-evoked nystagmus
- Neuromyotonia
- Retraction of the globe in Duane syndrome
- Superior oblique myokymia
- Synkinetic movements with cyclical oculomotor palsy and with aberrant reinnervation of the oculomotor nerve (see Chapter 70).

mechanism of cyclical spasms is unclear but is discussed elsewhere (Loewenfeld, 1999).

Gaze-evoked phenomena such as end-point nystagmus, the oculoauricular phenomenon, and orbicularis oculi myokymia are physiological or benign. Others, such as gaze-evoked nystagmus or tinnitus, are pathological (**Box 35.21**) and may be the result of damage to the horizontal NI (Lockwood et al., 2001).

Eye Movement Recording Techniques

Oculographic techniques provide clinicians and researchers with objective and quantitative means of analysis that have led to a better understanding of eye movement neurophysiology and ocular motility disorders. Quantitative oculography can measure saccadic latency, velocity, accuracy, pursuit and VOR gain, and nystagmus slow-phase velocity; it can detect unsuspected oscillations and intrusions and identify different nystagmus waveforms. Oculography is used to record both spontaneous and induced eye movements to a target, such as a projected light in front of the subject, or to vestibular and optokinetic stimuli.

Electro-oculography, also known as *electronystagmography* (Chapter 37), is a popular method of quantitative oculography but has a limited range and is unreliable for vertical eye movements because of eyelid artifact. Infrared oculography is more accurate but not ideal for vertical eye movements. The most quantitatively accurate technique involves the scleral search coil. Details of all the recording techniques are found in Dell'Osso and Daroff (1999b).

References

The complete reference list is available online at www.expertconsult.com.

Neuro-ophthalmology: Afferent Visual System

Matthew J. Thurtell, Robert L. Tomsak

From a conceptual standpoint, it is useful to consider vision as having two components: *central* or *macular* vision (high acuity, color perception, light adapted) and *peripheral* or *ambulatory* vision (low acuity, poor color perception, dark-adapted). Light, refracted by the cornea and lens, then focuses on the retina. For the best possible vision, the object of regard must focus on the *fovea*, which is the most sensitive part of the macula. The cone photoreceptors, which mediate central and color vision, are greatest in density at the fovea. The cone system functions optimally in conditions of light adaptation. Visual acuity and cone density fall off rapidly as eccentricity from the fovea increases. For example, the retina 20 degrees eccentric to the fovea can only resolve objects equal to Snellen 20/200 (6/60 metric) optotypes or larger. Rod photoreceptors are present in highest numbers approximately 20 degrees from the fovea and are more abundant than cones in the more peripheral retina; rods function best in dim illumination. The total extent of the normal peripheral visual field in each eye is approximately 60 degrees superior, 60 degrees nasal, 70 to 75 degrees inferior, and 100 degrees temporal to fixation (**Fig. 36.1**) (see Chapter 14).

Each eye sends visual information, transduced by the retina, to both hemispheres of the brain by the optic nerves, each of which contains over 1 million axons. Axons that arise from the ganglion cells of the nasal retina of each eye cross in the optic chiasm to the contralateral optic tract. Axons from the temporal retina do not decussate at the chiasm. The percentages of crossed and uncrossed axons in the human optic chiasm

are approximately 53% and 47%, respectively. Because of the optical properties of the eye, the nasal retina receives visual information from the temporal visual field, while the temporal retina receives visual information from the nasal visual field (see **Fig. 36.1**). Similarly, the superior retina receives information from the inferior visual field, and vice versa. These points are clinically important in evaluating visual loss (see Chapter 14).

Visual information stratifies further in the lateral geniculate nucleus (LGN), which is the only way station between the retinal ganglion cells and the primary visual cortex. The LGN, a portion of the thalamus, has six layers. Axons from ipsilateral retinal ganglion cells synapse in layers 2, 3, and 5; contralateral axons synapse in layers 1, 4, and 6. Layers 1 and 2 of the LGN are the *magnocellular layers* and receive input from M retinal ganglion cells. The magnocellular pathway is concerned mainly with movement detection, detection of low contrast, and dynamic form perception. After projecting to the primary visual cortex (visual area 1, V1, or Brodmann area 17), information from the M pathway is distributed to V2 (part of area 18) and V5 (junction of areas 19 and 37). Layers 3 to 6 of the LGN are the *parvocellular layers* and receive input from retinal P cells, which are color selective and responsive to high contrast. Information from the P pathway is distributed to V2 and V4 (fusiform gyrus) (Trobe, 2001). Superior fibers that leave the LGN go straight back to the primary visual cortex; inferior fibers loop anteriorly around the temporal horn of the lateral ventricles (*Meyer loop*). Since these fibers pass close to the tip

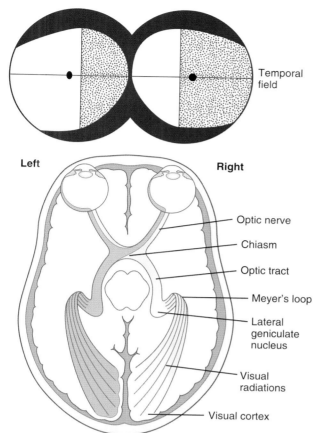

Fig. 36.1 Visual pathways.

Labels: Temporal field; Left; Right; Optic nerve; Chiasm; Optic tract; Meyer's loop; Lateral geniculate nucleus; Visual radiations; Visual cortex

of the temporal lobe, temporal lobectomy sometimes damages these fibers causing a "pie in the sky" homonymous visual field defect.

The primary visual cortex (striate cortex, area V1, or Brodmann area 17) is in the occipital lobe. Fibers from the macula project to the visual cortex closest to the occipital poles (each fovea appears to project to both occipital lobes), while fibers from the peripheral retina project to the visual cortex lying more anteriorly. The nonoverlapping part of the most peripheral temporal visual field (*monocular temporal crescent*) arises from unpaired crossed axons from the nasal retina that project to the most anteromedial part of the visual cortex. The primary visual cortex has interconnections with visual association areas concerned with color, motion, and object recognition (Trobe, 2001).

Neuro-ophthalmological Examination of the Afferent Visual System

The neuro-ophthalmological examination makes use of ophthalmic tools and techniques but aims at neurological diagnosis. Since many neurologists are not familiar with ophthalmic examination techniques, and ophthalmologists are often not experienced with neurological localization, the neuro-ophthalmological subspecialty provides a bridge between the two disciplines.

Examination of Visual Acuity

Visual acuity is the spatial resolution of vision. Visual acuity should always be measured with each eye individually and with the best possible optical correction (i.e., with the patient's glasses); other optical means such as the pinhole device or a refraction may be needed (Wall and Johnson, 2005). The resultant measure, called *best-corrected visual acuity*, is the only universally interpretable measurement of central visual function. Ideally, always measure vision both at a standard distance (usually 20 feet or 6 m) and at near (usually 0.33 m). The notation *20/20* (6/6 metric) means the patient (numerator) is able to see the optotypes seen by a normal subject at 20 feet (denominator). A vision of 20/60 (6/18 metric) means that the patient sees an optotype at 20 feet that a normal person would see at 60 feet.

A disparity between the best-corrected distance and near visual acuities is often indicative of a specific problem. For example, the most common cause of better distance than near acuity is uncorrected presbyopia. Common causes of better near than distance acuity are myopia and congenital nystagmus. In the latter disorder, convergence needed for near vision dampens the nystagmus.

When measuring near vision, the reading card should be held at the specified distance of 14 inches (or 0.33 m) to control for variation in image size on the retina. The medical record should clearly specify if a nonstandard distance is used. Two types of near cards are readily available; one has numbers and the other has written text (**Fig. 36.2**). Both are useful, but in neurological practice, a near card with text measures not only visual acuity but also reading ability to some degree. A disparity between the measurements from the two types of near card might suggest a disturbance of some other cortical function such as language function (see Chapter 11).

Contrast Vision Testing

Contrast vision, the ability to distinguish adjacent areas of differing luminance, can be evaluated by assessing the perception of lines or optotypes of different sizes (spatial frequencies) with varying degrees of contrast. Contrast vision can be impaired in numerous diseases of the eye (e.g., cataract) and retrobulbar visual pathways (e.g., optic neuropathy and Alzheimer disease). Special charts—the Pelli-Robson chart (sensitivity) and Sloan chart (acuity)—are required to measure contrast sensitivity and acuity.

Light-Stress Test

In some disorders of the macula, abnormalities are undetectable with the direct ophthalmoscope. The light-stress (or photo-stress) test is a useful method for determining whether reduced visual acuity is a consequence of macular dysfunction (Wall and Johnson, 2005). Prior to the test, the best-corrected visual acuity is measured in each eye. Then, with the eye with decreased vision occluded, the other eye is exposed to a bright light for 10 seconds. Immediately thereafter, the patient is instructed to read the next larger line on the eye chart, and the recovery period is timed. The same procedure is followed for the eye with decreased vision, and the results are compared. Fifty seconds is the upper limit of normal for visual

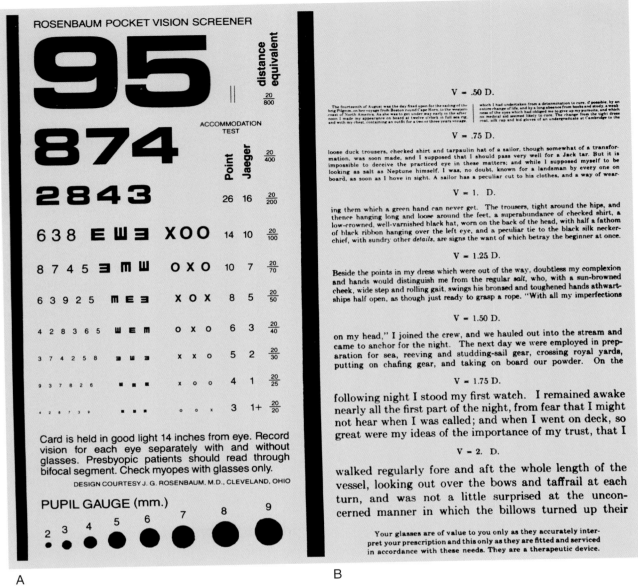

Fig. 36.2 A, Rosenbaum-style near vision card. **B,** Near vision card with written text.

recovery, although most normal subjects recover within several seconds. In patients with macular disease, the recovery period often takes several minutes.

Color Vision Testing

Dyschromatopsia, especially if asymmetrical between the eyes, is a good indication of optic nerve dysfunction, but it can also occur with retinal disease (Almog and Nemet, 2010). Symmetrical acquired dyschromatopsia might indicate a retinal degeneration, such as a cone-rod dystrophy. Congenital dyschromatopsia occurs in about 8% of men and 0.5% of women.

Techniques for assessing color vision range from the simple to the sophisticated. A gross color vision defect is identifiable at the bedside by assessing for red desaturation. The clinician holds a bright red object in front of each of the patient's eyes individually, and then asks for a comparison of both brightness and color intensity. Asking for a comparison of red saturation on each side of fixation sometimes detects a subtle hemianopia. Formal measurements of color vision can be obtained with pseudoisochromatic color plates (e.g., Ishihara or Hardy-Rand-Rittler plates) or with sorting tests (e.g., Farnsworth-Munsell test).

Examination of the Pupils

Examination of the pupils involves assessing pupil size and shape, direct and consensual reactions to light, near reaction, and the presence or absence of a relative afferent pupillary defect (RAPD). If a difference in pupil size (*anisocoria*) is noted, look for ptosis and ophthalmoplegia, keeping in mind the possibility of a Horner syndrome or third cranial nerve palsy. Record findings in an easily understood format (**Table 36.1**).

information necessary for making specific diagnoses. We also include details on testing and management of these patients.

Historical Background

Accounts of dizziness and vertigo can be found in the writings of ancient Egyptian and Greek physicians. However, prior to the late 19th century, not much was known about the causes of dizziness or hearing loss, and as a result quackery was commonplace. Patients complaining of dizziness or vertigo were usually grouped together with epileptic seizures and stroke under the rubric of "apoplectiform cerebral congestion," meaning too much blood to the brain. As a result, common treatments included bleeding, leeching, cupping, and purging. In 1861, Prosper Meniere was the first to recognize the association of vertigo with hearing loss and thus to localize the symptom to the inner ear (Baloh, 2001). Although not well received initially, his discovery provided the basis for later studies on the physiology and pathology of the vestibular system.

Caloric testing, the most widely used test of the vestibulo-ocular reflex (VOR), was introduced by Robert Barany in 1906. He was later awarded the Nobel prize for proposing the mechanism of caloric stimulation. Barany also provided the first clinical description of benign paroxysmal positional vertigo (BPPV) in 1921. Endolymphatic hydrops was identified in postmortem specimens of patients with Meniere disease in 1938. A method for measuring eye movements in response to caloric and rotational stimuli (electronystagmography) was introduced in the 1930s, and in the 1970s, digital computers began to be used to quantify eye movement responses.

The advent of modern neuroimaging in the late 1970s and 1980s greatly expanded our understanding of causes of dizziness and vertigo. Prior to this time, stroke was considered an exceedingly rare cause of vertigo (Fisher, 1967). Though it remains a controversial topic even today, infarctions within the cerebellum and brainstem have been identified on imaging studies in patients with isolated vertigo. Imaging studies continue to lead to new discoveries of causes of vertigo, as demonstrated by the recently described disorder of superior canal dehiscence (SCD). But the most common causes of vertigo—Meniere disease, BPPV, and vestibular neuritis—still have no identifiable imaging characteristics.

Over the last 25 years, our understanding of the mechanisms for the common neuro-otological disorders has been greatly enhanced. BPPV can now be readily identified and cured at the bedside with a simple positional maneuver, and variants have also been described (Aw et al., 2005; Fife et al., 2008). The head-thrust test can be used at the bedside to identify a vestibular nerve lesion, and because of this it has particular utility in helping distinguish vestibular neuritis from a posterior fossa stroke (Halmagyi and Curthoys, 1988; Kattah et al., 2009; Newman-Toker et al., 2008; Nuti et al., 2005). Controversies regarding Meniere disease have been clarified, and medical and surgical treatments have improved (Minor et al., 2004). It is now clear that patients with recurrent episodes of vertigo without hearing loss, a condition once called *vestibular Meniere disease*, do not actually have Meniere disease.

Migraine is now recognized as an important cause of dizziness, even in patients without simultaneous headaches.

In fact, benign recurrent vertigo (patients with recurrent episodes of vertigo without accompanying auditory symptoms or other neurological features) is usually a migraine equivalent (Oh et al., 2001b). The disorder of SCD was only recently described and provides important insight into the physiology of the vestibular system (Minor, 2005). A more detailed description of the rotational vertebral artery syndrome has led to appreciation of the high metabolic demands of the inner ear and its susceptibility to ischemia (Choi et al., 2005). Genetic research has identified ion channel dysfunction in disorders such as episodic ataxia and familial hemiplegic migraine, and patients with these disorders also commonly report vertigo (Jen et al., 2004a). It is hoped that identifying specific genes causing vertigo syndromes will lead to a better understanding of the mechanisms and also create the opportunity to develop specific treatments in the future.

Epidemiology of Vertigo, Dizziness, and Hearing Loss

A recent population-based telephone survey in Germany showed nearly 30% of the population had experienced moderate to severe dizziness (Neuhauser et al., 2005). Though most subjects reported nonspecific forms of dizziness, nearly a quarter had true vertigo. Dizziness is more common among females and older people and has important healthcare utilization implications; up to 80% of patients with dizziness seek medical care at some point. In the United States, the National Centers for Health Statistics report 7.5 million annual ambulatory visits to physician offices, hospital outpatient departments, and emergency departments (EDs) for dizziness, making it one of the most common principal complaints (Burt and Schappert, 2004).

Hearing loss affects approximately 16% of adults (age >18 years) in the United States (Lethbridge-Cejku et al., 2006). Men are more commonly affected than women, and the prevalence of hearing loss increases dramatically with age, so that by age 75, nearly 50% of the population reports hearing loss. Hearing loss is an important cause of disability. The most common type of hearing loss is sensorineural, and both idiopathic presbycusis and noise-induced forms are common etiologies. Bothersome tinnitus is less frequent in the U.S. population, with about 3% reporting it, although this increases to about 9% for subjects older than 65 (Adams et al., 1999). The most common type of tinnitus is a high-pitched ringing in both ears.

Normal Anatomy and Physiology

The inner ear is composed of a fluid-filled sac enclosed by a bony capsule with an anterior cochlear part, central chamber (vestibule), and a posterior vestibular part (**Fig. 37.1**). Endolymph fills up the fluid-filled sac and is separated by a membrane from the perilymph. These fluids primarily differ in their composition of potassium and sodium, with the endolymph resembling intracellular fluid with a high potassium and low sodium content, and perilymph resembling extracellular fluids with a low potassium and high sodium content. Perilymph communicates with the cerebrospinal fluid (CSF) through the cochlear aqueduct.

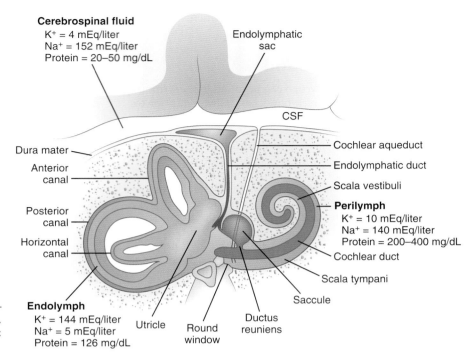

Cerebrospinal fluid
K⁺ = 4 mEq/liter
Na⁺ = 152 mEq/liter
Protein = 20–50 mg/dL

Endolymphatic sac

CSF

Dura mater

Anterior canal

Posterior canal

Horizontal canal

Cochlear aqueduct

Endolymphatic duct

Scala vestibuli

Perilymph
K⁺ = 10 mEq/liter
Na⁺ = 140 mEq/liter
Protein = 200–400 mg/dL

Cochlear duct

Scala tympani

Saccule

Ductus reuniens

Round window

Utricle

Endolymph
K⁺ = 144 mEq/liter
Na⁺ = 5 mEq/liter
Protein = 126 mg/dL

Fig. 37.1 Anatomy of the inner ear. *CSF,* Cerebrospinal fluid. *(From Baloh, R.W., 1998. Dizziness, Hearing Loss, and Tinnitus. F.A. Davis Company, Philadelphia, Figure 6, p. 16.)*

The cochlea senses sound waves after they travel through the external auditory canal and are amplified by the tympanic membrane and ossicles of the middle ear (Baloh and Kerber, 2011). The stapes, the last of three ossicles in the middle ear, contacts the oval window, which directs the forces associated with sound waves along the basilar membrane of the cochlea. These forces stimulate the hair cells, which in turn generate neural signals in the auditory nerve. The auditory nerve enters the lateral brainstem at the pontomedullary junction and synapses in the cochlear nucleus. The trapezoid body is the major decussation of the auditory pathway, but many fibers do not cross to the contralateral side. Signals then travel to the superior olivary complex. Some projections travel from the superior olivary complex to the inferior colliculus through the lateral lemnisci, and others terminate in one of the nuclei of the lateral lemniscus. Next, fibers travel to the ipsilateral medial geniculate body, and then auditory radiations pass through the posterior limb of the internal capsule to reach the auditory cortex of the temporal lobe.

The peripheral vestibular system is composed of three semicircular canals, the utricle and saccule, and the vestibular component of the eighth cranial nerve (Baloh and Kerber, 2011). Each semicircular canal has a sensory epithelium called the *crista*; the sensory epithelium of the utricle and saccule is called the *macule*. The semicircular canals sense angular movements, and the utricle and saccule sense linear movements. Two of the semicircular canals (anterior and posterior) are oriented in the vertical plane nearly orthogonal to each other; the third canal is oriented in the horizontal plane (horizontal canal). The crista of each canal is primarily activated by movement occurring in the plane of that canal. When the hair cells of these organs are stimulated, the signal is transferred to the vestibular nuclei via the vestibular portion of cranial nerve VIII. Signals originating from the horizontal semicircular canal then pass via the medial longitudinal fasciculus along the floor of the fourth ventricle to the abducens nuclei in the middle brainstem and the ocular motor complex in the rostral brainstem. The anterior (also referred to as the *superior*) and posterior canal impulses pass from the vestibular nuclei to the ocular motor nucleus and trochlear nucleus triggering eye movements roughly in the plane of each canal. A key feature is that once vestibular signals leave the vestibular nuclei they divide into vertical, horizontal, and torsional components. As a result, a lesion of central vestibular pathways can cause a pure vertical, pure torsional, or pure horizontal nystagmus.

The primary vestibular afferent nerve fibers maintain a constant baseline firing rate of action potentials. When the baseline rate from each ear is symmetrical (or an asymmetry has been centrally compensated), the eyes remain stationary. With an uncompensated asymmetry in the firing rate, either resulting from increased or decreased activity on one side, slow ocular deviation results. By turning the head to the right, the baseline firing rate of the horizontal canal is physiologically altered, causing an increased firing rate on the right side and a decreased firing rate on the left side (**Fig. 37.2**). The result is a slow deviation of the eyes to the left. In an alert subject, this slow deviation is regularly interrupted by quick movements in the opposite direction (nystagmus) so the eyes do not become pinned to one side. In a comatose patient, only the slow component is seen because the brain cannot generate the corrective fast components.

The plane in which the eyes deviate as a result of vestibular stimulation depends on the combination of canals that are stimulated (**Table 37.1**). If only the posterior semicircular canal on one side is stimulated (as occurs with BPPV), a vertical-torsional deviation of the eyes can be observed, which is followed by a fast corrective response generated by the conscious brain in the opposite direction.

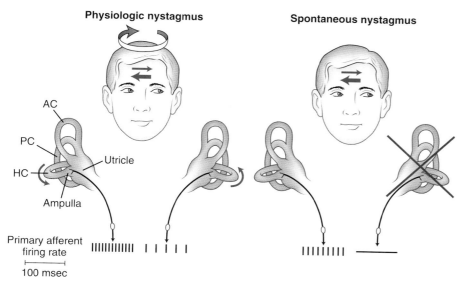

Fig. 37.2 Primary afferent nerve activity associated with rotation-induced physiological nystagmus and spontaneous nystagmus resulting from a lesion of one labyrinth. Thin straight arrows indicate the direction of slow components; thick straight arrows indicate the direction of fast components; curved arrows show the direction of endolymph flow in the horizontal semicircular canals. *AC*, Anterior canal; *HC*, horizontal canal; *PC*, posterior canal. (*From Baloh, R.W., 1998. Dizziness, Hearing Loss, and Tinnitus. F.A. Davis Company, Philadelphia, Figure 16, p. 36.*)

Table 37.1 Physiological Properties and Clinical Features of the Components of the Peripheral Vestibular System

Localization	Component(s)	Triggered Eye Movements	Common Clinical Conditions	Localizing Features
SEMICIRCULAR CANALS				
Posterior canal	PC	Vertical, torsional	BPPV-PC	Nystagmus
Anterior canal	AC	Vertical, torsional	BPPV-AC, SCD	Nystagmus, fistula test
Horizontal canal	HC	Horizontal ≫ torsional	BPPV-HC, fistula	Nystagmus, fistula test
VESTIBULAR NERVE				
Superior division	AC, HC, utricle	Horizontal > torsional	VN, ischemia	Nystagmus, head-thrust test
Inferior division	PC, saccule	Vertical, torsional	VN, ischemia	Nystagmus
Common trunk (cranial nerve 8)	AC, HC, PC, utricle, saccule	Horizontal > torsional	VN, VP, ischemia	Nystagmus, head thrust test, auditory findings
LABYRINTH	AC, HC, PC, utricle, saccule	Horizontal > torsional	EH, labyrinthitis	Nystagmus, auditory findings

AC, Anterior canal; *BPPV*, benign paroxysmal positional vertigo; *EH*, endolymphatic hydrops; *HC*, horizontal canal; *PC*, posterior canal; *SCD*, superior canal dehiscence; *VN*, vestibular neuritis; *VP*, vestibular paroxysmia.

However, if the horizontal canal is the source of stimulation (as occurs with the horizontal canal variant of BPPV), a horizontal deviation with a slight torsional component (because this canal is slightly off the horizontal plane) results. If the vestibular nerve is lesioned (vestibular neuritis) or stimulated (vestibular paroxysmia), a horizontal greater than torsional nystagmus is seen that is the vector sum of all three canals—the two vertical canals on one side cancel each other out.

Over time, an asymmetry in the baseline firing rates either resolves (the stimulation has been removed), or the central nervous system (CNS) compensates for it. This explains why an entire unilateral peripheral vestibular system can be surgically destroyed and patients only experience vertigo for several days to weeks. It also explains why patients with slow-growing tumors affecting the vestibular nerve, such as an acoustic neuroma, generally do not experience vertigo or nystagmus.

History of Present Illness

The history and physical examination provide the most important information when evaluating patients complaining of dizziness (Colledge et al., 1996; Lawson et al., 1999). Often, patients have difficulty describing the exact symptom experienced, so the onus is on the clinician to elicit pertinent information. The first step is to define the symptom. No clinician should ever be satisfied to record the complaint simply as "dizziness." For patients unable to provide a more detailed description of the symptom, the physician can ask the patient to place their symptom into one of the following categories: movement of the environment (vertigo), lightheadedness, or strictly imbalance without an abnormal head sensation. Because patient descriptions about dizziness can be unreliable and inconsistent (Newman-Toker et al., 2007), other details about the symptom become equally important. The physician should

Table 37.2   Distinguishing Among Common Peripheral and Central Vertigo Syndromes

Cause	History of Vertigo	Duration of Vertigo	Associated Symptoms	Physical Examination
PERIPHERAL				
Vestibular neuritis	Single prolonged episode	Days to weeks	Nausea, imbalance	"Peripheral" nystagmus, positive head thrust test, imbalance
BPPV	Positionally triggered episodes	<1 minute	Nausea	Characteristic positionally triggered burst of nystagmus
Meniere disease	May be triggered by salty foods	Hours	Unilateral ear fullness, tinnitus, hearing loss, nausea	Unilateral low frequency hearing loss
Vestibular paroxysmia	Abrupt onset; spontaneous or positionally triggered	Seconds	Tinnitus, hearing loss	Usually normal
Perilymph fistula	Triggered by sound or pressure changes	Seconds	Hearing loss, hyperacusis	Nystagmus triggered by loud sounds or pressure changes
CENTRAL				
Stroke/TIA	Abrupt onset; spontaneous	Stroke, >24 hours; TIA, usually minutes	Brainstem, cerebellar	Spontaneous "central" nystagmus; gaze-evoked nystagmus; usually focal neurologic signs
MS	Subacute onset	Minutes to weeks	Unilateral visual loss, diplopia, incoordination, ataxia	"Central" types or rarely "peripheral" types of spontaneous or positional nystagmus; usually other focal neurologic signs
Neurodegenerative disorders	May be spontaneous or positionally triggered	Minutes to hours	Ataxia	"Central" types of spontaneous or positional nystagmus; gaze-evoked nystagmus; cerebellar, extrapyramidal and frontal signs
Migraine	Onset usually associated with typical migraine triggers	Seconds to days	Headache, visual aura, photo-/phonophobia	Normal interictal exam; ictal examination may show "peripheral" or "central" types of spontaneous or positional nystagmus
Familial ataxia syndromes	Acute-subacute onset; usually triggered by stress, exercise, or excitement	Hours	Ataxia	"Central" types of spontaneous or positional nystagmus Ictal, or even interictal, gaze-evoked nystagmus; ataxia; gait disorders

BPPV, Benign paroxysmal positional vertigo; *MS,* multiple sclerosis; *TIA,* transient ischemic attack.

also ask the following questions: Is the symptom constant or episodic, are there accompanying symptoms, how did it begin (gradual, sudden, etc.), and were there aggravating or alleviating factors? If episodic, what was the duration and frequency of attacks, and were there triggers? **Table 37.2** displays the key distinguishing features of common causes of dizziness. One key point is that any type of dizziness may worsen with position changes, but some disorders such as BPPV only occur after position change.

Physical Examination

General Medical Examination

A brief general medical examination is important. Identifying orthostatic blood pressure can be diagnostic in the correct clinical setting, so blood pressure should be checked

for this pattern in any patient with orthostatic symptoms. Orthostatic hypotension is probably the most common general medical cause of dizziness among patients referred to neurologists. Identifying an irregular heart rhythm may also be pertinent. Other general examination measures to consider in individual patients include a visual assessment (adequate vision is important for balance) and a musculoskeletal inspection (significant arthritis can impair gait).

General Neurological Examination

The general neurological examination is very important in patients complaining of dizziness, because dizziness can be the earliest symptom of a neurodegenerative disorder (de Lau et al., 2006) and can also be an important symptom of stroke, tumor, demyelination, or other pathologies of the nervous system.

The cranial nerves should be thoroughly assessed in patients complaining of dizziness. The most important part of the examination lies in evaluating ocular motor function (described in more detail in the neurotology exam section). One should ensure that the patient has full ocular ductions. A posterior fossa mass can impair facial sensation and the corneal reflex on one side. Assessing facial strength and symmetry is important because of the close anatomical relationship between the seventh and eighth cranial nerves. The lower cranial nerves should also be closely inspected by observing palatal elevation, tongue protrusion, and trapezius and sternocleidomastoid strength.

The general motor examination determines strength in each muscle group and also assesses bulk and tone. Increased tone or cogwheel rigidity could be the main finding in a patient with an early neurodegenerative disorder. The peripheral sensory examination is important because a peripheral neuropathy can cause a nonspecific dizziness or imbalance. Temperature, pain, vibration, and proprioception should be assessed. Reflexes should be tested for their presence and symmetry. One must take into consideration the normal decrease in vibratory sensation and absence of ankle jerks that can occur in elderly patients. Coordination is an important part of the neurological examination in patients with dizziness because disorders characterized by ataxia can present with the principal symptom of dizziness. Observing the patient's ability to perform the finger-nose-finger test, the heel-knee-shin test, and rapid alternating movements adequately assesses extremity coordination.

Neuro-otological Examination

The neuro-otological examination is a specialty examination expanding upon certain aspects of the general neurological examination and also includes an audio-vestibular assessment.

Ocular Motor

The first step in assessing ocular motor function is to search for spontaneous involuntary movements of the eyes. The examiner asks the patient to look straight ahead while observing for nystagmus or saccadic intrusions. Nystagmus is characterized by a slow- and fast-phase component and is classified as either spontaneous, gaze-evoked, or positional. The direction of nystagmus is conventionally described by the direction of the fast phase, which is the direction it appears to be "beating" toward. Recording whether the nystagmus is vertical, horizontal, torsional, or a mixture of these provides important localizing information. Spontaneous nystagmus can have either a peripheral or central pattern. Although central lesions can mimic a "peripheral" pattern of nystagmus (Lee and Cho, 2004; Newman-Toker et al., 2008), some very unusual and unlikely circumstances are required for peripheral lesions to cause "central" patterns of nystagmus. A peripheral pattern of spontaneous nystagmus is unidirectional, that is, the eyes beat only to one side (Video 37.1). Peripheral spontaneous nystagmus never changes direction. It is usually a horizontal greater than torsional pattern because of the physiology of the asymmetry in firing rates within the peripheral vestibular system whereby the vertical canals cancel each other out. The prominent horizontal component results

from the unopposed horizontal canal. Other characteristics of peripheral spontaneous nystagmus are suppression with visual fixation, increase in velocity with gaze in the direction of the fast phase, and decrease with gaze in the direction opposite of the fast phase. Some patients are able to suppress this nystagmus so well at the bedside, or have partially recovered from the initiating event, that spontaneous nystagmus may only appear by removing visual fixation. Several simple bedside techniques can be used to remove the patient's ability to fixate. Frenzel glasses are designed to remove visual fixation by using +30 diopter lenses. An ophthalmoscope can be used to block fixation. While the fundus of one eye is being viewed, the patient is asked to cover the other eye. Probably the simplest technique involves holding a blank sheet of paper close to the patient's face (so as to block visual fixation) and observing for spontaneous nystagmus from the side.

Saccadic intrusions are spontaneous, unwanted saccadic movements of the eyes, without the rhythmic fast and slow phases characteristic of nystagmus. *Saccades* are fast movements of the eyes normally under voluntary control and used to shift gaze from one object to another. Square-wave jerks and saccadic oscillations are the most common types of saccadic intrusions. *Square-wave jerks* refer to small-amplitude, involuntary saccades that take the eyes off a target, followed after a normal intersaccadic delay (around 200 ms) by a corrective saccade to bring the eyes back to the target. Square-wave jerks can be seen in neurological disorders such as cerebellar ataxia, Huntington disease (HD), or progressive supranuclear palsy (PSP), but they also occur in normal individuals. If the square-wave jerks are persistent or of large amplitude (macro–square wave jerks), pathology is more likely.

Saccadic oscillations refer to back-to-back saccadic movements without the intersaccadic interval characteristic of square-wave jerks, so their appearance is that of an oscillation. When a burst occurs only in the horizontal plane, the term *ocular flutter* is used (Video 37.2). When vertical and/or torsional components are present, the term *opsoclonus* (or so-called dancing eyes) is used. The eyes make constant random conjugate saccades of unequal amplitude in all directions. Ocular flutter and opsoclonus are pathological findings typically seen in several different types of CNS diseases involving brainstem-cerebellar pathways. Paraneoplastic disorders should be considered in patients presenting with ocular flutter or opsoclonus.

Gaze Testing

The patient should be asked to look to the left, right, up, and down; the examiner looks for gaze-evoked nystagmus in each position (Video 37.3). A few beats of unsustained nystagmus with gaze greater than 30 degrees is called *end-gaze nystagmus* and variably occurs in normal subjects. Gaze-evoked downbeating nystagmus (Video 37.4), vertical nystagmus that increases on lateral gaze, localizes to the craniocervical junction and midline cerebellum. Gaze testing may also trigger saccadic oscillations.

Smooth Pursuit

Smooth pursuit refers to the voluntary movement of the eyes used to track a target moving at a low velocity. It functions to keep the moving object on the fovea to maximize vision.

Though characteristically a very smooth movement at low frequency and velocity testing, smooth pursuit inevitably breaks down when tested at high frequencies and velocities. Though smooth pursuit often becomes impaired with advanced age, a recent study found no significant decline in smooth pursuit in a group of healthy elderly individuals (>75 years) tested yearly for at least 9 years (Kerber et al., 2006). Patients with impaired smooth pursuit require frequent small saccades to keep up with the target, thus the term *saccadic pursuit* is used to describe this finding (see Video 37.3). Abnormalities of smooth pursuit occur as the result of disorders throughout the CNS and with tranquilizing medicines, alcohol, inadequate concentration or vision, and fatigue. Patients with diffuse cortical disease, basal ganglia disease, or diffuse cerebellar disease consistently have bilaterally impaired smooth pursuit. Patients with early or mild cerebellar degenerative disorders may have markedly impaired smooth pursuit with mild or minimal truncal ataxia as the only findings.

Saccades

Saccades are fast eye movements (velocity of this eye movement can be as high as 600 degrees per second) used to quickly bring an object onto the fovea. Saccades are generated by the burst neurons of the pons (horizontal movements) and midbrain (vertical movements). Lesions or degeneration of these regions leads to slowing of saccades, which can also occur with lesions of the ocular motor neurons or extraocular muscles. Severe slowing can be readily appreciated at the bedside by instructing the patient to look back and forth from one object to another. The examiner observes both the velocity of the saccade and the accuracy. Overshooting saccades (missing the target and then needing to correct) indicates a lesion of the cerebellum (Video 37.5). Undershooting saccades are less specific and often occur in normal subjects.

Optokinetic Nystagmus and Fixation Suppression of the Vestibulo-ocular Reflex

Optokinetic nystagmus (OKN) and fixation suppression of the vestibulo-ocular reflex (VOR suppression) can also be tested at the bedside. OKN is a combination of fast (saccadic) and slow (smooth pursuit) movements of eyes and can be observed in normal individuals when, for example, watching a moving train. OKN is maximally stimulated with both foveal and parafoveal stimulation, so the proper laboratory technique for measuring OKN uses a full-field stimulus by having the patient sit stationary while a large rotating pattern moves around them. This test can be approximated at the bedside by moving a striped cloth in front of the patient, though this technique only stimulates the fovea. Patients with disorders causing severe slowing of saccades will not be able to generate OKN, so their eyes will become pinned to one side. VOR suppression can be tested at the bedside using a swivel chair. The patient sits in the chair and extends his or her arm in the "thumbs-up" position out in front. The patient is instructed to focus on the thumb and to allow the extended arm to move with the body so the visual target of the thumb remains directly in front of the patient. The chair is then rotated from side to side. The patient's eyes should remain locked on the thumb, demonstrating the ability to suppress the VOR stimulated by rotation of the chair. Nystagmus will be observed during the rotation movements in patients with impairment of VOR suppression, which is analogous to impairment of smooth pursuit. Both OKN and VOR suppression can also be helpful when examining patients having difficulty following the instructions for smooth pursuit or saccade testing.

Vestibular Nerve Examination

Often omitted as part of the cranial nerve examination in general neurology texts, important localizing information can be obtained about the functioning of the vestibular nerve at the bedside. A unilateral or bilateral vestibulopathy can be identified using the *head-thrust test* (Halmagyi et al., 2008) (**Fig. 37.3** and Video 37.6). To perform the head-thrust test, the physician stands directly in front of the patient, who is seated on the exam table. The patient's head is held in the examiner's hands, and the patient is instructed to focus on the examiner's nose. The head is then quickly moved about 5 to 10 degrees to one side. In patients with normal vestibular function, the VOR results in movement of the eyes in the direction opposite the head movement. Therefore the patient's eyes remain on the examiner's nose after the sudden movement. The test is repeated in the opposite direction. If the examiner observes a corrective saccade bringing the patient's eyes back to the examiner's nose after the head thrust, impairment of the VOR in the direction of the head movement is identified. Rotating the head slowly back and forth (the doll's eye test) also induces compensatory eye movements, but both the visual and vestibular systems are activated by this low-velocity test, so a patient with complete vestibular function loss and normal visual pursuit will have normal-appearing compensatory eye movements on the doll's eye test. This slow rotation of the head, however, is helpful in a comatose patient who is not able to generate voluntary visual tracking eye movements. Slowly rotating the head can also be a helpful test in patients with impairment of the smooth-pursuit system, because smooth movements of the eyes during slow rotation of the head indicates an intact VOR, whereas continued saccadic movements during slow rotation indicates an accompanying deficit of the VOR (Migliaccio et al., 2004).

Positional Testing

Positional testing can help identify peripheral or central causes of vertigo. The most common positional vertigo, BPPV, is caused by free-floating calcium carbonate debris, usually in the posterior semicircular canal, occasionally in the horizontal canal, or rarely in the anterior canal. The characteristic burst of upbeat torsional nystagmus is triggered in patients with BPPV by a rapid change from an erect sitting position to supine head-hanging left or head-hanging right (the Dix-Hallpike test) (Video 37.7). When present, the nystagmus is usually only triggered in one of these positions. A burst of nystagmus in the opposite direction (downbeat torsional) occurs when the patient resumes the sitting position. A repositioning maneuver can be used to liberate the clot of debris from the posterior canal. We use the modified Epley maneuver (**Fig. 37.4** and Video 37.8), which is more than 80% effective in treating patients with posterior canal BPPV, compared to

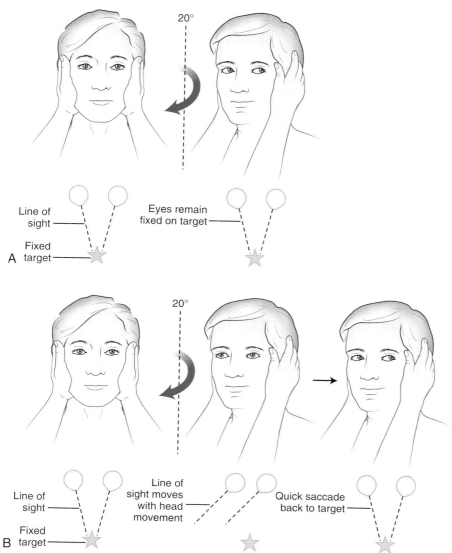

Fig. 37.3 Head-Thrust Test. The head thrust test is a test of vestibular function that can be easily done during the bedside examination. This maneuver tests the vestibulo-ocular reflex (VOR). The patient sits in front of the examiner and the examiner holds the patient's head steady in the midline. The patient is instructed to maintain gaze on the nose of the examiner. The examiner then quickly turns the patient's head about 10-15 degrees to one side and observes the ability of the patient to keep the eyes locked on the examiner's nose. If the patient's eyes stay locked on the examiner's nose (i.e., no corrective saccade) **(A)**, then the **peripheral vestibular system is assumed to be intact.** If, however, the patient's eyes move with the head **(B)** and then the patient makes a voluntary eye movement back to the examiner's nose (i.e., corrective saccade), then this **indicates a lesion of the peripheral vestibular system and not the central nervous system (CNS).** Thus, when a patient presents with the acute vestibular syndrome, the test result shown in **A** would suggest a CNS lesion (because the VOR is intact), whereas the test result in **B** suggests a peripheral vestibular lesion on the right side (because the VOR is not intact). *(From: Edlow JA, Newman-Toker DE, Savitz SI, 2008. Lancet Neurology 7, 951-964.)*

10% effectiveness of a sham procedure (Fife et al., 2008). The key feature of this maneuver is the roll across in the plane of the posterior canal so that the clot rotates around the posterior canal and out into the utricle. Once the clot enters the utricle, it may reattach to the membrane, dissolve, or may even remain free-floating in the utricle, but the debris no longer disrupts semicircular canal function. Recurrences are common, however.

If the debris is in the horizontal canal, direction-changing horizontal nystagmus is seen. Patients are tested for the horizontal canal variant of BPPV by turning the head to each side while lying in the supine position. The nystagmus can be either paroxysmal geotropic (beating toward the ground) or persistent apogeotropic nystagmus (beating away from the ground). In the case of geotropic nystagmus, the debris is in the posterior segment (or "long arm") of the horizontal canal, whereas the debris is in the anterior segment (or "short arm") when apogeotropic nystagmus is triggered. When geotropic nystagmus is triggered, the side with the stronger nystagmus is the involved side. However, when apogeotropic nystagmus

is observed, the involved side is generally opposite the side of the stronger nystagmus. With the geotropic variant, the debris can be removed from the canal by rolling the patient (barbecue fashion) toward the normal side. Other repositioning maneuvers for horizontal canal BPPV include the Gufoni maneuver and the "forced prolonged position" (Fife et al., 2008; Vannucchi et al., 1997). In cases of the apogeotropic variant, performing the barbeque maneuver toward the affected side can convert the nystagmus to geotropic because it moves the particles from the short arm of the canal to the long arm. Once the nystagmus is converted to geotropic, the typical treatments for the geotropic variant are used.

Positional testing can also trigger central types of nystagmus (usually persistent downbeating), which may be the most prominent examination finding in patients with disorders like Chiari malformation or cerebellar ataxia (Kattah and Gujrati, 2005; Kerber et al., 2005a). Central positional nystagmus can mimic the nystagmus of horizontal canal BPPV. Positional nystagmus may also be prominent in patients with migraine-associated dizziness (von Brevern et al., 2005).

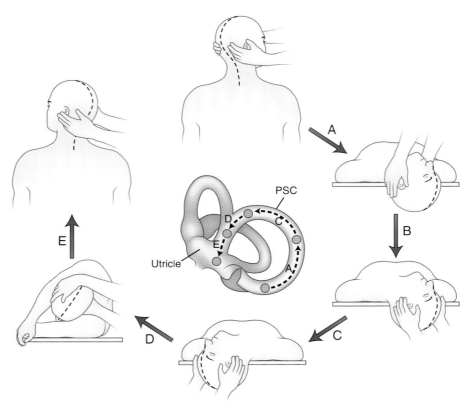

Fig. 37.4 Treatment maneuver for benign paroxysmal positional vertigo affecting the right ear. Procedure can be reversed for treating the left ear. Drawing of labyrinth in the center shows position of the debris as it moves around the posterior semicircular canal (PSC) and into the utricle (UT). **A,** Patient is seated upright with head facing examiner, who is standing on the right. **B,** Patient is then rapidly moved to head-hanging right position (Dix-Hallpike test). This position is maintained until nystagmus ceases. Examiner moves to the head of the table, repositioning hands as shown. **C,** Patient's head is rotated quickly to the left, with right ear upward. This position is maintained for 30 seconds. **D,** Patient rolls onto the left side while examiner rapidly rotates the head leftward until the nose is directed toward the floor. This position is then held for 30 seconds. **E,** Patient is then rapidly lifted into the sitting position, now facing left. The entire sequence should be repeated until no nystagmus can be elicited. Following the maneuver, the patient is instructed to avoid head-hanging positions to prevent the debris from reentering the posterior canal. *(From Baloh, R.W., 1998. Dizziness, Hearing Loss, and Tinnitus. F.A. Davis Company, Philadelphia, Figure 69, p. 166.)*

Fistula Testing

In patients reporting sound- or pressure-induced dizziness, a defect of the bony capsule of the labyrinth can be tested for by pressing and releasing the tragus (small flap of cartilage that can be used to occlude the external ear canal) and observing the eyes for brief associated deviations. Pneumatoscopy (introducing air into the external auditory canal through an otoscope) or Valsalva against pitched nostrils or closed glottis can also trigger associated eye movements. The direction of the triggered nystagmus helps identify the location of the fistula.

Gait

Casual gait is examined for initiation, heel strike, stride length, and base width. Patients are then observed during tandem walking and while standing in the Romberg position (with eyes open and closed). A decreased heel strike, stride length, flexed posture, and decreased arm swing suggests PD. A wide-based gait with inability to tandem walk is characteristic of truncal ataxia. Patients with acute vestibular loss will veer toward the side of the affected ear for several days after the event. Patients with peripheral neuropathy or bilateral vestibulopathy may be unable to stand in the Romberg position with eyes closed.

Auditory Examination

The bedside examination of the auditory system begins with otoscopy. The tympanic membrane is normally translucent; changes in color indicate middle ear disease or tympanosclerosis, a semicircular crescent or horseshoe-shaped white plaque within the tympanic membrane. Tympanosclerosis is rarely associated with hearing loss but is an important clue to past infections. The area just superior to the lateral process of the malleus should be carefully inspected for evidence of a retraction pocket or cholesteatoma. Findings on otoscopy are usually not associated with causes of dizziness because the visualized abnormalities typically do not involve the inner ear.

Finger rubs at different intensities and distances from the ear are a rapid, reliable, and valid screening test for hearing loss in the frequency range of speech (Torres-Russotto et al., 2009). If a patient can hear a faint finger rub stimulus at a distance of 70 cm (approximately one arm's length) from one ear, then a hearing loss on that side—defined by a gold-standard audiogram threshold of greater than 25 dB at 1000, 2000, and 4000 Hz—is highly unlikely. On the other hand, if a patient cannot hear a strong finger rub stimulus at 70 cm, a hearing loss on that side is highly likely. The whisper test can also be used to assess hearing at the bedside (Bagai et al., 2006). For this test, the examiner stands behind the patient to prevent lip reading and occludes and masks the non–test ear, using a finger to rub and close the external auditory canal. The examiner then whispers a set of three to six random numbers and letters. Overall, the patient is considered to have passed the screening test if they repeat at least 50% of the letters and numbers correctly. The Weber and Rinne tests are commonly used bedside tuning fork tests. To perform these, a tuning fork (256 Hz or 512 Hz) is gently struck on a hard rubber pad, the elbow, or the knee about two-thirds of the way along the tine. To conduct the Weber test, the base of the vibrating fork is placed on the vertex (top or crown of the head), bridge of the nose, upper incisors, or forehead. The patient is asked if the sound is heard and whether it is heard in the middle of the head or in both ears equally, toward the left, or toward the right. In a patient with normal hearing, the tone is heard centrally. In asymmetrical or a unilateral hearing impairment, the tone lateralizes to one side. Lateralization indicates an element of conductive impairment in the ear in which the sound localizes, a sensorineural impairment in the contralateral ear, or both. The Rinne test compares the patient's hearing by air conduction with that by bone conduction. The fork is first held against the mastoid process until the sound fades. It is then placed 1 inch from the ear. Normal subjects can hear the fork about twice as long by air as by bone conduction. If bone is greater than air conduction, a conductive hearing loss is suggested.

Specific Disorders Causing Vertigo

Peripheral Vestibular Disorders

Peripheral vestibular disorders are important for neurologists to understand because they are common, readily identified at the bedside, and often missed by frontline physicians (see **Table 37.2**).

Vestibular Neuritis

A common presentation to the ED or outpatient clinic is the rapid onset of severe vertigo, nausea, vomiting, and imbalance. The symptoms gradually resolve over several days, but some symptoms can persist for months. The etiology of this disorder is probably viral, because the course is generally benign and self-limited, it occurs in young healthy individuals, and occasionally occurs in epidemics. Histopathological studies provide evidence of a peripheral vestibular localization and support the etiology of a viral cause. A viral etiology is also the likely cause of most cases of Bell palsy and sudden sensorineural hearing loss. The key to the diagnosis of vestibular neuritis is recognizing the peripheral vestibular pattern of nystagmus and identifying a positive head-thrust test in the setting of a rapid onset of vertigo without other neurological symptoms. Magnetic resonance imaging studies (MRIs) are usually normal in patients with vestibular neuritis (Strupp et al., 1998b). The course of vestibular neuritis is self-limited, and the mainstay of treatment is symptomatic. A recent study of patients with vestibular neuritis showed improvement of peripheral vestibular function, as measured by caloric testing at 1 year, after receiving methylprednisolone within 3 days of onset, compared to placebo (Strupp et al., 2004). A formal vestibular rehabilitation program can help patients compensate for the vestibular lesion (Strupp et al., 1998a).

Benign Paroxysmal Positional Vertigo

Benign paroxysmal positional vertigo may be the most common cause of vertigo in the general population. Patients typically experience brief episodes of vertigo when getting in and out of bed, turning in bed, bending down and straightening up, or extending the head back to look up. As noted earlier, the condition is caused when calcium carbonate debris dislodged from the otoconial membrane inadvertently enters a semicircular canal. The debris can be free-floating within the affected canal (canalithiasis) or stuck against the cupula

(cupulolithiasis). Repositioning maneuvers are highly effective in removing the debris from the canal, though recurrence is common (see **Fig. 37.4**) (Fife et al., 2008). Once the debris is out of the canal, patients are instructed to avoid extreme head positions to prevent the debris from reentering the canal. Patients can also be taught to perform a repositioning maneuver should they have a recurrence of the positional vertigo.

Meniere Disease

Meniere disease is characterized by recurrent attacks of vertigo associated with auditory symptoms (hearing loss, tinnitus, aural fullness) during attacks. Over time, progressive hearing loss develops. Attacks are variable in duration, most lasting longer than 20 minutes, and are associated with severe nausea and vomiting. The course of the disorder is also highly variable. For some patients, the attacks are infrequent and decrease over time, but for others they can become debilitating. Occasionally, auditory symptoms are not appreciated by the patients or identified by interictal audiograms early in the disorder, but inevitably patients with Meniere disease develop these features, usually within the first year. Thus the term *vestibular Meniere disease*, previously used for patients with recurrent episodes of vertigo but no hearing loss, is no longer used. Though usually a disorder involving only one ear, Meniere disease becomes bilateral in about one-third of patients.

Endolymphatic hydrops, or expansion of the endolymph relative to the perilymph, is regarded as the etiology, though the underlying cause is unclear. Additionally, the characteristic histopathological changes of endolymphatic hydrops have been identified in temporal bone specimens of patients with no clinical history of Meniere disease (Merchant et al., 2005). Some patients with well-documented Meniere disease experience abrupt episodes of falling to the ground, without loss of consciousness or associated neurological symptoms. Patients often report the sensation of being pushed or thrown to the ground. The falls are hard and often result in fractures or other injuries. These episodes have been called *otolithic catastrophes of Tumarkin* because of the suspicion that they represent acute stimulation of the otoliths. The bedside interictal examination of patients with Meniere disease may identify asymmetrical hearing, but the head-thrust test is usually normal. Treatment is initially directed toward an aggressive low-salt diet and diuretics, though the evidence for these treatments is poor. Intratympanic gentamicin injections can be effective and are minimally invasive. Sectioning of the vestibular nerve or destruction of the labyrinth are other procedures (Minor et al., 2004). Autoimmune inner ear disease presents as a fulminate variant of Meniere disease. Another variant is so-called delayed endolymphatic hydrops. Patients with this disorder report recurrent episodes of severe vertigo without auditory symptoms developing years after a severe unilateral hearing loss caused by a viral or bacterial infection.

Vestibular Paroxysmia

Vestibular paroxysmia is characterized by brief (seconds to minutes) episodes of vertigo, occurring suddenly without any apparent trigger (Hufner et al., 2008). The disorder may be analogous to hemifacial spasm and trigeminal neuralgia, which are felt to be due to spontaneous discharges from a partially damaged nerve. In patients with vestibular paroxysmia, unilateral dysfunction can sometimes be identified on vestibular or auditory testing. Like the analogous disorders, it is conceivable that a normal vessel could be compressing the cranial nerve, and surgical removal of the vessel might seem to be a treatment option. However, many asymptomatic subjects have a normal vessel lying on the eighth nerve (usually the anterior inferior cerebellar artery), and most vestibular paroxysmia patients have a favorable course with conservative or medication management (Hufner et al., 2008), so the decision to operate in this delicate region is rarely indicated. Medications associated with a reduction in episodes include carbamazepine, oxcarbazepine, and gabapentin (Hufner et al., 2008; Moon and Hain, 2005).

Vestibular Fistulae

Superior canal dehiscence was first described in 1998 (Minor et al., 1998). As the name implies, dehiscence of the bone overlying the superior canal results in a fistula between the superior canal and the middle cranial fossa. Normally the semicircular canals are enclosed by the rigid bony capsule, so these vestibular structures are unaffected by sound pressure changes. The oval and round windows direct the forces associated with sound waves into the cochlea and along the spiral basilar membrane. A break in the bony capsule of the semicircular canals can redirect some of the sound or pressure to the semicircular canals causing vestibular activation, a phenomenon known as *Tullio phenomenon*. Prior to the discovery of SCD, fistulas were known to occur with rupture of the oval or round window or erosion into the horizontal semicircular canal from chronic infection. Pressure changes generated by increasing intracranial pressure (ICP) (Valsalva against closed glottis) or increasing middle ear pressure (Valsalva against pinched nostrils or compression of the tragus) triggers brief nystagmus in the plane of the affected canal. Surgically repairing the defect can be attempted if the patient is debilitated by the symptoms, but many patients do well with conservative management. Patients with SCD may have hypersensitivity to bone-conducted sound and bone-conduction thresholds on the audiogram lower than the normal 0 dB hearing levels, even though air conduction thresholds remain normal (Minor, 2005). Other vestibular fistulae can result from trauma or erosion of a cholesteatoma into the horizontal semicircular canal.

Other Peripheral Disorders

There are many other peripheral vestibular causes of vertigo, but most are uncommon. Vertigo often follows a blow to the head, even without a corresponding temporal bone fracture. This so-called labyrinthine concussion results from the susceptibility of the delicate structures of the inner ear to blunt trauma. Vestibular ototoxicity, usually from gentamicin, can cause a vestibulopathy that is usually bilateral but rarely can be unilateral (Waterston and Halmagyi, 1998). A bilateral vestibulopathy can also occur from an immune-mediated disorder (e.g., autoimmune inner ear disease, Cogan syndrome), infectious process (e.g., meningitis, syphilitic labyrinthitis), structural lesion (bilateral acoustic neuroma), or a genetic disorder (e.g., neurodegenerative or isolated vestibular). The bilateral vestibular loss often goes unrecognized because the vestibular symptoms can be overshadowed by auditory or other symptoms. Although the most prominent vestibular symptoms of bilateral vestibulopathy are oscillopsia and imbalance, some nonspecific dizziness and vertigo attacks may occur as well. Acoustic neuromas, vestibular schwannomas, typically present with slowly progressive unilateral hearing loss, but rarely vertigo can occur. Because the tumor growth is slow, the vestibulopathy is compensated by the CNS. Finally, any disorder affecting the skull base, such as sarcoidosis, lymphoma, bacterial and fungal infections, or carcinomatous meningitis, can cause either unilateral or bilateral peripheral vestibular symptoms.

Central Nervous System Disorders

The key to the diagnosis of CNS disorders in patients presenting with dizziness are the presence of other focal neurological symptoms or identifying central ocular motor abnormalities or ataxia. Because central disorders can mimic peripheral vestibular disorders, the most effective approach in patients with isolated dizziness is first to rule out common peripheral causes.

Brainstem or Cerebellar Ischemia/Infarction

Ischemia affecting vestibular pathways within the brainstem or cerebellum often causes vertigo. Brainstem ischemia is normally accompanied by other neurological signs and symptoms, because motor and sensory pathways are in close proximity to vestibular pathways. Vertigo is the most common symptom with Wallenberg syndrome, infarction in the lateral medulla in the territory of the posterior inferior cerebellar artery (PICA), but other neurological symptoms and signs (e.g., diplopia, facial numbness, Horner syndrome) are invariably present. Ischemia of the cerebellum can cause vertigo as the most prominent or only symptom, and a common dilemma is whether the patient with acute-onset vertigo needs an MRI to rule out cerebellar infarction. Computed tomography (CT) scans of the posterior fossa are not a sensitive test for ischemic stroke (Chalela et al., 2007). Abnormal ocular motor findings in patients with brainstem or cerebellar strokes include: (1) spontaneous nystagmus that is purely vertical, horizontal, or torsional, (2) direction-changing gaze-evoked nystagmus (patient looks to the left and has left-beating nystagmus, looks to the right and has right-beating nystagmus), (3) impairment of smooth pursuit, and (4) overshooting saccades. Rarely, central causes of nystagmus can closely mimic the peripheral vestibular pattern of spontaneous nystagmus (Lee et al., 2006b; Newman-Toker et al., 2008). Patients with brainstem or cerebellar infarction need immediate attention because herniation or recurrent stroke can occur. However, because of the rarity of ischemia causing isolated vertigo, MRI need only be considered in patients with significant stroke risk, factors such as older age, known history of stroke, transient ischemic attacks (TIAs), coronary artery disease, or diabetes.

Multiple Sclerosis

Dizziness is a common symptom in patients with multiple sclerosis (MS). Vertigo is the initial symptom in about 5% of patients with MS. A typical MS attack has a gradual onset, reaching its peak within a few days. Milder spontaneous episodes of vertigo, not characteristic of a new attack, and positional vertigo lasting seconds are also common in MS patients. The key to the diagnosis is to find lesions disseminated in time and space within the nervous system. Nearly all varieties of central spontaneous and positional nystagmus occur with MS, and occasionally patients show typical peripheral vestibular nystagmus when the lesion affects the root entry zone of the vestibular nerve. MRI of the brain identifies white matter lesions in about 95% of MS patients, although similar lesions are sometimes seen in patients without the clinical criteria for the diagnosis of MS.

Posterior Fossa Structural Abnormalities

Any structural lesion of the posterior fossa can cause dizziness. With the Chiari malformation, the brainstem and cerebellum are elongated downward into the cervical canal, causing pressure on both the caudal midline cerebellum and the cervicomedullary junction. The most common neurological symptom is a slowly progressive unsteadiness of gait, which patients often describe as dizziness. Vertigo and hearing loss are uncommon, occurring in about 10% of patients. Spontaneous or positional downbeat nystagmus is particularly common with Chiari malformations, but other forms of central nystagmus also occur. Dysphagia, hoarseness, and dysarthria can result from stretching of the lower cranial nerves, and obstructive hydrocephalus can result from occlusion of the basilar cisterns. MRI is the procedure of choice for identifying Chiari malformations; midline sagittal sections clearly show the level of the cerebellar tonsils. The most common CNS tumors in the posterior fossa are gliomas in adults and medulloblastoma in children. Ocular motor dysfunction (impaired smooth pursuit, overshooting saccades), impaired coordination, or other central findings occur in these patients. An early finding of patients with cerebellar tumors can be central positional nystagmus. Vascular malformations (arteriovenous malformations [AVMs], cavernous hemangiomas) can similarly cause dizziness but generally are asymptomatic until bleeding occurs, at which time they can be life threatening.

Neurodegenerative Disorders

It is not uncommon for a patient with the main complaint of dizziness to have or later develop typical features of PD, a parkinsonian syndrome (PSP, multiple systems atrophy), or a progressive ataxia disorder (de Lau et al., 2006). However, dizziness in these patients is usually better clarified as imbalance. Positional downbeat nystagmus occurs in patients with spinocerebellar ataxia type 6 (SCA6) and other progressive ataxia disorders (Kattah and Gujrati, 2005; Kerber et al., 2005a).

Epilepsy

Vestibular symptoms are common with focal seizures, particularly those originating from the temporal and parietal lobes. The key to differentiating vertigo with seizures from other causes of vertigo is that seizures are almost invariably associated with an altered level of consciousness. Episodic vertigo as an isolated manifestation of a focal seizure is a rarity if it occurs at all.

Vertigo in Inherited Disorders

The clinical evaluation of patients presenting with dizziness has traditionally hinged on the history of present illness and examination. However, with the recent rapid advances in molecular biology, it has become apparent that many causes of vertigo have a strong genetic component. Because of this, obtaining a complete family history is very important, particularly in patients without a specific diagnosis for their dizziness. Since the symptoms of these familial disorders are often not debilitating and can be highly variable, simply asking the patient about a family history at the time of the appointment may not be adequate. The patient should be instructed to specifically interview other family members regarding the occurrence of these symptoms.

Migraine

Migraine is a heterogeneous genetic disorder characterized by headaches in addition to many other neurological symptoms. Several rare monogenetic subtypes have been identified. Linkage analysis has identified a number of chromosomal loci in common forms of migraine, but no specific genes have been found. Dizziness has long been known to occur among patients with migraine headaches, and benign recurrent vertigo is usually a migraine equivalent because no other signs or symptoms develop over time, the neurological exam remains normal, and a family or personal history of migraine headaches is common, as are typical migraine triggers. Interestingly, some patients with benign recurrent vertigo (BRV) also report auditory symptoms similar to patients with Meniere disease, and a mild hearing loss may also be seen on the audiogram (Battista, 2004). The key distinguishing factor between migraine and Meniere disease is the lack of progressive unilateral hearing loss in patients with migraine. Other types of dizziness are common in patients with migraine as well, including nonspecific dizziness and positional vertigo (von Brevern et al., 2005). The cause of vertigo in migraine patients is not yet known, but the diagnosis of migraine should be entertained in any patient with chronic recurrent attacks of dizziness of unknown cause. Long-standing motion sensitivity including carsickness, sensitivities to other types of stimuli, and a clear family history of migraine help support the diagnosis. Also, some patients have a typical migraine visual aura or other focal neurological symptoms associated with headache. Though the diagnosis of migraine-associated dizziness remains one of exclusion, little else can cause recurrent episodes without any other symptoms over a long period of time. In a genome-wide linkage scan of BRV patients (20 families) linkage to chromosome 22q12 was found, but genetic heterogeneity was evident (Lee et al., 2006a). Testing linkage using a broader phenotype of BRV and migraine headaches weakened the linkage signal. Thus, no evidence exists at this time that migraine is allelic with BRV, even though migraine has a high prevalence in BRV patients.

Familial Bilateral Vestibulopathy

Familial bilateral vestibulopathy (FBV) patients typically have brief attacks of vertigo (seconds) followed by progressive loss of peripheral vestibular function leading to imbalance and oscillopsia, usually by the fifth decade. The recurrent attacks of vertigo may somehow cause damage to vestibular structures, leading to progressive vestibular loss. Quantitative rotational testing shows gains greater than 2 standard deviations below the normal mean for both sinusoidal and step changes in angular velocity. Caloric testing is insensitive for identifying bilateral vestibulopathy because of the wide range of normal caloric responses. The bedside head-thrust test may show bilateral corrective saccades when vestibulopathy is severe. As the vestibulopathy becomes more severe, attacks of vertigo become less frequent and eventually cease. Despite the high prevalence of familial hearing loss and enormous progress in identifying the genetic basis of deafness, to date no gene mutations have been identified that lead to isolated bilateral vestibulopathy in humans. Only a few FBV families have been described (Brantberg, 2003; Jen et al., 2004b). Given the high prevalence and genetic diversity of familial hearing loss, it seems reasonable to suspect that bilateral vestibulopathy would have a similar prevalence and genetic diversity. The huge disparity in knowledge about genetic deafness and genetic vestibulopathy might stem from our inadequacy to identify vestibulopathy rather than the rareness of the disorder. It is much more straightforward for healthcare providers to identify the symptoms of hearing loss than the symptoms of vestibular loss. Adequate laboratory testing for hearing loss is also much more readily available than it is for vestibular loss. Increased knowledge and use of the bedside head-thrust test, however, has the potential to substantially enhance the identification of bilateral vestibular loss.

Familial Hearing Loss and Vertigo

Familial progressive vestibular-cochlear dysfunction was first identified in 1988. Linkage to chromosome 14q12-13 was later found, and the disorder was designated DFNA9 (DFNA = deafness, familial, non-syndromic, type A [autosomal dominant]) (Manolis et al., 1996). Using an organ-specific approach, mutations within COCH were found to cause DFNA9 (Robertson et al., 1998). This disorder of progressive hearing loss is unique because no other autosomal dominant genetic hearing loss syndromes have vertigo as a common symptom. Progressive hearing loss is the most prominent symptom of DFNA9. Vertigo occurs in about 50% of DFNA9 patients. When present, vertigo may be spontaneous in onset or positionally triggered (Lemaire et al., 2003). Age of onset is variable, with some patients developing symptoms in the second to third decade and others developing symptoms later. Vertigo attacks last minutes to hours and can be accompanied by worsening of hearing, aural fullness, or tinnitus, thus closely mimicking Meniere syndrome. Vertigo episodes can precede or accompany onset of hearing loss. In addition to severe progressive hearing loss, eventually DFNA9 patients develop progressive loss of vestibular function and corresponding symptoms of imbalance and oscillopsia. Because some patients have attacks closely resembling Meniere syndrome, the COCH gene was screened for mutations in idiopathic Meniere disease patients, but none were found. No studies report the use of effective treatments for vertigo attacks, but like FBV patients, these attacks generally only last a few years and then become less frequent, presumably due to loss of vestibular function. Of the many autosomal dominant genes that cause hearing loss, DFNA11 is the only other one associated with vestibulopathy.

Enlarged vestibular aqueduct syndrome (EVA), designated *DFNB4* (DFNB = deafness, familial, non-syndromic, type B [autosomal recessive]), is characterized by early-onset hearing loss with enlargement of the vestibular aqueduct best seen on temporal bone CT. Normally, the vestibular aqueduct is less than 1.5 mm in diameter, but in EVA it is much larger. The mechanism leading to hearing loss and vertigo is unclear. The vestibular aqueduct contains the endolymphatic duct, which connects the medial wall of the vestibule to the endolymphatic sac and is an important structure in the exchange of endolymph. Enlargement may cause increased transmission of ICPs to the inner ear structures. However, the Valsalva maneuver—which increases ICP—does not trigger symptoms in EVA patients. Vertigo attacks last 15 minutes to 3 hours and are not associated with changes in hearing. Vertigo attacks may begin at the onset of hearing loss (early childhood) or years later and can be triggered by blows to the head or vigorous spinning (Oh et al., 2001a). Quantitative vestibular testing may be normal in EVA patients or reveal mild to moderate loss of vestibular function. Enlargement of the vestibular aqueduct has also been observed in Pendred syndrome (PS), branchio-oto-renal syndrome, CHARGE (*c*oloboma of the eye, *h*eart defects, *a*tresia choanae, *r*etardation of growth or development, *g*enitourinary anomalies, and *e*ar abnormalities or hearing impairment), Waardenburg syndrome, and distal renal tubular acidosis with deafness. EVA syndrome is allelic to PS, which is characterized by developmental abnormalities of the cochlea in combination with thyroid dysfunction and goiter.

Familial Ataxia Syndromes

Vestibular symptoms and signs are common with several of the hereditary ataxia syndromes including SCA types 1, 2, 3, 6, and 7, Friedreich ataxia, Refsum disease, and episodic ataxia (EA) types 2, 3, 4, and 5. In most of these disorders, the symptoms are slowly progressive, with the cerebellar ataxia and incoordination overshadowing the vestibular symptoms. Head movement–induced oscillopsia commonly occurs because the patient is unable to suppress the VOR with fixation. Attacks of vertigo may occur in up to half of patients with SCA6 (Takahashi et al., 2004), many of which are positionally triggered (Jen et al., 1998). Persistent downbeating nystagmus is often seen after placing patients into the head-hanging position; the positional vertigo and nystagmus can even be the initial symptom in these patients. Most of the episodic ataxia syndromes have onset before the age of 20 (Jen et al., 2004a). The attacks are characterized by extreme incoordination leading to severe difficulty walking during attacks. Vertigo can occur as part of these attacks, and migraine headaches are common in these patients as well. In fact EA2, SCA6, and familial hemiplegic migraine type 1 are all caused by mutations with the same gene, CACNA1A. An additional feature of EA2 and EA4 is the eventual development of interictal nystagmus and progressive ataxia. Patients with EA2 often have a dramatic response to treatment with acetazolamide.

Common Causes of Nonspecific Dizziness

Patients with nonspecific dizziness are probably referred to neurologists more frequently than patients with true vertigo. These patients are usually bothered by lightheadedness (wooziness), presyncope, imbalance, motion sensitivity, or anxiety. Side effects or toxicity from medications are common causes of nonspecific dizziness. Bothersome lightheadedness can be a direct effect of the medication itself or the result of lowering of the patient's blood pressure. Ataxia can be caused by antiepileptic medications and is usually reversible once the medication is decreased or stopped. Patients with peripheral neuropathy causing dizziness report significant worsening of their balance in poor lighting and also the sensation that they are walking on cushions. Drops in blood pressure can be caused by dehydration, vasovagal attacks, or as part of an autonomic neuropathy. Patients with panic attacks can present with nonspecific dizziness, but their spells are invariably accompanied by other symptoms such as sense of fear or doom, palpitations, sweating, shortness of breath, or paresthesias. Other medical conditions such as cardiac arrhythmias or metabolic disturbances can also cause nonspecific dizziness. In the elderly, confluent white matter hyperintensities have a strong association with dizziness and balance problems. Presumably the result of small vessel arteriosclerosis, decreased cerebral perfusion (Marstrand et al., 2002) has been identified in these patients even when blood pressure taken at the arm is normal. Patients with dizziness related to white matter hyperintensities on MRI usually feel better sitting or lying down and typically have impairment of tandem gait. Since many elderly patients are taking blood pressure medications, at least a trial of lowering or discontinuing these medications is warranted.

Common Presentations of Vertigo

Patients present with symptoms rather than specific diagnoses. The most common presentations of vertigo are the following.

Acute Severe Vertigo

The patient presenting with new-onset severe vertigo probably has vestibular neuritis but stroke should also be a concern. An abrupt onset and accompanying focal neurological symptoms, particularly those that can be related to the posterior circulation, suggests an ischemic stroke. If no significant abnormalities are noted on the general neurological examination, attention should focus on the neuro-otological evaluation. If no spontaneous nystagmus is observed, a technique to block visual fixation should be applied. The direction of the nystagmus should be noted and the effect of gaze assessed. If a peripheral vestibular pattern of nystagmus is identified, a positive head-thrust test in the direction opposite the fast phase of nystagmus is highly localizing to the vestibular nerve. By far the most common cause of this presentation is vestibular neuritis. A central vestibular lesion (e.g., ischemic stroke) becomes a serious concern if there are "red flags" such as other central signs or symptoms, direction-changing nystagmus, vertical nystagmus, a negative head-thrust test (i.e., no corrective saccade after the head-thrust test to the direction opposite

the fast phase of spontaneous nystagmus), or substantial stroke risk factors (Kattah et al., 2009; Lee et al., 2006b). Vertebral artery dissection can lead to an acute vertigo presentation, but the most common symptom is severe, sudden-onset occipital or neck pain, with additional neurological signs and symptoms (de Bray et al., 1997). If hearing loss accompanies the episode, labyrinthitis is the most likely diagnosis, but auditory involvement does not exclude the possibility of a vascular cause, because the anterior inferior cerebellar artery supplies both the inner ear and brain. When hearing loss and facial weakness accompany the acute onset of vertigo, one should closely inspect the outer ear for vesicles characteristic of herpes zoster (Ramsay Hunt syndrome). An acoustic neuroma is a slow-growing tumor, so only rarely is it associated with acute-onset vertigo. Migraine can mimic vestibular neuritis, though the diagnosis of migraine-associated vertigo hinges on recurrent episodes and lack of progressive auditory symptoms.

Recurrent Attacks of Vertigo

In patients with recurrent attacks of vertigo, the key diagnostic information lies in the details of the attacks. Meniere disease is the likely cause in patients with recurrent vertigo lasting longer than 20 minutes and associated with unilateral auditory symptoms. If the Meniere-like attacks present in a fulminate fashion, the diagnosis of autoimmune inner ear disease should be considered. Transient ischemic attacks (TIA) should be suspected in patients having brief episodes (minutes) of vertigo, particularly when vascular risk factors are present and other neurological symptoms are reported. Case series of patients with rotational vertebral artery syndrome demonstrate that the inner ear and possibly central vestibular pathways have high energy requirements and are therefore susceptible to levels of ischemia tolerated by other parts of the brain (Choi et al., 2005). Crescendo TIAs can be the harbinger of impending stroke or basilar artery occlusion. As with acute severe vertigo, accompanying auditory symptoms do not exclude the possibility of an ischemic disorder. Migraine and the migraine equivalent, BRV, are characterized by a history of similar symptoms, a normal examination, family or personal history of migraine headaches and/or BRV, other migraine characteristics, and typical triggers. Attacks are otherwise highly variable, lasting anywhere from seconds to days. If the attacks are consistently seconds in duration, the diagnosis of vestibular paroxysmia should be considered. Multiple sclerosis may be the cause when patients have recurrent episodes of vertigo and a history of other attacks of neurological symptoms, particularly when fixed deficits such as an afferent pupillary defect or internuclear ophthalmoplegia are identified on the examination.

Recurrent Positional Vertigo

Positional vertigo is defined by the symptom being *triggered*, not simply worsened, by certain positional changes. Vestibular neuritis is often confused with BPPV because vestibular neuritis patients can often settle into a relatively comfortable position and then experience dramatic worsening with movement. The patient complaining of recurrent episodes of vertigo triggered by certain head movements likely has BPPV, but this is not the only possibility. BPPV can be identified and treated at the bedside, so positional testing should be performed in any patient with this complaint. Positional testing can also uncover the other causes of positionally triggered dizziness (Bertholon et al., 2002). The history strongly suggests the diagnosis of BPPV when the positional vertigo is brief (<1 minute), has typical triggers, and is unaccompanied by other neurological symptoms. A burst of vertical torsional nystagmus is specific for BPPV of the posterior canal (Aw et al., 2005). If the Dix-Hallpike test is negative, the examiner should search for the horizontal canal variant of BPPV. Central positional nystagmus occurs as the result of disorders affecting the posterior fossa, including tumors, cerebellar degeneration, Chiari malformation, or MS. The nystagmus of these disorders is typically downbeating and persistent, though a pure torsional nystagmus may occur as well. Patients with loss of one vertebral artery may develop vertigo or significant dizziness after head turns to the direction opposite the intact artery because the bony structures of the spinal column can pinch off the remaining vertebral artery (Choi et al., 2005). Central types of nystagmus develop as a result, and vertigo can be the most prominent symptom. Finally, migraine can also closely mimic BPPV and central positional nystagmus (von Brevern et al., 2005). Patients with migraine as the cause typically report a longer duration of symptoms once the positional vertigo is triggered, and the nystagmus may be of a central or peripheral type. The mechanisms are not clear, but the disorder is benign because it is usually self-limited and not progressive. Associations between migraine and typical BPPV have also been made, but the link between these disorders is unclear.

Hearing Loss

Neurologists generally do not encounter patients principally bothered by auditory symptoms such as hearing loss or tinnitus, as opposed to patients with dizziness, who are frequently referred for evaluation. Nevertheless, an understanding of the auditory system, certain disorders causing auditory symptoms, and audiograms can enhance the diagnostic abilities of the neurologist.

Conductive Hearing Loss

Conductive hearing loss results from lesions involving the external or the middle ear. The tympanic membrane and ossicles act as a transformer, amplifying the airborne sound and effectively transferring it to the inner-ear fluid. If this normal pathway is obstructed, transmission can occur across the skin and through the bones of the skull (bone conduction) but at the cost of significant energy loss. Patients with a conductive hearing loss can hear speech in a noisy background better than a quiet background, since they can understand loud speech as well as anyone. The most common cause of conductive hearing loss is impacted cerumen in the external canal. The most common serious cause of conductive hearing loss is otitis media, which can result from either infected fluid (suppurative otitis) or noninfected fluid (serous otitis) accumulating in the middle ear and impairing conduction of airborne sound. With chronic otitis media, a cholesteatoma may erode the ossicles. Otosclerosis produces progressive conductive hearing loss by immobilizing the stapes with new bone growth in front of and below the oval window. Other common causes of conductive hearing loss are trauma, congenital mal-

formations of the external and middle ear, and glomus body tumors.

Sensorineural Hearing Loss

Sensorineural hearing loss results from lesions of the cochlea, the auditory division of the acoustic nerve, or both and results in inability to normally perceive both bone- and air-conducted sound. The spiral cochlea mechanically analyzes the frequency content of sound. For high-frequency tones, only sensory cells in the basilar turn are activated, but for low-frequency tones, all sensory cells are activated. Therefore, with lesions of the cochlea and its afferent nerve, the hearing levels for different frequencies are usually unequal, and the phase relationship between different frequencies may be altered. Patients with sensorineural hearing loss often have difficulty hearing speech that is mixed with background noise, and they may be annoyed by loud speech. Distortion of sounds is common with sensorineural hearing loss. A pure tone may be heard as noisy, rough, or buzzing, or it may be distorted so that it sounds like a complex mixture of tones.

Central Hearing Loss

Central hearing loss results from lesions of the central auditory pathways. These lesions involve the cochlear and dorsal olivary nuclear complexes, inferior colliculi, medial geniculate bodies, auditory cortex in the temporal lobes, and interconnecting afferent and efferent fiber tracks. As a rule, patients with central lesions do not have impaired hearing levels for pure tones, and they understand speech so long as it is clearly spoken in a quiet environment. If the listener's task is made more difficult with the introduction of background or competing messages, performance deteriorates more markedly in patients with central lesions than it does in normal subjects. Lesions involving the eighth nerve root entry zone or cochlear nucleus (demyelination or infarction in the lateral pontomedullary region), however, can cause unilateral hearing loss for pure tones. Because about half of afferent nerve fibers cross central to the cochlear nucleus, this is the most central structure in which a lesion can result in a unilateral hearing loss.

Specific Disorders Causing Hearing Loss

Meniere Disease

Auditory symptoms in Meniere disease consist of a fluctuating sense of fullness and pressure along with tinnitus and decreased hearing in one ear. In the early stages, the hearing loss is completely reversible, but in later stages a residual hearing loss remains. Tinnitus may persist between episodes but usually increases in intensity immediately before or during the acute episode. It is typically described as a roaring sound like the sound of the ocean or a hollow seashell. The hearing loss on the audiogram appears in the early stages as a low-frequency loss. However, as the disorder progresses, a more complete hearing loss occurs. In a small number of patients, the disorder becomes bilateral. Eventually, severe permanent hearing loss develops, and the episodic nature spontaneously disappears. When the progression of hearing loss (particularly when bilateral) is fulminant and rapidly progressive, the diagnosis of autoimmune inner ear disease should be considered. Also see the section on Meniere disease under Specific Disorders Causing Vertigo.

Cerebellopontine Angle Tumors

Acoustic neuromas (vestibular schwannoma) account for about 5% of intracranial tumors and more than 90% of cerebellopontine angle tumors. These tumors usually begin in the internal auditory canal, producing symptoms by compressing the nerve in its narrow confines. As the tumor grows, it protrudes through the internal auditory meatus, stretches adjacent nerves over the surface of the mass, and deforms the cerebellum and brainstem. By far the most common symptoms associated with acoustic neuromas are slowly progressive unilateral hearing loss and tinnitus from compression of the cochlear nerve. Rarely, acute hearing loss occurs, apparently from compression of the labyrinthine vasculature. Vertigo occurs infrequently, but approximately half of patients with an acoustic neuroma complain of mild imbalance or disequilibrium. An epidermoid tumor, meningioma, facial nerve schwannoma, or metastatic disease can also cause mass lesions within the cerebellopontine angle. The audiometric pattern is variable; however, patients with cerebellopontine angle tumors causing hearing loss usually have poor speech discrimination, acoustic reflex decay, and pure tone decay rather than a marked asymmetry of pure tones.

Superior Canal Dehiscence

Patients with SCD may experience conductive hyperacusis (hearing their eye move or the impact of their feet during walking or running) and autophony (hearing their own breath and voice sounds) in the affected ear. An air/bone gap is often identified on standard audiograms. The Weber tuning fork test typically lateralizes to the affected ear, and the Rinne turning fork test may show bone conduction greater than air conduction (see Specific Disorders Causing Vertigo).

Otosclerosis

Otosclerosis is a metabolic disease of the bony labyrinth that usually manifests by immobilizing the stapes, thereby producing a conductive hearing loss. A positive family history for otosclerosis is reported in 50% to 70% of cases. Bilateral involvement is usual, but about one-fourth of cases are unilateral. Although conductive hearing loss is the hallmark of otosclerosis, a combined conductive-sensorineural hearing loss pattern is frequent. Although otosclerosis is primarily a disorder of the auditory system, vestibular symptoms and signs are more common than generally appreciated.

Noise-Induced Hearing Loss

Noise-induced hearing loss is extremely common in our industrialized society. About one-third of individuals with hearing loss can attribute at least part of the loss to noise exposure. The loss almost always begins at 4000 Hz, creating the typical notched appearance on the audiogram, and does not affect speech discrimination until late in the disease process. Typically, levels of noise exposure greater than 85 dB

are required to cause the changes in the ear induced by loud noise. Examples of noise greater than 85 dB that are common sources of exposure include motorcycles, firecrackers, factory machinery, and music concerts.

Genetic Disorders

Many genetic causes of hearing loss have been identified, including syndromic and nonsyndromic phenotypes and inheritance types that are autosomal dominant, autosomal recessive, and mitochondrial. Typically these disorders start early in life and cause profound hearing loss. Vestibular symptoms are not common but may not be thoroughly assessed in affected individuals.

Ototoxicity

The most common medications causing hearing loss are aminoglycoside antibiotics, loop diuretics, and cisplatin. Impaired elimination of these drugs, such as occurs in patients with renal insufficiency, predisposes to ototoxicity. Patients receiving high-dose salicylate therapy frequently complain of hearing loss, tinnitus, and dizziness. These symptoms and signs are rapidly reversible after cessation of the salicylate ingestion.

Common Presentations of Hearing Loss

Asymmetrical Sensorineural Hearing Loss

Evaluation of patients identified as having an asymmetrical sensorineural hearing loss is primarily the search for a tumor in the area of the internal auditory canal or cerebellopontine angle, or more rarely other lesions of the temporal bone or brain. With an asymmetry of hearing defined as 15 dB or greater in two or more frequencies or a 15% or more asymmetry in speech discrimination scores, approximately 10% of patients will have lesions identified on MRI (Cueva, 2004). Acoustic neuromas are by far the most common abnormality found. Other causative lesions may include glomus jugulare tumors, ectatic basilar artery with brainstem compression, or petrous apex cholesterol granuloma. Auditory brainstem response testing shows a sensitivity and specificity around 70%, with a false-positive rate of 77%, but a false-negative rate of 29% (Cueva, 2004).

Sudden Sensorineural Hearing Loss

The etiology of sudden sensorineural hearing loss is similar to both Bell palsy and vestibular neuritis in that a viral cause is presumed in the majority of cases, but proof of a viral pathophysiology in a given case is difficult to obtain. The hearing loss can abruptly develop or evolve over several hours. Acoustic neuromas may be found in around 5% of patients with this presentation (Aarnisalo et al., 2004), but one should also be aware of false-positive MRIs, particularly for lesions smaller than 6 mm (Arriaga et al., 1995). Focal ischemia to the cochlea, cochlear nerve, or the root entry zone can also cause an abrupt loss of hearing over several minutes. In the setting of a patient at risk for stroke, this cause should be considered early, because it can be the harbinger of basilar artery occlusion (Toyoda et al., 2002). Sudden-onset bilateral hearing loss can rarely result from bilateral lesions of the primary auditory cortex in the transverse temporal gyri of Heschl. Deficits can range from auditory agnosia for speech or nonspeech sounds, with relatively normal hearing thresholds, to rare cases of cortical deafness characterized by markedly elevated pure-tone thresholds.

Hearing Loss with Age

The bilateral hearing loss commonly associated with advancing age is called *presbycusis*. It is not a distinct entity but rather represents multiple effects of aging on the auditory system. It may include conductive and central dysfunction, but the most consistent effect of aging is on the sensory cells and the neurons of the cochlea. The typical audiogram appearance in patients with presbycusis is that of symmetrical hearing loss, with the tracing gradually sloping downward with increasing frequency. The most consistent pathology associated with presbycusis is a degeneration of sensory cells and nerve fibers at the base of the cochlea.

Tinnitus

Tinnitus is a noise in the ear that is usually audible only to the patient, although occasionally the sound can be heard by the examining physician. It is a symptom that can be associated with a variety of disorders that may affect the ear or the brain. The most important piece of information is whether the patient localizes it to one or both years or if it is non-localizable. As a general rule, tinnitus localized to one ear will have an identifiable cause, but when localized to both ears or nonlocalizable, often it will not. The characteristics of the tinnitus should be described by the patient, as this can provide helpful information. For an example, the typical tinnitus associated with Meniere disease is described as a roaring sound like listening to a seashell. The tinnitus associated with an acoustic neuroma is typically a high-pitched ringing or like the sound of steam blowing from a teakettle. If the tinnitus is rhythmic, the patient should be asked whether it is synchronous with the pulse or with respiration. Recurrent rhythmic or even nonrhythmic clicking sounds in one ear can indicate stapedial palatal myoclonus. However, the most common form of tinnitus is a bilateral high-pitched sound that is usually worse at night when it is quiet and there is less background noise to mask it. Tinnitus can be worse when the patient is under stress or with the use of caffeine.

Laboratory Investigations in Diagnosis and Management

Dizziness and Vertigo

The history and physical examination should determine what diagnostic tests if any are necessary in patients presenting with dizziness or vertigo. Studies have repeatedly shown that MRI, audiogram, and vestibular tests are no different in unselected patients complaining of dizziness when compared to age-matched controls (Colledge et al., 1996; Colledge et al., 2002; Hajioff et al., 2002; Lawson et al., 1999; Yardley et al., 1998). Many disorders causing dizziness can be diagnosed and even treated at the bedside, with no further diagnostic tests indicated.

General Tests

General tests such as blood work, chest x-ray, or electrocardiograms are only indicated when searching for a specific abnormality. If a patient has otherwise unexplained nonspecific dizziness, ruling out metabolic causes is indicated.

Imaging

Brain imaging is commonly ordered in patients complaining of dizziness. Though a CT scan can rule out a large mass, smaller lesions can not be excluded because of artifact and poor resolution in the posterior fossa (Chalela et al., 2007). MRI is the imaging modality of choice but is expensive and generally a much less practical test than CT. Determining what patients should have an MRI can be difficult, which is why an understanding of the common peripheral vestibular disorders is important. Patients identified as having BPPV, vestibular neuritis, or Meniere disease do not require an imaging study. Additionally, patients with normal neurological and neuro-otological examinations reporting episodes of dizziness dating back more than several months are highly unlikely to have a relevant abnormality on MRI. Though studies show improved hearing preservation after surgery in patients with acoustic neuromas when diagnosed early, this does not mean that every patient complaining of dizziness requires an MRI to exclude this cause. Acoustic neuromas are rare, whereas dizziness and vertigo are extremely common. On the other hand, for any patient experiencing focal neurological symptoms or having unexplained neurological deficits or an otherwise rapid, unexplained progression of symptoms, an MRI should be strongly considered to rule out a mass lesion, stroke, structural abnormality, or MS. In dizzy patients with gradually progressive hearing loss, MRI may also be helpful.

Vestibular Testing
EYE MOVEMENT RECORDING
Methods of Recording Eye Movements

The earliest measures of eye movement recording were made using electro-oculography (EOG). This technique utilizes the potential difference between the cornea and retina, known as the *corneal-retinal potential*, which acts as an electric dipole oriented in the direction of the long axis of the eye (Baloh and Kerber, 2011). When electrodes are placed in the vicinity of the eyes, it becomes more positive when the eye rotates toward it and less positive when it rotates in the opposite direction. Recordings are made with a three-electrode system using differential amplifiers. Two of the (active) electrodes are placed on either side of the eye, and the reference (ground) electrode is placed somewhere remote from the eye. The two active electrodes measure a potential change of equal amplitude but opposite in direction. The difference in potential between these electrodes is amplified and used to control the displacement of a pen-writing recorder or similar device to produce a permanent record. Because the emphasis was initially on recording nystagmus, this test is also referred to as *electronystagmography* (ENG).

More recently, newer techniques for recording eye movements have been developed. One of these, video-oculography (VOG), is becoming popular in clinical use, while the other, the magnetic search coil technique, remains primarily a research tool. Each of these techniques has advantages and disadvantages. EOG is still probably the most widely used technique for recording eye movements. The equipment is less expensive to purchase, and the test provides reliable clinical information when individuals with proper training use it (Furman et al., 1996). Artifacts from lid movements or muscle action potentials are common, thus the "noise" is greater in ENG than either VOG or the magnetic search coil technique, and measuring torsional eye movements is difficult. Probably the main clinical advantage of VOG is the ability to go back and observe the actual video recording of the eye movements. This becomes particularly helpful when trying to distinguish an actual eye movement from an artifact such as a blink. Measuring torsional eye movements is also possible with VOG, although systems for doing so are still being developed. Disadvantages of VOG are the inability to measure eye movements with the eyes closed and difficulties stabilizing the head gear. The magnetic search coil technique uses a contact lens embedded with two coils of wire. One coil is wound in the frontal plane to sense horizontal and vertical movements and the other is wound in the sagittal plane to sense torsional eye movements. When the subject sits in a magnetic field, voltages are induced in these search coils that can be used to measure eye position. The magnetic search coil technique is the gold standard for measuring eye movements because it allows measurement of eye rotations around all three axes, with high sensitivity and low noise. This technique can be particularly helpful in obtaining accurate measures in patients who cannot reliably direct their gaze at calibration targets, since the device can be precalibrated. The main disadvantage of the magnetic search coil technique is the invasive nature of using the contact lens, which can cause discomfort for the patient or (rarely) corneal abrasion. Because of these factors, the magnetic search coil technique is generally only used in research laboratories. Newer versions of VOG systems with high-frequency sampling rates now rival the degree of precision of the magnetic search coil technique (Houben et al., 2006) and are thus being incorporated into more research laboratories. Though increased precision of VOG and the magnetic search coil technique is a clear advantage over EOG in research studies, it remains to be shown whether these tests enhance clinical diagnostic capabilities or change the management of patients when compared to EOG (Schmid-Priscoveanu and Allum, 1999).

EYE MOVEMENT SUBTESTS

A standard test battery includes a search for pathological nystagmus or saccadic intrusions with fixation and with eyes open in the darkness, tests of visual ocular control (saccades, smooth pursuit, OKN), and the bithermal caloric test (Baloh and Kerber, 2011). Administration of these subtests usually proceeds in a manner similar to the bedside evaluation. By convention, for horizontal recordings, eye movements to the right result in an upward deflection of the tracing and those to the left result in downward deflection. For vertical recordings, upward and downward eye movements produce upward and downward deflections.

RECORDING PATHOLOGICAL SPONTANEOUS EYE MOVEMENTS

Once the equipment has been set up and calibrated, the patient is asked to look straight ahead, both when fixating on a target and in darkness with eyes open (removing fixation). In this manner, spontaneous nystagmus or saccadic intrusions can be recorded. Patients are then instructed to look about 30 degrees from the midline in each direction, maintaining gaze for about 10 to 20 seconds in each direction. Gaze-evoked nystagmus is demonstrated when nystagmus not seen in the primary position appears with gaze. The most common type of gaze-evoked nystagmus has approximately equal amplitude in all directions and results from either medication toxicity or cerebellar dysfunction. In patients with a partially compensated peripheral vestibular lesion, nystagmus in one direction may be present. Small-amplitude nystagmus with gaze more than 30 degrees is typically a physiological nystagmus appearing in normal individuals and is referred to as *end-gaze nystagmus.* Positional testing using both the head-hanging positions and supine positions is used to search for positional nystagmus. A characteristic burst of nystagmus is seen in patients with BPPV. Persistent positional nystagmus (i.e., no burst) is a common finding when recordings are made with eyes open in darkness. When the average slow-phase velocity exceeds 4 degrees/sec, it is abnormal but non-localizing. When patients are able to suppress this nystagmus when presented with a visual target, a peripheral cause is suggested.

VISUAL OCULAR MOTOR CONTROL
Saccades

By presenting the patient with visual targets that move 10 to 30 degrees in the horizontal and vertical planes, measurements of saccade onset, velocity, and accuracy can be made. Patients are instructed to "jump" from target to target. Normal subjects, elderly and young alike, achieve a highly reproducible pattern of saccadic velocity that has a nonlinear relationship between peak velocity and amplitude of the eye movement. Velocities initially increase from about 5-degree to 30-degree movements, and then a maximum velocity is achieved. Saccade velocity remains intact through late age in individuals without focal neurological disease. Slowing of saccades can occur with lesions anywhere in the diffuse central pathways involved in generating saccades, but the most pronounced slowing occurs with lesions affecting the brainstem (pretectal and paramedian pontine gaze centers or ocular motor neurons) and the extraocular muscles. Typical disorders with slowing of saccades are PSP and HD. Slowing can also result if the patient has taken tranquilizing drugs. A lesion of medial longitudinal fasciculus results in slowing of the adducting eye, often more easily appreciated with quantitative measures than bedside testing. Normal subjects consistently undershoot target jumps larger than 20 degrees and will require a small corrective saccade to achieve the final position. Overshooting saccades, however, are rare and do not consistently occur in normal patients. Overshooting saccades typically are seen in patients with cerebellar dysfunction.

Smooth Pursuit

Recordings of smooth pursuit are made by having the patient follow a target back and forth. By convention, most laboratories do this using a target that moves in a sinusoidal fashion. The accuracy of smooth pursuit is quantified by repeatedly sampling eye and target velocities and plotting the two velocities against each other. A computer algorithm makes the comparison between eye and target velocity after saccade waveforms have been removed. The slope of this eye/target velocity relationship represents the gain of the smooth pursuit system, which depends on the velocity and frequency of the target movements. Higher velocity and frequency testing results in lower gains. Though each laboratory must establish normal values, typically normal subjects have very high mean gains (0.92 ± 0.05 at 0.2 Hz, 22.6 degrees/sec). Though a patient's age is typically considered when interpreting results, a recent study shows smooth-pursuit gains can be well maintained in subjects well into their ninth decade (Kerber et al., 2006).

Optokinetic Nystagmus

Laboratory testing of OKN uses a full-field visual stimulus (typically a patterned drum) that moves at a constant velocity and frequency around the subject, who is either instructed to follow the target (resulting in large-amplitude nystagmus) or stare through it (resulting in small-amplitude nystagmus). This stimulus also causes a sensation of self-rotation called *circular vection* even though the peripheral vestibular system is not being stimulated. The OKN gain is measured by comparing the slow-component velocity of the eye movement to the target velocity. As with smooth-pursuit testing, gain drops off with increasing frequency and velocity of the target in normal subjects. The normal and abnormal EOG appearance of saccades, smooth pursuit, and OKN are demonstrated in (**Fig. 37.5**).

BITHERMAL CALORIC TESTING

With the bithermal caloric test, each ear is irrigated alternately for a fixed duration (30 to 40 seconds) with a constant flow of water that is either 7°C above body temperature or 7°C below body temperature. The external auditory canal should first be inspected to make sure that cerumen does not occlude it and that the tympanic membrane is intact. The different temperatures of the water induce a movement of the endolymph mainly within the horizontal semicircular canal, because this canal is anatomically closest to the tympanic membrane. The resulting temperature gradient from one side of the canal to the other causes flow of the endolymph that triggers a very low frequency stimulus of the horizontal canal. The advantages of this test method are that the endolymph can be triggered to flow in both directions (ampullopetal and ampullofugal), each ear can be stimulated separately, and the test is tolerated by most patients. Limitations include the need for constant temperature baths and plumbing to maintain continuous circulation of the water through the infusion hose, the interindividual variability of caloric vestibular responses, and only being able to apply a single frequency stimulus.

The conventional method for measuring caloric stimulation is to compare the maximum slow-phase velocities achieved on one side to that of the other side, using the vestibular paresis formula:

$$\frac{(R30° + R44°) - (L30° + L44°)}{(R30° + R44° + L30° + L44°)} \times 100$$

Directional preponderance is also calculated using the following formula:

$$\frac{(L30° + R44°) - (L44° + R30°)}{(L30° + R44° + L44° + R30°)} \times 100$$

Dividing by the total response normalizes the measurements to remove the large variability in absolute magnitude of normal caloric responses. Typically, the finding of significant vestibular paresis of 25% to 30% with bithermal caloric stimulation suggests a lesion in the vestibular system that is located anywhere from the end-organ to the vestibular nerve root entry zone in the brainstem. This finding is a strong indicator of a unilateral peripheral lesion, but it must be placed in the context of the patient's clinical history and bedside examination; a caloric paresis can also occur in central vestibular disorders. A recent study found a high rate of significant vestibular

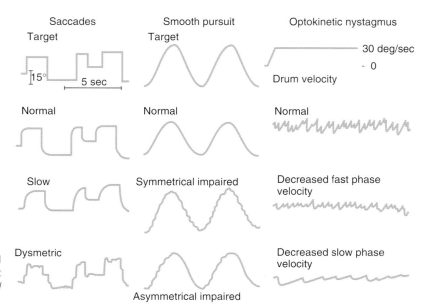

Fig. 37.5 Electronystagmographic recordings of normal and abnormal saccades, smooth pursuit, and optokinetic nystagmus. *(From Baloh, R.W., 1998. Dizziness, Hearing Loss, and Tinnitus. F.A. Davis Company, Philadelphia, Figure 37, p. 84.)*

paresis (as measured by the caloric test) in patients with acute vertigo presentations caused by stroke (Newman-Toker et al., 2008). It is also common to find a caloric asymmetry in control subjects without dizziness (particularly those with migraine or diabetes) who undergo this test. A significant directional preponderance on caloric testing (>30%) indicates an imbalance in the vestibular system but is nonlocalizing, occurring with both peripheral and central lesions.

ROTATIONAL TESTING

Rotational testing requires use of a motorized chair. The patient is placed in the chair that rotates under the control of a computer, and the patient's head and body move in unison with the chair. The chair is in a dark room, so fixation is removed. Eye movements induced by the vestibular system stimulating movements of the patient's head and body within the chair are recorded using any of the previously mentioned eye recording techniques. The computer precisely controls the velocity and frequency of rotations so that the VOR can be measured at multiple frequencies in a single session. Sinusoidal and step (impulse) changes in angular velocity are routinely used (**Fig. 37.6**). In clinical testing, generally only rotations about the vertical axis are used, which maximally stimulates the horizontal canals. Off-vertical rotation can be used to measure the function of the vertical semicircular canals and otoliths as well, but typically this is only done in research studies. For sinusoidal rotations, results are reported

as gain (peak slow-component eye velocity divided by peak chair velocity) and phase (timing between the peak velocity of eye and head) at different frequencies.

Because both inner ears are stimulated at the typically low velocities and frequencies used, rotational testing is most effective at determining a bilateral peripheral vestibular hypofunction that leads to a decreased gain and increased phase. Unilateral vestibular hypofunction can be suggested by a normal gain with increased phase on standard testing or a decreased unilateral gain with shortened time constant on impulse (rapid movement) testing. Normal rotational testing results in gains around 0.5 at low-frequency rotation (0.05 Hz), with gains approaching 1.0 at higher-frequency rotations (>1 Hz). Even patients with partial loss of bilateral vestibular function may have gains in the normal range at the higher frequency rotations, probably owing to the contribution of additional sensory systems (Jen et al., 2005; Wiest et al., 2001). The main disadvantage of rotational chair testing is the expense associated with setting it up. As a result, this vestibular test is typically only available at large academic centers. Because of this, portable devices using either passive (examiner-generated) head rotations or active (patient-generated) head turns have been developed, but the quality of evidence to support the use of these tests is low (Fife et al., 2000).

Rotational chair testing can also be used to measure the patient's ability to suppress the VOR and a combined

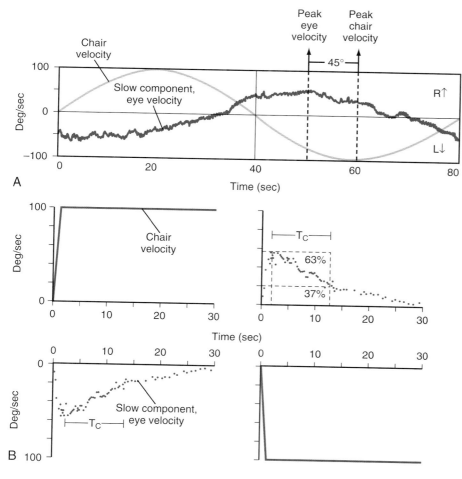

Fig. 37.6 Plots of slow-component eye velocity versus time for nystagmus induced by sinusoidal angular rotation in the horizontal plane at 0.0125 Hz and a peak velocity of 100 degrees/sec **(A)** and by step changes in angular velocity of 100 degrees/sec occurring with an acceleration of approximately 140 degrees/sec² **(B)**. Subject is seated on a motorized rotating chair with eyes open in darkness. Eye movements are recorded with electronystagmography. Fast components are identified and removed, and slow component eye velocity is measured every 20 msec. The gain of the response (peak slow-component eye velocity/peak chair velocity) is about 0.6 for both types of stimulation. The phase lead with sinusoidal stimulation is the difference in timing between the peak eye velocity and peak chair velocity (in this case 45 degrees). The time constant (T_C) is the time required for the response to decay to 37% of its initial value (about 10 seconds in **B**). (*From Baloh, R.W., 1998. Dizziness, Hearing Loss, and Tinnitus. F.A. Davis Company, Philadelphia, Figure 36, p. 81.*)

measure of both OKN and rotational testing (visual VOR).

POSTUROGRAPHY

Body sway is a normal phenomenon that occurs in everyone. Excessive sway is more common in older than in younger people and more common in patients with balance problems than in age-matched controls. Because the magnitude of sway tends to be small when subjects stand on a stable platform, moving platforms (dynamic posturography) have been developed in an attempt to increase test sensitivity. The platform can be tilted or linearly displaced, and the sway can be measured immediately after the movement or during the movement. Furthermore, in a effort to dissect the different sensory contributions to the maintenance of balance, systems have been developed to selectively manipulate somatosensation and vision. With these devices, the angle of sway is fed back to a dynamic platform or to a movable visual surround so that movement of the visual surround is sway-referenced.

Posturography is a method for quantifying balance. It is not a diagnostic test and is of little use for localizing a lesion. It can be helpful for following the course of a patient and may serve as a quantitative measure of the response to therapy or in research studies. As noted earlier, sway increases in older people, and several studies have shown that the frequency of falls increases as sway increases, suggesting that posturography may be a clinical tool for identifying older people at risk for falling, though whether it is better at this than a careful clinical assessment is unclear (Piirtola and Era, 2006). Posturography may be helpful in identifying patients with factitious balance disorders (Gianoli et al., 2000).

VESTIBULAR EVOKED MYOGENIC POTENTIALS

It has long been known that the sacculus, which during the course of its evolution functioned as an organ of hearing and still does in primitive vertebrates, can be stimulated by loud sounds. As a result of this stimulation, a signal travels via the inferior trunk of the vestibular nerve to cranial nerve VIII and into the brainstem. From there, inhibitory postsynaptic potentials travel to the ipsilateral sternocleidomastoid muscle (SCM), essentially allowing the individual to reflexively turn towards the sound. To generate this vestibular evoked myogenic potential (VEMP) response, intense clicks of about 95 to 100 dB above normal hearing level (NHL) are required (Welgampola and Colebatch, 2005). The response is measured from an activated ipsilateral SCM. Tonic contraction of the muscle is required to demonstrate the inhibitory response. The amplitude of the response and also the threshold needed to generate it are measured. Because the absolute amplitudes vary greatly from patient to patient, the more reliable abnormality is detecting a side-to-side difference in an individual. Additionally, responses are unreliable in subjects older than 60 years and in patients with middle ear abnormalities. Abnormal VEMP responses can be detected in most disorders affecting the peripheral vestibular system, but this test can be particularly helpful in identifying patients with vestibular neuritis selectively affecting the inferior vestibular nerve (Halmagyi et al., 2002) or SCD (Minor, 2005). Because caloric and rotational testing mainly stimulate the horizontal semicircular canal (which sends afferent responses via the superior vestibular nerve), the rare disorder affecting only the inferior vestibular nerve will not be identified with these tests. In patients with SCD, VEMP testing leads to increased amplitudes and lowered thresholds due to the low-impedance pathway created by the third window.

Hearing Loss and Tinnitus
Auditory Testing

Audiological assessment is the basis for quantifying auditory impairment. Most neurologists rely on bedside assessments of hearing. In defining an auditory abnormality, tuning forks are no substitute for a complete audiological battery. Audiological testing is most reliable in defining peripheral or cochlear auditory disturbances and often may provide useful information, based on subtests, to diagnose retrocochlear disorders such as an acoustic neuroma. Tests for central auditory dysfunction are more difficult and poorly understood. Detailed descriptions of audiological tests, both peripheral and central, are provided in standard texts (Katz et al., 2009).

The basic audiological evaluation establishes the degree and configuration of hearing loss, assesses ability to discriminate a speech signal, and provides some insight into the type of loss and possible cause. The test battery consists of pure-tone air- and bone-conduction thresholds, speech thresholds, speech discrimination testing, and immittance measures.

PURE-TONE TESTING

Pure-tone air-conduction thresholds provide a measure of hearing sensitivity as a function of frequency and intensity. When a hearing loss is present, the pure-tone air conduction test indicates reduced hearing sensitivity. Pure tones are defined by their frequency (pitch) and intensity (loudness). Normal hearing levels for pure tones are defined by international standards. Brief-duration pure tones at selected frequencies are presented through earphones (air conduction) or a bone-conduction oscillator on the mastoid bone (bone conduction). The audiogram indicates the lowest intensity at which a person can hear at a given frequency and displays the degree (in decibels) and configuration (sensitivity loss as a function of frequency) of a hearing loss. Thresholds in audiology are usually defined as the lowest-intensity signal a person can detect approximately 50% of the time during a given number of presentations. Bone-conduction tests are intended to be a direct measure of inner ear sensitivity. Pure-tone bone-conduction thresholds are obtained when a stimulus is presented by bone conduction.

Comparison of air- and bone-conduction thresholds establishes the type of hearing loss. Conductive loss results from disorders in the outer or middle ear. The audiogram of patients with SCD may also have an air/bone gap, even though there is no abnormality of the outer or middle ear. This exception results from the third window created by the dehiscence which increases bone conduction. Sensorineural loss is associated with disorders of the cochlear and eighth cranial nerves. Mixed loss is a conductive and sensorineural loss coexisting in the same ear. Typical audiogram pure-tone pattern seen in patients with four common causes of sensorineural hearing loss are shown in (**Fig. 37.7**).

SPEECH TESTING

The speech reception threshold (SRT) is the lowest-intensity level at which the listener can identify or understand two-syllable spoken words 50% of the time. This test provides

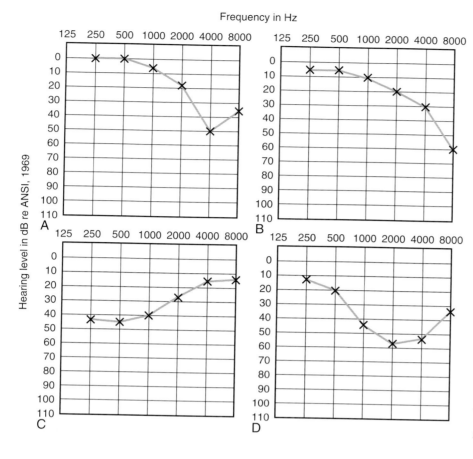

Fig. 37.7 Audiograms illustrating four characteristic patterns of sensorineural hearing loss. **A,** Notched pattern of noise-induced hearing loss. **B,** Downward-sloping pattern of presbycusis. **C,** Low-frequency trough of the Meniere syndrome. **D,** Pattern of congenital hearing loss. *(From Baloh, R.W., 1998. Dizziness, Hearing Loss, and Tinnitus. F.A. Davis Company, Philadelphia, Figure 39, p. 95.)*

a check on the validity of the pure-tone test, as it should agree (±5 dB) with an average of the two best pure-tone thresholds in the speech range (500-2000 Hz). Once the SRT is determined, the audiologist measures speech discrimination ability by presenting a standardized list of 50 phonetically balanced monosyllabic words at volume levels approximately 35 to 40 dB above SRT. The speech discrimination score is reported as the percentage of words the subject can correctly repeat back to the audiologist.

Pure tone, SRT, and speech discrimination testing comprise the major routine measures of hearing. Considering these tests together can also provide localizing information. In patients with retrocochlear lesions, speech discrimination can be severely reduced even when pure-tone levels are normal or near normal, whereas in patients with cochlear lesions, discrimination tends to be proportional to the magnitude of hearing loss.

MIDDLE EAR TESTING

Immittance measures assess the status of the middle ear and confirm information obtained in other tests of the battery. The basic immittance battery consists of tympanometry, static immittance, and acoustic reflex thresholds. Data from the tympanogram permit determination of the static compliance of the middle ear system. A result of "type A tympanogram" means that mobility of the tympanic membrane and middle ear structures is within normal limits.

ACOUSTIC REFLEX TESTING

Acoustic reflex measures the contraction of the stapedius muscle (innervated by the seventh cranial nerve) in response to a loud sound. The afferent limb of the reflex arch is through the auditory portion of the eighth cranial nerve, and the efferent portion of the reflex arch is through the seventh cranial nerve. The stapedius muscle normally contracts on both sides when an adequate sound is presented in one ear. As a result of contraction of the stapedius muscle, the tympanic membrane tightens or stiffens, thereby increasing the impedance or resistance of the eardrum to acoustic energy and resulting in a slight attenuation of sound transmitted through the middle ear system. In a normal subject, the acoustic reflex occurs in response to a pure tone between 70 and 100 dB above hearing level or when a white noise stimulus is presented at 65 dB above hearing level. Patients with conductive hearing loss do not have reflexes because the lesion prevents a change in compliance with stapedius muscle contraction. With cochlear lesions, the acoustic reflex may be present at sensation levels less than 60 dB above the auditory pure-tone threshold, which is a form of abnormal loudness growth or recruitment. Cochlear hearing losses must be moderate or severe before the acoustic reflex is lost. In contrast, patients with retrocochlear or eighth cranial nerve lesions often have abnormal acoustic reflexes with normal hearing. The reflex may be absent or exhibit an elevated threshold or abnormal decay. Reflex decay is present if the amplitude of the reflex

Table 37.3 Pattern of Acoustic Reflex Measurements with Unilateral Lesions

	Stimulus Presented			
	C	I	C	I
	Reflex Measured			
Type of Lesion	I	C	C	I
Cochlear (<85 dBHL)	+	+	+	+
Conductive (>30 dBHL)	–	–	+	–
Cranial nerve VIII	+	–	+	–
Cranial nerve VII	–	+	+	–

+, Reflex present; –, reflex absent; *C*, contralateral to lesion; *dBHL*, decibels hearing loss; *I*, ipsilateral to lesion.

decreases to half its original size within 10 seconds of stimulation at 1000 Hz, 10 dB above reflex threshold. This abnormality occurs in approximately 80% of patients with acoustic neuromas. Observation of the pattern of acoustic reflex testing, along with hearing evaluation, permits inferences to support the presence of a cochlear, conductive, or retrocochlear lesion of the seventh or eighth cranial nerves (**Table 37.3**).

EVOKED POTENTIALS

Brainstem auditory evoked potentials are also known as *brainstem auditory evoked responses* or *auditory brainstem responses* (ABRs). These physiological measures can be used to evaluate the auditory pathways from the ear to the upper brainstem. In addition, ABR threshold testing, although not a test of hearing sensitivity, may be used to determine behavioral threshold sensitivity in infants or uncooperative patients. The most consistent and reproducible potentials are a series of five submicrovolt waves that occur within 10 milliseconds of an auditory stimulus. These potentials are recorded by averaging 1000 to 2000 responses from click stimuli by use of a computer system and amplifying the response. The anatomical correlates of the five reliable potentials have been only roughly approximated. Wave I of the brainstem auditory evoked potential is a manifestation of the action potentials of the eighth cranial nerve and is generated in the distal portion of the nerve adjacent to the cochlea. Wave II may be generated by the eighth cranial nerve or cochlear nuclei. Wave III is thought to be generated at the level of the superior olive, and waves IV and V are generated in the rostral pons or in the midbrain near the inferior colliculus. The complex anatomy of the central auditory pathway, with multiple crossing of fibers from the level of the cochlear nuclei to the inferior colliculus, makes interpretation of central disturbances in the evoked responses difficult.

Abnormal interwave latencies (I-III or I-V) are seen with retrocochlear lesions (cerebellopontine angle tumors) and can even be seen when only mild or no hearing loss is detected on pure tone audiometry. However, compared to brain MRI with gadolinium, the sensitivity of the ABR test is low, particularly with small tumors (Cueva, 2004). The least specific finding is the absence of all waves. This occurs in some patients with acoustic neuroma and in some with cerebellopontine angle meningiomas. Such patients often have marked hearing deficits with poor discrimination, suggesting retrocochlear disease. The absence of all waves should not occur unless a severe hearing loss exists.

OTHER TESTS

Electrocochleography is a method of recording the stimulus-related electrical potentials associated with the inner ear and auditory nerve, including the cochlear microphonic, summating potential (SP), and compound action potential (AP) of the auditory nerve. The amplitude of the SP and compound AP is measured; an increased SP/AP ratio suggests increased endolymphatic pressure. This test is sometimes used in an attempt to distinguish Meniere disease from other causes of dizziness and hearing loss but lacks a rigorous analysis of its usefulness when there is clinical uncertainty.

Management of Patients with Vertigo

Treatments of Specific Disorders

The treatment of patients with dizziness and vertigo hinges on making a specific diagnosis. BPPV can be diagnosed and treated at the bedside, requiring no further treatment. Once repositioning is confirmed to be successful (see **Fig. 37.4**), patients are instructed to avoid head-hanging positions such as those used by dentists and hairdressers. These positions can cause the particles to reaccumulate in the posterior semicircular canals. For patients with horizontal canal BPPV, the "barbeque" rotation, Gufoni maneuver, or forced prolonged position can be used (Fife et al., 2008; Tirelli and Russolo, 2004; Vannucchi et al., 1997) can be used. The management of patients with vestibular neuritis is primarily symptomatic. After a couple of days, patients should be encouraged to move around and begin vestibular rehabilitation exercises that force the brain to compensate. Improved vestibular recovery measured by caloric responses has been shown in patients treated within 3 days for vestibular neuritis with methylprednisolone (Strupp et al., 2004), though it is not known whether this translates to improved functional or symptomatic recovery. Prolonged use of sedating medications to treat symptoms is not recommended, because it can slow down the vestibular compensation process. The early treatment of Meniere disease continues to be a low-salt diet and diuretics, though the evidence for these is not great (Minor et al., 2004). Minimally invasive intratympanic gentamicin injections can be used for patients with debilitating symptoms. Surgical ablation of the labyrinth or sectioning of the vestibular nerve are other options. Patients with vestibular paroxysmia may benefit from carbamazepine or a similar antiepileptic medication (Hufner et al., 2008). The third window in patients with SCD can be surgically repaired, but this is usually only recommended in patients debilitated by the symptoms (Minor, 2005).

Patients identified as having a small infarction in the posterior fossa should be closely monitored, as herniation or recurrent stroke can occur. Patients identified within 3 hours of an infarction are candidates for intravenous tissue plasminogen activator (tPA). There are some case reports of patients with recurrent vertigo caused by severe stenosis of the basilar artery who are cured by endovascular stenting (Kerber et al., 2005b), but this remains an experimental procedure. Patients identified with demyelinating lesions may be candidates for disease-modifying treatments even after presenting with a clinically isolated syndrome. Patients with episodic ataxia are typically highly responsive to treatment with acetazolamide, and there is anecdotal evidence of benefit of the use of acetazolamide in patients with BRV, a migraine equivalent. Patients with migraine-associated dizziness should first attempt to identify and eliminate triggers of their symptoms and also obtain adequate sleep and cardiovascular exercise. If these general measures are not adequate in controlling symptoms, a migraine prophylactic medication could be tried. Small trials of triptan medications in patients with migrainous vertigo suggest safety of these medicines but no significant benefit (Neuhauser et al., 2003).

Symptomatic Treatment of Vertigo

The commonly used antivertiginous drugs and their dosages are listed in **Table 37.4** (Huppert et al., 2011). It is often difficult to predict which drugs or combinations of drugs will be most effective in individual patients, and large trials are lacking. Additionally, the mechanisms of these medications are not specific to the vestibular system, so side effects are common. Anticholinergic or antihistamine drug are usually effective in treating patients with mild to moderate vertigo, and sedation is minimal. If the patient is particularly bothered by nausea, the antiemetics prochlorperazine and metoclopramide can be effective and combined with other antivertiginous medications. For severe vertigo, sedation is often desirable, and drugs such as promethazine and diazepam are particularly useful, though prolonged use is not recommended.

Management of Patients with Hearing Loss and Tinnitus

Hearing aids continue to become more effective and better designed for patient comfort and acceptance, although cost remains the major limiting factor in their more widespread

Table 37.4   Medical Therapy for Symptomatic Vertigo*

Class	Dosage[†]
ANTIHISTAMINES	
Meclizine	25 mg PO q 4-6 h
Dimenhydrinate	50 mg PO or IM q 4-6 h, or 100 mg suppository q 8 h
Promethazine	25-50 mg PO or IM or as a suppository q 4-6 h
ANTICHOLINERGIC AGENT	
Scopolamine	0.2 mg PO q 4-6 h, or 0.5 mg transdermally q 3 days
BENZODIAZEPINES	
Diazepam	5 or 10 mg PO, IM, IV q 4-6 h
Lorazepam	0.5-2 mg PO, IM, IV q 6-8 h
PHENOTHIAZINE	
Prochlorperazine	5 or 10 mg PO or IM q 6 h, or 25 mg suppository q 12 h
BENZAMIDE	
Metoclopramide	5 or 10 mg PO, IM, or IV q 4-6 h

IM, intramuscular; *IV* intravenous; *PO*, oral.
*Huppert et al., 2011.
[†]Usual adult starting dosage; maintenance dosage can be increased by a factor of 2-3. The most common side effect is drowsiness.

use. Cochlear implants have revolutionized the approach to treatment of profound sensorineural loss. The management of tinnitus remains difficult, and specific treatments are often ineffective. Patients with a specific cause for the problem usually have the most potential for improvement. Idiopathic high-pitched tinnitus may diminish with avoidance of caffeine, other stimulants, and alcohol. A masking device used in quiet environments may also provide some relief. For patients with intolerable idiopathic tinnitus, a trial of a tricyclic amine antidepressant may be of benefit.

References

The complete reference list in available online at www.expertconsult.com.

Chapter **38**

Neurourology

Jalesh N. Panicker, Clare J. Fowler, Ranan DasGupta

Urogenital dysfunction can result from a wide range of neurological conditions, and the importance of this problem to the patient's health and its negative impact on quality of life and loss of dignity is now widely recognized. The investigations and management of disorders of urogenital function was formerly regarded as the preserve of urologists. But as neurologists and rehabilitation specialists become aware of the range of possible effective nonsurgical treatments and increasingly inquire after patients' complaints of disordered urogenital function, they are taking a more active interest in *uroneurology*—bladder dysfunction viewed from a neurological perspective. This chapter describes what a neurologist needs to know for the management of patients with neurogenic urogenital problems. Urodynamic, neurophysiological, and radiological investigations and available medical treatments are described.

Lower Urinary Tract and Its Neurological Control

The lower urinary tract consists of the bladder and urethra and has two roles: storage of urine and voiding at appropriate times. Control of the detrusor and urethral sphincter muscles in these two mutually exclusive states is dependent upon both local spinal reflexes and central cerebral control. The pontine micturition center, which receives input from higher centers

(including the periaqueductal gray of the midbrain, hypothalamus, and cortical areas such as the medial prefrontal cortex) is responsible for switching between the two states. The frequency of micturition in a person with a bladder capacity of 400 to 600 mL is once every 3 to 4 hours. Voiding takes 2 to 3 minutes, so this means that for more than 98% of life, the bladder is in a storage phase. Switching to a voiding phase is initiated by a conscious decision triggered by the perceived state of bladder fullness and an assessment of the social appropriateness of doing so. To effect both storage and voiding, connections between the pons and the sacral spinal cord must be intact, as must the peripheral innervation that originates from the most caudal segments of the cord. During the storage phase, sympathetic- and pudendal-mediated contraction of the internal and external urethral sphincters, respectively, maintains continence. Inhibition of the parasympathetic outflow prevents detrusor contractions (Fowler et al., 2008). When it is deemed appropriate to void, the pontine micturition center is no longer tonically inhibited, and reciprocal activation-inhibition of the sphincter-detrusor reverses. Relaxation of the pelvic floor and external and internal urethral sphincters, accompanied by parasympathetic-mediated detrusor contraction, results in effective bladder emptying. Intact neural circuitry between the pontine micturition center and bladder ensures coordinated activity between the detrusor and sphincter muscles. **Fig. 38.1** reviews the innervation of the bladder.

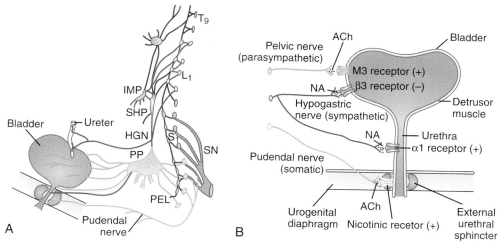

Fig. 38.1 Innervation of lower urinary tract. **A,** Sympathetic fibers *(shown in blue)* originate in T11-L2 spinal cord segments and run through inferior mesenteric ganglia (inferior mesenteric plexus [IMP]) and hypogastric nerve (HGN) or through the paravertebral chain to enter pelvic nerves at base of bladder and urethra. Parasympathetic preganglionic fibers *(shown in green)* arise from S2-S4 spinal segments and travel in sacral roots and pelvic nerves (PEL) to ganglia in the pelvic plexus (PP) and bladder wall. This is where the postganglionic nerves that supply parasympathetic innervation to the bladder arise. Somatic motor nerves *(shown in yellow)* that supply striated muscles of external urethral sphincter arise from S2-S4 motor neurons and pass through pudendal nerves. **B,** Efferent pathways and neurotransmitter mechanisms that regulate lower urinary tract. Parasympathetic postganglionic axons in pelvic nerve release acetylcholine (ACh), which produces bladder contraction by stimulating M3 muscarinic receptors in bladder smooth muscle. Sympathetic postganglionic neurons release noradrenaline (NA), which activates β_3-adrenergic receptors to relax bladder smooth muscle and activates β_1-adrenergic receptors to contract urethral smooth muscle. Somatic axons in pudendal nerve also release Ach, which produces contraction of external sphincter striated muscle by activating nicotinic cholinergic receptors. *L1,* First lumbar root; *S1,* first sacral root; *SHP,* superior hypogastric plexus; *SN,* sciatic nerve; *T9,* ninth thoracic root. *(From Fowler, C.J., Griffiths, D., de Groat, W.C., 2008. The neural control of micturition. Nat Rev Neurosci 9, 453-466.)*

Functional brain imaging studies have demonstrated that neurological control of the bladder in humans is essentially similar to that demonstrated in experimental animals. A number of positron emission tomography (PET) and, more recently, functional magnetic resonance imaging (fMRI) studies have investigated human control of urinary storage and voiding. The initial PET experiments of Blok and colleagues identified the brain centers activated during attempted micturition (Blok et al., 1997, 1998). In those able to void during the scanning , activity was shown in a region of the medioposterior pons called the *M-region*. In those subjects unable to void, a distinct region in the ventrolateral pontine tegmentum was activated, the *L-region*. Although it had been demonstrated in cats that separate pontine nuclei exist for the storage and voiding phases of bladder activity, subsequent experiments have failed to consistently demonstrate activity in this distinct L-region. In the cortex, the PET scans showed significant activity in the right inferior frontal gyrus and the right anterior cingulate gyrus during voiding that was not present during the withholding phase. Nour and associates then corroborated these findings with their own PET study of 12 healthy male volunteers, showing activity in a number of brain areas including the cerebellum (Nour et al., 2000). Other areas that show activation in fMRI during bladder filling include the anterior cingulate gyrus and right insula; fMRI has shown that the medial prefrontal cortex, responsible for complex cognitive and socially appropriate behavior, plays an important role in voiding. A recent article reviews the functional imaging studies evaluating bladder functions and their contributions to our understanding of bladder control (Fowler and Griffiths, 2010).

Bowel and Its Neurological Control

Similar to the bladder, the lower bowel also exists mostly in the storage mode. Continence is maintained by a combination of the acute anorectal angle, maintained by puborectalis contraction, and internal anal sphincter tone, determined by sympathetic activity. In health, defecation can be delayed if necessary by contraction of the external anal sphincter and pelvic floor musculature, which requires sensory feedback from the anorectum. The process of defecation involves a series of neurologically controlled actions that begin in response to the conscious sensation of a full rectum. When this is perceived and if judged to be appropriate, defecation is initiated by maneuvers to raise the intraabdominal pressure and by straining down, causing descent of the pelvic floor. The internal anal sphincter pressure falls as a result of the rectoanal inhibitory reflex, and the pubococcygeus and striated external sphincter muscles relax. Functional imaging has been applied to evaluate central processing of different types of gastrointestinal (GI) stimulation. Hobday and associates used fMRI to identify the brain centers involved in the processing of anal (somatic) and rectal (visceral) sensation in healthy adults (Hobday et al., 2001). Rectal stimulation produced activation of somatosensory cortex, insula, anterior cingulate, and prefrontal cortex (PFC); anal canal stimulation produced similar regions of activity, although anterior cingulate activity was absent, and the primary somatosensory activation was slightly more superior in location. The activation of cingulate cortex with rectal stimulation may signify the function of the limbic system in the processing of visceral stimuli.

The processing of rectal sensation is relevant in bladder function because unlike other gut organs, it has an important sensory role, and the rectum is a visceral organ that contains both unmyelinated C fibers and thinly myelinated Aδ afferents. In contrast, the anal canal has somatic innervation from the pudendal nerve. The study by Hobday and associates has highlighted the differences in its cortical representation from that of the rectum. The various brain imaging studies of visceral stimulation, including the foregoing report, have been reviewed (Derbyshire, 2003). When different visceral stimuli—esophageal distension, esophageal pain, rectal distension, or the mechanisms operative in irritable bowel syndrome—were analyzed, esophageal stimulation was found to activate the insula most consistently, with other commonly involved areas including somatosensory and motor cortices. Considerable variation was observed in whether the periaqueductal gray was activated or not. Lower GI stimuli predominantly activated the prefrontal and orbitofrontal cortices as well as the insula, with variability in cingulate activation. Overall, esophageal stimulation involved a more central sensory and motor neural circuit, whereas lower GI stimulation activated areas with projections to autonomic and affective control centers such as the brainstem and amygdala.

Sexual Function and Its Neurological Control

Physiological sexual response in men and women has been divided classically into four phases: excitement, plateau, orgasm, and resolution. Excitation occurs in response to either physical or psychological stimulation and results in penile or clitoral tumescence and erection or vaginal lubrication. The plateau phase is accompanied by the various physical changes of high sexual arousal in anticipation of orgasm. Orgasm, an intensely sensory event, usually is associated with rhythmic contraction of the pelvic floor and culminates with ejaculation in men. During resolution, the increased genital blood flow resolves. A modification of this model of sexual response was the three-phase model proposed by Kaplan, consisting of desire, arousal, and orgasm.

Much remains to be discovered about cortical control of sexual function. Although it is thought that cerebral processing determines libido and desire, the ability to effect a sexual response is determined by spinal autonomic reflexes. Libido is hormone dependent with a major hypothalamic component, and loss of libido may be the earliest symptom of a pituitary tumor. In experimental animals, the deep anterior midline structures that form the limbic system have been shown to be important for sexual responses, and the medial preoptic–anterior hypothalamic area has an integrating function (Andersson, 2001). Functional brain imaging experiments including five PET studies and seven fMRI studies have highlighted the key areas of brain activity associated with sexual functioning—for example, the role of the hypothalamus in reproductive function, regulation of human sexuality, and regulation of erection through medial preoptic area, or the roles of the insula and claustrum in autonomic regulation and visceral sensory processing. The aspects of sexual function covered include penile sexual stimulation (Arnow et al., 2002; Georgiadis and Holstege, 2005), male

ejaculation (Holstege et al., 2003), and visual sexual stimuli (Karama et al., 2002).

Male Sexual Response

Erection results from increased blood flow into the corpora cavernosa caused by relaxation of the smooth muscle in the cavernosal arteries and a reduction in venous return. The major peripheral innervation determining this is parasympathetic, which arises from the S2-S4 segments and travels to the genital region in the pelvic nerves. Sympathetic input is also important: sympathetic innervation of the genital region originates in the thoracolumbar chain (T11-L2) and travels through the hypogastric nerves to the confluence of nerves that lies on either side of the rectum and the lower urinary tract—the pelvic plexus.

The pelvic plexus also receives input from the pelvic nerves. It is from the pelvic plexus that the cavernous nerves arise and innervate the corpora cavernosa. Although erection is induced by parasympathetic activity, nitric oxide has been identified as important in causing relaxation of the corporeal blood vessels and the increase in penile blood flow that causes erection. Psychogenic erection requires cortical activation of spinal pathways, and the preservation of this type of responsiveness in men with low spinal cord lesions suggests that sympathetic pathways can mediate it. Reflex erections occur as the result of cutaneous genital stimulation. Preservation of reflex erections in men with lesions above T11 indicates that the response is the result of spinal reflexes, with afferent signals conveyed in the pudendal nerve and S2-S4 roots, and efferent signals through the same sacral roots. In health, reflex and psychogenic responses are thought to reinforce one another. In men, orgasm and ejaculation are not the same process; ejaculation is the release of semen, and orgasm consists of the sensory changes accompanied by pelvic floor contractions. Ejaculation involves emission of semen from the vas and seminal vesicles into the posterior urethra and closure of the bladder neck. The latter processes are under sympathetic control, whereas contraction of the pelvic floor muscles is under somatic nerve control, innervation being from the perineal branch of the pudendal nerve. After ejaculation, a period of resolution is necessary before sexual activity can be reinitiated.

Female Sexual Response

The neurological control of sexual function in women is less well understood than that in men, but similarities exist. The main parasympathetic innervation is from the pelvic nerves, sympathetic innervation from the hypogastric nerves, and bilateral somatic innervation from the pudendal nerves. The finding of acetylcholinesterase-positive nerves around blood vessels in the vagina points to parasympathetic control of vaginal vasodilation and secretomotor function. It seems likely that increased vaginal blood flow, erection of the cavernous tissue of the clitoris and around the outer part of the vagina, and lubrication are brought about through neural mechanisms similar to those that control erection in men. The lubrication that occurs as part of sexual arousal results from transudation through the vaginal walls and fluid from Bartholin glands.

During orgasm, a series of synchronous contractions of the sphincter and vaginal muscles may occur. As many as

Table 38.1   Diagnostic Findings in Patients with Suspected Neurogenic Bladder Dysfunction

	Suprapontine Lesion	Infrapontine- Suprasacral Lesion	Infrasacral Lesion
Examples	Stroke, PD	SCI, MS	Conus medullaris tumor, cauda equina syndrome, peripheral neuropathy
History/bladder diary	Urgency, frequency, urgency incontinence	Urgency, frequency, urgency incontinence, hesitancy, interrupted stream	Hesitancy, interrupted stream
PVR urine	PVR urine <100 mL	±Elevated PVR	PVR urine >100 mL
Uroflowmetry	Normal flow	Interrupted flow	Poor/absent flow
Urodynamics	Detrusor overactivity	Detrusor overactivity Detrusor sphincter dyssynergia	Detrusor underactivity, sphincter insufficiency

From Panicker, J.N., Fowler, C.J., 2010. The bare essentials: uro-neurology. Pract Neurol 10, 178-185.
MS, Multiple sclerosis; *PD*, Parkinson disease; *PVR*, postvoid residual; *SCI*, spinal cord injury.

20 consecutive contractions have been registered, lasting for 10 to 50 seconds. The accompanying sensory experiences generally are described as an intensely pleasurable pelvic event.

Neurogenic Bladder Dysfunction

Lesions of the nervous system, central or peripheral, can result in characteristic patterns of bladder dysfunction depending upon the level of the lesions in the neurological axis (Panicker et al., 2010). The storage function of the bladder is affected following suprapontine or infrapontine/suprasacral lesions. This results in involuntary spontaneous or induced contractions of the detrusor muscle (detrusor overactivity), which can be identified during the filling phase of urodynamics. The voiding function of the bladder can be affected by infrapontine lesions. Following spinal cord damage, there is simultaneous contraction of the external urethral sphincter and detrusor muscle, *detrusor-sphincter dyssynergia*, which results in incomplete bladder emptying and abnormally high bladder pressures. Following lesions of the conus medullaris or cauda equina, voiding dysfunction can be due to poorly sustained detrusor contractions and possibly non-relaxing urethral sphincters (**Table 38.1**).

Cortical Lesions
Bladder Dysfunction

It has been known since the 1960s that anterior regions of the frontal lobes are critical for bladder control. Among patients with disturbed bladder control, various frontal lobe disturbances have been reported: intracranial tumors, damage after rupture of an aneurysm, penetrating brain wounds, and prefrontal lobotomy (leukotomy). The typical clinical picture of frontal lobe incontinence is a patient with severe urgency and frequency of micturition and urge incontinence but without dementia; the patient is socially aware and embarrassed by the incontinence. Micturition is normally coordinated, indicating that the disturbance is in the higher control of these processes. Urinary retention also has been described in patients with brain lesions. A small number of case histories have described patients with right frontal lobe disorders who had urinary retention and in whom voiding was restored when the frontal lobe disorder was treated successfully (Fowler, 1999).

Urinary incontinence develops in some patients after stroke. Urodynamic studies in incontinent patients have been carried out, and the general conclusion drawn from studying patients with disparate cortical lesions is that voiding mostly is normally coordinated. The most common cystometric finding is that of detrusor overactivity. It has not been possible to demonstrate a correlation between any particular lesion site and urodynamic findings. Urinary incontinence at 7 days following stroke predicts poor survival, disability, and institutionalization independent of level of consciousness. It has been suggested that incontinence in such cases is the result of severe general loss of function, or that persons who became incontinent may be less motivated to recover both continence and general function. Patients with hemorrhagic stroke are more likely to have detrusor underactivity in urodynamics compared to patients with ischemic stroke, who more often have detrusor overactivity (Han et al., 2010). Small-vessel disease of the white matter (*leukoaraiosis*) is associated with urgency incontinence, and it is increasingly becoming apparent that this is an important cause for incontinence in the functionally independent elderly (Tadic et al., 2010).

The cause of urinary incontinence in dementia is probably multifactorial. Not all incontinent older adults are cognitively impaired, and not all cognitively impaired older adults are incontinent. In a study of patients with progressive cognitive decline, incontinence was observed to occur in more advanced stages of Alzheimer disease (AD), whereas it could occur earlier on in the course of patients with dementia with Lewy bodies (DLB) (Ransmayr et al., 2008).

A much less common cause of dementia is normal-pressure hydrocephalus, where incontinence is a cardinal feature. Improvement in urodynamic function has been demonstrated within hours of lumbar puncture (LP) in patients with this disorder.

Bowel Dysfunction

In patients with frontal lobe disorders, defecation is generally affected much less often than micturition. Cases of impaired defecation are always described with accompanying urinary dysfunction. A lone study concerned primarily with the anorectal abnormalities associated with frontal lobe damage of various types found that the frontal lobe is involved in neurological control of anorectal motility, as it is for bladder function. The lack of correlation between urinary and anorectal abnormality in individual cases, however, suggests that these functions depend on distinct areas of the frontal lobes.

Sexual Dysfunction

Before functional imaging experiments, all that was known about human cerebral control and sexuality came from observations of patients with brain lesions, particularly those affecting temporal or frontal regions. These areas can be involved by disorders that cause epilepsy or by trauma, tumors, cerebrovascular disease, or encephalitis. It has long been observed that sexual dysfunction is more common in men and women with epilepsy. Although various sexual perversions and occasionally hypersexuality have been described in patients with temporal lobe epilepsy (TLE), the picture most commonly seen is that of sexual apathy. From studies comparing sexual dysfunction in generalized epilepsy with that in focal TLE, the evidence is sufficient to suggest that the deficit is a result of the specific temporal lobe involvement rather than a consequence of epilepsy, psychosocial factors, or antiepileptic medication. The problem usually is that of a low or absent libido, of which patients may not complain.

The role of hormonal dysfunction has yet to be fully determined. On the basis of measurements of sex hormones and pituitary function, it has been suggested that the hyposexuality of TLE results from a subclinical hypogonadotropic hypogonadism, and that dysfunction of medial temporal lobe structures may dysmodulate hypothalamopituitary secretion (Murialdo et al., 1995). Erectile dysfunction (ED) with preservation of libido can occur in men with temporal lobe damage with or without epilepsy and may be characterized by loss of nocturnal penile tumescence. Surgery for epilepsy rarely restores erectile function, although a survey of operated patients showed a higher level of satisfaction with sexual function among those who were free of seizures. Sexual dysfunction is common after head injury, particularly in patients who demonstrate cognitive damage. Hypersexual behavior may occur after frontal lobe damage. Lesions of the frontal lobes, the basal-medial part in particular, may lead to loss of social control, which also may affect sexual behavior.

Basal Ganglia Lesions
Bladder Dysfunction

Bladder symptoms in Parkinson disease (PD) correlate with neurological disability (Araki and Kuno, 2000) and stage of disease; both findings appear to support a link between dopaminergic degeneration and symptoms of urinary dysfunction. In line with current thinking about staging of PD in terms of underlying neuropathology (Braak et al., 2004), it appears that bladder dysfunction does not occur until some years after the onset of motor symptoms, and the dysfunction is correlated with the extent of dopamine depletion (Sakakibara et al., 2001b). This means that the underlying pathological process is likely to have extended into the neocortex and explains why the clinical context in which bladder dysfunction is seen in PD

is common in patients with cerebral symptoms, as well as with adverse effects of long-standing treatment with dopaminergic agents.

The most frequent complaints are of nighttime frequency, urgency, and difficulty voiding (Sakakibara et al., 2001a), and the most common abnormality in urodynamic studies is detrusor overactivity (Araki et al., 2000). Of the several possible explanations for this finding, the hypothesis most widely accepted is that in healthy persons, the basal ganglia has an inhibitory effect on the micturition reflex, and with neuronal loss in the substantia nigra, detrusor overactivity develops. Studies on anesthetized cats demonstrated that rhythmic bladder contractions were inhibited by intracerebroventricular administration of a dopamine D_1 receptor agonist but were not affected by a D_2 receptor agonist. From this evidence, it was concluded that the D_1 receptor provides the main inhibitory influence on the micturition reflex (Yoshimura et al., 2003). Clinical studies that have looked at the effect of L-dopa or apomorphine on bladder behavior in patients with PD have, however, produced conflicting results. In patients demonstrating the on/off phenomenon, cystometry done after taking L-dopa showed improvement of overactivity in some and worsening in others. The unpredictable effect of antiparkinsonian medications on urinary symptoms has not been definitively shown to correlate with age or stage of disease (Winge and Fowler, 2006). Many patients with PD have nocturnal polyuria as well, which contributes to bladder symptoms and would not be expected to improve with antimuscarinics. In addition to neurogenic bladder dysfunction, benign prostatic obstruction may occur concomitantly in some men with PD and contribute to bladder dysfunction. A recent study suggests that contrary to previous teaching, transurethral prostate resection may be successful in carefully selected PD men and is associated with minimal risk of incontinence (Roth et al., 2009).

In a patient with severe urinary symptoms but mild parkinsonism, a diagnosis of multiple system atrophy (MSA) should be considered. The onset of urogenital symptoms in MSA may precede overt neurological involvement; ED and bladder symptoms begin on average 4 to 5 years before diagnosis and 2 years before more specific neurological symptoms appear. The neuronal degeneration of MSA affects the central nervous system (CNS) at several locations that are important for bladder control, which probably explains why urinary complaints occur so early and are so severe in this condition. It is thought that detrusor overactivity is caused by neuronal loss in the pontine region, whereas incomplete bladder emptying is caused by loss of parasympathetic innervation of the detrusor after neuronal degeneration in the intermediolateral cell columns of the spinal cord. In addition, anterior horn cell loss in the Onuf nucleus results in denervation of the urethral sphincter so that the patient has a combination of detrusor overactivity, incomplete bladder emptying, and a weak sphincter. Bladder dysfunction may change during the progression of MSA, and serial studies have shown that the mean postmicturition residual volume increases as the condition progresses (Ito et al., 2006). Bladder symptoms in other parkinsonian syndromes are less prominent than in MSA, and although they may occur as part of the patient's general disability, they rarely are as severe as in MSA and do not occur at a stage of the disease when a neurological cause is not evident.

Bowel Dysfunction

Constipation is now thought to be a preclinical manifestation of PD, and a symptom questionnaire showed that this was considered to be the most bothersome nonmotor symptom for PD patients (Sakakibara et al., 2001a). Several possible causes for constipation are recognized: a slow colonic transit time has been demonstrated in a number of studies; this finding may be secondary to a reduction in dopaminergic myenteric neurons. An abnormality of the defecation process has also been demonstrated in some patients with PD, with paradoxical contraction of the external anal sphincter and pubococcygeus causing outlet obstruction. This phenomenon can result in anismus and is thought to be a form of focal dystonia. Bowel dysfunction appears earlier and progresses faster in patients with MSA than in those with PD (Stocchi et al., 2000).

Sexual Dysfunction

Experimental evidence from animals and humans shows that dopaminergic mechanisms are involved in determining libido and inducing penile erection. In animal studies, the medial preoptic area of the hypothalamus has been shown to regulate sexual drive, and selective stimulation of dopamine D_2 receptors in this region increases sexual activity in rats (Andersson, 2001). An increase in libido in some patients with PD treated with dopamine agonists and L-dopa as part of the "hedonistic homeostatic dysregulation" syndrome (Giovannoni et al., 2000) is a well-recognized phenomenon, although its incidence is uncertain. The cause of ED in PD is unclear, but it is a significant problem and in one study was shown to affect 60% of a group of men with PD, compared with 37.5% of age-matched healthy men. ED usually affects men later in the course of PD, with onset years after the diagnosis of neurological disease has been established. A survey of relatively young patients with PD (mean age, 49.6 years) and their partners revealed a high level of sexual dysfunction, with the most severely affected couples being those in which the patient was male.

ED may be the first symptom in men with MSA, predating the onset of any other neurological symptoms by several years. The disorder appears to be chronologically distinct from the development of postural hypotension. The reason for the apparently early selective involvement of neural mechanisms for erection is not known. Preserved erectile function in a man with parkinsonism strongly contradicts the diagnosis of MSA. The available literature on female sexual problems in movement disorders is limited (Jacobs et al., 2000; Oertel et al., 2003).

Brainstem Lesions

Voiding difficulty is a rare but recognized symptom of a posterior fossa tumor and has been reported in series of patients with brainstem disorders (Fowler, 1999). In an analysis of urinary symptoms of 39 patients who had had brainstem strokes, lesions that resulted in micturition disturbance usually were dorsally situated (Sakakibara et al., 1996)—a finding consistent with the known location of the brainstem centers involved in bladder control. The proximity in the dorsal pons between the pontine micturition center and medial longitudinal fasciculus means that a disorder of eye movements, such as an internuclear ophthalmoplegia (INO), is highly likely in patients with a pontine disorder causing a voiding difficulty.

Spinal Cord Lesions
Bladder Dysfunction

Spinal cord disorders are the most common cause for neurogenic bladder dysfunction. Transspinal pathways connect the pontine micturition centers to the sacral cord. Intact connections are necessary to effect the reciprocal activity of the detrusor and sphincter needed to switch between storage and voiding. After disconnection from the pons, this synergistic activity is lost, resulting in detrusor-sphincter dyssynergia.

Initially after acute SCI, there usually is a phase of neuronal shock of variable duration, characterized clinically by complete urinary retention and urodynamics demonstrating an acontractile detrusor. Gradually over the course of weeks, new reflexes emerge to drive bladder emptying and cause detrusor contractions in response to low filling volumes. The neurophysiology of this recovery has been studied in cats, and it has been proposed that after spinal injury, C fibers emerge as the major afferents, forming a spinal segmental reflex that results in automatic voiding. It is assumed that the same pathophysiology occurs in humans. In support of this assumption is the observed response to intravesical capsaicin (a C-fiber neurotoxin) in patients with acute traumatic spinal cord injury (SCI) or chronically progressive spinal cord disease from multiple sclerosis (MS). The abnormally overactive, small-capacity bladder that characterizes spinal cord disease causes patients to experience urgency and frequency. However, patients with complete transection of the cord may not complain of urinary urgency. If detrusor overactivity is severe, incontinence is highly likely. Poor neural drive on the detrusor muscle during attempts to void, together with an element of detrusor-sphincter dyssynergia, contributes to incomplete bladder emptying. This difficulty may exacerbate the symptoms of the overactive bladder. Although the neurological process of voiding may have been as severely disrupted as the process of storage, the symptoms of difficulty emptying can be minor compared with those of urge incontinence. Only on direct questioning may the patient admit to having difficulty initiating micturition, an interrupted stream, or possibly a sensation of incomplete emptying.

Because bladder innervation arises more caudally than innervation of the lower limbs, any form of spinal cord disease that causes bladder dysfunction is likely to produce clinical signs in the lower limbs as well, unless the lesion is limited to the conus. This rule is sufficiently reliable to be of great value in determining whether a patient has a neurogenic bladder caused by spinal cord disease.

Spinal Cord Injury

After SCI, bladder dysfunction can be of such severity as to cause ureteric reflux, hydronephrosis, and eventual upper urinary tract damage. Before the introduction of modern treatments, renal failure was a common cause of death after SCI. The bladder problems of persons with SCI, therefore, must be managed aggressively to lessen the possibility of upper tract disease and to provide the patient with adequate bladder control for a fully rehabilitated life. People with SCI often are young and otherwise fit, and it may be best for them to undergo surgery on the lower urinary tract with a view to fulfilling these two aims, rather than to be treated medically.

Multiple Sclerosis

The pathophysiological consequences of progressive MS affecting the spinal cord for the bladder are similar to those of SCI, but the medical context of increasing disability is such that management must be quite different. Estimates of the proportion of patients with MS who have lower urinary tract symptoms vary according to the severity of the neurological disability in the group under study, but a figure of about 75% is frequently cited (Marrie et al., 2007). Several studies have shown that urinary incontinence is considered to be one of the worst aspects of the disease; 70% of a self-selected group of patients with MS responding to a questionnaire classified the impact bladder symptoms had on their life as "high" or "moderate" (Hemmett et al., 2004). A strong association between bladder symptoms and the presence of clinical spinal cord involvement, including paraparesis and UMN signs, has been recognized on examination of the lower limbs in patients with MS. This observation has also been made in patients with a similar condition, acute disseminated encephalomyelitis (ADEM) (Panicker et al., 2009).

The most common urinary symptom is urgency; all series of urodynamic studies in patients with MS have shown that this is due to detrusor overactivity. Hesitancy of micturition may be a symptom patients volunteer or admit on direct questioning, but the more disabled may find themselves unable to initiate micturition voluntarily, emptying their bladders only with an involuntary hyperreflexic contraction and an interrupted urinary flow. Evidence of incomplete emptying may come not from a sensation of continued fullness after voiding but rather from the need to pass urine again within 5 to 10 minutes (double voiding).

As the neurological condition progresses, bladder dysfunction may become more difficult to treat. However, unlike with the bladder dysfunction that follows SCI, progressive neurological diseases such as MS rarely result in upper urinary tract involvement. This is the case even when long-standing MS has resulted in severe disability and spasticity. The reason for this sparing of the upper urinary tract is not known, but it means that in such patients, management should emphasize symptomatic relief (Fowler, 1999).

A particular problem in MS is that neurological symptoms may deteriorate acutely when the patient has an infection and pyrexia, including urinary tract infection (UTI). As MS progresses, recurrent infections are likely to result in deficits that accumulate and lead to progressive neurological deterioration (Buljevac et al., 2002).

Bowel Dysfunction

Half of all patients need help with bowel management. A questionnaire survey of patients with SCI found that bowel dysfunction was a major problem, rated as only slightly less serious than loss of mobility (Glickman and Kamm, 1996). Bowel management may be equally problematic for patients with progressive spinal cord disease such as MS,

with prevalence rates for bowel dysfunction reported at 30% to 50% (DasGupta and Fowler, 2003). The loss of rectal sensation and the normal urge to defecate means that bowel emptying must be induced at a convenient time by digital anal stimulation, use of suppositories or enemas, or manual evacuation. The consequence of losing the ability to postpone bowel emptying because of impaired sensation of impending defecation and inability to voluntarily contract the anal sphincter is that fecal incontinence is common.

Sexual Dysfunction
MALE SEXUAL DYSFUNCTION

The level and completeness of a spinal cord lesion determine erectile and ejaculatory capability after SCI (Bors and Comarr, 1960). With a complete cervical lesion, psychogenic erections are lost, but the capacity for spontaneous or reflex erections may be intact. With low spinal cord lesions, particularly if the cauda equina is involved, little or no erectile capacity may be retained. Theoretically, a lesion below spinal level L2 leaves psychogenic erections intact, but in practice it is uncommon for men with such a lesion to have erections adequate for intercourse. Psychogenic erections are more likely to be preserved in incomplete lesions. Preservation of ejaculation function after a spinal cord lesion is unusual (Sipski, Alexander, and Gómez-Marín, 2006). Although earlier studies indicated a much lower figure, it is now known that 60% to 65% of men with MS have ED, often coexisting with urinary symptoms, with urodynamically demonstrable overactivity in a majority of those affected. Typically, in the early stages of MS, the chief complaint is difficulty sustaining an erection for intercourse. With advancing neurological disability, erectile function may cease, and difficulty with ejaculation may develop. A study of pudendal evoked potentials in men with MS found that those with severely delayed latencies (i.e., with more severe spinal cord disease) were more likely to be unable to ejaculate (Betts et al., 1994). Though it has been said that a diagnosis of MS should be considered in a young man presenting with impotence, this possibility seems unlikely in the absence of clinical spinal cord disease. In one series, only a single patient had erectile difficulties at the time of the first symptoms of MS, and neurological disease did not develop subsequently in any of the men who presented with ED.

FEMALE SEXUAL DYSFUNCTION

Studies of women with SCI at different levels, both complete and incomplete, have advanced current understanding of the neural pathways involved in female sexual response. It has been hypothesized that the sensory experience of orgasm may have an autonomic basis because orgasmic capacity is preserved in a proportion of affected women, particularly with higher cord lesions (Sipski et al., 2001); fMRI studies in SCI patients suggest preservation of vagal pathways. Sexual dysfunction in women with MS is common, affecting 50% to 60%, although probably underdiagnosed, with the incidence increasing with worsening disability. Neurogenic problems during intercourse include decreased lubrication and reduced orgasmic capacity. A double-blind, randomized, placebo-controlled crossover study of sildenafil citrate in treating females with sexual dysfunction due to MS showed no overall benefit with the drug, shown to be far more effective in men with MS (DasGupta et al., 2004). In women with advanced disease, additional problems may include lower limb spasticity, loss of pelvic sensation, genital dysesthesia, and fear of incontinence (Hulter and Lundberg, 1995).

Impaired Sympathetic Thoracolumbar Outflow

The fibers that travel from the thoracolumbar sympathetic chain emerge from the T10-L2 spinal levels and course through the retroperitoneal space to the bifurcation of the aorta, from which they enter the pelvic plexus. Loss of sympathetic innervation of the genitalia causes disorders of ejaculation, with either failure of emission or retrograde ejaculation; ability to experience the sensation of orgasm may be retained. Sympathetic thoracolumbar fibers are particularly likely to be injured by the procedure of retroperitoneal lymph node dissection or surgeries involving an anterior approach to the lumbar spine, and complaints of loss of ejaculation are common after these surgeries.

Conus and Cauda Equina Lesions

The cauda equina contains the sacral parasympathetic outflow together with the somatic efferent and afferent fibers. Damage to the cauda equina leaves the detrusor decentralized rather than denervated because the postganglionic parasympathetic innervation is unaffected. This distinction may explain why bladder dysfunction after a cauda equina lesion is unpredictable and why even detrusor overactivity has been described (Podnar and Fowler, 2010).

Inability to evacuate the bowel may be a severe problem, and manual evacuation may be necessary for the long term. Additional denervation of the anal sphincter can result in incontinence of flatus and feces. Damage to the cauda equina results in sensory loss, and both men and women complain of perineal sensory loss and loss of erotic genital sensation, for which no effective treatment is available. In men, ED is also a complaint (Podnar et al., 2006).

Impairment of bladder, bowel, and sexual function is particularly difficult for patients to bear psychologically when they are otherwise ambulant and mobile. Although a number of series have reported the urodynamic changes that can occur after a cauda equina lesion, no analysis has been performed to assess the effect of a cauda equina lesion on quality of life. The levels of compensation awarded in medicolegal cases reflect the fact that loss of control of the pelvic organs is a catastrophe.

For most patients, contact with other persons similarly affected may prove supportive.

Disturbances of Peripheral Innervation
Diabetic Neuropathy

Bladder involvement once was considered an uncommon complication of diabetes, but the increase in use of techniques for studying bladder function has shown that such involvement is common, although often asymptomatic. Bladder dysfunction does not occur in isolation, and other symptoms and signs of generalized neuropathy are necessarily present in affected patients. The onset of the bladder dysfunction is insidious, with progressive loss of bladder sensation and impairment of bladder emptying over years, eventually culminating in chronic low-pressure urinary retention (Hill et al., 2008). Urodynamic studies demonstrate impaired detrusor contractility, reduced urine flow, increased postmicturition residual volume, and reduced bladder sensation. It seems likely that vesical afferent and efferent fibers are involved, causing reduced awareness of bladder filling and decreased bladder contractility.

Diabetes is the most common cause of ED. Surveys of andrology clinics have found that 20% to 31% of men attending are diabetic. The prevalence of ED increases with age and duration of diabetes, and the problem is known to be associated with severe retinopathy, a history of peripheral neuropathy, amputation, cardiovascular disease, raised glycosylated hemoglobin, and the use of antihypertensives such as beta-blockers. A large population study of men with early-onset diabetes found that 20% had ED. Whether its pathogenesis in diabetic patients results mainly from neuropathy or involves a significant microvascular contribution, or whether the two processes are codependent, is not yet resolved. Age-matched studies of women with and without diabetes suggest that diabetic women also may be affected by specific disorders of sexual function including decreased vaginal lubrication and capacity for orgasm.

Amyloid Neuropathy

Autonomic manifestations are common in amyloid neuropathy and include ED, orthostatic hypotension, bladder dysfunction, distal anhidrosis and abnormal pupils. Lower urinary tract symptoms generally appear early on and are present in 50% of patients within the first 3 years of the disease. Patients most often complain of difficulty in bladder emptying and incontinence (Andrade, 2009). Often, however, bladder dysfunction may be asymptomatic and uncovered only during investigations. Urodynamic studies have demonstrated reduced bladder sensations, underactive detrusor, poor urinary flow, and opening of the bladder neck. Bladder wall thickening may be seen on ultrasound scan. Some 10% of patients with familial amyloidotic polyneuropathy (FAP) type I may proceed to end-stage renal disease (Lobato, 2003) and may complain of polyuria. Urinary incontinence has been shown to be associated with higher post–liver transplant mortality (Adams et al., 2000).

Bowel dysfunction results in alternating constipation and diarrhea. This occurs concomitantly with other manifestations such as episodic nausea, vomiting, and malnutrition. Anorectal physiology studies have demonstrated prolonged colonic transit time, low anal pressure at rest, and loss of spontaneous phasic rectal contractions during squeeze, suggesting an enteric neuropathy. Reduced libido and ED are common, and phosphodiesterase inhibitors may have the adverse effect of accentuating orthostatic hypotension and should therefore be used with caution.

Immune-Mediated Neuropathies

Approximately one-fourth of patients with Guillain-Barré syndrome have bladder symptoms. These symptoms usually occur in those patients with more severe neuropathy and appear after limb weakness is established. Both detrusor areflexia and bladder overactivity have been described.

Autoimmune Autonomic Ganglionopathy

Patients with autoimmune autonomic ganglionopathy present with rapid onset of severe autonomic failure, with orthostatic hypotension, GI dysmotility, anhidrosis, bladder dysfunction, ED, and sicca symptoms and may have ganglionic acetylcholine receptor (AChR) antibodies. Bladder dysfunction generally manifests with voiding difficulty and incomplete emptying. Severity and distribution of autonomic dysfunction appear to depend upon the level of antibody titers (Gibbons and Freeman, 2009).

Pure Autonomic Failure

Pure autonomic failure (PAF) is a degenerative postganglionic autonomic disorder. There is now evidence to suggest that the underlying basis is a synucleinopathy, with Lewy bodies confined primarily to the autonomic ganglia neurons. Nocturia and voiding dysfunction are common, and bladder emptying is often affected. Bladder dysfunction in PAF appears to be as common but less severe than in MSA, and this could possibly reflect slower progression of the disease (Sakakibara et al., 2000). ED and constipation are common.

Myotonic Dystrophy

Although myotonic activity has not been found in the sphincter or pelvic floor of patients with myotonic dystrophy, bladder symptoms may be prominent and difficult to treat, presumably because bladder smooth muscle is involved. With advancing disease, megacolon and fecal incontinence also may become intractable problems.

Urinary Retention in Young Women

Urinary retention or symptoms of obstructed voiding in young women in the absence of overt neurological disease have long puzzled urologists and neurologists alike, and in the absence of any convincing organic cause, the condition was once said to be "hysterical." The typical clinical picture is that of a young woman in the age range of 20 to 30 years who presents with retention and a bladder capacity greater than 1 L. Although patients retaining such quantities may be uncomfortable, they do not have the sensation of extreme urgency that might be expected. Many affected women have previously experienced interruption of the urinary stream but are unaware that this is abnormal, so a voiding history can be misleading unless taken carefully. Other clinical neurological features or findings on laboratory investigations that would support a diagnosis of MS are lacking, and MRI of the brain, spinal cord, and cauda equina are normal. The lack of sacral anesthesia makes a cauda equina lesion improbable. An association between this syndrome and polycystic ovaries was described in the original description of the syndrome.

In some young women with urinary retention, concentric needle electrode examination of the striated muscle of the urethral sphincter reveals complex repetitive discharges and myotonia-like activity, decelerating bursts. Known as *Fowler syndrome*, it could until recently only be managed symptomatically. However, it is now known that these patients respond particularly favorably to sacral neuromodulation.

Diagnostic Evaluation

History

History forms the cornerstone for evaluation and should address both storage and voiding dysfunction. Patients with storage dysfunction complain of frequency for micturition, nocturia, urgency, and urgency incontinence. Urgency, frequency, and nocturia, with or without incontinence, is called *overactive bladder syndrome*, *urge syndrome*, or *urgency-frequency syndrome* (Abrams et al., 2002). Patients experiencing voiding dysfunction report hesitancy for micturition, a slow and interrupted urinary stream, the need to strain to pass urine, and double voiding. Patients may be in complete urinary retention. The history of voiding dysfunction is often unreliable, and patients may be unaware of incomplete bladder emptying. Therefore, the history should be supplemented by a bladder scan (see later discussion).

Bladder Diary

The bladder diary supplements history taking and records the frequency for micturition, volumes voided, episodes of incontinence, and fluid intake over the course of a few days (**Fig. 38.2**).

Physical Examination

Findings on clinical examination are critical in deciding whether a patient's urogenital complaints are neurological in origin. Because the spinal segments that innervate the bladder and genitalia are distal to those that innervate the lower limbs, bladder disturbances generally have been shown to correlate with lower-limb deficits. The possible exceptions are lesions of the conus medullaris and cauda equina, where findings may be confined to saddle anesthesia and absence of sacral cord–mediated reflexes such as the anal reflex or bulbocavernosus reflex. Akinetic rigidity, cerebellar ataxia, and postural hypotension should raise the suspicion of MSA in conditions characterized by early and severe urinary incontinence and ED.

Examination for evidence of peripheral neuropathy is important. Peripheral neuropathy, notably diabetic, is the most common cause for male ED, and as neuropathy progresses, abnormalities and innervation of the detrusor muscle also develop. Clear evidence for peripheral neuropathy is likely before innervation of the bladder is involved.

		Time / Volume (mL)					Total Fluid Intake	Episodes of leakage
Day 1 26/4/2009	Time	6 AM	10 AM	12:30 PM	3:30 PM	5 PM	1700	4
	Volume	160	120	130	190	140		
Time out of bed (am) – 6 AM	Time	7 PM	8:45 PM	2:30 AM	4 AM			
	Volume	150	170	200	180			
Time to bed (pm) – 9 PM	Time							
	Volume							

Fig. 38.2 Bladder diary recorded over 24 hours, demonstrating increased daytime and nighttime urinary frequency, low voided volumes, and incontinence. These findings are seen in patients with detrusor overactivity. *(From Panicker, J.N., Kalsi, V., de Seze M., 2010. Approach and evaluation of neurogenic bladder dysfunction, in: Fowler, C.J., Panicker, J.N., Emmanuel, A, (Eds.), Pelvic Organ Dysfunction in Neurological Disease: Clinical Management and Rehabilitation. Cambridge University Press, New York.)*

The neurological examination is complete only after an inspection of the lumbosacral spine. Congenital malformations of the spine can sometimes present with pelvic organ symptoms in adulthood; dimpling, a tuft of hair, or a nevus or sinus in the sacral region may prove to be relevant.

If the neurological examination reveals normal findings in a patient with bladder complaints, detailed investigation with imaging and neurophysiology is unlikely to reveal relevant underlying neurological pathology.

Investigations
Screening for Urinary Tract Infections

It is advisable for patients presenting with bladder symptoms to be screened for UTIs. Combined rapid tests of urine using reagent strips ("dipstick" test) have a negative productive value of 98% for excluding UTI. However, the positive predictive value for confirming infection is only 50% (Fowlis et al., 1994), and hence if abnormal, a urine sample should be sent off to the lab for culture.

Bladder Scan

Because the extent of incomplete bladder emptying cannot be predicted from history or clinical examination, it is pertinent to estimate the postvoid residual urine by ultrasonography. This is most commonly carried out using a portable bladder scanner (**Fig. 38.3**), or by "in-out" catheterization, especially in patients who perform intermittent self-catheterization. It is recognized that a single measurement of a postvoid residual is often not representative; if possible, a series of measurements should be made over the course of 1 or 2 weeks.

Ultrasound Scan

In patients known to be at risk for upper tract disease, surveillance ultrasonography should be performed periodically to evaluate for evidence of damage such as upper urinary tract dilatation or renal scarring. Ultrasound may also detect complications of neurogenic bladder dysfunction such as bladder stones.

Urodynamic Studies

Urodynamic studies examine the function of the lower urinary tract. Included in this aspect of evaluation are measurements of urine flow rate and residual volume, cystometry during both filling and voiding, videocystometry, and urethral pressure profilometry. The term *urodynamics* is often used incorrectly as a synonym for *cystometry*. From the patient's point of view, urodynamic studies can be divided into noninvasive investigations and those requiring urethral catheterization.

NONINVASIVE BLADDER INVESTIGATIONS

Uroflowmetry is a valuable noninvasive investigation, particularly when combined with an ultrasound measurement of the postvoid residual volume. A commonly used design for a flow meter consists of a commode or urinal into which the patient passes urine as naturally as possible. In the base of the collecting system is a spinning disc, and flow of urine onto this disc

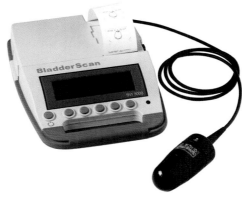

Fig. 38.3 A small portable ultrasound machine can be used to measure postvoid residual urine.

tends to slow its speed of rotation, which a servomotor holds constant. The urinary flow is calculated based upon the power necessary to maintain the rotation speed. A graphic printout of the urinary flow is obtained, and time taken to reach maximum flow, maximum and average flow rates, and voided volume are analyzed (**Fig. 38.4**). It is important that the patient performs the test with a comfortably full bladder containing, if possible, a volume of at least 150 mL; privacy is essential insofar as a spurious result may be obtained if the individual is not fully relaxed.

A significant neurogenic bladder disorder is unlikely if a patient has good bladder capacity, normal urine flow rate, and empties to completion, all of which may be noninvasively demonstrated.

INVESTIGATIONS REQUIRING CATHETERIZATION

Cystometry evaluates the pressure/volume relationship during nonphysiological filling of the bladder and during voiding. The detrusor pressure is derived by subtraction of the abdominal pressure (measured using a catheter in the rectum) from the intravesical pressure (measured using a catheter in the bladder). The rate of filling is recorded by the machine, which pumps sterile water or saline through the catheter in the bladder. For speed and convenience, most laboratories use filling rates of between 50 and 100 mL/min. This nonphysiological rapid filling does mean that the full bladder capacity can be reached usually within 7 or 8 minutes. The first sensation of bladder filling may be reported at around 100 mL, and full capacity is reached between 400 and 600 mL. In healthy persons, the bladder expands to contain this amount of fluid without an increase of pressure more than 15 cm H_2O. A bladder that behaves in this way is said to be "stable." The main abnormality sought during filling cystometry in patients with a neurological disease is the presence of detrusor overactivity (**Fig. 38.5**). This is a urodynamic observation characterized by involuntary detrusor contractions that may be spontaneous or provoked. It should be emphasized that on urodynamics, detrusor overactivity of neurogenic origin is indistinguishable from other causes for detrusor overactivity. When bladder filling has been completed, the patient voids into the flow meter, with the bladder and rectal lines still in place. Valuable information can be obtained by measuring detrusor pressure and urine flow simultaneously.

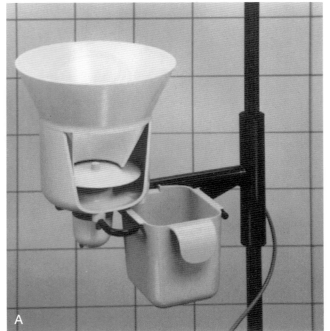

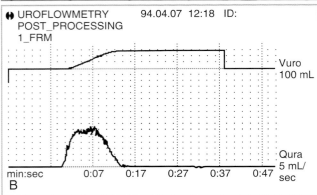

Fig. 38.4 A, Urinary flow meter. Side of uroflow transducer has been cut away to show disk at base of funnel, which rotates as urine passes into collecting vessel. **B,** Normal printout from uroflowmeter. A total of 290 mL was voided *(upper trace),* with a maximum flow rate of 30 mL per second *(lower trace). (Reprinted with permission from Dantec Medical A/S, Copenhagen.)*

When cystometry is carried out using a contrast filling medium and the procedure visualized radiographically, the technique is known as *videocystometry.* This gives additional information about morphological changes that may occur consequent to neurogenic bladder dysfunction and the presence of vesicoureteric reflux. Urologists and urogynecologists have found videocystometry useful for detecting sphincter or bladder neck incompetence in genuine stress incontinence, and the opportunity to inspect the outflow tract during voiding is of great value in patients with suspected obstruction.

A general criticism of cystometric studies is that valuable as they may be in demonstrating the underlying pathophysiology of a patient's urinary tract, the findings contribute little to elucidating the underlying cause of the disorder. A "urodynamic diagnosis" is therefore a meaningless term. The study provides information about the safety and efficiency of bladder filling and emptying. It is valuable for assessing risk factors for upper urinary tract damage and planning management. In addition, it is helpful in identifying concomitant urological conditions such as bladder outflow obstruction or stress incontinence.

Whether it is necessary to perform a complete urodynamic study in all patients with a suspected neurogenic bladder is a subject of debate. Patients with spinal cord injury, spina bifida, and possibly advanced MS should undergo urodynamic studies because of the higher risk for upper tract involvement and renal impairment, although ultrasound is a less invasive method for monitoring. Guidelines underlying the key role of urodynamics for baseline evaluation, management, and follow-up of a neurogenic bladder in these patient groups have been published. However, in other conditions such as early MS, stroke, and PD, some authors have recommended restricting the initial evaluation to noninvasive tests, on the basis that the risk for upper urinary tract damage is less (Fowler et al., 2009). In the absence of evidence-based medical data comparing these two models of management, the decision for performing complete baseline urodynamics would depend upon local resources and recommendations.

Urethral pressure profile is measured using a catheter-mounted transducer that is run slowly through the urethra by a motorized armature. The test can be performed in men or

Fig. 38.5 Filling cystometry demonstrating detrusor over-activity. Red trace (Pabd) is the intraabdominal pressure recorded by the rectal catheter, dark blue trace (Pves) is the intravesical pressure recorded by the bladder catheter. Pink trace (Pdet) is the subtracted detrusor pressure (Pves-Pabd). Green traces represent volume infused (Vinf) during the test and volume voided (Vura); orange trace represents urinary flow (Qura). Black arrow demonstrates detrusor overactivity, and black arrowhead indicates associated incontinence. *(From Panicker, J.N., Fowler, C.J., 2010. The bare essentials: uro-neurology. Pract. Neurol. 10, 178-185.)*

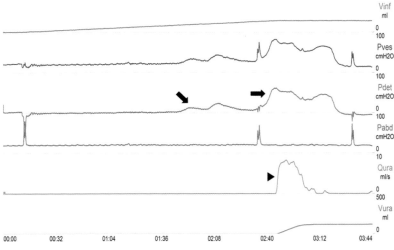

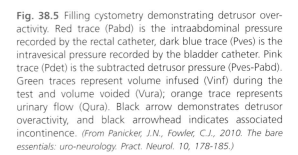

women and is called *static* if no additional maneuvers such as coughing or straining are performed. It has been found to be helpful in the assessment of women with obstructed voiding or urinary retention, some of whom have abnormally high urethral pressures.

Uroneurophysiology

Various neurophysiological investigations of the pelvic floor have been developed for assessing the innervation of muscles that are difficult to test clinically. These tests have been used by neurologists, urologists, andrologists, urogynecologists, and colorectal surgeons.

Electromyography

Pelvic floor electromyography (EMG) was first introduced as part of urodynamic studies to assess the extent of relaxation of the urethral sphincter during voiding, with the aim of recognizing detrusor-sphincter dyssynergia. However, it is now rarely recorded for several reasons. First, it is often technically difficult to obtain a good-quality EMG signal from a site as inaccessible as the urethral sphincter, particularly in the hostile recording environment in which urodynamic studies are performed. The best signal is obtained using a needle electrode, but the discomfort from the needle itself is likely to impair normal relaxation of the pelvic floor. Surface recording electrodes have been used, but they may record a considerable amount of noise, which makes interpretation of the results difficult. In addition to the difficulties of making a meaningful recording, the value of the information the procedure provides is limited. Video screening allows the outlet tract to be seen, and hence the indications for kinesiological sphincter EMG recording is now limited. One situation in which it is helpful is evaluating men with suspected dysfunctional voiding. These are usually young men who present with voiding difficulties and have otherwise normal neurological findings on examination and investigation. Recording electrical silence from the urethral sphincter during voiding would exonerate the external sphincter as the cause for voiding dysfunction.

Concentric needle EMG studies of the pelvic floor performed separately from urodynamics have been useful to assess innervation in certain scenarios. EMG has been used to demonstrate changes of reinnervation in the urethral or anal sphincter in a few neurogenic disorders. The motor units of the pelvic floor and sphincters fire tonically, so they may be conveniently captured using a trigger and delay line and subjected to individual motor unit analysis. Well-established values exist for the normal duration and amplitude of motor units recorded from the sphincter muscles.

SPHINCTER ELECTROMYOGRAPHY IN THE EVALUATION OF SUSPECTED CAUDA EQUINA LESIONS

Lesions of the cauda equina are an important cause for pelvic floor dysfunction. Most often, EMG of the external anal sphincter demonstrating changes of chronic reinnervation with a reduced interference pattern and enlarged polyphasic motor units (>1 mV amplitude) can be found in patients with long-standing cauda equina syndrome (Podnar et al.,

2006). Though EMG may demonstrate pathological spontaneous activity 3 weeks or more after injury, these changes of moderate to severe partial denervation or complete denervation often become lost in the tonically firing motor units of the sphincter.

SPHINCTER ELECTROMYOGRAPHY IN THE DIAGNOSIS OF MULTIPLE SYSTEM ATROPHY

Neuropathological studies have shown that anterior horn cells in the Onuf nucleus are selectively lost in MSA, and this results in changes in the sphincter muscles that can be identified by EMG. The anal sphincter is once again most often studied, and compared to the changes of chronic reinnervation in patients with cauda equina syndrome described earlier, the changes of reinnervation in MSA tend to result in prolonged-duration motor units, presumably because the progressive nature of that disease precludes motor unit "compaction." These changes can be detected easily, but it is important to include measurement of the late components of the potentials (**Fig. 38.6**).

Although the value of sphincter EMG in the differential diagnosis of parkinsonism has been widely debated, a body of opinion exists that maintains that a highly abnormal result in a patient with mild parkinsonism is of value in establishing a

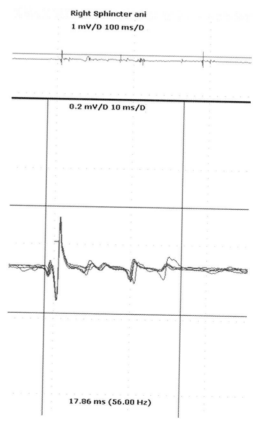

Fig. 38.6 Concentric needle electromyography (EMG) of external anal sphincter from a 64-year-old male presenting with parkinsonism and urinary retention. Duration of the motor unit is 17.9 msec (normal < 10 msec); prolonged motor units suggest chronic reinnervation. Mean duration of motor unit potentials (MUPs) during study was 22.9 msec; EMG is compatible with a diagnosis of multiple system atrophy.

diagnosis of probable MSA (Vodusek, 2001). This correlation is important not only for the neurologist but also for the urologist because inappropriate surgery for a suspected prostate enlargement as the cause for bladder troubles can then be avoided.

SPHINCTER ELECTROMYOGRAPHY IN THE INVESTIGATION OF URINARY RETENTION IN YOUNG WOMEN

Isolated urinary retention in young woman has long been an enigma; the neurological examination is typically normal, and investigations such as MRI exclude a neurological cause for voiding dysfunction. A characteristic abnormality, however, can be found on urethral sphincter EMG: complex repetitive discharges akin to the "sound of helicopters" and decelerating bursts, a signal somewhat like myotonia and akin to the "sound of underwater recording of whales." It has been proposed that this abnormal spontaneous activity results in impairment of relaxation of the urethral sphincter, which may cause urinary retention in some women and obstructed voiding in others. This condition, nowadays known as *Fowler syndrome*, is also characterized by elevated urethral pressures.

PENILOCAVERNOSUS REFLEX

The nomenclature of the various reflex responses that can be recorded from pelvic structures in response to electrical stimulation was recently revised so that the term used gives an indication of the site of stimulation and recording. The *penilocavernosus reflex*, formally known as the *bulbocavernosus reflex*, assesses the sacral root afferent and efferent pathways. The dorsal nerve of the penis (or clitoris) is electrically stimulated, and recordings are made from the bulbocavernosus muscle, usually with a concentric needle. It may be of value in patients with bladder dysfunction suspected to be secondary to cauda equina damage or damage to the lower motor neuron pathway. However, a normal value does not exclude the possibility of an axonal lesion.

PUDENDAL NERVE TERMINAL MOTOR LATENCY

The only test of motor conduction for the pelvic floor is the pudendal nerve terminal motor latency (PNTML). The pudendal nerve is stimulated either rectally or vaginally adjacent to the ischial spine using the St. Mark electrode, a finger-mounted device with a stimulating electrode at the fingertip and a surface EMG receiving electrode 7 cm proximal, around the base of the finger. This records from the external anal sphincter. Prolongation was initially considered evidence for pudendal nerve damage, although a prolonged latency is a poor marker of denervation. This test has not proved contributory in the investigation of patients with suspected pudendal neuralgia.

PUDENDAL SOMATOSENSORY EVOKED POTENTIALS

Pudendal somatosensory evoked potentials can be recorded from the scalp following electrical stimulation of the dorsal nerve of penis or clitoral nerve. Although this may be abnormal when a spinal cord lesion is the cause of sacral sensory loss or neurogenic detrusor overactivity, such pathology is usually apparent from the clinical examination. Results are compared to latencies of the tibial evoked potentials.

Complications Arising from Neurogenic Bladder Dysfunction

Detrusor overactivity and reduced bladder-wall compliance may result in raised intravesical pressure, which can in turn lead to structural changes in the bladder wall such as trabeculations and diverticuli. The upper urinary tract (kidney and ureter) can also show changes such as vesicoureteric reflux and hydronephrosis, renal impairment, and even end-stage renal disease. For reasons that are unclear, upper urinary tract damage and renal failure are surprisingly unusual in MS. On the other hand, patients with SCI and spina bifida have an increased risk for upper urinary tract damage and renal disease. The risk for upper urinary tract damage is highest in patients who have raised intravesical pressure due to detrusor overactivity, low bladder compliance, and a competent bladder neck. Patients with a neurogenic bladder are also prone to a variety of genitourinary tract infections such as cystitis, pyelonephritis, and epididymo-orchitis, and also to bladder stones.

Management of Neurogenic Bladder Dysfunction

The pattern of lower urinary tract symptoms and findings from relevant bedside investigations such as uroflowmetry and bladder scan are useful in the localization of neurological lesions (see **Table 38.1**). Variations from these expected patterns of symptoms and findings should warrant a search for additional urological conditions that may be occurring concomitantly and alter the pattern of lower tract dysfunction.

The goals one would wish to achieve when managing neurogenic bladder dysfunction are urinary continence, preventing UTIs, and preserving upper urinary tract function (Stohrer et al., 2009). Attaining these goals would help improve quality of life of patients with neurological disease. The management of neurogenic bladder dysfunction must address both voiding and storage dysfunction.

General Measures

Nonpharmacological measures are generally effective in the early stages when symptoms are mild. A fluid intake of around 1 to 2 L a day is suggested, although this should be individualized; it is often helpful to assess fluid balance by means of a bladder diary (Hashim and Abrams, 2008). Caffeine reduction may reduce urgency and frequency, especially for patients who drink coffee or tea in excess. Bladder retraining, whereby patients void by the clock and voluntarily "hold on" for increasingly longer periods, aims to restore the normal pattern of micturition. If voiding dysfunction has been excluded, pelvic floor exercises and neuromuscular stimulation may play a role in ameliorating overactive bladder symptoms.

Voiding Dysfunction

Knowledge of a patient's postvoid residual volume is critical in planning treatment of bladder symptoms. There is no consensus regarding the figure of residual volume at which intermittent self-catheterization should be initiated. However, in general, because patients with a neurogenic bladder have reduced bladder capacity, a volume of more than 100 mL or more than one-third of bladder capacity is taken as the amount of residual urine that contributes to bladder dysfunction (Fowler et al., 2009). The widespread use of intermittent self-catheterization has greatly improved management of neurogenic bladder dysfunction. Incomplete emptying can exacerbate detrusor overactivity, and an overactive bladder constantly stimulated by a residual volume responds by contracting and producing symptoms of urgency and frequency, thus making antimuscarinic medications less effective. Sterile intermittent catheterization was first introduced in the 1960s, but subsequently a clean rather than sterile technique was found to be adequate. Intermittent catheterization is best performed by patients themselves, who should be taught by someone experienced with this method, such as nurse continence advisors. Neurological lesions affecting manual dexterity, weakness, tremor, rigidity, spasticity, impaired visual acuity, and cognitive impairment may make it impossible for the patient to self-catheterize, in which case it may be performed by the partner or care assistant. The incidence of symptomatic UTIs is low when performed regularly.

Reflex voiding using trigger techniques and the Credé maneuver (nonforceful, smooth, even pressure applied from the umbilicus toward the pubis) are usually not recommended, as they may result in high detrusor pressure and incomplete bladder emptying during voiding (Fowler et al., 2009). Suprapubic vibration using a mechanical "buzzer" has been demonstrated to be effective in patients with MS with incomplete bladder emptying and detrusor overactivity, but its effect is limited (Prasad et al., 2003). Alpha-blockers relax the internal urethral sphincter in men, and there is evidence that they improve bladder emptying and reduce postvoid residual volumes (O'Riordan et al., 1995). However, this is not consistently seen in clinical practice unless there is concomitant bladder outlet obstruction. Botulinum toxin injections into the external urethral sphincter may improve bladder emptying in patients with SCI who have significant voiding dysfunction (Naumann et al., 2008).

Storage Dysfunction
Antimuscarinic Medications

Detrusor overactivity is a major cause for incontinence in patients with neurogenic bladder disorders. The sensation of urgency is experienced as the detrusor muscle begins to contract, and if the pressure continues to rise, the patient senses impending micturition. Antimuscarinic medications are the mainstay of treatment for detrusor overactivity. **Table 38.2** lists the medications available in the United Kingdom. Oxybutynin was one of the earlier drugs introduced, and subsequently several newer agents have been marketed. Meta-analyses suggest that efficacy is similar between these medications. Adverse events arise owing to their nonspecific anticholinergic action and include dry mouth, blurred vision for near objects, tachycardia, and constipation. These drugs can also block central muscarinic M1 receptors and cause impairment of cognition and consciousness in susceptible individuals. This may be mitigated by medications that have low selectivity for the M1 receptor, such as darifenacin, or restricted permeability across the blood-brain barrier (BBB), such as trospium. The postvoid residual urine may increase following treatment, and it should be monitored by repeat bladder scans, especially if initial beneficial effects are short lasting. In many patients, there may also be underlying voiding dysfunction, and the judicious use of antimuscarinic medication coupled with clean intermittent self-catheterization (CISC) often proves most effective for managing neurogenic bladder dysfunction (Fowler et al., 2009) (**Fig. 38.7**).

Desmopressin

Desmopressin, a synthetic analog of arginine vasopressin, temporarily reduces urine production and volume-determined detrusor overactivity by promoting water reabsorption at the distal and collecting tubules of the kidney. It is useful for treating urinary frequency or nocturia in patients with MS, providing symptom relief for up to 6 hours (Bosma et al., 2005). It is also helpful in managing nocturnal polyuria, characterized

Generic Name	Trade Name	Dose (mg)	Frequency
Darifenacin	Emselex	7.5-15	Once daily
Fesosterodine	Toviaz	4-8	Once daily
Oxybutynin IR	Ditropan, Cystrin	2.5-20	bid-qid
Oxybutynin ER	Lyrinel XL	5-20	Once daily
Oxybutynin transdermal	Kentera	36 mg (3.9 mg/24 h)	One patch twice weekly
Propantheline	Pro-Banthine	15-120	tid (1 hour before food)
Propiverine	Detrunorm	15-60	Once daily-qid
Solifenacin	Vesicare	5-10	Once daily
Tolterodine IR	Detrusitol	2-4	bid
Tolterodine ER	Detrusitol XL	4	Once daily
Trospium	Regurin	20-40	bid (before food)

Table 38.2 Antimuscarinic Medications Available in the United Kingdom

From Fowler, C.J., Panicker, J.N., Drake, M., et al., 2009. A UK consensus on the management of the bladder in multiple sclerosis. J Neurol Neurosurg Psychiatry 80, 470-477.

ER, Extended release; IR, immediate release; bid, twice daily; qid, four times daily; tid, three times daily.

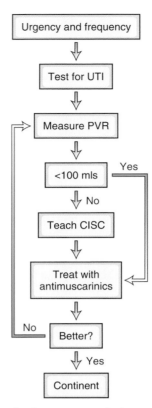

Fig. 38.7 Algorithm for the management of neurogenic lower urinary tract dysfunction. *(From Fowler, C.J., Panicker, J.N., Drake, M., et al., 2009. A UK consensus on the management of the bladder in multiple sclerosis. J Neurol Neurosurg Psychiatry 80, 470-477.)*

by increased production of urine in the night. This may be seen in patients with PD and also various neurological conditions associated with dysautonomia and orthostatic hypotension. However, it should be prescribed with caution in patients over the age of 65 or with dependent leg edema, and it should not be used more than once in 24 hours for fear of hyponatremia or congestive heart failure.

Cannabinoids

Positive anecdotal reports on the effect of cannabis in controlling bladder symptoms in MS patients and identification of the cannabinoid receptor in animal and human studies led to studies of cannabis-based medicinal extracts in this group. An open-label study in patients with advanced MS produced promising results, with diminished frequency, nocturia, and incontinence (Freeman et al., 2006). A license was recently granted in the United Kingdom for the use of a cannabis-based medicine to treat spasticity in MS, but this does not cover bladder dysfunction.

Botulinum Toxin

Botulinum toxin type A injected into the detrusor muscle under cystoscopic guidance appears to be a highly promising, although at the time of writing an unlicensed treatment, for intractable detrusor overactivity. The effect lasts 9 to 13 months and significantly improves storage symptoms and quality of life (Kalsi et al., 2007), though patients often have

to perform CISC afterwards. Studies also suggest that patients receiving botulinum toxin injections have fewer UTIs and reduced catheter bypassing (urethral leakage when using an indwelling catheter). Botulinum toxin was introduced on the theoretical basis that it blocks synaptic release of acetylcholine from the parasympathetic nerve endings and produces a paralysis of detrusor muscle (and indeed a demonstrable increase in bladder capacity has been reported in the various studies). However, accumulating evidence indicates that the mechanism of action is more complex and may actually involve the afferent innervation as well.

Vanilloids

Despite initial enthusiasm for their use, intravesical vanilloid therapy, capsaicin, and resiniferatoxin generally have been superseded by botulinum toxin therapy. Because only a few centers worldwide offer resiniferatoxin treatment, this treatment is not discussed further here.

Sacral Neuromodulation

An extradural sacral nerve stimulator can be highly effective in lessening detrusor overactivity that is resistant to antimuscarinic medication. It seems highly likely that the mechanism of action of this device is associated with stimulation in the presacral region of the pelvic afferents, which are known to have an inhibitory effect on the detrusor. Implanting the stimulator is a two-stage procedure, the first being a test phase with a stimulating lead inserted through the S3 foramen and connected to an external stimulator. During this test phase, it is noted whether the patient's symptoms diminish significantly, as judged by bladder diaries and measurement of residual volumes; if so, the patient is eligible for a permanent stimulator. This is implanted in a subcutaneous pocket and connected to the stimulating lead. The stimulator is continuously active, although its efficacy can be maintained at a subsensory level so that patients are not aware of its chronic action. The permanent stimulators are expensive, and patient selection is crucial in order to minimize the need for revision procedures. Evidence suggests that there is only a limited role for sacral neuromodulation in patients with progressive neurological conditions such as MS.

Nerve Root Stimulators

In patients who have suffered a complete spinal cord transection but in whom the caudal section of the cord and its roots are intact, implantation of a nerve root stimulator should be considered. This device was pioneered by Professor Giles Brindley and his collaborators, and several thousand have now been implanted worldwide. Stimulating electrodes are placed around the lower sacral roots (S2 to S4) and activated by an external switching device. The stimulating electrodes are usually applied intrathecally to the anterior roots, and the posterior roots are cut at the same time. After the implant, adjustments are made to the stimulation parameters so that the patient obtains maximum benefit in terms of making the bladder contract for voiding, assisting defecation, or even producing a penile erection. Although such devices are highly effective in selected cases, the additional neurological deficit caused by the need for sectioning of the dorsal roots and consequent loss of reflex erections has reduced its acceptance. The stimulators are suitable only for patients with complete spinal cord lesions, rather than partial cord lesions or progressive neurological disease.

Surgery

Various urological surgeries can be carried out to treat incontinence and are summarized in **Table 38.3**. A surgical procedure to rectify a disorder causing incontinence in an otherwise fit and healthy person often is highly successful. Even after SCI, a surgical option might be the best solution for long-term bladder management. This, however, does not apply to patients with progressive neurological disease causing incontinence. For example, at a time when the bladder is becoming unmanageable by intermittent catheterization and an antimuscarinic medication, the patient with MS may only just be managing to remain independent. This is not the moment to suggest major urological surgery, and in practice few patients with progressive neurological disease affecting bladder control opt for surgery. With the advent of botulinum toxin for the bladder, some of these debilitating symptoms can now be better controlled.

Permanent Indwelling Catheters

There comes a point when the patient is no longer able to perform self-catheterization, or when incontinence is refractory to management. It is at this stage that an indwelling catheter becomes necessary. The most immediate solution is an indwelling Foley catheter held in place by an inflatable balloon in the bladder, proximal to the catheter opening. The long-term ill effects of these devices are well known. One of the major problems may be catheter bypassing, which occurs when strong detrusor contractions produce a rapid urine flow that cannot drain sufficiently quickly. A common response to this would be to use a wider-caliber catheter, with the adverse effect that the bladder closure mechanism becomes progressively stretched and destroyed. The detrusor contraction may be of sufficient intensity to extrude the 10- or 20-mL balloon from the bladder, causing further damage to the bladder neck and resulting in a totally incompetent outlet. Bladder stones and recurrent infections are also more likely in patients with an indwelling catheter.

A preferred alternative to an indwelling urethral catheter is a suprapubic catheter. This can be inserted by a urologist, but

extreme care is required because these patients often have small, contracted bladders, contributing to the risk of bowel perforation during catheter placement. Although by no means a perfect system, a suprapubic catheter is a better long-term alternative to a urethral catheter, since it preserves urethral integrity and helps promote perineal hygiene and sexual functions.

The option of intermittent bladder drainage using a catheter valve, as opposed to continuous drainage into a leg bag, depends upon whether the bladder has a reasonable capacity to store urine.

External Devices

If incontinence is the major problem and the bladder empties completely, some men are able to wear an external device such as a penile sheath.

Stepwise Approach to Neurogenic Bladder Dysfunction

The treatment options offered to a patient should reflect the severity of bladder dysfunction, which generally parallels the extent of neurological disease (**Fig. 38.8**). However, beyond a certain point, incontinence may become refractory to all treatment options, and it is at this stage that a long-term indwelling catheter should be offered. Although most patients can be managed along these lines, there are specific situations where specialist urology services should be involved earlier on in the disease course (**Box 38.1**).

Table 38.3 **Urological Procedures That May Be Performed to Treat Various Causes for Incontinence**	
Stress incontinence: pelvic floor weakness	Bladder neck suspension TVT TOT
Stress incontinence: sphincter incompetence	Artificial sphincter
Urgency incontinence (detrusor overactivity)	Botulinum toxin Sacral neuromodulation Augmentation cystoplasty ?Myomectomy
Intractable incontinence	Urinary diversion with stoma

TOT, Transobturator tape; *TVT*, tension-free vaginal tape.

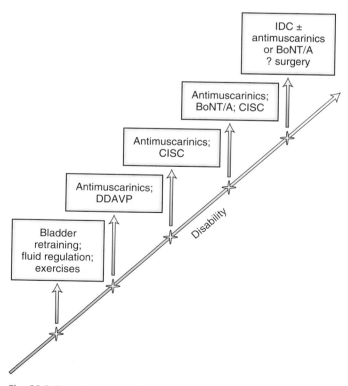

Fig. 38.8 Stepwise approach to neurogenic bladder dysfunction and its relation with progression of disabilities (see text for details). *BoNT/A*, Botulinum toxin A; *CISC*, clean intermittent self-catheterization; *DDAVP*, desmopressin; *IDC*, indwelling catheter.

Urinary Tract Infections

The presence of asymptomatic bacteria alone in a patient performing intermittent self-catheterization should not be an indication for antibiotics (Fowler et al., 2009). The usual indication would be presence of associated symptoms (local or systemic) and certainly if involvement of the upper urinary tract (pyelonephritis) occurs. In an individual with recurrent UTIs (more than 2 in 6 months or more than 3 in a year), the catheterization technique should be reviewed and if optimal, it is worthwhile to exclude a urological cause such as a bladder stone. In individuals with proven recurrent UTIs and when no urological structural abnormality has been identified, it is reasonable to start prophylactic low-dose antibiotics for a finite duration. Rotation of antibiotics is one approach to minimize antibiotic resistance developing. It is also important to distinguish relapsing from remitting infections and ensure that undertreatment of a causative organism is not the underlying cause of the symptoms. There is debate about the pros/cons of introducing CISC as a preventive measure against UTIs, as well as the threshold above which CISC should be recommended (e.g., a residual of 150 mL). The input of a specialist nurse in lower urinary tract dysfunction who teaches CISC is particularly helpful here.

The value of cranberry juice in preventing UTIs in neurogenic patients is debatable.

Management of Neurogenic Sexual Dysfunction

The first step in approaching sexual dysfunction of neurogenic origin is providing an opportunity for patients and their partners to openly discuss their sexual dysfunction. The topic can often be broached during the consultation while discussing concomitant bladder or bowel troubles. An explanation of the neurological basis for sexual dysfunction often relieves anxiety about the problem and removes assumptions that the problem is essentially psychological in origin.

Sexual dysfunction in neurological disease can be due to several different causes (Foley and Werner, 2000) (**Box 38.2**). *Primary sexual dysfunction* results from the actual neurological lesions directly affecting the neural pathways for sexual functions. For example, lesions in the spinal cord may cause loss of tactile sensations from the genitalia. Physical disabilities such as spasticity or pain resulting from the neurological disease can interfere with sexual functions as well. This is known as *secondary sexual dysfunction.* Sexual dysfunction arising from the psychological, emotional, or cultural impact of living with a neurological disease is known as *tertiary sexual dysfunction.* A holistic approach to managing sexual dysfunction involves identifying all these contributory factors.

Management of Erectile Dysfunction

Sexual dysfunction in men most commonly manifests with ED. The evidence generally points to spinal cord involvement as the major cause of ED in neurological conditions such as MS. Cord involvement may initially result in a partial deficit so that ED is variable, with preserved nocturnal penile erections and erections on morning waking. It is only in the last 10 to 20 years that neurological teaching has recognized the error of the view that "if a man can get an erection at any time, ED is likely to be psychogenic." With increasing neurological disability, there may be a total failure of erectile function and also difficulty with ejaculation. Few men with complete SCI can ejaculate, and difficulty with ejaculation may become apparent when ED is successfully treated. The treatment of ED was transformed by the introduction of phosphodiesterase type 5 inhibitors. These act to increase nitric oxide release in the corpora cavernosa and thereby induce penile erections; the first such agent was sildenafil (Viagra). Clinical studies have demonstrated that the optimal dose should be taken up to 1 hour before anticipated sexual activity. These are not aphrodisiacs, and it must be remembered that for medications to be effective, they must be accompanied by intimacy and stimulation, which promote nitric oxide release. The medications appear to have few side effects, and those that exist relate to its vasodilator action. In some patients, they produce headaches, flushing, dyspepsia, and nasal congestion. Given their known pharmacology, these medications increase the hypotensive effects of organic nitrates, leading to excessive vessel dilatation and therefore hypotension; *they are absolutely contraindicated in patients receiving nitrates to treat angina.* Of relevance to neurological patients, they should be avoided in patients with orthostatic hypotension.

After the introduction of sildenafil, two other medications with a similar mechanism of action have been introduced. All three medications are generally well tolerated, but there are some differences to be considered. Sildenafil and vardenafil are effective after 30 to 60 minutes from administration, respectively, and last for up to 4 hours. By contrast, tadalafil is effective from 30 minutes after administration, buts its peak efficacy is expected after approximately 2 hours. Efficacy is maintained for up to 36 hours and may, therefore, mean less planning and pressure to have sexual intercourse to a schedule. A fatty meal may affect the absorption of sildenafil and vardenafil, with potential bearing on efficacy. Specific characteristics of the three currently available phosphodiesterase 5 inhibitors are shown in **Table 38.4**.

Sublingual apomorphine hydrochloride is a dopamine D_1/D_2 receptor agonist that acts centrally. However, intact spinal cord pathways are required for its action, and the initial promise of this agent as an alternative therapeutic option to phosphodiesterase type 5 inhibitors have not been reflected in clinical practice.

Although the use of oral agents is now established as first-line treatment for most patients, alternative approaches are available if required. Prostaglandin E_1 (alprostadil) can be injected directly into the penis. It acts by relaxing the smooth muscle of the cavernosal vessels. Adverse effects include penile pain, groin pain, hypotension, prolonged erection (priapism), and in some instances, penile fibrosis when used long term. Intraurethral therapy of alprostadil (medicated urethral system for erection [MUSE]) was introduced to obviate the need for self-injection. Efficacy rates of 75% to 69% have been reported, but adverse effects include burning and irritation of the urethra, making the therapy unpopular.

Vacuum constriction devices are overall the most economical therapy for ED. A plastic tube is placed around the penis, and air is pumped out of the chamber, creating a vacuum, thereby drawing blood into the penis and resulting in penile engorgement. Tumescence is maintained by placing one or more tension bands around the base of the turgid penis. These bands may be left in situ for as long as 30 minutes, and the device may be reused. Though highly efficacious, satisfaction rates are generally only 55%. They are cumbersome and give an unnatural erection. They also require manual dexterity, and the patient may have to shave his pubic hair to facilitate the creation of a seal for the vacuum. Side effects include petechiae, pain, numbness or coldness, delayed ejaculation, and sense of trapped ejaculate. Generally, this type of therapy is preferred for older patients who are in stable relationships.

Rarely, implantation of a penile prosthesis can be offered. However their use in patients with neurological disease is limited because with increasing sensory loss, there is a risk of erosion of the prosthesis. Also, they may interfere with the management of concomitant lower urinary tract dysfunction.

Management of Ejaculation Dysfunction

Impaired ejaculation is a problem for many men with spinal cord lesions. There is as yet no medical intervention that restores ejaculatory function, although a small proportion of patients report some improvement of "erotic sensitivity" with yohimbine. This is an alkaloid derived from the bark of the African tree, *Pausinystalia yohimbe*, and the South American herb, quebracho, *Aspidosperma quebracho-blanco*. Available as an oral preparation, it is principally a monoamine oxidase inhibitor (MAOI) that stimulates release of norepinephrine. Yohimbine can be used 1 to 2 hours before intercourse. Its main side effects include rise in blood pressure and increased frequency of micturition. It may also have an anxiogenic effect. Midodrine, an α_1-agonist, has recently been shown to improve ejaculation in men with SCI (Soler et al., 2007).

Infertility caused by ejaculatory failure can be managed by means quite different from those that would be suggested for ejaculatory difficulties. Patients should be referred to a center that specializes in this problem; such centers usually exist in association with a spinal cord unit.

Sexual Dysfunction in Women

Until recently, sexual dysfunction in women has been generally neglected by mainstream clinical practice. Sexual dysfunction has significance on both the affected woman and her partner and often is an underlying strain in a relationship. The success of sildenafil in treating ED in men led to a placebo-controlled randomized study of its effect in women (Dasgupta et al., 2004). The only benefit seemed to be a slight but significant improvement in vaginal lubrication, explained by the vasodilatory action of sildenafil. However, this was not associated with an improvement in orgasmic function or on quality of life. Anesthetic gels or pain modulation may be useful for women with dyspareunia.

Management of Fecal Incontinence

Coordinated lower-bowel function depends less on the integrity of the spinal cord than bladder function. This is likely to be due to the well-developed enteric nervous system, which serves as the "little brain" of the gut. Consequently, fecal

Table 38.4 Phosphodiesterase Type 5 Inhibitors for the Treatment of Erectile Dysfunction			
Generic Name	**Sildenafil**	**Vardenafil**	**Tadalafil**
Available doses	25, 50, 100 mg	5, 10, 20 mg	10, 20 mg
Starting dose	50 mg/d	10 mg/d	10 mg/d
Time to onset of action	30-60 min	30 min	30 min
Duration of effect	4 h	4 h	36 h
Interaction with fatty meals	Yes	Yes	No

incontinence is much less common than urinary incontinence in patients with neurological disease. The first step in management of fecal incontinence is to establish the cause. The history usually will establish whether the complaint is due to diarrhea or urgency for defecation, and if so, the patient should be referred to a gastroenterologist for investigation. If no cause can be found and the problem persists, symptomatic treatment with an anticholinergic agent that reduces lower-bowel motility, such as loperamide, may be helpful.

Constipation is a common problem in patients with neurological disease. It may arise secondary to slow colonic transit or difficulties with evacuation. Problems with slow transit are more common, and management strategies include optimizing fiber and fluid intake and use of bulk laxatives or stool softeners. The osmotic laxative, polyethylene glycol, has been shown to be effective in managing constipation in neurological patients. Transanal bowel irrigation is a way of facilitating the evacuation of feces from the bowel by introducing water (or other fluids) into the colon via the anus in a quantity sufficient to reach beyond the rectum. It is thought to result in an emptying of the descending colon as well as the sigmoid and rectum and is found to be of particular benefit in managing refractory constipation of neurogenic origin.

Pelvic floor incompetence can occur in the context of a cauda equina lesion or as a result of more selective neurological injury to the pudendal nerves. Referral to a colorectal surgeon may be necessary for consideration of sphincter repair.

References

The complete reference list is available online at www.expertconsult.com.

Neuroepidemiology

Mitchell T. Wallin, John F. Kurtzke

A useful definition of *epidemiology* is "the science of the natural history of diseases." This concept is based on the Greek roots of the word: *logos*, from *legein*, "to study"; *epi*, "[what is] on"; *demos*, "the people." In epidemiology, the unit of study is a person affected with a disorder of interest. Therefore, a definitive diagnosis is the essential prerequisite. This is why the neurologist must be part of any inquiry into the epidemiology of neurological diseases.

After diagnosis, the most important question is the frequency of a disorder. Much of this type of information has been based on case series—that is, the series of cases encountered by individual practitioners, clinics, or hospitals. With such data, however, whether taken as numerator alone (case series) or compared with all admissions (relative frequency), it is difficult to ensure that what has been included is representative of the total population. Accordingly, case material has to be referenced to its proper denominator, its true source: the population at risk.

Population-Based Rates

Ratios of cases to population, together with the period to which they refer, constitute the population-based rates. Those commonly measured are the incidence rate, the mortality rate, and the so-called prevalence rate. They ordinarily are expressed in unit-population values. For example, a total of 10 cases among a community of 20,000 represents a rate of 50 per 100,000 population, or 0.5 per 1000.

The *incidence or attack rate* is the number of new cases over a defined study period divided by the population at risk. This usually is given as an annual incidence rate in cases per 100,000 population per year. The date of onset of clinical symptoms typically dictates the time of accession, although occasionally the date of first diagnosis is used. The *(point) prevalence rate* is more properly called a *ratio*, but it refers to the number of those affected, both old and new cases, at one point in time within the community per unit of population. The *lifetime prevalence rate* refers to the proportion of persons manifesting a disorder of interest during the period of their life up to the survey date. It typically is reported per 1000 of the population at risk. If no change in case-fatality ratios occurs over time and no change in annual incidence rates (and no migration) occurs, then the average annual incidence rate times the average duration of illness in years equals the point prevalence rate. When numerator and denominator for a rate each refer to an entire community, their quotient is a crude rate, for all ages. When both terms of the ratio are delimited by age or sex, these are age-specific or sex-specific rates, respectively. Such rates for consecutive age groups, from birth to the oldest group of each sex, provide the best description of a disease within a community. In comparing morbidity or mortality rates between two communities for an age-related disorder (such as stroke or epilepsy), differences in crude rates may be observed solely because of differences in the age distributions of the denominator populations. This can be avoided by comparing only the individual age-specific rates between the two, but this approach rapidly becomes unwieldy. Methods exist for adjusting the crude rates for all ages to permit such comparisons. One such method involves taking community age-specific rates and multiplying them by the proportion of a

DOI: 10.1016/B978-1-4377-0434-1.00049-9

687

"standard" population within the same age group. The sum of all such products provides an age-adjusted (to a standard) rate, or a rate for all ages adjusted to a standard population. One common standard in the United States is its population for a given census year. The *mortality* or *death rate* is the number of deaths in a population in a period with a particular disease as the underlying cause, such as an annual death rate per 100,000 population. Deaths by cause are provided by official government agencies, based on standard death certificates. At times, deaths listed as other than underlying cause on the certificate are added to give a count of total deaths for the disease. The standardized mortality ratio (SMR) is the observed number of deaths in the study group of interest divided by the expected number of deaths based on the standard population rates applied to the study group. The great advantage of death rates is their current availability over time and geographical area for many disorders, whereas morbidity rates require specific community surveys. Geographical distributions from death data are especially informative because most population studies available are, of necessity, spot surveys that may tell little about areas that were not investigated. Most often, too, the numbers are larger by orders of magnitude than those that prevalence studies can provide. The principal disadvantage, and it is a major one, is the question of diagnostic accuracy. In clinical practice, the diagnostic code used for mortality rates is a three- or four-digit number representing a specific diagnosis in the *International Statistical Classification of Diseases, Injuries and Causes of Death* (ICD), which is revised periodically. The changes in the 10th revision (ICD-10) were major. ICD-10 was published in 1992 and adopted for use in the United States in 1999. It introduced the innovation of an alphanumerical coding scheme of one letter followed by three numbers (e.g., I63.1, cerebral infarction due to thrombosis of precerebral arteries). One drawback of the ICD system of classification is that different diseases frequently are subserved under the same primary code. To provide a more refined classification for individual diseases, several disciplines have published specialty-related expansions of the primary ICD structure. ICD-10-NA is the expansion of the codes relating to neurological diseases, so that virtually every known neurological disease or condition has a unique alphanumerical identifier (van Drimmelen-Krabbe et al., 1998; World Health Organization, 1997). In the United States, the Department of Health and Human Services has mandated conversion to ICD-10 for all healthcare organizations by 2013. Lack of space here precludes attention to community survey methods, risk factors and analytic epidemiology, treatment comparisons, and statistical methods—all intrinsic aspects of epidemiology. This chapter highlights the descriptive epidemiological analysis for a few major neurological diseases selected as representative of those most likely to be encountered in clinical neurology.

Cerebrovascular Disease

Stroke (see Chapter 51) is the third leading cause of death and a major cause of disability in the United States (Miniño et al., 2009). Most recent epidemiological studies have subdivided stroke into subarachnoid hemorrhage (SAH), intracerebral hemorrhage, and cerebral infarction. Subdural hemorrhage is not included in this category. Cerebral infarction is the most common type of stroke in developed countries, making up more than 70% of cases. Intracerebral hemorrhages account for approximately 10% to 15% of strokes, and SAHs make up less than 5%, while the remainder are of undetermined etiology.

Mortality Rates

Since the late 1960s, U.S. stroke death rates have declined by 60% overall (Howard et al., 2001). The largest declines in stroke mortality were seen in white men and the smallest in black men. Similar decreasing rates in stroke mortality are reported for other countries including Japan, Australia, New Zealand, Canada, and all of Western Europe. Recent annual age-standardized mortality rates in Europe ranged between 26 and 50 per 100,000 for men and between 18 and 23 per 100,000 for women. Reported mortality rates over recent decades have actually increased for Eastern Europe (Sarti et al., 2003).

The geographic differences in stroke mortality within the United States are notable, with the highest rates in the southeastern region since the 1940s. The so-called stroke belt states of Georgia, North Carolina, and South Carolina have consistently demonstrated mortality rates above the U.S. average. The Reasons for Geographic and Racial Difference in Stroke (REGARDS) Study was launched in 2001 to better understand demographic differences in stroke. Recent data from this project have shown that geographic differences in risk factors contribute little to explaining geographic variations in stroke mortality (Howard et al., 2009).

In general, age-specific death rates for stroke exhibit a logarithmic increase with increasing age. Racial and ethnic disparities in mortality from stroke have been recorded in many studies in the United States. The Centers for Disease Control and Prevention (CDC) examined this issue by evaluating 2002 U.S. mortality and death certificate data. During 2002, 12% of all stroke deaths occurred among persons younger than 65 years of age (Centers for Disease Control and Prevention [CDC], 2005). Age-specific death rates were notably higher in blacks than in whites by factors of 2.5, 3.5, 2.8, and 1.9 for the successive age groups 0 to 44, 45 to 54, 55 to 64, and 65 to 74 years. For all other groups (Asian/Pacific Islanders, American Indians/Native Americans, Hispanics), little consistent difference from the whites was observed in any age group (**Fig. 39.1**). United States racial and ethnic disparities in mortality by stroke type have been reported for the period 1995 to 1998 (Ayala et al., 2001). National Vital Statistics death certificate data were used to calculate age-standardized rates for ischemic stroke, intracerebral hemorrhage, and SAH among Hispanics, blacks, American Indians/Alaska Natives, Asians/Pacific Islanders, and whites. For ischemic stroke, the ratio of the age-standardized death rate among blacks (96 per 100,000) compared with whites was 1.30; all other groups had lower rates than the whites. Death rates for intracerebral hemorrhage were highest for blacks (23 per 100,000) and Asian/Pacific Islanders (20 per 100,000), with corresponding risk ratios compared with whites of 1.70 and 1.52. Subarachnoid hemorrhage death rates were higher in whites than for all minority groups.

Morbidity Rates

Like mortality rates, stroke incidence has declined rapidly over the past 50 years. Within the past 2 decades, however, the incidence rates have seemed to plateau or decrease only slightly

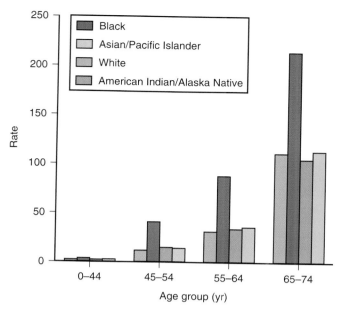

Fig. 39.1 Age-specific annual death rates per 100,000 population for stroke among persons younger than 75 years, by race and age group—United States, 2002. *(Data from Centers for Disease Control and Prevention, 2005. Regional and racial differences in prevalence of stroke—23 states and District of Columbia, 2003. MMWR Morb Mortal Wkly Rep 54, 481-484.)*

in industrialized countries (Kleindorfer et al., 2010). Stroke incidence increases logarithmically with increasing age but with a lesser increase beyond age 74. Average annual age-adjusted incidence rates by sex show a modest, but possibly increasing, male excess. In recent years, the annual stroke incidence rate in Europe and North America has been between 100 and 300 per 100,000 population, and mostly near 150.

The most recent trends in stroke incidence were reported from population-based stroke registries in six European countries (Heuschmann et al., 2009). Total stroke incidence for any first stroke between 2004 and 2006 and adjusted to the European population was 141 per 100,000 for men and 95 per 100,000 for women. Stroke incidence ranged in men from 101 per 100,000 in Sesto Fiorentino to 239 per 100,000 in Kaunas; and in women, from 63 per 100,000 in Sesto Fiorentino to 159 per 100,000 in Kaunas. The median age for first stroke was 73 years, with 51% occurring in females. On average, the highest rates were observed in Eastern Europe and the lowest in Southern Europe. Incidence rates in the United States for blacks remain higher than those for whites. The Greater Cincinnati and Northern Kentucky Stroke Study was the first large metropolitan-based study of stroke trends among blacks (Kleindorfer et al., 2010). The incidence for stroke between 1993 and 2005 decreased significantly for whites but was stable for blacks. These changes were driven by a drop in ischemic stroke among whites but stable ischemic stroke rates among blacks. Case fatality ratios did not differ by race. In the United States, age-, race-, and sex-adjusted stroke prevalence rates increased from 1.41% in the period 1971 to 1975 to 1.87% in the period 1988 to 1994 (Muntner et al., 2002). This corresponded with an increase of 930,000 noninstitutionalized stroke survivors, with increases observed in all age, race, and gender groups. With decreasing mortality trends and relatively

stable stroke incidence rates during the 1980s, these data point to a decreasing stroke case-fatality ratio as a major reason for the increasing prevalence.

Transient Ischemic Attacks

Although clearly a subset of cerebrovascular disease, transient ischemic attacks (TIAs) generally have been excluded from most morbidity and mortality surveys of stroke. As with stroke incidence and prevalence rates, a marked increase in TIA rates occurs with age. The Oxford Vascular Project found a slight increase in the incidence of TIAs between 1981 and 1984 and between 2002 and 2004, with overall rates rising from 0.33 per 1000 to 0.51 per 1000 (Rothwell et al., 2004). TIAs in persons older than 65 years of age accounted for the major part of this rate increase between time periods. This trend was also confirmed in a community-based study of older adults in Korea, where an age- and education-adjusted prevalence of TIA of 8.9% (age 65+) was found (Han et al., 2009).

The new tissue-based definition for TIA takes into account recent neuroimaging findings, as well as providing a much shorter duration for the diagnosis (Albers et al., 2002). If the new definition were to be used in epidemiological studies, the estimated annual incidence of TIA would be lowered by 33% and the incidence of ischemic stroke increased by 7% (Ovbiagele et al., 2003). However, a major underascertainment of TIA is probable in all surveys, with undefined differences among them. This also may give spuriously high frequencies for completed stroke after TIA because in many studies of stroke, only a retrospective history of TIA occurrence is given.

Primary Neoplasms

Three large centralized U.S. databases have been created that provide descriptive epidemiological data on primary brain tumors (see Chapter 52A). These databases include the Central Brain Tumor Registry of the United States (CBTRUS); the Surveillance, Epidemiology and End Results (SEER) database; and the National Cancer Database (NCDB). According to the CBTRUS database, a total of 158,088 persons were diagnosed with a primary brain or central nervous system (CNS) tumor in the United States in the years 2004-2006 (CBTRUS, 2010). The lifetime risk of developing a CNS tumor is estimated to be 0.65% for men and 0.50% for women (Ries et al., 2005). Little is known of the causes of most primary brain tumors, but their epidemiological features may provide clues for more definitive studies.

Within the CNS, approximately 85% of primary tumors have been intracranial and 15% intraspinal. For the brain, the major groupings are the gliomas (40% to 50%, of which approximately half are glioblastomas) and the meningiomas (15% to 20%). Pituitary adenomas plus schwannomas, especially acoustic, add another 15% to 20%. The most common spinal cord tumors are neurofibroma and meningioma, followed by ependymoma and angioma.

Mortality Rates and Survival

In the United States for 1995-1999, malignant CNS tumor deaths by age showed a steep rise from very low rates in early adult life to a peak of approximately 20 per 100,000 per year by age 75, followed by a steep decline with further increasing age (Davis et al., 2001). These rates presumably are chiefly for glioblastoma multiforme. A notable excess of whites over non-whites was seen in this group, with rates two to three times higher in the white patients. An excess of male deaths occurred in all racial groups.

Reported 5-year survival ratios have been approximately 60% for clinically diagnosed meningioma and 20% for gliomas as a group. When these two tumor types are taken together, median survival for benign brain tumors may be estimated at 6 years. The relative 5-year survival rate for children younger than 15 years of age with brain and other nervous system tumors is now 61%, compared with 35% some 20 years ago (Parker et al., 1997). Population-based data between 1990 and 2001 from the United Kingdom showed that 5-year survival rates for all CNS tumors for those 15 to 29 years of age were slightly worse than for those 0 to 14 years of age (62% versus 67%) (Feltbower et al., 2004). Glioblastoma is the most common primary brain tumor in adults, with a uniformly poor prognosis. Median survival for glioblastoma remains approximately 1 year after diagnosis. Several studies from cancer registries have indicated that the 5-year survival rate, typically reported at 4% to 10% over the past 3 decades, may be too optimistic (Tran and Rosenthal, 2010). Series from Canada, Sweden, and the United States that reviewed clinical and histological data from registries found that in half of all reported cases of glioblastoma, the tumor had been misclassified and on close inspection was found to be a less aggressive tumor (McLendon and Halperin, 2003). Corrected 5-year survival rates are more likely to be in the 2% to 3% range. Some positive news for a subgroup of glioblastoma patients with the MGMT (O^6-methylguanine-DNA methyltransferase) DNA repair gene was recently reported (Hegi et al., 2005). Irrespective of treatment, patients with glioblastoma with a methylated MGMT promoter survived approximately 55% longer than patients with an unmethylated MGMT promoter. The gain, although real, was therefore only some 6 months. The methylation of the MGMT promoter gene compromises DNA repair and triggers cytotoxicity. In addition, patients with glioblastoma and the MGMT promoter also demonstrated an improved treatment response to alkylating chemotherapy agents. The epidemiology of metastatic brain tumors is that of the primary cancer. Survival for patients with metastatic brain tumors is poor. Even after whole-brain irradiation, median survival is approximately 6 months (Andrews et al., 2004). Adjuvant therapy with sterotactic radiosurgery boost may extend survival for patients with a small number of metastases. Survival for 740 patients with brain metastases was reviewed by Hall and colleagues (2000). For all tumor types, the actuarial survival rate was 8.1% at 2 years, 4.8% at 3 years, and 2.4% at 5 years. At 2 years from diagnosis, ovarian carcinoma had the highest survival rate (23.9%) and small cell lung cancer (SCLC) the lowest (1.7%). Favorable prognostic variables for survival included a single metastatic lesion, surgical resection, and whole-brain irradiation.

Morbidity Rates

Average annual incidence rates for primary brain tumors in the more complete surveys have ranged mostly between 7 per 100,000 and 15 per 100,000 population, including pituitary tumor rates at 1 to 2 per 100,000. Primary tumors of the spinal cord are recorded at approximately 1 per 100,000; in one survey, peripheral nerve tumors had a rate of 1.5 per 100,000.

Using the SEER database, Gurney and Kadan-Lottick (2001) calculated incidence trends by age group for malignant brain tumors for 1975 to 1997 (**Fig. 39.2**). Incidence rates remained stable for persons 20 to 69 years of age during the period. A 35% increase in rates for children 0 to 14 years old was seen in the mid-1980s. A gradual increase in malignant tumor rates was observed for persons older than 70 years between 1975 and 1990. During the 1990s, the rates for most groups remained essentially stable. Increasing incidence trends must be interpreted with caution. At least some of these changes can be attributed to the dramatic improvements in neuroimaging seen from the 1980s on. In meningioma, age-specific rates continue to rise with age to the oldest group, and a female preponderance is found. The suspected excess in blacks was

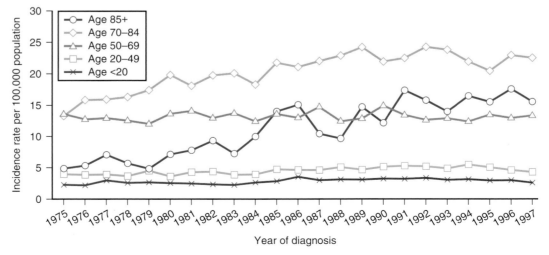

Fig. 39.2 Trends in central nervous system malignancy incidence rates by age (years) at diagnosis: surveillance, epidemiology, and end results (SEER) 1975-1997. Incidence rates are age standardized to the United States 2000 standard population. Central nervous system malignancies were classified as ICD-0-2 topography codes C70.0 and C75.1-75.3 and behavior code 3. *(Reprinted with permission from Gurney, J., Kadan-Lottick, N., 2001. Brain and other central nervous system tumors: rates, trends, and epidemiology. Curr Opin Oncol 13, 160-166.)*

borne out in a survey in the Los Angeles County Cancer Surveillance program. Age-adjusted average annual incidence rates for meningiomas were 1.8 per 100,000 males and 2.7 per 100,000 females. Respective non-Hispanic white rates were 1.8 per 100,000 and 2.5 per 100,000; for blacks, they were 2.5 per 100,000 and 3.6 per 100,000. In Rochester, Minnesota, annual incidence rates were 4.9 per 100,000 males and 5.8 per 100,000 females for the years 1935 to 1977, but only 1.2 and 2.6 per 100,000 respectively for cases diagnosed before death.

The most recent overall incidence estimate for malignant intracranial tumors in the United States is 7.2 per 100,000 person-years population for 2004-2006 (CBTRUS, 2010). For benign brain tumors for the same period, the figure is 11.5 per 100,000 person-years, including 6.3 per 100,000 for meningiomas and 2.5 for tumors of the sella region.

Metastatic brain tumors are more common than primary malignant brain tumors, with incidence rates of approximately 10 per 100,000. The relative frequencies of brain metastases, called *incidence proportions* (IPs), in patients diagnosed in the Metropolitan Detroit Cancer Surveillance System between 1972 and 2001 were reported by Barnholtz-Sloan and associates (2004). Total IP of brain metastases was 9.6% for all primary sites combined, with highest IPs for lung (19.9%), melanoma (6.9%), renal (6.5%), breast (5.1%), and colorectal (1.8%) cancers. African Americans demonstrated higher IPs than other racial groups. This total IP is lower than in earlier reports, which had ranged from 20% to 50%.

Although some CNS tumors have a clear genetic character, less than 5% can be attributed to inheritance. Many risk factors have been implicated in human brain tumors, the vast majority of which are unsubstantiated by scientific evidence. High-dose irradiation leads to an increased incidence of primary brain tumors, but the association of higher brain tumor risk with low doses of radiation is more controversial. Prolonged cell phone use and risk for brain tumors has been the subject of several studies over the past decade, with mixed results (Ahlbom et al., 2009). Overall, cell phone use studies to date do not demonstrate an increased risk of brain tumors within 10 years. For slow-growing tumors such as meningiomas or acoustic neuromas, the absence of an association is less conclusive with such a limited observation period.

Recent epidemiological studies suggest prenatal and early childhood environmental factors that may alter the risk of brain tumors. Increased risk for brain tumors was identified in persons born in late fall through early spring in one report (Brenner et al., 2004) and has been associated with maternal smoking during pregnancy in another (Brooks et al., 2004). The protective effects of vitamin supplementation during pregnancy have been borne out in several studies (Preston-Martin et al., 1998).

Convulsive Disorders

Epilepsy is defined as recurrent seizures (i.e., two or more distinct seizure episodes) that are unprovoked by any immediate cause (see Chapter 67). The International League Against Epilepsy (ILAE) classification system divides the epilepsies into four broad groups: (1) localization-related; (2) generalized; (3) undetermined whether localized or generalized; and (4) special syndromes (Everitt and Sander, 1999). Within the localization-related and generalized groups, further

subdivisions into symptomatic (known cause), idiopathic (presumed genetic origin), and cryptogenic (no clear cause) are recognized. The major clinical types of seizures are *generalized tonic-clonic*, *absence*, *incomplete convulsive* (myoclonic), *simple partial* (focal), and *complex partial* (temporal lobe or psychomotor). *Status epilepticus* is defined as any seizure lasting for 30 minutes or longer, or recurrent seizures for more than 30 minutes during which the patient does not regain consciousness.

Epidemiological studies on epilepsy have often suffered from lack of agreement on definitions and classifications. Consensus guidelines have been published to assist in the standardization of such studies, but a new simplified, etiological-oriented classification system will likely be needed in light of new genetic and imaging developments.

Mortality Rates

Reported mortality rates with epilepsy are on average two to three times greater than those in the general population. Shackleton and colleagues performed a meta-analysis on 21 studies of epilepsy mortality and found overall SMRs between 1.2 and 9.3 (Shackleton et al., 2002). Population-based studies with long-term follow-up give SMRs between 2 and 4, which seem the more accurate estimates.

As to evaluating cause of death, the proportionate mortality (PMR) is frequently used. The PMR for conditions related to epilepsy range between 1% and 13% for population-based studies (Hitiris et al, 2007). Etiologies include status epilepticus and seizure-related causes (PMR 0% to 10%), sudden unexplained death in epilepsy (SUDEP; PMR 0% to 4%), suicide (PMR 0% to 7%), and accidents (0% to 12%). Causes of nonepilepsy-related death include ischemic heart disease (PMR 12% to 37%), cerebrovascular disease (PMR 12% to 17%), cancer (PMR 18% to 40%), pneumonia (PMR 0% to 7%), suicides (PMR 0% to 12%), and accidents (0% to 4%).

Overall death rates with epilepsy are greater for men then women in most studies. Mortality is increased in the early years after diagnosis, largely due to the underlying cause of symptomatic epilepsy. Mortality is also increased for all patients with refractory epilepsy.

Epilepsy-related mortality has peaks in early childhood and early adulthood, after which rates tend to stabilize before rising once again in old age. Patients with idiopathic and cryptogenic epilepsy have the lowest long-term mortality rates, with SMRs of approximately 2, whereas those with symptomatic epilepsy with underlying neurological disease have the highest mortality rates, with reported SMRs of 11 to 25. Deaths attributed to epilepsy itself account for less than 50% of those of any cause in persons with the disorder; specific etiological disorders or factors include status epilepticus, accidents due to seizures, treatment-related factors, suicide, aspiration pneumonia, and SUDEP.

SUDEP generally is considered to be the most common cause of epilepsy-related death, with a relative frequency of 1 per 1000 epilepsy cases (Opeskin and Berkovic, 2003). Risk factors that have been consistent across studies include male sex, generalized tonic-clonic seizures, early age of onset of seizures, refractory treatment, and being in bed at the time of death. Proposed mechanisms for SUDEP include central apnea, acute neurogenic pulmonary edema, and cardiac arrhythmia precipitated by seizure discharges acting via the autonomic nervous system. Other causes of death in epilepsy can be classified as those in which epilepsy is secondary to an underlying disease (cerebrovascular disease) or is an unrelated disorder (ischemic heart disease). Age-specific mortality rates for Rochester, Minnesota, are shown in **Fig. 39.3**. Graphed curves for mortality data were similar in configuration to those for age-specific prevalence data, but rates were 1000-fold lower. This finding suggests that each year, 0.1% of the patients with epilepsy die of causes directly related to their epilepsy. Status epilepticus affects 105,000 to 152,000 persons annually in the United States (DeLorenzo et al., 1996). Status epilepticus represents a neurological emergency, and despite improvements in treatment, the mortality rate is still high. Population-based studies have reported 30-day case-fatality ratios between 8% and 22%. Short-term fatality after status epilepticus is associated with the presence of an underlying acute etiological disorder. Fatality ratios are lowest in children (short-term mortality rate 3% to 9%) and highest in the elderly (short-term mortality rate 22% to 38%). Case-fatality ratios for those surviving the initial 30 days after status epilepticus are 40% within the next 10 years.

Morbidity Rates

Fig. 39.3 also shows morbidity measures for epilepsy in Rochester, Minnesota, by age group. Age-specific incidence of epilepsy was high during the first year of life, declined during childhood and adolescence, and then increased again after age 55. The cumulative incidence of epilepsy was 1.2% through age 24 and steadily increased to 4.4% through age 85 years. Age-specific prevalence increased with advancing age; nearly 1.5% of the population older than 75 years had active epilepsy.

Point prevalence and average age-adjusted annual incidence rates for epilepsy are available from a number of community

surveys (Banerjee et al., 2009). In general, the prevalence of convulsive disorders is about 3 to 9 per 1000 population in industrialized countries. Some of the variation can be attributed to methodological differences in studies. Developing countries have reported higher prevalence rates of up to 41 per 1000. In general, males have higher rates than females, and recent studies have found no significant racial predilection. The overall lifetime prevalence of a nonfebrile seizure, as opposed to active epilepsy, is 5% in both industrialized and developing countries. Average annual age-adjusted incidence rates for epilepsy are about 50 per 100,000, with a range of 16 to 70 per 100,000 population in industrialized countries. A slight male excess is reported, which averages about 1.2 to 1. Surveys from developing countries are fewer and less rigorous and report much higher incidence rates, ranging between 43 and 190 cases per 100,000 per year. Within industrialized countries, temporal trends in epilepsy over the past 30 years have shown a decrease in incidence in children and an increase in incidence rates for the elderly. Improved prenatal care and immunization may explain the changes for the former, and perhaps longer life expectancy with more concomitant CNS disease for the latter. Overall prognosis for controlling seizures is good, with more than 70% of patients achieving long-term remission. Age-specific incidence rates for epilepsy from several surveys showed a sharp decrease from maximal rates in infancy to adolescence and thereafter a slow decline for new cases throughout life. In other studies, rates were essentially constant after infancy or showed an irregular rise with age. In Rochester, Minnesota, however, the configuration was U-shaped, with a marked increase in incidence rates at the age of 75 and older (**Fig. 39.4**). This configuration reflects generalized tonic-clonic disorders, together with absence and myoclonic seizures for the left arm of the U and complex partial and generalized tonic-clonic epilepsies for the right

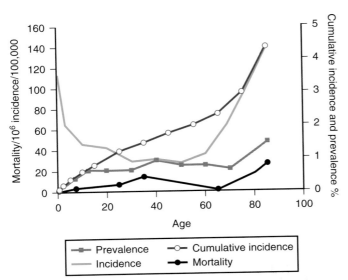

Fig. 39.3 Measures of epilepsy (Rochester, Minnesota, 1935-1984): age-specific incidence per 100,000 person-years; cumulative incidence (percent); age-specific prevalence (percent); and age-specific mortality per 100,000 person-years. *(Used with permission from Hauser, W.A., Annegers, J.F., Rocca, W.A., 1996. Descriptive epidemiology of epilepsy: contribution of population-based studies from Rochester, Minnesota. Mayo Clin Proc. 71, 576-586.)*

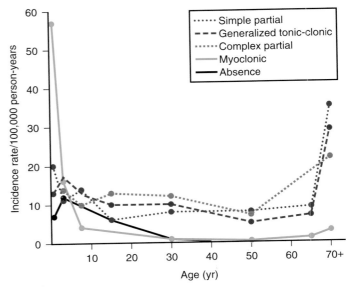

Fig. 39.4 Epilepsy. Average annual age-specific incidence rates per 100,000 population by clinical type of seizure—absence, myoclonic, generalized, simple, complex partial. *(Reprinted with permission from Kurtzke, J.F., Kurland, L.T., 2004. The epidemiology of nervous system disease, in: Baker and Joynt's Clinical Neurology on CD-ROM. Lippincott Williams & Wilkins, London.)*

arm. Myoclonic seizures were the major type diagnosed during the first year of life; they also were the most common in the 1 to 4 year age group but rarely occurred after 4 years of age. Absence (petit mal) seizures peaked in the 1 to 4 year age group and did not begin in patients older than 20. Complex partial and generalized tonic-clonic seizures both had fairly consistent incidence rates of 5 to 15 per 100,000 in persons 5 to 69 years of age, after low maxima at ages 1 to 4 years; for age 70 and older, the rates of each were sharply higher. Generalized tonic-clonic seizure rates had a similar configuration for both primary and secondary seizures. Simple partial seizures increased only slightly with age.

Febrile Seizures

In the United States and Europe, the risk of a child's developing febrile seizures has been about 2%, ranging between 1% and 4%. Surveys from Japan and the Mariana Islands showed rates of 7% and 11%, respectively. As with epilepsy in general, a male preponderance of 1.2 to 1 for febrile convulsions was observed. In most studies, recurrent febrile seizures occur in approximately one-third of the cases, and overall the risk of subsequent epilepsy is approximately 2% to 4% for simple and 11% for complex febrile seizures.

Multiple Sclerosis

Mortality Rates and Survival

Over the past 4 decades, mortality for multiple sclerosis (MS; see Chapter 54) declined steadily in North America and Western Europe and remained stable or increased in Eastern Europe. Data from Spain for the period 1981 to 1997 indicate annual age-adjusted mortality rates of 0.3 per 100,000 for men and 0.4 per 100,000 for women. A north-south gradient in age-adjusted mortality rates between 1971 and 1998 was observed in Spain. For both sexes, provinces with SMRs higher than the mean tended to be in the northern third of Spain, whereas those with SMRs lower than the mean were predominantly in the southern half (Llorca et al., 2005).

As to cause of death, many patients with MS die of complications related to their disease. Koch-Henriksen and colleagues (1998) in Denmark, as well as Smestad and colleagues (2009) in Norway, attributed more than half of all deaths in a large population cohort to MS or its complications. An overall SMR of 2.5 for all causes was calculated for the Norwegian cohort (Smestad et al., 2009). Infections were the most common cause of death; survival was age dependent and not related to disease course. As more patients with MS survive to older ages, however, a greater proportion of them can be expected to die of causes unrelated to MS and thus will not be coded as dying from MS (underlying cause). This last point is supported by analysis of contributory causes of death for patients with MS in Denmark and in the United States. The estimated 25-year survival of the population with MS in Rochester, Minnesota, was 76.2%, compared with 87.7% for the general U.S. white population of similar age and gender. Survival for men was less than for women. This survival figure was slightly greater than earlier estimates for Rochester. The Danish National MS Registry data provided a median survival of 30 years from onset of the disease. Median survival times for U.S. World War II veterans from

MS disease onset were 43 years (white females), 30 years (black males), and 34 years (white males) (Wallin et al., 2000). The male rates did not differ significantly, and when relative survival ratios were calculated, none of the three groups were significantly different, indicating the excess for the white females was more attributable to gender than to disease.

Morbidity Rates

Prevalence rates for Europe and the Mediterranean basin as of 1980 are plotted against geographical latitude in **Fig. 39.5**. The surveys then appeared to separate into clusters within two zones: one to the north, with rates of 30 per 100,000 and higher, considered to represent high frequency, and the other to the south, with rates less than 30 per 100,000 but greater than 4 per 100,000 population, classified as medium frequency.

The northernmost parts of Scandinavia and the Mediterranean basin were medium-prevalence regions in 1980. More recent surveys of Italy and its islands, however, have documented prevalence rates of 60 per 100,000 and higher; therefore, this country is now clearly within the high-frequency band (Kurtzke, 2005). This increase in prevalence appears to be recent, because some of the earlier Italian surveys with lower rates were well done. This change is not limited to Italy—indeed, all of Europe from northernmost Norway to the Mediterranean regions now fall in the high-frequency zone, as documented by Pugliatti et al. (2006) in **Fig. 39.6**.

Although clearly intra- and international diffusion of this disease has occurred in recent years, the general worldwide distribution of MS may still be described within three zones of frequency or risk. As of 2004, the high-risk zone, with prevalence rates of 30 per 100,000 population and above, included essentially all of Europe, the United States, Canada, Israel, and New Zealand, plus southeastern Australia and easternmost Russia. These regions are bounded by areas of medium frequency, with prevalence rates between 5 and 29 per 100,000, consisting now of Russia from the Ural mountains into Siberia, as well as the Ukraine. Also in the medium zone still fall most of Australia and perhaps Hawaii, all of Latin America, the North African littoral, and whites in South Africa; even northern Japan seems now to be of medium prevalence. Low-frequency areas, with prevalence rates below 5 per 100,000, still comprise all other known areas of Asia, Africa, Alaska, and Greenland (Kurtzke, 2005). MS clearly is a place-related disorder. All of the high- and medium-risk areas are found in Europe or the European colonies: Canada, the United States, Australia, New Zealand, Israel, South Africa, and probably Latin America. MS probably originated in northwestern Europe and was brought to the other lands by European settlers. In Europe itself, although the disease clearly has shown geographical clustering in some countries, there is evidence even within these clusters of diffusion over time, as well as the notable spread throughout the continent. The annual incidence rate for MS in high-risk areas at present is approximately 3 to 6 per 100,000 population, whereas in low-risk areas it is approximately 1 per 1,000,000. Medium-risk areas have an incidence near 1 per 100,000. In Denmark during the years 1939 to 1945, age-specific incidence rates rose rapidly, from essentially zero in childhood to a peak at about age 27 of more than 9 per 100,000 for females and almost 7 per 100,000 for males. Beyond age 40, little difference

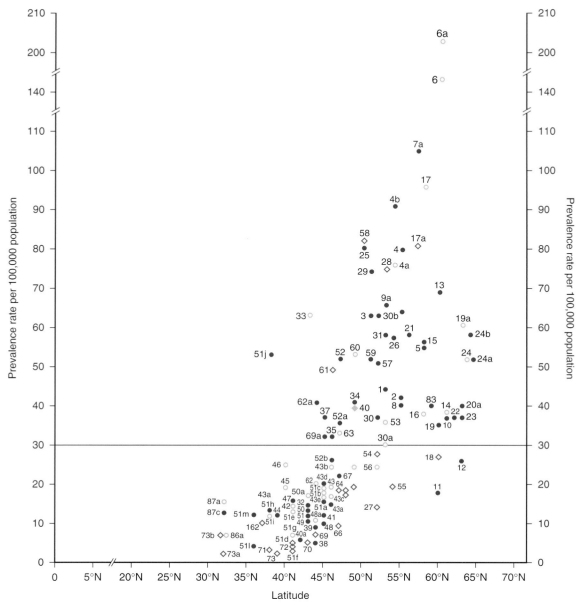

Fig. 39.5 Multiple sclerosis (MS). Prevalence rates per 100,000 population for probable MS in Europe and the Mediterranean area as of 1980, correlated with geographical latitude. Numbers identify studies in Kurtzke (1980). Solid circles represent class A (best) surveys; open circles, class B; open diamonds, class C; and closed diamonds, class E (MS–amyotrophic lateral sclerosis case ratios). Class C (poor) studies are listed only if no better-quality survey was available for the specific site. *(Reprinted with permission from Kurtzke, J.F., 1980. Geographic distribution of multiple sclerosis: an update with special reference to Europe and the Mediterranean basin. Acta Neurol Scand 62, 65-80. Copyright 1980, Munksgaard International Publishers Ltd., Copenhagen, Denmark.)*

between the sexes was seen; in both, rates declined equally to zero by age 65. The most recent evidence indicates that women of all races in the United States now have higher rates than white males, whereas black males have increased their risk to two-thirds that of the white males; men of other races still have but one-fourth the risk of white men (Wallin et al., 2004). The U.S. World War II veteran series showed a markedly elevated risk for residents who lived in the northern region of the country (**Fig. 39.7**). This was seen for both sexes among whites and for black men, with a north-to-south difference of almost 3 to 1. Veterans of the Vietnam War and later conflicts still showed a gradient, but it was much less. All southern states then were calculated to lie within the high-frequency zone, with prevalence rates that were estimated at well over 30 per 100,000 population. For all races and both sexes, the north-to-south difference was only 2 to 1. This is not a "regression to the mean" with a decreased prevalence in the north, but rather reflects an even greater increase in the south. This diffusion is in accord with the intra- and international changes for Europe as noted. MS is geographically a slowly spreading disease, the reason(s) for which must be environmental.

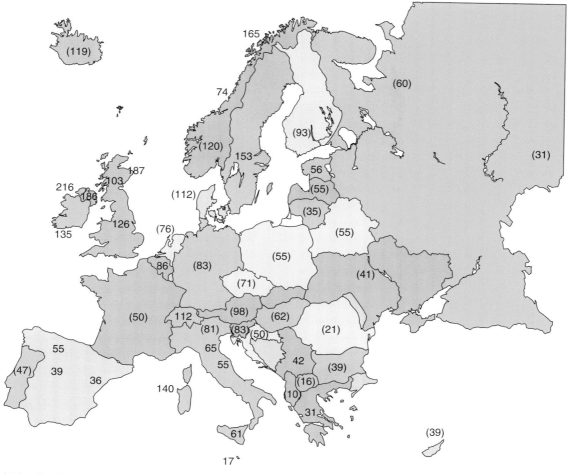

Fig. 39.6 Multiple sclerosis (MS) prevalence rates in Europe (adjusted to the 1966 European population; in brackets, crude rates when adjustment not possible). *(Reprinted with permission from Pugliatti, M., Rosati, G., Carton H., et al., 2006. The epidemiology of multiple sclerosis in Europe. Eur J Neurol 13, 709.)*

Genetic Studies

Family studies in MS have provided a means of assessing environmental factors against a set genetic background. Such studies have shown that the risk for multiple family members with MS is 3% to 4% for primary relatives and 20% to 30% for monozygotic twins. This finding is in contrast with the general population prevalence of approximately 0.1%. The increased family frequency may be related to shared environment, as opposed to shared genetic factors, because close relatives would be expected to share similar environmental influences. However, further evidence that MS is under some genetic control includes the following:

1. An excess of MS-concordant monozygous twins in most twin studies. The difference in concordance rates between monozygotic and dizygotic twins is attributable primarily to genetic factors. Moreover, a recent study found no evidence for genetic, epigenetic, or transcriptome differences in identical twins discordant for MS (Baranzini et al., 2010). The maximum concordance rate for MS in monozygotic twins in high-risk areas is approximately 30%. This indicates that although genes play a role in MS, the maximal effect of genes is at most 30%.

2. The association of HLA alleles (specifically the HLA DR2 haplotype) and MS, and the higher frequency of HLA sharing in affected sibling pairs. There is a dose effect of the DRB1*1501 on MS susceptibility.

3. Population groups relatively resistant to MS in high-frequency areas (Asians and Amerindians in North America, Lapps in Scandinavia, and Gypsies in Hungary).

Multiple sclerosis is a genetically complex disease that does not have a uniform mode of transmission. Genes are likely to play a role in both susceptibility and progression of MS. High linkage scores and significant allelic association with the HLA-DRB1*1501-DQB1*0602 haplotype have lent support to the major histocompatibility complex (MHC) region as the strongest genetic determinant of MS (Oksenberg et al., 2008). Large non-MHC genome-wide association studies have led to the discovery of several other MS susceptibility genes. These include the interleukin 2 (IL2RA) and interleukin 7 (IL7RA) receptor genes. Newer gene loci have relatively low risk ratios (<1.5) for determining MS susceptibility. Like other complex

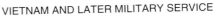

VIETNAM AND LATER MILITARY SERVICE

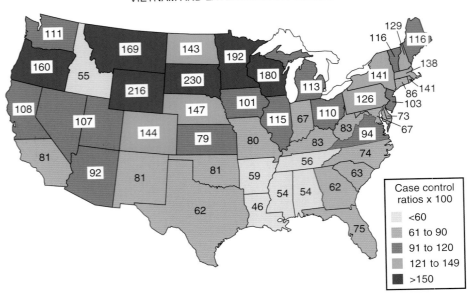

WWII–KOREAN CONFLICT

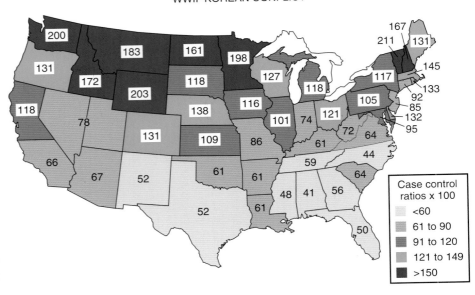

Fig. 39.7 Adjusted case-control ratios (×100) for white male U.S. veterans connected for multiple sclerosis by state of residence at entry into military service. *Top,* Vietnam War and later military service. *Bottom,* World War II and Korean conflict. *(Reprinted with permission from Wallin, M.T., Page, W.F., Kurtzke, J.F., 2004. Multiple sclerosis in United States veterans of Vietnam era and later military service. 1. Race, sex and geography. Ann Neurol 55, 68.)*

genetic diseases, many more genes will be discovered but likely not add significantly to the models of disease risk for individual patients.

Migration in Multiple Sclerosis

If the risk of MS is altered by moves to or from different risk areas, MS must have an acquired, exogenous, environmental cause or major precipitating factor. A number of studies of both morbidity and mortality in migrants show clearly that such moves do change the risk. Several identified a tendency for immigrants to retain much of, but not all, the risk of their birthplace if they came from high- or medium-risk areas. Evidence also surfaced that migrants from low-risk areas to

high-risk areas increased their risk for MS. A large case-control series among U.S. veterans clearly demonstrated a change in risk for MS by changing residence between birth and entry into military service. Those moving south decreased their risk; those moving north increased it. These findings also indicated that the time when such moves are critical is well after birth but also well before clinical onset, suggesting for the north-to-south moves an acquisition of the disease midway between birth and age at service entry, or at about age 10 to 15.

Kurtzke and associates (1998) identified North African immigrants among 7500 patients with MS in a nationwide survey in France in 1986. A total of 260 had immigrated from North Africa, mostly between 1960 and 1965. Two-thirds were from Algeria, where virtually its entire European population had emigrated in 1962 at the end of the Algerian war for independence. The migrants were younger at both prevalence day in 1986 and at onset of MS than the French-born persons with MS. The 225 with onset more than 1 year after migration presumably acquired their MS in France. They provided an age-adjusted (to the U.S. 1960 population) MS prevalence rate 1.5 times that for all of France. If the latter is 50 per 100,000 population, their estimated adjusted rate is 77. At each year of age at immigration, there was a mean interval of 13 years and a minimum of 3 years to clinical onset from either age 11 or age at immigration if that was older than 11. The other 27 migrants with presumed acquisition in North Africa had an estimated adjusted prevalence of 17 per 100,000, the same as expected in their native lands. Disease frequencies among immigrants that are higher than among natives are typical of their exposure to a new infection. The study also suggested that 3 years of exposure from age 11 were needed for immigrants from medium-risk areas to acquire MS, and that susceptibility extended to about age 45 or so.

Other studies of migrants from high- to low-risk areas also suggest a critical age for risk retention. This is exemplified by a series of north European immigrants to South Africa. Their MS prevalence rate for immigration under age 15 was 13 per 100,000, the same as for the native-born English-speaking white South Africans. For all older age groups at immigration, the prevalence rate was 30 to 80 per 100,000, the same as in their high-risk lands of birth. For those with onset after immigration, the intervals between immigration and clinical onset were some 20 to 30 years for those younger than 15 years of age and approximately 10 to 12 years for those 15 years or older. These findings support the existence of a long "incubation" or "latency" period between the acquisition of MS and clinical onset. They also indicate that young children are much less susceptible to MS, despite their living in high-risk areas such as northern Europe.

Epidemics of Multiple Sclerosis

The Faroe Islands are a semi-independent unit of the Kingdom of Denmark in the North Atlantic Ocean between Iceland and Norway. As of June 1999, we had found 70 native-born Faroese with onset of MS in the 20th century. Of these, 15 had lived more than 3 years off the islands after age 10 and before onset, and were excluded from the native resident series as having likely acquired their disease while living overseas in high–MS risk lands, a decision fostered by the finding that their periods of overseas residence correlated with age at onset. The remaining 55 comprised the native resident series: 14, most of whom had lived less than 2 years overseas, with such periods uncorrelated with time of onset; and 41 who had not lived off the islands before onset. Of the 55, no patient had clinical onset before July 1943, when symptoms began in one man. With a minimum exposure period of 2 years needed to acquire MS, 1941 was the most recent year for the disease to have been introduced into the Faroes. Between 1943 and 1949, 17 patients had symptom onset in this populace of 26,000. There were four others who were also at least age 11 by 1941, whose onsets occurred between 1950 and 1961. These 21 patients constituted a type 1 point source epidemic of MS. Annual incidence rates rose steeply from 0 to more than 10 per 100,000 in 1945 and 1946 and then fell almost as steeply with the short tail as

noted. Age at first exposure ranged from 11 to 45 and at onset 15 to 48.

We divided the other 33 patients (the 34th heralded a possible epidemic V) according to when they reached age 11, which then provided three more (type 2) epidemics of 10, 10, and 13 patients each—epidemics II, III, and IV (data as of 1991 are shown in **Fig. 39.8**) (Kurtzke and Heltberg, 2001).

We concluded that the disease was introduced into the Faroe Islands by the British troops who had occupied the islands for 5 years starting in April 1940, and most of whom had been billeted within the villages scattered across most of the islands where the patients had lived during the war. What was probably introduced was an infection that was transmitted to the Faroese population at risk from a large proportion of the British troops (because of its scattering), who were asymptomatic carriers (because they were healthy troops). We called this infection the *primary MS affection* (PMSA), which we defined as a single, specific, widespread, systemic but unknown infectious disease (that may be totally asymptomatic). PMSA produces clinical neurological MS (CNMS) in

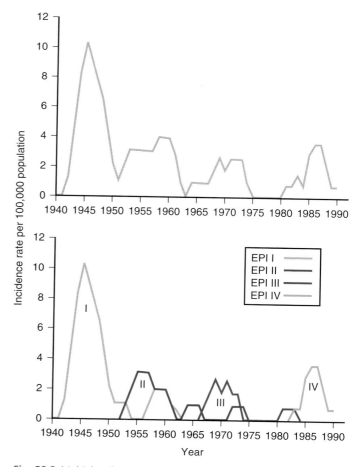

Fig. 39.8 Multiple sclerosis in the Faroes as of 1991: annual incidence rates per 100,000 population calculated as 3-year centered moving averages for four epidemics (EPI) defined by time when patients were age 11, by 1941 or later. *Top,* Total series. *Bottom,* rates by epidemic. *(Reprinted with permission from Kurtzke, J.F., Hyllested, K., Heltberg, K., et al., 1993. Multiple sclerosis in the Faroe Islands. 5. The occurrence of the fourth epidemic as validation of transmission. Acta Neurol Scand 88, 161-173. Copyright 1993, Munksgaard International Publishers Ltd., Copenhagen, Denmark.)*

only a small proportion of the affected population after an incubation period averaging 6 years in virgin populations and perhaps 12 years in endemic areas. Using this hypothesis, transmissibility is limited to part or all of this systemic phase, which ends by the usual age at onset of MS symptoms. After the British left the islands in 1945, any further disease would have had to have been transmitted from Faroese. The PMSA-affected persons of the first population cohort of Faroese transmitted the disease to the next Faroese population cohort, those who reached age 11 in the period when the first cohort was transmissible. Included in the second Faroese cohort were the epidemic II cases of CNMS, and this cohort similarly transmitted PMSA to the third population cohort with its own (epidemic III) cases, and from them to the fourth cohort with its epidemic IV. Thus, PMSA seems to be a geographically delimited, specific (but unknown), age-limited, transmissible, persistent infection that is acquired principally during the hormonally active years of age, and one that only rarely leads to clinical MS.

Movement Disorders

Movement disorders as a group (see Chapters 21 and 71) span multiple unique conditions within neurology. The most common adult-onset movement disorder is essential tremor. A recent review estimated the pooled prevalence of essential tremor to be 0.9% for all ages (Louis and Ferreira, 2010). There was a marked increase in essential tremor with increasing age, with a pooled rate of 4.6% for individuals older than 65 years.

Parkinson disease (PD) has received the most attention in epidemiological studies among movement disorders and will be the focus of this section. Idiopathic PD must be distinguished from other neurodegenerative diseases and parkinsonism related to other causes. An accurate diagnosis of PD can be made clinically and is based on symptomatic bradykinesia, muscular rigidity, rest tremor, and postural instability.

The cause of PD remains unclear. Age is the most important risk for developing the disease. Genetic studies have linked dopa-responsive parkinsonism to a variety of mutations in seven genes (Lees et al., 2009). Environmental risk factors that appear to be protective in developing PD include intake of caffeine and smoking. Weaker associations have been shown between PD and head injury, consumption of well water, and exposure to pesticides.

Morbidity Rates

The prevalence of PD ranges between 100 and 200 per 100,000 population in most studies from Western nations. Prevalence increases with increasing age, with rates for those older than aged 80 between 3% and 6%. In terms of age at onset, a population-based study from the United Kingdom reported 5.4% of PD cases had onset at younger than 50 years of age, and 33% at younger than 65 (Wickremaratchi et al., 2009). The sex ratio for PD prevalence has been mixed, with some studies showing a higher proportion of males with the disease and some showing no significant sex difference.

Recent prospective incidence studies have reported PD age-adjusted annual rates per 100,000 population between 9 and 22.5 (Linder et al., 2010). Incidence rates are slightly higher for men than women in many Western country studies, with a male-to-female rate of about 1.5. The rates by sex

for PD among Asian countries have been similar. Like prevalence rates, incidence rates for PD rise exponentially with increasing age.

Incidence rates have been relatively stable in studies that have tracked trends over several decades. In Olmsted County, Minnesota, the incidence of PD remained stable between 1935 and 1990 (Rocca et al., 2001). For the most recent period, 1976 to 1990, incidence rates in men ranged between 10.6 and 15.9 per 100,000 person-years, and for women between 7.3 and 11.6. There were no significant birth cohort effects in this population. These results suggest there were no major environmental risk agents introduced into the population during the period of study.

Mortality Rates

Parkinson disease has been generally shown to increase mortality in a number of studies, with risk ratios for death between 0.8 and 3.5. Studies evaluating incident PD with long follow-up have produced the best data on mortality. Recent studies with follow-up extending beyond 10 years have shown relative risk for death of PD ranging between 1.5 and 2.5. Patients who developed PD in the Physicians Health Study had a 2.3 relative risk of dying after adjustment for age at onset and smoking (Driver et al., 2008). This study matched controls on comorbidities and found PD patients were at increased risk for dying from stroke, psychiatric disease, and cardiac disease but were less likely to die from cancer. The risk of PD death was apparent across all categories of PD duration. This is in contrast to data from a European mortality study showing that the mortality burden in PD increased only after the first decade of the disease (Diem-Zangerl et al., 2009). Standardized mortality ratios in this study at 5 years after disease onset was 0.9, and by 20 to 30 years after onset was 1.3. Overall, PD independently increases the risk for death. Confirming modifiable risk factors for mortality will be important in the preventive care of patients with PD.

Selected Infections and Neurological Disease

Human Immunodeficiency Virus Infection

Human immunodeficiency virus (HIV; see Chapter 53A) infection has become a global epidemic since it was first identified in 1981 as the cause of the acquired immunodeficiency syndrome (AIDS). The virus is a member of the retrovirus family and selectively infects T-helper cells (T_H4, $CD4^+$), causing a defect in cell-mediated immunity. It is spread through contact with blood and bodily fluids. After acute infection, most people enter an asymptomatic period of 8 to 10 years before the virus infection manifests clinically through immune dysregulation (Harrison and McArthur, 1995).

Despite recent advances in treatment and prevention, the scope of the HIV epidemic remains daunting. As of 2008, 33 million people worldwide were living with HIV, and 2.7 million more were infected (UNAIDS, 2010). The infection killed 2 million in 2008 and has been the cause of death for greater than 20 million since the first AIDS cases were identified (UNAIDS, 2010). Sixty-eight percent of HIV cases occur in sub-Saharan Africa, where some 22 million persons are affected. During the first 6 months of 1996, the first reported decline in AIDS mortality rates occurred in the United States (CDC, 1997). Compared with estimates for the period January to June of 1995 (24,900), a 13% drop in AIDS deaths was observed in January to June of 1996 (22,000). This decline occurred in all racial and ethnic groups and in all regions of the United States. Mortality rates have continued to decline in many HIV-infected cohorts after the introduction of highly active antiretroviral therapy (HAART) in 1996. For example, Crum et al. (2006) noted an 80% decrease in deaths between 1990 and 2003 in their Department of Defense HIV cohort. Median survival times after HIV seroconversion in 1994-1996 were 8 years compared with 12 years during the late HAART era. Infections remained the leading cause of death in AIDS, followed by cancer. HIV disease can produce a variety of effects on both the CNS and the peripheral nervous system (PNS) (Price, 1996). A useful way of classifying these complications is to use the temporal profile of HIV infection on the immune system. **Box 39.1** illustrates a simplified classification scheme. Early neurological complications include acute aseptic meningitis, acute and chronic demyelinating polyneuropathy, and multiple mononeuropathy. These early complications are autoimmune in nature and occur at CD4$^+$ cell counts greater than 200 cells/mm^3. Late complications typically appear when a severe depression in cellular immunity occurs, with CD4$^+$ counts less than 200 cells/mm^3. Most of these disorders are opportunistic infections (cryptococcal meningitis) or represent reactivation of a prior infection (toxoplasmosis and progressive multifocal leukoencephalopathy [PML]). In the late 1980s and early 1990s, we also had personally encountered notable frequencies of tuberculosis and neurosyphilis among AIDS patients; these excesses have since disappeared. In sub-Saharan Africa, tuberculosis and malaria remain at excessively high frequencies among the HIV infected. HIV dementia, distal sensory polyneuropathy, and vacuolar myopathy are directly related to late stages of HIV infection itself. Other complications affecting the nervous system involve metabolic and toxic effects of treatment, including zidovudine myopathy and nucleoside neuropathy. Six AIDS-indicator neurological illnesses are defined by the CDC: HIV dementia, CNS crypto-

coccal infection, cytomegalovirus (CMV) infection, primary CNS lymphoma, CNS toxoplasmosis, and PML. The CDC records data on these illnesses primarily if they are the initial AIDS diagnosis. Occurrence of these illnesses during the course of HIV infection must therefore be studied in other series. One such population is the HIV Outpatient Study, which is a prospective cohort study of 7155 patients in 10 U.S. HIV clinics. Hospitalization rates for HIV-infected patients declined for the years 1994-2005, due predominantly to reductions in AIDS opportunistic infections including neurological illnesses (Buchacz et al., 2008). Compared to the years 1994-1997, patients in the era of HAART were hospitalized with higher CD4$^+$ cell counts and more frequent chronic end-organ conditions. Brodt and co-workers (1997) reported on the changing incidence of AIDS-defining illnesses in the Frankfurt AIDS Cohort Study, consisting of approximately 1000 homosexual men. The major illnesses decreased between 1992 and 1996 (**Fig. 39.9**). Included in the decline were toxoplasmic encephalitis, CMV disease, PML, and AIDS encephalopathy, all of which reached attack rates of less than 5 per 100 patient-years. Treatment with combination antiretroviral therapy and with protease inhibitors increased during the study period. Undoubtedly, these new combination therapies have had a role in the declining incidence rates in this cohort.

West Nile Virus Infection

The West Nile virus (WNV) is a mosquito-borne flavivirus that initially was isolated in 1937 from a symptomatic patient in Uganda (Tyler, 2009). The virus was rarely studied until 1999, when it first appeared in New York City as the cause of a naturally acquired meningitis and encephalitis. Over the next several years, a dramatic westward spread of WNV across the United States has been recognized. Most human infections occur through the bite of an infected mosquito of the *Culex* genus during the summer months. Wild birds, particularly crows, sparrows, and jays, serve as the natural reservoir. Symptoms begin after an average incubation period of approximately 1 week. WNV is now the leading cause of arboviral encephalitis in the United States.

A spectrum of clinical presentations may be seen with WNV infection, but approximately 80% of cases remain asymptomatic. Among symptomatic cases, West Nile fever is the most common illness. This traditionally has been characterized by fever, rash, and lymphadenopathy. Headache, fatigue, and gastrointestinal (GI) symptoms also are variably present. In a proportion of symptomatic cases, neurological illness develops, which may manifest as aseptic meningitis, encephalitis, or acute flaccid paralysis. A follow-up survey of New York City residents with WNV meningitis or encephalitis found that only 37% achieved a full recovery at 1 year (Klee et al., 2004). Deficits were found in physical, cognitive, and functional performance.

In 2009, the incidence of WNV neuroinvasive disease in the United States was 0.13 per 100,000 population, the lowest reported since 2001 (CDC, 2010). Between 2004 and 2007, WNV neuroinvasive disease incidence stabilized at 0.4 per 100,000 population. Evidence for WNV human disease continues to be detected in all geographic regions of the United States, with the highest rates in west-central states. The two major risk factors for neuroinvasive disease are increasing age and immunosuppression. Therapy for WNV infection is

---

Box 39.1 Neurological Complications of Human Immunodeficiency Virus Infection

Early Complications (CD4$^+$ Count >200 Cells/mm^3)

Acute aseptic meningitis
Demyelinating polyneuropathy (acute and chronic)
Mononeuritis

Late Complications (CD4$^+$ Count <200 Cells/mm^3)

Cryptococcal meningitis
CMV encephalitis or polyradiculopathy
Cerebral toxoplasmosis
PML
Primary CNS lymphoma
HIV dementia
Sensory neuropathy
Vacuolar myelopathy

CMV, Cytomegalovirus; *CNS,* central nervous system; *HIV,* Human Immunodeficiency virus; *PML,* progressive multifocal leukoencephalopathy.

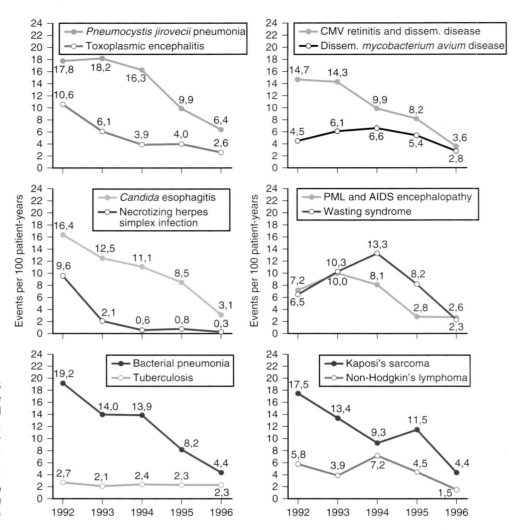

Fig. 39.9 Annual events of various acquired immunodeficiency syndrome (AIDS)-defining diseases, calculated as events per 100 patient-years. *CMV,* Cytomegalovirus; *PML,* progressive multifocal leukoencephalopathy. *(Reprinted with permission from Brodt, H.R., Gute, P., Kamps, P.S., et al., 1997. Changing incidence of AIDS-defining illnesses in the era of antiretroviral combination therapy. AIDS 11, 1731-1738.)*

Table 39.1 Neurocysticercosis: Overview of Large Case Series (United States, 1980-2004)

Study	Location	Case Collection Period	Number of Cases	Sex Ratio (M:F)	Average Age Range*
Loo, 1982	San Diego, CA	1972-1982	23	2.8	33 yr (19 mo-58 yr)
McCormick, 1982/ McCormick, 1985	Los Angeles, CA	1966-1982	230	1.2	— (10 to >60 yr)
Richards, 1985	Los Angeles, CA	1973-1983	497	1.2	31 yr (3-86 yr)
Earnest, 1987	Denver, CO	1976-1986	35	2.2	30 yr (2-59 yr)
Mitchell, 1988	Los Angeles, CA	1980-1986	52	—	— (21 mo-20 yr)
Scharf, 1988	Los Angeles, CA	1981-1986	238	1.4	35 yr (2-82 yr)
Ehnert, 1992	California	1989-1990	112	1.5	27 yr (*mdn*) (20 mo-64 yr)
Shandera, 1994	Houston, TX	1985-1991	112	1.2	28 yr (1-84 yr)
Rosenfeld, 1996	Chicago, IL	1986-1994	47	0.6	8 yr (1-15 yr)
Stamos, 1996	Chicago, IL	1988-1993	54	—	28 mo[†] (13 mo-6 yr)
Cuetter, 1997	El Paso, TX	1990-1995	33	3.5	34 yr (16-70 yr)
Townes, 2004	Oregon	1995-2000	61	1.9	24 yr (*mdn*) (2-79 yr)

Modified from Wallin, M.T., Kurtzke, J.F., 2004. Neurocysticercosis in the United States: review of an important emerging infection. Neurology 63, 1559-1564.
*Average age refers to mean unless noted; two studies reported only median age (*mdn*).
[†]This figure represents the average age of the seven patients for whom age data were available.

Table 39.2 Most Common Neurological Disorders: Incidence*

Disorder	Rate
Herpes zoster	400
Migraine	250
Brain trauma	200
Other severe headache	200[†]
Acute cerebrovascular disease	150
Head injury without brain trauma	150[†]
Transient postconcussive syndrome	150
Lumbosacral herniated nucleus pulposus	150
Lumbosacral pain syndrome	150[†]
Neurological symptoms (with no defined disease)	75
Epilepsy	50
Febrile fits	50
Dementia	50
Meniere disease	50
Transient ischemic attacks	40
Mononeuropathies	40
Polyneuropathy	50
Bell palsy	25
Single seizures	20
Parkinsonism	20
Cervical pain syndrome	20[†]
Persistent postconcussive syndrome	20
Alcoholism	20[†]
Meningitides	15
Encephalitides	15
Sleep disorders[‡]	15
Subarachnoid hemorrhage	15
Cervical herniated nucleus pulposus	15
Peripheral nerve trauma	15
Blindness	15
Metastatic brain tumor	10
Benign brain tumor	10
Deafness	10

Modified from Kurtzke, J.F., 1982. The current neurologic burden of illness and injury in the United States. Neurology 32, 1207-1214.

*Approximate average annual incidence rates per 100,000 population, all ages.

[†]Cited rates are 10% of actual rates, as proportions of patients likely to need care by a physician competent in neurology.

[‡]Narcolepsies and hypersomnias (with sleep apnea).

Table 39.3 Less Common Neurological Disorders: Incidence*

Disorder	Rate*
Cerebral palsy	9.0
Congenital malformations of central nervous system	7.0
Malignant primary brain tumor	7.0
Mental retardation, severe	6.0
Mental retardation, other	6.0[†]
Metastatic cord tumor	5.0
Tic douloureux	4.0
Multiple sclerosis	3.0[‡]
Optic neuritis	3.0[†]
Dorsolateral sclerosis	3.0
Functional psychosis	3.0[†]
Spinal cord injury	3.0
Motor neuron disease	2.0
Down syndrome	2.0
Guillain-Barré syndrome	2.0
Intracranial abscess	1.0
Benign cord tumor	1.0
Cranial nerve trauma	1.0
Acute transverse myelopathy	0.8
All muscular dystrophies	0.7
Chronic progressive myelopathy	0.5
Polymyositis	0.5
Syringomyelia	0.4
Hereditary ataxias	0.4
Huntington disease	0.4
Myasthenia gravis	0.4
Acute disseminated encephalomyelitis	0.2
Charcot-Marie-Tooth disease	0.2
Spinal muscular atrophy	0.2
Familial spastic paraplegia	0.1
Wilson disease	0.1
Malignant primary cord tumor	0.1
Vascular disease of cord	0.1

Modified from Kurtzke, J.F., 1982. The current neurologic burden of illness and injury in the United States. Neurology 32, 1207-1214; and from Kurtzke, J.F., Kurland, L.T., 1983. The epidemiology of neurologic disease, In: Baker A.B., Baker, L.H. (Eds.), Clinical Neurology, vol. 4. Harper & Row, Philadelphia.

*Approximate average annual incidence rates per 100,000 population, all ages.

[†]Cited rates are 10% of actual rates, as proportions of patients likely to need care by a physician competent in neurology.

[‡]Rate for high-risk areas.

primarily supportive because no treatment has been found to be effective in altering morbidity or mortality rates. Preventive efforts constitute the major focus of controlling this illness. These involve environmental control of mosquito breeding areas, wearing insect repellants and protective clothing, and screening the blood supply. Horses remain the major animal vector for WNV, and an effective vaccine has been in use for several years. Vaccine trials for human WNV are underway, and a safe and effective vaccine for humans is expected to be developed soon. In view of the high recurrence rates from 1999 to 2004, the transmission of WNV will continue to be an issue for many years to come.

Table 39.4   Most Common Neurological Disorders: Prevalence*

Disorder	Rate
Migraine	2,000[†]
Other severe headache	1,500[‡]
Brain trauma	800
Epilepsy	650
Acute cerebrovascular disease	600
Lumbosacral pain syndrome	500[‡]
Alcoholism	500[‡]
Sleep disorders[§]	300
Meniere disease	300
Lumbosacral herniated nucleus pulposus	300
Cerebral palsy	250
Dementia	250
Parkinsonism	200
Transient ischemic attacks	150
Febrile fits	100
Persistent postconcussive syndrome	80
Herpes zoster	80
Congenital malformations of central nervous system	70
Single seizures	60
Multiple sclerosis	60[¶]
Benign brain tumor	60
Cervical pain syndrome	60[‡]
Down syndrome	50
Subarachnoid hemorrhage	50
Cervical herniated nucleus pulposus	50
Transient postconcussive syndrome	50
Spinal cord injury	50

Modified from Kurtzke, J.F., 1982. The current neurologic burden of illness and injury in the United States. Neurology 32, 1207-1214.

*Approximate point prevalence rates per 100,000 population, all ages.

[†]Cited rate is 20% of actual prevalence rate, as a proportion of patients likely to need care by a physician competent in neurology.

[‡]Cited rates are 10% of actual rates, as proportions of patients likely to need care by a physician competent in neurology.

[§]Narcolepsies and hypersomnias (with sleep apnea).

[¶]Rate for high-risk areas.

Table 39.5   Less Common Neurological Disorders: Prevalence*

Disorder	Rate
Tic douloureux	40
Neurological symptoms without defined disease	40
Mononeuropathies	40
Polyneuropathies	40
Dorsolateral sclerosis	30
Peripheral nerve trauma	30
Other head injury	30[†]
Acute transverse myelopathy	15
Metastatic brain tumor	15
Chronic progressive myelopathy	10
Benign cord tumor	10
Optic neuritis	10
Encephalitides	10
Vascular disease of spinal cord	9
Hereditary ataxias	8
Syringomyelia	7
Motor neuron disease	6
Polymyositis	6
Progressive muscular dystrophy	6
Malignant primary brain tumor	5
Metastatic cord tumor	5
Meningitides	5
Bell palsy	5
Huntington disease	5
Charcot-Marie-Tooth disease	5
Myasthenia gravis	4
Familial spastic paraplegia	3
Intracranial abscess	2
Cranial nerve trauma	2
Myotonic dystrophy	2
Spinal muscular atrophy	2
Guillain-Barré syndrome	1
Wilson disease	1
Acute disseminated encephalomyelitis	0.6
Dystonia musculorum deformans	0.3
Primary malignant cord tumor	0.1

Modified from Kurtzke, J.F., 1982. The current neurologic burden of illness and injury in the United States. Neurology 32, 1207-1214; and from Kurtzke, J.F., Kurland, L.T., 1983. The epidemiology of neurologic disease, In: Baker A.B., Baker, L.H. (Eds.), Clinical Neurology, vol. 4. Harper & Row, Philadelphia.

*Approximate point prevalence rates per 100,000 population, all ages.

[†]Cited rate is 10% of actual rate, as a proportion of patients likely to need care by a physician competent in neurology.

Neurocysticercosis

Neurocysticercosis (NCC) is caused by an infection of the human CNS by the larval stage of the pork tapeworm, *Taenia solium* (Garcia and Del Brutto, 2005). Currently, the most common parasitic disease of the human CNS, NCC has become a major public health problem for most of the developing world, as well as in industrialized countries with a high immigration rate of people from endemic countries in Latin America, Asia, and Africa. It is the most common cause of symptomatic epilepsy worldwide.

Neurocysticercosis has become an increasingly important emerging infection in the United States. The number of cases of imported NCC is higher in the United States than in all other developed countries combined. These numbers have been driven largely by the influx of immigrants from endemic regions into the United States and ease of international travel, while widespread access to neuroimaging has permitted easier diagnosis. A total of 1494 patients with NCC were reported in the United States between 1980 and 2004 among large case series (i.e., N >20) (Wallin and Kurtzke, 2004). **Table 39.1** lists the 13 largest case series that have been published on NCC within the United States over this period. These reports are largely concentrated in the southwestern United States but include NCC cases from every region of the country. Among the case series, a slight male bias was observed, and the average age ranged between 24 and 35 years. Common onset symptoms for NCC patients within the United States include seizures (66%), hydrocephalus (16%), and headaches (15%). A majority of patients present with parenchymal disease (91%); ventricular cysts, subarachnoid cysts, and spinal cysts are the presenting manifestations in the remaining patients. Treatment with antiparasitic drugs has been shown to be beneficial in the early stages of parenchymal NCC. Seizures typically are controlled with standard anticonvulsants. Therapy directed at the parasite, however, varies according to the stage, location, and number of parasites within the CNS. An increasing number of NCC cases have been reported in the U.S. literature over the past 50 years. Currently, California and Oregon are the only states with mandatory reporting requirements. A national reporting network would be helpful in the control and eventual elimination of this disease. Because neurologists often are involved with the diagnosis and management of NCC in the United States, they must become familiar with the disorder.

Overview of the Frequency of Neurological Disorders

What follows are the best estimates of the numerical impact of neurological diseases. The data refer primarily to whites in western countries. Some modifications of the cited references have been made, but the authors have not found reasons to change most of these figures. For the 66 disorders listed in **Tables 39.2 and 39.3**, the average annual incidence rates add up to greater than 2500 per 100,000 population, or 2.5%. Included in these tables are eight disorders for which only one-tenth of the incident cases were thought to require neurological attention: the two vertebrogenic pain syndromes, nonmigrainous headache, head injury without brain trauma, alcoholism, psychosis, nonsevere mental retardation, and deafness. Total blindness numbers were taken as an estimate for the proportion of all visually impaired patients the neurologist might encounter. Even if all headaches, trauma, vertebrogenic pain, vision loss, deafness, and psychosis are excluded from consideration, it is estimated that more than 1100 new cases of neurological disease will appear each year in every 100,000 of the population, or more than 1 case for every 100 people (**Tables 39.4 and 39.5**).

Neurological practice, of course, varies widely among countries and even within the United States. The concept of the neurologist as a physician directly responsible for both acute and chronic care of patients with neurological diseases has evolved only over the last 3 decades in the United States. But such responsibilities, as well as provisions for continuity of care, are explicit statements in the current special requirements for residency training programs in neurology and child neurology. Regardless of the type of practice a given country deems appropriate for neurologists, patients with neurological disease will continue to require care. The data in **Tables 39.2 through 39.5** could therefore well serve as at least a basis for rational allocation of available resources for teaching, research, and care of patients with neurological disorders in any country.

References

The complete reference list is available online at www.expertconsult.com.

Clinical Neurogenetics

Brent L. Fogel, Daniel H. Geschwind

Genetics in Clinical Neurology

Since the discovery of the structure of deoxyribonucleic acid (DNA) and the elucidation of the genetic mechanisms of heredity, clinical neurology has benefited from advances in genetics and neuroscience. This clinically relevant basic research has permitted dissection of the cellular machinery supporting the function of the brain and its connections while establishing causal relationships between such dysfunction, human genetic variation, and various neurological diseases. In the modern practice of neurology, the use of genetics has become widespread, and neurologists are confronted daily with data from an ever-increasing catalogue of genetic studies relating to conditions such as developmental disorders, dementia, ataxia, neuropathy, and epilepsy, to name but a few. The use of genetic information in the clinical evaluation of neurological disease has expanded dramatically over the past decade. More efficient techniques for discovering disease genes has led to a greater availability of genetic testing in the clinic. Approximately one-third of pediatric neurology hospital admissions are related to a genetic diagnosis, and there are many dozens of genetic tests available to the practicing neurologist, including several related to common diseases. This number will surely continue to increase rapidly (**Fig. 40.1**).

As neuroscience and genetic research have progressed, we have been led to a deeper understanding of the sources and nature of human genetic variation and its relationship to clinical phenotypes. In the past there has been a tendency to consider genetic traits as either present or absent, and correspondingly, patients were either healthy or diseased; this is the traditional view of Mendelian, or single gene, conditions. Although certain relatively rare neurological diseases—Friedreich ataxia or Huntington disease (HD), for example—can be traced to a single causal gene, the common forms of other diseases such as Alzheimer dementia, stroke, epilepsy, or autism usually arise from an interplay of multiple genes, each of which increases disease susceptibility and likely interacts with environmental factors. Subsequently, the realm of the "sporadic" and the "idiopathic" has been challenged by the identification of genetic susceptibility factors, which has sparked a flurry of investigation into a variety of genes and genetic markers that confer a risk of illness yet are not wholly causative. Disease status may lie on the end of a continuum of individual variation and thus can be considered a quantitative rather than purely qualitative trait (Plomin et al., 2009). So, rather than using what might be considered an arbitrary cutoff point, such as a specific number of senile plaques or neuritic tangles that define affected or unaffected

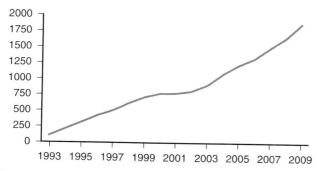

Fig. 40.1 Rapid growth of clinical testing for genetic disease. This graph plots the number of genetic diseases for which clinical testing was available over the period of 1993-2009, illustrating an approximate 20-fold increase in the number of testable disorders. *(Data from GeneTests: Medical Genetics Information Resource. Available at* http://www.ncbi.nlm.nih.gov/sites/GeneTests/.)

patients, one might instead think in terms of a continuum of pathology that relates to different levels of burden or susceptibility.

As we continue to discover more genes involved either directly or indirectly in neurological disease pathogenesis, the amount of information available to the clinician grows, as do the challenges in interpreting this in a meaningful way for an individual patient. Much of this information, particularly with respect to genetic risk, is not a matter of a positive or negative result, but instead is a feature to be incorporated into the clinical framework supporting an overall diagnosis. While modern neurologists need not also be geneticists, it is essential that they possess a firm understanding of the basics of human genetics in order to be fully prepared to confront the litany of diagnostic information available today. In this chapter we will discuss these essential basics and present examples of how genetic information has informed our understanding of disease definition and etiology, show how it is utilized in the practice of neurology today, and how it may be used in the future. Given the massive acceleration in technology, from microarrays to the methods enabling complete and efficient human genome sequencing, this future is likely closer than most realize.

Gene Expression, Diversity, and Regulation

The basic principles of molecular genetics are outlined in **Fig. 40.2** and **Table 40.1**, and more detailed descriptions can be found elsewhere (Alberts et al., 2008; Griffiths et al., 2002; Lodish et al., 2008; Strachan and Read, 2003). To briefly summarize, deoxyribonucleic acid (DNA), found in the nucleus of all cells, comprises the raw material from which heritable information is transferred among individuals, with the simplest heritable unit being the gene. DNA is composed of a series of individual nucleotides, all of which contain an identical pentose (2'-deoxyribose)-phosphate backbone but differ at an attached base that can be either adenine (A), guanine (G), thymine (T), or cytosine (C). A and G are purine bases and pair with the pyrimidine bases T and C, respectively, to form a double-stranded helical structure which allows for semiconservative bidirectional replication, the

means by which DNA is copied in a precise and efficient manner. In total, there are approximately 3.2 billion base pairs in human DNA. By convention, a DNA sequence is described by listing the bases as they are expressed from the 5′ to 3′ direction along the pentose backbone (e.g., 5′-ATGCAT-3′…etc.), as this is the order in which it is typically used by the cellular machinery, also called the *sense strand* (compare to RNA, later). The opposite paired, or *antisense*, strand is arranged antiparallel (3′ to 5′) and can also be referred to when discussing sequence; however, by convention this is generally not done unless that strand is also transcribed into RNA.

The expression of a gene is tightly and coordinately regulated (see **Fig. 40.2**), an important consideration for understanding the molecular mechanisms of disease. The typical gene contains one or more *promoters*, DNA sequences that allow for the binding of a cellular protein complex that includes RNA polymerase and other factors that faithfully copy the DNA in the 5′ to 3′ direction in a process known as *transcription*. The resulting single-stranded molecule contains a ribose sugar unit in its backbone and, thus the resulting molecule is termed *ribonucleic acid*, or RNA. RNA also differs from the template DNA by the incorporation of uracil (U) in place of thymine (T), as it also pairs efficiently with adenine, and thymine serves a secondary role in DNA repair that is not necessary in RNA. The sequence of the RNA matches the sense DNA strand and is therefore complementary to (and hence derived from) the antisense strand.

Transcribed coding RNA must be processed to become protein-encoding *messenger RNA* (mRNA), a term used to differentiate these RNAs from all other types of RNA in the cell. To become mature, RNA is stabilized by modification at the ends with a 7-methylguanosine 5′ cap and a long poly-A 3′ tail. A further critical stage in the maturation of the RNA molecule involves a rearrangement process termed *RNA splicing* (**Fig. 40.3**). This is necessary because the expressed coding sequences in DNA, called *exons*, of virtually every gene are discontinuous and interspersed with long stretches of generally non-conserved intervening sequences referred to as *introns*. This, along with other mechanisms, likely plays an evolutionary role in the development of new genes by allowing for the shuffling of functional sequences (Babushok et al., 2007). Nascent RNA molecules are recognized by the *spliceosome*, a protein complex that removes the introns and rejoins the exons. Not every exon is utilized at all times in every RNA derived from a single gene. Exons may be skipped or included in a regulated manner through alternative splicing, which occurs in nearly 95% of all genes to create different isoforms of that mRNA. The dynamic nature of this observation is critical to a complete understanding of cellular gene expression. DNA is essentially a storage molecule, and with few exceptions in the absence of mutagens, its sequence remains static and, aside from a few epigenetic events, is therefore limited to a genetic regulatory role as a transcriptional rheostat. Current estimates place the number of individual human genes at just over 22,000 (Pertea and Salzberg, 2010), so it is difficult to reconcile biological and clinical diversity with simple variations in expression. Alternative splicing provides a means of dramatically elevating this diversity by enabling a single gene to encode multiple proteins with a wide array of functions. Supporting this, recent analysis of RNA complexity in human tissues suggest that there are at least seven

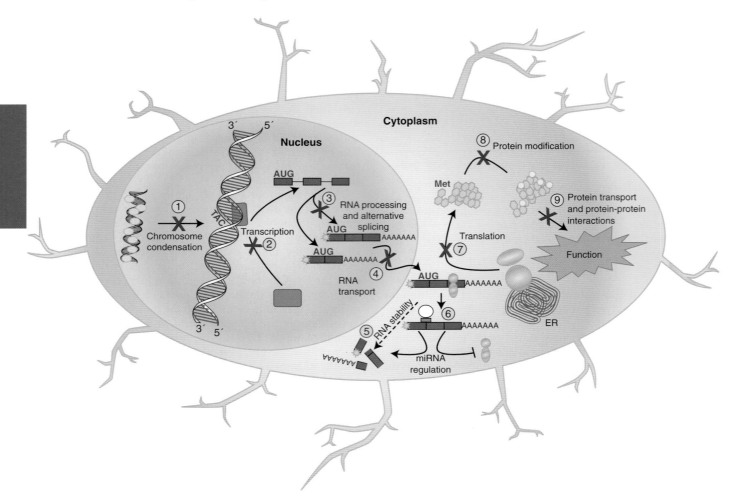

Fig. 40.2 Neuronal gene expression and regulation. A generic human neuron is depicted. **(1)** DNA bound to histones forms transcriptionally inactive chromatin, which can be relieved through the action of various proteins and enzymes. **(2)** Active DNA is bound by RNA polymerase in a process regulated by protein factors, and the genetic information contained within the DNA is converted to RNA via the process of transcription. An example of a three-nucleotide codon *(red)* is shown on the antisense DNA strand being converted to its complement on the sense strand of the RNA. **(3)** Nascent RNA undergoes processing to become messenger RNA (mRNA) with the addition of a 5′ cap structure *(green)* and a poly-A tail, as well as undergoing RNA splicing which removes noncoding sequences and can generate transcript diversity through the use of alternative exons (see text). **(4)** Mature mRNA is exported from the nucleus to the cytoplasm and/or to a specific subcellular location. **(5)** Over time, mRNA is subject to degradation within the cell, and its inherent stability can be dynamic, changing in relation to the state of the cell. **(6)** Short noncoding RNAs, called *micro-RNAs* (miRNAs) *(pink)*, can target cellular protein complexes *(white)* to specific mRNAs and regulate their activity by promoting degradation or blocking translation (see text). **(7)** The mRNA is bound by ribosomes (either free or associated with the endoplasmic reticulum) and undergoes translation into protein. The three-nucleotide codon *(red)* directs the incorporation of a single amino acid into the newly synthesized protein (in this example methionine, met). **(8)** The protein undergoes posttranslational chemical modifications *(blue)* to generate a functional protein for use by the cell. **(9)** Mature protein interacts with other proteins and/or is transported to its site of activity within the cell. All direct steps in this pathway are potential sites for disease-modifying therapies *(red X's)*, depending on the gene in question.

alternative splicing events per multi-exon gene, generating over 100,000 alternative splicing events (Pan et al., 2008). Because alternative splicing and other forms of RNA processing can be subject to complex layers of temporal and spatial regulation, particularly in the human brain (Licatalosi and Darnell, 2010; Ward and Cooper, 2010), it is a robust source for both biological diversity and disease-causing mutations (see Polymorphisms and Point Mutations).

DNA to RNA to Protein

The central dogma of genetics has been that DNA is transcribed into RNA that is than translated into protein—the "business" end of the process. So, following its transcription

from DNA in the nucleus, mRNA is transported out of the nucleus to the cytoplasm, and possibly to a specific subcellular location depending on the mRNA, where it can be deciphered by the cell. This takes place via interaction with a complex known as the *ribosome*, which binds the mRNA and converts its genetic information into protein via the process of *translation*. The ribosome initiates translation at a pre-encoded start site and converts the mRNA sequence into protein until a designated termination site is reached. Sequence information is read in three-nucleotide groups called *codons*, each of which specifies an individual amino acid. With the four distinct bases, there are mathematically 64 possible codons, but these have an element of redundancy and code for only 20 different amino acids and 3 termination signals (UAG, UGA, and

Table 40.1 Glossary of Genetic Terminology

Allele	Alternate forms of a locus (gene)
Anticipation	Earlier onset and/or worsening severity of disease in successive generations
Antisense	Nucleic acid sequence complementary to mRNA
Chromosome	Organizational unit of the genome consisting of a linear arrangement of genes
Cis-acting	A regulatory nucleotide sequence present on the molecule being regulated
Codon	A three-nucleotide sequence representing a single amino acid
Complex disease	Disease exhibiting non-Mendelian inheritance involving the interaction of multiple genes and the environment
De novo	A mutation newly arising in an individual and not present in either parent
Diploid	A genome having paired genetic information, half-normal number is haploid
DNA	Deoxyribonucleic acid; used for storage, replication, and inheritance of genetic information
Dominant	Allele that determines phenotype when a single copy is present in an individual
Endophenotype	Subset of phenotypic characteristics used to group patients manifesting a given trait
Exome	Portion of the genome representing only the coding regions of genes
Exon	Segment of DNA that is expressed in at least one mature mRNA
Expressivity	The range of phenotypes observed with a specific disease-associated genotype
Frameshift	DNA mutation that adds or removes nucleotides, affecting which are grouped as codons
Gene	Contiguous DNA sequence that codes for a given messenger RNA and its splice variants
Genome	A complete set of DNA from a given individual
Genotype	The DNA sequence of a gene
Haplotype	A group of alleles on the same chromosome close enough to be inherited together
Hemizygous	Genes having only a single allele in an individual, such as the X chromosome in males
Heteroplasmy	A mixture of multiple mitochondrial genomes in a given individual
Heterozygous	Genes having two distinct alleles in an individual at a given locus
Homozygous	Genes having two identical alleles in an individual at a given locus
Intron	Segment of DNA between exons that is transcribed into RNA but removed by splicing
Kilobase	1000 bases or base-pairs
Linkage disequilibrium	The co-occurrence of two alleles more frequently than expected by random chance, suggesting they are in close proximity to one another
Locus	Location of a DNA sequence (or a gene) on a chromosome or within the genome
Lyonization	The process of random inactivation of one of the pair of X chromosomes in females
Marker	Sequence of DNA used to identify a gene or a locus
Megabase	1,000,000 bases or base-pairs
Meiosis	Process of cellular division that produces gametes containing a haploid amount of DNA
Mendelian	Obeying standard single-gene patterns of inheritance (e.g., recessive or dominant)
Microarray	A glass or plastic support (e.g., slide or chip) to which large numbers of DNA molecules can be attached for use in high-throughput genetic analysis
Missense	DNA mutation that changes a given codon to represent a different amino acid
Mitosis	Process of cellular division during which DNA is replicated
Nonsense	DNA mutation that changes a given codon into a translation termination signal
Penetrance	The likelihood of a disease-associated genotype to express a specific disease phenotype
Phenotype	The clinical manifestations of a given genotype
Polymorphism	Sequence variation among individuals, typically not considered to be pathogenic
Probe	DNA sequence used for identifying a specific gene or allele
Promoter	DNA sequences that regulate transcription of a given gene
Protein	Functional cellular macromolecules encoded by a gene
Recessive	Allele that determines phenotype only when two copies are present in an individual
Relative risk	The ratio of the chance of disease in individuals with a specific genetic susceptibility factor over the chance of disease in those without it
Resequencing	A method of identifying clinically relevant genetic variation in a candidate gene of interest by comparing the sequence in individuals with disease to a reference sequence
RNA	Ribonucleic acid; expressed form of a gene, called messenger or mRNA if protein coding
Sense	Nucleic acid sequence corresponding to mRNA
Silent	DNA mutation that changes a given codon but does not alter the corresponding amino acid
SNP	Single nucleotide polymorphism
Splicing	RNA processing mechanism where introns are removed and exons joined to create mRNA; in alternative splicing, exons are utilized in a regulated manner within a cell or tissue
Trans-acting	A regulatory protein that acts on a molecule other than that which expressed it
Transcription	Cellular process where DNA sequence is used as template for RNA synthesis
Transcriptome	The complete set of RNA transcripts produced by a cell, tissue, or individual
Translation	Cellular process where mRNA sequence is converted to protein

CONSTITUTIVE AND ALTERNATIVE SPLICING

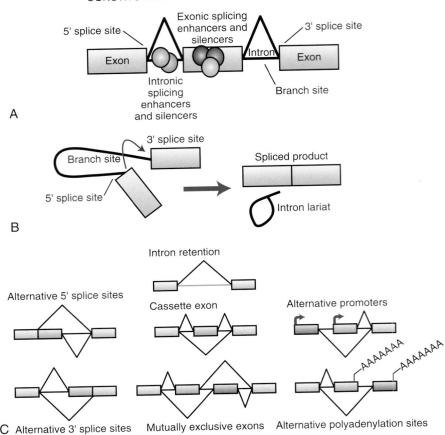

Fig. 40.3 RNA splicing. **A,** A generic precursor RNA is shown, consisting of three exons *(blue)* with intervening introns *(dark lines)*. Representative sequences recognized by the protein complexes that mediate splicing are shown (5′ and 3′ splice sites and the branch site). Binding of these complexes may be influenced either positively or negatively by regulatory sequences and their associated proteins *(circles)* located in either the introns or exons. Splicing pattern is shown by angled lines spanning introns. **B,** Splicing occurs via the complex-mediated association of the 5′ splice site and the branch site, with subsequent attack of the 3′ splice site by the upstream exon *(arrow)*, which joins it to the downstream exon and releases the intron. **C,** Possible alternative splicing patterns for various mRNAs are shown. Constitutive exons are in blue. Alternatively utilized exons are shown in orange or purple. A retained intron is shown by an orange line.

UAA), also called *stop codons*. The *start codon* is ATG and codes for methionine. These amino acids are joined by the ribosome to synthesize a protein. This protein, which may undergo further modification, will ultimately carry out a programmed biological function in the cell. Regulation of this process is highly coordinated and important in learning, for example, where activity-dependent translation at the synapse underlies some aspects of synaptic plasticity, which may go awry in certain disorders such as fragile X syndrome and autism (Morrow et al., 2008).

Over the last decade, the discovery of several classes of functional non–protein coding RNAs has added additional complexity to our understanding of how the genetic code is manifest at the level of cellular function. Of these, microRNAs (miRNAs) are increasingly being recognized as vital players in gene regulation and neurological disease (Weinberg and Wood, 2009). Nascent miRNA molecules are processed to form short (approximately 22-nucleotide) RNA duplexes that target endogenous cellular machinery to specific coding RNAs and induce posttranscriptional gene silencing through a diverse repertoire including RNA cleavage, translational blocking, transport to inactive cell sites, or promotion of RNA decay (Filipowicz et al., 2008; Weinberg and Wood, 2009). Depending on the cell and the context, miRNA activity can result in specific gene inactivation, functional repression, or more subtle regulatory effects and may involve multiple RNAs in a given biological pathway (Flynt and Lai, 2008). Estimates suggest that miRNAs may regulate 30% of protein-coding

genes, implicating these molecules as important targets for future research into the biology of neurological disease (Filipowicz et al., 2008; Weinberg and Wood, 2009).

For a specific disease-related gene, the DNA sequence present within an individual is referred to as their *genotype*, and the expression of that code often results in a feature (or features) that can be observed or measured, known as the *phenotype*. Genes are further organized into higher-order structures termed *chromosomes*, which together comprise the entire set of DNA, or *genome*, of the individual. The human genome is diploid, meaning we possess 23 pairs of chromosomes, 22 autosomes and 1 sex chromosome. Consequently, normal individuals possess two copies (or alleles) of every autosomal gene, one from the mother and one from the father. Because there are two distinct sex chromosomes, X and Y, genes on these chromosomes are expressed in a slightly different manner, discussed in more detail later for the sex-linked disorders.

It is important to emphasize that most genes are not simply "on" or "off." In reality, cells maintain strict regulatory control over their genes. Some genes, such as those required for cell structure or maintenance, must be expressed constitutively, but genes with specific precise functions may only be needed in certain cells at certain times under certain conditions. Potential levels of regulation are depicted in **Fig. 40.2** and include virtually every stage of gene expression. Initially, genes can be regulated at the level of transcription, ranging from the regulated binding of histone proteins, which leads to chromosome condensation, inactivating genes, to the coordinated activity of protein factors that activate or repress gene transcription in response to cell state, environmental conditions, or other factors. Once expressed, the RNA is subject to processing regulation, particularly through alternative splicing as already discussed. Transport of the mRNA and its translation provide additional steps for cellular regulation. Lastly, the final protein can be subject to control via posttranslational modifications or interactions with other proteins. To operate, all these levels of regulation require *trans-acting* factors, such as proteins, which stimulate or repress a particular step, as well as *cis-acting* elements, sequences recognized and bound by the regulatory factors.

These detailed levels of regulation provide a dynamic and expansive capability to precisely control cellular function, essential for growth, development, and survival in an unpredictable environment. However, this also provides many potential points at which disease can arise from disrupted regulation. Consequently, a defective gene could cause disease directly through its own action or indirectly by disrupting regulation of other cellular pathways. For example, the forkhead box P2 (FOXP2) transcription factor regulates the expression of genes thought to be important for the development of spoken language (Konopka et al., 2009). Mutations in this gene cause an autosomal dominant disorder characterized by impairment of speech articulation and language processing (Lai et al., 2001). However, other mutations in this gene are responsible for approximately 1% to 2% of sporadic developmental verbal dyspraxia (MacDermot et al., 2005), likely via downstream effects. Mutation of the methyl-CpG-binding protein 2 (MECP2), which regulates chromatin structure, causes the neurodevelopmental disorder, Rett syndrome, but other mutations in this gene can cause intellectual disability or autism (Gonzales and LaSalle, 2010). Similarly, the FOX1 protein (also called ataxin 2 binding protein 1, or A2BP1), a neuron-specific RNA splicing factor (Underwood et al., 2005) predicted to regulate a large network of genes important to neurodevelopment (Yeo et al., 2009; Zhang et al., 2008), causes autistic spectrum disorder when disrupted (Martin et al., 2007) but has also been implicated as a susceptibility gene associated with both primary biliary cirrhosis (Joshita et al., 2010) and hand osteoarthritis (Zhai et al., 2009), presumably due to downstream effects or specific effects in non-neural tissues. This concept of genes acting on other genes will be further explored later (see Common Neurological Disorders and Complex Disease Genetics).

In addition to the complexity of regulatory mutations that affect gene expression by altering RNA or protein levels or by disrupting RNA splicing, there are certain mutations that do not cause protein dysfunction, but instead have effects restricted to the RNA itself. For example, RNA inclusions are found in several forms of triplet repeat disorders (see Repeat Expansion Disorders) including myotonic dystrophy type 1 and the fragile X–associated tremor/ataxia syndrome (FXTAS) (Garcia-Arocena and Hagerman, 2010; Orr and Zoghbi, 2007). The latter is particularly interesting from a genetic standpoint, because a disorder of late-onset progressive ataxia, tremor, and cognitive impairment occurs in carriers of FMR1 alleles of intermediate sizes, which are not full fragile X–causing mutations (Garcia-Arocena and Hagerman, 2010). FXTAS is a dominant gain-of-function disease that occurs via an entirely different mechanism than the recessive loss-of-function

disease, fragile X syndrome (Garcia-Arocena and Hagerman, 2010; Penagarikano et al., 2007). Primary disorders of RNA still represent relatively uncharted territory, and it is likely that more RNA-specific diseases will be identified. This is particularly exciting for many reasons, not the least of which is that certain classes of these disorders may be amendable to therapy (Nakamori and Thornton, 2010; Wheeler et al., 2009).

Types of Genetic Variation and Mutations

Rare versus Common Variation

As dictated by the principles of natural selection, most genetic variation is not deleterious, and the induced phenotypic variability can be beneficial as a source on which evolution may act. From a clinical standpoint, it is helpful to dichotomize genetic variation into common and rare variation, while accepting that genetic variation is likely a continuum, and the choice of cutoff could be considered arbitrary. Rare genetic variants are of low frequency in the population (<1% frequency), either because they are deleterious and selected against, or because they are new and most often benign. Common genetic variation (>1% to 5% population frequency), on the other hand, is either adaptive, neutral, or not deleterious enough to be subject to strong negative selection; such variants are referred to as *polymorphisms*. The preeminent genetic model has been that common disease susceptibility is related to common genetic variation, and more rare forms of disease are caused by rare genetic variants, so-called mutations, which act in a Mendelian fashion. In contrast, common variants or polymorphisms may increase susceptibility for disease, but alone are not sufficient to cause disease (see Common Neurological Disorders and Complex Disease Genetics).

Polymorphisms and Point Mutations

The most prevalent form of genetic polymorphism is the *single nucleotide polymorphism* (SNP), which occurs on average every 300 to 1000 base pairs in the human genome. Most of these SNPs are relatively benign on their own and do not directly cause disease, so for the purposes of this initial discussion, we will concern ourselves primarily with mutations: rare genetic variants sufficient to cause disease. Pathogenic mutations can occur in numerous ways and vary from single nucleotide changes to gross rearrangements of chromosomes (**Fig. 40.4**). Owing to the large volume of DNA in the human genome, heritable mutations can arise spontaneously in the germline over time through errors in DNA replication or from DNA damage by metabolic or environmental sources despite the constant surveillance of extensive cellular preventive proofreading and repair mechanisms. Thus, mutations can be inherited from the parent or occur *de novo* in the germline. An example of a common de novo variant is trisomy 21, which causes Down syndrome (discussed further in Chromosomal Analysis and Abnormalities). The smallest pathogenic alterations, termed *point mutations*, involve a change in a single nucleotide within a DNA sequence. A point mutation can result in one of three possible effects with respect to protein: (1) a change to a different amino acid, called a *missense mutation*, (2) a change to a termination codon, called a *nonsense mutation*, or (3) creation of a new sequence that is *silent* with regard to protein sequence but alters some aspect of gene regulation, such as RNA splicing or transcriptional expression levels. Nonsense mutations can cause premature truncation of a protein, whereas a missense mutation can affect a protein in different ways depending on the chemical properties of the new amino acid and whether the change is located in a region of functional importance.

It should be emphasized that not all point mutations are disease-causing variants, although until recently, many considered that a premature stop codon was a "smoking gun." Whole genome sequencing demonstrates that more than 100 such nonsense mutations may exist per genome, and the vast majority are expected to be relatively benign (Lupski et al., 2010; see Whole Genome/Exome Sequencing in Disease Gene Discovery). So in many cases, the pathogenicity of rare variants is not immediately discernable, and without strong statistical or functional evidence, labeling such genetic variation a mutation is premature and may be misleading. It is likely that most of these, including some variants thought previously to cause rare Mendelian diseases, may simply be benign genetic variation. This is because even a complete knockout of one allele caused by a premature stop codon *(haploinsuf-*

ficiency) may have no discernable effect on gene function for a majority of genes in the human genome (Lupski et al., 2010; Ng et al., 2009; Yngvadottir et al., 2009).

Occasionally, silent coding mutations or point mutations in noncoding regions may be significant for disease if they damage sequences important for gene expression (e.g., transcriptional and/or RNA processing regulatory elements). It has been estimated that up to half of all disease-causing mutations impact RNA splicing, which can have dire consequences given the importance of splicing to regulated gene expression. Such is the case for frontotemporal dementia with parkinsonism linked to chromosome 17 (FTDP-17), where in some populations, the most common mutations disrupt splicing, causing a pathogenic imbalance in tau isoforms (D'Souza and Schellenberg, 2005). As for noncoding mutations, given the large volume of such sequences in the human genome—perhaps up to 96%—and our still imprecise ability to predict sequences required for regulation or to interpret identified sequence changes without direct experimentation, the majority of these mutations likely go unrecognized. It is hoped that the next generation of sequencing and bioinformatic technologies will allow for a better understanding of the role of these types of mutation in human disease.

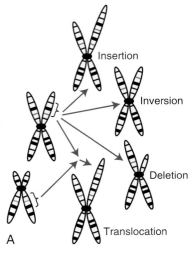

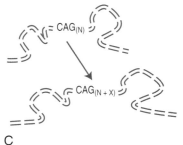

Normal

Protein	Ser - Val - Ile - Asp - Arg - Ser - Pro - Cys - Leu - Gln - Ala
RNA	AGC - GUA - AUC - GAU - CGC - UCU - CCG - UGC - UUG - CAG - GCU
DNA	TCG - CAT - TAG - CTA - GCG - AGA - GGC - ACG - AAC - GTC - CGA

Point mutation - missense

Protein	Ser - Val - Ile - Asp - **Gly** - Ser - Pro - Cys - Leu - Gln - Ala
RNA	AGC - GUA - AUC - GAU - **GGC** - UCU - CCG - UGC - UUG - CAG - GCU
DNA	TCG - CAT - TAG - CTA - **CCG** - AGA - GGC - ACG - AAC - GTC - CGA

Point mutation - nonsense

Protein	Ser - Val - Ile - Asp - Arg - Ser - Pro - **STOP**
RNA	AGC - GUA - AUc - GAU - CGC - UCU - CCG - **UGA** - UUG - CAG - GCU
DNA	TCG - CAT - TAG - CTA - GCG - AGA - GGC - **ACT** - AAC - GTC - CGA

Point mutation - silent

Protein	Ser - Val - Ile - Asp - Arg - Ser - Pro - Cys - Leu - Gln - Ala
RNA	AGC - GUA - AUC - GAU - CGC - **UCG** - CCG - UGC - UUG - CAG - GCU
DNA	TCG - CAT - TAG - CTA - GCG - **AGC** - GGC - ACG - AAC - GTC - CGA

Frameshift - insertion

Protein	Ser - Val - Ile - Asp - Arg - Ser - **Ser** - **Val** - **Leu** - **Ala** - **Gly**
RNA	AGC - GUA - AUC - GAU - CGC - UCC - **UCC** - **GUG** - **CUU** - **GCA** - **CCC** - **U**
DNA	TCG - CAT - TAG - CTA - GCG - AGG - **AGG** - **CAC** - **GAA** - **CGT** - **CCG** - **A**

Frameshift - deletion

Protein	Ser - Val - Ile - Asp - Arg - Ser - **Arg** - **Ala** - **Cys** - **Arg** - —
RNA	AGC - GUA - AUC - GAU - CGC - UC-C - **CGU** - **GCU** - **UGC** - **AGG** - **CU**
DNA	TCG - CAT - TAG - CTA - GCG - AG-G - **GCA** - **CGA** - **ACG** - **TCC** - **GA**

Fig. 40.4 Genetic mutations. **A,** Categories of chromosomal aberrations. Paired homologous chromosomes are shown, with various anomalies indicated. An insertional translocation is depicted; other common types include reciprocal translocations and centric fusions (Robertsonian translocations). **B,** Types of point mutations. A generic DNA sequence is shown *(boxed)* along with its corresponding mRNA sequence. Codons are indicated, as are their translation into protein (designed by the standard three-letter code). Mutations are in purple, as are the corresponding alterations in the mRNA and protein if present. Note that silent point mutations do not alter the protein sequence. **C,** Repeat expansion disorders. An example mRNA is shown with a CAG-codon (polyglutamine) repeat region indicated. In the expanded form, an additional number of repeats are present which may perturb the function of the protein produced and/or lead to cell damage via the expanded polyglutamine region (see text for details).

Structural Chromosomal Abnormalities and Copy Number Variation

Small deletions and insertions can occur through slippage and strand mispairing at regions of short, tandem DNA repeats during replication. If the deletion or insertion is not a multiple of three, a *frameshift* will result, which leads to the translation of an altered protein sequence from the site of the mutation. On a larger scale, errors of chromosomal replication or recombination can result in inversions, translocations, deletions, duplications, or insertions (Stankiewicz and Lupski, 2010). When the region of deletion or duplication is greater than 1 kb, this is referred to as a *copy number variation* (CNV). Copy number variation is far more common than previously suspected, and it is estimated that at least 4% of the human genome varies in copy number (Conrad et al., 2010; Redon et al., 2006), much of which is commonly observed in the population and benign (Conrad et al., 2010). However, some rare CNVs such as the recurrent chromosome 17p12 duplication underlying most cases of Charcot-Marie-Tooth type 1A (Shchelochkov et al., 2010) or the alpha-synuclein triplication that can cause Parkinson disease (PD) (Singleton et al., 2003) are pathogenic and act in a Mendelian fashion. Even though such changes may be extensive, they may not be pathogenic if they do not disrupt expression of any key genes. This is particularly true for balanced translocations where genetic material is rearranged between chromosomes, yet no significant portion is actually lost. Although an individual with such a condition may be normal, if the germline is affected, their offspring may receive unbalanced chromosomal material and consequently develop a clinical phenotype (Kovaleva and Shaffer, 2003). CNVs will be discussed in greater detail when we consider common and complex disease genetics (see Copy Number Variation and Comparative Genomic Hybridization).

Repeat Expansion Disorders

Most mutations thus far discussed pass from parent to offspring unaltered, and in large affected families, the identical mutation can potentially be traced back generations. In contrast, there is a specific class of mutation, the repeat expansion (Orr and Zoghbi, 2007) (**Table 40.2**), which is unstable and can present with earlier onset and increasing severity in successive generations, a process known as *anticipation*. There are several examples of diseases caused by expanded repeats in coding sequence (e.g., most spinocerebellar ataxias, HD), as well as examples in noncoding sequence (e.g., fragile X syndrome, myotonic dystrophy) and within an intron (e.g., Friedreich ataxia). Interestingly, virtually all these disorders show neurological symptoms that can include such features as ataxia, intellectual disability, dementia, myotonia, or epilepsy, depending on the disease. The most common repeated sequence seen in these diseases is the CAG triplet, which codes for glutamine and expansion of which is seen in a variety of the spinocerebellar ataxias (SCAs) including SCA types 1, 2, 3, 6, 7, 17, and dentatorubropallidoluysian atrophy (DRPLA). In addition to protein-specific effects, these disorders likely share a common pathogenesis due to the presence of the polyglutamine repeat regions. In some disorders, the phenotype can be quite different depending on the number of repeats, such as in the FMR1 gene, where more than 200 CCG repeats causes fragile X syndrome, but repeats in the premutation range of 60 to 200, from which fully expanded alleles arise, can result in FXTAS or premature ovarian failure (Oostra and Willemsen, 2009). Although in general, the underlying mutation is similar, each specific repeat expansion has distinct effects on its corresponding gene, and thus in addition to varying phenotypes, they may also show very different inheritance patterns as illustrated later (see Disorders of Mendelian Inheritance).

Chromosomal Analysis and Abnormalities

The DNA coding for an individual gene is generally too small to be visualized microscopically, but it is possible to observe the chromosomes as they condense during mitosis as part of cell division (Griffiths et al., 2002; Strachan and Read, 2003). Traditionally, various staining techniques (e.g., Giemsa) are applied, producing a detailed pattern of banding along the chromosomes that are then photographed and aligned for comparative analysis. This arrangement and analysis of the chromosomes is known as a *karyotype* (**Fig. 40.5**). Through these methods, it is possible to visually identify large chromosomal deletions, duplications, or rearrangements. If high-resolution banding techniques are employed, structural alterations on the order of as small as 3 Mb (3 million base pairs) can be detected. More sophisticated techniques can also be employed, such as fluorescent in situ hybridization (FISH). In this method, a short DNA sequence, or probe, that corresponds to a chromosomal region of interest is hybridized with the patient's DNA and detected visually via excitation of a fluorescent label. FISH can improve on visual resolution by 10- to 100-fold and is in common use for detection of a large number of well-defined genetic syndromes (Speicher and Carter, 2005) such as 15q duplication syndrome, DiGeorge syndrome (22q11 deletion), and Smith-Magenis syndrome (17p11 deletion).

More recent technological developments involving microarray technology (Geschwind, 2003) permit screening of the entire genome at high resolution (from kilobase to single nucleotide level) and are rapidly replacing techniques based on microscopic analysis. This technology is responsible for the emerging appreciation for the structural chromosomal variation in humans mentioned earlier, most of which is submicroscopic. For this section, we will focus on chromosomal alterations that can be detected microscopically, since the clinical implications of many small or rare structural variants identified are not yet clear (see Copy Number Variation and Comparative Genomic Hybridization).

The most common chromosomal abnormalities encountered clinically involve sporadic aneuploidy, either a deletion leaving one chromosome, or a monosomy, or a duplication leaving three chromosomes, or a trisomy (Strachan and Read, 2003). This occurs most frequently via nondisjunction, whereby chromosomes fail to separate during meiosis in the production of the gametes. The majority of aneuploidies are lethal, although there are a few that are viable and will be briefly discussed. Monosomy X (45,XO), also called Turner syndrome, is seen in approximately 1 of every 5000 births and results in sterile females of small stature with a variety of mild physical deformities including webbing of the neck, multiple

Table 40.2 Selected Repeat Expansion Disorders

Disease	Locus	Gene Symbol	Protein Name	Protein Function	Normal Repeat*	Repeat Location†	Expanded Repeat‡
DM1	19q13.2-q13.3	DMPK	dystrophia myotonica protein kinase	Ser/Thr protein kinase	≤34 CTG	3′ UTR	≥50
DM2	3q13.3-q24	ZNF9	zinc finger protein 9	Translational regulation	≤26 CCTG	Intronic	≥75
DRPLA	12p13.31	ATN1	atrophin-1	Transcription	≤35 CAG	Coding	≥48
FRAXA FXTAS§	Xq27.3	FMR1	fragile-X mental retardation protein	Translational regulation	≤40 CGG	5′ UTR	>200 60-200§
FRDA	9q13	FXN	frataxin	Mitochondrial metabolism	≤33 GAA	Intronic	≥66
HD	4p16.3	HTT	huntington	Unknown	≤26 CAG	Coding	≥36
SBMA	Xq11-q12	AR	androgen receptor	Transcription	≤34 CAG	Coding	≥38
SCA1	6p23	ATXN1	ataxin-1	Transcription	≤38 CAG	Coding	≥39
SCA2	12q24	ATXN2	ataxin-2	RNA processing	≤31 CAG	Coding	≥32
SCA3	14q24.3-q31	ATXN3	ataxin-3	Protein quality control	≤44 CAG	Coding	≥52
SCA6	19p13	CACNA1A	Ca$_V$2.1	Calcium channel	≤18 CAG	Coding	≥20
SCA7	3p21.1-p12	ATXN7	ataxin-7	Transcription	≤19 CAG	Coding	≥36
SCA8‖	13q21	ATXN8 ATXN8OS	ataxin-8 none	Unknown Unknown	≤50 CAG ≤50 CTG	Coding Noncoding	≥80 ≥80
SCA10	22q13	ATXN10	ataxin-10	Unknown	≤29 ATTCT	Intronic	≥800
SCA12	5q31-q33	PPP2R2B	protein phosphatase 2 regulatory subunit B, beta	Mitochondrial morphogenesis	≤32 CAG	5′ UTR	≥51
SCA17	6q27	TBP	TATA box-binding protein	Transcription	≤42 CAG	Coding	≥49

*In some instances, normal/abnormal repeat length is an estimate due to adjacent polymorphic sequences.

†Location of repeat region within the expressed mRNA.

‡Does not include alleles with known incomplete penetrance.

§Premutation alleles for FRAXA result in the FXTAS phenotype.

‖SCA8 involves bi-directional expression from two overlapping reading frames.

DM, Myotonic dystrophy; *DRPLA*, dentatorubral-pallidoluysian atrophy; *FRAXA*, fragile X syndrome; *FRDA*, Friedreich ataxia; *FXTAS*, fragile X–associated tremor/ataxia syndrome; *HD*, Huntington disease; *SBMA*, spinal and bulbar muscular atrophy; *SCA*, spinocerebellar ataxia; *UTR*, untranslated region.

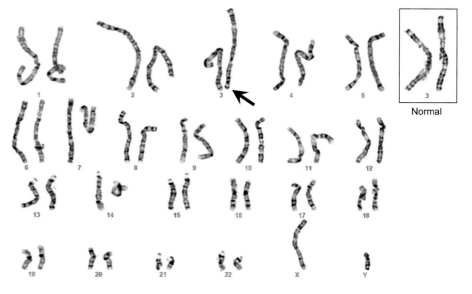

Fig. 40.5 Abnormal male karyogram. Patient is a male child with a clinical diagnosis of autism. Metaphase chromosomes were isolated from peripheral blood leukocytes and high-resolution GPG banding was performed to visualize structural features. A deletion of the telomeric region of the long arm of chromosome 3 was detected *(arrow)*, consistent with a diagnosis of 3q29 microdeletion syndrome. A normal chromosome 3 pair is shown for comparison *(insert)*. Analysis of the parents showed this to be a de novo deletion. *(Photo courtesy F. Quintero-Rivera, UCLA Clinical Cytogenetics Laboratory.)*

nevi, and hand and elbow variations, with a very specific cognitive profile in patients with the full deletion (Strachan and Read, 2003). Individuals with additional copies of the X chromosome are also seen. While both females (47,XXX) and males (47,XXY) may have varying degrees of learning disabilities, especially involving language and attention (Geschwind et al., 2000), the males are referred to as having Klinefelter syndrome (KS) due to a phenotype also involving gynecomastia and infertility. XYY males have cognitive profiles similar to XXY males but several studies have suggested more severe social and behavioral problems in some individuals, especially increased aggression, which is rare in KS. Trisomy 21 (47, +21), or Down syndrome, includes profound intellectual impairment, flat faces with prominent epicanthal folds, and a predisposition to cardiac disease. At 1 in approximately 700 births, this is the most common genetic cause of intellectual disability and is associated with advanced maternal age at the time of conception. The other aneuploidies which can survive to term (trisomy 13 [47, +13], Edwards syndrome; trisomy 18 [47, +18], Patau syndrome) have much more severe phenotypes with drastically decreased viability, and death generally occurs within weeks to months after birth.

Disorders of Mendelian Inheritance

In this section we will consider genetic disorders caused by mutation of a single gene. Associating a clinical disease phenotype to the mutation of a specific gene has long been the goal of clinically based, or translational, neuroscience. It is expected that gene identification will eventually lead to an understanding of the disease etiology as well as more accurate diagnosis and better treatments. The ability to determine the genetic nature of most single-gene disease is ultimately based upon the laws of inheritance devised by Mendel in the late 1800s (Griffiths et al., 2002). To summarize these findings in a clinical context, the assumption is made that a phenotypic trait (or in this example, a disease) is caused by the alteration of a single gene. It is important to emphasize that this assumption does not always hold true, particularly for the more complex genetic diseases, as we will discuss later, but it is still true for many diseases seen by neurologists, and more than 3000 Mendelian conditions have been identified to date (OMIM, 2010). Now, if we accept the premise that a given disease is caused by a single gene, we know that for any individual, the gene exists as a pair of alleles with one copy from each parent. However, the alleles may not be equal, and one member of the pair may control the phenotype despite the presence of the other copy. In this case, we say that allele is *dominant* over the other, the latter of which is labeled as *recessive*. Depending on the gene and the mutation, as discussed later, a disease allele may be either dominant or recessive. Next, during the development of the gametes, these alleles segregate randomly in a process independent from all other genes. Therefore, the chance of a child receiving a particular allele is entirely random. If these laws all hold true, the observed inheritance of the clinical disease in families will follow a specific pattern that can be used to identify the nature of the causative gene. Although diseases showing Mendelian inheritance are either rare conditions or rare forms of common conditions (e.g., early-onset Alzheimer dementia or PD), identification of such genes are seminal biological advances

that can have enormous impact on our understanding of these neurological conditions.

Autosomal Dominant Disorders

Diseases involving autosomal genes that require mutation of only one allele are defined as dominant. In most cases, the affected individual has two distinct alleles of a gene (in this case, one normal and one pathogenic) and is described as being *heterozygous*. Often these pathogenic mutations impart new functionality, referred to as a *toxic gain of function*, meaning that the phenotype is produced as a result of the expression of the mutated protein. Other disease mechanisms in dominantly inherited conditions include: (1) *haploinsufficiency*, where inactivation of a single allele is sufficient to produce disease despite the presence of another normal copy, and (2) *dominant negative* effects, where a mutated protein disrupts function of the normal protein transcribed from the other nonmutant allele.

Autosomal dominant inheritance is characterized by direct transmission of the disorder from parent to child (**Fig. 40.6**). Affected individuals are seen in all generations, and a vertical line can be drawn on the pedigree to illustrate the passage of the disorder. Since only one deleterious copy of the disease gene is necessary, risk of transmission from an affected parent is 50%. Since the disorder is autosomal, there is no sex preference, and both males and females can present with the disease. One caveat involves the concept of *penetrance*, or the percent likelihood that a trait will manifest in a person with

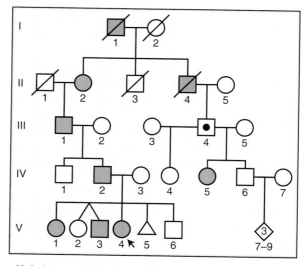

Fig. 40.6 Autosomal dominant inheritance. A pedigree diagram is shown, using standard nomenclature. Generations are numbered consecutively on the left, and individuals are numbered within each generation. Males are depicted as squares and females as circles. Affected persons are indicated by filled icons. Death is indicated by a diagonal line. A union producing offspring is indicated by horizontal lines. A diamond represents individuals (n) of unknown sex. A triangle represents a spontaneous abortion. Individuals V-2 and V-3 illustrate the diagramming of dizygotic twins. The proband of the pedigree is indicated by an arrow. An autosomal dominant pedigree demonstrates vertical transmission of disease without a sex preference. On average, 50% of offspring are affected. Individual III-4 represents a case of incomplete penetrance (dark circle) where the individual carries the mutation but does not manifest disease. Anticipation (see text) would be illustrated by increasing severity/onset in patients III-1, IV-2, and V-4.

Table 40.3 Selected Online Clinical Neurogenetics Resources	
Disease-specific and gene-specific resources	GeneReviews at GeneTests University of Washington, Seattle, WA USA US National Center for Biotechnology Information http://www.ncbi.nlm.nih.gov/sites/GeneTests/
	Locus Specific Mutation Databases Human Genome Variation Society, Australia http://www.hgvs.org/dblist/glsdb.html
	Neuromuscular Disease Center Washington University, St. Louis, MO USA http://neuromuscular.wustl.edu/
	Online Mendelian Inheritance in Man Johns Hopkins University, Baltimore, MD USA US National Center for Biotechnology Information http://www.ncbi.nlm.nih.gov/omim/
Clinical genetic testing and clinical trials	ClinicalTrials.gov US National Institutes of Health http://clinicaltrials.gov/
	GeneTests University of Washington, Seattle, WA USA US National Center for Biotechnology Information http://www.ncbi.nlm.nih.gov/sites/GeneTests/
Genomic variation and other genome resources	Alternative Splicing and Transcript Diversity Database European Molecular Biology Laboratory—European Bioinformatics Institute http://www.ebi.ac.uk/astd/
	Catalog of Published Genome-Wide Association Studies US National Human Genome Research Institute http://www.genome.gov/gwastudies/
	Ensembl Databases European Molecular Biology Laboratory—European Bioinformatics Institute Wellcome Trust Sanger Institute, UK http://www.ensembl.org/
	Database of Genomic Variants The Centre for Applied Genomics, Canada http://projects.tcag.ca/variation/
	International HapMap Project http://hapmap.ncbi.nlm.nih.gov/index.html
	Single Nucleotide Polymorphism Database US National Center for Biotechnology Information http://www.ncbi.nlm.nih.gov/projects/SNP/
	1000 Genomes Project http://www.1000genomes.org/

a specific genotype. A dominant gene is considered to have complete penetrance if all individuals with a given mutation develop disease. In practice, however, many autosomal dominant genes show varying degrees of penetrance or expressivity, most likely due to the influence of other genes and environmental factors.

There are over 400 examples of diseases with neurological phenotypes that show autosomal dominant inheritance (OMIM, 2010). These conditions include hyperkalemic periodic paralysis (voltage-gated sodium channel $Na_V1.4$ on chromosome 17, often caused by missense mutations), HD (Huntington on chromosome 4, caused by CAG repeat expansion), SCA type 3 (ataxin-3 on chromosome 14, caused by CAG repeat expansion), Charcot-Marie-Tooth type 1B (myelin protein zero on chromosome 1, often caused by missense mutations), early-onset familial Alzheimer disease (AD) (presenilin-1, often caused by missense mutations), frontotemporal dementia with parkinsonism (microtubule-associated protein tau on chromosome 17, often caused by missense or splicing mutations), tuberous sclerosis type 1 (hamartin on chromosome 9, often caused by nonsense mutations and frameshifts), neurofibromatosis type 1 (neurofibromin on chromosome 17, caused by point mutations, frameshifts, and splicing mutations), and familial amyotrophic lateral sclerosis (ALS) (superoxide dismutase-1 on chromosome 21, caused by missense mutations), to name a few. Even rare Mendelian forms of more common syndromes such as epilepsy or sleep disorders (e.g., familial advanced sleep-phase syndrome) have been identified. More detailed lists can be found using the recommended online resources (**Table 40.3**).

Autosomal Recessive Disorders

Disease involving autosomal genes that require mutation of both alleles is defined as *recessive*. An unaffected individual who harbors one disease-causing allele is referred to as a *carrier* of that allele. For some disorders, a mild phenotype can be seen in these individuals, who are then described as symptomatic carriers. An individual with two identical alleles (in this case both pathogenic) is described as being *homozygous*. Alternatively, if they possess two different pathogenic alleles this is described as being *compound heterozygous*. In general, autosomal recessive mutations modify the function of the protein in a negative way, meaning that the phenotype is produced because of the absence of the mutated protein. This is referred to as a *loss of function*.

Autosomal recessive inheritance is characterized by lack of intergenerational transmission, in contrast to dominantly inherited disorders (**Fig. 40.7**). Affected individuals are seen in single generations, often separated by one or more unaffected generations. Because two deleterious copies of the disease gene are necessary, transmission requires both parents to be either affected or carriers. In the most common scenario when both parents are carriers, the risk of an affected child is 25% (50% from each parent). As with all autosomal disorders, there is no sex preference, and both males and females can present with the disease. In families showing this mode of inheritance, it is important to ask about consanguinity. In rare cases of families with considerable inbreeding, recessive alleles may be so common as to cause disease in successive generations, creating a *pseudodominant* pattern of inheritance.

As mentioned for the autosomal dominant disorders, diseases that share this mode of inheritance may have very distinct types of underlying mutations. Upwards of 600 disorders with autosomal recessive inheritance show neurological symptoms (OMIM, 2010). Examples include Friedreich ataxia (frataxin on chromosome 9, caused by intronic GAA repeat expansion), spinal muscular atrophy type 1 (survival of motor neuron 1 on chromosome 5, caused by deletion of exon 7), Wilson disease (ATPase, Cu^{++} transporting, beta-polypeptide on chromosome 13, often caused by missense mutations), Tay-Sachs disease (hexosaminidase A on chromosome 15, commonly caused by frameshift, splicing, or nonsense mutations), glycogen storage type II or Pompe disease (acid alpha-glucosidase gene on chromosome 17, often caused by point mutations, splicing mutations, and exon deletions), phenylketonuria (phenylalanine hydroxylase on chromosome 12, often caused by missense mutations), and ataxia-telangiectasia (ataxia-telangiectasia mutated on chromosome 11, often caused by point mutations and splicing mutations). More detailed lists can be found using the recommended online resources (see **Table 40.3**).

Sex-Linked (X-Linked) Disorders

The sex chromosomes in humans are referred to as the X and Y chromosomes, the latter of which programs the individual to be male. There are as yet no known Y-linked diseases, so we will focus on the X chromosome. As males only possess a single X chromosome, they are *hemizygous* for all its genes, and consequently any pathogenic mutation is expressed by default. Because of this, dominance of X-linked genes applies with respect to whether female carriers express disease. This is complicated by the observation that although females possess two X chromosomes, no single cell expresses genes from both; instead, one chromosome is randomly and permanently inactivated during development via a process known as *lyonization*. Therefore, all women inherently possess cells of two different genotypes, or are *mosaic*, for the X chromosome. This can be clinically relevant insofar as disproportionate activation of an abnormal X chromosome could potentially lead to clinical phenotypes in female carriers of recessive X-linked disorders. Usually though, skewing occurs, so that the pathogenic allele is less expressed than the other normal allele.

Recessive X-linked transmission is characterized by the presence of disease in males only (**Fig. 40.8**). Affected males cannot pass the disease on to their sons, but all their daughters must inherent the abnormal X chromosome and are, therefore, *obligate carriers*. A carrier female has a 50% chance of passing the disease allele to a child, but all males receiving it will be affected. Dominant X-linked transmission (see **Fig. 40.8**) is similar, except carrier females are affected and transmit the disease to 50% of their children irrespective of their sex. Affected males usually show a more severe phenotype, or may even exhibit lethality, and transmit the disease to all of their daughters and none of their sons.

Over 100 X-linked disorders with neurological phenotypes are known (OMIM, 2010). The majority of these X-linked disorders are recessive, and as seen for the autosomal diseases, mutation type varies widely among the different disorders. Some examples include X-linked adrenoleukodystrophy (ATP-binding cassette subfamily D member 1, commonly caused by missense and frameshift mutations), Duchenne muscular dystrophy (dystrophin, commonly caused by deletions), Emery-Dreifuss muscular dystrophy-1 (emerin, often caused by nonsense mutations), Menkes disease (ATPase, Cu^{++}-transporting, alpha-polypeptide, commonly caused by frameshifts, nonsense mutations, and splicing mutations), Fabry disease (alpha-galactosidase A, commonly caused by point mutations, gene rearrangements, and splicing

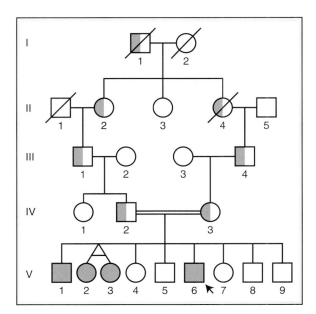

Fig. 40.7 Autosomal recessive inheritance. A pedigree diagram is shown, using standard nomenclature as described in **Fig. 40.6**. Carriers of disease are indicated by half-filled icons. Individuals V-2 and V-3 illustrate the diagramming of monozygotic twins. Consanguineous mating is indicated by a doubled line. An autosomal recessive pedigree demonstrates indirect transmission of disease without a sex preference, often in a single generation (occasionally described as horizontal). On average, 25% of offspring of two carriers are affected.

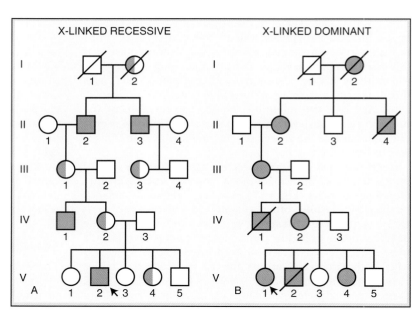

Fig. 40.8 X-linked inheritance. **A,** X-linked recessive disease. A pedigree diagram is shown using standard nomenclature as described in **Fig. 40.6**. Carriers of disease are indicated by half-filled icons. Disease manifests only in hemizygous males. Fathers cannot pass the disease to their sons, but all daughters of an affected male are obligate carriers of disease. Carrier females have a 50% chance to pass on the disease gene and can have affected sons. In some cases, a female carrier can be mildly symptomatic, usually due to non-random lyonization. **B,** X-linked dominant disease. A pedigree diagram is shown using standard nomenclature as described in **Fig. 40.6**. Disease manifests in heterozygous females (although severity may be affected by lyonization). The mutant gene is either lethal in males (as shown here) or has a much more severe phenotype. Affected females pass on the disease 50% of the time.

mutations), and Pelizaeus-Merzbacher disease (proteolipid protein-1, often caused by duplications and missense mutations). X-linked dominant disorders include Rett syndrome (methyl-CpG-binding protein-2, often due to missense and nonsense mutations), incontinentia pigmenti (inhibitor of kappa light polypeptide gene enhancer in B cells, kinase gamma [IKBKG], often due to deletions), and Aicardi syndrome (gene unknown). More detailed lists can be found using the recommended online resources (see **Table 40.3**).

Mendelian Disease Gene Identification by Linkage Analysis and Chromosome Mapping

As mentioned previously, patterns of inheritance can be utilized to locate genes responsible for disease. Traditionally, genes showing Mendelian patterns of inheritance can be physically mapped and identified through linkage analysis (Altshuler et al., 2008; Pulst, 2003) (**Fig. 40.9**). In this technique, one attempts to find a known region of DNA, termed a *marker*, which is co-inherited (segregates) with the disease being studied and subsequently uses the location of that marker to find the disease gene. Although in principle, two points on the same chromosome theoretically segregate independently from one another, the recombination process that mediates this (termed *crossing-over* because maternal and paternal chromosomes swap segments during gamete formation) is statistically more likely to separate points that are far apart from one another than those that are close. Segments of DNA that segregate together are described as being linked. If the degree of linkage exceeds that expected by chance, the regions are said to be in *disequilibrium* and are therefore in close proximity. By using naturally occurring DNA polymorphisms as locational markers, the physical mapping of an unknown disease gene is possible, although the mapped region will likely contain other genes as well. Depending on the size of the family, the generational distance of affected individuals sampled, and the density of the markers being used, the region containing the disease gene is narrowed down to a size more amenable to further detailed analysis. Subsequent analysis, usually DNA sequencing of likely candidate genes, is then performed to locate a mutation that segregates with the affected members of the original family. Many genes important to neurological disease have been identified in this way, including the genes for HD, Duchenne muscular dystrophy, Wilson disease, neurofibromatosis type 1, Von Hippel-Lindau syndrome, torsion dystonia 1, Friedreich ataxia, myotonic dystrophy type 1, hyperkalemic periodic paralysis, familial advanced sleep-phase syndrome, and many others. Although still useful clinically for large families, utilization of this technique is not possible for many diseases because of small family sizes and/or lack of power due to insufficient generational separation between affected individuals in the pedigree.

Non-Mendelian Patterns of Inheritance

In rare instances, pedigree analysis of affected families has revealed patterns of inheritance that do not conform to the classic Mendelian patterns thus far described and therefore must result from other mechanisms. In this section, we will discuss the more common and clinically relevant ways in which single-gene disorders can be transmitted in a non-Mendelian fashion: mitochondrial inheritance, imprinting, and uniparental disomy. It is important to recognize that this is not all inclusive. Other examples exist, such as developmental events that can potentially lead to disease or syndromic conditions through formation of a mosaic, an individual with cells of different genotypes derived from a common cell, or a *chimera*, an individual who contains cells of different distinct genotypes (e.g., from separate fertilizations). Such rare events will not be discussed further. Additionally, the non-Mendelian heritability of diseases that are polygenic, or involve multiple genes, and other forms of complex disorders will be discussed in later sections.

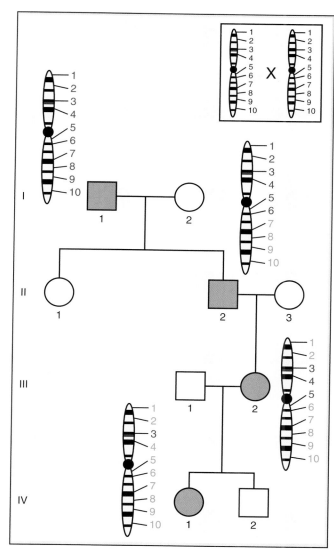

Fig. 40.9 Linkage analysis. A pedigree is depicted as in **Fig. 40.6**, showing autosomal dominant inheritance of disease *(filled icons)*. Transmission of the chromosome containing the mutant gene *(purple line)* is illustrated for all affected individuals. Numbers represent the location of specific chromosomal markers (e.g., single nucleotide polymorphisms or other sequences). Purple numbers represent markers originally from the mutant chromosome in individual I-1. With each mating, there is potential crossing over between regions of homologous chromosomes *(insert)*, likely resulting in the separation of markers spaced far apart along the chromosome. In this example, examination of all affected individuals shows the disease segregates with marker 3, and the two are therefore in linkage disequilibrium, suggesting they are near one another. Once identified, the marker location can be used to select candidate genes for sequencing to identify the causative gene and mutation in the family.

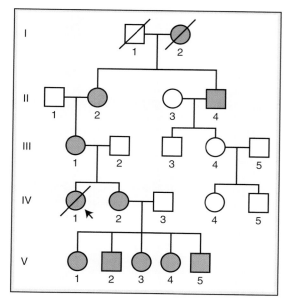

Fig. 40.10 Mitochondrial (maternal) inheritance. A pedigree diagram is shown using standard nomenclature as described in **Fig. 40.6**. As the mutant gene is carried in the mitochondrial genome, disease is passed on to all the offspring of affected females (see text). Males can be affected but cannot pass on disease. Severity and onset of the disease may be affected by heteroplasmy, the proportion of abnormal mitochondria per cell, as illustrated by a severe phenotype seen in patient IV-1.

Mitochondrial Disorders

Mitochondria are double-membraned organelles responsible for energy production within the cell via the process of oxidative phosphorylation, which relies on the transfer of electrons through a chain of protein complexes within the inner mitochondrial membrane. Disruption of mitochondrial function can lead to a variety of diseases with multisystem involvement, including prominent neurological symptoms (DiMauro and Hirano, 2009; Zeviani and Carelli, 2007). Mitochondria possess their own genome with 37 genes. Because mitochondria are cytoplasmic and the majority of cytoplasm within the zygote is derived from the egg and not the sperm, disorders involving mitochondrial DNA are inherited through the maternal line (**Fig. 40.10**). A single cell contains many mitochondria which all replicate independently of the nuclear DNA, so it is possible that a mutation in the mitochondrial genome may be present in some of the mitochondria but not others, a condition termed *heteroplasmy*. This proportion can affect whether a disease is expressed and, if so, what tissues are affected if a minimum threshold of abnormal mitochondria is reached. Heteroplasmy may also change over time as cells divide and the mitochondria are redistributed. Some examples of such disorders include MELAS (mitochondrial encephalomyopathy, lactic acidosis, and stroke-like episodes, caused by point mutations within the gene encoding mitochondrial tRNA[LEU]), MERRF (myoclonic epilepsy with ragged red fibers, caused by point mutations within the gene encoding mitochondrial tRNA[LYS]), and LHON (Leber hereditary optic neuropathy, most often caused by point mutations in either of two mitochondrial genes encoding complex I subunits, ND4 or ND6).

Because the mitochondria themselves contain only a few genes, the majority of mitochondrial proteins, including the machinery responsible for the replication and repair of the mitochondrial genome, are all encoded by nuclear genes. Since these genes are located within the nuclear genome, despite the fact that their mutation gives rise to dysfunctional mitochondria, the disease will show a Mendelian pattern of inheritance. Some examples include infantile-onset SCA (twinkle on chromosome 10, autosomal recessive, caused by missense mutations), progressive external ophthalmoplegia A2 (adenine nucleotide translocator 1 on chromosome 4, autosomal dominant, caused by missense mutations), and Charcot-Marie-Tooth type 2A2 (mitofusin-2 on chromosome 1, autosomal dominant, often caused by missense mutations). Interestingly, various mutations, commonly missense, of the nuclear gene DNA polymerase gamma (POLG) on chromosome 15, which encodes the polymerase responsible for both replication and repair of the mitochondrial genome, cause a wide variety of diverse phenotypes with different modes of inheritance (Hudson and Chinnery, 2006). These include the autosomal recessive Alpers syndrome of encephalopathy, seizures, and liver failure, an autosomal dominant form of chronic progressive external ophthalmoplegia, and autosomal recessive phenotypes of cerebellar ataxia and peripheral neuropathy, among others.

Imprinting

For most genes, expression is controlled by distinct cellular processes that operate irrespective of the gene's parental origin. However, for some genes, expression in the offspring differs depending on whether the allele was maternally or paternally inherited, and such genes are described as being imprinted (Spencer, 2009). *Imprinting* arises from epigenetic modifications such as DNA or histone methylation, which are parent-specific alterations that do not change the actual DNA sequence (**Fig. 40.11**). One example of this is sex-specific DNA methylation that occurs for some genes during the formation of gametes. In the offspring, the methylated gene is bound by histone proteins forming transcriptionally inactive heterochromatin. This allows all gene expression to be driven by the allele derived from the other parent. This can be dynamic depending on the gene, and the magnitude of differential expression between the alleles can vary based on stage of development, tissue type, and possibly other factors. Deletion of an imprinted region or defective imprinting in gametogenesis can lead to disease as illustrated by observations involving chromosome 15q (Lalande and Calciano, 2007). In this example, differential methylation affects the expression of multiple genes, and loss of maternal patterning can lead to Angelman syndrome, characterized by intellectual impairment, epilepsy, ataxia, and inappropriate laughter, while loss of the paternal pattern causes Prader-Willi syndrome, associated with intellectual impairment, obesity, and behavioral problems. The most common mechanism involves de novo deletion of the imprinted region from one parent, although in some cases, defective imprinting can also occur during gametogenesis. In the majority of cases, defective imprinting occurs spontaneously and is therefore unlikely to recur in families; however, imprinting defects can rarely be due to small deletions involving sequences important for regulating parent-specific methylation.

Uniparental Disomy

Uniparental disomy arises when pairs of chromosomes are inherited from the same parent, either in their entirety or in large segments due to segregation errors or chromosomal rearrangement (Kotzot, 2008) (see **Fig. 40.11**). The uniparentally inherited chromosomes can be identical (isodisomic) or

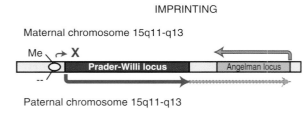

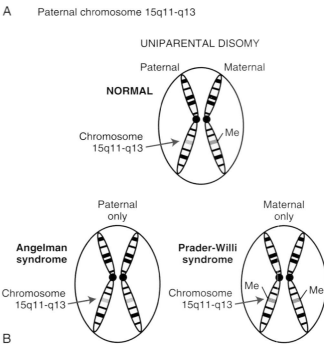

Fig. 40.11 Epigenetics in human disease. **A,** Imprinting. Gene expression on human Chromosome 15q11-q13 is subject to epigenetic regulation via imprinting. The region contains the loci for two neurological diseases, Prader-Willi syndrome and Angelman syndrome (see text). When inherited from the father, gene expression occurs from the Prader-Willi locus *(blue arrow)*, and this also inactivates genes at the Angelman locus via a presumed antisense-RNA mechanism *(dashed arrow)*. In contrast, when inherited from the mother, a specific site on the chromosome called the *imprinting center (circle)* becomes methylated (Me). This methylation causes transcriptional inactivation of the genes within the Prader-Willi locus *(X)*, which correspondingly allows transcription from genes at the Angelman locus *(pink arrow)*. If imprinting does not properly occur, either Angelman or Prader-Willi syndrome will arise depending on whether the maternal or paternal expression pattern is absent. **B,** Uniparental disomy. During gamete/zygote formation, errors in chromosomal segregation or chromosomal rearrangement can result in retention of all or part of a chromosome inherited from the same parent. Although there is no loss of genetic information, the epigenetic imprinting pattern is lost, and therefore correct gene expression patterns are not retained. For chromosome 15q11-q13, for example, this can give rise to Angelman or Prader-Willi syndrome depending on whether the duplicated chromosome is that of the father or the mother, respectively.

different (heterodisomic). In families where the parents lack underlying chromosomal abnormalities, these events usually occur spontaneously and are unlikely to recur. Disease can result from effects related to loss of chromosomal imprinting, pairing of an autosomal recessive mutation, pairing of an X-linked recessive mutation in a female child, or from the generation of a mosaic trisomy. The disorders most commonly associated with this mechanism are the Prader-Willi and Angelman syndromes, discussed previously for imprinting disorders, which can arise from maternal and paternal uniparental disomy, respectively, due to a loss of the imprinting pattern from the missing parental allele. Down syndrome can also rarely result from a mosaic trisomy. There are several examples in the literature of single cases where an autosomal recessive disease arose in a child from uniparental disomy pairing an abnormal allele from a carrier parent, including disorders such as abetalipoproteinemia, Bloom syndrome, autosomal recessive deafness-1A, spinal muscular atrophy, cystic fibrosis, and others (Zlotogora, 2004).

Common Neurological Disorders and Complex Disease Genetics

To this point, we have focused on Mendelian neurological disease, in which mutations of a single gene are sufficient to cause disease. Neurological diseases with Mendelian inheritance are rare in most populations, and account for less than 5% of those with common conditions such as Alzheimer dementia. Yet, many of the common neurological diseases seen worldwide have significant genetic contributions (**Table 40.4**). For example, twin studies have shown high heritability (≥60%) for Alzheimer dementia (Gatz et al., 2006) and autism (Abrahams and Geschwind, 2008; Freitag, 2007), increased relative risk is seen in first-degree relatives of probands with ALS (approximately 10-fold) (Fang et al., 2009) and epilepsy (about 2.5-fold) (Helbig et al., 2008), and a variety of studies support a degree of heritability in PD (Belin and Westerlund, 2008) and cerebrovascular disease (Matarin et al., 2010). But even when family history is present, the mode of inheritance is not clear, and no major disease-causing Mendelian mutations are usually identified in the majority of cases. So in contrast to the single-gene Mendelian disorders previously discussed, these common complex genetic conditions appear to be genetically heterogeneous and multifactorial, likely involving interplay between multiple genes, each with small effect size, and environmental factors, none of which are

sufficient to be causal, but each of which increases susceptibility to the disorder. This is the basis of the "common disease–common variant" (CDCV) model, which has driven most research into common genetic diseases (Schork et al., 2009). The alternative model is that rather than common SNPs, multiple inherited rare variants of small to intermediate effect size or de novo mutations with large effect size underlie genetic risk for common disorders. The difficulty with assessing this latter proposition is that until the very recent advent of efficient whole genome or whole exome sequencing, genome-wide identification of such rare variants was not feasible. In contrast, efficient genome-wide assessment of common variation has been possible for several years and has been applied to numerous neurological disorders (**Table 40.5**). Still, the true nature of the type of genetic variation underlying most complex disease is not known, but major advances are being made. Here we discuss the strategies currently being used, starting with genome-wide screening for common variation.

Common Variants and Genome-Wide Association Studies

As already discussed, genetic linkage provides a means of localizing a disease gene to a specific region of a chromosome by using a DNA marker that tracks with affected individuals within families. Linkage analysis, while not without value in genetically complex disease, is less powered than genetic association studies for identification of common variation in complex genetic disease. Genetic association studies assess whether one or more of a defined set of genetic variants are increased or decreased in a disease versus a control population. If a genetic variant is observed in individuals with disease significantly more often or less than expected by chance, that variant is said to be associated with the disease. When one or a few genes are studied, this is a candidate gene association study. When common variants from across the entire genome are studied in this manner, the result is a genome-wide association study, or GWAS (Mullen et al., 2009; Simon-Sanchez

Table 40.4 Estimated Heritability of Selected Neurological Diseases

Disease	Heritability*	Method	Reference
Alzheimer dementia	60%-80%	Twin studies	(Gatz et al., 2006)
Amyotrophic lateral sclerosis	9.7 RR[†]	Familial aggregation data	(Fang et al., 2009)
Autism	70%-90%	Twin studies	(Abrahams and Geschwind, 2008)
Epilepsy	80%[‡]	Twin study	(Kjeldsen et al., 2003)
Frontotemporal dementia	42%[§]	Family history data	(Rohrer et al., 2009)
Ischemic stroke	1.75 RR	Family history data	(Flossmann et al., 2004)
Multiple sclerosis	25%-76%	Twin studies	(Hawkes and Macgregor, 2009)
Parkinson disease	6 RR (onset ≤ 50 years)	Twin study	(Vaughan et al., 2001)
Restless legs syndrome	40%-90%	Twin studies	(Caylak, 2009)

RR, Relative risk among family members.

*Unless otherwise indicated, percent heritability refers to the proportion of variation attributable to genetic causes.

[†]Among first degree relatives.

[‡]Varies per syndrome.

[§]Estimation based on likelihood of having an affected family member.

Table 40.5 Selected Genome-Wide Association Studies of Neurological Disease

Year	Study	PubMed ID	Discovery Cohort Cases/Controls	Replication Cohort Cases/Controls	Genotyping Platform	Total SNPs*	Locus	Associated SNP†	P Value	Closest Gene(s)‡	Minor Allele Frequency§	Odds Ratio‖	95% CI‖
ALZHEIMER DEMENTIA													
2010	Seshadri et al.	20460622	3006 / 14,642	6505 / 13,532	Affymetrix and Illumina	2.5 million	19q13.32	rs2075650	1.00×10^{-295}	APOE	0.14	2.53	[2.41-2.66]
2009	Harold et al.	19734902	3941 / 7848	2023 / 2340	Illumina	529,000	19q13.32	rs2075650	1.80×10^{-157}	APOE TOMM40	0.15	2.53	[2.37-2.71]
							8p21.1	rs11136000	8.50×10^{-10}	CLU	0.40	0.84	[0.79-0.89]
							11q14.2	rs3851179	1.30×10^{-09}	PICALM	0.37	0.85	[0.80-0.90]
2009	Lambert et al.	19734903	2032 / 5328	3978 / 3297	Illumina	537,000	1q32.2	rs6656401	3.50×10^{-09}	CR1	0.19	1.21	[1.14-1.29]
							8p21.1	rs11136000	7.50×10^{-09}	CLU	0.38	0.86	[0.81-0.90]
AMYOTROPHIC LATERAL SCLEROSIS													
2009	Van Es et al.	19734901	2323 / 9013	2532 / 5940	Illumina	293,000	19p13.11	rs12608932	2.50×10^{-14}	UNC13A	0.34	1.25	[NR]
							9p21.2	rs2814707	7.45×10^{-09}	MOBKL2B	0.23	1.22	[NR]
AUTISM													
2009	Weiss et al.	19812673	1553 affected of 1031 families	1755 trios	Affymetrix	365,000	5p15.2	rs10513025	$2.10 \times 10^{-07¶}$	SEMA5A	0.04	0.55	[NR]
2009	Wang et al.	19404256	3101 members of 780 families, 1204 / 6491	1390 members of 447 families, 108 / 540	Illumina	474,000	5p14.1	rs4307059	2.10×10^{-10}	CDH10 CDH9	0.38	1.19	[NR]
EPILEPSY (PARTIAL)													
2010	Kasperaviciute et al.	20522523	3445 / 6935	NR¶	Illumina	529,000	6q14.1	rs346291	$3.34 \times 10^{-07¶}$	AL132875.2	0.37	0.83	[0.77-0.89]
FRONTOTEMPORAL DEMENTIA													
2010	Van Deerlin et al.	19812673	515 / 2509	89 / 553	Illumina	500,000	7p21.3	rs1990622	1.08×10^{-11}	TMEM106B	0.44	0.61	[0.53-0.71]
MULTIPLE SCLEROSIS													
2010	Sanna et al.	20453840	882 / 872	1775 / 2005	Affymetrix	6.6 million	3q13.11	rs9657904	1.60×10^{-10}	CBLB	0.83	1.4	[1.27-1.57]
2009	Bahlo et al.	19525955	1618 / 3413	2256 / 2310	Illumina	302,000	6p21.32	rs9271366	7.00×10^{-184}	HLA-DRB1 METTL1	0.16	2.78	[NR]
							12q14.1	rs703842	5.40×10^{-11}	CYP27B1	0.33	0.81	[NR]

Year	Study	PMID	Discovery (cases / controls)	Replication (cases / controls)	Platform	SNPs*	Locus	SNP†	P value	Gene‡	MAF§	OR‖	95% CI
2009	De Jager et al.	19525953	2624 / 7220	2215 / 2116	Affymetrix and Illumina	2.6 million	6p21.32	rs3135388	3.80×10^{-225}	HLA-DRB1	0.22	2.75	[2.46-3.07]
							6p22.1	rs2523393	1.00×10^{-17}	HLA-B	0.41	0.78	[0.72-0.85]
							12p13.31	rs1800693	1.59×10^{-11}	TNFRSF1A	0.45	1.20	[1.10-1.31]
							1p13.1	rs2300747	3.10×10^{-10}	CD58	0.12	0.77	[0.68-0.88]
							16q24.1	rs17445836	3.73×10^{-09}	IRF8	0.19	0.80	[0.72-0.89]
							11q12.2	rs17824933	3.79×10^{-09}	CD6	0.25	1.18	[1.07-1.30]
2007	Hafler et al.	17660530	931 trios, 2431 controls	2322 / 2987	Affymetrix	335,000	6p21.32	rs3135388	8.94×10^{-81}	HLA-DRA	0.23	1.99	[1.84-2.15]
NARCOLEPSY													
2009	Hallmayer et al.	19412176	807 / 1074	1057 / 1104	Affymetrix	550,000	14q11.2	rs1154155	1.90×10^{-13}	TRA-alpha TRAJ10	0.14	1.69	[1.52-1.88]
PARKINSON DISEASE													
2009	Satake et al.	19915576	988 / 2521	612 / 14,139 321 / 1614	Illumina	435,000	4q22	rs11931074	7.35×10^{-17}	SNCA	0.42	1.37	[1.27-1.48]
							1q32	rs947211	1.52×10^{-12}	PARK16	0.48	1.30	[1.21-1.39]
							4p15	rs4538475	3.94×10^{-09}	BST1	0.36	1.24	[1.16-1.34]
2009	Simon-Sanchez et al.	19915575	1713 / 3978	3361 / 4573	Illumina	463,000	4q22.1	rs2736990	2.24×10^{-16}	SNCA	0.51	1.23	[NR]
							17q21.31	rs393152	1.95×10^{-16}	MAPT	0.18	0.77	[NR]
RESTLESS LEGS SYNDROME													
2008	Schormair et al.	18660810	628 / 1644	1835 / 3111	Affymetrix	209,000	9p23	rs4626664	5.91×10^{-10}	PTPRD	0.12	1.44	[1.31-1.59]
2007	Stefansson et al.	17634447	306 / 15,664	311 / 1895	Illumina	307,000	6p21.2	rs3923809	2.00×10^{-12}	BTBD9	0.66	1.8	[1.50-2.10]
2007	Winkelmann et al.	17637780	401 / 1644	1158 / 1178	Affymetrix	237,000	2p14	rs2300478	3.41×10^{-28}	MEIS1	0.24	1.74	[1.57-1.92]
							6p21.2	rs9296249	3.99×10^{-18}	BTBD9	0.24	1.67	[1.49-1.89]
							15q23	rs12593813	1.06×10^{-15}	MAP2K5	0.33	1.5	[1.36-1.66]
STROKE													
2009	Ikram et al.	19369658	1544 / 19,602	215 / 2430 652 / 3613	Affymetrix and Illumina	2.2 million	12p13.33	rs12425791	1.10×10^{-09}	NINJ2	0.19	1.29	[1.19-1.41]

Data obtained from a public database (Hindorff, L.A., Junkins, H.A., Hall, P.N., et al., 2010. A Catalog of Published Genome-Wide Association Studies. Available at: www.genome.gov/gwastudies/. Accessed July 2010.), as well as review of the primary publications. Studies are listed by year of publication and first author. Studies without replication cohorts and SNPs whose P values were not below an arbitrary threshold of 1.0×10^{-08} were excluded. Multiple discovery and replication cohorts are separated by commas. Note that some authors of more recent studies did not report significant associations with well-established loci, so readers are referred to the original publications to confirm any lack of association.

*Approximate number of SNPs used for association analysis following quality control filtering.

†If multiple SNPs from a single locus were significantly associated with disease, only the strongest is shown.

‡Closest gene as suggested by study authors.

§When multiple allele frequencies were reported, the minor allele frequency for largest control population is listed.

‖When multiple odd ratios were reported, the ratio for the combined discovery and replication groups is listed.

¶Included because of high interest within their respective fields.

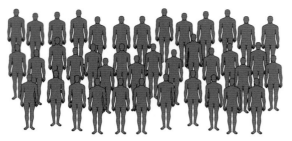

#1 Select population (cases and controls) for study

#2 Genotyping

Single Nucleotide Polymorphism (SNP)
...ACGTCAGTGGCATA...Major allele
...ACGTCAGTCGCATA...Minor allele

#3 Analysis – Is either SNP associated with disease phenotype?

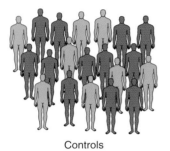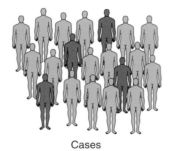

Controls   Cases

Patients with major allele are more likely to have disease
odds ratio > 1.0

Fig. 40.12 Genome-wide association study (GWAS). A GWAS for disease is performed by genotyping a selected population of cases and controls using microarray or other technology for single nucleotide polymorphisms (SNPs) across the genome. In this example, a sample SNP is depicted, with major and minor alleles illustrated as green or red, respectively. Detailed computational analysis is performed to determine whether any individual SNPs are associated with the disease state greater than by chance. In this example, the major allele *(green)* is associated with the disease and more likely to be present in cases than controls, reflected in an odds ratio above 1.0. Note that while the SNP in question may be involved in the disease, it may also be a marker near an involved gene.

the interplay of effects caused by common polymorphisms in multiple genes, as well as environmental and other factors. The aim of a GWAS is to identify these *common variants* that correlate to risk for the disease in question but do not alone cause the disease. Because the effect size, or increase in odds for a disease, is expected to be small (negative selection would have removed strongly deleterious variants from the population), and many independent genetic markers are tested, large sample sizes are needed to have power to detect genome-wide association. This is further compounded by two of the many major factors challenging GWASs of common neurological diseases, phenotypic and genetic heterogeneity. *Phenotypic heterogeneity* describes the wide and variable clinical spectrum patients with a particular neurological disorder or syndrome (e.g., frontotemporal dementia, epilepsy, multiple sclerosis, autism) manifest. *Genetic heterogeneity* refers to the notion that even in those with a relatively homogeneous phenotype, many different genetic factors may be contributing in different individuals to lead to the same phenotype. Both of these forms of heterogeneity require large samples to have adequate power to detect genetic risk factors of even moderate size. The smaller the effect of any given genetic variant, the larger the sample size needed to detect that variant. One strategy that may increase power is to study intermediate phenotypes, or *endophenotypes*, that may be more related to individual genetic risk factors than the broad clinical diagnosis of a disorder, such as specific measures of language or social behavior in autism (Abrahams and Geschwind, 2008; Alarcon et al., 2008; Vernes et al., 2008). Alternatively, such phenotypes can be used to identify more homogeneous subgroups of patients, such as those with specific forms of pathology, as in TAR DNA-binding protein (TDP-43) inclusion-positive frontotemporal dementia (FTD), which may have improved power in a recent FTD GWAS by reducing heterogeneity (Van Deerlin et al., 2010).

Efficiently generating the extensive genotype data necessary for a GWAS has been made possible using microarray technology (Coppola and Geschwind, 2006; Geschwind, 2003). In this type of experiment, specific fragments of DNA corresponding to the sequences of the target SNPs are immobilized in a grid pattern across a glass slide, termed the *array*. Genomic DNA from individual cases and controls is fluorescently labeled, hybridized to the slide, and the signals from laser-induced dye excitation are collected. The readout will be a map of the SNP pattern for each patient. Data cleaning, quality control, and statistical analysis are performed to determine whether any SNPs are associated with patients more than controls. Given the large number of independent tests performed in a GWAS, statistical significance is commonly set at 5×10^{-8} (McCarthy et al., 2008; Wellcome Trust Case Control Consortium, 2007) to correct for multiple comparisons. It is now also considered standard to demonstrate that any statistically significant association identified is present in more than one study population, providing an independent replication of the initial finding. Study power and replication may also both be aided by the availability of shared GWAS data (**Box 40.1**).

Recently published genome-wide association studies of interest involving neurological disease are shown in **Table 40.5**. One example illustrating the use of a GWAS in complex disease is from a 2009 study by Ikram and colleagues, who performed a GWAS using a population of 19,602 white persons, of whom 1544 had strokes (Ikram et al., 2009). They

and Singleton, 2008) (**Fig. 40.12**). Original genetic association studies were conducted with a small number of candidate genes, but advances in technology have permitted GWAS in thousands of subjects in a wide variety of human diseases, including dozens of neurological conditions (see **Table 40.5**). Although the SNPs themselves may directly influence the disease under study, most often this is not the case, and SNPs are best thought of as markers for the location of a gene(s) or region relevant to the disease. In fact, most alleles of the second major type of common genetic variation, CNVs, are mostly captured by SNPs (Conrad et al., 2010) and can be identified by the common SNP genotyping platforms, allowing GWASs to evaluate the contribution of common inherited CNVs as well as SNPs.

The model that underlies the value of GWAS is based on the concept that common disease is predicted to arise from

Box 40.1 **Genetic Data Repositories and Data Sharing**

Sharing genetic data is very important, and this is emphasized clearly in relation to genome-wide association study (GWAS) data which, because it is produced on common platforms typing essentially the same genetic variation in multiple populations, has great value beyond its original intended purpose. By sharing this data, other researchers have the opportunity to virtually perform GWAS analysis on populations they would not necessarily be able to evaluate. Since large sample sizes increase the power of GWAS, and few single groups can recruit enough patients for a well powered GWAS, this permits pooling and reanalysis of data collected in many laboratories on a single neuropsychiatric disease such as schizophrenia (e.g., Purcell et al., 2009; The International Schizophrenia Consortium at http://pngu.mgh.harvard.edu/isc/). It also permits study across diseases that may share common etiologies, such as amyotrophic lateral sclerosis and frontotemporal dementia (van Es et al., 2009) or autism and schizophrenia (e.g., Cantor and Geschwind, 2008; Psychiatric GWAS Consortium at https://pgc.unc.edu/index.php).

Additionally, the population could be resorted based on other known variables, SNPs could be excluded or grouped during analysis, different methods of analysis could be applied to the raw data, or data from individual members could be extracted for use in other studies (Purcell et al., 2009). Because of the benefits of this versatility, many funding organizations, including the National Institutes of Health, and major scientific journals, such as Nature and Science, have policies in place for investigators to make GWAS data available to other researchers. In some cases, disease-specific repositories have been established for the purpose of sharing both the biomaterials and genetic information, such as the Autism Genetic Resource Exchange (AGRE at http://www.agre.org/) and the NIMH Human Genetics Initiative repository (https://www.nimhgenetics.org/nimh_human_genetics_initiative/).

identified two intergenic SNPs on chromosome 12p13 with significant genome-wide association for total stroke implicating the NINJ2 gene, which is a cell-adhesion molecule found in radial glia (Ikram et al., 2009). Replication in an independent cohort confirmed the association of one SNP with a combined hazard ratio of 1.29 for ischemic stroke in white persons (Ikram et al., 2009). The mechanism of how NINJ2 increases risk for ischemic stroke is unclear at this time, but the results of this GWAS open up a new avenue of research by highlighting it as a candidate for future molecular and cellular studies into stroke etiology.

GWASs can also contribute to the discovery of biological pathways relevant to disease, as seen in a recent study of FTD patients grouped pathologically by the presence of TDP-43 inclusions. The study identified a susceptibility locus on chromosome 7p21.3 that contained a previously uncharacterized transmembrane protein, TMEM106B (Van Deerlin et al., 2010).

Similarly, for the most common neurodegenerative dementia, Alzheimer dementia, recent GWASs have benefited from large numbers of available cases and expanded the loci known to be associated with disease beyond the apolipoprotein E locus to include other neuronal molecules such as BIN1 and

PICALM, which are involved in clathrin-mediated endocytosis and intracellular trafficking, and the apolipoprotein, CLU (Harold et al., 2009; Lambert et al., 2009; Seshadri et al., 2010). In Parkinson disease, recent GWASs in large cohorts of European and Japanese patients identified alpha-synuclein (SNCA) and LRRK2 as susceptibility loci (Edwards et al., 2010; Satake et al., 2009; Simon-Sanchez et al., 2009), which is notable because both genes also give rise to autosomal dominant forms of parkinsonism. The tau protein (MAPT), another gene responsible for autosomal dominant forms of parkinsonism, was also found to be associated with disease in European populations (Edwards et al., 2010; Simon-Sanchez et al., 2009). Together these results suggest a commonality between Mendelian and sporadic forms of this disorder.

It is important that physicians have a clear understanding of the meaning of GWAS results so as to be able to differentiate common variants associated with disease from disease-causing mutations. A potential error to be avoided in the clinical interpretation of GWAS data is directly equating the findings to the future development of the disease. It must be reiterated that the finding of an association with a common variant does not equal the finding of a disease gene. By definition, these common variants must have low penetrance, otherwise they would not be so common in normal individuals, and they would likely act in a more Mendelian way. Furthermore, such variants might be associated with disease modifiers—for example, genes acting either upstream or downstream in pathways where disruption or dysregulation can lead to the disease, or perhaps genes involved in the production or regulation of factors involved in such pathways. Instead of directly causing disease, such modifier genes confer a risk of disease, the magnitude of which is sometimes not directly quantifiable because it involves interaction with other genes and the environment. Therefore, for most conditions, reported GWAS information cannot be directly translated into a clinical setting, because the presence of the variant does not necessarily lead to the disease in most cases, particularly for the more rare disorders. As an example, one of the strongest and best-known identified associations, the apolipoprotein E ε4 allele detected in sporadic AD, with an odds ratio of 4 (Coon et al., 2007), has such an inconsistent predictive value that it is not recommended for routine use in disease prediction nor as a typical part of most clinical dementia evaluations (Knopman et al., 2001). Despite this, some commercial organizations have begun to create direct-to-consumer tests for genetic variation associated with disease. As the public has become more aware of the impact of genetics on health and disease, there has been a growing desire for preemptive screening, particularly for individuals with family members afflicted with common disease. In response to this need, genetic variation screening tests are often marketed as a means of assessing the potential for future development of disease. Given the caveats discussed, there is no definitive means at present to accurately define an individual's risk of disease based on the presence of one or more associated common variants. It is important for the physician to be aware of this insofar as patients may contact them regarding such testing, and it should be emphasized that any positive results would have unclear predictive value.

Perhaps even more vexing is the fact that most genetic risk factors identified in GWASs are of very small effect sizes, ranging from a relative risk of 1.1 to 1.3, so the clinical consequences of having such a single variant in an individual patient is likely minor. The hope is that by combining many such variants, a clinically relevant risk profile can be developed.

There are examples of clinically important allelic variants identified by other methods, so such expectations for GWAS in neurological disease are not unfounded. One such illustration is the variation seen in the cytochrome P450 isoenzyme, CYP2C9, which is responsible for the metabolism of a number of clinically relevant pharmaceutical agents, in particular the anticoagulant, warfarin (Sanderson et al., 2005). The major allele, CYP2C9*1, is seen in more than 95% of Asian and African populations, but multiple variants commonly exist in European and Caucasian populations, including CYP2C9*2 and CYP2C9*3, both of which reduce warfarin metabolism (Sanderson et al., 2005). In one study, 20% of patients carried either CYP2C9*2 or CYP2C9*3 and required a mean reduction of their warfarin dosage by 27% to maintain an optimal therapeutic range, reflected by an increased relative risk of bleeding of about 2.3 (Sanderson et al., 2005). Although the relative risk in this example is still greater than typically seen in most GWASs, it demonstrates how common variant risk information can potentially affect the care of an individual patient. As we discover more regarding the nature of complex genetic disease, new ways of utilizing this information clinically will likely be determined. In the meantime, the value of GWAS data, especially from a pharmacogenomic research perspective, is significant; it can help identify new genes, pathways, and biological networks related to disease that may have therapeutic benefit (**Box 40.2**).

Rare Variants and Candidate Gene Resequencing

So far, common variation is only able to explain a small percentage of genetic risk for common neurological disease. The other major model that attempts to explain what is currently referred to as the missing heritability (Manolio et al., 2009) in complex genetic disease implicates rare variants with medium to high penetrance instead of more common ones with low penetrance (Schork et al., 2009) (**Fig. 40.13**). *Rare variants* are defined as DNA alterations that are found in less than 1% of most populations or, in some cases, are "private" and only seen in specific affected families. In this model, one or more rare variants, alone or in combination with common variants, produce the disease in question. A GWAS is not well suited to detect these variants, because they are rare and most likely to be relatively recent mutations that do not segregate on common haplotypes measured in these studies. Even when they do, they do not occur in high enough frequency in the general population to provide statistical power for their detection using current sample sizes. Detection generally requires resequencing of potentially involved candidate genes in a defined population of patients and controls. One major difficulty of such investigations is that the baseline level of rare variation among normal humans is not clearly established. Studies such as the 1000 Genomes Project (http://www.1000genomes.org/) are attempting to catalog normal human variation within the 0.1% to 1% range, so researchers will be able to better define this class of rare

variants and develop more effective strategies for their detection.

An example of this approach involves the developmental disorder, autism, where sequencing of the gene, contactin-associated protein-like 2 (CNTNAP2), in 635 patients with autism spectrum disorder (ASD) and 942 controls found 13 rare variants unique to patients, including one which was seen in 4 patients from 3 unrelated families (Bakkaloglu et al., 2008). Recessively inherited mutations in CNTNAP2 in an Amish family with a syndromic form of autism with epilepsy provided the most convincing evidence for the causal role of mutations in this gene (Strauss et al., 2006). Interestingly, this same gene illustrates that the common disease–rare variant and common disease–common variant hypotheses are not mutually exclusive, since common variants in this gene modulate language function in ASD and other conditions (Alarcon et al., 2008; Vernes et al., 2008). Exciting advances in DNA sequencing (see Whole Genome/Exome Sequencing in Disease Gene Discovery) will allow us to finally analyze many whole genomes and understand to what extent common and/or rare variants contribute to many common neurological diseases.

Box 40.2 **Pharmacogenetics and Personalized Medicine**

In addition to contributing to disease susceptibility, genetic variation can have other medically applicable roles. One of the most highly anticipated benefits for genetic research is the capability of tailoring medical or pharmacological therapies to target a patient's disease based on their individual genotype, the so-called concept of personalized medicine. The initial application of this concept is in the optimization of drug effects and minimization of toxic side effects based on genotype, termed pharmacogenetics (Holmes et al., 2009). Although this field has not yet advanced to the point of routine clinic use, there are examples of the potential utility and the benefit to patients we may hope to see in the near future. In the management of stroke, genetic variation has been found to impact patient response to antiplatelet agents and anticoagulants (Meschia, 2009; see main text) and influence statin-associated myopathy (Link et al., 2008; Meschia, 2009). In a recent GWAS analysis, 85 patients with myopathy were identified from an initial group of over 12,000 patients taking simvastatin, and association was demonstrated in both this cohort and a large replication cohort with a SNP in the SLCO1B1 gene (Link et al., 2008). SLCO1B1 encodes a membrane protein that mediates liver uptake of various drugs including statins, and in the presence of the associated SNP, the odds ratio for myopathy was 4.3 when heterozygous and 17.4 when homozygous (Link et al., 2008), clearly reflecting a need to modify statin treatment in such patients.

A number of practical issues will have to be solved before such testing can achieve widespread use in the clinic, particularly determinations of the clinical benefit and cost-effectiveness in specific diseases and populations (Holmes et al., 2009; Meschia, 2009; Swen et al., 2007); however, recent rapid advancements in technology, such as next-generation DNA sequencing, may prove beneficial in this arena.

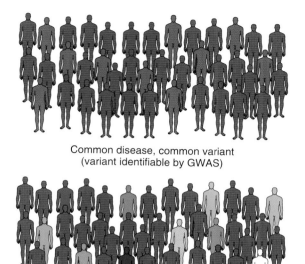

Common disease, common variant
(variant identifiable by GWAS)

Common disease, rare variant
(variant too rare to be identifiable by GWAS)

Fig. 40.13 Models of causal variants in complex disease. In the common disease–common variant model, risk of disease is imparted by the presence of one or more gene variants present in 5% or more of the population *(red)*. Such variants are amendable to detection by genome-wide association studies (GWAS). Conversely, in the common disease–rare variant model, disease is caused by rare genetic variants present in less than 1% of the population or only in specific families *(various colors)*. Such variants would not be amendable to detection by GWAS, since they would not be represented in large enough numbers to generate statistical significance. Note that both models are not mutually exclusive, and both may contribute to common disease.

Copy Number Variation and Comparative Genomic Hybridization

The majority of variation and disease-causing mutations discussed to this point have centered around single base pair changes in DNA sequence. However, as previously described in Structural Chromosomal Abnormalities and Copy Number Variation, the CNV (Beckmann et al., 2007; Stankiewicz and Lupski, 2010; Wain et al., 2009; Zhang et al., 2009) (**Fig. 40.14**) actually represents more total real estate in our genome. Advances in methods such as the advent of the microarray

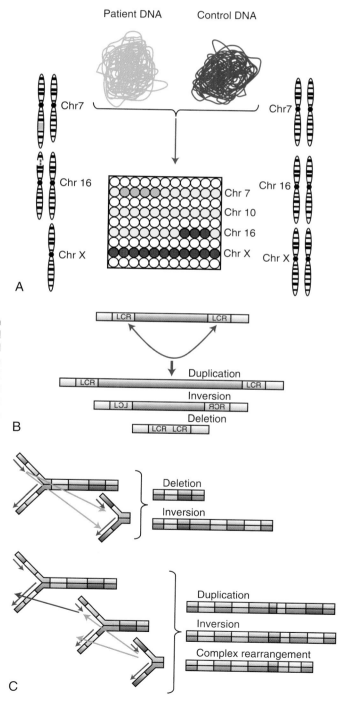

Fig. 40.14 Copy number variation (CNV). **A,** Copy number variation can be detected via comparative genomic hybridization or chromosomal microarray analysis, shown here. In this example, patient genomic DNA and an equal amount of control DNA is hybridized to a microarray platform containing representative probes spanning the genome at a specified resolution, usually at the kilobase level. In the illustration, patient DNA is fluorescently labeled green, and control DNA is labeled red. Following hybridization, regions present in equal amounts are yellow, whereas regions duplicated in the patient are green, and deletions are red. In this example, the patient possesses two CNVs, a duplication on chromosome 7 (illustrated by the increased green signal at that locus on the array) and a deletion on chromosome 16 (with corresponding increased red signal at the locus). The patient also has Turner syndrome (monosomy X) reflected by the increased red signal across the entire chromosome. Chromosome 10 is shown as an example of a chromosome that does not differ between the samples *(yellow)*. **B,** Introduction of CNV by the nonallelic homologous recombination (NAHR) mechanism. NAHR occurs when genomic instability is introduced by the presence of low copy repeat (LCR) regions greater than 1 kilobase in size with more than 90% homology. Pairing of nearby regions during DNA replication can lead to deletions, duplications, or inversions as illustrated. **C,** Introduction of CNVs by the fork stalling and template switching (FoSTeS) mechanism. FoSTeS occurs when replication on the lagging strand stalls during DNA replication and resumes at an adjacent replication fork. The structural variation introduced depends on whether the reinitiation occurs upstream or downstream of the original fork and whether it occurs on the lagging or leading strand. Examples of how deletions, duplications, or inversions might result are shown *(orange arrows)*. Furthermore, if more than one FoSTeS event occurs *(purple arrow)*, a complex structural rearrangement could result.

indicate that such changes occur quite commonly (at 10^{-4} to 10^{-6} per locus per generation) compared to single nucleotide changes (10^{-8} per base pair per generation on average) (Lupski, 2007). Overall, CNVs are estimated to represent at least 4% (Conrad et al., 2010) and potentially up to 13% of the total human genome (Redon et al., 2006; Stankiewicz and Lupski, 2010). The high frequency of these events may reflect an evolutionary advantage of CNVs as a mechanism for producing genetic diversity (Zhang et al., 2009) but also implies that clinically relevant CNVs are quite likely to occur de novo more frequently than point mutations (**Table 40.6**). CNVs can potentially cause disease in numerous ways, including disruption of a gene's coding region (which could cause a dominant effect or release a recessive effect on the homologous allele) or by altering regulated gene expression via positive or negative dosage effects. If the CNV itself results in the disease phenotype, it could be transmitted as a Mendelian disorder, as is the case for Charcot-Marie-Tooth type 1A. Such CNVs may be examples of rare variants in the common disease model. Alternatively, their contribution may be more subtle and insidious, with low penetrance and variable expressivity contributing to the risk of a complex genetic disease, such as in autism (Bucan et al., 2009).

CNVs can be detected via essentially the same microarray technology used to detect SNPs, with only a few minor adjustments. In this case, DNA probes corresponding to specific chromosomal regions are placed on an array and hybridized with differentially fluorescent-labeled genomic DNA from the individual being studied and from a reference genomic DNA sample, a technique termed *array comparative genomic hybridization* (CGH) (also called *chromosomal microarray analysis*) (see **Fig. 40.14, A**). The average ratio of fluorescence is normalized across the array and then evaluated for each probe. If both samples hybridize to a given probe equally, the corresponding DNA region is present equally in both samples. However, if the DNA sample being studied hybridizes more or less intensely than the reference sample, it must contain either more or less of the chromosomal region in question, thus indicating a copy number variation at that location. The minimum size of a CNV that can be detected by this method is limited to the genomic distance between the minimum number of probes needed to observe a statistically significant signal change, but is usually on the order of kilobases for the highest resolution arrays. The same microarrays used to genotype SNPs in GWASs may also be used to detect CNVs, incorporating both intensity and inheritance data. Array CGH essentially produces a molecular karyotype capable of detecting genomic structural changes with much finer detail than routine microscopic methods. In most major diagnostic labs, this method has replaced microscopic karyotyping and FISH, the latter of which is now used for confirmation.

Some examples of clinically relevant copy number variations are seen in Mendelian disorders including adult-onset autosomal dominant leukodystrophy (autosomal dominant, caused by duplication of the lamin B1 gene on chromosome 5), Charcot-Marie-Tooth type 1A (autosomal dominant, most frequently caused by duplication of the peripheral myelin protein 22 on chromosome 17), hereditary liability to pressure palsies (autosomal dominant, most commonly due to deletion of the peripheral myelin protein 22 on chromosome 17), spastic paraplegia type 4 (autosomal dominant, occasionally caused by deletion of the spastin gene on chromosome 2),

juvenile PD 2 (autosomal recessive, occasionally caused by deletions or duplications in parkin on chromosome 6), and Williams syndrome (autosomal dominant, caused by deletion of several contiguous genes on chromosome 7).

CNVs are also particularly important for neurodevelopmental disorders, with de novo CNVs present in more than 5% of patients with intellectual disability (ID) (Koolen et al., 2009) or ASD (Bucan et al., 2009; Marshall et al., 2008; Pinto et al., 2010; Sebat et al., 2007). Based on these findings, array CGH is now clinically indicated in children with a wide range of neurodevelopmental disabilities including ID and ASD (Miller DT et al., 2010). These studies also revealed several potential new autism candidate genes as well as novel biological pathways for future study of disease pathogenesis (Bucan et al., 2009; Pinto et al., 2010). Remarkably, de novo CNVs are also associated with schizophrenia (Stefansson et al., 2008; Walsh et al., 2008), especially childhood-onset forms, and some of the same CNVs observed in ASD are also observed in schizophrenia (Cantor and Geschwind, 2008), suggesting some shared liability between what were previously considered clinically distinct conditions.

Whole Genome/Exome Sequencing in Disease Gene Discovery

The identification of disease genes and their mutations hinges on the capability to sequence DNA to assess for detrimental alterations. The standard method of DNA sequencing technology currently in use is called *Sanger sequencing*. Although effective and accurate, the high throughput of this method is severely limited by reaction time and length of read, which is less than 1 kilobase. Recently, another new technology has been developed, termed *next-generation sequencing* (NextGen) (Metzker, 2010), that can rapidly generate large amounts of high-quality DNA sequence information in a relatively inexpensive and efficient manner (**Table 40.7**). The sequence of the human genome was derived using Sanger sequencing over a 13-year period, and subsequent Sanger sequencing of human genomes took roughly a year, but next-generation sequencing can currently accomplish the same feat in weeks. Therefore, it is now possible to rapidly interrogate an individual patient's DNA on a genome-wide level for unknown disease-causing mutations. Several different technologies exist under the next-generation sequencing umbrella and cannot be fully described here (for details, see Metzker, 2010). The same technology can also be applied to mRNA to study gene expression and/or alternative splicing on a genome-wide basis. This technology has dramatically reduced the cost of sequencing an entire genome to less than 1% of the cost of Sanger technology (Metzker, 2010), and this is expected to reach a level comparable to current clinical testing, such as Sanger sequencing–based genetic panels, in the near future. Questions regarding data storage, analysis, and quality control, as well as translation to a clinical setting, still remain but will hopefully be answered soon, allowing the integration of the technology into the clinician's repertoire (Geschwind and Konopka, 2009). The clinical utility of this approach was demonstrated recently by Lupski and colleagues, who sequenced the whole genome of the proband in a family with a previously undiagnosed form of Charcot-Marie-Tooth (CMT) disease type 1 (Lupski et al., 2010). By comparing the proband's genome sequence to

Table 40.6   Selected Neurologic Diseases Caused by Copy Number Variation

Disease	Locus	Variation	Gene*	Inheritance†
Alzheimer dementia	21q21	Duplication	APP	Complex
Amyotrophic lateral sclerosis	5q12.2-q13.3	Deletion	SMN1	Complex
Angelman syndrome	15q11-q12	Maternal deletion	UBE3A	Sporadic
Aniridia	11p13	Deletion	AN	Sporadic
Ataxia with oculomotor apraxia type 2	9q34.13	Deletion	SETX	Mendelian
Autism spectrum disorder	2p16.3	Deletion	NRXN1	Complex
	15q11-q13	Deletion or duplication	Many	Complex, sporadic
	16p11.2	Deletion or duplication	Many	Complex, sporadic
	22q13.3	Deletion	SHANK3	Complex
	Xp22.33	Deletion	NLGN4	Complex
Autosomal dominant leukodystrophy	5q23.2	Duplication	LMNB1	Mendelian
Charcot-Marie-Tooth type 1A	17p12	Duplication	PMP22	Mendelian
Charcot-Marie-Tooth type 4B2	11p15.4	Deletion	SBF2	Mendelian
CHARGE syndrome	8q12.1	Deletion	CHD7	Sporadic
Cri du chat syndrome	5p15.2-p15.3	Deletion	Many	Sporadic
DiGeorge and velocardiofacial syndrome	22q11.2	Deletion	Many	Sporadic
Duchenne/Becker muscular dystrophy	Xp21.2	Deletion or duplication	DMD	Mendelian
Epilepsy	15q13.3	Deletion	CHRNA7	Complex
Hereditary neuropathy with liability to pressure palsies	17p12	Deletion	PMP22	Mendelian
Miller-Dieker syndrome	17p13.3	Deletion	LIS1	Sporadic
Neurofibromatosis type 1	17q11.2	Deletion or duplication	NF1	Sporadic
Parkinson disease	4q21	Duplication or triplication	SNCA	Mendelian
Pelizaeus-Merzbacher disease	Xq22.2	Deletion or duplication	PLP1	Mendelian
Potocki-Lupski syndrome	17p11.2	Duplication	RAI1	Sporadic
Prader-Willi syndrome	15q11-q12	Paternal deletion	Many	Sporadic
Rett syndrome & variants	Xq28	Deletion or duplication	MECP2	Sporadic
Rubinstein-Taybi syndrome	16p13.3	Deletion or duplication	CREBBP	Sporadic
Schizophrenia	2q31.2	Deletion	RAPGEF4	Complex
	2q34	Deletion	ERBB4	Complex
	5p13.3	Deletion	SLC1A3	Complex
	12q24	Deletion	CIT	Complex
Silver-Russell syndrome	11p15	Duplication	Many	Complex
Smith-Magenis syndrome	17p11.2	Deletion	RAI1	Sporadic
Sotos syndrome	5q35	Deletion	NSD1	Sporadic
Spinal muscular atrophy	5q13	Deletion	SMN1	Mendelian
Tuberous sclerosis	16p13.3	Deletion or duplication	TSC2	Sporadic
WAGR syndrome	11p13	Deletion	Many	Sporadic
Williams-Beuren syndrome	7q11.23	Deletion	ELN	Sporadic
Other microdeletion/duplication syndromes with developmental delay and/or mental retardation	1q41-q42	Deletion	Many	Sporadic
	2q37	Deletion	Many	Sporadic
	3q29	Deletion or duplication	Many	Sporadic
	7q11.23	Duplication	Many	Sporadic
	17q21.3	Deletion or duplication	Many	Sporadic
	22q11.2	Duplication	Many	Complex

Table adapted from Fanciulli et al., 2010; Lee and Scherer, 2010; Stankiewicz and Lupski, 2010; Wain et al., 2009. Additional data accessed July 2010 from the Database of Genomic Variants available at http://projects.tcag.ca/variation/; GeneTests: Medical Genetics Information Resource available at http://www.ncbi.nlm.nih.gov/sites/GeneTests/; OMIM: Online Mendelian Inheritance in Man available at http://www.ncbi.nlm.nih.gov/omim/.

*If a single causative or strong candidate gene is known. If multiple genes are suspected to be involved, this is indicated.

†Inheritance is described as sporadic if the variation typically arises de novo in patients, complex if it most commonly increases disease susceptibility (rare familial mutations may also occur), and Mendelian if it is typically inherited.

Table 40.7   Comparison of DNA-Sequencing Technologies for Genome Sequencing

	Sanger	Current Next-Generation	Projected Next-Generation
Technology	Dye-terminator	Massively parallel*	Massively parallel, single molecule
Approximate read length (bases)	500-800	50-100[†]	>1000
Current clinical use	Gene mutation analysis	Research only	Research only
Number of individual genomes sequenced and published[‡]	1[§]	10	0
Estimated cost per genome	$Millions (US)	~$10,000 (US)[‖]	~$1000 (US)
Estimated time per genome	Years	~Weeks[‖]	Days
Predicted future clinical use	Single gene mutation analysis	Whole genome/ exome sequencing	Whole genome/ exome sequencing

*A number of commercial platforms exist which utilize variations in this technology.
[†]Most common, varies per specific platform used.
[‡]As of July 2010.
[§]Not including the Human Genome Project reference genome.
[‖]Best available as of this writing.

the human genome reference sequence, over 3.4 million SNPs and 234 CNVs were detected and subsequently paired down using a more detailed analysis until compound heterozygous mutations were identified in the SH3TC2 gene on chromosome 5, a gene previously shown to cause a different form of CMT, CMT type 4C (Lupski et al., 2010). The new mutations identified within this single family revealed an unexpected level of complexity in this Mendelian disorder, suggesting that such comprehensive sequencing methods may be clinically necessary to identify novel disease-causing mutations in known disease genes if they lead to phenotypic variation.

Although extremely powerful, the challenges of data interpretation and analysis may slow the arrival of whole genome sequencing to the clinic. As an initial step in the transition of this technology to the clinical arena, a significant reduction in cost, data volume, and degree of analysis can be achieved by selecting only genomic regions containing protein-coding information for sequencing, a process called *exome sequencing* (Choi et al., 2009; Hedges et al., 2009; Ng et al., 2009). These coding sequences are initially enriched from a pool of total genomic DNA and then subjected to next-generation sequencing. Although this would be unable to detect relevant noncoding or structural events such as copy number variation, it should prove useful as a means of evaluating Mendelian dis-

orders caused by coding mutations. This has been illustrated by recent reports using this technology to detect novel mutations causing distal arthrogryposis type 2A (Freeman-Sheldon syndrome) (Ng et al., 2009), to confirm an unanticipated diagnosis of congenital chloride diarrhea (Choi et al., 2009), and to elucidate the gene underlying postaxial acrofacial dysostosis (Miller syndrome) (Ng et al., 2010).

In addition to identification of Mendelian mutations, this technology also allows for a more detailed exploration of complex genetic variation. In studies of common disease, it may prove a more effective means of assessing the contributions of rare variants than other methods such as a GWAS (Cirulli and Goldstein, 2010). Additionally, it may also identify novel types of variation such as double- and triple-nucleotide polymorphisms, which generate amino acid changes more than 90% and 99% of the time, respectively, and occur at 1% the density of SNPs (Rosenfeld et al., 2010). Future studies will have to further assess the contribution of such novel DNA changes to human disease, but the current findings confirm that next-generation sequencing technology will be able to uncover new types of functional genomic variation.

Lastly, whole genome sequencing may also provide new information regarding environmental contributions to disease. Recently, whole genome sequencing was reported from a pair of monozygotic twins who were discordant for multiple sclerosis (Baranzini et al., 2010). No significant genomic, transcriptional, or epigenetic changes were found to explain disease disconcordance among these twins (Baranzini et al., 2010), suggesting there may be other critical genetic or epigenetic factors not examined by this study, or that key differences may lie in other cell types, or that as-yet-undetermined environmental factors are contributing to disease—conclusions which would not be possible to establish without next-generation sequencing technology.

Future Role of Systems Biology in Neurogenetic Disease

The complex relationship between genetic risk variants, even when they are inherited in a Mendelian fashion, and clinical features, or the relationship of these mutations to disease pathophysiology, presents significant challenges to the use of genetics for diagnosis and therapeutics. Furthermore, the majority of studies investigating genetic disorders have focused on the discovery and molecular analysis of the disease genes themselves, as these would intuitively appear to be the most immediately useful in diagnosis and potential treatment. There are some examples, such as metabolic disease and enzyme replacement therapy (Beck, 2010), which support this practice. However, for many more diseases, including virtually all neurodegenerative disorders, knowledge of the specific causative gene has not immediately yielded new curative therapies but has instead raised many new questions regarding the underlying molecular etiology of the disease. The hope is that research into these underlying mechanisms will uncover new therapeutic targets; toward that goal, the technologies discussed have made greater amounts of information available for scientific analysis than ever before. For example, microarrays can be used to study not only genome-wide genetic variation via SNPs as described earlier but also variations in gene expression (**Fig. 40.15**). For this method, the array platform

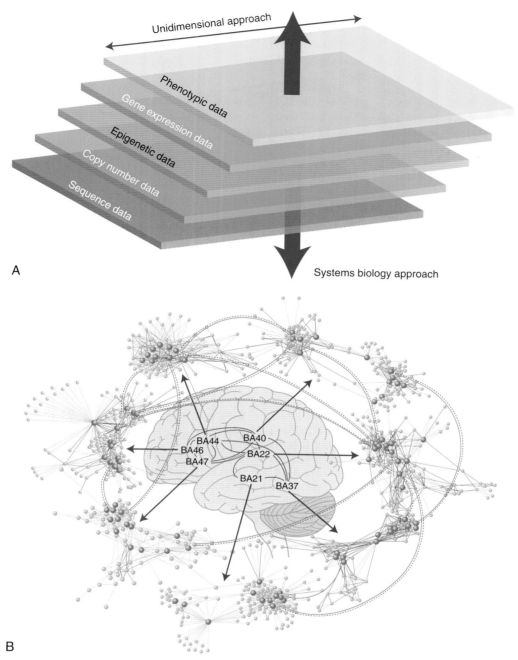

Fig. 40.15 A systems biology approach to human disease allows integration of multiple layers of data. **A,** Typical experimental approaches to neurological diseases are one dimensional, and most commonly, efforts focus on a single layer of information such as genetic data (e.g., sequence variants), genomic data (e.g., gene expression changes), or clinical data (e.g., phenotypes). The systems biology approach considers all these aspects simultaneously using comprehensive databases to explore the relationships between the individual data sets by identifying higher-level structure. This multidimensional use of the data sets (e.g., via network analysis) links the different types of information. **B,** An example using a systems-based approach to study regional gene expression in the brain, using network-based analysis and imaging data to provide insights into brain connectivity. This is a stylized visualization of the combination of diffusion tensor imaging of language areas, with gene expression and weighted gene coexpression network analysis (WGCNA) to reveal integration of gene coexpression across brain areas (BA, Brodmann area), as well as novel brain region wiring. The green lines and dashed red lines indicate information flow in both directions and can be extrapolated to suggest excitatory and inhibitory interconnections. Each gene is depicted as a node *(green or purple)*, with hub genes (those with the most connections to other genes) represented by purple nodes. Blue lines indicate positive correlations, and red lines indicate negative correlations. Lines between Brodmann areas indicate real and potential interactions through white matter tracts. This integration of network analysis, gene expression data, and imaging demonstrates relationships among key genetic factors in distinct regions and their role in regional brain connectivity in both normal individuals and those with disease. *(Originally published as Figure 3 in Geschwind, D.H., Konopka, G., 2009. Neuroscience in the era of functional genomics and systems biology. Nature 461, 908-915.)*

contains probes that are complementary to genome-wide mRNA sequences, and the study is performed by hybridizing the array with fluorescently labeled mRNA collected from either patients or controls. The intensity of the fluorescent signal can be used to determine and compare the relative levels of expression for each gene across the samples. Similar techniques can also be used to evaluate RNA splicing with probes that correspond to all the exons in a given gene and then assessing samples for their alternative usage in cases and controls. With the availability of this genome-wide data, encompassing both genetic variation and gene expression in clinically-evaluated patients and controls, it becomes possible to incorporate and synthesize the totality of this information together in ways which assess phenotype, genetic variation, and gene expression simultaneously in a more comprehensive way. This field of study, known as *systems biology*, strives to use these sets of information to develop detailed genetic pathways to identify related genes and genetic programs relevant to disease (Geschwind and Konopka, 2009) (see **Fig. 40.15**). Such integrative analysis has begun to accelerate our understanding of disease pathogenesis and generate new insights into more effective treatment strategies, which will only improve as we learn more and the techniques improve.

One example of this type of systems biology approach involves using gene expression data, such as from microarray studies, to group individual genes according to their degree of coexpression, forming functionally related gene expression modules. These modules are then graphed according to the interconnectivity of their members which produces a network of correlations centered around one or more key genes, termed *hubs*, which functionally drive the association either directly or indirectly. Further assessment of these hub genes and their connections can identify potentially important genes and biological pathways affected in disease. Such techniques have already been applied to dementia (Miller JA et al., 2008; Miller JA et al., 2010), schizophrenia (Torkamani et al., 2010), and ALS (Saris et al., 2009). These early systems biology studies illustrate the versatility of such an approach and the potential impact these studies can have on research into complex disease pathogenesis.

Environmental Contributions to Neurogenetic Disease

Although this chapter has principally dealt with the molecular aspect of neurogenetic disease, the contributions of the environment cannot be overlooked, particularly for complex genetic disease. Aside from perhaps the few Mendelian disorders with complete penetrance, all genetic disorders are likely either influenced directly by environmental factors or indirectly by the influence of the environment on other aspects of the patient's genetic background. Despite this, we still know very little regarding the precise role of the environment in the development of neurogenetic disease, and this is therefore an important area requiring further study (Reis and Roman, 2007). Monozygotic twin studies and animal studies have both indicated that environmental influences can affect the development/severity of Mendelian genetic disease, as well as more complex disorders, but precisely how this occurs in a genetically susceptible individual remains a mystery. Many suggestions have been postulated for various disorders, including exposures to diverse physical, chemical, or biological insults, but an overall comprehensive picture has yet to develop. For example, multiple sclerosis (MS) is a complex neurological disease that likely results from a combination of genetic susceptibility and environmental contributions (Handel et al., 2010) and is one of the most well-studied neurological disorders for environmental influence. Several environmental factors have been postulated to play a role in the development of multiple sclerosis. These include vitamin D levels, which may explain epidemiological findings that MS risk is associated with geographical location in childhood and month of birth; exposure to Epstein-Barr virus, which is associated with increased MS risk if it occurs after the age of 15 years; and smoking, which appears to increase MS risk and can worsen established disease course (Handel et al., 2010). If such environmental influences could be linked to specific molecular and/or cellular events that may trigger disease in genetically susceptible individuals, it would have a dramatic impact on our understanding of disease pathogenesis, our treatment of established patients, and our recommended preventive strategies to reduce disease. The influx of new genetic information identifying risk factors for complex disease is expected to stimulate research into the impact of the environment on these variants (Traynor, 2009), ideally translating into improvements in our understanding of the environmental effects on neurogenetic disease.

Genetics and the Paradox of Disease Definition

Research into the genetics of neurological disease has established an alternative standard to the clinical or pathological definition of a disease, the genetic diagnosis. However, these standards are not equivalent, and to fully understand the difference, we must consider the meaning of a genetic diagnosis. Currently, pathology is thought of as a gold standard for diagnosis, but it is not available antemortem in many cases. A clinical diagnosis is limited by the homogeneity of the disease in question and the sensitivity and specificity of its clinical features. Although genetic testing can often provide a definitive answer to diagnosis, one of the potential paradoxes that has emerged from our identification of disease genes, and subsequent clinical and pathological correlations, is that the relationship between genetic susceptibility and clinical diagnosis is far from simple. This is true for virtually all Mendelian diseases and becomes even more complicated when complex diseases are considered.

In Mendelian disorders, X-linked adrenoleukodystrophy is a prime example of this paradox. In a single family, all with the same mutation, neurological phenotypes may range from an inflammatory cerebral demyelination to a noninflammatory distal axonopathy to a behavioral phenotype similar to attention deficit hyperactive disorder or autism spectrum disorder (Moser et al., 2005), despite all family members carrying the identical genetic diagnosis. With regard to complex disease, frontotemporal dementia spectrum disorders provide another salient example, as families with the same mutations can have vastly different clinical features ranging from purely psychiatric to motor neuron disease, parkinsonism, cortical basal degeneration, progressive supranuclear palsy, or dementia, either singly or in combination (van Swieten and Heutink, 2008). A similar scenario can be observed in epilepsy, where broad seizure phenotypes are seen in some familial forms of epilepsy (Helbig et al., 2008). Conversely, identification of Mendelian mutations can lead to a broadening of disease definition, as has been the case in Friedreich ataxia, where adults with a distinct late-onset phenotype are now frequently identified (Bhidayasiri et al., 2005), or in adult polyglucosan body disease, a progressive myeloneuropathy discovered to be the adult form of glycogen storage disease type IV, which can lead to fatal liver complications in children (Lossos et al., 2009). What is further remarkable is that genetic findings in certain Mendelian forms of PD question the notion of pathology as the gold standard. Here, certain families with mutations in the LRRK2 gene lack Lewy body pathology, yet have clear dopamine-responsive PD (Zimprich et al., 2004). This raises the question as to what *is* the gold standard, as the absence of Lewy bodies would not be consistent with a pathological PD diagnosis. Seen from this perspective, it is clear that neither pathology, genetic findings, nor clinical phenotypes can be interpreted in isolation, and it is the combination of these characteristics that define a disease. As we gather more genetic information about neurological disorders in the coming years, our definitions of these diseases will certainly expand and change. Identifying disease-causing mutations and/or establishing a genetic risk profile will provide further knowledge regarding disease etiology, with implications for counseling, further diagnostic workup, and eventually for treatment—described in greater detail next.

Clinical Approach to the Patient with Suspected Neurogenetic Disease

In this chapter we have outlined the current state of clinical neurogenetics and the techniques available to neuroscientists to better understand and study genetic disease for the benefit of patients. A consistent theme has been that, in the near future, most neurological diseases will be described on a genomic level, and large amounts of detailed genetic information will become available to the clinician, particularly with the availability of whole exome and whole genome sequencing. This raises the important question of how the clinical neurologist is to synthesize all this newly available genetic information regarding Mendelian disorders and common disease and apply that to patients in the clinic on a daily basis. We hope this overview will provide some basic tools to utilize and interpret such information in a meaningful way. In this section, we will deal with the four major clinical areas impacted most by this new genetic knowledge: (1) evaluation and diagnosis, (2) genetic counseling, (3) prognosis, and (4) treatment.

Evaluation and Diagnosis

Evaluation and diagnosis benefit from the arsenal of genetic testing available for single gene disorders and for genomic variation. Many commercial laboratories offer testing for Mendelian disease genes, and in some settings, genetic testing has become as routine as other common blood tests. However, because genetic testing carries additional implications for a patient and their family, particularly with regard to heritability

Table 40.8 The Neurogenetic Evaluation and the Clinical Utilization of Genetic Testing

Establish the phenotype	All patients in whom a genetic diagnosis is suspected require a thorough physical examination and clinical history including a detailed family history. Differential diagnosis is established based on phenotype. Genetic etiologies should be considered in all cases where there is a positive family history of disease.
Rule out non-genetic etiologies	With the exception of suspected genetic diseases with known disease-modifying treatments, patients should be fully evaluated for non-genetic causes of disease prior to the initiation of genetic testing, as these are generally more amenable to treatment.
Order genetic testing based on phenotype	Genetic testing should not be used as a screening tool. Physicians suspecting a hereditary disorder but unable to arrive at a diagnostically useful clinical phenotype should refer these patients for further evaluation at a tertiary center specializing in such cases.
Use disease biomarkers when available	Cost management should be maintained through the use of biomarker testing whenever possible, with genetic testing as the confirmatory step in diagnosis to obtain the genotype for clinical trials, research studies, and genotype-phenotype clinical correlations.
Avoid genetic panels	Disease- or inheritance-based multigene panels should be discouraged in routine clinical practice, as these are not a cost-effective use of patient resources. There may, however, be a role for small focused panels in specific disorders with heterogeneous phenotypes.
Provide genetic counseling	Genetic counseling (by a physician, geneticist, or genetic counselor) should be provided to all patients for whom genetic testing is recommended. Follow-up counseling should be provided to all patients with a positive gene test and offered to family members who may be at risk or disease carriers. Any and all ethical concerns should be fully addressed.
Utilize new technology in challenging cases	Whole genome and/or exome sequencing, when clinically available, could potentially be an appropriate consideration for patients with suspected genetic disease and complete negative genetic and non-genetic evaluations.

of disease, it is important that it be used appropriately and that patients be fully educated prior to such testing. Important points to consider for genetic testing are summarized in **Table 40.8**. Although how the testing is incorporated into a clinical evaluation strategy will vary by disease, a general principle is that most genetic disease is diagnosed clinically via a thorough history (including family history) and physical examination. A complete evaluation for nongenetic causes should be performed as appropriate prior to any genetic testing so that possible treatments can be initiated in a timely manner. Genetic testing should only be used to confirm a clinical suspicion, not for screening purposes, because currently this is low yield and not cost-effective in the majority of cases. Specialist referral to a tertiary center is appropriate for all cases where a diagnostically useful clinical phenotype cannot be established. Genetic counseling (see later) should be provided, either by a physician or a licensed genetic counselor, prior to testing to ensure that patients understand the nature of the test and the possible results. When testing is ordered, it should be based on phenotype and supported by mode of inheritance if this can be determined. Testing of an asymptomatic minor is never indicated for a genetic disease where there is no treatment or cure. Knowledge of the disease status without chance for treatment may have many negative consequences.

Many companies now offer broad genetic panels based on general phenotypes or modes of inheritance for a particular symptom, which have appeal because they are simple to order and often advertised as a molecular means of differentiating between overlapping phenotypes. Unfortunately this does a disservice to the patient, since these panels can be quite costly (up to $15,000 or more) and despite being billed as complete, often test disorders with such diverse phenotypes as to make it impossible to consider both in the same individual, or they test genes so rare that only a few families are even known to possess them. The clinical examination should be used to precisely define the patient's phenotype, which will in turn suggest the most high-yield conditions for genetic testing. This systematic approach is of immense benefit in resource management.

The types of single-gene testing available vary per laboratory and gene (**Table 40.9**). The most comprehensive (and expensive) testing type is full gene sequencing, where all coding regions, as well as approximately 50 bases in each intron/exon junction, are sequenced for the presence of mutation. This will detect all coding point mutations and splice-site mutations as well as small insertions and deletions but will miss more detailed structural variation. Importantly, novel coding mutations can be detected in this way. Targeted sequence analysis (also called *select exon testing*) consists of specific sequencing reactions designed to only detect one or a few previously identified mutations. This will not detect any sequence variations outside of the limited region of the gene being searched. For repeat disorders, there are specific tests to identify the relevant expansions using either polymerase chain reaction (PCR) or Southern blotting, a hybridization-based DNA sizing technique. Larger deletions or duplications (e.g., copy number variations) can be detected by quantitative PCR methods or by comparative genomic hybridization. It is important to be aware of the type of testing being ordered; in some cases, such as select exon testing, a negative result does not exclude mutations elsewhere in the gene being tested. Interpretation of these genetic results may be straightforward, for example, if no mutations are present or if known pathogenic changes are found. In contrast, interpretation may be complicated if novel sequence variants of unknown pathological significance are identified. Inconclusive results may require interpretation by a specialist and/or further testing to determine the likelihood of pathogenicity.

Common diseases must be approached in a different manner, because detailed phenotype alone cannot always predict the mutation to test for, particularly when assessing genomic variation. Still, the goal remains to develop strategies incorporating known genetic information into a systematic

Table 40.9	Types of Genetic Testing	
Type of Test	**Sequence Variant(s) Identified**	**Sequence Variant(s) Missed or Not Accurately Determined**
Gene sequencing	Point mutations* Frameshifts Splicing mutations[†] Polymorphisms	Noncoding variants[‡] Copy number variations[§] Repeat expansions[¶]
Select exon sequencing (Targeted mutation analysis)	Known predefined variants *Target region only*[¶,#] Point mutations* Frameshifts Splicing mutations[†] Polymorphisms	*Variants outside target region*[#] Point mutations* Frameshifts Splicing mutations[†] Polymorphisms Noncoding variants[‡] Copy number variations[§] Repeat expansions[¶]
Repeat expansion testing[‖] (Targeted mutation analysis)	Repeat expansion in the specific gene tested	Point mutations* Frameshifts Splicing mutations[†] Polymorphisms Noncoding variants[‡] Copy number variations[§]
Gene copy number variation (Deletion/ duplication testing)	Copy number variation[§] of gene tested	Point mutations* Frameshifts Splicing mutations[†] Polymorphisms Noncoding variants[‡] Repeat expansions[¶]
Chromosomal microarray analysis** (Comparative genomic hybridization)	Genome-wide copy number variations[††]	Point mutations* Frameshifts Splicing mutations[†] Polymorphisms Noncoding variants[‡] Repeat expansions[¶]
Whole exome sequencing**,[‡‡]	Point mutations* Frameshifts Splicing mutations[†] Polymorphisms	Noncoding variants[‡] Copy number variations[§] Repeat expansions[¶]
Whole genome sequencing**,[‡‡]	Point mutations* Frameshifts Splicing mutations[†] Polymorphisms Noncoding variants[‡] Copy number variations[§]	Repeat expansions[¶]

*Includes missense, nonsense, and silent mutations.

[†]Includes only those involving splice sites and exonic splicing regulatory sequences.

[‡]Includes promoter mutations and noncoding splicing regulatory elements.

[§]Arbitrarily defined here as any deletion/duplication/insertion larger than detectable by Sanger sequencing.

[‖]Targeted mutation analysis using either polymerase chain reaction (PCR) and/or Southern blot is preferred, as sequencing may be inaccurate due to the large size of many repeat regions.

[¶]Only detectable if sequencing is performed as opposed to individual mutation-specific detection methods.

[#]Size and number of region(s) targeted varies per individual test.

**Genome-wide testing method.

[††]Minimum size of CNVs detected and density of genomic coverage varies per test.

[‡‡]Not yet available clinically.

protocol designed to maximize diagnostic capability while minimizing cost and unnecessary testing (Lintas and Persico, 2009). Tests such as chromosomal microarray analysis are clinically available to search genome-wide for disease-causing CNVs and are recommended for sporadic causes in disorders such as intellectual disability or autism where CNVs have been found responsible for a reasonable percentage of disease (Geschwind and Spence, 2008; Miller DT et al., 2010). Use of such testing in sporadic adult-onset disease is less clear, so the physician is advised to refer to current published guidelines for the disease in question before ordering. For more specific phenotypes, other available tests include those assessing for CNVs (often called simply *deletions/duplications*) involving individual genes or specific chromosomal regions. Overall, interpretation of CNV results can be challenging, particularly if the CNV was previously unreported. Here, the parents will often need to be evaluated to determine whether the CNV in question is inherited or de novo. As already discussed for DNA sequence changes, such findings may require interpretation by a specialist and/or further testing to determine the likelihood of pathogenicity.

Whole genome and/or whole exome sequencing are not yet routinely available in the clinic but are predicted to arrive within the next 5 years or sooner. Whole genome sequencing is the more comprehensive of the two and capable of detecting more types of mutation, as well as structural variation, but its use will hinge on the development of accurate and efficient bioinformatic techniques for translating the expected massive genomic variation per patient (millions of SNPs and hundreds of CNVs across the whole genome) into clinically meaningful results. How such a pipeline would operate has not yet been established, but we expect that the cost should be equivalent to that of an MRI study within 5 years. Incorporation of such testing into a clinical evaluation will also depend on other elements such as cost of testing and time of analysis, but these factors are not expected to vary much from methods of genetic testing currently in use.

Genetic Counseling

Establishing a precise genetic diagnosis will definitively establish the means of inheritance of a disorder and is extremely useful in genetic counseling and family planning, particularly for disorders that show incomplete penetrance. However, unlike other tests typically ordered by physicians, a positive diagnosis carries implications not only for individual patients but for the entire family. Genetic counseling, therefore, should be provided in all cases where genetic testing is recommended, either by an experienced neurologist, a geneticist, or a licensed genetic counselor. Follow-up counseling should also be provided to all patients with a positive test result and, in many cases, offered to other family members who may be at risk for disease or as carriers. Physicians must be aware of the various ethical implications involved in such testing (Ensenauer et al., 2005). One area of particular importance in this regard involves considerations of genetic testing in asymptomatic individuals, especially minors. This stems in part from concerns that have been raised regarding risks of depression and suicide in asymptomatic individuals diagnosed with fatal genetic disease, although this is not well established, and further study will be important for determining best practices. For minors, standard practice dictates that unless there is

disease-modifying therapy available for them, they should not be tested if asymptomatic until they reach an age to consent to such testing and are properly counseled as to the implications. Counseling regarding prenatal testing and assisted reproduction are other topics of relevance to patients of reproductive age. Current reproductive medicine techniques such as in vitro fertilization and preimplantation genetic testing, by assuring that offspring will not harbor the mutation in question, can aid couples concerned about the risk for passing on inherited conditions. Other ethical considerations may also apply, depending on the disease and specific family/patient circumstances.

Prognosis and Treatment

A confirmed genetic diagnosis can contribute clinically useful data concerning patient prognosis, as it allows information from published case studies to be utilized in the care of an individual patient. This can aid in the identification of specific clinical features to focus on for surveillance in the development of a particular genetic disorder, such as cognitive decline in a patient with isolated chorea found to have HD or cardiac testing in an autistic patient with chromosome 15q duplication. A genetic diagnosis may also alert the clinician to potential life-threatening comorbidities such as adrenal insufficiency in X-linked adrenoleukodystrophy or cardiomyopathy in Friedreich ataxia. Review of case studies in a particular disorder may help answer questions regarding life expectancy or future disability, such as years of disease prior to loss of ambulation in the various SCAs Lastly, there are important positive psychological aspects to establishing a definitive diagnosis, particularly for patients who have undergone many fruitless clinical evaluations.

Although the majority of genetic diseases are not curable, therapies do exist for many of them. Defining the genetic etiology of a patient's disease allows for utilization of the published literature on symptomatic treatments and pharmacotherapy that may benefit a specific condition. Phenylketonuria is an excellent example of this, since dietary restriction of phenylalanine initiated soon after birth will prevent cognitive impairment and enable virtually normal development (Burgard et al., 1999). More importantly, new clinical trials are being developed frequently and can be offered to patients with an established diagnosis. Many disease-based patient registries exist to facilitate this.

The ultimate goal of translational neuroscience is to utilize advances in our understanding of disease at the molecular level to aid in the treatment of patients in the clinic. Recent new treatments, which take advantage of the molecular aspects of these disorders, show promise in the clinic and the laboratory. Such treatments include enzyme replacement therapy for metabolic disorders such as the severe fatal glycogen storage disorder Pompe disease, where use of recombinant acid α-glucosidase in 18 infants prior to 6 months of age enabled all to live to the age of 18 months, a 99% reduction in death, as well as reduced their risk of death or invasive ventilation by 92% compared to historical controls (Kishnani et al., 2007). Work in animal models has suggested potential new pharmacological treatments, such as a recent research study which demonstrated that the use of histone-deacetylase inhibitors can unsilence expanded frataxin alleles in a Friedreich ataxia mouse model, restoring wild-type gene expression levels and reversing cellular transcription changes associated with frataxin deficiency (Rai et al., 2008). Targeted molecules have been designed to correct specific disease-causing biological defects, as shown by recent work where antisense oligonucleotides were used to block mutations that promote splicing defects in the ataxia-telangiectasia mutated (ATM) gene in cell lines from patients with ataxia-telangiectasia, leading to restoration of functional protein (Du et al., 2007). Such newer techniques may markedly exceed the therapeutic benefit of current options, such as in Duchenne muscular dystrophy where patients can expect only moderate short-term benefit (up to 2 years) from the gold standard, glucocorticosteroid treatment (Manzur et al., 2008; Wood et al., 2010). Newer molecular strategies such as dystrophin splice-modulation, which promotes exon skipping via antisense oligonucleotides to bypass point mutations or frameshifts, may potentially resolve the primary defect and has shown promising results in early clinical trials (Wood et al., 2010). Novel treatments aimed at genetic modification of disease are also in development, as was seen in a recent study where investigators used RNA interference techniques to specifically degrade and thus silence the disease allele in a rat model of SCA type 3, resulting in a reduction in neuropathological changes in the brain (Alves et al., 2008). New technologies such as next-generation sequencing and the use of systems biology approaches to disease are expected to lead to additional new innovations. With these advances, the future of clinical neurogenetics is full of promise and stands poised to answer the challenge stated most eloquently by Bernard Baruch (1870-1965): *"There are no such things as incurables; there are only things for which [medicine] has not found a cure."*

References

The complete reference list is available online at www.expertconsult.com.

Neuroimmunology

Tanuja Chitnis, Samia J. Khoury

The past decade has seen a rich interaction between the fields of neurology and immunology. This has provided further insight into the mechanisms of immunologically-mediated neurological diseases and given rise to new therapies for many neuroimmunological diseases, including multiple sclerosis (MS). To understand and effectively employ these emerging neuroimmunologically based therapies, a solid grasp of immunology is required. Here we provide an overview of the major components of the immune system and highlight important advances in the field of neuroimmunology, with a focus on relevant disease processes and treatment strategies.

Immune System

The function of the immune system is to protect the organism against infectious agents and prevent reinfection by maintaining immunological memory. Additionally, the immune system performs tumor surveillance, promotes healing, and prevents damage mediated by dying cells.

The immune system normally does not react to self-antigens, a state known as *tolerance*, except in the setting of autoimmune disease. An overactive immune system may mediate ongoing immune-mediated damage, so a delicate balance must be maintained between the protective effects of the immune system and potential deleterious effects.

The normal functions of the immune system and the disorders resulting from its dysfunction are listed in **Box 41.1**.

Adaptive and Innate Immunity

The immune system has two functional divisions: the innate immune system and the adaptive immune system. The innate immune system acts nonspecifically as the body's first line of defense against pathogens. However, this type of response, if perpetuated, would result in unwanted nonspecific damage to the host. Therefore a secondary, antigen-specific response develops and leads the attack. This is mediated by T cells and B cells, which are equipped with antigen-specific receptors. The effector cells release mediators and trigger other components of the immune system to eliminate the target. Subpopulations of T and B cells develop and maintain immunological memory, which facilitates a more rapid response in the case of recurrent infection.

The innate immune system consists of the following components:

1. Skin—The exterior surface of the body, primarily the skin, is the body's primary defense against foreign pathogens. Many inflammatory cells and

DOI: 10.1016/B978-1-4377-0434-1.00041-4

antigen-presenting cells (APCs) line the epidermis and serve as the first line of defense.

2. Phagocytes are cells capable of phagocytosing foreign pathogens. They include polymorphonuclear cells, monocytes, and macrophages. These cells are present in the blood as well as in organs. Phagocytes recognize cell components or pathogen-associated molecular patterns (PAMPs) of a variety of microorganisms through families of pattern recognition receptors (PRRs) expressed on their cell surface. PRRs allow phagocytes to attach nonspecifically and phagocytose pathogens, which are then killed via intracellular lysosomes. Families of PRRs include the Toll-like receptors (TLRs) and the nucleotide-binding oligomerization domain (NOD) receptors.

3. Natural killer (NK) cells—NK cells recognize cell surface molecules on virally infected or tumor cells. They subsequently bind to the infected cells and kill them via cell-mediated cytotoxicity.

4. Acute-phase proteins—C-reactive protein is a model acute-phase protein whose concentration increases in response to infection. C-reactive protein binds to cell surface molecules on a variety of bacteria and fungi and acts as an opsonin, essentially increasing recognition of pathogens by phagocytic cells.

5. Complement system—The complement system is a cascade of serum proteins whose overall function is to enhance and mediate inflammation. The complement system has the intrinsic ability to lyse the cell membranes of many cells including bacteria. It functions in concert with components of both the innate and adaptive immune systems and can also act as an opsonin, facilitating phagocytosis. The complement cascade can be directly activated by certain microorganisms through the alternative pathway, or it can be activated by particular antibody subtypes through the classical pathway.

The adaptive immune response consists of the following components:

1. Antibodies—Otherwise known as *immunoglobulins* (Igs), antibodies are able to specifically recognize a variety of free antigens. Igs are produced by B cells and are present on their cell surface. In addition, Igs are secreted in large amounts in the serum. Antibodies recognize specific microbial and other antigens through their antigen-binding sites and bind phagocytes via their Fc receptors, thereby facilitating antigen removal. Some subclasses of Ig are capable of activating complement via their Fc portion, thereby lysing their targets.

2. B cells—The primary function of B cells is to produce antibody. Antigen binding to B cells stimulates proliferation and maturation of that particular B cell, with subsequent enhancement of antigen-specific antibody production, resulting in the development of antibody-secreting plasma cells. Most B cells express class II major histocompatibility complex (MHC) antigens and have the ability to function as APCs.

3. T cells, or thymus-derived cells, have the ability to recognize specific antigens via their T-cell receptors (TCRs). T cells may be classified into two main groups, T-helper (T_H) cells expressing CD4 antigen on their cell surface and T-cytotoxic (T_C) cells expressing CD8 on their surface. CD4 T cells recognize antigen presented in association with MHC class II on the surface of APCs. CD4 T cells help to promote B-cell maturation and antibody production and produce factors called *cytokines* to enhance the innate or nonspecific immune response. CD8 T cells recognize antigen in association with MHC class I antigen on the surface of most cells and play an important role in eliminating virus-infected cells. Cytotoxic T cells are capable of damaging target cells via the release of degrading enzymes and cytokines. Responses in which the T cell plays a major role are termed *cell-mediated immunity* (CMI). T cell–macrophage interactions often lead to delayed reactions, termed *delayed-type hypersensitivity* (DTH).

4. APCs are required to present antigen to T cells. They are found primarily in the skin, lymph nodes, spleen, and thymus. Unlike B cells that can recognize free antigen, T cells are only capable of recognizing antigen in the context of self-MHC molecules. APCs process antigen intracellularly and present antigen peptide in the groove of their MHC class II molecules. The primary APCs are macrophages, monocytes, dendritic cells, and Langerhans cells.

Principal Components of the Immune System

Cells of the immune system arise from the pluripotent stem cells in the bone marrow and diverge into the lymphoid or myeloid lineages. The myeloid lineage primarily contains cells with phagocytic functions such as neutrophils, basophils, eosinophils, and macrophages. The lymphoid lineage consists of T cells, B cells, and NK cells.

Monocytes and Macrophages

Bone marrow–derived myeloid progenitor cells give rise to monocytes (mononuclear phagocytes of the reticuloendothelial system) that serve important immune functions. They constitute about 4% of the peripheral blood leukocytes and are morphologically identified by an abundant cytoplasm and a kidney-shaped nucleus. Their cytoplasm contains many enzymes, which are important for killing microorganisms and processing antigens. Monocytes differentiate into tissue-specific macrophages including Kupffer cells of the liver and brain microglia.

Natural Killer Cells

Natural killer cells make up about 2.5% of peripheral blood lymphocytes and are synonymous with large granular lymphocytes because of their large intracytoplasmic azurophilic granules and high cytoplasm-to-nucleus ratio. NK cells are activated primarily in response to interferons and are involved in the elimination of virally infected host cells; they also play a role in tumor immunity. Unlike cytotoxic CD8+ T cells, NK cells lack immunological memory and have the ability to kill a wide variety of tumor and virus-infected cells without MHC restriction (see the discussion of the function of MHC genes) or activation. NK cells lack the cell surface markers present on B cells and T cells. NK1.1+ T cells are a subset of cells sharing characteristics of both NK cells and T cells. These cells express the α/β TCR and the NK1.1 receptor and secrete large amounts of IFN-γ or interleukin 4 (IL-4) in response to TCR stimulation.

T Lymphocytes

T cells originate from the thymus. Differentiation of T cells occurs in the thymus, and every T cell that leaves the thymus is conferred with a unique specificity for recognizing antigens. T cells that recognize self-antigens are generally either deleted or rendered tolerant within the thymus, a process called *central tolerance.*

T cells may be divided into two groups on the basis of expression of either the CD4+ or CD8+ marker. Functionally, CD4+ T cells are involved in delayed-type hypersensitivity (DTH) responses and also provide help for B-cell differentiation (and hence are termed *helper T cells*). In contrast, CD8+ T cells are involved in class I restricted lysis of antigen-specific targets (and hence are termed *cytotoxic T cells*). T cells with suppressor or regulatory activity can express either CD4 or CD8.

T-Cell Receptors

The TCR consists of two glycosylated polypeptide chains, alpha (α) and beta (β), of 45,000 and 40,000 dalton molecular weight, respectively. This heterodimer of an α and β chain is linked by disulfide bonds. Amino acid sequences show that each chain consists of variable (V), joining (J), and constant (C) regions closely resembling Igs (**Fig. 41.1**). There are about 10^2 TCR-variable genes grouped by homology into a small number of families, compared with 10^3 or greater for Igs (see later discussion). The principles governing generation of diversity in the TCR are very similar to those for Ig genes. T cells can only recognize short peptides that are associated with MHC molecules. In contrast, the Ig receptor can recognize peptides, whole proteins, nucleic acids, lipids, and small chemicals.

T cells also express a variety of nonpolymorphic antigens on their surfaces. The most abundantly expressed is CD45, comprising 10% of lymphocyte membrane proteins. CD45

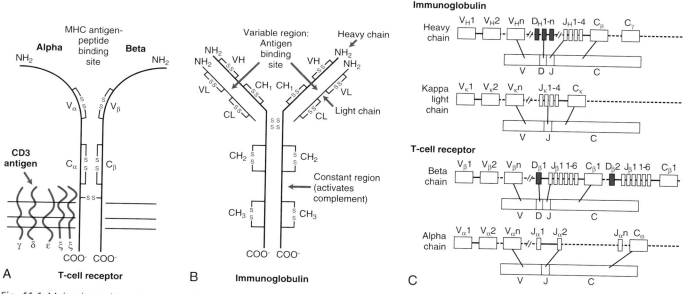

Fig. 41.1 Molecular and genetic organization of the T-cell receptor (TCR) and immunoglobulin (Ig) molecule. **A-B,** Structural organization of the TCR and Ig molecule. The TCR is a heterodimer consisting of two chains, a and b; the Ig molecule consists of two heavy and light chains. Both molecules are stabilized by interchain and intrachain disulfide bonds. Variable-region domains are located at the amino terminal, and constant-region domains are located on the carboxy terminal. The antigen-binding site on the Ig molecule is located between the variable-region domains of the heavy and light chains. The variable region of the TCR recognizes foreign peptides in the context of self-MHC (major histocompatibility complex) molecules. The TCR is also associated with the CD3 antigen (consisting of g, d, e, and z-z chains) to form the TCR complex. **C,** Organization of the gene families of Ig and TCR. The common feature of the four gene pools is that they contain a number of variable (V) gene segments that are separated from the constant (C) region genes by the joining (J) genes. In the case of the TCR b chain and the Ig heavy-chain gene, additional diversity (D) genes are present. During ontogeny, one of the V gene segments is juxtaposed to the J segment through a process of chromosomal rearrangement to form the V(D)J gene. This, along with the constant region genes, is transcribed to form messenger RNA and then protein.

exists as a number of isoforms that differ in the molecular weight of their extracellular domains as a result of RNA splicing. These isoforms can be distinguished serologically. The low molecular weight (CD45RO) isoforms define activated, or memory, T-cell populations.

B Lymphocytes

B cells are the precursors of antibody-secreting cells. The cells develop in the bone marrow and during their ontogeny acquire Ig receptors that commit them to recognizing specific antigens for the rest of their lives. B cells normally express IgM on their cell surfaces but switch to other isotypes as a consequence of T-cell help, while maintaining antigen specificity (see later discussion). Following antigenic challenge, T lymphocytes assist (help) B cells directly (cognate interaction) or indirectly by secreting helper factors (noncognate interaction) to differentiate and form mature antibody-secreting plasma cells.

Immunoglobulins

Immunoglobulins are glycoproteins that are the secretory product of plasma cells. Their biochemical structure and genomic organization is shown in **Fig. 41.1**. All Ig molecules share a number of common features. Each molecule consists of two identical polypeptide light chains (kappa [κ] or lambda [λ]) linked to two identical heavy chains. The light and heavy chains are stabilized by intrachain and interchain disulfide bonds. According to the biochemical nature of the heavy chain, Igs are divided into five main classes: IgM, IgD, IgG, IgA, and IgE. These may be further divided into subclasses depending on differences in the heavy chain.

Each heavy and light chain consists of variable and constant regions. The amino terminus is characterized by sequence variability in both the light and the heavy chain, and each variable heavy- and light-chain unit acts as the antigen-binding site (the Fab portion). The carboxy terminal of the heavy chain (also known as the *Fc portion*) is involved in binding to host tissue and fixing complement. This part of the molecule is important for antibody-dependent, cell-mediated cytotoxicity by cells of the reticuloendothelial system and for complement-mediated cell lysis.

Classes of Igs differ in their ability to fix complement. In humans, IgM, IgG1, and IgG3 antibodies are capable of activating the complement cascade. Different Ig classes also differ in their transport properties and ability to bind to phagocytes. Fc binding to Fc receptors (FcR) present on macrophages, dendritic cells, neutrophils, NK cells, and B cells initiates signaling within the cell only when the receptors are cross-linked by immune complexes containing more than one IgG molecule. Different Fc receptors (FcR) mediate different cellular responses, some being predominantly stimulatory, while others are inhibitory.

Genetics of the Immune System
Antigen Receptor Gene Rearrangements

During B- and T-cell development, multiple gene rearrangements occur to form their respective antigen receptors, the Ig and the TCR. Diversity of the antigen receptors is due to

diversity in their principal components, the variable (V) gene segment and the joining (J) gene segments. One of the many V gene segments is juxtaposed by chromosomal rearrangements with one of the J segments (and when present, with the diversity [D] segment) to form the complete variable region gene. Recombinational inaccuracies at the joining sites of the V, D, and J regions further increase the diversity of the antigen receptors.

Constant (C) gene segments are present in all receptors. The V, D, J, and C gene segments along with the intervening noncoding gene segments between the J and C regions are initially transcribed into mature RNA. Through a process of RNA splicing, the noncoding gene segments are excised, and the V(D)JC messenger RNA (mRNA) is translated into protein. After binding antigen, B cells undergo somatic mutations that further increase the diversity and the affinity of antigen binding (affinity maturation). This phenomenon does not occur in T cells. During isotype switching in B cells, further rearrangements lead to recombination of the same variable region gene with new constant region genes (see **Fig. 41.1**).

Major Histocompatibility and Human Leukocyte Antigens

Major histocompatibility complex gene products or the human leukocyte antigens (HLAs) serve to distinguish self from nonself. In addition, they serve the important function of presenting antigen to the appropriate cells. The MHC class I gene product contains an MHC-encoded α chain, and a smaller non-MHC-encoded β_2-microglobulin chain. The MHC class II gene product consists of two polypeptide chains, α and β, which are noncovalently linked. Both class I and class II proteins are stabilized by intrachain disulfide bonds. Class I antigens are expressed on all nucleated cells, whereas class II antigens are constitutively expressed only on dendritic cells, macrophages, and B cells and are also expressed on a variety of activated cells including T cells, endothelial cells, and astrocytes.

In humans, class I molecules are HLA-A, B, and C, whereas the class II molecules are HLA-DP, DQ, and DR. Several alleles are recognized for each locus; thus the HLA-A locus has at least 20 alleles, and HLA-B has at least 40. The number of alleles for the D region appears to be as extensive as that for HLA-A, HLA-B, and HLA-C. In view of the extensive polymorphisms present, the chances of two unrelated individuals sharing identical HLA antigens are extremely low. The reason for the extensive diversity and evolutionary pressure that lead to this are not fully understood.

Class I antigens regulate the specificity of cytotoxic CD8$^+$ T cells, which are responsible for killing cells bearing viral antigens or foreign transplantation antigens (**Fig. 41.2**). The target cells share class I MHC genes with the cytotoxic cell. Thus the cytotoxic cell that is specific for a particular virus is capable of recognizing the antigenic determinants of the virus only in association with a particular MHC class I gene product. The function of class II MHC gene products appears to be to regulate the specificity of T-helper cells, which in turn regulate DTH and antibody response to foreign antigens. Similarly, an immunized T-cell population will recognize a foreign antigen only if it is presented on the surface of an APC that shares the same class II MHC antigen specificity as the immunized T-cell population. Thus the functional specificity of the T-cell population is restricted by the MHC molecules they recognize. CD8$^+$ T cells (cytotoxic) and CD4$^+$ T cells (helper) are referred to as *MHC class I* and *MHC class II restricted T cells*, respectively (**Fig. 41.3**).

The analysis of the three-dimensional structure of the class I and class II molecules has confirmed the notion that these molecules are carriers of immunogenic peptides that are processed by APCs and presented on the cell surface (**Fig. 41.4**). Both MHC class I and class II molecules share similarities in crystal structure that allow them to accept and retain immunogenic peptides in grooves, or pockets, and present them to T cells.

Organization of the Immune Response

Initiation of the Immune Response
Antigen Presentation

One of the crucial initial steps in the immune response is the presentation of encountered antigens to the immune system. Antigens are carried from their site of arrival in the periphery by way of lymphatics or blood vessels to the lymph nodes and spleen. There, antigens are then taken up by cells of the monocyte-macrophage lineage and by B cells, processed intracellularly, and presented not as whole molecules but as highly immunogenic peptides.

Accessory Molecules for T-Cell Activation

The interaction of MHC-peptide complex with T cells, although necessary, is insufficient for T-cell activation. Other classes of molecules are involved in T-cell antigen recognition, activation, intracellular signaling, adhesion, and trafficking of

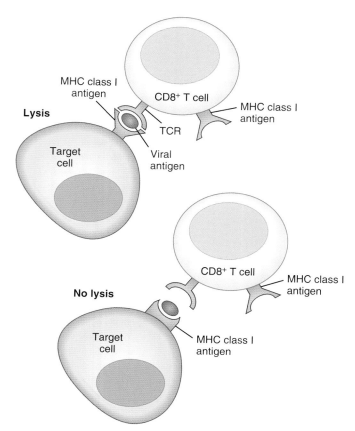

Fig. 41.2 The phenomenon of major histocompatibility complex (MHC) restriction. For antigen-specific cytolysis of virus-infected targets to occur, T cells should be sensitized to the virus and share the same class I human leukocyte antigen (HLA) with the target cell. In the lower part of the figure, the MHC class I antigen expressed on the CD8$^+$ T cell is different from the MHC class 1 antigen expressed on the target cell; therefore lysis does not occur. *TCR*, T-cell receptor.

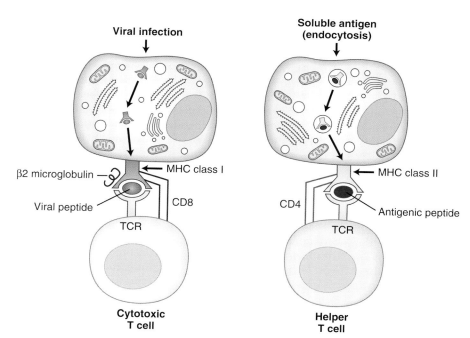

Fig. 41.3 Antigenic recognition of cytotoxic and helper T cells. The cytotoxic T cell recognizes viral peptides associated with human leukocyte antigen-A (HLA-A), HLA-B, or HLA-C molecules. The coreceptor for the helper T cell is the CD4 molecule. *MHC*, Major histocompatibility complex; *TCR*, T-cell receptor.

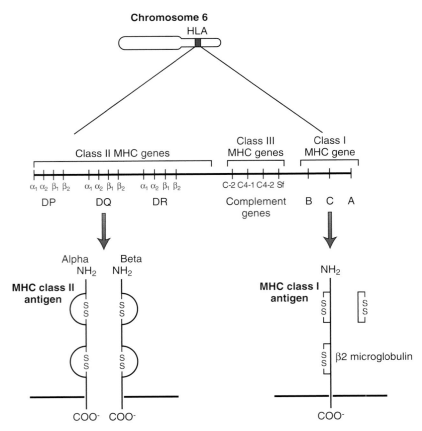

Fig. 41.4 Schematic diagram of the human leukocyte antigen (HLA) complex in humans, located on chromosome 6. The HLA class I gene (HLA-A, -B, and -C) codes for a single heavy-chain molecule. The β_2-microglobulin is coded by genes on a different chromosome. The HLA class II genes (DR, DP, and DQ) form the $\alpha\beta$ heterodimer. The HLA class III genes include those encoding for members of the complement family of proteins. *MHC*, Major histocompatibility complex.

T cells to their target organs. The distinction between the functions of these classes of molecules is not absolute, and many may be involved in interactions between other cells of the immune system.

CD3

Molecules whose primary role is signaling include the CD3 molecule. The CD3 molecule is part of the TCR complex. Although the TCR interacts with the MHC-peptide complex on APCs, the signals for the subsequent enactment of T-cell activation and proliferation are delivered by the CD3 antigen. The cytoplasmic tail of the CD3 proteins contains one copy of a sequence motif important for signaling functions, called the *immunoreceptor tyrosine-based activation motif* (ITAM). Phosphorylation of the ITAM initiates intracellular signaling events. In experimental situations, anti-CD3 antibodies can nonspecifically activate these intracellular signals, producing activated T cells in the absence of antigen.

CD4 AND CD8

CD4 or CD8 antigens are expressed on mature T cells and serve an accessory role in signaling and antigen recognition. CD4 binds to a nonpolymorphic site on the MHC class II β chain, and CD8 binds to the $\alpha3$ domain of the MHC class I molecule. Signals for cell division that are delivered to the nucleus are mediated by second messengers. When the receptor binds its ligand, it causes the activation of protein kinases. These kinases add phosphate groups to other proteins that ultimately signal the cell to divide. CD4, CD8, and CD3 on T

cells and CD19 on B cells are examples of receptors that are linked to kinases. CD4 is the cell surface receptor for human immunodeficiency virus (HIV-1), and the fact that certain non-T cells such as microglia and macrophages can express low levels of CD4 may explain the propensity of the virus for the central nervous system (CNS).

COSTIMULATORY MOLECULES

Costimulatory molecules serve as a "second signal" to facilitate T-cell activation. Costimulatory pathways that are critical for T-cell activation include the B7-CD28 and CD40-CD154 pathways. Members of the integrin families including vascular cell adhesion molecule 1 (VCAM-1), intercellular adhesion molecule (ICAM-1), and leukocyte function antigen 3 (LFA-3) can provide costimulatory signals, but they also play critical roles in T-cell adhesion, facilitate interaction with the APCs, mediate adhesion to nonhematopoietic cells such as endothelial cells, and guide cell traffic (**Fig. 41.5**).

The B7-CD28 interaction is one of the most extensively studied costimulatory systems. The B7 molecules are expressed on antigen-presenting cells, and their expression is induced in activated cells. There are two forms of B7, B7-1 (CD80) and B7-2 (CD86), that share some homology but have different expression kinetics. The B7 molecules interact with their ligand, CD28, which is constitutively expressed on most T cells. Binding of the CD28 molecule mediates intracytoplasmic signals that increase expression of the growth factor, IL-2, and enhance expression of the anti-apoptotic molecule, Bcl-x$_L$. An alternate ligand for B7 is CTLA-4, which is homologous to CD28 in structure, but in contrast to CD28,

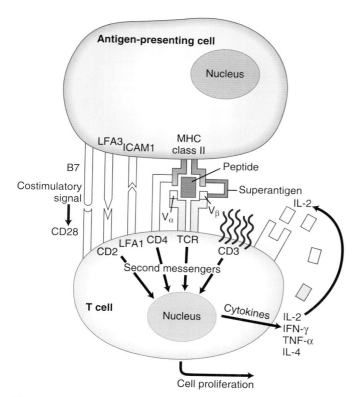

Fig. 41.5 Antigen-driven activation of helper T cells. Proliferation of T cells requires the delivery of a number of concordant signals. Along with stimulation through the T-cell receptor–CD3 complex, the presence of appropriate costimulatory signals via CD28 antigen, adhesion molecules, leukocyte function antigen 1 (LFA1) and CD2, and the coreceptor molecule CD4 are essential for T-cell activation and proliferation. The membrane events of antigen recognition lead to activation of second messengers. The second messengers signal the nucleus and cell to divide and secrete cytokines. Interleukin 2 (IL-2) acts as an autocrine growth stimulator, thereby amplifying the response. *ICAM*, Intercellular adhesion molecule; *IFN-γ*, interferon γ; *MHC*, major histocompatibility complex; *TCR*, T-cell receptor; *TNF*, tumor necrosis factor.

CTLA-4 functions to inhibit T-cell activation. Costimulatory molecules may deliver either a stimulatory (positive) or inhibitory (negative) signal for T-cell activation (Brunet et al., 1987). Examples of molecules delivering a positive costimulatory signal for T-cell activation include the B7-CD28, CD40-CD154 pathways. Examples of molecular pathways delivering a negative signal for T-cell activation include B7-CTLA4 and PD1-PD ligand (Khoury and Sayegh, 2004). The delicate balance between positive and negative regulatory signals can determine the outcome of a specific immune response.

CELL MIGRATION

Molecules primarily involved in cell migration into tissues include chemokines, integrins, selectins, and matrix metalloproteinases (MMPs). Chemokines constitute a large family of chemoattractant peptides that regulate the vast spectrum of leukocyte migration events through interactions with chemokine receptors. The integrin family includes VCAM-1, ICAM-1, LFA-3, CD45, and CD2 and mediates adhesion to endothelial cells and guiding cell traffic. L-selectins facilitate

the rolling of leucocytes along the surface of endothelial cells and function as a homing receptor to target peripheral lymphoid organs. The MMPs are a family of proteinases secreted by inflammatory cells; MMPs digest specific components of the extracellular matrix, thereby facilitating lymphocyte entry through basement membranes including the blood-brain barrier (BBB).

Accessory Molecules for B-Cell Activation

Like T cells, B cells require accessory molecules that supplement signals mediated through cell-surface Igs. Signaling molecules whose functions are likely to be analogous to CD3 are linked to Ig. Unlike T cells that may only respond to peptide antigens, B cells can respond to proteins, peptides, polysaccharides, nucleic acids, lipids, and small chemicals. B cells responding to peptide antigens are dependent on T-cell help for proliferation and differentiation, and these antigens are termed *thymus-dependent* (T-dependent), and these antigens do not require T-cell help to induce antibody production and are therefore T-independent.

The interaction between B cells and T-helper (CD4[+]) cells requires expression of MHC class II by B cells and is antigen dependent. In addition, a number of other molecules mediate adhesion between T and B cells and induce signaling for B-cell activation. These include B7 expressed on B cells interacting with CD28 on T cells and CD40 on B cells interacting with CD154. Interaction of T-helper and B cells occurs in the peripheral lymphoid organs, initially in the primary follicles and later in the germinal centers of the follicle. Activation of B cells induces activation of transcription factors (c-Fos, JunB, NFκB, and c-Myc), which in turn promote proliferation and Ig secretion. Cytokines elicited from the T-helper cell induce isotype switching in B cells, producing stronger and long-lived memory responses, in contrast to weak IgM responses to T-independent antigens.

Further generation of high-affinity antibody-producing B cells and memory B cells occurs in the germinal center of lymphoid follicles through a process called *affinity maturation*. As the amount of available antigen lessens, B cells that do not express high-affinity receptors for antigen are eliminated by apoptosis. Some B cells lose the ability to produce Ig but survive for long periods and become memory B cells.

Regulation of the Immune Response
Cytokines

Cytokines play a major role in regulating the immune response. Cytokines are broadly divided into the following categories, which are not mutually exclusive: (1) growth factors: IL-1, IL-2, IL-3, and IL-4 and colony-stimulating factors; (2) activation factors, such as interferons (α, β, and γ, which are also antiviral); (3) regulatory or cytotoxic factors, including IL-10, IL-12, transforming growth factor beta (TGF-β), lymphotoxins, and tumor necrosis factor alpha (TNF-α); and (4) chemokines that are chemotactic inflammatory factors, such as IL-8, MIP-1α, and MIP-1β.

Cytokines are necessary for T-cell activation and for the amplification and modulation of the immune response. A limited representation of the cytokines that participate in the immune response is shown in **Table 41.1**. Secretion of

Table 41.1 **An Abridged List of Cytokines Involved in Interactions Between the Immune and Nervous Systems**

Cytokine	Cell Source	Cells Principally Affected	Major Functions
IL-1	Most cells; macrophages, microglia	Most cells; T cells, microglia, astrocytes, macrophages	Costimulates T- and B-cell activation Induces IL-6, promotes IL-2 and IL-2R transcription Endogenous pyrogen, induces sleep
IL-2	T cells	T cells, NK cells, B cells	Growth stimulation
IL-3	T cells	Bone marrow precursors for all cell lineages	Growth stimulation
IL-4	T cells	B cells, T cells, macrophages	MHC II up-regulation Isotype switching (IgG1, IgE)
IL-6	Macrophages, endothelial cells, fibroblasts, T cells	Hepatocytes, B cells, T cells	Inflammation, costimulates T-cell activation MHC I up-regulation, increases vascular permeability Acute phase response (Schwartzman reaction)
IL-10	Macrophages, T cells	Macrophages, T cells	Inhibition of IFN-γ, TNF-α, IL-6 production Down-regulation of MHC expression (macrophages)
IL-12	Macrophages, dendritic cells	T cells, NK cells	Costimulates B-cell growth, CD4$^+$ T$_H$1 cell differentiation, IFN-γ synthesis, cytolytic function
IL-17	T cells	Neutrophils, T cells, epithelial cells, fibroblasts	Host defense against gram-negative bacteria, induction of neutrophilic responses Induction of proinflammatory cytokines
IFN-γ	T cells, NK cells	Astrocytes, macrophages, endothelial cells, NK cells	MHC I and II expression Induces TNF-α production, isotype switching (IgG$_2$) Synergizes with TNF-α for many functions
TNF-α	Macrophages, microglia (T cells)	Most cells, including oligodendrocytes	Cytotoxic (e.g., for oligodendrocytes), lethal at high doses Up-regulates MHC, promotes leukocyte extravasation Induces IL-1, IL-6, cachexia; endogenous pyrogen
Lymphotoxin (TNF-β)	T cells	Most cells (shares receptor with TNF-α)	Cytotoxic (at short range or through contact) Promotes extravasation
TGF-β	Most cells; macrophages, T cells, neurons	Most cells	Pleiotropic, antiproliferative, anticytokine Promotes vascularization, healing

IFN, Interferon; *Ig,* immunoglobulin; *IL,* interleukin; *MHC,* major histocompatibility complex; *NK,* natural killer; *TGF,* tumor growth factor; *TNF,* tumor necrosis factor.

IL-1 by macrophages results in stimulation of T cells. This leads to synthesis of IL-2 and IL-2 receptors and finally to the clonal expansion of T cells. Only activated T cells express the IL-2 receptor (CD25); therefore the cytokine-induced expansion favors antigen-activated cells only. T-cell activation causes secretion of interferon gamma (IFN-γ), which induces expression of MHC class I and class II molecules on many cell types including APCs. This in turn increases the T-cell response to the antigen. Secretion of IL-2 also results in activation of NK cells that mediate lysis of tumor cell targets. In addition, IL-3 is released, resulting in stimulation of hematopoietic stem cells. The signal for differentiation of B cells to form antibody-secreting cells involves clonal expansion and differentiation of virgin memory B cells. IL-4 and B-cell differentiation factors secreted by T cells induce differentiation and expansion of committed B cells to become plasma cells.

IFN-α and IFN-β are both type I interferons. IFN-α is produced by macrophages, whereas IFN-β is produced by fibroblasts. Both inhibit viral replication by causing cells to synthesize enzymes that interfere with viral replication. They also can inhibit the proliferation of lymphocytes by unknown mechanisms.

Although the emphasis has been on factors that cause expansion and differentiation of lymphocytes, there are cytokines that can down-regulate immune responses. Thus IFN-α and IFN-β, in addition to possessing antiviral properties, can modulate antibody response by virtue of their antiproliferative properties. Similarly, TGF-β (a cytokine produced by T cells and macrophages) can also decrease cell proliferation. IL-10, a growth factor for B cells, inhibits the production of IFN-γ and thus may have antiinflammatory effects.

CD4$^+$ T-helper cells differentiate into T$_H$1 or T$_H$2 phenotypes, as well as a recently described T$_H$17 subset, which secrete characteristic cytokines and stimulate specific functions. T$_H$1 cells secrete IFN-γ, IL-2, and TNF-α. These cytokines exert proinflammatory functions and, in T$_H$1-mediated diseases such as MS, promote tissue injury. IL-2, TNF-α, and IFN-γ mediate activation of macrophages and induce DTH. T$_H$1 cell differentiation is driven by IL-12, a cytokine produced by monocytes and macrophages. In contrast, the T$_H$2 cytokines IL-4, IL-5, IL-6, IL-10, and IL-13 promote antibody production by B cells, enhance eosinophil functions, and generally suppress cell-mediated immunity (CMI). T$_H$3 cells secrete TGF-β, which inhibits proliferation of T cells and inhibits activation of macrophages. Cytokines of the T$_H$1 type may inhibit production of T_H2 cytokines and vice versa. More recently, a subset of T cells that predominantly produce IL-17 have been described (Yao et al., 1995). These cells are believed to represent a distinct subset from IFN-γ-producing T_H1 cells, evidenced by the dependence of T_HIL-17 cells on IL-6 and TGF-β for differentiation (Bettelli et al., 2006; Mangan et al., 2006; Veldhoen et al., 2006) and IL-23 for expansion (Aggarwal et al., 2003; Langrish et al., 2005), as opposed to T_H1 cells, which are dependent on IL-12 and IL-2, respectively, for differentiation and expansion. Both T_H1 and T_H2 cytokines have been shown to suppress the development of T_H17 cells (Harrington et al., 2005; Park et al., 2005). T_HIL-17 cells facilitate the recruitment of neutrophils and participate in the response to gram-negative organisms. These cells may also play a role in the initiation of autoimmune disease. Another effector T-cell subset, T_H9 cells, has recently been described (Dardalhon et al., 2008; Veldhoen et al., 2008). Driven by the combined effects of TGF-β and IL-4, T_H9 cells produce large amounts of IL-9 and IL-10. It has been shown that IL-9 combined with TGF-β can contribute to T_H17 cell differentiation, and T_H17 cells themselves can produce IL-9 (Elyaman et al., 2009).

Traditionally, T_H cell subsets have been distinguished by their patterns of cytokine production, but identification of distinguishing surface molecule markers has been a major advance in the field. Tim (T cell, immunoglobulin and mucin-domain containing molecules) represent an important family of molecules that encode cell-surface receptors involved in the regulation of T_H1 and T_H2 cell–mediated immunity. Tim-3 is specifically expressed on T_H1 cells and negatively regulates T_H1 responses through interaction with the Tim-3 ligand, galactin-9, also expressed on CD4$^+$ T cells (Monney et al., 2002; Sabatos et al., 2003; Zhu et al., 2005). Tim-2 is expressed on T_H2 cells (Chakravarti et al., 2005), and appears to negatively regulate T_H2 cell proliferation, although this has not been fully established. Tim-1 is expressed on T_H2 cells > T_H1 cells, and interacts with Tim-4 on APCs to induce T-cell proliferation (Meyers et al., 2005).

Chemokines

Chemokines are a recently discovered and extensively studied group of molecules that aid in leukocyte mobility and directed movement. Chemokines may be grouped into two subfamilies based on the configuration and binding of the two terminal cysteine residues. If the two residues participating in disulfide bonding are adjacent, they are termed the *C-C family* (e.g., MCP, MIP-1α, RANTES). Those separated by one amino acid, are C-X-C family members (e.g., IL-8), where X indicates a nonconserved amino acid. An important recent discovery is that two chemokine receptors, CCR-5 and CXCR-4, can act as coreceptors for strains of HIV. Chemokines are produced by a variety of immune and nonimmune cells. Monocytes, T cells, basophils, and eosinophils express chemokine receptors, and these receptor-ligand interactions are critical to the recruitment of leukocytes into specific tissues.

Termination of an Immune Response

The primary goal of the immune response is to protect the organism from infectious agents and generate memory T- and B-cell responses that provide accelerated and high-avidity secondary responses on reencountering antigens. It is desirable to terminate these responses once an antigen has been cleared. In parallel, the immune system must constantly function to prevent autoimmune activation and maintain self-tolerance. A number of systems operate to prevent uncontrolled responses. Here we discuss termination of individual components of the immune response. Following is a discussion of the mechanisms that maintain self-tolerance, many of which are also involved in immune-response termination.

B-Cell Inhibition

In most instances, an antigen is cleared either by cells of the reticuloendothelial system or through the formation of antigen-antibody complexes. These complexes can themselves result in the inhibition of B-cell differentiation and proliferation through binding of the Fc receptor to the CD32 (FcγRIIB) receptor on the surface of the B cell.

Immunoglobulin

The variable regions of the Ig and the TCR molecule represent novel proteins that can act as antigens. Antigenic variable regions are called *idiotopes*, and responses against such antigens are called *anti-idiotypic*. Niels Jerne's network hypothesis postulates that anti-idiotypic responses serve to regulate the immune response; however, the extent to which this operates is unclear.

T Cells

Termination of the T-cell immune response is mediated by several mechanisms including anergy, deletion, and suppressor cell activity. Anergy or functional unresponsiveness occurs when there is insufficient T-cell activation. Repeated stimulation of T cells may lead to activation-induced cell death through apoptosis. Cytokine-mediated regulation can also serve to terminate the immune response, notably by secretion of T_H2 and T_H3 cytokines. Regulatory cells generally inhibit the immune response through secretion of cytokines, through cytotoxic mechanisms, or by modulation of the function of APCs. A combination of these mechanisms cooperate to maintain self-tolerance, particularly peripheral tolerance, and are discussed later.

Self-Tolerance

An organism's ability to maintain a state of unresponsiveness to its own antigens is termed *self-tolerance*. Self-tolerance is maintained through three principal mechanisms: deletion, anergy, and suppression. Self-tolerance may be broadly categorized as either central or peripheral tolerance. Similar mechanisms may also be used to induce tolerance to a foreign antigen or terminate an immune response.

Central Tolerance

Bone marrow stem cells migrate to the thymus, thereby becoming thymocytes, or T cells. In this location, T-cell VDJ germline genetic elements recombine to create α and β chains, which in turn form the TCR. Thymocytes then undergo a process of education that involves positive and negative selection. Positive selection of thymocytes occurs in the thymus cortex when the cells are in the double negative stage, CD4⁻ CD8⁻. The cortex contains dendritic and epithelial cells that present MHC antigens to the developing thymocytes. T cells with receptor having no affinity to MHC will fail to receive signals needed for maturation and will die in situ. Those with low affinity toward MHC survive and become single-positive thymocytes depending on their affinity toward MHC I (CD8⁺) or MHC II (CD4⁺). In the thymus medulla, thymocytes that display a high affinity toward self-antigen are deleted by apoptosis, a process called *negative selection*. Most T-cell education occurs in the thymus; however, extrathymic sites may exist.

Peripheral Tolerance

Self-reactive lymphocytes may escape central tolerance; therefore peripheral mechanisms exist to maintain self-tolerance. This is termed *peripheral tolerance*. Peripheral tolerance is maintained through clonal anergy or clonal deletion. It is not clear to what extent each of these mechanisms functions in maintaining human self-tolerance; however, extensive research has been done to elucidate the mechanisms through which anergy and deletion work. In addition, self-tolerance may be maintained despite the presence of antigen-responsive lymphocytes. It is postulated that this is due to the presence of suppressor T cells or other factors that may interfere with a successful lymphocyte response.

Anergy Due to Failure of T-cell Activation

In normal circumstances, an APC presents antigen as a peptide + MHC complex (signal one). In the absence of signal one, the T cell dies because of neglect. If signal one is presented in the absence of costimulatory signals (signal two), the T cell

becomes anergic. An example of this situation occurs when an antigen is presented by nonprofessional APCs that lack the appropriate costimulatory molecules (**Fig. 41.6**). However, when a T cell is activated, it up-regulates the expression of an alternate costimulatory molecule, CTLA-4. CTLA4 engagement by CD80 and CD86 on the surface of APCs sends a negative signal to the T cell, inhibiting cell growth and proliferation. Animals deficient for CTLA-4 expression on their T lymphocytes have an uncontrolled lymphoproliferative phenotype with autoreactivity (Waterhouse et al., 1995).

Apoptosis

Apoptosis is the process in which a cell undergoes programmed cell death. As opposed to necrosis, when interruption of the supply of nutrients triggers cell death, apoptosis may be triggered by various signals including withdrawal of growth factors, cytokines, exposure to corticosteroids, and repeated exposure to antigens. Mediators of apoptosis include the Bcl family of genes, which are mostly antiapoptotic, and the Fas family of genes, which are proapoptotic. Activated T cells also express Fas ligand (CD95L or FasL) and Fas (CD95); ligation of Fas and FasL induces apoptosis of the T cells.

Repeated stimulation with an antigen may also induce apoptosis via the Fas/FasL pathway, a process termed *activation-induced cell death* (AICD). Therefore an autoreactive T lymphocyte may encounter large doses of self-antigen in the periphery and consequently may be deleted by AICD. Mice lacking Fas or FasL develop a lupus-like syndrome (Zhou et al., 1996), and mutations in the Fas gene were associated with an autoimmune disease with lymphoproliferation in humans (Drappa et al., 1996).

IL-2 is the prototypical growth factor, inducing clonal expansion of antigen-stimulated lymphocytes; paradoxically, disruption of the IL-2 gene leads to accumulation of activated lymphocytes and autoimmune syndromes (Sadlack et al.,

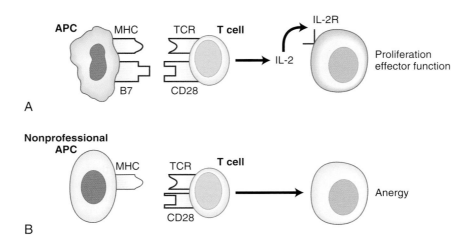

Fig. 41.6 A two-signal model of T-cell activation. Activation of the T-cell receptor (TCR) by an antigen major histocompatibility complex (MHC) provides signal 1, which is sufficient to induce the T cell to enter the cell cycle and begin blast transformation, which is characterized by an increase in cell size. Signal 2, the costimulatory signal, can be provided to the T cell through interaction of CD28 with molecules of the B7 family found on the surface of bone marrow–derived antigen-presenting cells (APCs). **A,** In this instance, TCR signals are complemented, enabling the T cell to proliferate, produce cytokines, and develop mature effector functions. **B,** In the absence of a second signal, T-cell activation is abortive, and the cell becomes anergic. Signal 2 might not be delivered if the APC does not express a costimulatory ligand on its surface, perhaps because a nonprofessional APC, such as an epithelial cell, is presenting antigen. *IL,* Interleukin.

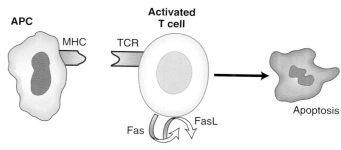

Fig. 41.7 Activation of the T cell leads to coexpression of the death receptor Fas (CD95) and its ligand (FasL), resulting in death of the cell and neighboring cells. *APC,* Antigen-presenting cell; *MHC,* major histocompatibility complex; *TCR,* T-cell receptor.

1993). This is because IL-2 induces the transcription and surface expression of Fas ligand (FasL). Interactions of Fas with FasL lead to cell death (**Fig. 41.7**). Therefore IL-2 plays a dual role in T-cell regulation, reflecting a possible role for cytokine concentration and timing of exposure. Other cytokines that mediate apoptosis and cell death are TNF-α and IFN-γ. Complete absence of either of these cytokines results in deficient T-cell apoptosis, inability to terminate the immune response, and uncontrolled autoimmune disease.

Regulatory T Cells

Regulatory T cells (T_{reg}) function to down-regulate CD4 and CD8 T-cell responses. Regulatory T cells can be of the CD4+ or CD8+ subtypes. Regulatory T cells have been found in several animal models of disease, and some are antigen specific. In vitro they can be generated under similar conditions used to generate anergic cells, and it has been postulated that they are the same entity (Lombardi et al., 1994). Several populations of regulatory or suppressor T cells have been described in humans. These include CD4+CD25+Foxp3 regulatory T cells (Baecher-Allan et al., 2001; Dieckmann et al., 2001; Levings et al., 2001; Stephens et al., 2001; Yagi et al., 2004), CD8+CD28− T cells (Koide and Engleman, 1990), IL-10-producing T_H2 cells (Bacchetta et al., 1994), and TGF-β producing T_H3 cells (Kitani et al., 2000; Roncarolo and Levings, 2000). In humans, there is little evidence for antigen-specific suppressor cell responses. Regulatory T cells suppress T-cell proliferation through a variety of mechanisms, including the production of immunosuppressive cytokines (T_H2 or TGF-β) or through T-T cell interactions, including the expression of inhibitory molecules such as CTLA-4. Regulatory cells play an important role in the control of the immune response in autoimmune disorders, and the function of regulatory T cells may be enhanced by immunomodulatory therapies.

Immune System and Central Nervous System

Immune Privilege in the Central Nervous System

Immunological reactions in the CNS differ from those in the rest of the body because of its unique architecture, cellular composition, and molecular expression. The CNS has been termed an *immunologically privileged site* because of the relative improved survival of allografts within this region. Indeed, the same factors that play a role in immunological tolerance in the CNS play a role in immune-mediated diseases involving the CNS, infections of the CNS, tumor survival, and therapies.

Important factors relevant to immunological responses in the CNS are: (1) absence of lymphatic drainage, limiting the immunological circulation; (2) the blood-brain barrier (BBB), which limits the passage of immune cells and factors; (3) the low level of expression of MHC factors, particularly MHC II in the resident cells of the CNS; (4) low levels of potent APCs, such as dendritic or Langerhans cells; and (5) the presence of immunosuppressive factors such as TGF-β (Wilbanks and Streilein, 1992) and CD200 (Webb and Barclay, 1984).

Because of the lack of a lymphatic system, antigens drain along perivascular spaces. Monocyte-derived CNS resident cells, termed *microglia*, play an important role in immune surveillance in these areas. The BBB is composed of tight junctions between endothelial cells and a layer of astrocytic foot processes that prevent entry of inflammatory cells and other factors into the CNS. Entry of inflammatory cells across the BBB is facilitated by upregulation of adhesion molecules ICAM-1 and VCAM-1 on endothelial cells. T cells must be activated before crossing the BBB. Entry is facilitated by expression of receptors for adhesion molecules, including α4-integrin.

The CNS houses cells that are capable of antigen presentation under certain conditions in vitro, but to what extent this occurs in vivo remains under debate. In the CNS, endogenous expression of MHC class I and class II on APCs such as microglia is low, and in oligodendrocytes and astrocytes, it is almost undetectable. Neurons express MHC class I only when damaged and in the presence of IFN-γ (Neumann et al., 1995). Expression of MHC antigens on both microglia and astrocytes are enhanced by the presence of cytokines, TNF-α, and IFN-γ. Under certain conditions, microglial cells may play a role as APCs in the nervous system (Perry, 1994). More recently, populations of perivascular dendritic cells capable of antigen presentation have been identified in rodents (Greter et al., 2005), with analogous populations demonstrated in humans; however, their role in human disease is unclear.

Immune privilege in the CNS is also influenced by the constitutive expression of a number of immunoregulatory factors, some of which are common to immune privilege in the anterior chamber of the eye. Anterior chamber immune privilege is due in part to expression of TGF-β in the aqueous of the eye. In the CNS, TGF-β is produced by astrocytes and microglia and may play a role in down-regulating immune responses locally. Neurons are also capable of producing TGF-β, which in animal models has been shown to facilitate the differentiation of regulatory T cells (Liu et al., 2006). Increased expression of Fas ligand in the CNS compared with the peripheral nervous system (PNS) may increase apoptosis of T cells, thereby down-regulating the immune response (Moalem et al., 1999). Some CNS tumors express large amounts of TGF-β, which may play a role in protecting them from immune surveillance. CNS tumors may also express Fas or Fas ligand, facilitating protection from immune surveillance. Some populations of neurons express a cell surface marker named *CD200*. CD200 is a nonsignaling molecule but serves to inhibit activation of cells including microglia and macrophages that express the CD200 receptor (CD200R) (Hoek et al., 2000; Wright et al., 2000). CD200 has been shown to down-regulate inflammatory responses in models of MS (Liu et al., 2010) and uveitis (Banerjee and Dick, 2004; Broderick et al., 2002). Fractalkine (CXCL1) is a chemokine that is constitutively expressed on some populations of neurons. Interaction with its receptor, CX3CR1, present on microglia and NK cells, serves to down-regulate microglial-mediated neurotoxicity both in vitro and in animal models of Parkinson disease and ALS (Cardona et al., 2006). In the animal model of MS, absence of fractalkine or its receptor resulted in a reduction of NK cells in the CNS and exacerbation of disease, supporting the view that NK cells play an inhibitory role in CNS inflammation (Huang et al., 2006).

Neuroglial Cells and the Immune Response

Neuroglial cells including microglia and astrocytes participate in immune responses within the CNS, and there is increasing evidence that these cells play a central role in initiating and propagating immune-mediated diseases of the CNS.

Microglia are derived from bone marrow cells during ontogeny (Hickey and Kimura, 1988) and reside within the CNS as three principal types of cells: perivascular microglia, parenchymal microglia, and Kolmer cells, which reside in the choroid plexus. Microglia have mitotic potential and can differentiate from bone marrow–derived cells to perivascular microglia and parenchymal microglia. Compared to macrophages, microglia are relatively radioresistant. Microglia may exist either in a resting (ramified) form or activated or phagocytic forms within the CNS. Activated microglia express higher levels of MHC class II and produce higher levels of proinflammatory cytokines including TNF-α, IL-6, and IL-1, as well as nitric oxide and glutamate. Microglia express chemokine receptors and various pattern recognition receptors (PRRs) including Toll-like receptors. PRRs recognize pathogen-associated molecular patterns (PAMPs) expressed by a variety of microbes, and interaction results in microglial activation. The primary functions of microglia are immune surveillance for foreign antigens and phagocytic scavengers of cellular debris. Microglia, particularly perivascular microglia, may also participate in antigen presentation within the CNS under certain conditions. Microglia play a role in regulating the programmed elimination of neural cells during brain development and, in some cases, enhance neuronal survival by producing neurotrophic and antiinflammatory cytokines. Microglia may also play a role in neuroregeneration and repair. However, there is overwhelming evidence that microglia play a deleterious role in several neurodegenerative diseases: MS, ALS, Parkinson disease and HIV-associated dementia. Their role in Alzheimer disease (AD) is less clear. Overactivation of microglia, possibly by microbes or other environmental factors through PRRs, may result in chronic proinflammatory milieu in the CNS, leading to progressive neurodegeneration. Strategies to down-regulate such responses are under investigation (Block et al., 2007).

Astrocytes play multiple roles in the CNS, including their role in the glia limitans at the BBB and physical support of neuronal and axonal structures, as well as provision of growth factors. Astrocytes secrete cytokines including TGF-β and are also influenced by IL-1 and interferons to divide and express proteins such as costimulatory molecules and Toll-like receptors on their surfaces. There is increasing evidence against the role of astrocytes in antigen presentation within the CNS. Astrocytes play a critical role in converting glutamate to glutamine, a less toxic substance, so impairment of astrocyte function may result in increased glutamate-mediated neurotoxicity. Astrocytes also produce chemokines including stromal-derived factor-1 (SDF-1), which plays a significant role in HIV-associated dementia.

Cells of the CNS not only respond to inflammatory stimuli but are also capable of producing cytokines and other inflammatory factors, often directly under the influence of lymphocytes. These observations led to the conclusion that the brain is not an immunologically sequestered organ but that it interacts, produces immunologically active factors, and is closely involved with the systemic immune response.

Putative Mechanisms of Human Autoimmune Disease

Why does autoimmune disease occur? It largely results as a culmination of interactions between genetic predisposition, environmental factors, and failure of self-tolerance maintenance mechanisms. Some diseases such as MS are termed *immune-mediated* because no definitive autoantigen has been demonstrated. Other diseases are clear cases of molecular mimicry such as Gd1b-mediated axonal neuropathy, in which the self-antigen attacked by the immune system is similar to that of an environmental antigen (in this case the Penner O:19 serotype of *Campylobacter jejuni*). Thus autoimmune diseases may be mediated by heterogeneous mechanisms, and in some cases more than one mechanism may be operating.

Autoimmune diseases may be classified as T- or B-cell mediated. Some, such as myasthenia gravis (MG), are mediated through a combination of both. In many B-cell mediated diseases, an autoantigen has been identified, to which the B cell produces autoantibodies. Examples are MG, in which sera from patients contain antibodies to the α subunit of the acetylcholine receptor, and Lambert-Eaton syndrome, in which symptoms are caused by antibodies targeting calcium channels. In contrast to T cell–mediated diseases, identification of autoantigens in antibody-mediated diseases may be easier, because B cells react to whole proteins, whereas the determinants recognized by T cells tend to be APC-processed small peptides of 10 to 20 amino acids. Thus for T cell–mediated diseases such as MS, inflammatory demyelinating polyneuropathy, and polymyositis, there is little evidence demonstrating a causal relationship between an autoantigen and autoimmune disease. In addition, T-cell reactivity to autoantigens does not necessarily guarantee disease, because autoreactivity to some self-antigens is seen in healthy individuals. Thus the only conclusive evidence that can indicate causality between an antigen and T cell–mediated autoimmune disease would be the reversal of the disease process by removal of the putative autoreactive T-cell repertoire. Although this has been feasible in some animal models, establishing the efficacy of such a strategy is difficult in most human T cell–mediated diseases.

Genetic Factors

Genetic makeup plays a role in susceptibility to autoimmune diseases. In particular, an association between certain MHC haplotypes and disease has been noted. MS is linked to the HLA-DR2 allele, and the relative risk of having this allele in the Northern European population is 3.8. MG has been linked to HLA-DR3. However, the presence of the allele does not guarantee disease. In general, the relative risk of developing disease among individuals who carry the antigen may be calculated by the following formula:

$$\frac{\left[\begin{array}{c}\text{number of patients carrying} \\ \text{the HLA antigen}\end{array}\right] \times \left[\begin{array}{c}\text{number of controls} \\ \text{lacking the antigen}\end{array}\right]}{\left[\begin{array}{c}\text{number of patients lacking} \\ \text{the HLA antigen}\end{array}\right] \times \left[\begin{array}{c}\text{number of controls} \\ \text{carrying the antigen}\end{array}\right]}$$

Association of a particular HLA haplotype with autoimmune disease may be due to the ability of a particular MHC molecule to bind and present autoantigen to the T cell, as in MS where the MHC class II allele, DRB1*1501, has been shown to be effective in presenting myelin basic protein (MBP peptide) to T-cell clones isolated from MS patients (Wucherpfennig et al., 1995; Wucherpfennig et al., 1997). Conversely, if an MHC molecule does not bind a particular self-antigen in the thymus, the developing T cell will not recognize that antigen as self and will escape negative selection. Therefore certain MHC haplotypes have an association with disease, whereas others protect against disease. Disease linkage tends to be with class II genes of the MHC rather than class I, suggesting a key role for T-cell autoimmunity.

Association of a particular HLA-haplotype with disease may be due to its linkage to another locus or disease susceptibility gene. *Linkage disequilibrium* refers to the increased chance of inheriting two alleles together because they are genetically linked, as opposed to inheriting them together as separate random events.

Sex is one of the most important genetic determinants associated with autoimmune disease. Many autoimmune diseases are more frequent in females; systemic lupus erythematosus (SLE) is 10 times more common in women, and MS twice as common. Evidence from animal models has shown that females are more resistant to infections and reject foreign skin grafts sooner than their male counterparts. This is especially true during periods of high estrogen availability. Estrogen levels decrease after ovulation or during pregnancy, and this is associated with a progesterone surge. The lowering of estrogen ensures immunological tolerance toward the sperm and subsequently toward the fetus. Therefore estrogen's effects on the immune system may predispose women toward autoimmune diseases. This is reflected in experimental disease models of autoimmunity. Only female (NZB × NZW)F1 mice develop the SLE-like disease, and this is abrogated by androgen treatment. Similarly, in experimental autoimmune encephalomyelitis (EAE), an experimental model for MS, female SJL mice are more susceptible to disease induction and are protected with testosterone (Dalal et al., 1997). Preliminary studies testing the effectiveness of a testosterone gel in males with MS have shown encouraging results but require additional validation. Initial studies investigating estriol effects in women with MS have shown a potent effect on

reduction of new lesion formation, evident on gadolinium-enhanced magnetic resonance imaging (MRI) (Sicotte et al., 2002).

Environmental Factors

Environmental factors may play a role in the pathogenesis of autoimmune diseases. Molecular mimicry is one of the mechanisms implicated. In this situation, an environmental antigen resembling a self-antigen elicits an immune response to both itself and the self-antigen. The environmental antigen involved in molecular mimicry may be a superantigen. Superantigens have the property of stimulating all T cells that express a given TCR variable gene family, regardless of their exact specificity, because of direct TCR-superantigen interaction. They are usually of bacterial or viral origin and bind as intact molecules to MHC.

In many cases of molecular mimicry, the environmental antigen is a pathogen, and autoimmune disease follows the pathogen-caused disease. The classic example of this is streptococcal-induced endocarditis. Neurological diseases caused by this mechanism include streptococcal-induced chorea, Gd1b axonal neuropathy, Semple rabies vaccine-induced encephalomyelitis, and the anti-Hu paraneoplastic syndrome. Several studies have demonstrated that both adult (Ascherio and Munger, 2007) and pediatric (Alotaibi et al., 2004; Banwell et al., 2007; Lunemann et al., 2008; Pohl et al., 2006) MS patients more frequently demonstrate evidence of a remote infection with Epstein-Barr virus (EBV) than controls, implicating a role for this virus in disease pathogenesis. Interestingly, epitopes of EBV resemble myelin basic protein (MBP), supporting a role for molecular mimicry in disease pathogenesis (Lang et al., 2002). Despite these associations, however, it is clear that the majority of persons are infected with EBV without autoimmune sequelae. Recent studies have integrated risk factors in the pathogenesis of MS and found that the relative risk of MS among DR15-positive women with elevated (>1:320) anti-EBNA-1 titers was ninefold higher than that of DR15-negative women with low (<1:80) anti-EBNA-1 titers (De Jager et al., 2008).

It is possible that once an inflammatory reaction proceeds, the tissue injury may expose other self-antigens that were previously unrecognized by the immune system. For unknown reasons, peripheral tolerance mechanisms may fail, and an autoimmune reaction ensues. The spreading of the autoimmune reaction from one antigen to another is termed *determinant spreading* or *epitope spreading*. Epitope spreading may play a role in perpetuating immune-mediated reactions and therefore in causing chronic diseases. Therapies that inhibit molecular mimicry or epitope spreading may be useful in preventing autoimmune diseases.

Neuroimmunological Diseases

Immune-mediated disorders occur at all levels of the nervous system. Disorders of the CNS and PNS, including the peripheral nerve, neuromuscular junction, and muscle have been described. Some of these disorders are clearly autoimmune, in that a clear autoantigen has been identified, whereas others are immune-mediated. In this section, we identify neurological immune-mediated diseases and highlight immunological features pertinent to pathogenesis and treatment. A full description of each disease may be found in other sections of this book.

Multiple Sclerosis

Multiple sclerosis is a heterogeneous disease and is characterized by neurological deficits disseminated in time and space. It is a major cause of disability in the adult population in North America. Women are predominantly affected, in a ratio of 2:1. The disease is characterized by a varying array of neurological deficits. There are four main disease types, classified on the basis of the clinical disease course: relapsing-remitting (RR), secondary progressive (SP), primary progressive (PP), and progressive relapsing (PR). RR disease affects 65% of patients and is characterized by onset of neurological deficits that remit over a period of weeks to months. After 15 years, most RR patients go on to have an SP form of disease in which neurological deficits become fixed and accumulate. PP patients accumulate permanent neurological deficits from the onset of disease, whereas patients with PR disease have a combination of progressive and stepwise deficits. Disease onset generally occurs in the early 20s for RR disease and in the mid-30s for PP disease, although childhood-onset MS is becoming increasingly recognized.

MS is a complex polygenic disease. Monozygotic twins carry a concordance rate of 27%, whereas dizygotic twins of the same sex display a 2.3% concordance rate. The incidence for first-degree relatives of MS patients is 2% to 5%, whereas the incidence for the general population is under 0.1%. Genetic linkage studies have been performed, and several regions of interest have been found, but the most robust association remains with the HLA region. There is an increased incidence of MS in patients with the HLA-DR2 (DR1501) haplotype (Haines et al., 1998; Sawcer and Goodfellow, 1998; Stewart et al., 1981). More recently, a large genome-wide study identified single nucleotide polymorphism of IL-2R and IL-7R alleles as risk alleles for MS (Hafler et al., 2007). MS remains most prevalent among people of Northern European descent. There is a lower prevalence in other populations, such as Arabic and Mediterranean people, but among those with disease, there is a higher incidence of other disease-associated haplotypes such as DR4 and DR6.

Although genetic factors play an important role in pathogenesis, migration and other studies have demonstrated that environment also plays a critical role. Epidemiological studies have shown that residence in certain geographical areas and migration to these areas before the age of 15 increases the incidence of MS. In addition, there is a diminishing north-to-south gradient in MS prevalence in the Northern Hemisphere, with an opposite trend in the Southern Hemisphere. This led to the hypothesis and demonstration of an inverse association between sunlight exposure and MS (van der Mei et al., 2003).

An extension of this hypothesis has led to exploration of the role of vitamin D in MS, since vitamin D is metabolized in the skin by ultraviolet (UV) irradiation. A prospective study in army recruits found that 25-hydroxyvitamin D levels in the highest quintile (above 99.1 nmol/L) were associated with a lower risk of MS (odds ratio [OR], 0.38) (Munger et al., 2006). Treatment of animal models of MS with vitamin D ameliorates disease, and several studies have shown that the active form of vitamin D, calcitriol, can down-regulate proinflammatory dendritic cells (DC) and reduce T_H1 lymphocyte

responses while promoting antiinflammatory T_H2 lymphocyte responses (Adorini et al., 2004; Griffin et al., 2001; Penna and Adorini, 2000; Penna et al., 2007). Studies exploring the therapeutic effects of vitamin D in MS are underway (Burton et al., 2010).

Pathologically, MS is characterized by inflammatory infiltrates in the CNS white matter, with resultant demyelination and axonal transections (Trapp et al., 1998) producing sclerotic plaques. Inflammation is generally perivenular, and lesions typically occur in the periventricular subcortical white matter, corpus callosum, optic nerve, brainstem, cerebellum, and spinal cord. Cortical lesions have also been described. The pathology of MS lesions has been classified into four distinct subtypes with the following predominant features: (1) cellular infiltration, (2) antibody deposition, (3) oligodendrocyte apoptosis, and (4) oligodendrocyte death without apoptosis (Lucchinetti et al., 2000). Observations to date show a single subtype of lesion in each patient, raising the possibility of distinct MS disease pathogenetic types. Activated microglia have been demonstrated in non-lesion, or otherwise normal-appearing white matter (NAWM) and may play a role in axonal damage and disease progression.

It is clear that the immune system plays a central role in mediating CNS damage in MS. Oligoclonal bands are commonly observed in the CNS of MS patients; however, the target of these antibodies has yet to be elucidated. Cell-mediated immunity, primarily involving T-helper cells, is believed to play an important role in initiating the disease, and immunological studies have substantiated the presence of activated T cells in MS. Most of the therapies for MS also target T cells. No clear autoantigen has been described in MS, and it therefore remains an immune-mediated disease rather than an autoimmune disease. Reactivity to various myelin antigens, including myelin basic protein (MBP), proteolipid protein (PLP), and myelin oligodendrocyte protein (MOG) has been investigated. MBP-reactive T cells are present in normal individuals; however, MS patients have a higher frequency of activated MBP-reactive T cells in the peripheral blood and the cerebrospinal fluid (CSF) (Zhang et al., 1994).

The immunopathogenesis of MS is thought to involve activation of myelin-specific T cells via molecular mimicry or by a superantigen presumably in the periphery. These cells are believed to predominantly be of the T_H1 phenotype, as evidenced by increased production of IL-12 (the major inducer of T_H1 cytokines) by APCs in the peripheral blood of MS patients with active disease, and the observation that a clinical trial of IFN-γ worsened MS. These cells then cross the BBB and get reactivated in the CNS when they are presented with their cognate antigen. Perivascular dendritic-like cells have been shown to play a role in T-cell reactivation in animal models of MS (Greter et al., 2005), but their role in the human disease is unclear. Adhesion molecules and their ligands are expressed on T cells and endothelial cells to facilitate passage through the BBB. VCAM-1 and its ligand, VLA-4, are up-regulated in T cells during chronic disease, thus perpetuating inflammation, and VLA-4 antibody therapy (natalizumab) has recently been shown to be effective in reducing MS relapses and lesion formation.

Invasion of activated T cells into the brain and reactivation within the CNS initiates a cascade of cytokines. IL-2, IFN-γ, and TNF-α activate macrophages, which in turn elicit nitric oxide and TNF-α. In experimental models, myelin damage is mediated by nitric oxide lipid peroxidation, direct TNF-α damage, and complement-induced pore formation. As mentioned previously, T_H2 cytokines can induce B-cell activation and antibody production that further damage myelin. Each of these steps in the pathogenesis may be targeted for therapeutic intervention.

There is mounting evidence indicating that T cells play a key role in the relapsing-remitting phase of MS. However, recent work has demonstrated that disease progression in MS may be due to distinct mechanisms (Weiner, 2009). Epitope spreading may occur within the CNS, and in animal models can be facilitated by microglia, macrophages, and dendritic cells (McMahon et al., 2005). Activated microglia are found in progressive forms of the disease and have been associated with axonal damage and demyelination (Kutzelnigg et al., 2005). B-cell follicles have been demonstrated at autopsy in patients with chronic MS (Serafini et al., 2004) and may play a role in facilitating an autonomous inflammatory response within the CNS. Cortical demyelination is also associated with progressive forms of MS (Kutzelnigg et al., 2005).

Neuromyelitis optica (NMO), or Devic disease, is a rare subtype of MS characterized by clinical episodes of optic neuritis and transverse myelitis and demonstration of contiguous lesions in the spinal cord (Wingerchuk et al., 2006). The presence of serum antibodies targeting the aquaporin-4 water channel present on the surface of the glia limitans at the BBB has been shown to be a sensitive and specific marker of NMO (Lennon et al., 2004). Injection of aquaporin-4 antibodies into animal models of disease have demonstrated enhanced complement deposition around blood vessels, loss of aquaporin-4, and astrocyte and myelin damage (Kutzelnigg et al., 2005). This study, as well as others, indicate increasing recognition of the role of glial pathology in MS.

A number of immune-mediated autoimmune disorders of the nervous system are available for study in laboratory animals. Besides allowing for the analysis of the immunoregulatory network, they have been critical in designing immunotherapies. Two major animal models exist that mimic the clinical manifestations of MS. These are experimental autoimmune encephalomyelitis (EAE) and Theiler murine encephalomyelitis virus-induced disease (TMEV-IDD). Although animal models are not identical to the human disease, each model may represent certain pathogenic aspects of MS.

EAE is a T cell–mediated autoimmune demyelinating disease of the CNS. The disease can be induced in a number of experimental laboratory animals, including primates, by subcutaneous injection of whole-brain homogenate or of a purified preparation of MBP, PLP, or MOG emulsified in adjuvant. By altering the immunization protocols and animal strains, a relapsing-remitting or a chronic form of the disease may be induced. Various EAE models have demonstrated that mice with a T_H1 cytokine profile are more susceptible to EAE than wild-type mice, whereas animals with a T_H2 (IL-4, IL-10) cytokine profile are generally resistant to disease development (Chitnis et al., 2001). Transfer of T_H17-producing cells induces a more severe form of EAE than transfer of T_H1 cells (Jager et al., 2009); the role of these cells in MS is starting to be elucidated.

TMEV-IDD is induced by injecting TMEV picornavirus into the cerebral hemisphere. The virus infects neurons and glial cells. In some strains of mice, the host is unable to clear the virus, resulting in encephalitis and death; in other cases, the virus is cleared completely, and the host is resistant to demyelination. In TMEV-IDD-susceptible strains of mice, the virus is partially cleared, saving the host from death but inciting an immune response that results in demyelination. Thus the damage induced by the virus is due to a failure of the host to mount a fully protective response, which predisposes the pathogen to persistence, resulting in immunopathology. TMEV-IDD is a T cell–mediated disease; although the exact immunological mechanisms inducing demyelination remain unclear, damage may be a result of epitope spreading (Miller et al., 1997). Studies in both EAE and TMEV have contributed vastly to our understanding of MS, and these models offer a system for testing new therapeutics.

Details of available therapies in MS are discussed in Chapter 60. Here, we discuss the immunological mechanisms of currently used medications, as well as experimental therapeutic strategies.

β-Interferon (IFN-β) therapy for MS is one of the most important advances in the treatment of this disease. It is available in three different forms: subcutaneous IFN-β-1b (Betaseron), subcutaneous IFN-β-1a (Rebif), or intramuscular IFN-β-1a (Avonex). Interferons have many properties, including suppressing proliferation of viruses and T cells. The mechanisms of IFN-β action in MS has been attributed to several different mechanisms. Interferon-associated increased production of IL-10 by macrophages down-regulates the number of T_H1 cells. IFN-β has also been shown to decrease production of IL-12 by dendritic cells, potential CNS APCs, further inhibiting T_H1 cell formation. In addition, IFN-β modulates adhesion molecule expression, primarily by facilitating the conversion of cell-associated VCAM-1 into soluble VCAM-1. These drugs also down-regulate costimulatory molecule expression, thus decreasing T-cell activation and migration to the CNS (Yong, 2002).

Glatiramer acetate (GA), also known as *copolymer-1* or *Copaxone*, is another class of drug used in the treatment of MS. In contrast to IFN-β, GA is a synthetic molecule that was originally designed to resemble MBP. It is composed of random repetitive sequences of the amino acids glutamic acid, lysine, alanine, and tyrosine (G-L-A-T). Its mechanism of action is unclear; however, it is thought to bind with high affinity to the MHC groove, leading to the generation of GA-specific T cells. Several studies have suggested that GA-specific T cells display a T_H2 bias (Duda et al., 2000), and animal models have demonstrated that these cells can migrate to the CNS and ameliorate EAE disease through a local down-regulation of the immune responses (Aharoni et al., 1997). It has also been demonstrated that GA-specific T cells protect from optic nerve crush injuries, possibly mediated by the production of brain-derived neurotrophic factor (BDNF) (Kipnis et al., 2000).

Altered peptide ligands (APL) resembling MBP have been used in phase 1 trials for MS with little success. Two concurrent trials were initiated using the same compound, CGP77116. One showed an increased number of lesions on MRI in some patients after the initiation of treatment (Bielekova et al., 2000). In the other trial, 9% of patients developed allergic-type reactions associated with a T_H2 deviation (Kappos et al., 2000). Both trials were stopped because of safety concerns.

Several new therapies for the treatment of MS are monoclonal antibodies targeting specific receptors on immune cell populations. Natalizumab, an $\alpha 4\beta 1$-integrin antibody (Tysabri), is approved for the treatment of relapsing forms of MS and effectively blocks T- and B-cell migration across the BBB. However, blockade of CNS immune surveillance has produced profound adverse effects, as evidenced by the development of progressive multifocal leukoencephalopathy (PML) with a frequency of approximately 1:1000. The experience with Tysabri has highlighted the importance of balancing potential adverse effects such as infection and tumor with therapeutic efficacy.

Campath-1H targets the CD52 receptor present on lymphocytes and monocytes. Phase 2 studies have shown potent effects in MS, with depletion of peripheral lymphocytes. However, a quarter of treated patients develop autoimmune thyroid disease, and rarely immune thrombocytopenic purpura, suggesting that Campath enhances immune dysregulation in a subset of patients (Coles et al., 2008; Jones et al., 2009). Daclizumab blocks the IL-2R α chain (CD25) present in the high-affinity IL-2 receptor on T cells, thus inhibiting T-cell replication and making more IL-2 available to the low-affinity CD25 receptor present on NK cells, which induces a regulatory NK cell population (Bielekova et al., 2006).

Rituximab, an antibody that primarily targets activated B cells, has recently been shown to reduce disease activity in relapsing-remitting (Hauser et al., 2008) and a subset of primary progressive MS patients (Hawker et al., 2009). Interestingly, open-label studies have suggested that rituximab treatment is effective in patients with neuromyelitis optica, which is increasingly thought of as an antibody-mediated disease. Another therapy currently under investigation is CTLA4Ig, which blocks B7-CD28 costimulatory signals on T cells and may induce T-cell anergy in vivo.

Many therapeutic strategies that have been used in the past nonspecifically target components of the immune response. Nonspecific strategies include cyclophosphamide, mitoxantrone, and cladribine, which depress bone marrow production of cells, including T cells. Cyclophosphamide may also function by inducing a cytokine switch, with a decrease in IL-12 and an increase in IL-4, IL-5, and TGF-β (Comabella et al., 1998). A novel strategy to suppress immune responses in MS is a small molecule, fingolimod, which targets the sphingosine-1-phosphate receptor, which is necessary for lymphocyte egress from lymph nodes (Comi et al., 2010).

Acute Disseminated Encephalomyelitis

Acute disseminated encephalomyelitis (ADEM) is a monophasic demyelinating disease associated with vaccination or a systemic viral infection; it can affect both adults and children. ADEM was originally described in association with rabies and smallpox vaccines, both of which were prepared with neural tissues, suggesting a parallel with EAE, the animal model of MS. These vaccines have since been modified, using non-neural human diploid cell lines. ADEM has not been associated with any vaccines that are currently administered in the United States. The parainfectious variant of ADEM has been associated with measles infection, rubella, mumps, and several other viruses. Viral or bacterial epitopes resembling myelin antigens have the capacity to activate myelin-reactive T-cell clones through molecular mimicry (Wucherpfennig, Hafler, and Strominger, 1995) and can

thereby elicit a CNS-specific autoimmune response. Thus, it has been suggested that microbial infections elicit a cross-reactive antimyelin response through molecular mimicry, resulting in ADEM. Myelin peptides have been shown to resemble several viral sequences, and in some cases, cross-reactive T-cell responses have been demonstrated. MBP is the prototypical inducer of EAE, but other myelin proteins like MOG and PLP have also been extensively studied. Examples of cross-reactive T cells with MBP antigens include HHV-6 (Tejada-Simon et al., 2003), coronavirus (Talbot et al., 1996), influenza virus hemagglutinin (Markovic-Plese et al., 2005), and EBV (Lang et al., 2002). PLP shares common sequences with *Haemophilus influenzae* (Olson et al., 2001). Semliki Forest virus (SFV) peptides mimic MOG (Mokhtarian et al., 1999).

The lesions in ADEM resemble those of MS. The CNS white matter contains perivascular inflammatory infiltrates as well as demyelination. The most likely mechanism by which this disease occurs is molecular mimicry. Experimental evidence has shown that T cells isolated from patients with ADEM are 10 times more likely to react with MBP than controls, likening this disease to EAE in animal models (Pohl-Koppe et al., 1998). We have recently found that 30% of patients with ADEM demonstrate serum antibodies to MOG, which were absent in MS patients (O'Connor K et al., 2007). Because of the monophasic nature of ADEM, it appears that the immunological response occurs acutely, but in contrast to MS, further amplification of inflammation within the CNS is suppressed.

MRI demonstrates multifocal white matter lesions involving the cerebrum, brainstem, cerebellum, and spinal cord, which may or may not enhance with gadolinium. Lesions generally resolve over time. CSF is characterized by normal pressure, moderately elevated cell count (5–100/μL), moderately elevated protein (40–100 mg/dL), and normal glucose. The presence of red blood cells may indicate a diagnosis of hemorrhagic leukoencephalitis. Oligoclonal bands may very rarely be present, and these cases should be followed for the development of MS.

Acute episodes of ADEM should be treated with intravenous corticosteroids. The usual dose is 1 g/day of methylprednisolone for 5 days in adults. Refractory cases have been treated with plasmapheresis or cyclophosphamide. Cases that are suspicious for MS should be followed with MRI.

Immune-Mediated Neuropathies

The immune-mediated neuropathies are a large and heterogeneous group of diseases. We shall focus on acute inflammatory demyelinating polyneuropathy (AIDP) and chronic inflammatory demyelinating polyneuropathy (CIDP), which may be defined by the time to peak disability; in the former, 4 weeks, and in the latter, 2 months. Although AIDP and CIDP share many characteristics, the question of whether one is a continuum of the other is still under debate. AIDP or Guillain-Barré syndrome (GBS) usually presents with symmetrical ascending weakness and may be associated with autonomic dysfunction and respiratory depression. Sensory systems may be involved and may present with paresthesias or numbness. Demyelination and axonal damage may be involved to varying degrees. If the patient's symptoms continue to progress beyond 4 weeks, the illness is termed *CIDP*.

AIDP is the most common acute paralytic disease in the Western world, with a mean annual incidence of 1.8 per 100,000 persons. There is an increasing incidence with age. Mortality was generally due to respiratory failure and has now been significantly reduced with the introduction of positive-pressure ventilation. Epidemics have been found, most notably in northern China, where a high incidence has been associated with *C. jejuni* infections (McKhann et al., 1993).

AIDP or GBS is characterized pathologically by an endoneurial lymphocytic, monocytic, and macrophage infiltrate. Several autoantibodies to myelin glycolipids have been identified, including GM1, GD1a, and GD1b. Antibody-mediated demyelination due to complement fixation has been identified in pathology specimens. In some cases, axonal damage is present and is believed to be a result of bystander damage. Activation of calcium-dependent processes within the nerve, including calpain activation, has been shown in animal models to augment axonal degeneration (O'Hanlon et al., 2003). GBS is primarily an antibody-mediated disease, as evidenced by the fact that many patients improve after treatment with plasmapheresis, and that serum from GBS patients causes demyelination after transfer into experimental animals and peripheral nerve cultures. The Miller-Fisher variant of GBS is characterized by ophthalmoplegia, ataxia, and areflexia and is associated with the presence of GQ1b antibodies in the serum.

The occurrence of AIDP has been linked to many infectious diseases, including *C. jejuni*, herpesvirus, *Mycoplasma pneumonia*, and many other bacterial and viral infections, as well as vaccinations. The incidence of infection has been reported to be 90% in the 30 days before occurrence of GBS. *C. jejuni* is one of the most commonly identifiable agents, and molecular mimicry and host susceptibility play a role in disease pathogenesis. Autoantibodies not present in controls have been identified in the sera of GBS patients associated with *C. jejuni*, including autoantibodies to the gangliosides GM1, GD1a, GD1b, and GQ1b (Sheikh et al., 1998).

In contrast to AIDP, in CIDP no specific autoantibodies have yet been discovered. The histopathological picture is similar to AIDP; however, most studies identify fewer inflammatory infiltrates. Nerve biopsy reveals mixed demyelination and axonal changes. Onion bulbs may be present, indicating attempts at remyelination. There is little laboratory evidence that this disease is antibody mediated, but paradoxically, patients do improve with plasmapheresis. There is indirect evidence that CIDP is T-cell mediated; however, this area is still under investigation.

Treatment of AIDP involves supportive care and cardiac and respiratory monitoring. Plasmapheresis or intravenous immunoglobulin (IVIG) have been used for acute treatment of AIDP and have been shown to be equally effective in shortening recovery time. Plasmapheresis is a short-term immunotherapy that nonspecifically removes antibodies from the circulation. IVIG is an immunomodulating agent commonly used in the treatment of allergic and autoimmune diseases. It works in part through the presence of Fc fragments that interact with the inhibitory Fc receptor, FcγRIIB, which is also induced on macrophages following IVIG administration (Samuelsson et al., 2001). Additionally, IVIG may displace low-affinity autoantibodies from the nerve. High-dose steroids have not been found to be effective in AIDP. In contrast to AIDP, CIDP responds well to high-dose oral corticosteroids. Both plasmapheresis and IVIG are also used

with success. Immunosuppressants such as cyclosporine A, cyclophosphamide, and azathioprine have had positive outcomes in refractory cases but require further testing in controlled studies. Future therapies for AIDP or CIDP may target complement activation or inhibition of axonal calpain activation.

Autoimmune Myasthenia Gravis

Myasthenia gravis is a disorder of the neuromuscular junction. It is an autoimmune disorder, and 80% to 90% of cases have detectable autoantibodies to the α subunit of the acetylcholine receptor (AChR). MG is characterized by fluctuating weakness and fatigability, primarily in muscles innervated by the cranial nerves, but may occur in skeletal and respiratory muscles. MG has a biphasic age distribution. Most cases occur in women between the ages of 20 to 40 years, the remainder in older patients, with an equal sex distribution. Thymomas occur in 10% to 15% of cases; most are in the older age group. Some 75% of patients will have a thymic abnormality, 85% being thymic hyperplasia. MG is often associated with other autoimmune diseases, thyroid disorders, rheumatoid arthritis (RA), pernicious anemia, and SLE. A similar syndrome, Lambert-Eaton, is associated with antibodies against the presynaptic voltage-gated calcium channel, generally in the setting of small cell cancer of the lung.

Autoimmune MG is caused by the presence of α_1 nicotinic acetylcholine receptor (nAChR) antibodies and is a B cell–mediated disease. Eighty percent to 90% of patients have detectable autoantibodies. These are polyclonal and may be of any IgG subtype. Transfer of serum from myasthenic patients to experimental animals results in neuromuscular blockade. The mechanism by which antibody mediates neurological symptoms is controversial. Possible mechanisms include neuromuscular blockade or damage to the AChR from complement-mediated damage after attachment of the IgG antibody. There is, however, poor correlation between serum antibody titers and disease course and severity.

Although the B cell is the effector cell producing antibodies, experimental evidence has shown that autoreactive T cells are necessary for the disease to occur (Yi and Lefvert, 1994). Removal of the thymus results in improvement of disease in 80% to 90% of myasthenic patients. The role of thymic abnormalities remains unclear, and patients with thymomas have antibodies to additional skeletal muscle proteins such as the ryanodine receptor and titin, as well as the neuromuscular junctional protein, MuSK. Patients may also display symptoms of neuromyotonia. Antibodies directed towards α_3-nAChR are associated with autoimmune autonomic neuropathy.

A large body of research is targeted at understanding the reasons for the failure of T-cell and subsequent failure of B-cell tolerance in MG. Both normal and myasthenic thymus glands contain myoid cells and epithelial cells that express the AChR. T cells expressing the $V_\beta 5.1^+$ TCRs are overrepresented, both in the core of germinal centers and in perifollicular areas of hyperplastic thymuses, suggesting a role in the autoimmune response (Truffault et al., 1997). Failure of central or thymic tolerance may play an important role in disease pathogenesis.

Genetic factors play a role in the pathogenesis of autoimmune MG, but monozygotic twins demonstrate less than 50%

concordance rate. There is a moderate association of MG with the HLA antigens B8 and DRw3 in young women. The stronger association with HLA-DQw2 remains controversial. There is an unusually high incidence of other autoimmune diseases such as SLE, RA, and thyroid diseases in first-degree relatives of myasthenic patients, suggesting the presence of shared autoimmune genes.

Therapies in MG are targeted toward alleviating symptoms with acetylcholinesterase inhibitors and using strategies to reduce the damage being done by the immune system. Thymectomy is recommended for patients 15 to 65 years old, with 80% to 90% remission rate (Durelli et al., 1991). The thymus plays an important role in T-cell education in the developing human; therefore prepubertal thymectomy is discouraged. A variety of anticholinesterase inhibitors provide temporary symptomatic relief in most patients. Pyridostigmine bromide (Mestinon) and neostigmine bromide (Prostigmin) are the most commonly used agents and must be taken daily.

MG is an antibody-mediated disease and therefore responds to therapies that nonspecifically target antibodies. Both plasmapheresis and treatment with IVIG are used for acute MG exacerbations or in preparation for surgery (Gajdos et al., 1997). Because the autoantigen is known in MG, investigational therapies may target specific molecules such as the B-cell surface Ig or the TCR and deliver immunotoxins.

Immunosuppressives such as cyclosporine, azathioprine, and mycophenolate are used to augment treatment when symptoms are not adequately controlled by the previously mentioned methods, but the decision to use such agents must balance the need and the side effects. Corticosteroids are used at various stages of treatment and have multiple effects on the immune system, including reducing AChR antibody levels.

Inflammatory Muscle Diseases

Polymyositis (PM), dermatomyositis (DM), and inclusion body myositis (IBM) are all inflammatory and presumably immune-mediated diseases of the muscle and the surrounding connective tissue. Each has its own unique clinical and immunohistological features. Both PM and DM are more common in females, whereas IBM is more common in males. DM in adults is associated with an increased risk of cancer, and therefore a full cancer screening should be part of patient management.

PM is thought to result from a multitude of causes, including systemic autoimmune connective-tissue disorders and viral and bacterial infections. PM is characterized histopathologically by an endomysial inflammatory infiltrate containing predominantly CD8[+] T cells. There is relative sparing of blood vessels. In one subtype of PM, T cells with $\gamma\delta$ receptors have been identified surrounding non-necrotic muscle fibers (Hohlfeld et al., 1991).

In contrast, DM is characterized by perifascicular atrophy. There is hypoperfusion and subsequent degeneration of the muscle fibers in the periphery of the fascicle, secondary to microvascular damage. Damage to capillaries, resulting in muscle fiber ischemia, is mediated by complement. Immunofluorescence studies have revealed immune-complex deposition within the endothelium, indicating that this is an antibody-mediated disease; therefore the disease differs from PM (Kissel et al., 1986).

As with PM, IBM is mediated by CD8[+] T cells. However, in contrast to PM, the muscle biopsy in IBM may also demonstrate the presence of characteristic autophagic "rimmed" vacuoles. Amyloid deposits may be demonstrated in the muscle, similar to those seen in AD, suggesting similarities in pathogenesis of these two diseases (Askanas et al., 1992).

Various autoantibodies directed against nuclear and cytoplasmic cell components are found in up to 30% of inflammatory myopathies. Most are nonspecific for connective-tissue disease. Viruses including coxsackie B are implicated in the pathogenesis of disease, and both PM and DM patients may have anti-Jo-1 antibodies to the viral enzyme, histidyl-tRNA synthetase (Mathews and Bernstein 1983). More recently, the presence of B cells, and in particular antibody-secreting plasma cells with V-D-J rearrangements, has been demonstrated in muscle biopsies from both IBM and PM and to a lesser extent in DM (Greenberg et al., 2005).

The mainstay of treatment of PM and DM is corticosteroids. Dosages may vary from 60 to 100 mg/day of prednisone, and duration is determined by clinical outcome. Alternative treatment options for the inflammatory myositis diseases include IVIG, methotrexate, azathioprine, cyclophosphamide, cyclosporine, and in extreme cases, total lymphoid or whole-body irradiation (Mastaglia et al., 1998). Mortality rates vary between 15% and 35% and are generally due to cardiac or respiratory failure. Because there is a higher incidence of malignancy with PM and DM, screening for breast, lung, hematological, ovary, stomach, and colon carcinoma should be performed on patients with these diagnoses. IBM may be more resistant to corticosteroid therapy and is often diagnosed after an assumed PM fails to respond to treatment.

Alzheimer Disease and Amyotrophic Lateral Sclerosis

It may seem strange to include AD and ALS in a chapter on neuroimmunology. These diseases have traditionally been considered neurodegenerative, but recent studies and therapies have suggested a role for the immune system in disease pathogenesis and protection.

β-Amyloid plaques and neurofibrillary tangles consisting of hyperphosphorylated tau protein are the hallmarks of AD. Clearance of amyloid plaques consisting of amyloid-β-fibrils is considered a primary goal of therapy. Amyloid plaques are often surrounded by activated microglia and reactive astrocytes, and are associated with complement activation, leading to the hypothesis that the immune response participates in the clearance of amyloid deposits. Further studies in animal models of AD demonstrated that immunization with amyloid-β peptide resulted in the induction of amyloid-β-specific antibodies, which enhanced the clearance of amyloid plaques (Janus et al., 2000; Morgan et al., 2000). Passive transfer of amyloid-β-specific antibodies yielded similar results. Amyloid plaque clearance is believed to occur through either microglial- and complement-mediated clearance or through direct antibody-amyloid interactions. These studies led to a clinical trial investigating an amyloid-β vaccine administered in conjunction with an adjuvant, which enhanced T_H1 responses. Although cognitive testing results were favorable, 6% of patients developed meningoencephalitis, which is generally believed to be a result of T-cell responses to amyloid-β (Gilman et al., 2005; Orgogozo et al., 2003). Thus, induction of an antibody and microglial-mediated clearance of amyloid in the absence of a prominent T_H1 response is the current goal of therapy. An intriguing study has recently demonstrated that nasal administration of glatiramer acetate (Copaxone), which induces a predominantly T_H2 cellular response, to a murine model of AD resulted in the clearance of amyloid-β plaques in association with activated microglia, but in the absence of antibody formation (Frenkel et al., 2005). Future immunotherapeutic strategies for AD include modified vaccines and strategies to induce activation of microglial cells in the absence of deleterious side effects.

In ALS, a new avenue of investigation has emerged: exploring the role of microglia in disease pathogenesis and, in particular, on disease progression. Pathological analysis and neuroimaging using positron electron tomography (PET) studies have demonstrated activated microglia in areas of severe motor neuron loss. Studies in the animal model of ALS have demonstrated that the presence of the SOD1 mutation in microglia enhanced disease progression (Boillee et al., 2006). Use of minocycline, which acts in part by inhibiting microglial activation, has shown some initial promise in the treatment of ALS. Cyclooxygenase-2 (COX-2) inhibitors have reduced disease severity in animal models of ALS but have been ineffective in humans. Lymphocytes, including T cells, do not appear to play a significant role in this disease, and this is reinforced by the failure of studies using T cell–targeted therapies including total lymphoid irradiation (TLI) or cyclophosphamide. Thus, possible future therapies for ALS include strategies to down-regulate microglial activation.

Immune Response to Infectious Diseases

The immune response within the CNS must carefully balance the need to eliminate the pathogen and the risk of inducing bystander damage to the delicate and vital nervous tissues. This is believed to be the reason the CNS immune response deviates from that in the rest of the body, and it remains an immune-privileged site. The result is that many pathogens are not completely eliminated and may persist to cause further symptoms. Examples of this are CNS syphilis, Lyme neuroborreliosis, herpes zoster, HIV, and *Mycobacterium tuberculosis.* Lyme *Borrelia* incites IFN-γ production, with correspondingly low levels of IL-4 in the CSF, thus predisposing the CNS tissue to bystander damage.

The portal of entry and site of replication of the pathogen plays a critical role in elimination of the infection. In the case of viral meningitis, the portal of entry is the mucosal membrane, usually the nasopharynx. This incites a strong local immune response to the proliferating organism, and by the time the virus disseminates to the leptomeninges, a sufficient immune response has been mounted in the periphery to eliminate the pathogen. However, in the case of viral encephalitis, the CNS invasion is so sudden that the peripheral immune system has insufficient time to react, and the weak CNS immune response is often inadequate, resulting in a poor outcome.

HIV-associated dementia (HAD) is a clinical disorder characterized by cognitive, behavioral, and motor dysfunction in AIDS patients. HIV infection of the brain is characterized by multinucleated giant cells, astrogliosis, microglial nodules, and neuronal loss in the cortex and basal ganglia. The HIV protein, gp120, can bind directly to CXCR4 on neurons, resulting in neuronal signaling and apoptosis. Neurodegeneration is also thought to occur through production of neurotoxic factors by HIV-infected microglia and astrocytes. HIV infection results in production of proinflammatory cytokines (IL-6, IL-1 and TNF-α), nitric oxide, and MMPs by microglia, aa well as increased glutamate by dysfunctional astrocytes. Astrocyte production of SDF-1 (CXCR4 ligand), which is subsequently cleaved by MMP-2 to produce a truncated protein, c-SDF, is neurotoxic in vitro. In summary, glial-mediated neurotoxicity plays a significant role in the pathogenesis of HAD and is an active area of investigation.

Tumor Immunology

The immunological response to tumors has elicited much interest in the past 10 years. This field provides opportunities for understanding the cause and immunological features of tumors and venues for treatment.

The body uses a mechanism called *tumor immunosurveillance* to prevent the formation of tumors or inhibit further growth. The main effector cells are CTLs, NK cells, and TNF-α-producing macrophages. Tumor-reactive antibodies have also been identified in patients but are thought to play a lesser role. It has been recognized that tumors express tumor-specific antigens that may be recognized by the previously mentioned cells. However, tumor cells may escape the body's natural surveillance mechanisms, resulting in cancer. Tumor cells escape surveillance mechanisms by masking or modulating antigens on their surface, down-regulating class I and II molecules (thereby inhibiting antigen presentation), and expressing immunosuppressant factors.

Tumors in the CNS have similar abilities to evade the immune system, and it has been shown that some gliomas produce high levels of TGF-β, an immunosuppressant. Down-regulation of class II MHC may also occur, but this is remains controversial. It has recently been established that gliomas may express high levels of FasL, allowing for local apoptosis of Fas-bearing cells including lymphocytes. Increased expression of the inhibitory costimulatory molecule, B7H1, on gliomas has been shown to play a role in down-regulating T-cell responses (Wintterle et al., 2003). Glioma patients have been shown to express increased frequencies of $CD4^+CD25^+Foxp3^+$ regulatory T cells. Treatment with daclizumab (anti-CD25 antibody) in a murine model of glioma reduced regulatory T-cell function and enhanced host tumor immunity, so daclizumab therapy in CNS tumors merits additional investigation.

Additional therapies are being designed to exploit the body's natural tumor immunosurveillance mechanisms. One avenue of research is vaccination with killed tumor cells or tumor antigens. Another technique employs genetic engineering to transfect tumors with plasmids bearing genes for costimulatory molecules to enhance the tumor APC ability. Injection of cytokines such as IL-2 and TNF-α, which enhance lymphocyte and NK function, has been attempted with variable results. Dendritic cells pulsed with tumor antigens to induce NK cell-mediated tumor killing is a promising new therapy for CNS gliomas and is under investigation.

Overall, strategies to enhance host tumor immunosurveillance and reduce inhibitory responses mediated by CNS tumors are promising new avenues of treatment.

Paraneoplastic Syndromes

Neurological paraneoplastic disorders are defined as neurological syndromes arising in association with a distant cancer. These are mediated by antibodies produced by the immune system in reaction to a tumor antigen, which cross-react with neural tissue. It is likely that aberrant, primitive, or hamartomatous antigens are expressed by the tumor cells. Enhanced cellular infiltrates are found in tumors associated with paraneoplastic syndrome compared to those not associated with a paraneoplastic syndrome. Therefore one can postulate that the immune system is more active in these situations. Cancers associated with paraneoplastic syndromes are generally associated with a better outcome. Several autoantibodies associated with paraneoplastic syndromes have been identified. The anti-Hu antibody arises in association with small-cell cancer of the lung and cross-reacts with neurons; it is linked to a syndrome of encephalomyelitis and/or sensory neuropathy. Similarly, anti-Yo antibody produces cerebellar degeneration due to cross-reactivity with Purkinje cell cytoplasm and is associated with breast and ovarian cancer. Opsoclonus-myoclonus syndrome is associated with anti-Ri antibody and is found in cases of cancer of the ovary and breast. Cases of paraneoplastic and immune-mediated brainstem and limbic encephalitis have recently been reported to be caused by antibodies targeting LGI1, a neuronal-secreted protein that interacts with presynaptic ADAM23 and postsynaptic ADAM22 (Lai et al., 2010). NMDA receptor encephalitis typically presents with seizures and psychiatric symptoms, but a recent case report describes a patient presenting with optic neuritis and transverse myelitis mimicking neuromyelitis optica (Kruer et al., 2010). Antibodies directed against VGKC are also associated with acquired neuromyotonia, or Isaac syndrome, and Morvan syndrome, characterized by neuromyotonia and insomnia. Lambert-Eaton myasthenic syndrome is caused by antibodies directed against the P/Q type of voltage-gated calcium channels and is generally found in the setting of small-cell cancer of the lung. The same antibodies have also been associated with cases of lung cancer–associated cerebellar ataxia. Stiff person syndrome is associated with antibodies to glutamic acid decarboxylase (GAD), and both autoimmune and paraneoplastic forms, principally associated with breast cancer, have been described.

Antibody-Associated Neurological Syndromes

In the past 10 years, more sophisticated techniques have led to greater insights into the study of antibodies in CNS diseases. Antiphospholipid (APL) syndrome, or Hughes syndrome, results in CNS symptoms that include chorea, strokes, bleeding, migraine headaches, and epilepsy (Asherson, 2006). These result in part from the underlying systemic problems of coagulopathy and thrombocytopenia, but more direct effects of autoantibodies directed against neuronal antigens have been implicated both in APL syndrome and in CNS lupus. One study found that antibodies directed against the NR2A and NR2B subunits of the NMDA receptor were found in a subset of patients with CNS lupus and could facilitate apoptotic death of neurons (DeGiorgio et al., 2001).

Sydenham chorea is associated with *Streptococcus pyogenes* (β-hemolytic streptococcal) infections, and there is considerable evidence for a causative role of antibodies that cross-react with streptococcal antigens and neurons in the basal ganglia. This association has led to the postulation that molecular mimicry mechanisms related to streptococcal infections may result in other movement disorders, including Tourette syndrome and the clinical entity of pediatric autoimmune neuropsychiatric disorders associated with streptococcal infection (PANDAS), which encompasses tics and obsessive-compulsive disorder in children. Evidence for an immune-mediated mechanism is inconclusive (Harris and Singer, 2006).

Antibodies directed against glutamate receptor 3 (GluR3) are associated with Rasmussen encephalitis, a form of severe intractable epilepsy localized to one hemisphere and partially responsive to immunotherapy. The presence of antibodies directed against voltage-gated potassium channels in a small group of patients with intractable epilepsy has recently been demonstrated (Majoie et al., 2006) and raises the question of whether other immune-mediated forms of epilepsy may exist.

Immunology of Central Nervous System Transplant

Recently, there has been much research in the field of CNS transplantation, with the use of fetal dopaminergic striatal cells, various types of genetically engineered cells, and the potential of stem cell transplantation. A major factor in the survival of these grafts is their lack of immunogenicity in the relatively immune-privileged site of the CNS. Therefore transplant grafts in the CNS tend to have longer survival times than peripheral grafts; however, this is not absolute, and rejection can undoubtedly occur.

Factors that influence CNS graft survival are: type of graft (xenogenic, allogeneic, genetically modified tissue, or stem cell populations); location of the graft, with the periventricular areas being the most susceptible to rejection; presence of antigen-presenting cells within the graft, which can be eliminated in purified grafts; and host immunosuppression.

Immunosuppressive strategies currently under investigation include the immunophilins, daclizumab, and cyclosporine. Successful immunosuppression must be balanced against the risk of graft toxicity.

Neural stem cells (NSCs) are increasingly being investigated in neurodegenerative diseases. In addition to their effects on repair, studies in the animal model of MS found that these cells suppress disease (Einstein et al., 2003; Einstein et al., 2007; Pluchino et al., 2003; Pluchino et al., 2005; Yang et al., 2009) through immunomodulatory mechanisms. Some studies suggested that NSCs can directly inhibit T-cell proliferation in response to concanavalin A (ConA) or to MOG peptide (Einstein et al., 2003; Pluchino et al., 2005) by inducing T-cell apoptosis (Pluchino et al., 2005; Yang et al., 2009) or through nitric oxide– and PGE2-mediated T-cell suppression (Wang et al., 2009). Neural stem cells can express costimulatory molecules, CD80 and CD86, particularly after exposure to the proinflammatory cytokines, IFN-γ and TNF-α (Imitola et al., 2004). Thus, NSCs are not conventional immune cells, but under certain conditions, they can interact with immune cells.

Summary

The field of immunology has progressed significantly in the past 30 years. This knowledge is currently being applied to immune-mediated diseases in neurology. In this rich environ-ment, we can expect many advances in the field of neuroim-munology, including new therapies and better strategies for the treatment of neurological diseases.

References

The complete reference list is available online at www.expertconsult.com.

Neuroendocrinology

Paul E. Cooper

Neuroendocrinology is the study of the coordinated interaction of the nervous, endocrine, and immune systems to maintain the constancy of the internal milieu (homeostasis). In practical clinical terms, it concentrates mainly on the function of the hypothalamus and its interaction with the pituitary gland.

Neuropeptides, Neurotransmitters, and Neurohormones

One of the features of the neuroendocrine system is that it uses neuropeptides as both neurotransmitters and neurohormones. The term *neurotransmitter* is applied traditionally to a substance that is released by one neuron and acts on an adjacent neuron in a stimulatory or inhibitory fashion. The effect usually is rapid, brief, and confined to a small area of the neuron surface. In contrast, a *hormone* is a substance that is released into the bloodstream and travels to a distant site to act over seconds, minutes, or hours to produce its effect over a large area of the cell or over many cells. *Neuropeptides* can act in either fashion. For example, the neuropeptide, vasopressin, produced by the neurons of the supraoptic and paraventricular nuclei, is released into the bloodstream and has a hormonal action on the collecting ducts in the kidney. Vasopressin is also released within the central nervous system (CNS), where it acts as a neurotransmitter (Landgraf and

Neumann, 2004). Similarly, the neuropeptide, substance P, acts as a neurotransmitter in primary sensory neurons that convey pain signals, and more as a neurohormone in the hypothalamus.

The influence of neurohormones and neuropeptides on the brain can be divided into two broad categories: organizational and activational. *Organizational effects* occur during neuronal differentiation, growth, and development and bring about permanent structural changes in the organization of the brain and therefore brain function. An example of this is the structural and organizational changes brought about in the brain by prenatal exposure to testosterone. *Activational effects* are those that change preestablished patterns of neuronal activity, such as an increased rate of neuronal firing caused by exposure of a neuron to substance P.

Numerous neuropeptides are found in the brain, where they have a wide variety of effects on neuronal function (**Table 42.1**). Current understanding of all the actions of neuropeptides in the nervous system is far from complete.

Neuropeptides and the Immune System

It has been known for many years that stress, acting through the hypothalamic-pituitary-adrenal axis, modulates the function of the immune system (Tsigos and Chrousos, 2002;

Table 42.1 Neuropeptides Found in the Brain and Their Effects on Brain Function*

Neuropeptide	Central Nervous System Function
HYPOTHALAMIC PEPTIDES MODULATING PITUITARY FUNCTION	
Corticotropin (ACTH)-releasing hormone (CRH)	Regulation of ACTH secretion Integration of behavioral and biochemical responses to stress Modulatory effects on learning and memory
Growth hormone–releasing hormone (GHRH)	Regulation of growth hormone secretion
Growth hormone release–inhibiting hormone (somatostatin)	Regulation of growth hormone secretion
Ghrelin	Regulation of growth hormone secretion Regulation of feeding
Thyrotropin-releasing hormone (TRH)	Regulation of thyroid-stimulating hormone secretion May be involved in depression Enhances neuromuscular function (in the periphery)
Gonadotropin-releasing hormone (luteinizing hormone–releasing hormone) (GnRH)	Regulates gonadotropin secretion Controls sexual receptivity
Prolactin-releasing peptide	Stimulates prolactin secretion
Neurotensin	Endogenous neuroleptic Regulates mesolimbic, mesocortical, and nigrostriatal dopamine neurons Thermoregulation Analgesia
Neuropeptide Y	Satiety (induces obesity) and drinking Sexual behavior Locomotion Memory
Orexins (hypocretins)	Stimulates CRH and antidiuretic hormone (ADH) Inhibits GHRH Stimulates GnRH May stimulate preovulatory prolactin release Inhibits TRH release
PITUITARY PEPTIDES	
Prolactin	Maternal behavior Mood Anxiety
Growth hormone	
Thyroid-stimulating hormone	
Follicle-stimulating hormone	
Luteinizing hormone	Elevated levels may promote neurodegeneration
Pro-opiomelanocortin	
ACTH	
ACTH-like intermediate lobe peptides	
β-Endorphin	Analgesic mechanisms Feeding Thermoregulation Learning and memory
β-Lipotropic hormone	Skin tanning
Melanocyte-stimulating hormone (α- and γ-)	Weight loss Skin tanning Increased sexual desire Antiinflammatory effect Important mediator of leptin control on energy homeostasis
Oxytocin	Anxiety and mood Active/passive stress coping Maternal behavior, aggression Pair bonding

Continued

Table 42.1 **Neuropeptides Found in the Brain and Their Effects on Brain Function—cont'd**

Neuropeptide	Central Nervous System Function
Vasopressin	Active/passive stress coping Anxiety Spatial memory Social discrimination, social interaction Pair bonding
Neurophysins	
BRAIN–GASTROINTESTINAL TRACT PEPTIDES	
Vasoactive intestinal polypeptide	Cerebral blood flow Potent antiinflammatory factor
Somatostatin	
Insulin	Feeding behavior Modulatory effect on learning and memory Hunger
Glucagon	Inhibition of feeding
Pancreatic polypeptide	
Gastrin	
Cholecystokinin	Feeding behavior Satiety Modulates dopamine neuron activity Facilitation of memory processing (especially under stress)
Tachykinins (e.g., substance P)	Substance P co-localizes with serotonin and is involved in nociception
Secretin	Modulates motor and other functions in brain, facilitating GABA
Thyrotropin-releasing hormone	
Bombesin	Thermoregulation Inhibition of feeding Modulatory effect on learning and memory
Orexins (hypocretin)	Gastric and gastrointestinal motility and secretion Pancreatic hormone release Regulation of energy homeostasis Feeding behavior Locomotion and muscle tone Wakefulness/sleep
Galanin	Modulates release of gonadotropin-releasing hormone, prolactin, insulin, glucagons, growth hormone, and somatostatin Affects feeding, sexual behavior, and anxiety Potent anticonvulsant effects
Leptin	Satiety factor
GROWTH FACTORS	
Insulin-like growth factors (IGF) 1 and 2	
Nerve growth factors	Axonal plasticity
OPIOID FAMILY	
Endorphins	Analgesia
Enkephalins (met-, leu-)	Analgesic mechanisms Feeding Temperature control Learning and memory Cardiovascular control
Dynorphins	
Kytorphin	
NEUROPEPTIDES MODULATING IMMUNE FUNCTION	
ACTH	
Endorphins	
Interferons	

Table 42.1	Neuropeptides Found in the Brain and Their Effects on Brain Function—cont'd
Neuropeptide	**Central Nervous System Function**
Neuroleukins	
Thymosin	
Thymopeptin	
OTHER NEUROPEPTIDES	
Atrial natriuretic factors	?Role in cerebral salt wasting
Bradykinins	Cerebral blood flow
Migraine	
OTHER NEUROPEPTIDES	
Angiotensin	Hypertension
	Thirst
Synapsins	
Calcitonin gene–related peptide	Migraine and other vascular headaches
Calcitonin	
Sleep peptides	Regulation of sleep cycles
Orexins (hypocretin)	Sleep-wake regulation
	Narcolepsy
	Energy homeostasis
Carnosine	
PRECURSOR PEPTIDES	
Pro-opiomelanocortin	
Proenkephalins (A and B)	
Calcitonin gene product	
Vasoactive intestinal polypeptide gene product	
Proglucagon	
Proinsulin	

ACTH, Adrenocorticotropic hormone; *GABA*, γ-aminobutyric acid.
*This is only a partial list of all of the neuropeptides that have been found in the brain, and not all of the putative functions have been listed.

Wrona, 2006). Certain peptides and their receptors, once thought to be unique to either the immune or the neuroendocrine systems, actually are found in both.

Cytokines—interleukins (IL)-1, -2, -4, and -6 and tumor necrosis factor (TNF)—are synthesized by glial cells in the CNS in response to cell injury. IL-1 and the other cytokines, through their ability to stimulate the synthesis of nerve growth factor, may be important promoters of neuron damage repair. Circulating cytokines have been thought to play a role in the hypothalamus to activate the hypothalamic-pituitary-adrenal axis in response to inflammation elsewhere in the body (see Fever, later in this chapter) and inhibit the pituitary-thyroid and pituitary-gonadal axes in response to systemic disease.

Several other hormones and neuropeptides have modulatory effects on immune function. Similarly, immunocompetent cells contain hormones and neuropeptides that may affect neuroendocrine and brain cells (**Table 42.2**). Despite speculation about the ability of the psyche to influence immunological function and therefore disease outcome, conclusive evidence suggesting a clinically significant effect remains lacking (Padgett and Glaser, 2003).

Nonendocrine Hypothalamus

Temperature Regulation

The hypothalamus plays a key role in ensuring that body temperature is maintained within narrow limits by balancing the heat gained from metabolic activity and the environment with the heat lost to the environment. A theoretical schema of the mechanisms of hypothalamic temperature regulation is depicted in **Fig. 42.1**. Although numerous neurotransmitters and peptides alter body temperature, their physiological roles remain unclear.

Hypothalamic injury can cause disordered temperature regulation. One potentially serious consequence is the hyperthermia that may occur when the preoptic anterior hypothalamic area is damaged or irritated by ischemia, subarachnoid hemorrhage, trauma, or surgery. In some patients, the marked impairment of heat-loss mechanisms and the resulting hyperthermia may be fatal. In those individuals who survive, temperature control usually returns to normal over a period of days to weeks. Chronic hyperthermia of hypothalamic origin is extremely uncommon; it may occur with continued impairment of ability to dissipate heat adequately or with difficulty

Table 42.2 **Immunoregulatory Effects of Several Hormones and Peptides**

Hormone or Peptide	Immunocompetent Cell in which Hormone Is Found	Comments
INHIBITORY		
Glucocorticoids		Inhibit lymphokine synthesis, inflammation
Corticotropin (ACTH)	B lymphocytes	Stimulated by corticotropin-releasing hormone; inhibited by cortisol Macrophage activation, synthesis of IgG and γ-interferon
Chorionic gonadotropin	T cells	Stimulated by thyrotropin-releasing hormone; inhibited by somatostatin Activity of T cells and natural killer cells
α-Endorphin		IgG synthesis, T-cell proliferation
Somatostatin	Mononuclear leukocytes, mast cells	T-cell proliferation, inflammatory cascade
Vasoactive intestinal peptide	Mononuclear leukocytes, mast cells	T-cell proliferation and migration in Peyer's patches Potent antiinflammatory effect
α-Melanocyte-stimulating hormone		Fever, prostaglandin synthesis, secretion of interleukin 2 Impairs function of antigen-producing cells and T cells Antiinflammatory effects
STIMULATORY		
Estrogens		Lymphocyte proliferation and secretion
Growth hormone	T lymphocytes	Stimulated by growth hormone Thymic growth, lymphocyte reactivity
Prolactin	Mononuclear cells	Thymic growth, lymphocyte proliferation
STIMULATORY		
Thyrotropin (TSH)	T cells	Stimulated by thyrotropin-releasing hormone; inhibited by somatostatin IgG synthesis
β-Endorphin		Activity of T, B, and natural killer cells
Substance P		Proliferation of T cells and macrophages, inflammatory cascade
Corticotropin (ACTH)-releasing hormone		Lymphocyte and monocyte proliferation and activation
NOT KNOWN TO BE STIMULATORY OR INHIBITORY		
Enkephalins	B lymphocytes	
Vasopressin	Thymus	
Oxytocin	Thymus	
Neurophysin	Thymus	

Modified from Reichlin, S., 1993. Neuroendocrine-immune interactions. N Engl J Med 329, 1246-1253.
ACTH, Adrenocorticotropic hormone; IgG, immunoglobulin G; TSH, thyroid-stimulating hormone.

sensing temperature elevations. Chronic hypothalamic hyperthermia does not respond to salicylates and other antipyretics because it is not prostaglandin mediated. Both acute and chronic hypothermia can be due to hypothalamic injury, the most common causes being head trauma, infarction, and demyelination. Other entities to be considered in the differential diagnosis are severe hypothyroidism, Wernicke disease, and drug effect. Some patients with no apparent hypothalamic structural abnormalities may have episodes of recurrent hypothermia. The cause of this syndrome is unclear, although the response of some patients to anticonvulsant agents and of others to clonidine or cyproheptadine suggests a possible neurotransmitter abnormality. Agenesis of the corpus callosum in association with episodic hyperhidrosis and hypothermia (Shapiro syndrome) is caused in some individuals by an abnormally low hypothalamic set point. These symptoms may respond to clonidine (a centrally acting α_2-adrenergic agonist). A similar condition associated with hyperthermia (so-called reverse Shapiro syndrome) has been found to respond with normalization of temperature to low-dose L-dopa; higher doses cause hypothermia. Large lesions in the posterior hypothalamus may impair both heat production (by altering the set point) and heat loss (by damaging the outflow from the preoptic anterior hypothalamic area). This results in poikilothermia, a condition in which body temperature varies with the environmental temperature.

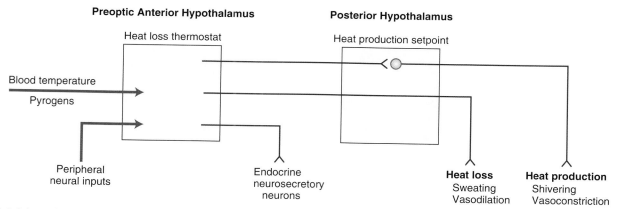

Fig. 42.1 Schematic representation of hypothalamic temperature regulation mechanisms. Preoptic anterior hypothalamus functions as a thermostat and contains mechanisms for regulation of heat loss. Posterior hypothalamus integrates heat production mechanisms. Lesions of the preoptic anterior hypothalamus result in hyperthermia; lesions of the posterior hypothalamus cause hypothermia or poikilothermia. *(Reprinted with permission from Cooper, P.E., Martin, J.B., 1983. Neuroendocrine disease, in: Rosenberg, R.N. (Ed.), The Clinical Neurosciences. Churchill Livingstone, New York.)*

Fever

Classical teaching has been that inflammatory cells in the periphery (primarily monocytes) released cytokines in response to infection and inflammation. These cytokines were thought to act on the hypothalamus to induce production of prostaglandin E_2 (PGE$_2$) and cause elevation of the body temperature set point. The body then used its normal physiological mechanisms of vasoconstriction, vasodilation, sweating, and shivering to maintain this new higher set point (i.e., fever). This view of the mechanism by which bacterial infections cause fever probably is incorrect. Bacterial endotoxic lipopolysaccharide (LPS) does appear to work in the periphery to cause macrophages to release a variety of factors; however, the initial signal to the brain probably travels by vagal afferents to the preoptic anterior hypothalamus via norepinephrine, which activates the cyclo-oxygenase isoenzyme, COX-2, to generate and release PGE$_2$. The slower or second febrile increase in PGE$_2$ is due to COX-2 activation by IL-1β produced locally in the brain, not to circulating factors (Blatteis et al., 2000). Interference with prostaglandins is probably how drugs such as acetylsalicylic acid and acetaminophen act to treat fever.

In otherwise healthy persons, extreme elevations of body temperature (as high as 41.1°C [106°F]) sometimes can be tolerated without serious effects. Hyperthermia associated with prolonged exertion, heatstroke, malignant hyperthermia, neuroleptic malignant syndrome, hyperthyroidism, pheochromocytoma crisis, and some drugs, however, may have serious and even fatal consequences. Exertional hyperthermia occurs with prolonged physical activity, particularly in hot, humid weather. It usually decreases athletic performance initially and can cause muscle cramps or heat exhaustion. When severe, it may result in heatstroke, a syndrome characterized by hyperthermia, hypotension, tachycardia, hyperventilation, and decreased level of consciousness.

Drug-Induced Hyperthermia

Drug-induced hyperthermic syndromes include anticholinergic poisoning, sympathomimetic poisoning, malignant hyperthermia, neuroleptic malignant syndrome, and serotonin syndrome. In *malignant hyperthermia*, a syndrome associated most often with the use of various general anesthetic agents and muscle relaxants, an inherited defect leads to excessive release of calcium from sarcoplasmic reticulum, stimulating severe muscle contraction (see Chapters 64 and 79). The *neuroleptic malignant syndrome* (NMS) is characterized by diffuse muscular rigidity, akinesia, and fever accompanied by a decreased consciousness level and evidence of autonomic dysfunction—namely, labile blood pressure, tachyarrhythmias, excessive sweating, and incontinence. NMS can be associated with administration of major tranquilizers (primarily those that work by blocking dopamine receptors), with rapid withdrawal from dopaminergic agents, including entacapone, and less commonly with administration of tricyclic antidepressants. It appears to result from an alteration of temperature control mechanisms in the hypothalamus. As part of treatment, withdrawal of all neuroleptics is mandatory. In addition to general supportive measures and cooling, the use of bromocriptine (2.5 to 10 mg 4 times daily, increasing by 7.5 mg daily in divided doses to a maximum of 60 mg daily) is helpful. Hypotension, psychosis, and nausea are possible side effects. An alternative is dantrolene (50 to 200 mg/day orally, or 2 to 3 mg/kg/day intravenously (IV), to a maximum of 10 mg/kg/day). The *serotonin syndrome* is characterized by mental status changes, neuromuscular symptoms, autonomic dysfunction, and gastrointestinal dysfunction. In addition to tremor and rigidity (seen also in NMS), other features may include shivering, myoclonus, and hyperreflexia. Nausea, vomiting, and diarrhea are common in serotonin syndrome but are uncommon in NMS. Treatment entails withdrawal from the offending drug and general supportive care.

Appetite

Given free access to food and water, most animals maintain their body weight within narrow limits. With a change in energy intake/expenditure (a change in the size or number of individual meals that is not balanced by an equal and opposite change in energy use), the animal experiences a change in weight. One possible model of nutrient balance is depicted in **Fig. 42.2**. The four components of energy balance are (1) the afferent system, (2) the CNS processing unit, (3) the efferent

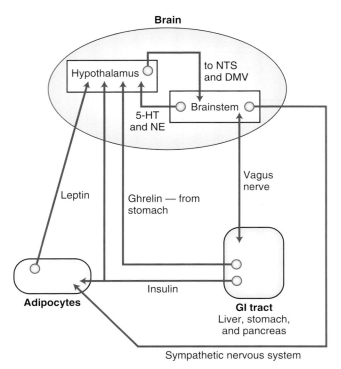

Brain

Fig. 42.2 Sympathetic nervous system. In the regulation of energy balance, the brain is the central processing unit. It receives afferent neuronal signals from the vagus nerve, via the brainstem and hormonal signals—ghrelin (from the stomach), insulin (from the pancreas), and leptin (from adipocytes). The brainstem also has input to the hypothalamus via norepinephrine (NE) (from the locus ceruleus) and serotonin, or 5-hydroxytryptamine (5-HT) (from the raphe nuclei). These afferent signals are interpreted both in the brainstem (in the nucleus of the tractus solitarius) and in the hypothalamus (in the ventromedial nucleus). The ventromedial nucleus of the hypothalamus communicates with the lateral hypothalamic area (LHA) and the paraventricular nucleus (PVN) by means of pro-opiomelanocortin-cocaine/amphetamine-regulated transcript (POMC-CART), an anorexigenic peptide (the release of which is stimulated by insulin and leptin), and by neuropeptide Y/agouti-related protein (NPY/AGRP), an orexigenic peptide (the release of which is stimulated by ghrelin and inhibited by leptin and insulin)—or through the parasympathetic nervous system. Output from the LHA and PVN is either via the sympathetic nervous system, which leads to energy expenditure through physical activity, activation of β₂-adrenergic receptors, and uncoupling proteins in the adipocyte to cause energy release through lipolysis, or through the parasympathetic nervous system. Output via the vagus nerve leads to increased insulin secretion, which causes adipogenesis and energy storage. For a more complete explanation of this control of energy balance, the interested reader is directed to the article by Lustig (2001). *DMV,* Dorsal motor nucleus of the vagus; *GI,* gastrointestinal; *NTS,* nuclear tractus solitarius.

system, and (4) the absorption of food from the gut and its metabolism in the liver. Defects at any point in these systems may lead to weight loss or weight gain (Wynne et al., 2005).

In response to a meal or to starving, hormonal and neural signals are generated in the periphery. Some are of short duration, and others are of long duration. Some relate to satiety, others relate to feeding behavior, and still others relate to "thinness and fatness." Ghrelin, a stimulator of growth hormone (GH) release, is released from the stomach in the fasting state. Ghrelin activates neuropeptide Y and agouti-related protein in the hypothalamus, leading to increased

feeding and deposition of energy into body fat. Peripheral insulin seems to mediate a satiety signal in the ventromedial hypothalamus. Leptin is the other component of the afferent system.

Destruction of the ventromedial hypothalamus, both in animals and in humans, leads to obesity. Lesions in the paraventricular nucleus have a similar effect. Overeating (hyperphagia) is only one of the mechanisms that produces hypothalamic obesity; more efficient handling of calories by the eater is probably another important factor. Hypothalamic lesions also can cause weight loss. Lesions in the dorsomedial nucleus lead to a reduction in body weight and fat stores, as do lesions in the lateral hypothalamus. Studies in the decerebrate rat suggest that oral motor and meal-size responses are dependent on centers in the caudal brainstem, on which the hypothalamus has only a modulatory effect (Grill and Kaplan, 2002).

Meal size and food intake are influenced by many different stimuli. Sensory cues such as the sight, aroma, and taste of food are major factors in dietary obesity. A decrease in blood glucose or a decrease in the oxidation of fatty acids in the liver stimulates the act of eating. Stomach distention gives rise to neural and hormonal signals that reduce food intake. Gastrointestinal peptides such as cholecystokinin, bombesin, and glucagon inhibit feeding by their actions on the autonomic nervous system, particularly the vagal nucleus. Increased fatty acid oxidation leads to higher levels of 3-hydroxybutyrate, which then acts on the hypothalamus to reduce food intake. Interference with any of these sensing systems in the CNS can lead to obesity. Neuropeptide Y infused into the ventromedial nucleus of the hypothalamus induces obesity, perhaps by inhibiting sympathetic drive and stimulating insulin release. Although this may explain obesity with hypothalamic lesions, obesity related to eating highly palatable food probably is not related to central changes in neuropeptide Y.

In animals, the ob, db, and fa genes play a role in the ability of adipose tissue to regulate feeding through a circulating factor. When the product of the ob gene, leptin, is administered peripherally to a genetically obese (ob/ob) mouse deficient in leptin, the animal reduces its intake of food, with a resulting decrease in body weight. The role of leptin in appetite regulation is complex. Leptin does not reverse the obesity seen in db/db mice and in obese humans. In these groups, serum leptin concentrations are higher than in subjects of normal weight, suggesting an insensitivity to endogenous leptin production.

When α-melanocyte-stimulating hormone (α-MSH) binds to its receptor in the hypothalamus, it causes satiety. Up to 5% of obese children have been found to have an abnormality of the α-MSH receptor, MC₄R, as a cause of their obesity (Lustig, 2001).

The orexins (hypocretins) are neuropeptides that play a role in energy balance and arousal (Ferguson and Samson, 2003). Narcolepsy is caused by failure of orexin-mediated signaling. Orexins are found in the hypothalamus, where they regulate sleep/wake cycles (Baumann and Bassetti, 2005), and in the GI tract, where they excite secretomotor neurons and modulate gastric and intestinal motility and secretion (Kirchgessner, 2002).

Anorexia nervosa and bulimia nervosa are clinical eating disorders of unknown etiology seen primarily in young women and girls. Anorexia nervosa is characterized by reduced caloric intake and increased physical activity associated with weight loss, a distorted body image, and a fear of gaining weight. Bulimia nervosa is characterized by episodic gorging followed by self-induced vomiting or laxative and diuretic abuse or dieting and exercise to reduce weight. Initially these syndromes were considered to be neuroendocrine in origin, then for many years, they were assumed to be purely psychiatric. Although malnutrition produces changes in neuroendocrine function, disturbances in corticotropin-releasing hormone (CRH), opioids, neuropeptide Y, vasopressin, oxytocin, cholecystokinin (CCK), and leptin as well as the monoamines—serotonin, dopamine, and norepinephrine—have been found in patients with eating disorders (Barbarich et al., 2003). These neurotransmitters play a role not only in appetite but in mood and impulse control. The abnormalities have been found to persist, in some instances, long after recovery. Furthermore, patients with anorexia nervosa seem to have an increased total daily energy expenditure because of their increased physical activity. All of this suggests a complex interaction between the psyche and the endocrine system as a cause for these syndromes.

Emotion and Libido

Experimental and clinical data support the hypothesis that interaction of the frontal and temporal lobes and the limbic system is necessary for normal emotional function. Lesion and stimulation experiments in cats have shown that rage reactions can be provoked from the hypothalamus. In humans, electrical stimulation of the septal region produces feelings of pleasure or sexual gratification, whereas lesions of the caudal hypothalamus or manipulation of this area during surgery may cause attacks of rage. The amygdala (with its rich input from polysensory areas and limbic-associated areas and its output to the hypothalamus) and other subcortical areas are important structures through which the external environment can influence and cause emotional responses. In depression, activation of the hypothalamic-pituitary-adrenal axis has been recognized, but the story is more complex than this simple observation. Data have shown that depressed patients with suicidal ideation have less activation of the hypothalamic-pituitary-adrenal axis, whereas those who commit suicide have a more active axis. Unfortunately, many of these data are derived from peripheral tests that primarily examine pituitary function rather than assessing true hypothalamic function.

Libido, like other feelings, requires the participation of both hypothalamic and extrahypothalamic sites. In most instances of hypothalamic disease, loss of libido is caused by impaired release of gonadotropin-releasing hormone (GnRH) and a subsequent decrease in testicular testosterone in men. In women, libido is related more to adrenal androgens, and in menstruating women to ovarian androgens. Adrenal androgen levels may be low in women with corticotropin (i.e., adrenocorticotropic hormone [ACTH]) deficiency and secondary adrenal insufficiency. Hypersexuality associated with hypothalamic disease is rare and may occur with or without a subjective increase in libido. The melanocortins (ACTH and α-, β-, and γ-MSH) may play a role in the motivational aspects of sexual behavior, as well as having a sildenafil-like effect on penile and vaginal blood flow, albeit through a central rather than a peripheral mechanism (Raffin-Sanson et al., 2003).

Current understanding of the human hypothalamus in relation to normal development, sexual differentiation, aging, and some degenerative neurological disorders is gradually expanding. The sexually dimorphic nucleus, or intermediate nucleus, of the preoptic area is twice the volume in male subjects compared to that in female subjects—although this finding is disputed by some investigators. Two other cell groups in the preoptic anterior hypothalamus are larger in males than in females. The size does not differ between homosexual and heterosexual men. Although the shape of the suprachiasmatic nucleus differs in male and female subjects, the vasopressin cell number and volume are similar in men and women. Homosexual men seem to have a larger suprachiasmatic nucleus containing twice as many cells as in heterosexual men (Swaab et al., 2001). The site of the central nucleus of the bed nucleus of the stria terminalis is perhaps involved in gender identity in transsexuals. At present, the significance of these observations is uncertain.

It has been known for some time that oxytocin, the classical posterior pituitary hormone, works in the brain to promote mother-infant bonding. Now, it has been shown that it can promote more appropriate social behavior and affect in patients with high-functioning autism or with Asperger syndrome (Andari et al., 2010).

Biological Rhythms

Most endocrine rhythms are circadian—that is, a complete cycle takes approximately 24 hours. Although longer and shorter cycles do occur, the circadian rhythms have been studied most extensively. In many animals, light plays an important role in regulating circadian rhythms. Nerve fibers project from the optic chiasm to the suprachiasmatic and arcuate nuclei of the hypothalamus. The hypothalamus is responsible for the hormonal rhythms, such as cortisol and GH secretion, and for the behavioral rhythms, such as sleep/wake cycles and estrous activity. Although patients with hypothalamic disease often have disturbances in their biological rhythms, these usually are of less clinical importance than other problems caused by such lesions, and this is seldom if ever a presenting complaint.

Endocrine Hypothalamus: The Hypothalamic-Pituitary Unit

Functional Anatomy

In humans, discernible hypothalamic-pituitary tissue begins to develop during week 5 of embryonic life. The Rathke pouch, a diverticulum of the buccal cavity, forms and expands dorsally to contact and invest the diverticulum that develops from the floor of the third ventricle. By week 11, the buccal tissue has lost its connection with the foregut and has flattened to form the primitive anterior pituitary, whereas the neural tissue from the floor of the third ventricle is forming the posterior pituitary. Residual Rathke pouch tissue is postulated to give rise to the craniopharyngiomas that can occur in this region. Rarely, ectopic functional pituitary tissue in the oropharynx can cause signs and symptoms of hyperpituitarism.

The hypothalamus, despite its small size, is the region of brain with the highest concentrations of neurotransmitters and neuropeptides. Beginning with the pioneering work of

Ernst and Berta Scharrer and Geoffrey Harris in the 1940s, the hypothalamus has been assigned a central role in regulating anterior pituitary function. In addition to the identified hypophysiotropic hormones (**Table 42.3**), other peptides with putative regulatory functions are found in high concentration in the hypothalamus: neurotensin, substance P, cholecystokinin, neuropeptide Y, vasoactive intestinal polypeptide, and the opioid peptides. The hypothalamus also is rich in acetylcholine, norepinephrine, dopamine, serotonin, histamine, and γ-aminobutyric acid (GABA). In many neurons, these neurotransmitters co-localize with peptides, although this co-localization and presumptive co-release have uncertain physiological significance. In patients with nonfunctioning pituitary or parapituitary tumors, symptoms produced by compression of neural structures adjacent to the pituitary gland are a common presentation. Understanding these symptoms requires knowledge of the anatomy of the region (**Fig. 42.3**).

Tumor erosion of the floor of the sella turcica may lead to cerebrospinal fluid (CSF) rhinorrhea. Conversely, sinusitis or sphenoid sinus mucocele can invade the sella, resulting in anterior pituitary dysfunction. Expansion of pituitary tumors into the cavernous sinus can produce a variety of upper cranial nerve palsies. The development of such deficits is especially common with the sudden expansion of pituitary tumors that occurs in pituitary apoplexy. Carotid aneurysms or ectatic carotid arteries in the cavernous sinus may expand medially and mimic pituitary adenomas by enlarging the sella and causing anterior pituitary hypofunction.

The dura overlying the sella is sensitive to pain, and stretching of this structure by expanding pituitary tumors gives rise to headache referred to the vertex and retro-orbitally. In some cases, especially if intracranial pressure is elevated, the dura may herniate into the sella, where continued pulsation of the CSF over time leads to remodeling and expansion of the sella. This produces the radiological finding of the empty sella syndrome, another cause of which is lymphocytic hypophysitis. The pituitary gland becomes a thin ribbon of tissue along the walls of the expanded sella, and the sella contains mostly CSF. Only rarely can evidence of impairment of pituitary function be found in such patients.

Expansion of pituitary tumors out of the sella tends to lead to compression of the anterior and inferior crossing fibers of the optic chiasm (see Chapters 14 and 36). These fibers subserve vision in the superior temporal quadrants. Therefore, pituitary adenomas typically cause bitemporal superior quadrantanopias. Lesions such as craniopharyngiomas that impinge on the posterior and superior fibers of the optic

Table 42.3 **Hypothalamic Peptides Controlling Anterior Pituitary Hormone Release**

Pituitary Hormone	Hypothalamic Factor
Growth hormone	Growth hormone–releasing hormone (GHRH) Growth hormone release–inhibiting hormone (somatostatin)
Prolactin	Prolactin-releasing factor(s) (PRF) Prolactin release–inhibiting factor: dopamine and possibly the precursor of gonadotropin-releasing hormone (GnRH)
Thyrotropin	Thyrotropin-releasing hormone (TRH) Thyrotropin release–inhibiting factor: somatostatin can do this but has not been confirmed to do so physiologically
Pro-opiomelanocortin is cleaved to form corticotropin (ACTH)	Corticotropin-releasing hormone (CRH)
Luteinizing hormone (LH) and follicle-stimulating hormone (FSH)	Gonadotropin-releasing hormone (GnRH)

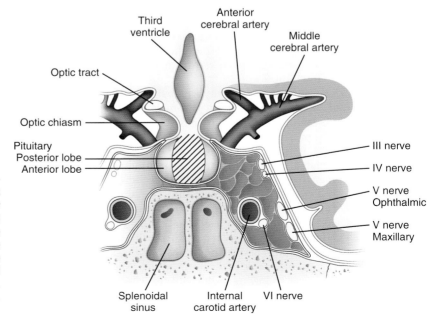

Fig. 42.3 Diagrammatic representation of the anatomical relations of the pituitary fossa and cavernous sinus. The lateral wall of the sella turcica is formed by the cavernous sinus. The sinus contains the carotid artery, two branches of the fifth cranial nerve (the ophthalmic and maxillary nerves), third nerve (oculomotor), fourth nerve (trochlear), and sixth nerve (abducens). The optic chiasm and optic tract are located superior and lateral, respectively, to the pituitary. *(Drawing by B. Newberg. Modified from Makwell, A.K., 1973. Gray's Anatomy, thirty-fifth ed. Saunders, Philadelphia.)*

chiasm tend to manifest with bitemporal inferior quadrantanopias. Nevertheless, owing to the variability of the positioning of the optic chiasm and the tendency for tumors to be asymmetrical in their growth, parasellar lesions result in a wide variety of field defects.

Blood Supply

The superior and inferior hypophysial arteries are the pituitary's major source of blood (**Fig. 42.4**). The posterior pituitary gland is supplied principally by the inferior hypophysial arteries and is drained by the inferior hypophysial veins. The superior hypophysial artery forms a primary capillary plexus in the median eminence of the hypothalamus. From here, blood flows into the long hypophysial portal veins, which carry it to the anterior pituitary. Although some blood from the anterior pituitary drains into the cavernous sinus, some drains into the posterior pituitary, and some returns to the median eminence by way of the long portal veins, which are capable of bidirectional blood flow. This vascular anatomy provides a potential mechanism for the important feedback loops necessary for regulation of hypothalamic-pituitary function.

Anterior Pituitary

Hypothalamic Control of Anterior Pituitary Secretion

The hypothalamus produces hypophysiotropic substances that control the secretion of anterior pituitary hormones. Five neuropeptides and one neurotransmitter (dopamine) are known to be important physiological regulators of pituitary function (see **Table 42.3**). In addition, several neurotransmitters affect pituitary hormone release, although their physiological role remains uncertain. Since their discovery in 1998, the orexins (hypocretins) have been found to regulate virtually all the hypothalamic-pituitary axes as well as participate in the coordination of anterior pituitary function with sleep, arousal,

and general metabolism. This is well reviewed in a recent article by López, Tena-Sempere and Diéguez (2010).

Abnormalities of Anterior Pituitary Function
Hypofunction

The causes of pituitary insufficiency are summarized in **Box 42.1**. In general, the symptoms of hypopituitarism (**Table 42.4**) are those of the secondary failure of end-organ function. Because the associated changes usually develop slowly and some autonomous end-organ function remains, the symptoms often are less severe than those that occur with primary end-organ disease. The term *Simmonds disease* is applied to panhypopituitarism. When this syndrome develops in the postpartum period after an episode of pituitary infarction, it is called *Sheehan syndrome*.

Intrauterine growth is independent of GH. Therefore, although GH-deficient children are of normal size at birth, they subsequently fail to grow. Insulin-like growth factors (IGF) 1 and 2 are important mediators in human somatic growth. IGF-1 production in the liver is GH dependent, whereas IGF-2 is relatively insensitive to GH. True GH deficiency is rare. It may manifest in an isolated fashion or as part of general pituitary failure. Apparent GH deficiency may result from an isolated deficiency of growth hormone–releasing hormone (GHRH) or from a lack of GH receptors in the liver, leading to failure of IGF-1 production (resulting in Laron dwarfism). GH is a contra-insulin hormone, and in children especially, its deficiency may be associated with episodes of fasting hypoglycemia.

Pituitary insufficiency in children may manifest as delayed or absent puberty. Onset of puberty depends to some extent on achievement of a critical body mass. Thus, anything that delays growth, such as GH deficiency or hypothyroidism, delays puberty. If breasts or sexual hair have not started to develop in girls by age 14, or if testicular enlargement and sexual hair growth have not occurred in boys by age 15, puberty should be considered delayed. Luteinizing hormone (LH) or follicle-stimulating hormone (FSH) deficiency may occur as part of generalized pituitary failure or as a result of

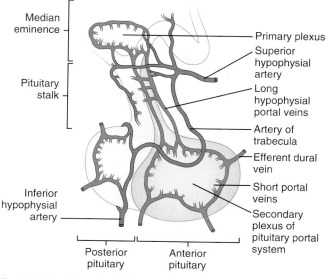

Fig. 42.4 Blood supply of the median eminence and pituitary gland. *(Reprinted with permission from Cooper, P.E., Martin, J.B., 1983. Neuroendocrine disease, in: Rosenberg, R.N. (Ed.), The Clinical Neurosciences. Churchill Livingstone, New York.)*

Figure labels: Median eminence, Pituitary stalk, Inferior hypophysial artery, Primary plexus, Superior hypophysial artery, Long hypophysial portal veins, Artery of trabecula, Efferent dural vein, Short portal veins, Secondary plexus of pituitary portal system, Posterior pituitary, Anterior pituitary

---

Box 42.1 **Causes of Pituitary Insufficiency**

Pituitary aplasia:
   Complete
   Monohormonal
Trauma:
   Head injury
   Surgery
   Radiotherapy
   Compression by cysts or tumors
Pituitary apoplexy
Pituitary infarction
Hypophysitis:
   Infection
   Granulomatous disease
   Autoimmune disease
Hypothalamic failure

Table 42.4   Clinical Syndromes of Anterior Pituitary Dysfunction

Hormone	Excess Secretion	Deficient Secretion
Growth hormone	*In children*: Gigantism *In adults*: Acromegaly	*In children*: Growth failure and tendency to hypoglycemia

Prolactin	*In children*: Delayed puberty
	In adults:
	    Women: Amenorrhea, galactorrhea, and infertility
	    Men: Impotence, infertility, and (rarely) galactorrhea
		In adults:
		    Women: Inability to breast-feed and possible infertility

Luteinizing hormone and follicle-stimulating hormone	*In children*: Precocious puberty *In adults*: Infertility, hypogonadism, polycystic ovary syndrome	*In children*: Delayed puberty *In adults*: Amenorrhea, infertility, erectile dysfunction
Thyrotropin (TSH)	Hyperthyroidism Hyperprolactinemia (due to excessive TRH stimulation)	Hypothyroidism
Pro-opiomelanocortin	Cushing disease, Nelson syndrome	Hypoadrenalism; glucocorticoids affected more severely than mineralocorticoids

high prolactin levels inhibiting their release from the pituitary or from GnRH deficiency.

One cause of hypopituitarism is *pituitary apoplexy*, a term that should be reserved for infarction of or hemorrhage into the normal pituitary gland or into a pituitary adenoma. To be classified as true apoplexy, the hemorrhage should be of sufficient severity to produce signs of compression of parasellar structures or evidence of meningeal irritation. The sudden expansion of the pituitary gland may lead to chiasmal compression or cranial nerve palsies. Rupture of the necrotic gland into the CSF may be clinically indistinguishable from subarachnoid hemorrhage due to rupture of a berry aneurysm or an arteriovenous malformation. Hypotension, aggravated by coexisting ACTH deficiency, may further complicate the picture. The diagnosis usually can be made readily by computed tomography (CT) scanning or magnetic resonance imaging (MRI). Treatment includes general supportive measures, corticosteroid replacement, and if necessary, surgical decompression.

Hyperfunction
PRECOCIOUS PUBERTY

Development of secondary sexual characteristics before age 8 in girls and age 9 in boys is considered abnormal. In approximately one-fifth of affected girls and half of affected boys, the cause of precocious puberty is a neurological lesion. A variety of tumors have been associated with the development of precocious puberty, including hamartoma, teratoma, ependymoma, optic nerve glioma, glioma, and neurofibroma, either alone or as part of von Recklinghausen syndrome. Tumors are most commonly located in the posterior hypothalamus, pineal gland, or median eminence, or they put pressure on the floor of the third ventricle. The cause of precocious puberty under these circumstances has not been clearly delineated. Some of these tumors, however, may be an ectopic source of GnRH or of human chorionic gonadotropin, a placental peptide with LH- and FSH-like activity.

In the investigation of precocious puberty, LH and FSH levels should be measured, as well as human chorionic gonadotropin. An MRI study of the head is mandatory. If LH and

FSH levels are in the adult range and the head imaging result is negative, it is most likely that the precocious puberty is idiopathic. High human chorionic gonadotropin levels suggest ectopic production. If LH and FSH levels are low, adrenal, ovarian, testicular, or exogenous causes must be sought.

Chronic administration of long-acting analogs of GnRH results in an initial stimulation of LH and FSH secretion, followed by complete inhibition. This effect on LH and FSH release can be used to stop and prevent progression of hypothalamic precocious puberty.

HYPERPROLACTINEMIA

Probably the most common abnormality of pituitary function encountered by the neuroendocrinologist is hyperprolactinemia (Wand, 2003); causes are summarized in **Box 42.2**. Prolactin levels in excess of 200 ng/mL (normal, <25ng/mL) are almost always due to excessive production of the hormone by a pituitary adenoma. In premenopausal women, the development of amenorrhea secondary to direct inhibition of LH and FSH by prolactin leads to early investigation and diagnosis of tumors at the microadenoma (<10 mm in diameter) stage. In men, the insidious onset of erectile dysfunction and reduced libido usually means that these tumors are found late, often only after they have produced signs and symptoms of optic nerve compression. Galactorrhea is a common accompaniment of elevated prolactin in women and a rare finding in men.

Serum prolactin levels increase after generalized tonic-clonic seizures and complex partial seizures but show no change after virtually all cases of psychogenic, absence, or simple partial seizures or complex partial seizures of frontal lobe origin. After a seizure, prolactin levels peak at 15 to 20 minutes and then decrease to baseline levels within 60 minutes. The increase should be at least two times baseline. Caution should be exercised in interpreting early-morning prolactin levels, because a 50% to 100% increase in prolactin is normal just before waking. Furthermore, prolactin elevations are far from specific for epilepsy, and some tendency for the elevation to attenuate in patients with frequent seizures has been observed.

Because prolactin secretion is under strong inhibitory control by the hypothalamus, anything that interferes with the

Box 42.2 Causes of Hyperprolactinemia

Drugs:
  Dopamine receptor blockers
  Phenothiazines such as chlorpromazine
  Butyrophenones such as haloperidol
  Metoclopramide
  Reserpine
  α-Methyldopa
  Monoamine oxidase inhibitors
  Tricyclic antidepressants (unusual, probably idiosyncratic)
  Benzodiazepines (unusual, probably idiosyncratic)
  Verapamil
  Cocaine
  Fluoxetine
  Amoxapine
Hormones:
  Estrogens
  Thyrotropin-releasing hormone (as can occur in primary hypothyroidism)
  Pituitary tumor
  Prolactin-secreting adenoma
  Interference of flow of dopamine down the pituitary stalk by large pituitary or parapituitary tumor
Chest wall stimulation
Chronic skin disease (e.g., severe acne)
Tumors of chest wall
Chronic renal failure
Cirrhosis
Ectopic production
Hypothalamic disease
Pseudocyesis
Idiopathic

Box 42.3 Common Clinical Signs and Symptoms of Acromegaly

Headache—nonspecific, tension-type like, felt at the vertex and behind the eyes
Impaired glucose tolerance or diabetes mellitus
Enlargement of hands and feet
Enlargement of the jaw, with increased spacing between the teeth and malocclusion
Hypertension
Menstrual irregularities
Soft-tissue growth:
  Thick skin
  Doughlike feel to palm (e.g., during handshake)
  Carpal tunnel syndrome
Arthralgia and osteoarthritis
Proximal muscle weakness
Hyperhidrosis

free flow of blood down the pituitary portal veins can reduce the exposure of the pituitary to the dopamine released by the hypothalamus. This results in raised peripheral blood prolactin levels. In patients with this condition, prolactin levels commonly range from 50 to 150 ng/mL (usually <100 ng/mL; normal, <25 ng/mL); such elevations can be seen, for example, in patients with granulomatous disease involving the pituitary stalk. However, probably the most common situation in which this occurs is in patients in whom the pituitary stalk is "kinked" by a pituitary adenoma. In such circumstances, this may lead to the erroneous assumption that the pituitary adenoma is secreting prolactin, and long-term therapy with bromocriptine might be undertaken. We have seen such patients whose prolactin levels became normal but whose tumors continued to grow. The mistake with these patients is to assume that a macroadenoma would result in a moderately elevated prolactin level, when in reality, microprolactinomas usually produce prolactin levels in excess of 200 ng/mL, and patients with macroadenomas that secrete prolactin would be expected to have much higher levels, often in excess of 1000 ng/mL.

Patients taking neuroleptic medications also may have elevated prolactin levels, and occasionally the elevation is enough to cause galactorrhea or amenorrhea. In such patients, it may be uncertain whether symptoms are secondary to drug-induced hyperprolactinemia or to a microadenoma. Our practice is to perform an MRI study of the pituitary to look for a tumor and to perform dynamic pituitary testing with thyrotropin-releasing hormone and metoclopramide. In most patients, drug-induced hyperprolactinemia responds normally to stimulation with these agents. The treatment of drug-induced hyperprolactinemia is difficult if the causative drug cannot be stopped. Some patients may benefit from the use of atypical antipsychotics with reduced or no action at dopamine receptors (at normal therapeutic doses).

GIGANTISM AND ACROMEGALY

Presence of excessive amounts of circulating GH before closure of the epiphyses leads to gigantism. If the epiphyses have closed, only tissue still capable of responding to GH will grow, leading to the clinical syndrome of acromegaly; its clinical features are summarized in **Box 42.3**. Of particular note for the neurologist and the neurosurgeon is the frequent complaint of headache and symptoms related to carpal tunnel syndrome. It is not uncommon to find patients with acromegaly in whom surgery for carpal tunnel release was performed 3 to 5 years before diagnosis of their disease.

Most cases of gigantism and acromegaly are due to excess GH production by a pituitary adenoma. Rare cases of ectopic GH production have been described; for example, excessive GHRH production by pancreatic tumors can cause acromegaly. Excess production of GHRH by the hypothalamus could theoretically cause an identical clinical syndrome.

CUSHING DISEASE AND NELSON SYNDROME

The term *Cushing syndrome* refers to the clinical picture resulting from exposure to excessive corticosteroids, either endogenous or exogenous. If the clinical manifestations are caused by excessive production of ACTH from the pituitary, the condition is referred to as *Cushing disease*. Common clinical features of Cushing disease are listed in **Box 42.4**. The syndrome of hyperpigmentation and local compression of parapituitary structures that occurs in approximately 10% of patients with Cushing disease who have been treated with bilateral adrenalectomy is called *Nelson syndrome*. Given the generally good results from surgery on the pituitary gland in Cushing disease, Nelson syndrome is now quite uncommon.

Box 42.4 Common Clinical Features of Cushing's Disease

Truncal obesity—arms and legs tend to be thin; excess fat deposition in preauricular and supraclavicular fat pads
Hypertension
Impaired glucose tolerance and diabetes mellitus
Menstrual irregularities or amenorrhea
Excessive hair growth
Acne
Proximal myopathy
Abdominal striae (purplish)
Osteoporosis
Thin skin with excessive bruising

The diagnosis of Cushing syndrome, although simple in theory, often is quite difficult in practice (Findling and Raff, 2005). It is also often difficult for tests to distinguish between true Cushing syndrome and so-called pseudo-Cushing syndrome due to alcoholism, depression, and eating disorders.

As a screening test, the most sensitive and specific screening tool is an 11 PM salivary cortisol determination. Unfortunately, this test may not be readily available in all clinical centers, and 24-hour urine collections for urinary free cortisol are still used. The sensitivity and specificity of the 24-hour collection can be increased by doing two collections on consecutive days. For years now, the dexamethasone suppression test has been pivotal in the diagnosis of Cushing disease. For this test, 0.5 mg of dexamethasone is given every 6 hours for 8 doses; during the second 24 hours of administration, the normal response is suppression of cortisol production, as reflected by reduced urinary levels of 17-ketogenic steroids or urinary free cortisol. Patients with Cushing disease usually show a similar suppression only when the dose of dexamethasone is increased to 2 mg every 6 hours for 8 doses. The formal dexamethasone suppression test is cumbersome, requiring 6 consecutive days of collection of urine for urinary free cortisol levels. Various modifications of this test may be useful and less cumbersome. More detailed discussion can be found in the literature, both for screening (Findling and Raff, 2005) and for diagnosis (Lindsay and Nieman, 2005) of Cushing syndrome.

In Cushing disease, ACTH levels usually are in the normal range or moderately elevated. Failure to suppress on high-dose dexamethasone and unmeasurable ACTH levels are seen with primary adrenal problems such as adenoma or carcinoma. Ectopic ACTH production usually is insuppressible, and the ACTH levels tend to be much higher than those seen in typical pituitary Cushing disease, although many exceptions to these rules have been found. In well-documented cases of ectopic ACTH production and primary adrenal problems, dexamethasone suppression test results have been compatible with a diagnosis of pituitary ACTH production. Intermittent excess ACTH production also can give rise to false-negative results in patients who actually have Cushing disease.

Even when all test results point to a pituitary source for the excessive ACTH production, care must still be taken in diagnosing the patient as having Cushing disease. An abnormality of the sella may or may not be present on CT or MRI. Intermediate-lobe cysts or clefts may mimic the appearance of adenoma on CT or MRI. In such cases, simultaneous sampling from the petrosal sinuses bilaterally and from the inferior vena cava can help localize the excessive ACTH production.

The pituitary glands of some patients with biochemical Cushing disease do not show adenoma formation but demonstrate evidence of hyperplasia of the cells that secrete ACTH. Although this picture can be due to ectopic production of CRH, the hypothalamic peptide that stimulates release of ACTH, or to excessive release of CRH from the hypothalamus, such etiologies affect less than 0.3% of patients with Cushing disease who have pituitary surgery.

EXCESSIVE SECRETION OF THYROID-STIMULATING HORMONE

Elevated levels of thyroid-stimulating hormone (TSH) are seen most commonly with primary hypothyroidism. The resulting pituitary hypertrophy infrequently can be of sufficient magnitude to cause visual field defects. Hyperthyroidism due to excessive TSH secretion is a rare (accounting for less than 1% of all pituitary tumors) but well-recognized entity, and these tumors are usually large and readily visible on CT scans.

Pituitary resistance to thyroid hormone also may produce a clinical picture of hyperthyroidism with high-normal or mildly elevated TSH levels. Unlike in the case of TSH-secreting tumors, which are relatively autonomous, the TSH levels in patients with pituitary resistance usually respond well to stimulation with thyrotropin-releasing hormone or to suppression with dexamethasone or dopamine.

GONADOTROPIN-SECRETING TUMORS

Many pituitary tumors formerly classified as nonfunctioning are actually gonadotropin- or gonadotropin subunit–producing tumors. The usual presentation is a macroadenoma in an elderly man; however, they occur in persons of all ages and both sexes, with a male preponderance.

Many of these tumors secrete only FSH, and only rarely do they secrete LH alone. Some may secrete both LH and FSH, and others secrete biologically inactive gonadotropin subunits: the α subunit, LH-αβ subunit, or FSH-β subunit. Most clinical radioimmunoassays used to measure LH and FSH require the α and β subunits to be associated before they register in the assay. As a result, subunit secretion is not detected in such assays. FSH levels usually are elevated in patients with FSH-secreting tumors, and testosterone or estradiol levels almost always are low. In patients with LH-secreting tumors, LH levels usually are elevated, and estradiol or testosterone levels may be high. Despite high sex steroid levels, these patients often are clinically hypogonadal. Patients with tumors that secrete both LH and FSH usually have normal or high sex steroid levels, but again, they are clinically hypogonadal. Because subunits are biologically inactive, they do not interfere directly with hormonal function, although by means of pressure effects on the pituitary, subunit-secreting tumors can cause hypopituitarism.

Long-standing primary hypogonadism that is not replaced adequately may cause pituitary enlargement secondary to gonadotroph hyperplasia. Rarely, this may lead to gonadotroph tumor development. Most of the time, the pituitary enlargement is asymptomatic and regresses in response to sex steroid replacement.

An overall review of pituitary dysfunction can be found in the article by Levy (2004).

Pituitary Tumors and Pituitary Hyperplasia

Pituitary tumors account for approximately 15% of all intracranial tumors. Although most are benign, they can be locally invasive. Only rarely is true malignancy evidenced by metastases. The old classification of pituitary adenomas into chromophobe, acidophil, and basophil has been supplanted by a more functional classification based on findings of immunological and electron microscopic examinations (**Table 42.5**). Hyperplasia of various cellular elements of the pituitary is relatively rare and usually only seen in cases of ectopic hypothalamic-releasing hormone production (Ironside, 2003).

Most pituitary tumors that have been removed surgically and examined have been found to be monoclonal in origin. This finding suggests that a majority of pituitary tumors arise from a single cell in which a mutation either activated a proto-oncogene or inactivated a tumor suppressor gene. Almost half of pituitary tumors show aneuploidy (usually more or [rarely] fewer than the normal number of chromosomes). The significance of this to tumor formation is uncertain. The cell cycle inhibitory proteins, p14ARF and p16[INK4a], are coded for by the CDKN2A (cyclin-dependent kinase inhibitor) gene. This gene has been found to have reduced expression in a majority of human pituitary tumors. PTTG (pituitary tumor–transforming gene) expression is increased in certain human pituitary tumors, but whether these changes in gene expression play a role in tumor induction or whether they are the result of tumor formation is unclear.

The G proteins are a family of proteins comprising α, β, and γ subunits that bind to guanine nucleotides. A variety of mutations involving single amino acid substitutions in the portion of the Gs gene that encodes the Gs α subunit have been identified in nearly 40% of GH-secreting tumors. These mutations inhibit the breakdown of the α subunit, thereby mimicking the effect of specific growth factors and leading to increased adenylate cyclase activity and elevated intracellular cyclic adenosine monophosphate levels. Nevertheless, no single mutation or alteration of function seems to explain tumor formation in more than the occasional case. Somatostatin inhibits both GH and cyclic adenosine monophosphate production, and this may be the mechanism by which it shrinks GH-secreting pituitary tumors.

Table 42.5 Classification of Pituitary Adenomas	
Tumor	**Frequency (%)**
Growth hormone cell adenoma	14.0
Prolactin cell adenoma	27.2
Growth hormone–prolactin cell adenoma	8.4
Corticotroph cell adenoma	8.1
Thyrotroph cell adenoma	1.0
Gonadotroph cell adenoma	6.4
Clinically nonfunctioning adenoma	31.2
Plurihormonal adenoma	3.7

Modified with permission from Thapar, K., Kovacs, K., Muller, P.J., 1995. Clinical-pathological correlations of pituitary tumours. Clin Endocrinol Metab 9, 243-270.

Levy and Lightman (2003) suggest that although some pituitary tumors may be due to genetic abnormalities, it is possible that a majority of pituitary tumors are not "tumors" in the usual sense but rather represent an overresponse to normal trophic factors that has failed to normalize once the growth stimulus has returned to normal.

Other Tumors

Gliomas, meningiomas, chordomas, teratomas, and dermoid and epidermoid tumors all can occur in the region of the sella turcica, and local compressive effects may produce a clinical picture resembling that of primary pituitary tumors. The pituitary gland is the site of metastatic deposits in 4% of cancer patients. Usually these metastases are asymptomatic; when symptoms do occur, however, they most often are related to disturbance of posterior pituitary function.

Craniopharyngiomas are only one-third as common as pituitary tumors. They are thought to arise from residual rests of Rathke pouch tissue. Most commonly found in a suprasellar location, they also occur anywhere along the pituitary-hypothalamic axis, including within the sella. Craniopharyngiomas can appear at any age; however, approximately a third of cases arise before the age of 15 years. Because these tumors produce no hormones, patients usually present with signs of local compression, especially of the visual system, or with hypothalamic dysfunction such as growth failure or diabetes insipidus (DI). Almost half of affected children show evidence of growth failure. Three-fourths of patients, both adults and children, have visual symptoms.

Hypophysitis

Hypophysitis from infection or granulomatous disease such as sarcoidosis can result in hypopituitarism. Lymphocytic hypophysitis, a sterile inflammation of the pituitary of probable autoimmune origin, is seen almost exclusively in women, particularly during pregnancy. Usually it causes hypopituitarism, although it can cause hyperprolactinemia and may be a cause of the empty sella syndrome.

Posterior Pituitary

Physiology
Vasopressin

Vasopressin, or antidiuretic hormone (ADH), an essential hormone in fluid and electrolyte homeostasis, is synthesized in the magnocellular neurons of the supraoptic and paraventricular nuclei as a large precursor molecule, which is cleaved enzymatically to yield vasopressin and neurophysin. The function of this latter peptide is unknown.

Four vasopressin-containing pathways have been recognized in the brain: (1) hypothalamo-neurohypophysial, (2) paraventricular nucleus to the zona incerta of the median eminence, (3) paraventricular nucleus to the limbic system (amygdala), and (4) paraventricular nucleus to the brainstem and spinal cord. The best-characterized of these is the hypothalamo-neuro-hypophysial (hypophysial-portal) pathway. Virtually all of the neurons from the supraoptic nuclei contribute to this pathway, whereas only a portion of paraventricular nuclei terminate in the posterior pituitary.

Some of the vasopressin-containing fibers from the paraventricular nuclei appear to be more involved in ACTH regulation than in fluid balance. Vasopressin-containing fibers also project widely outside the hypothalamus, where (as some evidence suggests) they may participate in memory.

Oxytocin

Oxytocin, like vasopressin, is synthesized in magnocellular neurons of the supraoptic and paraventricular nuclei as a large precursor molecule that is cleaved into oxytocin and a specific neurophysin. Many of the physiological stimuli of vasopressin also result in oxytocin release, and although in supraphysiological doses, oxytocin does have ADH-like properties, its physiological role in these circumstances remains obscure. The only specific stimulus that causes the release of oxytocin but not vasopressin is suckling. Oxytocin's role in normal lactation and parturition in the human remains to be defined clearly. Oxytocin receptors are found in the limbic system, particularly in the amygdala, and for this reason oxytocin has been implicated in emotion. Lim and Young (2006) have shown that in mammals it plays a role in a variety of complex social behaviors as well as helping regulate the response to stress.

Thirst and Drinking

Certain cells of the anterior hypothalamus are sensitive to changes in the osmolality of the blood bathing them and respond by signaling the cells of the supraoptic and paraventricular nuclei to alter their secretion of vasopressin. These cells are most sensitive to osmotic substances that do not diffuse freely into cells, such as sodium, sucrose, and mannitol. Substances such as urea produce less osmotic stimulation because they diffuse freely. Glucose, in addition to diffusing freely, actually inhibits ADH release. These cells respond with marked increases in ADH secretion not only to increased osmolality, and hence dehydration, but also to hypotension.

Water homeostasis cannot be maintained by antidiuresis alone but also requires thirst and the drinking behavior induced by it. A drinking center is thought to be located near the feeding center in the lateral hypothalamus. Angiotensin may play an important role in stimulating drinking in humans and animals.

Sodium Homeostasis and Atrial Natriuretic Peptide

Sodium homeostasis is extremely important for normal functioning of the organism. Most of the regulation of body sodium takes place in the kidney. Sodium reabsorption is under control of the renin-angiotensin-aldosterone system. Under normal physiological circumstances, aldosterone, the principal mineralocorticoid produced by the adrenal gland, is affected in only a minor way by ACTH.

The human heart has been shown to synthesize and secrete atrial natriuretic peptide, which has diuretic, natriuretic (serving to increase urinary sodium excretion), and vasorelaxant properties. In addition to atrial natriuretic peptide, the brain contains brain natriuretic peptide and C-type natriuretic peptide. Judging from the pattern of their distribution in the brain, these substances may have important roles in the central control of the cardiovascular system. The natriuretic peptides seem to act as natural antagonists to the central actions of angiotensin II.

Diabetes Insipidus

Diabetes insipidus (DI) is a clinical syndrome characterized by severe thirst, polydipsia, and polyuria. Central DI must be distinguished from nephrogenic DI (an inability of the kidney to respond to ADH) and from compulsive water drinking (Baylis, 1995). Distinguishing among these entities normally is done using a water deprivation test. A urine osmolality of greater than 750 mmol/L after water deprivation excludes the diagnosis of DI. Central DI is characterized by an increase in osmolality to greater than 750 mmol/L after administration of desamino-D-arginine-vasopressin (DDAVP). In nephrogenic DI, little change in osmolality occurs after DDAVP administration. The polyuria induced by chronic compulsive water drinking may produce a renal tubular concentrating defect because of medullary washout—that is, the loss of sodium and other solutes from around the loops of Henle. This can make it difficult to differentiate partial DI of central or renal cause from polydipsia. Treatment by gradual fluid restriction, with or without DDAVP, can be used to reverse the medullary washout, thereby increasing the sensitivity of the test.

The water deprivation test must be strictly supervised by a physician familiar with the technique. Severe and potentially fatal dehydration can occur rapidly in patients with complete DI, especially children. Similarly, patients with compulsive water drinking given DDAVP and allowed access to water can drink themselves into hyponatremic coma.

Etiology

Approximately a third of patients with central DI have no demonstrable disease of the hypothalamic-posterior pituitary unit. The remaining patients have damage to the supraoptic-hypophysial-portal pathway from trauma, surgery, tumors, inflammatory lesions (which may be granulomatous or infectious), or vascular lesions. In patients with polyuria, the urine should be examined to ensure that a solute diuresis, as with hyperglycemia, has not occurred, or that a type of nephrogenic DI has not been induced by hypokalemia, hypercalcemia, or lithium carbonate therapy. In the acute care setting on a neurosurgical ward, administration of mannitol may be one of the more common causes of polyuria. The investigation of DI has been well summarized by Diederich and colleagues (2001).

Management

Patients with DI excrete mainly water, and therefore water replacement alone is the mainstay of their management. Patients who are alert and have intact thirst mechanisms should be given free access to water. Only if urine output exceeds 7 L/day is treatment necessary. In most circumstances, DDAVP given as a nasal solution or as an oral tablet is the treatment of choice. To avoid water intoxication, underreplacement is preferable in these patients, who should be allowed to modulate their water balance by drinking.

The unconscious patient can present a problem in management. When calculating such a patient's fluid needs, the clinician should be aware that the urine in DI is electrolyte poor. Thus, the electrolyte requirements of such a patient are little different from those of other patients. The bulk of the urinary replacement should be given as 5% dextrose in water. The administration of 5% dextrose in 0.2 NaCl or solutions with even higher salt concentrations presents a high solute load to the kidney and tends to exacerbate the polyuria.

Syndrome of Inappropriate Antidiuretic Hormone Secretion

Etiology and Pathophysiology

The syndrome of inappropriate ADH secretion (SIADH) is characterized by low serum sodium, high urine sodium, and relative or absolute hyperosmolarity of urine to serum. Before making the diagnosis, the physician must exclude all of the following: (1) dehydration, (2) edema-forming states such as congestive cardiac failure, (3) primary renal disease, (4) adrenal or thyroid insufficiency, and (5) use of medications that cause salt loss in urine (e.g., diuretics).

The initial clue to the diagnosis of SIADH is the low serum sodium (Reynolds et al., 2006). Measured serum osmolality also must be low to exclude the artifactual hyponatremia that occurs with hyperlipidemia and hyperproteinemia, in which the sodium concentration in the plasma water actually is normal. The urine osmolality in SIADH is not always above the serum osmolality, but the urine is less than maximally dilute, which excludes the dilutional hyponatremia of water intoxication. Causes of SIADH are listed in **Box 42.5**.

Clinical Features

The clinical features of SIADH are nonspecific and are related to the hypo-osmolality of the body fluids. The more rapidly this condition develops, the more symptomatic the patient. Serum sodium less than 115 mmol/L almost always is associated with confusion or obtundation, and seizures can occur. With milder hyponatremia, the symptoms may be nonspecific, including fatigue, general malaise, loss of appetite, and some clouding of consciousness (Bhardwaj, 2006).

Treatment

For asymptomatic or mildly symptomatic SIADH-induced hyponatremia, the mainstay of treatment is restriction of fluid. Intake should be reduced to insensible losses (approximately 800 mL/day). Obtundation by itself does not necessitate more aggressive treatment of hyponatremia. In patients with severe hyponatremia complicated by seizures, however, a more rapid *partial* correction can be undertaken. Diuresis is induced with furosemide (1 mg/kg IV), and urinary losses are replaced with 3% sodium chloride through a central line at a rate of 0.1 mL/kg/min, to which appropriate amounts of potassium are added (to counter urinary losses). Considerable controversy exists over the rate at which serum sodium can be raised safely. Some clinicians suggest that active correction be by no more than 20 to 25 mmol/L during the first 48 hours, to a level no higher than 130 mmol/L, and that the *rate* of replacement is not important. Patients must be monitored carefully to avoid acute elevation to hypernatremic or even normonatremic levels, and to avoid a change of more than 25 mmol/L in 48 hours, which seems to be dangerous and can cause the syndrome of osmotic demyelination, one form of which is central pontine myelinolysis (Tisdall et al., 2006).

Box 42.5 Causes of Syndrome of Inappropriate Antidiuretic Hormone Secretion (SIADH)

Disorders of the nervous system:
  Tumor, usually parapituitary and large
  Trauma, often to the pituitary stalk
  Surgery in the region of the pituitary/hypothalamus
  Metabolic encephalopathy
  Infections (meningitis, encephalitis)
  Vascular (e.g., stroke)
  Subdural hematoma
  Hydrocephalus
  Guillain-Barré syndrome
  Acute intermittent porphyria
Drugs:
  Carbamazepine
  Chlorpromazine
  Chlorpropamide
  Cisplatinum
  Clofibrate
  Cyclophosphamide
  Oxytocin
  Selective serotonin reuptake inhibitors (SSRIs)
  Thiazide diuretics
  Tricyclic antidepressants
  Vasopressin (e.g., in overtreatment of diabetes insipidus)
  Vinblastine
  Vincristine
Disorders of the chest:
  Pneumonia
  Tuberculosis
  Cystic fibrosis
  Pneumothorax
  Empyema
  Asthma
Endocrine causes:
  Hypoadrenalism
  Hypothyroidism—unusual cause of SIADH
Ectopic production of antidiuretic hormone:
  Carcinoma—lung, gastrointestinal tract, and genitourinary tract (especially kidney)
  Mesothelioma
  Lymphoma and leukemia
  Thymoma
  Sarcoma
  Idiopathic

Prolonged fluid restriction often is poorly tolerated by patients, who may quickly become noncompliant. In cases in which the underlying cause of the SIADH cannot be eliminated or corrected, the drug demeclocycline, a tetracycline, in a dose of 300 to 600 mg twice a day can be used to induce a temporary nephrogenic DI, alleviating the necessity for fluid restriction. Antagonists of the vasopressin receptor in the kidney (e.g., lixivaptan and tolvaptan—still investigational vasopressin receptor antagonists) may be more effective than demeclocycline at managing SIADH. Conivaptan, a vasopressin receptor antagonist has been approved recently by the FDA for the treatment of hyponatremia caused by SIADH. To date, it seems to have low side effects and good efficacy.

Cerebral Salt Wasting

Some patients with hyponatremia do not have SIADH secretion with resultant retention of renal free water. Instead, they have an inappropriate natriuresis. Hyponatremia, accompanied by renal sodium loss and volume depletion, occurs in patients with primary cerebral tumors, carcinomatous meningitis, subarachnoid hemorrhage, head trauma, and after intracranial surgery and pituitary surgery. Unlike patients with SIADH, these patients respond to vigorous sodium and water replacement, and their condition actually is worsened by fluid restriction. This inappropriate natriuresis that accompanies intracranial disease (so-called cerebral salt wasting) may be caused either by a natriuretic hormone such as atrial natriuretic peptide or by an alteration of the neural input to the kidney.

It is critical to distinguish between these patients and those with SIADH, because the treatment for SIADH worsens the hyponatremia of cerebral salt wasting. Differentiation is best done by a careful assessment of volume status using clinical and laboratory examinations to detect signs of volume depletion. If the diagnosis is uncertain, fluid restriction should be instituted. Then, if the natriuresis persists in the face of volume restriction, the syndrome of cerebral salt wasting should be suspected and appropriate therapy initiated. Because either syndrome can develop in patients undergoing pituitary surgery, it is very helpful to know the patient's presurgical weight. This makes it much easier to determine their postsurgical volume status.

Approach to the Patient with Hypothalamic-Pituitary Dysfunction

History and Physical Examination

Patients with suspected hypothalamic or pituitary disorders should be questioned specifically about dysfunction of the nonendocrine aspects of the hypothalamus: appetite, body temperature, sleep/wake cycles, emotion, libido, and autonomic nervous system function. Such symptoms may point to a hypothalamic rather than a pituitary location. A careful functional inquiry also should cover clinical aspects of the hyperfunction and hypofunction of each of the anterior and posterior pituitary hormones.

Because of the proximity of the optic nerves to the hypothalamic-pituitary unit, a careful examination of the visual fields is essential (see Chapters 14 and 36).

Assessment by Imaging Studies

Magnetic resonance imaging has generally replaced CT scanning as the investigation of choice in the diagnosis of pituitary and parapituitary lesions. The use of MRI with gadolinium contrast is associated with a detection rate for pituitary tumor of 82% to 94%. With use of two-dimensional techniques, it is important to obtain thin (1- to 2-mm) coronal slices of the sella to achieve the best results. Cerebral angiography is rarely required, because large cerebral aneurysms mimicking pituitary adenomas are readily picked up by MRI. Angiography is reserved primarily to demonstrate the blood supply of suspected meningiomas, and very often this information can be gathered from CT angiography.

Endocrinological Investigation

Not every patient with hypothalamic-pituitary disease requires a full battery of pituitary tests. In general, the endocrinological investigation is aimed at determining the extent of pituitary functional damage if any and—in patients whose blood levels of hormones are elevated or in whom excessive hormonal secretion is suspected on the basis of clinical features—determining whether the hormones in question respond normally to physiological suppressors and stimulators.

No single endocrine test can provide all the answers about pituitary function. Conclusions are based on a synthesis of evidence gained from clinical examination, endocrine tests, and MRI. Endocrine testing is used to determine residual pituitary function after surgery or radiotherapy. The return of biochemical markers of abnormal pituitary secretion or their failure to resolve can be used to gauge the success of surgery and aid in differentiating scar tissue from tumor recurrence on postoperative MRI scans. **Table 42.6** summarizes some of the more common pituitary tests and their use.

Table 42.6 **Common Tests of Pituitary Function**	
Test	**Comments**
Insulin hypoglycemia (Regular insulin, 0.1 unit/kg of body weight IV, fasting)	Adequate hypoglycemia is associated with a rise in growth hormone, ACTH, and to a lesser extent, prolactin. It probably is the most physiological stressor of the hypothalamic-pituitary-adrenal axis. The test should not be used in patients with epilepsy or unstable angina.
Gonadotropin-releasing hormone (2 µg/kg IV to a maximum of 100 µg)	Stimulates LH and FSH release directly at the pituitary. May be used to test LH and FSH reserve. Cannot reliably distinguish between pituitary and long-standing hypothalamic problem.
Thyrotropin-releasing hormone (7 µg/kg IV to a maximum of 400 µg)	Stimulates release of thyroid-stimulating hormone and prolactin from pituitary. Failure of prolactin to respond to thyrotropin-stimulating hormone is very suggestive of autonomous secretion by an adenoma, but exceptions do occur.
Metyrapone test (750 mg every 4 hours for 6 doses; collect 24-hr urine the day before, day of, and day after the test)	Metyrapone blocks the production of cortisol in the adrenal gland, resulting in increased ACTH secretion. This test is an alternative to insulin hypoglycemia as a test of the hypothalamic-pituitary-adrenal axis.
l-Dopa (500 mg PO)	l-Dopa can be used to stimulate growth hormone release (probably by increasing growth hormone–releasing hormone). It is a less potent stimulus than insulin-induced hypoglycemia but can be used as an alternative.
Corticotropin-releasing hormone (CRH) (1 µg/kg or 100 µg IV)	Stimulates release of cortisol and ACTH. ACTH is sampled at −5, 0, 15, and 30 minutes and cortisol at −5, 0, 30, and 45 minutes.

ACTH, Adrenocorticotropic hormone (corticotropin); *FSH,* follicle-stimulating hormone; *IV,* intravenously; *LH,* luteinizing hormone; *PO,* orally.

Treatment of Pituitary Tumors
Medical Management
PROLACTINOMA

Hyperprolactinemia of whatever cause often can be suppressed by a dopamine agonist, but such suppression is not diagnostic of a prolactinoma. Bromocriptine (2.5 to 7.5 mg/day in divided doses) or cabergoline (0.5 mg once or twice a week) usually normalizes serum prolactin. In up to 25% of patients on bromocriptine and 10% to 15% on cabergoline, however, prolactin levels will fail to normalize, and a 50% or greater reduction in tumor size will not be achieved. Maximum shrinkage of tumors occurs within 6 months—often within 6 to 8 weeks. Experience indicates that bromocriptine is safe to use to restore fertility. Once pregnancy occurs, the bromocriptine can be stopped with little risk of expansion of the prolactinoma during the remainder of the pregnancy and immediate postpartum period. Bromocriptine appears to cause growth of fibrous tissue in prolactinomas. This fibrous tissue may make such tumors more difficult to remove surgically, resulting in lower rates of surgical success. Use of bromocriptine and cabergoline at high doses in patients with Parkinson disease has been associated with valvular fibrosis of the heart. This does not seem to be an issue with the usual low-dose treatment of pituitary tumors but should be kept in mind if higher doses are used or if symptoms of this condition develop. Baseline echocardiography with regular follow-up can be used to achieve early detection of any cardiac valve abnormalities.

CUSHING DISEASE

Results with long-term medical therapy of Cushing disease have been disappointing. Cyproheptadine temporarily lowers ACTH levels in some patients, but it is rarely effective for long and commonly associated with somnolence and increased appetite. Drugs such as metyrapone and ketoconazole, which block corticosteroid synthesis, can be used to lower cortisol levels and improve the patient's clinical status before surgery. Ketoconazole can be used to control cortisol levels over the long term, but patients must be monitored closely for side effects. Recently, mifepristone (RU-486) in high dose has been shown to provide good control of Cushing disease that had been refractory to other medications.

ACROMEGALY

Until the development of a long-acting somatostatin analog (octreotide), the outcome of medical therapy for acromegaly, like that for Cushing disease, was disappointing. Bromocriptine in doses of 20 to 60 mg/day could reduce GH levels and cause tumor shrinkage, but it seldom normalized GH levels. Octreotide can normalize GH levels when given by subcutaneous injection every 8 hours or when used in a long-acting form given once monthly. The analog can be combined with bromocriptine if necessary to achieve maximal suppression and tumor shrinkage. For those patients who fail to respond to long-acting octreotide, pegvisomant (a growth hormone receptor blocker) can be added to the regimen to normalize growth hormone and IGF-1 levels (Cook et al., 2004). Most patients treated with pegvisomant will require continuing therapy with octreotide to prevent enlargement of the pituitary tumor when pegvisomant is used alone.

THYROID-STIMULATING HORMONE–SECRETING AND GONADOTROPIN-SECRETING TUMORS

Most patients with TSH-secreting and gonadotropin-secreting tumors are treated surgically, sometimes followed by radiotherapy. TSH-secreting tumors respond to octreotide with a decrease in hormone production; however, little if any tumor shrinkage is achieved. Early reports suggest that octreotide can reduce levels of α-subunit secretion in gonadotropin-secreting tumors, as can bromocriptine. Although some tumor shrinkage may occur with bromocriptine, it is unclear whether long-term octreotide use will have the same effect.

Surgery

In a medically fit patient with an accessible lesion, surgery is the treatment of choice for all nonsecretory pituitary and parapituitary lesions that are causing symptoms or signs or are showing signs of growth on serial imaging. For secretory tumors, surgery offers the possibility of rapid and complete cure. It is the preferred treatment when serious compression of parapituitary structures occurs. Surgical cure rates have been reported to be more than 80% in cases of microadenoma, although these rates may well be lower when strict endocrine criteria for cure are applied and with follow-up periods of 15 years. In the hands of an experienced neurosurgeon, pituitary surgery is associated with low morbidity and mortality rates. In tumors that secrete prolactin or growth hormone, medical management is now achieving results that are sometimes better than those being achieved by surgery. Depending on the availability of surgery and the skill of the surgeon, for prolactinomas and growth-hormone secreting tumors, surgery may no longer be the first choice but used only in those patients who fail medical therapy.

Radiotherapy

Conventional radiotherapy is used primarily as an adjunct to surgery and medical therapy, most commonly in the treatment of acromegaly, although octreotide and pegvisomant are reducing its need. It also is used frequently in surgical failures in cases of Cushing disease. It is rarely used in treating microprolactinoma in North America, although it can be used with larger tumors. Recurrence of nonsecreting adenomas after partial removal is effectively prevented by radiotherapy. The major problems with conventional radiotherapy are the long delay in onset of its effect (often 18 months or longer), its tendency to incomplete efficacy in secretory tumors, and the high frequency of eventual development of panhypopituitarism.

Proton beam therapy, external beam radiation therapy using a linear accelerator (LINAC), and the Gamma Knife permit a dose of radiation to be given at the pituitary gland that is 20 to 25 times greater than with conventional radiotherapy techniques. At the same time, radiation doses to other brain areas are limited. Unfortunately, these techniques are available in only a few centers. Furthermore, the tumor must be farther than 5 mm from the chiasm. The reported results compare favorably with those of transsphenoidal surgery, but the tumors that are best for this type of treatment are also those that are the best candidates for transsphenoidal surgery.

Treatment of Hypopituitarism

Vasopressin, ACTH, and TSH are the pituitary hormones critical to health and well-being. The management of vasopressin deficiency has been discussed already. ACTH deficiency is managed by glucocorticoid replacement; mineralocorticoid supplementation is seldom necessary in patients with ACTH deficiency. Most patients require 5 mg of prednisone (or 20 mg of hydrocortisone) each morning, and some require an additional 2.5 mg of prednisone (or 10 mg of hydrocortisone) in the evening. With the development of mild intercurrent illness, the dose of steroid should be doubled. Corticosteroid replacement in the glucocorticoid-deficient patient with serious illness or undergoing surgery consists of hydrocortisone sodium succinate, 10 mg/h IV around the clock. As the patient recovers, the dose is slowly tapered to maintenance levels.

Thyroid-stimulating hormone deficiency is managed by levothyroxine (L-thyroxine) replacement. Suppression of elevated TSH cannot be relied on to determine the adequacy of replacement in patients with pituitary-hypothalamic disease. Resolution of the clinical signs and symptoms of hypothyroidism is the important goal. In patients who receive adequate replacement, so that triiodothyronine (T_3) levels in the upper half of the therapeutic range are achieved, thyroxine (T_4) levels often are at or above the upper limit of normal.

Gonadotropin deficiency usually is managed by administration of testosterone or estrogen. This therapy, however, does not restore fertility. In patients for whom fertility is sought, a consultation with a reproductive endocrinologist and administration of various substitution therapies for LH and FSH may allow induction of fertility.

Growth hormone deficiency in children is treated by the administration of synthetic GH. GH-deficient adults currently do not routinely receive GH replacement. The evidence suggests that muscle strength, wound healing, and lean body mass all are improved by treatment with synthetic GH. Unfortunately, these studies have been short term, and the dose of GH required for long-term replacement is unknown. Because of the potentially deleterious effects of excessive levels of GH, studies are underway to determine appropriate replacement doses. No therapy is available for prolactin deficiency.

Neuroendocrine Tumors

Many endocrine cells distributed throughout the body are capable of taking up and decarboxylating amine precursors and synthesizing biogenic amines and polypeptide hormones. These cells are referred to as *APUD* (*a*mine *p*recursor *u*ptake and *d*ecarboxylation) cells. APUD cells are found in the pituitary gland, adrenal gland, peripheral autonomic ganglia, lung, GI tract, pancreas, gonads, and thymus. Tumors arising from APUD cells, as a class, generally produce symptoms through the secretion of biogenic amines (norepinephrine, epinephrine, dopamine, serotonin) or hormones. APUD cell tumors—insulinomas, gastrinomas, vasoactive intestinal polypeptide–secreting tumors, medullary carcinomas of the thyroid, pheochromocytomas, and carcinoid tumors—can manifest as clinical emergencies. Of these, only pheochromocytomas and carcinoid tumors are discussed here.

Pheochromocytomas

Pheochromocytomas are rare tumors that arise most commonly (85% to 90% of the time) from the catecholamine-producing cells of the adrenal medulla; they also can arise from extraadrenal chromaffin tissue in the cervical and thoracic regions and in the abdomen. A majority of these tumors develop spontaneously; however, they can be part of other syndromes such as multiple endocrine neoplasia types II and IIb, von Hippel-Lindau disease, neurofibromatosis, ataxia-telangiectasia, tuberous sclerosis, and Sturge-Weber syndrome.

Pheochromocytomas secrete predominantly norepinephrine, epinephrine, and some dopamine. These compounds are responsible for the most common signs and symptoms of pheochromocytoma: throbbing headache, sweating, palpitations, pallor, nausea, vomiting, and tremor. Pheochromocytomas also are capable of secreting other neuropeptides that can be responsible for different clinical symptoms. Pheochromocytoma should be suspected in patients with progressive or malignant hypertension, hypertension of early onset without family history, hypertension resistant to conventional therapy, paradoxical worsening of hypertension in response to treatment with beta-blockers, and a history of pressor response provoked by anesthesia, labor or delivery, or angiography. We screen for pheochromocytoma by collecting two consecutive 24-hour urine specimens and having them analyzed for vanillylmandelic acid, norepinephrine, epinephrine, metanephrine, normetanephrine, and dopamine. Ideally, these collections should be done around the time when the patient is symptomatic, because periodic hormone secretion does occur, and levels may at times be normal. The completeness of the 24-hour collection should be confirmed by an analysis of urinary creatinine. Sensitivity and specificity of testing can be enhanced by adding an assay of plasma catecholamines.

Tumor localization usually can be achieved by CT scanning of the adrenals. If a wider search is necessary, MRI may be more helpful. Radiolabeled metaiodobenzyl guanidine (^{123}I-MIBG), an iodinated guanethidine derivative, is taken up by chromaffin tissue, and its use with single-photon emission computed tomography (SPECT) can be helpful in localizing nonadrenal tumors and metastases. Some centers have been using indium 111–labeled pentetreotide, an analog of somatostatin, to localize somatostatin receptors on these tumors; 6-^{18}F-fluorodopamine and [^{11}C]hydroxyephedrine PET scanning also are complementary techniques for tumor localization (Eriksson et al., 2005).

Patients with pheochromocytoma should be managed in centers with previous experience in treating this type of tumor. Suitable preoperative preparation is necessary to prevent hypertensive or hypotensive crisis during surgery. For benign tumors, complete surgical removal is the treatment of choice. For malignant tumors, palliative management is indicated using a variety of treatments.

Carcinoid Tumors

Carcinoid tumors arise from enterochromaffin cells in the GI tract, pancreas, or lungs and only rarely from the thymus or gonads. When carcinoid tumors release biogenic amines directly into the systemic circulation, bypassing the liver, the *carcinoid syndrome* results. This syndrome is characterized by episodes of flushing, often with accompanying diarrhea or asthma. Later in the syndrome, fibrosis of the endomyocardium develops. Carcinoid tumors may be a source of ectopic ACTH, CRH, or GHRH secretion.

The diagnosis is made by finding elevated urinary 5-hydroxyindoleacetic acid levels. As in pheochromocytoma, carcinoids also secrete peptides (e.g., kallikrein, substance P, neurotensin) and other amines (e.g., histamine, dopamine), and some of these substances may be responsible for the flushing that occurs in the syndrome. To localize these tumors, $[^{11}C]$5-hydroxytryptophan and $[^{11}C]$l-dihydroxyphenylalanine can be useful in PET scans.

Surgery is the treatment of choice, but by the time the tumors become symptomatic, they often are incurable, because liver metastases are required for the appearance of symptoms. Serotonin antagonists may be used to relieve some of the symptoms, and octreotide may successfully manage carcinoid crisis. Radiolabeled octreotide is being used in some centers for palliative management of these tumors.

References

The complete reference list is available online at www.expertconsult.com.

Chapter 43

Management of Neurological Disease

Robert B. Daroff, Gerald M. Fenichel, Joseph Jankovic, John C. Mazziotta

How an experienced neurologist uses the history of the patient's illness, the neurological examination, and investigations to diagnose neurological disease is discussed in Chapters 1 and 31. This chapter presents some general principles guiding the management of neurological disease. Chapters 44 to 48 cover individual areas of neurological management such as pain management, neuropharmacology, intensive care, neurosurgery, and neurological rehabilitation. Details about the management of specific neurological diseases are presented in Chapters 49 to 82. Many aspects of management are common to all neurological disorders; these management considerations are the subject of this chapter.

Principles of Neurological Management

As in all medical disciplines, many neurological diseases are, at present, "incurable." This does not mean, however, that such diseases are not treatable and that nothing can be done to help the patient. Help that can be provided short of curing the disease ranges from treating the symptoms, to providing support for the patient and family, to end-of-life care (**Box 43.1**). Healthcare professionals are so committed to the scientific understanding of diseases and their treatment that the natural tendency of the clinician is to feel guilty when confronted with a patient with an incurable disease. The number of neurological diseases that *are* curable or arrestable is constantly expanding thanks to research.

Unfortunately, a physician who is fixated on the need to cure disease may simply strive to make the diagnosis of an as-yet incurable disease and then give no thought to patient management. Such a physician will tell the patient that he or she has an incurable disease, so coming back for further appointments is pointless ("diagnose and adios"). The aphorism "To cure sometimes, to relieve often, to comfort always" originated in the 1800s with Dr. Edward Trudeau, founder of a tuberculosis sanatorium. Any other attitude not only is an abrogation of the physician's responsibility to care for the patient, but also leaves the patient without the many modalities of assistance that can be provided even to those with incurable diseases. The neurologist who accepts the responsibility for treating the patient will review with the patient and family all the issues listed in **Box 43.1**. In fact, it usually is necessary to spend *more* time with the patient with an incurable disease than with one for whom effective treatment is available. In addition to providing all practical help available, the compassionate neurologist should share the grief and provide consolation for the patient and family; both are essential aspects of patient management.

Evidence-Based Medicine in Neurology

Recent emphasis on evidence-based medicine is appropriate. No treatment should be given to a patient without a good rationale. The scientific management of disease has always involved using all of the information available in the literature, so evidence-based medicine is not new. Although considered to be the standard method of analysis of benefit, double-blind placebo-controlled studies have some serious limitations.

Subjects selected for these studies often are strictly defined by inclusion/exclusion criteria, and they may not represent the population for whom the treatment will eventually be prescribed. Such patients, for example, may not necessarily have exactly the same demographics or clinical characteristics as those of the well-defined study population, and they may be taking other medications that could affect the response. For these and other reasons, the findings from controlled trials often may not be generalizable. Furthermore, most double-blind placebo-controlled drug trials are relatively short-term studies, and it is not until a long-term open-label trial that efficacy and adverse effects become better understood. Moreover, the cumulative experience of a seasoned physician whose clinical judgment relies not only on the published evidence-based literature but also on personal and often empirical experience can be of great importance in the management of a specific patient. It would be wrong if this resource were to be disregarded in areas where the literature is not definitive or available. Absence of evidence (usually because the appropriate studies have not yet been done or published) does not mean that support for a specific intervention or application is lacking. This applies at least as much to neurology as it does to other disciplines.

Goals of Treatment

In defining the goals of treatment, it is important to separate neurological impairment, disability, and handicap. *Neurological impairment* (presence of abnormal neurological signs) allows a diagnosis to be made. Impairment may cause *disability*, which in turn produces a *handicap.* For instance, a stroke may cause a hemiplegia, which is the impairment. The hemiplegia may cause difficulty in walking, which is the disability. The difficulty in walking may make it impossible for the patient to leave the house, which is the handicap. The patient does not care about the abnormal neurological signs but wants correction of the disability and relief from the handicap. It may not be possible to correct the underlying stroke lesion or reverse the hemiparesis, but symptomatic treatment such as providing physical therapy, a walker, and a wheelchair can help alleviate the handicap. Improvement in the functional state of a stroke patient resulting from neurological rehabilitation is gratifying when compared with the state of untreated patients.

Amyotrophic lateral sclerosis (ALS) is perhaps the disease that epitomizes the role of symptomatic care. Patients with ALS often report being told by their doctor that they have ALS, they are likely to die within 3 years, and because nothing can be done for them, they should go home, put their affairs in order, and prepare to die. A doctor who dispenses such advice not only is uncaring but also leaves the patient without hope and the symptomatic treatment that can help circumvent the disabilities and handicaps that attend the disease. The psychological support of a caring neurologist who is familiar with the disease can be of great help to the patient and family. An increasing number of lay organizations and support groups are available to provide information and services. Patients often will have found these by searching the Internet, but the physician should keep available the addresses and contact information of key organizations to give to patients.

Symptomatic treatment depends on the nature of the disease. It can consist of arresting an attack in a disease such as multiple sclerosis (MS); circumventing the effects of the disease, such as with antispasticity medications; or end-of-life care for a patient approaching death. The latter sometimes is called *palliative care,* but in fact every treatment short of cure, even in the early stages of a disease, is palliative. There is no "cookbook" approach to the management of any neurological disorder; therapy must be individualized, and the selection of the therapeutic strategy must be guided by the specific impairment and tailored to the needs of the patient.

Arresting an Attack

Many neurological diseases cause episodic attacks. These include strokes, migraine, MS, epilepsy, paroxysmal dyskinesias, and periodic paralyses, and in some of these diseases, treatment may prevent or halt the attacks. Although it does not cure the underlying disease, aborting the attacks is of great help to the patient. Triptan-class drugs generally arrest a migraine, and valproate, a beta-blocker, or a calcium channel blocker will reduce the frequency of the attacks (see Chapter 69). Status epilepticus usually can be arrested by intravenous antiepileptic drugs, and the frequency of epileptic attacks can be reduced by the use of chronic oral anticonvulsant drugs (see Chapter 67). Intravenous and intraarterial thrombolytics may terminate and potentially reverse an otherwise disastrous "brain attack" (cerebral ischemia) (see Chapter 51A).

Slowing Disease Progression

Examples of treatments that slow the progress of neurological disease are numerous. A malignant cerebral glioma is almost universally fatal, but high-dose corticosteroids, neurosurgical debulking, radiotherapy, and chemotherapy may slow tumor growth and prolong survival (see Chapters 52E and 52F). The β-interferons, glatiramer, natalizumab, or mitoxantrone may reduce relapses and slow the progress of MS (see Chapter 54). Liver transplantation in familial amyloid polyneuropathy may slow or arrest disease progression (see Chapter 76). Riluzole may slow the progress of ALS (see Chapter 74). Despite many efforts to slow the progression of Parkinson disease (PD), no neuroprotective therapy has proved to be effective, although certain monoamine oxidase B inhibitors and dopamine agonists delay the onset of levodopa-related motor complications.

Relieving Symptoms

Symptomatic treatment is available for many neurological diseases. Relief of pain, although not curative, is the most important duty of the physician and can be accomplished in many ways (see Chapter 44). Baclofen and tizanidine can reduce spasticity, particularly in spinal cord disease, without affecting the disorder causing it. Injections of botulinum toxin provide marked relief in patients with dystonia, spasticity, and other disorders manifested by abnormal muscle contractions. High-dose corticosteroid therapy reduces the edema surrounding a brain tumor, temporarily relieving headache and neurological deficits without necessarily affecting tumor growth. In PD, dopaminergic drugs partly or completely relieve symptoms for a period, without affecting the progressive degeneration of substantia nigra neurons (see Chapter 71). The physician-patient relationship and the placebo response both are important tools used by the experienced neurologist in helping to relieve a patient's symptoms.

Circumventing Functional Disability

In neurological diseases such as Alzheimer disease, PD, and ALS, the clinical course usually is progressive. Other disorders, such as stroke and spinal cord injury, have an acute onset, and the damage occurs before the neurologist first sees the patient. Although some recovery is expected, substantial functional deficits often persist. In both situations, many ways to circumvent the functional disability and the resultant handicap are available.

Neurological rehabilitation is the discipline that concentrates on restoration of function (see Chapter 48). Physical and occupational therapy help the patient to strengthen weak muscles, retrain the nervous system to compensate for lost function, increase mobility, and reduce spasticity. Some authorities believe that cognitive or behavioral therapy may similarly reeducate undamaged cortical areas to compensate for the effects of brain injury and stroke. Orthopedic procedures can be beneficial for rehabilitation; transfer of the tibialis posterior tendon to the dorsum of the foot can correct a footdrop in appropriate cases. Surgical release of Achilles tendon and iliotibial contractures in boys with Duchenne muscular dystrophy can delay the loss of ability to walk by 2 years or more.

Aids and appliances such as ankle-foot orthoses to prevent footdrop, canes, walkers, and wheelchairs can increase mobility and limit handicap. Changes to the home and work environment—a ramp or stair lift, widening of doors to allow wheelchair access, rails for the bath and toilet, replacement of the bath with a shower and shower chair—can be of great help to the patient. Only the ingenuity of clinicians and biomechanical engineers, the availability of technology, and the cost limit the scope of such appliances. Cochlear implants are already in clinical use for persons who were born deaf. Computer-controlled motorized body and lower-limb braces may allow paraplegic patients to walk.

The range of options available to help a patient with a severe, chronic neurological disease can be illustrated by reference to ALS. In the early stages, the patient may simply need enlarged handles on tools, pens, and utensils to compensate for a weak hand grip, or a cane to help with walking. Later, the patient may need a wheelchair and home adaptation.

Speech therapy, a communication board, or a computer with specialized software can help when speech is severely impaired. Weight loss and choking from dysphagia may necessitate a percutaneous gastrostomy. An incentive spirometer and an artificial cough machine can protect respiratory function (see Respiratory Failure later in the chapter). If the patient decides not to use a ventilator, end-of-life counseling and hospice care are needed.

Management of disabilities in patients with progressive neurological diseases may tax the neurologist's knowledge and ingenuity, but the beneficial effect of symptomatic therapy on patients and families makes the effort worthwhile and demonstrates that no neurological disease is untreatable. Collaboration with colleagues in other fields (e.g., pulmonary medicine, physical therapy, biomedical engineering, hospice care) often can be extremely helpful.

Principles of Symptom Management

Treatment of Common Neurological Symptoms

Several symptoms, such as pain, weakness, dysphagia, and respiratory failure, are common to many different neurological diseases. This section outlines the general principles that govern management of these symptoms. Chapters 44, 45, and 48 provide more complete discussions. Specific treatment for individual diseases is found in the relevant chapters in Volume II of this book.

Pain

The first step in pain management is to diagnose the source of the pain and assess the prognosis of the disease (see Chapter 44). Consider, for example, a patient with incapacitating pain in one leg from carcinoma infiltrating the lumbosacral plexus on one side. This patient's life expectancy may be measured in weeks or months, and progressive plexus damage will produce leg paralysis. Destructive procedures and narcotics are justified in this situation. Surgical interruption of pain pathways is considered the final choice to relieve pain from carcinomatous infiltration of the lumbosacral plexus. Such procedures include surgical or chemical posterior rhizotomy, contralateral anterolateral spinothalamic tractotomy in the midthoracic region, and stereotactic contralateral thalamotomy. Tachyphylaxis for narcotics can occur, and the oral dose of narcotics required to control pain may rise rapidly in patients who live for several months. This does not appear to occur with morphine administered by an intrathecal or epidural spinal catheter using a subcutaneous infusion pump.

Narcotics should not be used for patients with nonmalignant chronic pain syndromes such as painful polyneuropathies or low back pain, because of the development of tachyphylaxis and the risk of producing drug dependency without pain control. Biofeedback, hypnosis, and acupuncture may help some patients control pain. Antidepressant drugs are of benefit in many chronic pain syndromes by blocking the neurochemical transmitter mechanisms of central nervous system pain pathways, as well as treating depression. Many patients are resistant to taking antidepressant drugs for pain because they insist that the pain is real and not from depression; the effectiveness of antidepressant drugs for pain control is a point that needs to be clarified in such instances. Sometimes a single drug may be effective, but frequently a combination of a selective serotonin reuptake inhibitor (SSRI) and a tricyclic antidepressant (TCA) is better.

Sensory Loss, Paresthesias, and Burning Pain

Occasionally, sensory loss produces an intolerable positive sensation termed *anesthesia dolorosa* that may respond to a combination of a TCA with either carbamazepine, gabapentin, pregabalin, or an SSRI. Paresthesias generally result from damage to the large-diameter myelinated axons in the peripheral nerves or posterior columns of the spinal cord. Patients who complain of burning sensations from small-fiber peripheral neuropathies often are helped by a TCA, an SSRI, or pregabalin, or a combination of these.

Weakness

The management of weakness, considered more fully in Chapter 48, is a major component of neurological rehabilitation. Choice of treatment depends on the extent, severity, and prognosis of the patient's weakness. For example, weakness of flexion of the ankle due to Charcot-Marie-Tooth disease may be treated with a triple arthrodesis of the foot. Such a procedure, however, would not be appropriate to overcome the footdrop caused by a more rapidly progressive condition such as ALS. For such patients, an ankle-foot orthosis is best. Most neuromuscular conditions are benefited by exercise, although fatigue limits the amount of exercise that can be tolerated. Myasthenia gravis, however, is worsened by exercise. Weakness due to upper motor neuron disease can be addressed by physical and occupational therapy to promote the use of alternative neuronal pathways. Medications such as baclofen, tizanidine, and botulinum toxin injections reduce spasticity and may improve function in upper motor neuron disorders.

Ataxia

Ataxia can result from cerebellar dysfunction or sensory deafferentation. A weighted cuff (wrist weight) placed on an ataxic limb may lessen kinetic tremor; the added inertia reduces the amplitude of the involuntary movement during feeding and other activities of daily living that require coordinated movement. Gait ataxia is best managed with the use of walking aids such as a cane, walker, wheelchair, and other measures designed to prevent fall-related injuries. Displacing the center of gravity forward improves the gait of elderly patients, whose loss of postural reflexes causes retropulsion and falls. Increasing the height of the heels on the shoes and lowering the walker so the patient must stoop forward displaces the center of gravity forward.

Slowness of Movement or Abnormal Involuntary Movements

Along with rest tremor and rigidity, slowness of movement (bradykinesia) is one of the clinical hallmarks of PD and other parkinsonian disorders. Bradykinesia usually responds to dopaminergic therapy. Conversely, excessive involuntary movements, such as chorea and stereotypies, typically decrease

with drugs that deplete dopamine or block dopamine receptors. Postural tremors (e.g., essential tremor) often remit with beta-blockers, primidone, and topiramate.

Botulinum toxin injections are considered the treatment of choice for most focal dystonias and also may be effective for movement disorders including tremors, tics, and conditions associated with abnormal muscle contractions. Stereotactic surgery, particularly high-frequency deep brain stimulation, is now an established therapeutic strategy in patients with severe movement disorders that continue to be troublesome or disabling despite optimal medical therapy.

Aphasia and Dysarthria

Treatment of language disorders is, in principle, very similar to that of limb weakness. Speech therapy can improve aphasia by retraining contralateral speech and nonspeech areas of the brain to compensate for the effects of damaged speech centers. If the lesion is limited, some aspects of language function may be preserved and so provide an immediate mechanism for communication. For instance, an aphasic patient may be able to communicate through writing. With speech therapy, dysarthric patients can learn to slow their delivery and emphasize words, thereby improving the clarity of speech.

Respiratory Failure

Respiratory failure may develop in several neurological diseases (**Box 43.2**; see also Chapter 45). Patients with chronic neuromuscular diseases often complain of respiratory distress when they are close to respiratory failure. Patients with a weak diaphragm experience dyspnea when lying supine, because the abdominal contents prolapse into the chest, thereby lowering the patient's vital capacity and tidal volume. A neurologist or a pulmonary specialist who is relatively inexperienced in neurological problems affecting respiration may underestimate the warning signs of potentially fatal respiratory failure. This is particularly true in myasthenia gravis and Guillain-Barré syndrome. Blood gas measurements do not change until late in the development of respiratory failure in chronic neuromuscular diseases. By the time evidence of hypoxia and hypercapnia appears in the blood, the patient may be bordering on acute respiratory collapse. Reduced vital capacity, patient distress, and a good knowledge of the disease are better ways of judging impending respiratory failure. A patient with Duchenne muscular dystrophy and a vital capacity of 600 mL may survive for several years without dyspnea. A patient with

---

Box 43.2 Types of Neurological Disease Associated with Respiratory Failure

Acute neurological disease
Brainstem damage
High cervical cord injury
Subacute or chronic neurological disease
Bulbar palsy with airway compromise
Motor neuron degenerations (e.g., amyotrophic lateral sclerosis)
Neuropathies (e.g., Guillain-Barré syndrome)
Neuromuscular junction diseases (e.g., myasthenia gravis)
Muscle diseases (e.g., muscular dystrophy)

myasthenia gravis who has a vital capacity of 1200 mL but is anxious, sweating, and complaining of dyspnea is at serious risk for the development of fatal respiratory paralysis. With borderline respiratory function, sleep or sedation may produce carbon dioxide retention and narcosis, leading to further respiratory suppression and death.

ETHICAL CONSIDERATIONS IN THE TREATMENT OF RESPIRATORY FAILURE

Respiratory failure was once invariably fatal but now is commonly treated by noninvasive positive-pressure ventilation in the early stages and by intubation and positive-pressure ventilation in the terminal stages. The treatment of chronic progressive respiratory failure in neuromuscular diseases such as ALS and muscular dystrophy is very challenging. Moreover, cultural differences in different countries must be recognized. For example, in Japan, it is established practice to provide the ALS patient with a tracheostomy and positive-pressure ventilation when signs of early respiratory failure appear. In Western countries, most patients consider life on a ventilator unacceptable, and the neurologist must discuss quality-of-life issues with the patient and family before intubation.

Ideally, decisions about life-support measures should be made long before the patient is in acute respiratory distress, because it is more difficult to make these decisions when death is imminent. Patients and families require considerable counseling by the neurologist and may benefit from speaking to others who have experienced the situation, such as patients on a ventilator or persons who have lost a relative to ALS. Many patients cannot make a definitive decision about life-support measures and so defer the decision until the emergency occurs.

In these matters, the decision of a competent patient or the healthcare surrogate (in cases of an incompetent patient or one with whom communication is impossible) holds primacy. For instance, a 40-year-old patient with ALS may request respiratory support to see a child graduate or marry, even though no likelihood of recovery exists. On the other hand, a request to continue ventilator support for a 90-year-old patient with cancer and severe dementia cannot be considered rational, and the physician should convey the hopelessness of the situation and the patient's unnecessary suffering to the next of kin. Patients who decide against ventilator support should provide a living will or terminal care document to their physician and next of kin and legally grant to a designated person (the healthcare surrogate) the power of attorney to make medical management decisions for them if they become incompetent. Even if patients have prepared a living will, they will be taken by emergency services to a hospital emergency department and be intubated unless proper arrangements are in place for end-of-life care at home, usually through hospice services.

For patients who decide to request ventilator support, health insurance and economic matters must be considered. Although the availability of insurance to cover the cost of ventilator care is paramount in the United States, in Japan the health insurance system pays for the costs of 24-hour home ventilatory care for all ALS patients.

Patients with a tracheostomy may still be able to talk using a valved tracheostomy tube or a partially inflated cuff, but many lose bulbar functions and need to use communication devices such as computers or letter boards. Many of the conditions listed in **Table 43.2** also cause limb paralysis, which further impairs the ability to communicate. Quality of life usually becomes an issue when ventilator dependency becomes permanent. In many patients, the prognosis becomes clear within a relatively short time, as with stroke and coma. Because the patient is unconscious, the healthcare surrogate or, if such a person is not designated, the next of kin must decide, with the advice of the doctor, whether to continue respiratory support. If the healthcare surrogate or family of an unconscious patient requests that respiratory support be discontinued, it is standard medical practice in most parts of the world to do so. The legal and ethical issues are more complex with an awake and competent patient who requests that the ventilator be switched off. Although the legal systems in many parts of the world accept that such requests fall under the right of the patient to refuse medical treatment, involvement of a hospital ethics committee is strongly recommended.

MANAGING TERMINAL RESPIRATORY FAILURE

If the patient opts for life-support measures, an elective tracheostomy and intermittent positive-pressure ventilation should be offered at the first signs of terminal respiratory failure. Patients who have respiratory insufficiency, whether or not they decide to opt for tracheostomy, often can be helped for a prolonged period by noninvasive positive-pressure ventilation through a nose mask or nasal "pillows." Patients who decide against respiratory support should be counseled *not to go to the hospital in a crisis*, because they will inevitably be intubated. They should be referred to home hospice services, and when terminal respiratory distress appears, home treatment with oxygen, morphine, and sedation will be provided, despite the risk that this may hasten death. Neurologists should learn to manage chronic respiratory failure due to neurological disease. Although neurologists must work collaboratively with the intensive care specialist and hospice doctors, they should assume an active role in management decisions.

Memory Impairment and Dementia

Alzheimer disease is the most common cause of progressive impairment of memory and dementia, and only symptomatic care is possible, which includes anticholinesterase inhibitors. Some causes of progressive dementia are curable (see Chapter 66), and their recognition important. Even if no specific curative treatment is available, the experienced neurologist can provide essential advice to the family of a patient with a condition like Alzheimer disease on how to anticipate problems and minimize them. This includes helping the patient to make shopping lists and checklists of things to do before leaving the kitchen or the house and before going to bed. For a period, these measures can prevent the patient from leaving the house unlocked, or from forgetting about a pot boiling on the stove. Inevitably, the patient will have difficulty managing a checkbook, and a family member should take over money management before financial disaster occurs. The patient eventually will need either a live-in companion or must move in with a family member or into a nursing home. Much of the neurologist's efforts are directed toward helping the patient and family circumvent problems and adjust to expected changes. Family members need access to books and publications by foundations and support groups such as the Alzheimer's Disease Association.

Treatment of Secondary Effects of Neurological Disease

Predictable reactions occur in a patient who is given the diagnosis of a chronic incurable neurological disease. These reactions progress at variable rates through the stages of anger, denial, "why me?," depression, and eventually acceptance, often with oscillation among these phases. The neurologist must provide support through this process of adjustment, sometimes with the assistance of a mental health professional.

The psychological, social, and economic impact of the disease on the family also must be considered. Family members caring for a patient with Alzheimer disease often say that it is like looking after a young child but with much more stress. The family of a boy with Duchenne muscular dystrophy will experience both mental and physical stress because the child eventually will lose the ability to walk and must be lifted into and out of chairs, bed, and bath. Mechanical lifting devices can help, but they are slow and clumsy. Often, home alterations are needed to allow one-level living and wheelchair access. Someone needs to get up several times a night to turn the patient in bed. Lack of sleep and increasing daytime care strain the family dynamics. Other children may be neglected and emotionally deprived; marital disharmony is common. The physician may need to refer such families for counseling or put them in touch with a family support group. School authorities need information and should be encouraged to keep the child in mainstream schooling. As the young man with Duchenne muscular dystrophy reaches maturity, he may consider college or employment, and the neurologist can provide information to assist the relevant authorities.

The neurologist caring for a patient with a progressive neurological disease plays an important role for both the patient and the family. Help from many other professionals often is required, but the neurologist must anchor the management team.

Explaining the Prognosis

Establishing the diagnosis is necessary for the neurologist to be able to define the prognosis for the patient and family. The physician should ascertain what the patient and family want to know and then provide answers at a rate they can accept. Some patients fear that they will die or become a "vegetable" within a few months and are greatly relieved to learn that they have several years of useful life ahead. Patients may wish to make financial arrangements or accelerate unfulfilled plans if the prognosis is poor. Patients may not always wish to be told the prognosis, but relatives generally want to know. The neurologist should always present the prognosis with some hopeful caveats, because the diagnosis may be wrong or the disease may not follow the expected course. Patients should always be given some hope; even ALS can arrest or remit. A useful way to cushion bad news is to say that the patient needs to *hope for the best but plan for the worst.*

Palliation and Care of the Terminally Ill Patient

Palliative care starts from the earliest stage of the doctor-patient relationship. Pain, depression, and anxiety are the three major symptoms that require palliation. The treatment of pain is considered in Chapter 44. Psychological reactions are treated with a range of pharmacological agents, including benzodiazepines for anxiety, neuroleptics for psychotic symptoms, and an ever-increasing list of medications for depression. The psychological support for the patient and family provided by the doctor, however, usually is more important than pharmacological therapy. The experienced neurologist provides help to the patient and family by drawing on lessons learned from treating many similar patients. Even though the disease and its effects cannot be arrested, the neurologist can help ease the emotional burden. When possible, the neurologist should discuss each new phase of the disease with the patient and family *before* it occurs. No patient likes to hear of impending deterioration, but if the neurologist clarifies the importance of anticipation, the patient is reassured that the doctor is ready to deal with change, when and if it occurs.

Genetic Counseling

Approximately 1 in 10 neurological conditions has a genetic basis. Rapid advances in molecular genetics require that the neurologist keep abreast of the many diseases that can be diagnosed by genetic testing (see Chapter 40). Genetic counseling should take into account the limitations and pitfalls of the various commercially available DNA tests, however, and the assistance of an experienced medical geneticist is invaluable. A parent with a neurological disease commonly fears that the disease will pass to the children. Hence, if a disease has no hereditary component, the parent should be reassured. If the disease has a hereditary tendency, the risk to offspring must be discussed. For instance, the chance of occurrence of MS in the offspring of a patient with MS is higher than that in the general population, but it is still only about 3%.

In Huntington disease (HD), however, the risk that each offspring will inherit the disease is 50%; at-risk persons may choose not to have children because of this. An offspring of a patient with HD can be advised about alternative ways to have a family—adoption, artificial insemination by donor when the husband is at risk, or surrogate gamete in vitro fertilization when the wife is at risk. In addition, an individual carrying a mutant gene who wishes to have a child can use the technique of embryo genotesting. After in vitro fertilization with the parents' ova and sperm, the embryo is allowed to grow to the 8- to 16-cell stage. A single cell is then removed for DNA testing; embryos bearing two normal huntingtin genes are accepted for implantation, and those with an abnormal huntingtin gene are discarded. Cost and availability of services limit the use of this procedure.

The neurologist should provide the patient and spouse with the available information about the mode of inheritance of the disease and, when relevant, the possibilities for prenatal and preclinical diagnosis. A couple's attitude to therapeutic termination of pregnancy should be part of the discussion. When a disease has an autosomal recessive mode of inheritance and the gene frequency in the population is low, children of an affected parent are at very little risk unless the patient marries a close relative. If the gene frequency in the general population is known, the risk of having an affected child can be quantified.

Each pregnancy of a parent with a fully penetrant autosomal dominant disorder has a 50% risk of resulting in an offspring bearing the mutant gene. If the proband is apparently a sporadic case, a risk approaching 50% must still be assigned because many apparently sporadic cases are in fact due to dominantly inherited mutations in which the proband was the product of undisclosed parentage or are due to new mutations.

In response to genetic counseling, some patients may make what the neurologist considers to be an irrational decision about having children. Some patients consider 50% quite good odds even when considering the risk of having a child with HD. On the other hand, some patients may decide against having children because of odds of 1 in 100. In both circumstances, the physician should provide as much information as possible about the meaning of the results of the genetic tests but must emphasize that the ultimate decision rests with the couple.

Genetic testing can reveal that an asymptomatic person will almost certainly develop the disorder. Asymptomatic patients who carry the mutation for the disease can be identified by the use of testing for the mutant gene. Huntington disease and myotonic dystrophy are two such examples. Because HD currently is not treatable and affected persons have a high suicide rate, the neurologist should be aware of the risks that accompany disclosure. The services of a qualified genetic counselor are very helpful for managing these problems. Before testing is begun, the genetic counselor will thoroughly review the hypothetical possibilities and potential management decisions with the patient and spouse. Although most people think they want to know their genetic status, after considering the implications, many conclude that a positive result on genetic testing would be too difficult to tolerate and, hence, forgo screening.

Legal Issues

There are serious practical and legal aspects patients and families must face when they or their relative are diagnosed with certain types of neurological disorders. Perhaps the most common is the question of whether the patient can drive. Most states have laws that govern particular circumstances. For example, some states require physicians to report to regulatory agencies (e.g., Department of Public Health, Motor Vehicle Department, etc.) any patient who has a seizure or alteration in consciousness, motor control, or vision if these symptoms are likely to recur. Failure to do so puts the patient and physician at risk for criminal and civil prosecution. As public debate on such matters evolves, there may soon be similar laws related to cognitive function and judgment. Certain types of employment also may have specific restrictions (e.g., airline pilots, commercial drivers, construction workers, etc.). Neurologists need to be completely familiar with these rules and policies in the state where they practice.

It is often very difficult for the physician to inform patients that they will be reported because of their diagnosis and/or symptoms. Frequently the patient will object and ask that this not be done, as it may result in significant practical and economic hardship. Losing the privilege of driving is also associated with a loss of personal freedom and independence. Nevertheless, it is the neurologist's responsibility and duty to explain the reasons for such decisions, the consequences of not doing so, and the associated risks. It is prudent to give examples. Tell the patient what could happen if he or she had a seizure while driving: that they or others could be injured or killed, and they and their family would be liable for the financial consequences. When realistic, indicate that with proper treatment, such restrictions may be dropped and the privilege reinstated.

Implications for Clinical Practice

The numerous and multifaceted aspects of modern management of neurological disease presented in this chapter serve to underscore an expanded role for the neurologist in clinical practice. Improved diagnostic methods identify affected persons more often and earlier, and patients with serious or even fatal disease are living longer, so that the physician-patient relationship may be prolonged. It is essential for today's clinical neurologists to recognize that their scope of practice involves much more than diagnosis. Although a correct diagnosis is essential, the clinician's proper focus is on treatment and management of the patient and the disease.

Principles of Pain Management

YiLi Zhou

Definition and Challenge

Chronic pain constitutes a major public health burden. Between 15% and 20% of the population in the United States suffers from chronic pain. The prevalence of persistent chronic pain increases with age, and between ages 35 and 54 years, the prevalence could be up to 29%. In those 55 years and older, the prevalence could be as high as 39%. Treatment of chronic headache, trigeminal neuralgia (TN), and pain conditions caused by damage or malfunction in the central and peripheral nerve systems are still a major task and challenge facing most neurologists in their daily work.

The International Association for the Study of Pain defines *pain* as an unpleasant sensory and emotional experience associated with actual or potential tissue damage, or described in terms of such damage, or both. Pain is classified as acute, chronic, or malignant. *Acute pain* is caused by injury, surgery, illness, trauma, or painful medical procedures. It generally lasts for a short period of time and usually disappears when the underlying cause has been treated or has healed. However, acute pain may lead to chronic pain problems that exist beyond an expected time for healing. *Chronic pain* is a persistent pain state not associated with malignancy or acute pain caused by trauma, surgery, infection, or other factors.

Malignant pain is associated with carcinoma. Pain in cancer patients can be caused by disease itself, treatment, or autoimmune antibodies associated with the malignancy.

Over the last 2 decades, an increasing number of healthcare professionals outside the field of neurology are devoting more effort to the research and management of headache and other chronic pain conditions. Among them are anesthesiologists, physiatrists, and psychiatrists, as well as physicians from other specialties. Neurologists are traditionally well trained in anatomical localization and differential diagnosis of a variety of neurological disorders. In terms of pain management, neurologists are probably in a better position to identify the pain sources. However, the field of pain management has developed rapidly. Successful treatment of chronic pain conditions not only requires an accurate diagnosis, it also requires the treating physician to be familiar with new techniques available for pain management. Multidisciplinary team care is now recognized to be crucially important in the management of chronic pain, and the word *multidisciplinary* implies not just the involvement of physicians from different specialties, but the utilization of various treatment modalities as well. These modalities include pharmacological therapy, physical therapy and rehabilitation, psychological care, interventional pain management, alternative medicine techniques, and surgical treatment.

DOI: 10.1016/B978-1-4377-0434-1.00051-7

In this chapter, we will first outline the anatomical basis of chronic pain conditions and some recent developments in molecular pain research. The second portion of the chapter will discuss some common pain conditions seen in daily neurology practice. The last section of the chapter will illustrate recent developments in pharmacological treatment, as well as interventional pain management techniques for treating common chronic pain conditions.

Anatomy and Physiology of the Pain Pathways

Nociceptor receptors are found in skin, connective tissue, blood vessels, periosteum, and most of the visceral organs. These nociceptors are formed by peripheral endings of sensory neurons with various morphological features. Noxious stimuli are transduced into depolarizing current by specialized receptors congregated in the nociceptor terminals. Cutaneous nociceptors include: (1) high-threshold mechanical nociceptors (HTMs) associated with small-diameter myelinated axons (Aδ fibers), (2) myelinated mechanothermal nociceptors (MTs) (Aδ fibers), and (3) polymodal nociceptors associated with unmyelinated axons (C fibers). Polymodal nociceptors respond to mechanical, chemical, and thermal stimuli. The afferent fibers that convey nociceptive information are thinly myelinated Aδ fibers with conduction velocities of about 15 m/sec and unmyelinated C fibers with conduction velocities of 0.5 to 2 m/sec. Stimulation of afferent Aδ nociceptive fibers causes a sharp, well-localized pain sensation. Activation of nociceptive C fibers is associated with a dull, burning, or aching and poorly localized pain. Because pain impulses are conducted by small, slowly conducting nerve fibers, conventional nerve conduction velocity (NCV) studies that measure the speed of conduction of large myelinated fibers are not sensitive to abnormal function of small-diameter fibers. It is very common that patients with small-fiber neuropathy have normal NCV tests.

Most primary afferent fibers that innervate tissues below the level of the head have cell bodies located in the dorsal root ganglion (DRG) of the spinal nerves. Visceral nociceptive afferent fibers (Aδ, C fibers) travel with sympathetic and parasympathetic nerves whose cell bodies are also found in the DRG.

Axons of DRG neurons send the primary nociceptive afferents through the dorsal roots to the most superficial layers of the dorsal horns (Rexed laminae I and II) and to some of the deep laminae (Rexed V). The Aδ fibers conveying input from HTMs and MTs terminate primarily in laminae I and V; C fibers mainly terminate in lamina II. Neurotransmitters related to pain conduction include excitatory amino acids and neuropeptides, particularly substance P (Geracioti et al., 2006). The second-order neurons in the dorsal horn include cells that respond only to noxious stimuli (nociceptive specific neurons) and others (wide dynamic range [WDR] neurons) that respond to both nociceptive and non-nociceptive sensory stimuli.

Axons of most of the second-order sensory neurons associated with pain sensation cross in the anterior white commissure of the spinal cord and ascend as the spinothalamic tract in the opposite anterolateral quadrant. This tract is somatotopically organized, with sacral elements situated posterolaterally and cervical elements more anteromedially. In humans, most of the spinothalamic tract projects to the ventral posterolateral (VPL) nucleus of the thalamus as the neospinothalamic pathway, which is related to fast and well-localized pain sensation. Axons from the third-order sensory neurons in the VPL directly project to the primary sensory cortex. Some of the fibers in the spinothalamic tract synapse with neurons of the periaqueductal gray (PAG, spinoreticular pathway) and other brainstem nuclei. Fibers from these brainstem neurons join with fibers from the spinothalamic tract to project to the central or laminar nuclei of the thalamus and constitute the paleospinothalamic tract, which is related to slow and poorly localized pain and emotional response to pain stimulation.

Multiple areas of the cerebral cortex are involved in the processing of pain sensation and the subsequent behavioral and emotional responses. Recent functional magnetic resonance imaging (fMRI) and positron emission tomography (PET) scan studies indicate that the primary and secondary somatosensory cortex, thalamus, periaqueductal gray matter, supplemental motor, inferior prefrontal, and insular cortex are activated in response to painful stimulation. It is now believed that primary sensory cortex (SI) seems to play a role in basic pain processing, while secondary sensory cortex (SII) and insula are involved in higher functions of pain perception. Emotional aspects of pain perception are mediated by the anterior cingulate cortex and the posterior insula and parietal operculum.

Central Modulation of Nociception

Nociceptive transmissions are modulated at the spinal level by both local neuronal circuits and descending pathways originating in the brainstem through the dorsal horns and the spinothalamic projections. Intrasegmental and intersegmental projections arising from cells located in the Rexed laminae I and II modulate both presynaptic and postsynaptic elements of primary nociceptive afferent terminals in the spinal cord. Activation of non-nociceptive afferent fibers may suppress nociceptive transmission in the dorsal horn. This is the major component of circuitry models referred to as the *gate control theory of pain transmission*. The development and widespread use of the spinal cord stimulator is based on this theory.

Descending inhibitory systems appear to have three functionally interrelated neurotransmitter mechanisms: the opioid, the noradrenergic, and the serotonergic systems. Opioid precursors and their respective peptides (β-endorphin, methionine [met]-enkephalin, leucine [leu-] enkephalin, and dynorphin) are present in the amygdala, hypothalamus, PAG, raphe magnus, and the dorsal horn. Noradrenergic neurons project from the locus caeruleus and other noradrenergic cell groups in the medulla and pons. These projections are found in the dorsolateral funiculus. Stimulation of these areas produces analgesia, as does the administration (direct or intrathecal) of α_2-receptor agonists such as clonidine (Khodayar et al., 2006). Many serotonergic neurons are found in the raphe magnus. These neurons send projections to the spinal cord via the dorsolateral funiculus. Administration of serotonin to the spinal cord produces analgesia, and pharmacological blockade or lesion of the raphe magnus can reduce the effects of morphine. The antinociceptive effects of antidepressants such as tricyclics and newer serotonin-norepinephrine reuptake inhibitors such as duloxetine and milnacipran are believed to reduce pain by increasing serotonin and norepinephrine concentrations in descending inhibitory pain pathways.

Opioid Receptors

Opioids are the core pharmacological treatment for acute pain. They act via receptors on cell membranes. Opioid receptors are coupled to G proteins and are thus able to effect protein phosphorylation via the second messenger system and change ion channel conductance. Presynaptically, activation of opioid receptors inhibits the release of neurotransmitters involved in pain, including substance P and glutamate. Postsynaptically, activation of opioid receptors inhibit neurons by opening potassium channels that hyperpolarize and inhibit the neuron.

Currently, there are five proposed classes of opioid receptors: μ, δ, κ, σ, and ε. μ Receptors are the main functional target of morphine and morphine-like drugs; they are present in large quantities in the periaqueductal gray matter in the brain and the substantia gelatinosa in the spinal cord. μ Receptors are also found in the peripheral nerves and skin. Activation of μ receptors results in analgesia, euphoria, respiratory depression, nausea, vomiting, and decreased gastrointestinal (GI) activity, as well as the physiological syndromes of tolerance and dependence. Two distinct subgroups of the μ receptors have been identified: μ_1, found supraspinally, and μ_2, found mainly in the spinal cord. The μ_1 receptor is associated with the pain-relieving effects of opioids, whereas μ_2 receptors mediate constipation and respiratory depression.

The δ receptor has similar central and peripheral distribution as the μ receptors. Studies have shown that δ-opioid agonists can provide relief of inflammatory pain and malignant bone pain. Meanwhile, peripherally restricted κ-opioid agonists have been developed to target κ-opioid receptors located on visceral and somatic afferent nerves for relief of inflammatory, visceral, and neuropathic chronic pain. The potential analgesic effects, combined with a possible lower abuse rate and fewer side effects than μ-receptor agonists, makes δ- and peripherally restricted κ-opioid receptor agonists promising targets for treating pain (Vanderah, 2010).

Peripheral Sensitization

Neurological systems may change their responses to various incoming stimuli. This process is called *neuroplasticity* and occurs in both the peripheral and central nervous systems. Peripheral sensitization may result in decreased threshold and increased responses after repeated stimuli to the peripheral nervous system. Most of the inflammatory mediators sensitize the peripheral nerve endings through posttranslational phosphorylation of the key receptor channels. For example, phosphorylation of tetrodotoxin-resistant voltage-gated sodium channels by protein kinase A and protein kinase C increases the sodium current to depolarize the nerve terminal, thereby producing greater excitation in the peripheral nerve and lowering the activation threshold of the neurons. A damaged C fiber therefore may begin to fire spontaneously. Changes in non-nociceptive afferents such as Aβ fibers also contribute to the process of sensitization. These fibers normally convey information about non-noxious mechanical stimuli. Following an injury, a pain-related neurotransmitter such as substance P may be released from terminals of Aβ fibers. These

alterations may explain the pain induced by non-nociceptive stimuli, such as allodynia.

Central Sensitization

Central sensitization plays a major role in the development of neuropathic pain syndromes. First, postsynaptic depolarization in the spinal cord in response to afferent stimulation can induce removal of magnesium blockade in N-methyl-D-aspartate (NMDA) receptors such that glutamate now induces a depolarization upon receptor binding. This process is short lasting and is called *wind up* (Katz and Rothenberg, 2005). It is responsible for the temporal summation of inputs. The second set of changes is related to phosphorylation of the NMDA receptor, which is a key process for longer-lasting changes in the excitability of the dorsal horn neurons that produce central sensitization. This posttranslational modification of the NMDA receptors results in dramatic changes in excitability due to removal of the voltage-dependent magnesium block in the absence of cell depolarization and also to changes in channel kinetics, such as channel opening time. NMDA receptor activation allows calcium influx into the cell, which further augments signal transduction within the dorsal horn neurons by activating a number of intracellular signal transduction kinases. As a result, relatively brief C-fiber inputs initiate very rapid changes in membrane excitability. This manifests both as a progressive increase in excitability during the course of the stimulus (wind up) and as post-stimulus changes that may last for several hours (central sensitization).

Clinically, the real meaning of *peripheral* and *central sensitization* is the enhanced and prolonged pain perception to minor stimulations, or sometimes without peripheral stimulation. Once peripheral and central sensitizations are involved, the pain is usually more difficult to treat. It is now believed that peripheral and central sensitization may be involved in a wide variety of chronic pain conditions such as reflex sympathetic dystrophy, tension headache, carpal tunnel syndrome, pain after spinal cord injury (Carlton et al., 2009), and even in pain conditions previously thought to be mainly nociceptive in nature such as fibromyalgia, epicondylalgia, and osteoarthritis (Gwilym et al., 2009). The challenge to the clinician is that when trying to make a diagnosis for a pain patient, we should not only try to localize the pain source—as most clinicians always do—we should also factor in the role of peripheral and central sensitization and what the best treatment strategy will be in each case.

Common Pain Syndromes

Trigeminal Neuralgia

Trigeminal neuralgia (TN), or *tic douloureux*, is characterized by paroxysmal lancinating attacks of severe facial pain. TN has an incidence of approximately 4/100,000, with a large majority of cases occurring spontaneously. Both genders experience TN, but there is a slight female predominance, and the diagnosis is most common over the age of 50. Classic TN is characterized by abrupt onset and termination of unilateral brief electric shock-like pain. Pain is often limited to the distribution of one or two (commonly the second and third) divisions of the trigeminal nerve. Trivial stimuli including washing, shaving, smoking, talking, and/or brushing the teeth (*trigger factors*) can evoke the pain. Some areas in the nasolabial fold and/or chin may be particularly susceptible to stimulation (*trigger areas*). In individual patients, pain attacks are stereotyped, recurring with the same intensity and distribution. Most TN patients are symptom free between attacks, and clinical examination is usually normal. Attacks of TN occur in clusters, and remissions can last for months.

The cause of TN pain attacks is unknown. Compression of the trigeminal nerve by benign tumors and vascular anomalies may play a role in the development of clinical symptoms. Studies of surgical biopsy specimens from TN patients who had presumed vascular compression demonstrate evidence of inflammation, demyelination, and close apposition of axons (leading to the possibility of ephaptic transmission between fibers). The *ignition hypothesis* of Devor proposes that a trigeminal nerve injury induces physiological changes that lead to a population of hyperexcitable and functionally linked trigeminal primary sensory neurons. The discharge of any individual neuron in this group can quickly spread to activate the entire population, resulting in a sudden synchronous discharge and a sudden jolt of pain characteristic of a TN attack.

The diagnosis of TN is based primarily on a history of characteristic paroxysmal pain attacks. The White and Sweet criteria are still commonly used worldwide (**Box 44.1**). In the majority of TN patients, the clinical examination, imaging studies, and laboratory tests are unremarkable (*classic TN*). In a smaller group, TN is secondary to other disease processes affecting the trigeminal system (*symptomatic TN*). Because a significant percentage of patients have symptomatic TN resulting from other disease processes, diagnostic MRI studies should be part of the initial evaluation of any patient with TN symptoms. Special attention should be paid to MS plaques, tumor, and subtle vascular anomalies that may be the source of root compression. Recent studies found that high-resolution three-dimensional (3D) MRI reconstruction and magnetic resonance cisternography may provide alternative tools to better identify the presence of neurovascular compression and even measure the volume of neurovascular compression at the cerebellopontine angle and predict the prognosis after initial treatment (Tanaka et al., 2009).

Carbamazepine is the first choice for treatment of TN; both controlled and uncontrolled studies confirm its clinical efficacy. Carbamazepine monotherapy provides initial symptom control in as many as 80% of TN patients. Of those initially responding to the drug, approximately 75% will continue to have long-term control of pain attacks. Controlled studies demonstrate that baclofen and lamotrigine are superior to placebo for treatments of TN. In the experience of many clinicians, baclofen is just as effective as carbamazepine and often

better tolerated. A recent study found that oxcarbazepine may be effective for those who were unresponsive to the treatment of carbamazepine (Gomez-Arguelles et al., 2008). Pregabalin may also be potentially effective. If a patient is not satisfied with single medication therapy, adding another oral medication may offer additional benefits. Intravenous (IV) lidocaine or phenytoin could be effective for some severe refractory cases of TN. However, these treatments carry additional risks and require close cardiovascular monitoring. Opioid analgesics have not been proven effective for TN and should be avoided.

Posterior fossa exploration and microvascular decompression (MVD) is assumed to directly treat the cause of TN. However, this is a complex and invasive therapy with a possibility of death. With the availability of other less-invasive procedures, MVD is infrequently used and is only reserved for younger and healthier patients. Several studies demonstrated trigeminal radiofrequency rhizotomy successfully controls symptoms in over 85% of TN cases. The technique is minimally invasive. To heat the gasserian ganglion, a radiofrequency needle is inserted through the foramen ovale under the guidance of fluoroscopy. The procedure can be finished in less than 30 minutes in experienced hands. A few patients experience sensory loss and dysesthesia (analgesia dolorosa) in the distribution of the damaged trigeminal fibers with this procedure. Stereotactic radiosurgery (SRS) employs computerized stereotaxic methods to concentrate ionizing radiation on the trigeminal root entry zone. Several studies have demonstrated the high clinical efficacy and relative safety of this new technique. It is currently recommended as a first-line noninvasive surgical technique in many pain centers, especially for frail or elderly patients (Zahra et al., 2009).

Low Back Pain

Low back pain (LBP) is the most common condition seen in pain clinics. Approximately 60% to 80% of the U.S. population will experience back pain some time during life. Neurologists are often consulted for the diagnosis and treatment of LBP. It is critical for clinicians to appropriately examine the patients and make a diagnosis before treatment is rendered. Common causes of LBP include muscle strain, lumbar disk herniation, lumbar radiculopathy, lumbar facet joint syndrome, sacroiliac joint syndrome, and lumbar spinal stenosis.

Patients with acute muscle strain in the low back often have histories of acute injury. Physical examination may reveal tenderness or muscle spasms. Nonsteroidal anti-inflammatory drugs (NSAIDs), muscle relaxants, massage therapy, physical therapy, or acupuncture often provide effective pain relief. However, many times muscle pain in the low back is secondary to injuries in deeper tissues, such as lumbar disk herniation or lumbar radiculopathy.

Acute lumbar disk herniation after injury may cause severe LBP. Patients often complain of severe shooting or stabbing pains in the low back, with frequent radiation pain down the dorsomedial part of the foot when the L5 nerve root is involved, or the lateral part of the foot or the small toe when the S1 nerve root is involved. The straight leg raising test is often positive. Detailed neurological examinations may find decreased sensation to pin prick in the area innervated by L5 and/or S1 nerve root(s). Patient may also have mild weakness

---

Box 44.1 **White and Sweet Criteria for Trigeminal Neuralgia**

1. The pain is paroxysmal.
2. The pain may be provoked by light touch to the face (trigger zones).
3. The pain is confined to the trigeminal distribution.
4. The pain is unilateral.
5. The clinical sensory examination is normal.

on the tibialis anterior (L5), or peroneus longus and brevis muscles (S1). These patients usually have severe tenderness and spasm over the lumbar paraspinal muscles. Lumbosacral MRIs may reveal disk herniation at L4-5 and/or L5-S1 level(s). Electromyography (EMG)/NCV tests may not detect a lumbar radiculopathy. NSAIDs, muscle relaxants, and physical therapy may help some patients with acute disk herniation and lumbar radiculopathy. If patients fail these treatments, lumbar epidural corticosteroid injections may offer fast and effective pain relief if the nerve roots are not severely mechanically compressed. Surgery is suggested for those with severe focal weakness of relevant muscles or incontinence. Surgery may also be indicated for severe pain that lasts for more than 3 months and does not respond to aggressive pain management if disk herniation is demonstrated by MRI or computed tomography (CT) studies.

Lumbar facet joint syndrome is found in up to 35% of patients with LBP. It is frequently associated with arthritis or injuries in lumbar facet joints. Patients may complain of pain in the low back, often on one side only. Pain may radiate down the back or front of the thigh. Physical examination may find positive tenderness over the lumbar paraspinal muscles and facet joints. Back extension and lateral rotation to the side of the pain often increases the back pain. Results of a straight leg raising test should be negative. Neurological examination should be normal unless there is a coexistent lumbar radiculopathy or other neurological condition. Diagnosis of facet joint syndrome is clinical. MRI and CT reports of facet joint arthropathy do not correlate with clinical findings. Often these changes are age related. NSAIDs should be tried for patients with lumbar facet joint syndrome before they are considered for diagnostic medial branch blocks or intra-joint corticosteroid injections.

Sacroiliac (SI) joint syndrome is another major source of LBP. The patient may have pain in one side of the low back, with pain radiation down to the hip or thigh. Pain is often increased when these patients try to walk upstairs. Physical examination may find tenderness over the SI joint, and the Patrick test or single-leg standing often exacerbate SI joint pain. NSAIDs are the first-line medication for SI joint inflammation. SI joint corticosteroid injection can provide temporary pain relief. Radiofrequency lesions to denervate the SI joint have been reported effective; however, more studies are needed to confirm clinical efficacy of this treatment.

Lumbar spinal stenosis is a common age-related change. The majority of seniors older than 60 years of age have varying degrees of spinal stenosis due to disk herniation, osteophytes, or degenerative spondylolisthesis. Preexisting congenital lumbar canal stenosis predisposes to the development of this syndrome. Fortunately, fewer than 30% of those with spinal stenosis have clinical pain. Patients often have pain in the low back, with pain radiation down the back of both legs. Standing or walking may worsen pain. Patients often walk with a hunched back and sit down after walking a short distance to relieve pain (neurogenic claudication). The pain usually takes minutes to disappear, compared to seconds with vascular claudication. On physical examination, patients often have less tenderness over the lumbar spine than those with acute lumbar disk herniation. A straight leg raising test may be normal. The condition must be distinguished from vascular claudication. Patients may try NSAIDs first. Lumbar epidural corticosteroid injections may provide pain relief for this group of patient for

weeks or even months. If a patient has severe pain and refuses surgery, chronic narcotic treatment often provides adequate pain control but runs a risk of the development of tolerance and addiction.

Cervicogenic Headache

Cervicogenic headache refers to head pain originating from pathology in the neck. It is believed that pain from the C2-C3 nerve dermatome can radiate to the head and face (**Fig. 44.1**). An earlier study found that pain from the C2-C3 and C3-C4 cervical facet joints also can radiate to the occipital area (**Fig. 44.2**). The term *cervicogenic headache* was first introduced by Sjaastad and colleagues in 1983. However, the concept of cervicogenic headache is controversial and not well accepted by the majority of neurologists. The International Headache Society (2004) published its first diagnostic criteria in 1998 and revised it 2004. Patients with cervicogenic headache often have histories of head and neck trauma. Pain may be unilateral or bilateral. Pain is frequently localized to the occipital area, but it may also be referred to the frontal, temporal, or orbital regions. Headaches may be triggered by neck movement or sustained neck postures. This headache is constant with episodic throbbing attacks like a migraine. Patients may have other symptoms mimicking a migraine, such as nausea, vomiting, photophobia, phonophobia, and blurred vision. Owing to significant overlap of the symptoms of cervicogenic headache and migraine without aura, cervicogenic headache is often misdiagnosed as migraine. Clinicians should always consider cervicogenic headache in the differential diagnoses when evaluating a headache patient. History of head/neck injury and detailed examination of the occipital and upper cervical area should be part of the evaluation for headache. Patients with cervicogenic headache may have tenderness over

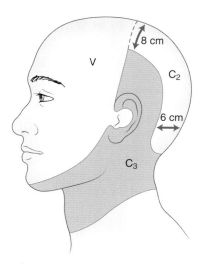

Fig. 44.1 Pain referral from C2 and C3 nerve roots. The C2 pain dermatome consists of an occipital parietal area 6 to 8 cm wide, extending paramedially from the subocciput to the vertex. The C3 pain dermatome is a craniofacial area, including the scalp around the ear, the pinna, the lateral cheek over the angle of the jaw, the submental region, and the lateral and anterior aspects of the upper neck. *(From Poletti, C.E., 1996. Third cervical nerve root and ganglion compression: clinical syndrome, surgical anatomy, and pathological findings. Neurosurgery 39, 941-948.)*

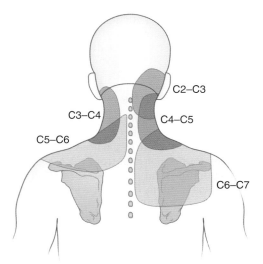

Fig. 44.2 Pain referral pattern from the cervical facet joints. Injection of contrast medium into the cervical facet joints in normal volunteers induced pain in the head, neck, and shoulder area. Of note, injection of C2-C3 facet joints can cause pain in the occipital area. *(From Dwyer, A., Aprill, C., Bogduk, N., 1990. Cervical zygapophyseal joint pain patterns. I: a study in normal volunteers. Spine 15, 453-457.)*

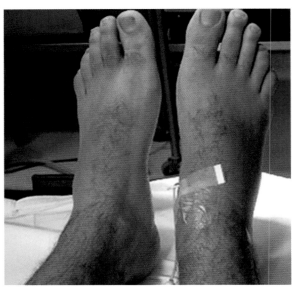

Fig. 44.3 Complex regional pain syndrome I. The right foot and ankle are mildly swollen and reddish in comparison with the left foot and ankle. The intravenous access was used for a Bier block.

the greater or lesser occipital nerve, cervical facet joints, and muscles in the upper or middle cervical region. Cervicogenic headache does not respond well to migraine medications. Treatment should be focused on removal of the pain source from the occipital-cervical junction. Initial therapy is directed to physical therapy modalities and NSAIDs. Interventional treatment such as greater occipital nerve block, cervical facet joint block, deep cervical plexus block, and botulinum toxin injections may provide effective pain relief (Zhou et al., 2010).

Complex Regional Pain Syndrome

Terminology describing the complex regional pain syndromes has evolved over the last century. The term *causalgia* was first coined by Weir Mitchell in the 1870s for severe progressive distal limb pain with major nerve injury. In 1946, Evans introduced the term *reflex sympathetic dystrophy* (RSD); it was later defined by the International Association for Study of Pain (IASP) as "continuous pain in a portion of an extremity after trauma, which may include fracture but does not involve a major nerve, associated with sympathetic hyperactivity." In 1994, the IASP introduced the term *complex regional pain syndrome* (CRPS), describing a painful condition that includes regional pain, sensory changes (e.g., allodynia), abnormalities of temperature, abnormal sudomotor activity, edema, and abnormal skin color changes that occur after an initiating noxious event such as trauma. Two types of CRPS have been recognized: *CRPS I* corresponds to RSD, in which no definable nerve lesion is found. *CRPS II* refers to the cases with a definable nerve lesion and corresponds to the earlier term of *causalgia*.

The mean age of CRPS patients ranges from 36 to 46 years, with women predominating (60%-81%). It is caused typically by an injury such as a fracture (16%-46%), strain or sprain (10%-29%), post surgery (3%-24%), and contusion or crush

injury (8%-18%). Clinical features of CRPS often include pain, edema, autonomic dysfunction such as change in temperature or color in the involved limbs, motor dysfunction, and psychological abnormalities such as depression (**Fig. 44.3**). Schwartzman and Maleki reported the pattern of spreading of CRPS in three stages. In the early stage, CRPS often involves only one limb with pain, minor edema, and increased skin temperature. CRPS may spread from one limb to the others. In the later stage, CRPS could involve the full body and the four extremities with severe pain, edema, cold and cyanotic limbs, joint contracture, and atrophy of muscles and bones.

Excruciating pain is the cardinal feature of CRPS. Pain is often described as burning, aching, pricking, or shooting. Severity of pain is not proportional to the initial injury, and pain is not limited to the area of the injury or a specific nerve distribution. Patients may feel severe pain to minor pain stimulation such as a safety-pin prick (hyperalgesia). A light touch to skin (innocuous stimulation) may cause severe long-lasting pain (mechanical allodynia). A cooling stimulus such as a drop of alcohol may be perceived as painful (thermal allodynia). Decreased temperature and pinprick sensations in the affected limb are common.

Edema of the affected limb is present in the majority of patients. It could be very mild in the early stage of CRPS, mimicking mild cellulitis. However, in the late stage, edema may be so severe that a Doppler test is needed to rule out the possibility of deep vein thrombosis.

Autonomic dysfunction may manifest as changes of skin color and temperature, as well as sweating abnormalities. The affected area may be reddish at one time and then become blue, purple, or pale over a course of minutes to hours. Livedo reticularis is common in CRPS. *Livedo* is a descriptive term used to describe the red, non-blanchable (i.e., does not turn white when pressed) network pattern (reticulated) in the skin. About 60% of patients may report excessive sweating in the affected limbs. Temperature asymmetry between the affected and unaffected sides may exceed 1°C.

Motor dysfunctions in CRPS include mild weakness, decreased range of motion, tremor, dystonia, and myoclonus. Dystrophic manifestations are seen in the form of increased or decreased nail and hair growth in the affected extremity, hyperkeratosis or thin glossy skin, and osteoporosis of the underlying bones.

Diagnosis of CRPS is clinical. According to IASP, if a patient has the above-mentioned features, a diagnosis of CRPS may be made if other clinical conditions such as infection or DVT are ruled out. EMG/NCV tests are not sensitive to CRPS and frequently cause severe pain to patients. A triple-phase bone scan may reveal abnormal absorption in the affected limbs (increased or decreased), though it is not a primary diagnostic procedure for CRPS.

The pathophysiology of CRPS is not completely understood. Multiple mechanisms are considered in the generation and maintenance of CRPS. Increased systemic calcitonin gene-related peptide (CGRP) levels may contribute to neurogenic inflammation, edema, vasodilatation, and increased sweating. Elevated neuropeptide concentrations may lead to pain and hyperalgesia. Immunological mechanisms (e.g., altered expressions of human leukocyte antigen [HLA], substance P, cytokines, and interleukins) are believed to contribute to the pathogenesis of clinical symptoms such as edema. Up-regulation of adrenergic receptors and functional coupling between sympathetic efferent and sensory afferent fibers may provide the basis of the sympathetic nervous system abnormalities in the pathogenesis of CRPS. The central mechanisms in CRPS may include central sensitization in the spinal cord, brainstem, or thalamus, cortical reorganization in the primary somatosensory cortex, and disinhibition of the motor cortex.

The goals of treatment for CRPS are pain relief, functional recovery, and psychological improvement. However, treatment of CRPS remains a challenge. There is little if any evidence for the efficacy of any treatment modality. In the early stages of CRPS treatment, occupational and physical therapies are often used. Occupational and physical therapies are supported by anecdotal data and have not been validated by randomized prospective trials.

Patients diagnosed with CRPS for over 2 months should also undergo a psychological evaluation—which includes psychometric testing—to identify and treat psychological disorders such as anxiety, depression, or personality disorders. Counseling, behavioral modification, biofeedback, relaxation therapy, group therapy, and self-hypnosis should be considered. The goal of psychotherapy is to improve patient motivation and coping skills.

Tricyclic antidepressants, antiepileptics, and narcotics such as methadone are commonly used empirically for CRPS, even though clinical controlled studies have not proven their efficacy. A recent review article summarized the evidence derived from randomized controlled trials pertaining to the treatment of CRPS. The review reported clinical improvement with dimethyl sulfoxide, steroids, epidural clonidine, and intrathecal baclofen. Only bisphosphonates appear to offer clear benefits for patients with CRPS (Tran de et al., 2010). NMDA receptor modulation is a major interest of current research. It has been reported that subanesthetic infusions of ketamine might offer a promising therapeutic

option in the treatment of appropriately selected patients with intractable CRPS (Schwartzman et al., 2009). A recent preliminary study reported that IV immunoglobulin treatment could potentially decrease pain in CRPS patients (Goebel et al., 2010). However, more studies are needed to further establish the safety and efficacy of these novel approaches.

Minimally invasive techniques have been used extensively for the treatment of CRPS. Techniques include sympathetic block, intravenous regional block (IVRB), somatic nerve block, epidural drug administration, intrathecal drug delivery, and neurostimulation. Stellate ganglion blocks in early-stage CRPS may significantly decrease pain and hasten clinical recovery. It may also prevent the recurrence of CRPS after reoperation of the affected extremity. In a double-blind study, IVRB with bretylium provided significantly longer analgesia than lidocaine. Good pain relief is reported with the use of epidural delivery of clonidine and ketamine and also with intrathecal baclofen and morphine. An early study with 2-year follow-up reported that spinal cord stimulation (SCS) results in a long-term pain reduction and improvement in health-related quality of life. However, a more recent randomized study with 5-year follow-up found no extra benefit in terms of pain relief for those with a combination of SCS and physical therapy, compared to those with physical therapy alone (Kemler et al., 2008). The author shares the same experience and opinion with the cited report. It seems that most RSD patients feel better immediately after the SCS implantation. However, the SCS itself may have difficulty stopping the spread of RSD, and once RSD spreads out of the area initially covered by the SCS, the pain is no longer "under control."

Post-Stroke Pain Syndrome

Lesions at any level of the neuroaxis (generally affecting spinothalamocortical afferent sensory pathways) including the medulla, pons, midbrain, thalamus, subcortical white matter, and the cortex may produce central post-stroke pain syndrome (PSP). However, the thalamus and brainstem are common sites for PSP; 8% to 16% of thalamic stroke may lead to chronic pain. The frequency of pain after a geniculothalamic artery stroke is even higher (13%-59%).

The pathogenesis of PSP is not yet known. However, it has been suggested that hyperexcitation in the damaged sensory pathways, damage to the central inhibitory pathways, or a combination of the two may be responsible for the onset of PSP. Pain is the cardinal symptom and is described as spontaneous, severe, paroxysmal, and burning. Patients with thalamic pain syndrome also have hyperalgesia and allodynia in the affected limbs. Right-sided lesions predominate among reported cases of the thalamic pain syndrome.

Patients reporting pain due to brainstem infarction usually have involvement of pontine or medullary structures. Patients with midbrain infarction seldom complain of pain. Transitory eye and nose pain may be an initial symptom of pontine infarction. About 25% patients with dorsolateral medullary infarction develop ipsilateral facial pain, especially when the lesion involves the spinal trigeminal tract. Facial allodynia is also common. Some patients may experience pain in the contralateral limbs and trunk.

Treatment of central post-stroke pain remains a challenge. Tricyclic antidepressants are still a choice of treatment.

Gabapentin and lamotrigine have been used to treat central post-stroke pain syndrome in open-labeled studies. Selective posterior rhizotomy has been reported to decrease painful spasticity in the lower limbs of hemiplegic patients after a stroke. It has been reported that chronic motor cortex stimulation therapy provides pain relief for some post-stroke patients (Brown and Pilitsis, 2006). Stereotactic radiosurgery of the pituitary and deep brain stimulation (DBS) have been used to treat PSP syndrome with some success (Pickering et al., 2009).

Some 40% to 60% of patients develop shoulder pain after a stroke. The mechanism of shoulder pain is not clear, but a strong association exists between pain and an abnormal shoulder joint examination, ipsilateral sensory abnormalities, and arm weakness. These patients usually have significant tenderness over the shoulder joint. It is postulated that the pain is due to inflammation in the joint secondary to immobilization and joint contracture (*frozen shoulder syndrome*). The majority of shoulder pain may be resolved or improved for 6 months following a stroke with intensive physical/occupational therapy. Antiinflammatory medications may be used. Suprascapular nerve or brachial plexus block can provide temporary pain relief to prepare for physical therapy. Proper positioning of the shoulder, range-of-motion activities, and avoidance of immobilization may further help prevent or alleviate shoulder pain.

Spinal Cord Injury and Pain

There are about 240,000 patients with spinal cord injuries (SCIs) in the United States; 86% of individuals with SCI report pain at 6 months post discharge, with 27% of these individuals reporting pain that impacts most of their daily activities. Patients can have pain both at and below the level of spinal injury. Pain intensity is not associated with the magnitude or location of the lesion, occurrence of myofascial pain syndrome, or onset of pain. However, pain is usually more severe in patients with gunshot injuries.

Pain after SCI originates from different sources including neuropathic, musculoskeletal, and visceral pain. Neuropathic pain after SCI is further divided into central and segmental pain. Central neuropathic pain often begins within weeks or months after injury. It is generally described as a burning, sharp, or shooting pain. Patients feel pain at or below the level of injury in areas where there is partial or complete loss of sensation to touch. Central pain is believed to be due to differentiation caused by SCI. Astrocytic activation in the spinal cord, up-regulation of chemokines, hyperexcitability of wide–dynamic range neurons in the spinal dorsal horn rostral to the lesion, and loss of γ-aminobutyric acid (GABA)ergic interneurons in laminae I-III of the spinal cord dorsal horn (Meisner et al., 2010) have been suggested to cause the neuropathic pain that follows SCI. Segmental pain often occurs around the border of injury and usually develops within the first few months after an injury. Allodynia and hyperalgesia are common. Nerve root entrapment could lead to severe segmental pain. Patients may describe stabbing or sharp pain or a band of burning pain at the level of injury. Syringomyelia with a cyst ascending from the level of the SCI may occasionally cause central pain.

Musculoskeletal pain in this group of patients may be due to muscle spasms below the level of SCI and arthritis in disused joints. Pain is generally described as dull or aching. It is usually worsened by movement and eased with rest. Visceral pain may begin a short time following SCI and could be related to constipation and urinary retention due to sphincter dysfunction. It may occur in the abdomen above or below the level of injury. This pain is often described as cramping, burning, and constant.

Pain management after SCI is difficult. Pharmacological and rehabilitative procedures are effective in only about 38% of patients. However, the initial workup should target identifying the pain source. Different kinds of pain may respond differently to treatments. For neuropathic pain, medications such as gabapentin, amitriptyline, and nortriptyline may ease the pain in some patients. Intravenous lidocaine may provide temporary pain relief. Intrathecal baclofen therapy may reduce chronic musculoskeletal pain associated with spasticity and improve the patient's quality of life. Intrathecal morphine and clonidine offer limited help to relieve the pain. DBS has been reported to be effective in some cases, but there is insufficient evidence to validate its routine use. Limited evidence exists for use of motor cortex stimulation (Previnaire et al., 2009). SCS lacks long-term efficacy for the relief of spasticity and pain in SCI and is believed not to be cost-effective. Dorsal root entry zone lesions and dorsal rhizotomy have also been used with limited success. Appropriate management of bowel or bladder dysfunction may help ease visceral pain. If an ascending syrinx is present, surgical drainage may be effective in relieving the pain.

Pain in Multiple Sclerosis

Pain is a common symptom in multiple sclerosis (MS). The prevalence of pain in this disease is higher than what was initially expected; some studies estimate it to be up to 86% (Bermejo et al., 2010), depending on the sample and specific questions used to assess the incidence and severity of pain. Osterberg et al. studied pain syndromes in 429 patients with definite MS, and 58% reported pain during the course of their disease; 100 (28%) had central pain, including 18 patients (5%) with trigeminal neuralgia. The majority of patients (87%) with central pain had symptoms located in the legs, while 31% were in the arms. Pain was mostly bilateral (76%) and constant. Aching, burning, and pricking were common qualities. Other reported pain syndromes in MS include the Lhermitte sign, dysesthetic pain, back pain, headache, and painful tonic spasms. Chronic pain in MS was found to have no significant relationship to gender, age of onset, disease duration, or disease course. Chronic pain can have a significant negative impact on functions in persons with MS, such as the ability to engage in household work and psychological functioning. Chronic pain is significantly related to anxiety and depression in females. In the long-term care facility, residents with MS are more physically disabled and experience more frequent pain and a higher prevalence of pressure ulcers and depression than residents without MS.

Though pain affects a high percentage of patients with MS, its pathophysiology is unknown, and few studies have been conducted to investigate the treatment of pain in MS. The following principles are currently recommended for treatment of MS related pain:

1. For pain directly related to MS, such as trigeminal neuralgia, carbamazepine is the first choice. Lamotrigine,

gabapentin, oxcarbazepine, and other anticonvulsants may also be used. Painful "burning" dysesthesia may be treated with tricyclic antidepressants or carbamazepine. Further options include gabapentin or lamotrigine.

2. Pain related to spasticity may improve with adequate physiotherapy. Drug treatment includes antispastic agents like oral baclofen or tizanidine. In severe cases, intrathecal baclofen and botulinum toxin injections merit consideration.

3. Pain due to subcutaneous injections of β-interferons or glatiramer acetate may be reduced by optimizing the injection technique and by local cooling. Systemic side effects of interferons (e.g., myalgias) could be reduced by paracetamol or ibuprofen.

Even though cannabis is not legally used in the United States to treat pain, European studies indicate that cannabis-based medicines are effective in reducing pain and sleep disturbance in patients with MS-related central neuropathic pain and are mostly well tolerated (Rog et al., 2005; Thaera et al., 2009). Oral ketamine, an NMDA receptor antagonist, has also been reported to be effective in the treatment of pain and allodynia associated with MS.

Phantom Limb Pain and Stump Pain

Phantom-limb pain describes the pain in a body part that is no longer present, which occurs in 50% to 80% of all amputees. Pain can have several different qualities, such as stabbing, throbbing, burning, or cramping. It seems to be more intense in the distal portions of the phantom limb. This pain may be related to a certain position or movement of the phantom and may be elicited or exacerbated by a range of physical factors (e.g., changes in weather or pressure on the residual limb) and psychological factors (e.g., emotional stress). It is more likely to occur if the individual had chronic pain before the amputation. Pain in the phantom is often similar to the pain felt in the limb before amputation. Phantom pain is most common after the amputation of an arm or leg, but it may also occur after the surgical removal of other body parts such as breast, rectum, penis, testicle, eye, tongue, or teeth. About 30% of persons with amputation report the feeling of *telescoping*, the retraction of the phantom towards the residual limb, and in many cases the disappearance of the phantom into the limb. This may be accompanied by a shrinking of the limb. Recent evidence suggests that telescoping is associated with more phantom-limb pain.

Phantom-limb pain is commonly confused with pain in the area adjacent to the amputated body part. This pain is referred to as *residual-limb* or *stump pain*. Patients may report severe "knife-stabbing" or sharp pain at the end of the amputated limb. Formation of a neuroma or pressure lesions of the stump may exacerbate stump pain. Physical examination may reveal the existence of a neuroma; it is usually very sensitive to touch or pressure. However, stump pain may coexist with phantom-limb pain.

Changes along the neuroaxis may contribute to the experience of phantom-limb pain. Spinal mechanisms are characterized by increased excitability of the dorsal horn neurons, reduction of inhibitory processes, and structural changes at the central nerve endings of the primary sensory neurons,

interneurons, and the projection neurons. Supraspinal changes related to phantom-limb pain involve the brainstem, thalamus, and cortex. Reorganization of the somatosensory cortex of the human cerebral cortex in amputees has been supported by findings from several imaging studies. People with arm or hand amputations show a shift of the mouth into the hand representation in the primary somatosensory cortex (Woodhouse, 2005). Studies in human amputees have shown that reorganizational changes also occur at the thalamic level and are closely related to the perception of phantom limbs and phantom-limb pain. Neuroma in the stump may be more responsible for stump pain than phantom-limb pain. However, abnormal input originated from a neuroma in the residual limb may increase the amount of central reorganization, enhancing the chance of phantom-limb pain. Psychological factors play a role in the modulation of phantom-limb pain; the pain may be exacerbated by stress. Patients who lack coping strategies, fear the worst, or receive less social support tend to report more phantom-limb pain.

Treatment for phantom-limb pain is difficult. Although tricyclic antidepressants and sodium channel blockers are treatments of choice for neuropathic pain, no controlled studies exist of these agents for phantom-limb pain. Opioids, calcitonin, and ketamine have proven to be effective in reducing phantom-limb pain in controlled studies. Transcutaneous nerve stimulation (TENS) may have a minor effect. A maximum benefit of about 30% has been reported from treatments such as local anesthesia, far-infrared rays, sympathectomy, dorsal root entry-zone lesions, cordotomy, rhizotomy, neurostimulation methods, or pharmacological interventions such as anticonvulsants, barbiturates, antidepressants, neuroleptics, and muscle relaxants. Use of a myoelectric prosthesis may alleviate cortical reorganization and phantom-limb pain, and DBS has also been reported to treat phantom-limb pain. Mirror therapy has been studied, but to date, there is only circumstantial evidence for the effectiveness of mirror therapy in treating phantom pain; more studies are needed to support its clinical use.

Pharmacological Management of Chronic Pain

In recent years, several different adjunct analgesics have been used to treat chronic pain syndromes, including NSAIDs, antidepressants, anticonvulsants, local anesthetics, topical agents, baclofen, and NMDA receptor antagonists. Tricyclic antidepressants and anticonvulsants are the first-line drugs in the treatment of neuropathic pain. If a patient does not respond to treatment with different agents within one drug class, agents from a second drug class may be added. When all first-line options have been exhausted, narcotic analgesics may provide some benefit, but with the risks of tolerance and addiction.

Nonsteroidal Antiinflammatory Drugs

Nonsteroidal antiinflammatory drugs, including aspirin, are the most widely used analgesics. Traditionally NSAIDs are considered weak analgesics and used extensively for headaches, arthritis, and a wide range of minor aches and post-surgical pain conditions.

Table 44.1   Commonly Used Oral Nonsteroidal Antiinflammatory Drugs

Generic Name	Trade Name	Adult Dosage
Acetaminophen	Tylenol	500-1000 mg q 4 h
Acetylsalicylic acid	Aspirin	325-650 mg q 4 h
Celecoxib	Celebrex	200 mg q 12 h
Choline magnesium trisalicylate	Trilisate	500-750 mg q 8-12 h
Diclofenac sodium	Voltaren	25-75 mg q 8-12 h
Diflunisal	Dolobid	250-500 mg q 8-12 h
Etodolic acid	Lodine	200-400 mg q 6 h
Fenoprofen calcium	Nalfon	200 mg q 4-6 h
Flurbiprofen	Ansaid	100 mg q 8-12 h
Ibuprofen	Motrin	400-800 mg q 6-8 h
Indomethacin	Indocin	25-50 mg q 8-12 h
Ketoprofen	Orudis	25-75 mg q 6-8 h
Ketorolac	Toradol	10 mg q 6-8 h
Meclofenamate sodium	Meclomen	50 mg q 4-6 h
Naproxen	Naprosyn	275-500 mg q 8-12 h
Phenylbutazone	Butazolidin	100 mg q 6-8 h
Piroxicam	Feldene	10-20 mg once daily
Salsalate	Disalcid	500 mg q 4 h
Sulindac	Clinoril	150-200 mg q 12 h
Tolmetin	Tolectin	200-600 mg q 8 h

Table 44.2   Tricyclic Antidepressants Commonly Used for Pain Management

Generic Name	Trade Name	Adult Dosage Range (mg/day)
Amitriptyline	Elavil	10-100
Clomipramine	Anafranil	25-200
Desipramine	Norpramin	10-200
Doxepin	Sinequan	10-200
Imipramine	Tofranil	10-200
Nortriptyline	Pamelor	10-150

tablets to prescription status and mandated new labeling on acetaminophen packaging (Krenzelok, 2009). Acetaminophen is a potential cyclooxygenase 2 (COX-2)–selective inhibitor. It may also increase cardiovascular risks.

Cardiovascular risks of NSAIDs, especially COX-2 inhibitors, have become a major focus of attention in recent years. Suggestions that the use of COX-2 inhibitors may decrease prostacyclin (PGI2) levels, with relatively unopposed platelet thromboxane A2 generation that may lead to increased thrombotic risk, have cautioned against the use of such agents. Rofecoxib (Vioxx) was withdrawn from the market in September 2004 owing to increased cardiovascular risks. A recent study found that the hazard ratio (95% confidence interval) for death was 1.70, 1.75, 1.31, 2.08, 1.22, and 1.28 for rofecoxib, celecoxib, ibuprofen, diclofenac, naproxen, and other NSAIDs, respectively (Gislason et al., 2009). Even though limited long-term data on cardiovascular risk associated with nonselective NSAIDs have been available, and some contradictory warnings and recommendations have been published recently by the American Heart Association, FDA, and independent experts (Gluszko and Bielinska, 2009), the general suggestion is that both NSAIDs and selective COX-2 inhibitors should be avoided or used with extreme caution if a patient has a high cardiovascular risks and a history of heart failure.

Antidepressants

Tricyclic antidepressants are probably the most commonly used adjunct analgesics in the management of chronic pain (Dworkin et al., 2010) (**Table 44.2**). The tertiary amines (amitriptyline, imipramine, doxepin, and clomipramine) and the secondary amines (nortriptyline and desipramine) both have analgesic properties. Amitriptyline is the prototype antidepressant used in this context. Clinical efficacy of tricyclics for neuropathic pain has been demonstrated by numerous well-controlled double-blind clinical studies for both neuropathic and somatic pain. Clinicians have to be familiar with the possible side effects of amitriptyline, especially in elderly patients. These adverse effects include sedation, dry mouth, constipation, urinary retention, glaucoma, orthostatic hypotension, and cardiac arrhythmias. Patients should be warned about the side effects before they start the medication. Amitriptyline should be avoided in patients with a history of heart disease (conduction disorders, arrhythmias, or heart failure) and closed-angle glaucoma. Amitriptyline should be started at a relatively low dose (10 mg) at bedtime and slowly titrated up

NSAIDs are powerful inhibitors of prostaglandin synthesis through their effect on cyclooxygenase (COX). Prostaglandins are not thought to be important pain mediators, but they do cause hyperalgesia by sensitizing peripheral nociceptors to the effects of various mediators of pain and inflammation such as somatostatin, bradykinin, and histamine. Thus, NSAIDs are used primarily to treat pain that results from inflammation and hyperalgesia. **Table 44.1** lists commonly used NSAIDs.

Acetaminophen is not strictly an antiinflammatory medication. Its peripheral and antiinflammatory effects are weak, but it shares many properties of NSAIDs. It readily crosses the blood-brain barrier, and its action resides primarily in the central nervous system (CNS), where prostaglandin inhibition produces analgesia and antipyresis.

Common side effects of NSAIDs include GI toxicity, stomach ulcers, and gastric bleeding. Renal dysfunction can occur with prolonged and excessive use of NSAIDs. Particularly at risk from excessive use of NSAIDs are elderly patients with renal dysfunction, congestive heart failure, ascites, or hypovolemia. Other adverse effects of NSAIDs include hepatic dysfunction or necrosis, asthma, vasomotor rhinitis, angioneurotic edema, urticaria, laryngeal edema, or even cardiovascular collapse. Because of the wide availability of acetaminophen and its potential toxicity (especially liver toxicity), in 2009 the U.S. Food and Drug Administration (FDA) proposed a decrease in the maximum daily dose of acetaminophen from 4000 mg to 3250 mg, reducing the maximum individual dose from 1000 to 650 mg. They relegated 500 mg

as tolerated. Most patients report improved sleep after taking amitriptyline. The onset of pain relief may precede the anticipated onset of antidepressant effects. In general, pain relief may be expected in 7 to 14 days. The dosage required for pain management is usually lower than for depression; 75 to 100 mg at bedtime is often effective. If the patient cannot tolerate this dose or is not a good candidate for amitriptyline, other tricyclics such as nortriptyline or desipramine may be considered. These secondary amines generally have fewer anticholinergic effects and are therefore better tolerated than tertiary amines. However, their clinical efficacy is not as well established as that for amitriptyline.

The main advantage of the selective serotonin reuptake inhibitors (SSRIs) is the favorable side-effect profile. However, SSRIs are clearly less effective than tricyclic antidepressants. The NNT (number needed to treat to reach 50% pain relief) is 6.7 versus 2.4 (Coluzzi and Mattia, 2005). It seems that selective serotonin/noradrenaline reuptake inhibitors (SNRI) are relatively more effective for pain management than most of the SSRIs. Venlafaxine is an SNRI for which randomized controlled trials showed good pain relief effect for painful polyneuropathy and neuropathic pain following treatment of breast cancer. Duloxetine has also been demonstrated to have significant analgesic effects in diabetic polyneuropathy and fibromyalgia. Milnacipran is another SNRI; randomized double-blind placebo-controlled studies found that milnacipran is effective in controlling pain and improving global status, fatigue, and physical and mental function in patients with fibromyalgia (Arnold et al., 2010). Nausea, hyperhidrosis, and headache are the most common adverse events.

Anticonvulsants

Anticonvulsants are believed to be particularly useful in treating lancinating, electrical, or tic-like pain. These medications may be also beneficial in patients with neuropathic pain who do not respond to antidepressants. The older generation of anticonvulsants includes carbamazepine, valproic acid, clonazepam, and phenytoin. Carbamazepine was perhaps the most popular agent used for trigeminal neuralgia. However, carbamazepine may cause serious side effects such as sedation, nausea, vomiting, bone marrow suppression, hyponatremia, hepatic dysfunction, and serious drug-drug interaction. Carbamazepine should be started at 100 mg at night and titrated up slowly, especially for the elderly.

Valproic acid has been proven to be effective in reducing the frequency of migraine attacks (Vikelis and Rapoport, 2010). Some studies found that valproates may provide significant pain relief in patients with post herpetic neuralgia and diabetic neuropathy. However, negative results have also been reported. Common side effects include tremor, ankle swelling, sedation, and GI discomfort. Weight gain and hair loss may be a major cosmetic concern, especially for younger patients. Valproate should not be used for children younger than 2 years of age because of hepatotoxicity. Generally, valproate is not the first-line choice for neuropathic pain.

Gabapentin modulates the function of the α_2-δ subunit of voltage-dependent calcium channels in the dorsal horn of the spinal cord to decrease the release of excitatory neurotransmitters such as glutamate and substance P. The analgesic efficacy of gabapentin has been demonstrated in several types of nonmalignant neuropathic pain. Its high safety profile, few

drug-drug interactions, and proven analgesic effect in several types of neuropathic pain have made gabapentin the recommended first-line co-analgesic for treating a variety of neuropathic pains, especially in the medically ill and in elderly patients. The most common adverse effects are drowsiness, dizziness, and unsteadiness. Gabapentin should be started at a dose of 100 to 300 mg at bedtime. If titrated carefully, gabapentin is usually well tolerated up to 3600 mg daily. However, gabapentin has a nonlinear pharmacokinetic profile: the rate of bioavailability decreases as the dose increases.

Pregabalin is a GABA analog with similar structure and mechanism of action as gabapentin. It has antiepileptic, analgesic, and anxiolytic activity. Pregabalin has been approved by the FDA for the management of neuropathic pain associated with diabetic neuropathy, postherpetic neuralgia, and fibromyalgia (Straube et al., 2010). Food does not significantly affect the extent of absorption. Pregabalin is not protein bound and exhibits a plasma half-life of about 6 hours. Hepatic metabolism is negligible, and most of the oral dose (95%) appears unchanged in the urine. At a dose of 300 mg/day, about 45% of diabetic neuropathy patients had 50% pain relief. This means that pregabalin has an NNT of 2.2 for diabetic neuropathy. Pregabalin seems to be more effective than gabapentin and other anticonvulsants for neuropathic pain. Common side effects of pregabalin include dizziness, sedation, dry mouth, and peripheral edema.

Oxcarbazepine is a ketoderivative of carbamazepine, with better tolerability. It can block sodium-dependent action potentials. The medication does not induce hepatic enzymes and has fewer drug-drug interactions than carbamazepine. Multiple open studies have suggested that oxcarbazepine may be effective for the treatment of neuropathic pain. However, a double-blind controlled study did not find significant difference between oxcarbazepine and placebo for the treatment of pain due to diabetic neuropathy (Grosskopf et al., 2006).

Lamotrigine is an antiepileptic drug that stabilizes neural membranes by blocking the activation of voltage-sensitive sodium channels and inhibiting the presynaptic release of glutamate. Multiple open studies have supported the use of lamotrigine in neuropathic pain. However, controlled studies found no efficacy of lamotrigine for the treatment of neuropathic pain (Breuer et al., 2007; Rao et al., 2008). Lamotrigine is ineffective for prevention of migraine.

Topiramate has proven its efficacy and safety in the prophylactic treatment of episodic migraine in a number of randomized controlled clinical trials (Naegel and Obermann, 2010). Even though open studies and case reports continue to support the use of topiramate in the treatment of various kinds of neuropathic pain, controlled studies failed to reveal any benefit of topiramate for the treatment of neuropathic pain. The mechanisms of action include blockade of sodium channels, enhancement of GABA inhibition, and attenuation of kainate-induced responses at glutamate receptors. The starting dose is usually small (e.g., 25 mg twice a day for an adult). It may be incrementally increased weekly by 50 mg up to 200 mg/day. Topiramate may induce memory loss, word-finding difficulties, disorientation, and sedation. The other common adverse affects are renal calculi, tremors, dizziness, ataxia, headaches, fatigue, and GI upset. Topiramate may also induce significant weight loss. This medication may be more helpful in obese pain patients.

Tiagabine, zonisamide, and levetiracetam are among the group of new anticonvulsants. Some uncontrolled and case studies have reported positive effects of these medications for neuropathic pain. However, controlled double-blind studies have not been reported.

Systemic Local Anesthetics

Systemic administration of local anesthetics has been used to treat neuropathic pain syndrome. Clinical trials have provided some evidence that lidocaine and mexiletine are superior to placebo for neuropathic pain (Carroll et al., 2008). Intravenous lidocaine is used for the treatment of neuropathic pain as a second-line therapy. If a patient has a positive response to IV lidocaine therapy, a trial of oral mexiletine may be considered. However, mexiletine has a relatively high rate of adverse effects such as nausea, vomiting, tremor, dizziness, unsteadiness, and paresthesias. Given the limited number of supportive studies, mexiletine and other oral local anesthetics should only be used as second-line agents for neuropathic pain that has failed to respond to anticonvulsants or antidepressants.

Topical Analgesics

Double-blind placebo-controlled studies have confirmed the efficacy of the 5% lidocaine patch for the treatment of postherpetic neuralgia (Lin et al., 2008) and for those patients with trigger points in myofascial pain syndrome (Affaitati et el., 2009). However, the lidocaine patch may not be effective in treating pain due to traumatic rib fractures (Ingalls et al., 2010). Minimal systemic absorption occurs. The patch is usually applied 12 hours per day, with minimal systemic side effects. Topical lidocaine ointment in various concentrations (up to a compounded formulation of 10%) may offer a cost-effective alternative.

Capsaicin is the spicy ingredient in chili pepper. It can deplete substance P from the terminals of afferent C fibers, potentially leading to decreased pain perception. Capsaicin creams are effective in reducing postsurgical pain in cancer patients. When applied topically, it may initially release substance P and cause severe burning pain. Pain related to the use of capsaicin gradually decreases over a few days if the cream is applied regularly. A lower-concentration cream (0.025%) or the application of a topical local anesthetic may help some patients decrease the initial burning pain and tolerate the medication better. A recent study found that topical capsaicin might effectively decrease pain in patients with chronic migraine (Papoiu and Yosipovitch, 2010). It is important to warn patients not to get any trace of the cream on mucous membranes, since this causes severe pain.

Miscellaneous Drugs

Baclofen is a GABA$_B$ receptor agonist with powerful antinociceptive effects in experimental animal models and established efficacy for chronic pain. It may be most useful in blocking the lancinating or episodic types of pain and reducing allodynia. It is commonly used for trigeminal neuralgia, together with carbamazepine. Baclofen may be started in doses of 5 mg, 2 to 3 times a day, and may be escalated to a maximum dose of 200 mg given in divided doses. Common side effects include CNS symptoms such as dizziness and drowsiness, as well as GI symptoms. Baclofen is a highly hydrophilic agent and has poor penetration of the blood-brain barrier. Intrathecal baclofen could be a promising adjuvant therapy to enhance the effect of other intrathecal medications such as morphine or clonidine or SCS for chronic pain.

N-Methyl-D-Aspartate Receptor Blockers

NMDA receptors are involved in the development of central sensitization associated with chronic refractory pain syndromes. NMDA antagonists may modulate CNS function, offering a novel approach to treating chronic neuropathic pain. Intravenous anesthetic doses of ketamine may induce serious side effects such as vivid hallucinations and psychosis. However, double-blind placebo-controlled studies have confirmed that low-dose IV ketamine may provide significant pain relief for CRPS type 1 without significant psychomimetic side effects (Sigtermans et al., 2009). Methadone has the property of both μ-opioid receptor agonist and NMDA antagonist. Evidence indicates that methadone has similar analgesic efficacy to morphine, but adverse effects due to prolonged half-life—particularly respiratory depression, cardiac arrhythmia, and sudden death—make it critical for providers to be familiar with methadone's pharmacological properties before considering methadone as an analgesic therapy for chronic pain. Amantadine is a noncompetitive NMDA antagonist. Dextromethorphan, the D-isomer of the codeine analog, levorphanol, is a weak, noncompetitive NMDA receptor antagonist. Memantine is an NMDA antagonist used for the treatment of Alzheimer disease. All three of these medications possess some analgesic properties. Current data are too scant or too weak, however, to recommend clinical use of any of these drugs for chronic pain management.

Opioid Analgesics

Opioids are the major class of analgesics used in the management of moderate to severe pain. These medications produce analgesia by binding to specific receptors both within and outside the CNS. However, their use in nonmalignant pain is still controversial. Opioid analgesics should be used with caution for chronic nonmalignant pain.

Opioids are classified according to the activity on the opioid receptors as full agonists, partial agonists, or mixed agonists-antagonists. Commonly used full agonists include hydrocodone, codeine, morphine, oxycodone, hydromorphone, methadone, and fentanyl. Buprenorphine is a partial agonist. It has lower intrinsic efficacy compared to other full opioid agonists and displays a ceiling effect to analgesia. Mixed agonist-antagonists include pentazocine, butorphanol tartrate, dezocine, and nalbuphine hydrochloride. These mediations block opioid analgesia at one type of receptor (μ) while simultaneously activating other opioid receptors (κ). Mixed agonist-antagonists should not be used together with full agonists, because they may cause withdrawal syndrome and increased pain. **Table 44.3** lists commonly used narcotics and their equi-analgesic dosage.

Equi-analgesic dosage means the dose of different narcotics needed to reach the same analgesic effects. The middle two columns of **Table 44.3**, for example, indicate that 7.5 mg of oral hydromorphone every 3 hours may have analgesic effects

Table 44.3   **Commonly Used Opioids**

| Generic Name | Trade Name | Equi-analgesic Dosage* | | Average Adult Dosage | |
		Oral	Parenteral	Oral or transdermal	Parenteral
Codeine		30 mg q 3-4 h	10 mg q 3-4 h	30 mg q 3-4 h	10 mg q 3-4 h
Fentanyl patch	Duragesic	N/A	N/A	25 µg/h patch q 72 h	N/A
Hydrocodone	Lortab, Lorcet	10 mg q 3-4 h	N/A	10 mg q 3-4 h	N/A
Hydromorphone	Dilaudid	7.5 mg q 3-4 h	1.5 mg q 3-4 h	6 mg q 3-4 h	1.5 mg q 3-4 h
Meperidine	Demerol	300 mg q 2-3 h	100 mg q 3 h	200 mg q 3 h	100 mg q 3 h
Methadone	Dolophine	20 mg q 6-8 h	10 mg q 6-8 h	10 mg q 6-12 h	5 mg q 8-12 h
Morphine		30 mg q 3-4 h	10 mg q 3-4 h	30 mg q 3-4 h	10 mg q 3-4 h
Morphine SR	MS Contin	N/A	N/A	15 mg q 12 h	N/A
Oxycodone	Percocet	N/A	N/A	5 mg q 3-4 h	N/A
Oxycodone	OxyContin	N/A	N/A	10 mg q 8-12 h	N/A

*The equi-analgesic dosage is the dose of different narcotics needed to achieve the same analgesic effects. Example, 7.5 mg of oral hydromorphone q 3 h has analgesic effects equal to 1.5 mg intravenous hydromorphone q 3-4 h or 30 mg oral morphine q 3-4 h.
N/A, Not applicable; *SR*, sustained release.

equal to 1.5 mg of IV hydromorphone every 3 to 4 hours or 30 mg of oral morphine every 3 to 4 hours.

Narcotics are also classified as mild to strong according to their potency. Codeine is the prototype of the mild opioid analgesics. The duration of action (2-4 hours) is similar to that of aspirin and acetaminophen. It is commonly used together with NSAIDs when NSAIDs alone have proven ineffective. Hydrocodone, oxycodone, propoxyphene, and meperidine are other mild opioid analgesics. Meperidine is likely to cause dysphoria, or less commonly to cause myoclonus, encephalopathy, and seizures. These toxic effects result from metabolites such as normeperidine that accumulate with repeated doses. Meperidine should be avoided in patients who require chronic treatment. Morphine and hydromorphone are the prototypes of high-potency opioid analgesics. Morphine has a relatively rapid onset, especially when administered parenterally, and a short duration of action, about 2 to 4 hours. Sustained-release oral preparations (e.g., MS Contin and Kadian, with duration of action of 12 hours and 24 hours, respectively) are useful for patients requiring chronic opioid therapy.

Route of administration is important to consider when choosing opioids. Oral administration of opioids is the preferred route, because it is the most convenient and cost-effective. Oral opioids are available in tablet, capsule, and liquid forms and in immediate and controlled-release formulations. Patients should be informed not to break the controlled-release tablets, since this can cause immediate release and cause a potential overdose. If patients cannot take medication orally, other less-invasive routes such as transdermal or rectal routes should be tried. Intramuscular administration of narcotics should be avoided because this route is often painful and inconvenient, and absorption is unreliable. Intravenous administration may be more expensive and is not practical for most chronic pain patients.

The advantage of transdermal administration is that it bypasses GI absorption. Both fentanyl and buprenorphine are commercially available for transdermal administration.

Fentanyl patches come in five sizes, delivering medication at 12, 25, 50, 75, and 100 µg/h. Each patch contains a 72-hour supply of fentanyl, passively absorbed through the skin during this period. Plasma levels rise slowly over 12 to 18 hours after the patch placement. This dosage form has an elimination half-life of 21 hours. Unlike IV fentanyl, transdermal administration of fentanyl is not suitable for rapid dose titration. It is often used for patients with chronic pain and already on opioids. As with other long-acting analgesics, all patients should be provided with oral or parenteral short-acting opioids for breakthrough pain.

Intrathecal analgesia may be considered when pain cannot be controlled by oral, transdermal, subcutaneous, or IV routes because side effects such as confusion and nausea further limit dose titration. Documentation of the failure of maximal doses of opioids and adjunct analgesics administered through other routes should precede consideration of intrathecal analgesia. For patients with chronic pain who have failed or cannot tolerate other treatment modalities, before implantation of a permanent pump, a trial is usually needed of single intrathecal injections, epidural injection, or continuous epidural administration. If there is significant pain relief without major side effects during the trial, the patient may be a candidate for permanent implantation of an intrathecal delivery system. Morphine is the most commonly used intrathecal drug used for pain relief. The main indication of the long-term intrathecal opioids is intractable pain in the lower part of the body. With proper selection and screening, good to excellent pain relief is expected in up to 90% of patients.

Physicians need to be familiar with side effects of opioids before prescribing these medications. Common side effects of opioids include constipation, sedation, nausea, vomiting, and respiratory depression due to overdoses. Occasionally, opioids may cause myoclonus, seizures, hallucinations, confusion, sexual dysfunction, sleep disturbances, and pruritus. Constipation is a common problem associated with opioid administration. Tolerance to the constipating effects of opioids hardly ever occurs during chronic therapy. Some patients are too embarrassed to tell the physician about constipation problems, so physicians should always ask patients about this. Mild constipation can usually managed by an increase in fiber consumption and the use of mild laxatives such as milk of magnesia. Severe constipation may be treated with a stimulating cathartic drug (e.g., bisacodyl, standardized senna concentrate, MiraLax, and similar drugs). Tapentadol is a novel centrally acting analgesic with two modes of action, μ-opioid agonist and norepinephrine reuptake inhibition. It was approved by the FDA for treatment of acute pain in the year 2008. Multiple double-blind controlled studies found tapentadol's analgesic effects similar to morphine and oxycodone. However, tapentadol has fewer GI side effects such as nausea and vomiting (Daniels et al., 2009; Smit et al., 2010). Owing to its dual mechanism of action and better GI tolerability, there is potential for off-label use in chronic pain.

Transitory sedation is common if opioid doses are increased substantially, but tolerance also usually develops rapidly. Reducing the opioid dose, switching to another opioid, or use of CNS stimulants such caffeine, dextroamphetamine, or methylphenidate may help increase alertness. Nausea and vomiting may be managed with antiemetics chosen according to the modes of action (e.g., metoclopramide, chlorpromazine, haloperidol, scopolamine, hydroxyzine). Patients receiving long-term opioid therapy usually develop tolerance to the respiratory-depressant effects of these agents. However, respiratory depression is often due to an overdose, or when pain is abruptly relieved and the sedative effect of the opioid is no longer opposed by the stimulating effect of pain. To reverse respiratory depression, opioid antagonists (e.g., naloxone) should be given incrementally in doses that improve respiratory function but do not reverse analgesia, to avoid reoccurrence of severe pain.

Accumulation of normeperidine, a metabolite of meperidine, may cause seizures, especially in patients with chronic renal insufficiency. Therefore, meperidine is only indicated for acute use; chronic use should be avoided. Tramadol is a synthetic narcotic, most commonly used for mild pain. Tramadol may decrease the seizure threshold and induce seizures, so it should be avoided in patients with a history of seizures. It should not be not be used with tricyclic antidepressants. The recommended maximum dosage of tramadol is 400 mg/day.

Tolerance and physical dependence should be expected with long-term opioid treatment and not confused with psychological dependence or drug abuse, which is characterized by compulsive use of narcotics. Patients may crave narcotics and continue to consume it despite physiological or social damage consequent to their use. *Tolerance* of opioids may be defined as the need to increase dosage requirements over a period of time to maintain optimum pain relief. For most pain patients, the first indication of tolerance is a decrease in the duration of analgesia for a specific dose. Patients with stable disease do not usually require increasing doses. Increasing the dosage requirement is most consistently correlated with a progressive disease that produces more intense pain. *Physical dependence* on opioids is revealed when opioids are abruptly discontinued or when naloxone is administered; it typically manifests as anxiety, irritability, chills and hot flashes, joint pain, lacrimation, rhinorrhea, diaphoresis, nausea, vomiting, abdominal cramps, and diarrhea. The mildest form of the *opioid abstinence syndrome* may be manifested as viral flu-like syndromes. For short-acting opioids (i.e., codeine, hydrocodone,

morphine, hydromorphone), the onset of withdrawal symptoms may occur within 6 to 12 hours and peak at 12 to 72 hours after discontinuation. For opioids with long half-lives (i.e., methadone and transdermal fentanyl), the onset of the withdrawal syndrome may be delayed for 24 hours or more after drug discontinuation. If a rapid decrease or a discontinuation of opioids is possible because the pain has been effectively eliminated, the opioid abstinence syndrome may be avoided by withdrawal of the opioid on a schedule that provides half the prior daily dose for each of the first 2 days and then reduces the daily dose by 25% every 2 days thereafter until the total dose (in morphine equivalent) is 30 mg/day. The drug may be discontinued after 2 days on the 30-mg/day dose, according to 1992 guidelines from the American Pain Society. Transdermal clonidine (0.1–0.2 mg/day) may reduce anxiety, tachycardia, and other autonomic symptoms associated with opioid withdrawal.

Diminishing opioid analgesic efficacy and increased pain during the course of opioid therapy is quite common. It is traditionally considered a result of opioid tolerance but could also be the result of opioid-induced hyperalgesia (OIH), which occurs when prolonged administration of opioids results in a paradoxical increase in atypical pain that appears to be unrelated to the original nociceptive stimulus. The mechanism of OIH is still unclear. However, opioid receptor desensitization, up-regulation of spinal dynorphin, and enhanced activity of excitatory transmitters such as NMDA are believed to be involved the pathogenesis of OIH (Silverman, 2009). Clinically, it is difficult to distinguish opioid tolerance and OIH. However, the issue of opioid-induced pain sensitivity should also be considered when an adjustment of opioid doses is being contemplated because opioid treatment is failing to provide the expected analgesic effects and/or there is an unexplainable pain exacerbation following a period of effective opioid treatment. Quantitative sensory testing of pain may offer the most appropriate way of diagnosing hyperalgesia. With OIH, an increased opioid dose is not always the answer. Office-based detoxification, reduction of opioid dose, opioid rotation, and the use of specific NMDA receptor antagonists are all viable treatment options for OIH.

Interventional Pain Management

Interventional pain management techniques have grown rapidly since 1990 and have become a major tool in treating acute and chronic pain. The American Society of Interventional Pain Physicians has developed evidence-based guidelines for improving compliance and the quality of care. Numerous reports have been published to investigate the long-term efficacy of interventional pain management techniques and have provided critical evidence indicating that these techniques may be useful (Manchikanti et al., 2009).

Traditionally, neurosurgeons have utilized surgical techniques to destroy part(s) of the peripheral and central nerve systems to interrupt conduction of painful information into the CNS. These techniques include resection of peripheral nerves, dorsal root ganglia, the dorsal root entry zone, the spinal thalamic tract, entire spinal cord, nuclei of the thalamus, and the sensory cortex, as well as the pituitary gland. Although these techniques may provide temporary pain relief, the pain may quickly become even worse than presurgical levels because of subsequent deafferent pain that is more difficult to treat than most somatic pain. As a result, surgical resection techniques are not commonly used any more. Instead, modern interventional pain management techniques emphasize the importance of accurate delivery of medications such as corticosteroids or local anesthetics to suppress inflammation and block conduction of painful information, respectively. Selective destruction of nerve tissue with heat generated by radiofrequency energy or freezing the nerve tissue with liquid nitrogen (cryotherapy) has largely replaced surgical resections. Nerve stimulation techniques have also evolved concomitant to neuroscientific developments in our understanding of the mechanisms of pain. **Table 44.4** lists commonly used interventional pain management techniques and their indications.

Greater Occipital Nerve Block

Greater occipital nerve block is indicated for occipital neuralgia, commonly seen in patients after whiplash injury, falls on the back of the head, and other closed-head injuries. Patients are often misdiagnosed as having tension headache

or migraine. These patients may have continuous headaches in the occipital, parietal, and sometimes the frontal region. The headaches may be increase several times a week and may be accompanied by nausea and vomiting. This condition is easily confused with migraine attacks, but physical examination may reveal positive tenderness over the greater occipital nerve. Palpation of the greater occipital nerve often makes the headache worse.

Greater occipital nerve block is the easiest interventional procedure for neurologists to perform in the office. For the procedure, one can palpate the posterior occipital protuberance, move 1.5 to 2 cm laterally, feel for the occipital artery pulsation and groove, then inject 2 to 3 mL of 0.5% bupivacaine with 20 mg of triamcinolone down to the bone and fan out (**Fig. 44.4**). According to this author's data, for patients with occipital neuralgia after whiplash injuries, a greater occipital nerve block may provide immediate headache relief in 90% of patients and last for an average of 28 days. More rigorous clinical trials are needed to confirm the clinical efficacy of occipital nerve block for occipital neuralgia and cervicogenic headache (Ashkenazi et al., 2010). More research and education are warranted to increase clinician awareness of the existence of occipital neuralgia and cervicogenic headache, inasmuch as most neurologists seem more interested and well trained in examining the 12 pairs of cranial nerves than the greater occipital nerves.

Anecdotally, this author was called to consult on a headache patient with "normal neurological examination and MRI findings." The patient was being treated with IV continuous hydromorphone, 2 mg/h, by a group of neurologists and residents at a major teaching university hospital in the United States. Examination revealed severe tenderness over the bilateral greater occipital nerves. Bilateral greater occipital nerve blocks immediately relieved the headache and made it possible to discontinue the IV hydromorphone. This patient reported that no one had touched her occipital area over several days of hospital stay, except for repeated MRI and CT scans, lumbar puncture, and multiple specialist consultations. The patient was discharged home with no headache. This case strongly suggests that examination of the greater occipital nerve should be a routine part of the physical examination of every headache patient.

Table 44.4 Commonly Used Interventional Pain Management Techniques and Indications

Name of Procedure	Indication
Celiac plexus block	Pancreatic cancer
Diskography	Diagnosis of anatomical localization of diskogenic pain
Epidural corticosteroid injection	Lumbar or cervical radiculopathy
Facet joint block	Lumbar or cervical facet joint syndrome
Facet joint rhizotomy	Lumbar or cervical facet joint syndrome
Gasserian ganglion block	Trigeminal neuralgia
Greater occipital nerve block	Greater occipital neuralgia
Intravenous regional block	Complex regional pain syndromes
Lumbar sympathetic block	Complex regional pain syndromes of the legs
Percutaneous disk decompression	Lumbar or cervical disk herniation
Sacroiliac joint injection	Sacroiliac joint pain
Sphenopalatine ganglion block	Headache and facial pain
Spinal cord stimulator	CRPS, PVD, low back pain, angina
Stellate ganglion block	CRPS of arm, neck, and head; headache
Suprascapular nerve block	Shoulder pain
Vertebroplasty	Vertebral fracture
Motor cortex stimulation	Neuropathic pain
Deep brain stimulation	Neuropathic pain

CRPS, Complex regional pain syndrome; *PVD,* peripheral vascular disease.

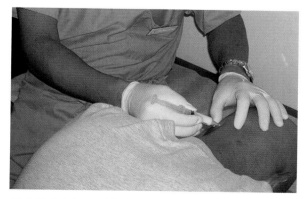

Fig. 44.4 Occipital nerve block. For block of the greater occipital nerve, the patient sits in a chair resting the head on the arms above a treatment table.

Sphenopalatine Ganglion Block for Headache and Facial Pain

The sphenopalatine ganglion is a small triangular structure located in the pterygopalatine fossa, posterior to the middle turbinate and inferior to the maxillary nerve. It is covered by a thin layer (about 1 to 5 mm) of connective tissue and mucous membrane. Anesthetization of the sphenopalatine ganglion can be accomplished via the transnasal approach. The patient is placed supine on the treatment table with the nose pointed at the ceiling. A cotton applicator soaked with 2% to 4% lidocaine is inserted into the nose on the side of headache. To avoid mechanical discomfort, the cotton applicator should not be inserted deeply into the upper posterior wall of the nasopharynx. A slow drip of 2 to 4 mL of lidocaine over a 2- to 4-minute period into the nose through the cotton applicator often achieves the goal of a sphenopalatine ganglion block, with the local anesthetic flowing down to the back of nasopharynx by gravity. Sphenopalatine ganglion blocks have been reported to be effective in the relief of a wide variety of pain conditions of the head including acute migraine attacks, cluster headache, atypical facial pain, head and facial RSD, and postdural puncture headache (Cohen et al., 2009). Intranasal sphenopalatine ganglion block is safe and easy to perform in the clinic and may be helpful for neurologists without special training in interventional pain management techniques to treat an acute headache attack. Other methods for sphenopalatine ganglion block such as a lateral approach with fluoroscopic guidance or endoscopic sphenopalatine ganglion block have also been used. However, special training and equipment are needed.

Gasserian Ganglion Lesions for Trigeminal Neuralgia

The first choice for treatment of trigeminal neuralgia is carbamazepine. It can be used with other medication such as baclofen. Gasserian ganglion lesions are indicated when patients fail other medication treatments. These procedures include radiofrequency thermocoagulation, balloon compression, and glycerolysis. Radiofrequency thermocoagulation is the most commonly used procedure. This procedure is often performed by neurosurgeons, interventional pain specialists, or interventional radiologists with special training. The treatment requires inserting a radiofrequency needle through the face and foramen ovale into the base of the skull under the guidance of fluoroscopy, CT, or CT fluoroscopy. After the needle reaches the gasserian ganglion, radiofrequency energy is applied to induce thermocoagulation; 87% to 91% of patients experience immediate pain relief. In a 5-year follow-up, 50% of patients still had good pain relief. Common side effects include corneal anesthesia, masticator weakness, and anesthesia dolorosa. Recently, stereotactic radiosurgery for trigeminal neuralgia has been used more widely because of its noninvasive nature. Significant pain relief was achieved in 73% at 1 year, 65% at 2 years, and 41% at 5 years follow-up (Kondziolka et al., 2010). However, this procedure may be more costly than other procedures already mentioned.

Stellate Ganglion Block

The stellate ganglion is a sympathetic ganglion innervating the ipsilateral upper extremity, the neck, and the head. The structure is usually located in front of the junction between the C7 vertebral body and the transverse process. Stellate ganglion block is primarily indicated for complex regional pain syndrome of the head, neck, and upper extremities. Uncontrolled clinical reports indicate this procedure provides effective pain relief or may even reverse the course of early-stage CRPS type I. Other indications include vascular insufficiency of the arm and acute herpes zoster infection.

Technically, this block is achieved by inserting a needle through the neck to the front of the junction between the C7 vertebral body and the transverse process. Traditional hand palpation technique without guidance of fluoroscopy bears significant risks of injecting local anesthetics into critical structures in the neck such as the carotid and vertebral arteries or intrathecal space. Incorrectly located injections of local anesthetics may lead to loss of consciousness, seizures, paralysis, cardiac arrest, and death. Current use of fluoroscopic guidance for stellate ganglion block dramatically decreases the possibility of serious side effects and increases the rate of success.

Epidural Corticosteroid Injection

Pain specialists have used epidural corticosteroid injection (ESI) for decades to treat back and neck pain. The procedure is further divided into cervical, thoracic, and lumbar ESI (LESI), with the purpose of treating pain originating from different spinal regions. By 1995, there were at least 12 so-called double-blind placebo-controlled studies investigating the clinical efficacy of LESI for LBP. Of these studies, only six yielded positive results, while the other studies did not support the use of LESI for LBP. Actually, several of these studies exhibited the critical flaw of treating "low back pain" as a single entity. It is now realized that LBP is a clinical syndrome that may be caused by a variety of pathologies in the lumbar spine and adjacent organs. It is not reasonable to treat LBP with ESI, regardless of the cause. More recent well-designed placebo-controlled studies have provided clinical evidence that LESI decreases lumbar radicular pain caused by lumbar disk herniation (Roberts et al., 2009). The pain-relieving effect of LESI may last up to 3 months. Corticosteroids appear to speed the rate of recovery and return of function, allowing patients to reduce medication levels and increase activity while waiting for the natural improvement expected in most spinal disorders. Recent studies also support the use of LESI for pain relief in patients with spinal stenosis (Lee et al., 2010).

Past the age of 60, more than 90% of the normal population has a variety of degenerative spine changes including disk herniation, spinal stenosis, and foraminal stenosis. The majority of persons with these changes, however, do not have pain. It is now believed that the pain in patients with disk herniation and associated radiculopathy is not purely due to mechanical compression but is more likely due to chemical inflammation. A recent study provided convincing evidence for the role of inflammatory mediators in the pathogenesis of lumbar radicular pain and LBP in patients with lumbar degenerative diseases. In the study, the immunoreactivity of an array of cytokines was measured in lavage samples and compared with clinical response to the therapeutic injection. Ten subjects underwent repeated epidural lavage sampling 3 months after the steroid injection. It was found that interferon gamma (IFN-γ) was the most consistently detected cytokine. IFN-γ

immunoreactivity was also highly correlated with reduction of pain 3 months after the epidural steroid injection. In subjects reporting significant pain relief (>50%) from the injection, mean IFN-γ immunoreactivity was significantly greater compared with patients experiencing no significant relief. The IFN-γ immunoreactivity in repeated lavage samples decreased to trace residual concentrations in patients who reported pain relief from the steroid injection. These results suggest that IFN-γ may be part of a biochemical cascade triggering pain in lumbar radicular pain (Scuderi et al., 2009). Other chemical substances such as phospholipase A_2, which is responsible for the liberation of arachidonic acid from cell membranes and starting the cascade of formation of inflammatory mediators such as prostaglandin E (PGE), is also believed to play a major role in pathogenesis of LBP. Epidural corticosteroid injection has been proven to suppress the functional activity of inflammatory mediators such IFN-γ and phospholipase A_2 (Scuderi et al., 2009) to decrease inflammation in the epidural space and surrounding nerve roots. With the support of evidence from both basic science and clinical studies, it is current common practice to offer patients with lumbar radicular pain due to disk herniation a trial of LESI before considering a surgical treatment for lumbar disk herniation. The procedure often prevents back surgeries. As long as pain is relieved and the patient is free of neurological deficits, a herniated disk should be left alone without further treatment.

Lumbar Facet Joint Block

The lumbar facet joint block procedure is indicated for lumbar facet joint pain syndrome. Lumbar facet joint syndrome may be found in up to 35% of patients with LBP. Clinically, this syndrome may mimic lumbar radiculopathy (sciatica). Patients may complain of LBP, often on one side, with pain radiating down the back or front of the thigh. Clinical examination may reveal tenderness on either or both sides of the lumbar spine over the lumbar facet joints. Lumbar spine extension and lateral rotation to the painful side may increase LBP because this maneuver increases pressure on the lumbar facet joints. The straight leg raising test is often negative. Traditionally, pain specialists have performed intrajoint corticosteroid injections, but over the last decade, this procedure has largely been replaced by a diagnostic medial branch (nerve innervating the lumbar facet joints) block with a small amount of local anesthetic. If the patient has significant pain relief (more than 50%) after two consecutive diagnostic medial branch blocks, facet joint rhizotomy with radiofrequency destruction of the medial branch will be performed to denervate the lumbar facet joints. A recent systematic literature review found moderate evidence to support the clinical efficacy and use of radiofrequency rhizotomy for lumbar facet joint syndrome (Datta et al., 2009).

Percutaneous Disk Decompression

Over 300,000 spine surgeries are performed each year in the United States. A majority of these surgeries are conducted for lumbar and cervical disk herniation. Traditional neurosurgical and orthopedic techniques for lumbar disk herniation include laminectomy, diskectomy, and fusion. A significant number of patients end up with so-called failed back surgery syndrome. Recurrent disk herniation, epidural abscess, scar tissue formation around nerve roots, facet joint syndrome, and muscle spasm may contribute to the clinical features of this syndrome. According to the recent literature, up to 100,000 new cases of failed back surgeries are produced every year in the United States alone as the result of spine surgeries. To avoid possible complications of open surgery, minimally invasive techniques for disk decompression have been developed. These techniques include chymopapain, the Nucleotome system, laser diskectomy, nucleoplasty, and disk Dekompressor.

Chymopapain is a proteolytic enzyme from the papaya fruit that may induce enzymatic decompression of the nucleus pulposus of a herniated disk. Initial clinical reports were highly positive, but serious side effects such as anaphylactic shock, transverse myelitis, and even death caused chymopapain to be largely replaced by other techniques.

Percutaneous Nucleotome was developed by a Japanese orthopedic surgeon, Dr. Hijikata, in 1975. This procedure inserts a 7-mm-diameter tube into the annulus and removes the disk material with specially designed forceps. The procedure has a reported success rate of 72%. However, because of the large diameter of the cannula, this technique is no longer commonly used. In 1986, Ascher and Choy introduced YAG laser diskectomy, a procedure still being used by spine surgeons, neurosurgeons, and some interventional pain specialists. This technique utilizes an 18-gauge probe and generates laser energy to evaporate part of the nucleus pulposus. It decreases the intradiscal pressure, with a reported success rate for back pain relief of 78% to 80%. Heat generated by the laser energy may cause patients to experience severe pain during the procedure and increased muscle spasm afterward.

Over the last decade, two new percutaneous disk decompression techniques have been reported. Introduced in 2000, DISC Nucleoplasty utilizes a unique plasma technology called *Coblation* to remove tissue from the center of the disk. During the procedure the DISC Nucleoplasty SpineWand is inserted into the center of the disk, where a series of channels are created to remove tissue from the nucleus. Disc DeKompressor was introduced in 2003. This procedure uses a 1.5-mm percutaneous lumbar diskectomy probe to aspirate the disk material. It is minimally invasive with less risk for nerve root damage. This technique is indicated for patients with contained disk herniation and lumbar radiculopathy. Observational studies suggest both Nucleoplasty and Disc DeKompressor may be potentially effective, minimally invasive treatments for patients with symptomatic contained disks. However, prospective randomized controlled trials are needed to confirm their clinical efficacy and to determine ideal patient selection for these procedures (Gerges et al., 2010).

Motor Cortex Stimulation

Motor cortex stimulation (MCS) has been used for the treatment of central and neuropathic pain syndromes since 1991. It has been used to treat medically unresponsive central and neuropathic pain including that due to thalamic, putaminal, and lateral medullary infarction, traumatic trigeminal neuropathy (not idiopathic trigeminal neuralgia), facial postherpetic neuralgia, brachial plexopathy, neuropathic pain after an SCI, phantom-limb pain, and CRPS. MCS has shown particular promise in the treatment of intractable neuropathic facial pain and central pain syndromes such as thalamic pain syndrome (Levy et al., 2010).

The MCS leads are surgically placed on the dura, with the target selected on the primary motor cortex based on somatotopic anatomical landmarks. The optimal stimulation level is that which provides the best pain relief yet does not cause a seizure, pain from dural stimulation, or EMG activity. Cortical stimulation is not indicated for patients with a history of seizures. Personality disorders such as severe depression or psychotic disorders must be screened out prior to using this procedure.

The precise mechanism for MCS in relieving pain remains unknown, but studies have demonstrated that it leads to an increase in cerebral blood flow in the ipsilateral thalamus, cingulate gyrus, orbitofrontal cortex, and midbrain. The extent of pain relief correlates best, however, with anterior cingulate gyrus blood flow. Rostroventromedial medulla (RVM) and the descending serotonergic pathway acting on the spinal 5-HT (1A) receptor may also contribute to spinal antinociception induced by M1 stimulation.

Spinal Cord Stimulation

Spinal cord stimulation (dorsal column stimulation) uses an array of electrodes placed in the epidural space immediately behind the spinal cord to stimulate the dorsal column of the spinal cord. The exact mechanism of SCS is unclear. However, it is believed that the gate-control theory of pain conduction plays a major role. When the dorsal column of the spinal cord is stimulated, it may attenuate the conduction of the pain signal on the spinothalamic tract through collateral inhibition. Inhibitory neurotransmitters such as GABA may also be involved.

As noted earlier in the chapter, patients should have a trial of SCS prior to permanent implantation. During the trial, a percutaneous lead is inserted through the skin into the epidural space. Once the tip of the lead reaches the appropriate level, it is connected to an external pulse generator. When the stimulator is turned on, the patient may feel tingling and numbness. If the painful area is covered by the stimulation, the pain is decreased by more than 50% and the patient is satisfied with the stimulation, a permanent implantation may be considered. The procedure of permanent implantation of the SCS is performed by pain specialists or neurosurgeons in an operating room. It requires percutaneous insertion of an electrode into the epidural space under the guidance of fluoroscopy. The tip of the electrode is threaded up to the T9-T11 level in the epidural space immediately behind the dorsal column for the treatment of low back and leg pain. The other end of the electrode is connected through a subcutaneous tunnel to an internal pulse generator buried under the skin in the low back or abdominal wall. The strength of the stimulation can be changed through a remote control. Common complications of SCS implantation include infection, migration of the electrodes, and failure of pain relief even after a "satisfied" trial. Serious complications such as spinal cord compression or epidural abscesses are rare.

SCS is indicated for failed back surgery syndrome, CRPS, and unremitting pain due to peripheral vascular disease. Multiple studies have found that SCS may also improve pain due to refractory angina and improve circulation in the coronary arteries. Some authors have reported treatment success with SCS for severe peripheral neuropathy, postherpetic neuralgia, chronic knee pain following total knee replacement, central pain in MS, and painful spasms of atypical stiff limb syndrome (Ughratdar et al., 2010). The value of SCS for amputation stump pain, phantom-limb pain, and SCI is yet to be established. Patients seeking SCS treatments usually have failed all other conservative treatments such as medication, physical therapy, and nerve blocks with anesthetics and/or corticosteroids. SCS is not indicated for severe depression and contraindicated for patients with a cardiac pacemaker or defibrillators.

Intrathecal Drug Delivery Systems

For patients with chronic severe pain, especially malignant pain, who are unable to tolerate the side effects of oral or IV medications, intrathecal delivery of medication offers a useful alternative. The technique of intrathecal delivery of medication has evolved since 1979. There are two kinds of pumps available in the United States: Codman and Medtronic intrathecal pumps. The pump is usually implanted subcutaneously in the abdominal wall. The pump contains about 18 to 50 mL of medication. It is connected to one end of a small-diameter tube that runs to the intrathecal space. The pump continuously delivers small amounts of medication directly into the lumbar cerebrospinal fluid. The Codman pump has fixed delivery rates of 0.5 ml or 1 ml/day. The concentration of medication has to be changed in order to change the daily dose of medication. Medtronic pumps are programmable with an external magnetic control to adjust the dosage and time of medication delivery.

Commonly used medications for pain management include morphine, hydromorphone, bupivacaine, clonidine, and ziconotide, a novel peptide that functions as a calcium channel blocker. Ziconotide was approved by the FDA in 2004 for treating intractable severe chronic pain, but its serious side effects have called the clinical use of this medication into question (Ziconotide, 2008). Baclofen is a GABA$_B$ agonist. It has been used through an intrathecal delivery system for the treatment of severe spasticity and may also decrease the pain related to spasticity. Even though intrathecal opioid treatment was initially approved by the FDA for the treatment of patients with malignant pain, over the last decade, intrathecal opioids have been used extensively for nonmalignant pain such as failed back surgery syndrome. A retrospective cohort study with 3-year follow-up found a favorable outcome for intrathecal opioids. Some patients are able to eliminate oral opioids, although some increase in intrathecal opioid dosing may be required (Atli et al., 2010).

Summary

Treatment of chronic pain conditions remains a challenge. However, recent advances in basic scientific research and clinical studies have provided clinicians with more insight regarding the mechanism and clinical features of chronic pain conditions. Advances in clinical technologies have provided new hope in the treatment of some refractory pain conditions previously regarded as impossible. With a combination of multidisciplinary pain treatment modalities, a majority of pain conditions may be alleviated or managed. The future of pain management requires more physicians, including neurologists, to contribute diagnostic and therapeutic skills to fulfill the need of patients.

References

The complete reference list is available online at www.expertconsult.com.

Principles of Neurointensive Care

Alejandro A. Rabinstein

Neurocritical care is a discipline devoted to the application of critical care principles to seriously ill patients with acute neurological or neurosurgical conditions. It has become one of the most rapidly growing subspecialties of neurology in recent years. Neurological-neurosurgical (or neuroscience) intensive care units (NICUs) are staffed by clinicians with solid knowledge of the principles of ICU management (mechanical ventilation, hemodynamic monitoring, nutrition, infection control and antibiotic prescription, general postoperative care, etc.) and specific interest in the treatment of acute neurological and neurosurgical diseases. In-depth knowledge of acute neurology is a sine qua non to master the job.

Patients admitted to a NICU have central or peripheral nervous system dysfunction as a consequence of a primary neurological condition or as a complication of systemic illness. The most common diagnoses encountered in the NICU are acute ischemic strokes, intracerebral hemorrhage (ICH), subarachnoid hemorrhage (SAH), traumatic brain injury (TBI), brain tumors, raised intracranial pressure (from any of the previous or other conditions), spinal cord injury, central nervous system infections (meningitis, encephalitis, brain abscesses), status epilepticus, neuromuscular respiratory failure, and postoperative care (either after open neurosurgery or an endovascular procedure). Management of each of these conditions demands specific training because they require approaches that focus on neurological recovery. Principles of general ICU care are applicable but must be adjusted accordingly.

Clinical Assessment of Critically Ill Neurological Patients

The practice of neurology in the ICU demands specific clinical skills for timely and effective patient assessment. Since it is often impossible to gather direct history from the patient, and the neurological examination must necessarily be more focused, attention to detail becomes crucial. Time for examination is very limited in neurological emergencies, and patients are often unconscious, sedated, acutely distressed, or confused and agitated. Physical findings may change rapidly, but a proficient physical examination remains central to determining diagnosis and prognosis in these critically ill patients.

The neurological examination for a NICU patient should always begin by defining the level and content of consciousness. *Level of consciousness* measures the degree of arousal or wakefulness of the patient. Scales are useful to facilitate communication and monitor changes over serial examinations; the Glasgow Coma Scale (GCS) is the most widely used (see Chapter 5, **Table 5.4**). However, it loses accuracy in patients who are intubated or develop cerebral ptosis (inability or only partial ability to open the eyes [by contracting the frontalis muscle] because a brain lesion impairs control of eye-opening mechanisms) and fails to provide information on brainstem function and respiratory status. A new scale (the FOUR score) that addresses these shortcomings has been validated in various patient populations and merits consideration as an alternative (Wijdicks et al., 2005) (**Fig. 45.1**). For patients with localized structural brain diseases, the National Institutes of Health (NIH) Stroke Scale may be used to grade and track focal neurological deficits.

In patients with altered consciousness, the results of one of these scales should be complemented with documentation of additional neurological features. Detailed description of the location and movements of the eyes, brainstem reflexes (pupillary light reactions, corneal, oculocephalic, oculovestibular, gag, cough), spontaneous movements and motor responses to pain, lateralizing signs, and breathing pattern must be recorded. In patients with delirium, the clinician must note the predominant behavioral abnormalities, degree of motor activity, and ability to interact with the environment. It is always important to dedicate special attention to any abnormal or adventitious movements, since seizures in critically ill patients may present with very subtle motor manifestations (e.g., nystagmoid eye movements). Fundoscopy may also offer valuable information and should be attempted; however, to avoid confounding future pupillary evaluations, mydriatic agents should not be administered. The reader is referred to Chapters 4 and 5 for further information relative to clinical evaluation of comatose and delirious patients.

Another essential aspect of the examination in critically ill patients is evaluating neuromuscular respiratory weakness. Timely recognition of signs of impending neuromuscular respiratory failure may avoid potentially devastating complications. Among them, use of accessory muscles and paradoxical breathing pattern are most indicative of problems. *Paradoxical breathing* is defined as the loss of synchronicity in chest and abdominal movements during respiration (i.e., abnormal sinking of the abdomen during inspiration) and represents an unequivocal sign of diaphragmatic failure (Rabinstein and Wijdicks, 2003b).

It is important to integrate the information provided by the neurological examination with data from the general systemic examination, vital signs monitoring, and other physiological variables. Alterations in heart rate, respiration, and blood pressure (BP), for example, often result from brain herniation.

Monitoring in the Neurointensive Care Unit

Systemic Monitoring

Systemic monitoring in the NICU typically includes cardiac telemetry, frequent scheduled noninvasive BP measurements (by automatic cuff inflation) or continuous invasive arterial BP recording, pulse oximetry, and core body temperature. Continuous arterial BP monitoring is accomplished by inserting an indwelling cannula into a medium-caliber artery (e.g., radial arterial line). The invasiveness of the procedure is justified by the precise real-time information it provides. Continuous arterial BP monitoring is especially recommended in patients treated with induced hypertension (e.g., symptomatic vasospasm after SAH), cases requiring very strict BP control

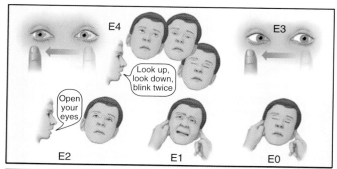
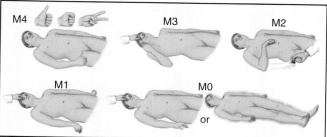
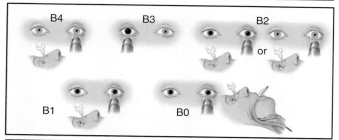
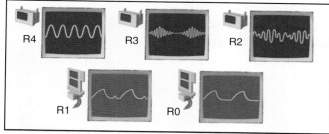

Fig. 45.1 FOUR score. Scale for assessing coma in the neurological-neurosurgical ICU. *E: eye examination.* E4, eyelids open or opened and eyes tracking and eyelids blinking to command; E3, eyelids open but eyes not tracking; E2, eyelids closed but open to loud voice; E1, eyelids closed but open to pain; E0, eyelids remain closed with pain. *M: motor response.* M4, thumbs-up, fist, or peace sign to command; M3, localizing to pain; M2, flexion response to pain; M1, extensor response to pain; M0, no response to pain or generalized myoclonic status. *B: brainstem reflexes.* B4, pupillary and corneal reflexes present; B3, one pupil dilated and fixed; B2, pupillary or corneal reflexes absent; B1, pupillary and corneal reflexes absent; B0, absent pupillary, corneal, and cough reflexes. *R: respiration.* R4, not intubated with regular breathing pattern; R3, not intubated with Cheyne-Stokes breathing pattern; R2, not intubated with irregular breathing pattern; R1, intubated breathing above the ventilator rate; R0, intubated breathing at ventilator rate or apnea.

to avoid hemorrhagic complications (e.g., ruptured arteriovenous malformations), and patients with hypotension (e.g., sepsis), compromised cerebral perfusion pressure (CPP) (e.g., TBI with raised intracranial pressure [ICP]), or autonomic instability (e.g., Guillain-Barré syndrome). Arterial lines provide the additional advantage of eliminating the need for repeated arterial punctures to measure arterial blood gases. However, although generally safe, placement of an arterial line may be complicated by local infection, leading to bacteremia and thrombosis with risk of digital ischemia. Careful attention to proper technique and adherence to strict sterile conditions during placement and manipulation of the catheter are mandatory (Tegtmeyer et al., 2006).

The most accurate method of measuring core body temperature is a pulmonary artery catheter thermistor, but since most patients in the NICU do not require pulmonary artery catheter insertion, bladder or rectal probes are most frequently used. Bladder and rectal probes correlate well with pulmonary artery catheter thermistor readings, but there is a lag in the detection of temperature changes by the probes. The site of temperature recording becomes particularly important in patients treated with cooling measures. Thus, monitoring esophageal temperatures is recommended when using certain intravascular cooling devices (De Georgia et al., 2004).

Central venous catheters allow monitoring of central venous pressure while providing access for fluid and drug administration. They are, however, a frequent source of infection. Rigorous sterile techniques at the time of catheter insertion, cutaneous antisepsis with chlorhexidine (rather than povidone-iodine), topical application of antiinfective ointment or a chlorhexidine-impregnated dressing to the insertion site, and catheters with an antiinfective surface may reduce the risk of catheter-related bloodstream infection (Safdar et al., 2002). The role of pulmonary artery catheters in ICUs is shrinking as studies consistently demonstrate that their use is associated with higher rates of complications (Sandham et al., 2003; Wheeler et al., 2006).

Brain Monitoring

Neurological examination may lack sensitivity in critically ill patients who have depressed levels of consciousness due to the brain disease or from the effect of sedative medications. Brain monitoring methods developed and refined over the past 25 years may provide additional valuable information in these cases. These techniques offer real-time data, unlike imaging modalities that represent only "snapshots" of the patient's condition at certain points in time. Therefore, brain monitoring techniques are better suited to dynamic assessment of the changes in neurological status of critical patients.

Multiple brain monitoring methods are now available. They are most useful when applied in combination, a practice known as *multimodality monitoring* (Diedler and Czosnyka, 2010). It is important to be aware, however, that the endpoints of most studies validating the use of brain monitoring methods modalities have been surrogate physiological measures rather than actual assessments of patients' functional outcome. In fact, there is no class I evidence proving that the use of multimodality brain monitoring results in improved clinical outcomes. Currently, the clinical application of brain monitoring techniques is restricted to large centers, especially those treating numerous TBI patients.

Methods for cerebral monitoring are divided into three main categories according to their spatial resolution: global, regional, and local brain monitoring (**Table 45.1**). Global brain monitoring techniques measure ICP, CPP, electrical potentials, and venous oxygen saturation. Regional and local

brain monitoring methods include cerebral blood flow (CBF), cerebral blood flow velocities (BFV), brain tissue metabolism, temperature, and oxygenation.

Global Brain Monitoring Techniques
Intracranial Pressure Monitoring

The intracranial space is occupied by three constituent compartments: the brain (accounting for 80% to 90% of the intracranial volume), the blood, and the cerebrospinal fluid (CSF). Because the skull is rigid, any expansion of one of these compartments must be compensated by a reduction in size of the others (a physiological principle known as the *Monro-Kellie doctrine*). When this compensation is insufficient, the ICP rises. Small increases in intracranial volume can be initially accommodated with little or no effect on the ICP, but as more volume is added, intracranial compliance falls until it reaches a critical point beyond which a minimal increase in volume causes an exponential rise in ICP. This pressure-volume relationship is depicted in **Fig. 45.2**. In other words, the initial physiological response to an increase in brain volume is a reduction in the CSF and venous blood volumes by shifting these fluids out of the intracranial space (except in the cases of hydrocephalus and venous thrombosis). Once these compensatory mechanisms are exhausted, the system becomes noncompliant, and further increments in brain volume compromise arterial blood flow and eventually lead to herniation of brain tissue.

Normal ICP in a supine individual is less than 10 mm Hg when measured at the level of the foramen of Monro (typically referenced to the tragus). Levels exceeding 20 mm Hg define raised ICP. Knowing the actual ICP is a prerequisite to determining CPP, which is defined by the relationship between ICP and mean arterial pressure (MAP) as follows:

$$CPP = MAP - ICP$$

It has also been argued that the main purpose of ICP monitoring is maintenance of normal CPP (normal, >70 mm Hg) because the latter may be more related to secondary ischemic injury (Rosner et al., 1995). The relative importance of ICP and CPP as main targets of therapy remains a matter of debate.

ICP is pulsatile and has systolic and diastolic components. In addition to the value of mean ICP, these components must also be evaluated carefully. The normal ICP waveform consists of a 3-peaked wave (**Fig. 45.3**). P1, the first and generally the tallest peak, is also known as the *percussion wave* and corresponds to the transmitted systolic BP; P2 (the tidal wave) and P3 (the dicrotic wave) are normally smaller peaks, and the notch between them corresponds to the dicrotic notch of the arterial waveform. As ICP increases, P2 and P3 rise and eventually surpass P1. Ultimately, with continued elevation of ICP, the waveform loses distinct peaks and assumes a triangular morphology. Intracranial pathology leading to sustained elevations of ICP may produce *plateau waves*, also known as *A-waves of Lundberg* (see **Fig. 45.3**). These waves reflect a sudden dramatic rise in ICP to levels of 40 to 100 mm Hg, often lasting 5 to 20 minutes. Plateau waves indicate critically low intracranial compliance leading to marked changes in ICP, even with very small variations in intracranial volume. Although their pathophysiology is not fully elucidated, experimental observations suggest that plateau waves

Table 45.1 Brain Monitoring Methods

Method	Spacial Resolution	Temporal Resolution	Purpose	Advantages	Disadvantages
ICP	Global	Continuous	Measure intracranial compliance	Reliable Quantitative Allows monitoring of CPP	Invasive Risk of infection Risk of hemorrhage
Jugular oximetry (SjvO$_2$)	Global	Continuous	Measure adequacy of hemispheric oxygenation	Quantitative Allows monitoring of AVDO$_2$ and O$_2$ER	Susceptible to artifacts Local complications (e.g., infection, thrombosis)
EEG	Global	Continuous	Monitoring electrical brain activity Detection of seizures	Technique well standardized Only method to diagnose nonconvulsive seizures	Qualitative Relatively insensitive to secondary insults
SSEP	Global	Continuous	Monitoring integrity of sensory pathways	Technique well standardized Simple	Qualitative Fairly insensitive to secondary insults
Bedside Xe-133 CBF	Regional	Discontinuous	Measure hemispheric CBF	Quantitative	Only accurate if radiotracer injected into carotid artery Radioactivity
Laser Doppler flowmetry	Local	Continuous	Measure cortical CBF	Accurate Dynamic information	Qualitative Invasive Susceptible to artifacts Only monitors 1-2 mm^3 of tissue
Thermal diffusion flowmetry	Local	Continuous	Measure cortical CBF	Simple Dynamic information	Qualitative Invasive Monitors small volume of tissue
TCD	Regional	Continuous	Measure CBF velocities	Simple Noninvasive Allows measuring PI, VMR	Qualitative and indirect assessment of CBF Difficult to keep probes in place
Brain tissue PO$_2$	Local	Continuous	Measure cerebral oxygenation	Quantitative Sensitive Probes also measure brain temperature	Invasive Susceptible to artifacts Monitors small volume of tissue
NIRS	Local	Continuous	Measure cerebral oxygenation	Noninvasive	Measures only relative changes Susceptible to artifacts
Microdialysis	Local	Discontinuous	Measure cerebral metabolism	Sensitive Quantitative	Invasive Complicated technique Labor intensive Unclear which is the best parameter to monitor

AVDO$_2$, Arteriovenous oxygen difference; *CBF,* cerebral blood flow; *CPP,* cerebral perfusion pressure; *EEG,* electroencephalogram; *ICP,* intracranial pressure; *NIRS,* near-infrared spectroscopy; *O$_2$ER,* oxygen extraction rate; *PI,* pulsatility index; *PO$_2$,* partial pressure of oxygen; *TCD,* transcranial Doppler; *SSEP,* somatosensory evoked potentials; *VMR,* vasomotor reactivity.

may be generated by brief episodes of systemic hypotension leading to exaggerated cerebral vasodilation in patients with abnormal vasomotor reactivity (Rosner and Becker, 1984).

ICP may be monitored using intraparenchymal, intraventricular, epidural, or subdural devices (Brain Trauma Foundation, 2007). Intraventricular monitoring remains the gold standard because of its precision. It consists of a ventricular catheter connected to an external transducer which allows continuous ICP readings. Advantages of this technique are providing reliable ICP measurements and allowing external drainage of CSF. Hence, ventricular monitoring is indicated in patients with hydrocephalus and often preferred in those with

refractory intracranial hypertension. Major drawbacks are higher risk of infection (rate of ventriculitis is 3% to 8% and increases with duration of the ventriculostomy) (Flibotte et al., 2004; Holloway et al., 1996; Martinez-Manas et al., 2000), risk of bleeding at the time of catheter placement (especially in patients with underlying coagulopathy or recent use of antithrombotics), and system malfunction (dampening of the waveform may be caused by apposition of the catheter tip against the ventricular wall or obstruction of the catheter by a blood clot or an air bubble). Risks may be minimized by careful placement of the catheter and maintenance of the system under strict sterile conditions, use of antibiotic

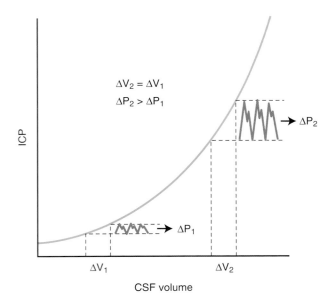

Fig. 45.2 Relationship between pressure and volume changes in the intracranial compartment. *CSF,* Cerebrospinal fluid; *ICP,* intracranial pressure; *P,* pressure; *V,* volume.

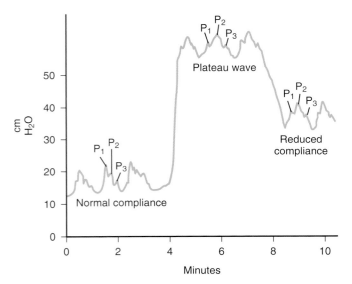

Fig. 45.3 Intracranial pressure tracings in the setting of normal and reduced compliance. Plateau wave (A wave of Lundberg) is seen in the center of the figure.

prophylaxis (e.g., cefotaxime 2 g every 6 hours from the time of catheter insertion until 24 to 48 hours after its removal) (Flibotte et al., 2004), and withdrawal of the catheter as soon as possible (Holloway et al., 1996). Exchange of the catheter every 5 days, although a common practice, does not appear to decrease the risk of infection (Holloway et al., 1996; Lozier et al., 2002); in fact, repeated catheter insertions have been found to be associated with higher risk of ventriculitis (Arabi et al., 2005).

Intraparenchymal fiberoptic monitors are also quite accurate. When compared with intraventricular catheters, the measurements provided by intraparenchymal monitors differ on average by ± 2 to 5 mm Hg. Advantages of this monitoring system include simple and safe insertion technique, easy

maintenance, relative lack of substantial drift (even after several days), and low risk of infection. Disadvantages include high cost, technical complications (e.g., breakage of the optical fiber), and most importantly, inability to drain CSF. Epidural and subdural monitors are less reliable and therefore rarely used but are a valuable option for patients with severe coagulopathy (e.g., liver failure with cerebral edema), given their lower risk of hemorrhagic complications (Vaquero et al., 2005).

ICP should be monitored in patients with severe TBI and a GCS sum score below 9 and an abnormal computed tomography (CT) scan, or a normal CT scan with two or more of the following criteria: age older than 40, unilateral or bilateral motor posturing, and systolic BP less than 90 mm Hg (Brain Trauma Foundation, 2007). It is difficult to extrapolate the value of these guidelines to patients with diagnoses other than trauma, owing to lack of specific data on ICP monitoring in those other conditions. Some experts advocate monitoring ICP in comatose patients with a large intracranial mass lesion (hematoma, abscess, large infarctions, etc.) causing radiologically documented tissue shift. Patients with SAH, ICH, or cerebellar ischemic or hemorrhagic strokes producing acute hydrocephalus typically have their ICP monitored once a ventriculostomy catheter has been placed primarily for drainage purposes.

Jugular Bulb Oximetry

Jugular bulb oximetry measures the oxygen saturation of venous blood returning from the brain (normal 50% to 65%) by means of a fiberoptic catheter (Feldman and Robertson, 1997). The main goal of jugular venous oxygen saturation ($Sjvo_2$) monitoring is to provide a continuous measure of the changing balance between cerebral oxygen delivery and cerebral oxygen consumption. Simultaneous determination of $Sjvo_2$ using the jugular bulb catheter and arterial oxygen saturation (Sao_2) allows for the calculation of the intracranial arteriovenous oxygen difference ($AVDo_2$) (normal 24%-42%). Cerebral oxygen consumption can be calculated as the product of $AVDo_2$ and CBF. The cerebral oxygen extraction rate (O_2ER) is derived from the ratio of cerebral oxygen consumption to cerebral oxygen delivery.

Jugular venous desaturations denote relative reductions of global cerebral oxygenation. $Sjvo_2$ below 50% for 15 minutes or more are deemed indicative of ischemia. $Sjvo_2$ monitoring has been mostly tested in patients with severe TBI. In these patients, jugular venous desaturations have been shown to correlate with the occurrence of secondary brain insults and poor outcome (Gopinath et al., 1994; Robertson et al., 1995). High $Sjvo_2$ should not simply be equated with hyperemia; it may also be associated with poor outcome in comatose patients, possibly indicating lack of oxygen utilization after extensive neuronal death (Cormio et al., 1999). Favorable experience with jugular bulb oximetry has been reported in patients with SAH and ICH (Heran et al., 2004; von Helden et al., 1993), but interpreting $Sjvo_2$ may be difficult in patients with severe hemispheric ischemic strokes (Keller et al., 2002). This technique is also used to monitor cerebral oxygenation during neurosurgical procedures.

Therapeutic interventions in response to information provided by jugular bulb oximetry have been proposed, including adjustment of the degree of hyperventilation, timing and intensity of osmotherapy, adjustment of MAP, and treatment of anemia (Macmillan and Andrews, 2000). There is no proof, however, that these interventions improve functional outcome. As shown by the negative results observed in studies testing therapies guided by pulmonary artery catheters, the clinical value of aggressive interventions aimed at optimizing physiological parameters must be proven before we incorporate these into clinical practice.

Advantages of the jugular bulb catheter as a monitoring modality include the practicality of continuous bedside monitoring, the capability of confirming the oximeter reading by drawing blood through the catheter, and the numerous physiological parameters that can be derived from the Sjvo₂ to ascertain cerebral oxygen balance. Disadvantages of the catheter include its susceptibility to positioning artifacts and the complications associated with catheter insertion, including carotid puncture, infection, accidental misplacement, and jugular thrombosis (Coplin et al., 1997; Coplin et al., 1998; Latronico et al., 2000).

Electroencephalography

Continuous bedside electroencephalography (EEG) monitoring is based on four of its major neurobiological features (Jordan, 1995): (1) its close relationship to cerebral metabolic rate; (2) its sensitivity in detecting hypoxic-ischemic neuronal dysfunction at an early stage; (3) its obvious primacy as a monitor of seizure activity; and (4) its value in cerebral localization. Continuous EEG recording has been advocated as a valuable routine tool to monitor critically ill neurosurgical and neurological patients.

Despite the fact that the technical aspects of EEG application in the NICU do not differ greatly from the standard routine EEG, some factors are relatively unique to the ICU setting. The main differences are the abundance of electrical artifact sources (ventilators, intravenous [IV] pumps, dialysis machines, suctioning equipment) and the inability of the patient to cooperate, secondary to various degrees of encephalopathy. In addition, continuous bedside EEG monitoring requires EEG interpreters available to view the recording frequently throughout the day and specially trained nurses capable of recognizing meaningful changes in the tracing.

Status epilepticus is the most common indication for EEG monitoring, because the clinical ascertainment of ongoing seizure activity is often obscured by the effect of sedatives and analgesic agents. The EEG is essential for monitoring the effects of treatment, especially when barbiturates or general anesthetics are administered to achieve a burst-suppression pattern. Detection of nonconvulsive seizures and nonconvulsive status epilepticus (NCSE) can only be accomplished by EEG monitoring. Timely diagnosis of NCSE is important because delayed recognition may be associated with increased mortality (Young et al., 1996).

Nonconvulsive seizures were reported in up to one-third of unselected NICU patients, frequently involving the presence of NCSE (Jordan, 1995). NCSE has also been noted in 8% of comatose patients in medical ICUs (Towne et al., 2000), and nearly a third of septic patients with encephalopathy may have electrographic seizures without obvious clinical manifestations (Oddo et al., 2009). Continuous EEG monitoring has documented nonconvulsive seizures after severe TBI, ischemic stroke, poor-grade SAH, ICH, and after termination of generalized convulsive status epilepticus (DeLorenzo et al., 1998; Dennis et al., 2002; Vespa et al., 1999). These events might exacerbate excitotoxic injury in vulnerable brains and have been associated with high mortality (Young et al., 1996). But while their prognostic value is fairly well established, the impact of aggressive treatment of nonconvulsive seizures on clinical outcome remains to be determined (Hirsch, 2004).

Continuous EEG monitoring has also been used as an aid for early detection of ischemia in patients with SAH at high risk for vasospasm. Although early experience is promising (Claassen et al., 2006; Vespa et al., 1997), it is too early to recommend continuous EEG for this indication. Intracortical EEG (based on the use of deep electrodes) may be substantially superior to scalp EEG for detecting changes related to secondary neurological insults in patients with various forms of acute brain injury (Waziri et al., 2009). Furthermore, recurrent cortical spreading depolarizations may exacerbate local brain hypoxia in patients with TBI or SAH (Bosche et al., 2010), but the value of monitoring for these changes with intracortical EEG remains to be conclusively determined.

Other applications of EEG in the ICU, especially in comatose patients, include evaluating metabolic encephalopathy (EEG serves to substantiate the diagnosis by showing diffusely slow, low-amplitude activity, and often triphasic waves, but does not distinguish between different causes of the condition), recognizing psychogenic unresponsiveness, and confirming brain death (Wijdicks, 2001). After cardiac arrest, near-complete suppression, burst-suppression, nonreactive alpha or theta rhythms (alpha or theta coma), status epilepticus and generalized periodic complexes are considered malignant patterns (Rossetti et al., 2007; Synek, 1990). Although valuable for the prognostication of anoxic-ischemic encephalopathy, EEG data should not be interpreted in isolation in these patients (Wijdicks et al., 2006).

Evoked Potentials

Evoked potentials have a more restricted role in the NICU (Moulton et al., 1998). The median nerve somatosensory evoked potential (SSEP) has been mostly used; technical details are discussed in Chapter 32A. Bilateral absence of the N20 response 1 to 3 days after cardiopulmonary resuscitation accurately predicts poor chances of recovery of awareness (Zandbergen et al., 2006). Unfortunately, presence of these responses after anoxic brain injury lacks meaningful prognostic value.

Continuous monitoring of brainstem evoked potentials and SSEP is now technically feasible. However, the very few studies conducted using these modalities failed to demonstrate any value in early recognition of secondary insults.

Regional/Focal Brain Monitoring Techniques

Regional Cerebral Blood Flow Monitoring

A major focus in neurointensive care is to ensure that patients maintain adequate CBF. Normal CBF in adult individuals ranges from 45 to 60 mL/100 g/min, and it is higher in the gray matter than in the white matter. Values below 10 mL/100 g/min are considered indicative of ischemia. Determinants of CBF include the status of brain metabolism,

Paco₂, systemic BP, hematocrit, and cardiac output. Most of these determinants can be therapeutically manipulated by interventions such as the use of sedatives, changes in the ventilator setting, volume expansion, administration of vasoactive agents, blood transfusions, and inotropic medications. When interpreting information offered by CBF monitoring techniques, it is essential to understand the concept that CBF may be inappropriately low (i.e., metabolic demands exceed supply of blood flow, resulting in ischemia), appropriately low (i.e., metabolic demands are reduced and result in a coupled reduction in blood flow and oxygen consumption), inappropriately high (i.e., cerebral hyperemia), or appropriately high (i.e., situations of increased metabolic demand, such as seizures or fever). There are regional and local techniques for CBF monitoring. Regional modalities include: (1) bedside xenon-133 IV injection technique, (2) stable xenon CT scan, (3) single-photon emission tomography (SPECT), (4) positron emission tomography (PET), (5) perfusion-weighted imaging by magnetic resonance imaging (PWI-MRI), and (6) CT perfusion scans.

The main disadvantage of most of these techniques is that they require transportation of the patient outside of the ICU to the location of the scanner. Consequently, they only provide information about the status of CBF at certain points in time, while CBF is a highly dynamic variable that may fluctuate extensively over time. The bedside xenon-133 technique is the only regional CBF monitoring modality that permits repeated testing in the NICU. However, it requires injection of small doses of the radioactive isotope. The xenon-CT technique involves transporting the patient to the CT scanner and administering non-radioactive xenon gas by inhalation. The inhaled gas can create a euphoric sensation, thus making this technique less desirable in agitated patients. SPECT, PET, MR perfusion, and CT perfusion are valid options for assessing brain perfusion at a certain point in time. PET also allows measurement of the oxygen extraction fraction, which is a reliable indicator of hemodynamic failure and early ischemia when elevated. MRI scanning provides greater anatomical information and the advantage of displaying areas of ischemia on diffusion-weighted imaging. CT perfusion is becoming increasingly available and offers quantifiable perfusion data. However, cumulative exposure to radiation limits the number of CT perfusion scans that can be safely performed for monitoring purposes.

Local CBF monitoring techniques include laser Doppler flowmetry and thermal diffusion flowmetry. Laser Doppler flowmetry is based on assessing the Doppler shift of low-power laser light captured by the moving red blood cells (red cell flux). It produces the continuous real-time flow output, which is linearly related to CBF, thus providing reliable information on local perfusion with excellent dynamic resolution. The main disadvantages of this technique, however, are its invasiveness (requires insertion of the probe via a burr hole), its susceptibility to movement artifact, its small sample volume (1 to 2 cubic millimeters), and the qualitative nature of the information provided (this technique does not allow quantification of CBF, and only relative changes can be assessed). Thermal diffusion flowmetry is used to estimate cortical blood flow by measuring changes in the temperature gradient between two cold plates within a probe applied to the cortex. Advantages include its simplicity and continuous measurement without using ionizing radiation. However, this technique does not provide absolute measures of CBF, and it has not been sufficiently standardized to be recommended for clinical practice.

Transcranial Doppler (TCD) ultrasonography and various brain oxygenation monitoring techniques represent indirect measures of CBF monitoring.

Transcranial Doppler Ultrasonography

TCD ultrasonography is a noninvasive technique used to evaluate mean CBF velocity in the large intracranial arteries at the level of the circle of Willis. TCD is easy to learn and use, noninvasive, and safe. It measures CBF velocity rather than CBF, and the linear relationship between CBF and BFV depends on the angle of insonation. Still, TCD provides a wealth of useful clinical information including the presence or absence of blood flow, its velocity (systolic, diastolic, and mean), and direction. It also allows calculation of the pulsatility index (PI = peak systolic velocity minus end diastolic velocity divided by mean BFV), which represents the downstream resistance to blood flow. Increases in BFV are observed in patients with cerebral vasospasm, hyperventilation (which produces vasoconstriction), and anemia. Cerebral vasospasm may be distinguished from hyperdynamic status by measuring the hemispheric index or Lindegaard ratio (ratio of middle cerebral artery to extracranial internal carotid artery mean BFV) (Lindegaard et al., 1989). A ratio greater than 3 is considered indicative of vasospasm; a low ratio is more suggestive of hyperemia. TCD also allows assessment of vasomotor reactivity (Ng et al., 2000). Impairment of vasomotor reactivity is a well-established poor prognostic factor in patients with TBI and may portend the occurrence of symptomatic vasospasm in patients with SAH (Czosnyka et al., 1997; Frontera et al., 2006b). TCD may also be used as a confirmatory test for the diagnosis of brain death (severely diminished mean cerebral BFV associated with absent diastolic flow, reversed flow, and severely elevated PI).

The diagnosis of cerebral vasospasm in patients with SAH remains the main indication of TCD monitoring in the NICU. The criteria for vasospasm in the middle cerebral artery territory is a mean BFV greater than 120 cm/sec with a hemispheric index greater than 3, or an increment greater than 50 cm/sec within a 24-hour period (Suarez et al., 2002). A specialized headset allows continuous monitoring of BFV and may be a useful adjunct in monitoring patients at high risk for vasospasm. TCD monitoring in patients with cerebral vasospasm has good correlation with angiographic vasospasm and is comparable to conventional angiography in the prognostication of delayed ischemia in these patient, although neither technique is uniformly diagnostic (Rabinstein et al., 2004).

Local Cerebral Oxygenation Monitoring Techniques

Brain tissue oxygen probes and near-infrared spectroscopy allow assessment of local oxygenation. Brain tissue oxygen may be measured by invasive probes such as the Licox catheter. Apart from tissue Po₂, this catheter allows measurement of brain temperature. Brain tissue Po₂ measures the diffusion of dissolved plasma oxygen across the blood brain barrier (rather than CBF, arterial delivery of oxygen, or brain metabolism) in a relatively small area of brain tissue (approximately 15 mm³) (Rosenthal et al., 2009). Factors that determine brain tissue Po_2 include Pao_2, arterial $Paco_2$, systemic BP, and CBF. Normal brain tissue Po_2 values range from 25 to 30 mm Hg. The major disadvantages of brain oxygen probes include their invasiveness, limited spatial resolution, and susceptibility to artifacts (due to inappropriate calibration and head movement, among other factors). Its use has been recommended by experts in various major centers for patients with severe head injuries and poor-grade SAH (Maloney-Wilensky et al., 2009). It is best used when applied in the setting of multimodality monitoring, along with jugular oximetry and perhaps microdialysis (Andrews et al., 2008) (**Fig. 45.4**).

Near-infrared spectroscopy (NIRS) is based on the property of a near-infrared light (700–1000 nm) to pass through tissues while being both scattered and absorbed. The absorption of a near-infrared light is proportional to the local concentration of certain chromophores, most notably hemoglobin. Thus, the absorption of near-infrared light changes according to the oxygenation state of hemoglobin. The probes illuminate up to a volume of 10 mL of brain tissue. All measurements are expressed as absolute concentration changes from a baseline zero at the start of the measurement. Normal values of oxygenated hemoglobin are reported to be 60% to 80%, and ischemic threshold is estimated to be below 47% saturation (Casati et al., 2006). However, the reliability of this technique has been questioned. It is susceptible to extraneous light, motion artifact, and signal drift. The measurement may also become unreliable when obtained through intracranial hematomas or through blood in the CSF.

Microdialysis

The basic concept of microdialysis involves inserting a fine catheter into the brain parenchyma, then perfusing the catheter with a physiological solution such as Ringer's lactate, thereby facilitating the exchange of molecules between the perfusate and the extracellular fluid across a dialysis membrane located within the catheter tip. The dialysate is sampled under sterile conditions at hourly or other regular intervals and put through a microdialysis analyzer at the bedside. Insertion artifacts make measurements unreliable for the first hour after placement (Bellander et al., 2004).

Microdialysis allows monitoring of brain pH, lactate and pyruvate, glucose, glycerol, glutamate, urea, and potentially other soluble molecules of interest (Bellander et al., 2004; Nilsson et al., 1999; Vespa et al., 1998). Changes in lactate concentration, lactate/pyruvate ratio, and glutamate concentration have been used as indices of cerebral ischemia. A lactate/pyruvate ratio greater than 25 is probably the best indicator of ischemia (Andrews et al., 2008; Bellander et al., 2004). Rises in glycerol are believed to reflect phospholipid breakdown as a result of cell membrane damage. Because of this, cerebral microdialysis has been employed in the NICU to monitor for cerebral vasospasm and delayed cerebral ischemia in SAH, to identify secondary insults after severe brain trauma, and to follow extracellular glutamate concentration peri-ictally in patients with epilepsy.

Several aspects of microdialytic analysis remain controversial, such as where to place the catheter (Andrews et al., 2008), whether the lactate/pyruvate ratio alone or in combination with other parameters is a better indicator of early cerebral ischemia, and why there has been no correlation between microdialysis measures and clinical outcome in some studies. Other problems are the invasiveness and labor intensiveness of the technique. It currently represents a valuable research tool, but its widespread clinical use cannot yet be recommended.

Principles of Managing Critically Ill Neurological Patients

Analgesia and Sedation

Analgesia and sedation are essential practices in neurointensive care. It is always challenging to avoid confounding the neurological examination while keeping the patient comfortable. Distinguishing agitation from the psychomotor manifestations of pain may be a difficult task in acutely ill neurological patients. Anxiety and pain lead to stress responses characterized by a hyperdynamic circulation, increased metabolic rate, and hyperkinesis. When pain is the cause of restlessness, the abnormal behavior may be more refractory to sedative medications. In those cases, appropriate and timely use of analgesics may result in correction of the abnormal behavior.

Whenever a patient is agitated in the NICU, an organic cause for the agitation should be sought. Confusion and restlessness are often seen in patients with acute strokes (especially

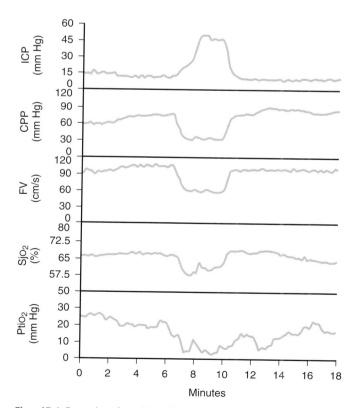

Fig. 45.4 Example of multimodality monitoring in a patient with traumatic brain injury. Notice the evidence of local and regional hypoxia with elevation of intracranial pressure leading to reduction in cerebral perfusion. *CPP,* Cerebral perfusion pressure; *FV,* flow velocities on transcranial Doppler; *ICP,* intracranial pressure; *PtiO2,* oxygen pressure in brain tissue; *SjO2,* oxygen saturation in jugular blood.

those involving the right parietal lobe or the left posterior cerebral artery territory), early after SAH, in TBI with bifrontal damage, and in certain postictal states. On the other hand, patients with neuromuscular respiratory failure may become extremely anxious as they fail to achieve adequate ventilation and gas exchange. Drug withdrawal and side effects from medications are other common causes of agitation in the NICU. Metabolic and endocrine derangements should also be investigated in agitated critically ill patients.

The ideal sedative agent in the NICU would be one that can achieve sedation rapidly and allow for fast and reliable reversal of its effect. Propofol is one of the most commonly used drugs because it fulfills the criteria to a great extent. Propofol crosses the blood-brain barrier within minutes of administration and is a markedly effective hypnotic agent. Another advantageous pharmacokinetic property of propofol is that its clearance is not significantly altered by liver or renal failure, which is often a problem with benzodiazepines and opiates. Propofol lacks amnestic properties, so adequate analgesia should always be ensured in patients receiving this drug.

Awakening is typically seen within minutes of discontinuation of the infusion, but time to awakening may be significantly prolonged when the drug has been used in large doses for several days, because propofol is redistributed to the fat tissue from where it is only slowly released. Hypotension is the most common side effect of propofol infusion, especially when administered as a bolus. Falls in BP are more frequent and pronounced in patients who are hypovolemic. Other adverse effects include caloric overload (1 mL of propofol contains 1 kilocalorie), hypertriglyceridemia, and withdrawal myoclonus (often confused with seizures). Propofol can also be used to treat elevated ICP and status epilepticus (Parviainen et al., 2006). However, administration of high doses of propofol for prolonged periods of time (i.e., >4-5 mg/kg/h for more than 48 hours) can cause the *propofol infusion syndrome* (Kam and Cardone, 2007). This is a serious complication characterized by metabolic acidosis, rhabdomyolysis, refractory bradycardia, myocardial depression, and when most severe, cardiac arrest (Iyer et al., 2009). Even strict surveillance for these manifestations may fail to prevent this life-threatening complication. Consequently, propofol should be used with great caution for the treatment of recalcitrant intracranial hypertension and status epilepticus, indications in which high doses of the medication are often necessary for up to several days to achieve the therapeutic goal.

Midazolam and lorazepam are the two most commonly used benzodiazepines in the NICU. The advantages of midazolam are its rapid effect and short duration of action (half-life 1.9 hours); it has only one active metabolite. Clearance is fast, but accumulation may occur after 3 days of continuous infusion. Patients who receive midazolam for several days can be expected to exhibit delayed awakening. Clearance of midazolam is diminished by hepatic and renal failure. Lorazepam has a much longer half-life (14 hours), which leads to a much slower emergence from sedation. However, continuous infusion of lorazepam can produce severe metabolic acidosis from propylene glycol toxicity (Arroliga et al., 2004). The main side effect of benzodiazepines is respiratory depression in patients who are not mechanically ventilated. They can also induce hypotension in patients with reduced intravascular volume. Risk of withdrawal symptoms is small. Benzodiazepines are effective in the treatment of status epilepticus,

but pharmacoresistance emerges over time and requires progressive increase in the rate of infusion of the drug. They do not have a significant effect on ICP.

Unlike propofol, benzodiazepines have an effective antidote in flumazenil, which is a benzodiazepine receptor antagonist with little or no agonist activity and a half-life of 0.5 to 1.3 hours. Its administration is free of negative cardiovascular effects but may be complicated by the occurrence of seizures. The risk of seizures after administration of flumazenil is relatively small, except in patients with a history of epilepsy or with a significantly reduced seizure threshold. Therefore, caution should be exercised when administering this medication to patients with acute brain disease.

Dexmedetomidine is a selective α_2-adrenergic receptor agonist. It produces effective sedation while preserving patient's alertness. Patients sedated with this medication are often easily aroused, so adequate neurological assessment may be performed without the need to temporarily discontinue the sedative infusion. Upon initial administration, this drug may produce transient mild hypertension followed by a temporary drop in BP. It has a short elimination half-life of approximately 2 hours, though this may be prolonged in patients with liver failure. Caution is recommended when using this medication in patients with severe bradycardia or abnormal cardiac conduction, in patients with a severely depressed cardiac ejection fraction, and in patients who are hypovolemic or hypotensive at the time of infusion.

Haloperidol is the drug of choice for patients with signs of psychosis. Intravenous doses of haloperidol may achieve successful control of agitated psychotic behavior within 20 minutes. The drug is fairly safe, but its use can be complicated by the appearance of extrapyramidal signs and (rarely) by neuroleptic malignant syndrome. Haloperidol should be used with caution in patients with prolongation of the QT interval. New-generation antipsychotics (atypical antipsychotics such as risperidone, olanzapine, and quetiapine) are also useful in the management of agitation and delirium. However, they can only be administered by the enteric route, and their therapeutic effect is slower, hence they should not be used to control acute severe agitation.

Opiates represent the mainstay of analgesic treatment in acutely ill neurological patients. Options include morphine, fentanyl, sufentanil, alfentanil, and codeine. They all produce analgesia, reduced level of consciousness, and respiratory depression. Hypotension may occur in hypovolemic patients or when using high doses of these medications. Fentanyl is preferred to morphine because it provokes fewer cardiovascular side effects and does not produce histamine release. Codeine is a much less potent agent, and its role is limited in the NICU. The action of opioids may be reversed by using naloxone, a competitive antagonist. Hypertension and cardiac arrhythmias are potential side effects of naloxone use. For milder forms of pain, nonsteroidal antiinflammatory agents (e.g., ketorolac), tramadol, and acetaminophen may be used. **Table 45.2** summarizes key pharmacokinetic and pharmacodynamic information for the most commonly used sedative and analgesic agents in the NICU.

Airway and Ventilatory Assistance

Acutely ill neurological patients typically develop respiratory failure because of inability to oxygenate or to sustain their

Table 45.2 Most Commonly Used Sedatives and Analgesics in the NICU

Drug	Therapeutic Class	Main Advantages	Main Disadvantages
Propofol	Sedative	Rapid sedation Rapid clearance Anticonvulsive Reduces ICP	Expensive Respiratory depression Accumulates over time Hypotension May lower CBF Hypertriglyceridemia Hypercaloric Lack of amnestic properties Infusion syndrome
Midazolam	Sedative	Rapid sedation Rapid clearance Anticonvulsive Amnestic and anxiolytic properties	Expensive Respiratory depression Clearance reduced in renal or liver failure Contraindicated in untreated glaucoma
Lorazepam	Sedative	Cheaper Otherwise similar to midazolam	Longer duration of action Risk of metabolic acidosis Otherwise similar to midazolam
Dexmedetomidine	Sedative	Relative preservation of arousal Minimal respiratory depression Analgesic and anxiolytic properties	Expensive Hypertension/hypotension Possible bradycardia
Haloperidol	Neuroleptic	Rapidly effective treatment for agitation No respiratory depression	Risk of extrapyramidal signs and NMS
Opioids	Analgesics	Rapidly effective analgesia	Respiratory depression Sedation Constipation Urinary retention Emesis Hypotension Histamine release (morphine)
NSAIDs	Analgesics	Lack of sedation Antiinflammatory	May increase risk of bleeding Possible renal toxicity
Tramadol	Analgesic	Less respiratory depression than opioids	Less potent than opioids May lower seizure threshold

CBF, Cerebral blood flow; *ICP,* intracranial pressure; *NICU,* neurological-neurosurgical intensive care unit; *NMS,* neuroleptic malignant syndrome; *NSAIDs,* nonsteroidal antiinflammatory drugs.

ventilatory needs. The most common causes for oxygenation failure in NICU patients are cardiogenic and neurogenic pulmonary edema. However, sudden hypoxia should always raise the suspicion for pulmonary embolism (PE). Aspiration pneumonia occurs frequently because of inability to protect the airway in patients with depressed level of consciousness and impaired cough reflex. Atelectasis may be a cause of hypoxia in patients with neuromuscular weakness. Hypercapnia is the hallmark of patients with ventilatory failure. Ventilatory insufficiency from upper airway collapse is encountered in patients with neuromuscular respiratory failure or coma.

At the time of endotracheal intubation, the two main complications in neurological patients are a rise in ICP and exacerbation of hypoxia. Rapid-sequence intubation is the safest approach for patients with increased ICP (Wijdicks and Borel, 1998). Rapid-sequence intubation proceeds in three phases: (1) preoxygenation to prevent worsening hypoxia during intubation—this can be achieved by providing effective bag-valve-mask (AMBU) ventilation; (2) pretreatment with drugs to mitigate the hemodynamic changes that may increase ICP upon intubation (e.g., lidocaine, thiopental); and (3) sequential administration of a potent sedative (e.g., propofol) and, when necessary, a rapidly acting nondepolarizing neuro-

muscular blocking agent (e.g., rocuronium, vecuronium). Succinylcholine should be avoided because it may increase ICP due to widespread muscle fasciculations, increased central venous pressure, and hypercarbia, and because it can produce dangerous hyperkalemia in patients with underlying muscle disease. In cases of TBI, it is also essential to maintain in-line stabilization of the cervical spine. When cervical spine injury is suspected, fiberoptic-assisted intubation is preferred.

The essential goal of mechanical ventilation is to assist the patient to achieve adequate gas exchange. There are two basic forms of mechanical ventilation: volume control and pressure control. *Volume-control ventilation* delivers a consistent preset volume of air with each ventilator breath. *Pressure-control ventilation* delivers a preset amount of pressure to the patient, with varying degrees of volume, depending on the amount of resistance in the system.

The modes of volume-control ventilation most frequently used in neurological and neurosurgical patients are assist/control (A/C) and synchronized intermittent mandatory ventilation (SIMV). In A/C ventilation, the ventilator will always deliver the preset air volume. In control mode, breaths are initiated by the machine and not influenced by the patient. The rate of these controlled breaths is determined in the ventilatory settings. In assist mode, the ventilator will deliver extra breaths of the same predetermined tidal volume every time the patient generates sufficient negative pressure during an attempted inspiration. In SIMV, the ventilator delivers breaths with full preset volume up to a prescribed rate. If the patient's inspiratory effort exceeds such preset rate, all additional breaths initiated by the patient (spontaneous breaths) will have a volume determined by the extent of the negative inspiratory pressure produced by the patient. The volume of this spontaneous breath may be adjusted by setting a support function on the ventilator called *pressure support*. Thus, pressure support is used in conjunction with SIMV to augment the patient's negative inspiratory force and increase the efficiency of the independent breaths produced by the patient. SIMV is well tolerated by patients and avoids deconditioning of respiratory muscles. Its main disadvantages include the possibility of developing high peak airway pressures, high rate of gas delivery in the early phase of inspiration (which may not be tolerated by agitated patients), and insufficient treatment of hypoxia in severely hypoxemic patients.

Pressure-control ventilation differs from volume control mode in that inspiratory and expiratory airway pressures are consistently regulated at the expense of variation in the delivered volume. Pressure-control ventilation is used most frequently in patients who are sedated and paralyzed. It requires setting the fraction of inspired oxygen (FIO_2), the ventilatory rate, and the pressure difference between inspiration and expiration.

In *pressure-support ventilation* (PSV), all breaths are triggered by the patient. The ventilator delivers a particular level of pressure support each time a breath is initiated; this pressure is delivered at the onset of inspiration. When the flow rate reaches 20% of its initial value, gas flow is terminated. This mode is often fairly comfortable for the conscious patient, as it closely approximates the flow characteristics of a normal breath. Since patients on a pressure-support ventilator may become hypopneic, they should be closely monitored with the help of adequately set apnea alarms.

Regardless of the ventilatory mode used, oxygenation depends upon the FIO_2 and the level of positive end-expiratory pressure (PEEP) provided. Increasing the FIO_2 increases the oxygen available for absorption by the pulmonary capillaries. Very high levels of FIO_2 (>0.5) may result in pulmonary oxygen toxicity. PEEP allows for tapering of the FIO_2 in many cases. The basic goal of PEEP is to prevent microatelectasis by keeping alveoli from collapsing at the end of expiration. This improves the efficiency of gaseous exchange by maximizing recruitment of lung units. The main danger of PEEP use is increasing intrathoracic pressure to levels that compromise venous return. This may result in hypotension unless intravascular filling pressures are augmented by volume expansion. High levels of PEEP may also produce tension pneumothorax. Finally, it is important to monitor the ICP when positive airway pressure is applied. Patients with decreased intracranial compliance may develop increases in ICP as intrathoracic pressure rises and imposes resistance to venous return. However, for the most part, relatively high levels of PEEP are well tolerated by euvolemic patients with intracranial hypertension.

Weaning from mechanical ventilation is usually achieved in critically ill neurological patients by decreasing the rate of mandatory breaths on SIMV or by using PSV. In fact, both methods can be combined in practice. A patient on SIMV can have the set rate decreased as clinical improvement occurs. If the patient has adequate spontaneous tidal volumes and no apneas, he or she may be switched to PSV, which consists of pressure support at the onset of inspiration and PEEP to prevent alveolar collapse and improve oxygenation. Subsequently, the amount of pressure support may be weaned until extubation is deemed safe.

In patients with acute brain disorders, level of consciousness may a limiting factor when considering extubation. Despite successful weaning, the stuporous patient may be considered unsafe for extubation because of concerns about airway safety. Keeping patients intubated once they have fulfilled the ventilatory criteria for extubation is a common but questionable practice. In patients with TBI, this practice may be associated with a higher risk of ventilator-associated complications (Coplin et al., 2000). Thus, safety of extubation in patients with adequate respiratory function but persistently depressed level of consciousness is a problem that demands further research (Manno et al., 2008).

Patients who fail extubation and those who are considered unsafe for an extubation trial require tracheostomy. The timing of a tracheostomy varies according to the patient's primary condition. Local airway complications increase with longer duration of endotracheal intubation. In addition, tracheostomy is more comfortable for patients than endotracheal intubation and provides better access for effective pulmonary toileting. The most common indications for tracheostomy in the NICU are persistent stupor or coma, severe impairment of cough reflex, and prolonged neuromuscular respiratory failure. Percutaneous tracheostomy has become the standard procedure in most ICUs. It is important to bear in mind that tracheostomies are reversible. Also, specially modified tracheostomy tubes that allow patients to vocalize and communicate are now available.

Pulmonary Complications

The main respiratory complications in critically ill neurological patients are pneumonia (either induced by aspiration or ventilator-associated), PE, atelectasis, and pulmonary edema (either cardiogenic or neurogenic). Aspiration is common in patients with depressed level of consciousness, seizures, or bulbar weakness. Patients who have been intubated for over 48 hours may develop ventilator-associated pneumonia, manifested by increased amount of thick secretions, fever, leukocytosis, new radiographic abnormalities, and increased PaO_2:FIO_2 ratio. Aspiration pneumonia should prompt coverage for anaerobes and gram-negative organisms. Coverage for ventilator-associated pneumonia will depend on the organisms and susceptibility most prevalent on each ICU.

Sudden development of unexplained hypoxia should be considered possible PE until proven otherwise. Patients with critical neurological illness are especially predisposed to the development of venous thromboembolism because of prolonged immobility. Tachypnea is often prominent in patients with PE. However, quadriparetic patients with high cervical lesions cannot develop this response, and oxygen desaturation associated with tachycardia may be the only manifestation in these patients. The differential diagnosis in cases of acute tachypnea and oxygen desaturation includes plugging of the airway by secretions. However, these patients typically also develop hypercapnia due to hypoventilation. If hypoxia is not resolved by airway suctioning and the situation remains unexplained after an emergent chest radiograph (to exclude new infiltrates, pneumothorax, or lobar collapse), the patient should undergo specific studies to rule out PE. At present, CT angiograms are the diagnostic modality of choice. The possibility of deep venous thrombosis (DVT) should also be investigated by venous Doppler of the lower extremities. The treatment of venous thromboembolism may be particularly challenging in acute neurological patients. Patients with large ischemic strokes or intracranial hemorrhages are at increased risk for complications from IV heparin. When systemic anticoagulation is deemed strictly contraindicated, insertion of a vena cava filter may be a reasonable alternative. Patients with massive PE may require endovascular maneuvers to mechanically remove the clot or intraarterial infusion of a thrombolytic agent.

Atelectasis is very common in patients receiving mechanical ventilation. Large areas of atelectasis or lobar collapse may produce profound hypoxia. Mucous plugging of the airway is common among critically ill patients. Increasing levels of PEEP are often used to treat collapsed lung regions. Physical measures including suctioning, postural drainage, and external percussion may be effective, but bronchoscopic suction and lavage are necessary in severe cases.

Interpretation of pulmonary edema is more complex in critically ill neurological patients than in the general population of ICU patients. While most cases of pulmonary edema will be due to cardiac failure, neurogenic pulmonary edema may occur after acute SAH, TBI, and other neurological catastrophes associated with massive surge of central sympathetic output. Neurogenic pulmonary edema is successfully treated using high levels of PEEP. Cardiogenic pulmonary edema should be treated by ameliorating cardiac workload (through diuresis and vasodilatation) and providing adequate levels of supplemental oxygen.

Cardiovascular Care and Blood Pressure Management

Cardiac disorders are common in critically ill neurological patients, and they may precede or accompany the neurological illness. They are often related to the massive catecholamine release associated with the acute brain insult (Banki et al., 2005). The most common forms of cardiac complications in the NICU are acute coronary syndrome, cardiac arrhythmias, and congestive heart failure.

Acute Coronary Syndrome

Electrocardiographic (ECG) and clinical abnormalities suggestive of myocardial ischemia are fairly common in patients with acute brain injury (e.g., large ischemic stroke, SAH, large intraparenchymal hematoma, TBI with contusions, status epilepticus). Typical ECG abnormalities in patients with acute brain damage include symmetrically inverted T waves (**Fig. 45.5**) and sometimes ST-segment elevation across all the precordial leads. Elevation of serum troponin levels should be considered indicative of myocardial injury, whereas elevation of serum creatinine kinase is much less specific in patients with acute brain damage (Woodruff et al., 2003). Yet, troponin elevation is seen in patients with SAH as an expression of

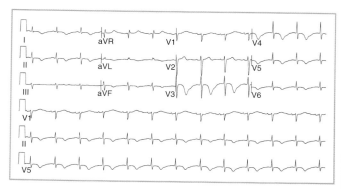

Fig. 45.5 Electrocardiographic changes in a patient with acute aneurysmal subarachnoid hemorrhage. Notice diffuse repolarization abnormalities in the precordial leads.

ventricular dysfunction secondary to the neurogenic (adrenergic-induced) injury (Deibert et al., 2003).

It is always difficult to define optimal hemodynamic goals in patients with coexistent myocardial ischemia and acute neurological conditions that require maintenance of adequate CPP, such as acute ischemic stroke and SAH at risk for vasospasm. In these patients, lowering the BP to the levels commonly used as goals in most patients with acute myocardial ischemia may further compromise cerebral perfusion and precipitate infarction in areas of ischemic penumbra. Anticoagulation or IV glycoprotein IIb/IIIa inhibitors may be contraindicated early after an extensive ischemic stroke, in patients with a large intraparenchymal hematoma, or shortly after a neurosurgical procedure. Percutaneous coronary angioplasty and stenting may be considered, but limitations on the use of aspirin and clopidogrel after the intervention may increase the risk of acute in-stent thrombosis. Induced diuresis is indicated to reduce afterload in patients with depressed left ventricular ejection fraction, but it should be closely monitored; hypovolemia may induce cerebral ischemia in patients with vasospasm or areas of ischemic penumbra.

Cardiac Arrhythmias

Cardiac arrhythmias in acute neurological patients may be due to preexisting cardiac disease. They may also be responsible for the acute neurological disorder, as occurs in patients with atrial fibrillation presenting with embolic stroke. On the other hand, arrhythmias and conduction abnormalities may be due to acute brain disease. Decreased high rate viability, increased risk for arrhythmias, and even increased risk for sudden death have been documented in patients with insular strokes (Abboud et al., 2006). Cardiac arrhythmias may also develop as a complication of seizures. Dysregulation of autonomic function may provoke life-threatening arrhythmias in patients with Guillain-Barré syndrome.

Profound bradycardia in the ICU may be seen in the context of autonomic dysreflexia, after carotid stenting (from stretching of the carotid body), and with increasing ICP (Cushing reflex). Cases of symptomatic bradycardia with hemodynamic compromise should be treated emergently with IV atropine. Immediately after controlling the emergency, treatment should be focused on the underlying cause of the bradycardia. *Autonomic dysreflexia* is a severe complication of high cervical spinal cord lesions, typically consisting of profound bradycardia and extreme hypertension, often precipitated by distension of the viscera, manipulations (e.g., bladder catheterizations), or a change in body position (e.g., turning). Autonomic dysreflexia caused by high spinal cord injuries does not have an effective treatment, so episodes of autonomic imbalance must be prevented by carefully avoiding the situations that precipitate them. The bradycardia observed after carotid stenting is transient, and in most cases hemodynamic stability may be preserved with adequate fluid therapy. Bradycardia due to increased ICP demands immediate treatment of the primary problem. The patient should be emergently assessed for the possibility of hydrocephalus. If the rise in ICP is secondary to cerebral edema, then osmotherapy, corticosteroids, or hyperventilation should be instituted as needed.

Tachycardias in the NICU are most commonly supraventricular. They include paroxysmal supraventricular tachycardia, atrial fibrillation, and atrial flutter. Treatment does not vary from that applied to other critically ill patients. When sustained ventricular tachycardia occurs, patients should be investigated for the possibility of myocardial ischemia, underlying cardiac disease, or prolonged QT interval.

Congestive Heart Failure

Administration of large amounts of IV fluids may precipitate volume overload and pulmonary edema in patients with underlying cardiac insufficiency. This is common among patients with SAH who receive hemodynamic augmentation therapy for symptomatic vasospasm. It is also a frequent complication in patients with acute ischemic stroke aggressively treated with fluids to maximize collateral flow in an attempt to preserve an area of ischemic penumbra. Cautious induced diuresis is indicated in these patients when the degree of pulmonary edema is severe enough to produce hypoxemia.

Apical ballooning syndrome is a characteristic form of cardiomyopathy seen after acute neurological insults (Lee et al., 2006). Sudden sympathetic hyperstimulation of the myocardium causes a specific pattern of myocardial stunning (Prasad et al., 2008), and its diagnosis depends on echocardiographic demonstration of apical hypokinesis or akinesis with sparing of basal segments. Consequently, the heart takes on the form of an octopus catcher pot (*takotsubo* in Japanese, hence the name *takotsubo cardiomyopathy* sometimes given to this condition). Patients with apical ballooning syndrome have reductions in left ventricular ejection fraction and may develop acute congestive heart failure with pulmonary edema. The presentation may also mimic myocardial ischemia. Cardiac function typically returns to baseline after 2 or 3 weeks (Lee et al., 2006; Prasad et al., 2008).

Blood Pressure Management

BP management represents one of the most crucial aspects of neurocritical care. The three main goals of BP management in critically ill neurological and neurosurgical patients are to ensure adequate cerebral perfusion, prevent intracranial bleeding, and avoid exacerbation of cerebral edema. These goals must often be balanced in individual cases in which the risk of hypoperfusion and worsening ischemia coexist with the danger of new or enlarging hemorrhage and progression of brain swelling. Although guidelines and practice

Table 45.3 Guidelines for Blood Pressure Management in the Most Common Conditions Treated in the NICU

Diagnosis	Recommendation
Acute ischemic stroke	Keep <180/110 mm Hg if thrombolysis Treat only BP >220/120 if no thrombolysis
Intracerebral hemorrhage	Keep SBP <180 and MAP <130 mm Hg (ideal SBP <160 and MAP <110 mm Hg)
Subarachnoid hemorrhage	Keep SBP <160 mm Hg before aneurysm treated Do not lower BP after aneurysm treated
Traumatic brain injury	Keep adequate MAP to maintain CPP >60 mm Hg

BP, Blood pressure; *CPP*, cerebral perfusion pressure; *MAP*, mean arterial pressure; *NICU*, neurological-neurosurgical intensive care unit; *SBP*, systolic blood pressure.

parameters have been published to guide BP treatment in various acute neurological conditions (**Table 45.3**), there are still areas of debate in regard to what should be considered optimal BP targets in patients with some of the most common disorders treated in the NICU.

ACUTE ISCHEMIC STROKE

Sudden and profound reductions of BP are associated with neurological decline in patients with acute ischemic stroke (Oliveira-Filho et al., 2003). This is likely related to insufficient perfusion in areas already affected by ischemic penumbra. In fact, elevation of BP appears to be a protective physiological response that occurs after occlusion of a cerebral vessel, as suggested by the spontaneous resolution of hypertension in patients who achieve successful recanalization (Mattle et al., 2005). Furthermore, low BP (diastolic BP <70, systolic BP <155, or MAP <100 mm Hg) on initial evaluation in the emergency department and greater BP fluctuations within the first 3 hours have been shown to correlate with increased 90-day mortality in patients with acute cerebral ischemic infarction (Stead et al., 2005; Stead et al., 2006).

Current practice guidelines advocate a very conservative approach to treating hypertension after acute ischemic stroke. In patients ineligible for thrombolysis, antihypertensive therapy is only recommended for patients with systolic BP higher than 220 mm Hg or diastolic BP higher than 120 mm Hg (Adams, Jr. et al., 2007). Intermittent doses of IV labetalol or continuous infusion of nicardipine are the preferred treatment options; when diastolic BP exceeds 140 mm Hg, sodium nitroprusside should be infused instead. The initial objective of treatment should be to reduce the BP by 10% to 15%. However, it is important to acknowledge that this permissive approach to hypertension is not based on direct evidence from randomized trials. In fact, preliminary data indicate that modest BP reduction early after cerebral ischemia could actually be beneficial (Potter et al., 2009), so this important clinical matter demands more investigation.

In patients eligible for thrombolytic therapy, BP management should be more aggressive to limit the risk of hemorrhagic complications associated with use of the fibrinolytic agent. The BP should be below 185/110 mm Hg before starting thrombolysis. After administration of the fibrinolytic drug, BP must be strictly maintained below 180/105 mm Hg. Failure to control the BP according to this parameter has been repeatedly shown to be associated with increased risk of symptomatic intracranial hemorrhagic and poor functional outcome.

There is limited but promising evidence suggesting that pharmacological elevation of BP may be beneficial for certain patients with acute ischemic stroke (Mistri et al., 2006). Further research is needed to determine the safety of this intervention and which patients could be optimal candidates for this type of aggressive hemodynamic treatment.

INTRACEREBRAL HEMORRHAGE

The treatment of hypertension in patients with spontaneous (hypertensive) intraparenchymal hematomas is more controversial. There is abundant (Fogelholm et al., 1997; Leira et al., 2004; Terayama et al., 1997) although not uniform (Brott et al., 1997; Jauch et al., 2006; Qureshi et al., 1999) evidence that extreme hypertension is associated with greater risk of hematoma expansion, a major determinant of poor outcome and increased mortality in ICH (Davis et al., 2006). Meanwhile, solid demonstration that areas of hypoperfusion are frequently present around parenchymal hematomas (Kidwell et al., 2001; Mayer et al., 1998; Rosand et al., 2002) has supported the argument that aggressive BP reduction could precipitate ischemia in these regions. This theoretical risk is, however, not substantiated by PET studies showing decreased oxygen extraction fraction in the hypoperfused perihematoma tissue (as opposed to the increased oxygen extraction that would be expected in areas of ischemic penumbra) (Zazulia et al., 2001) and preserved CBF in those regions after acute BP reduction (Powers et al., 2001).

There are valid arguments both in favor of and against aggressive BP reduction in acute ICH. Current guidelines advise keeping the SBP ideally below 160 mm Hg and the MAP ideally below 110 mm Hg unless there is suspicion of intracranial hypertension, in which case ICP monitoring is recommended to target therapy to maintain CPP between 60 and 80 mm Hg (Broderick et al., 2007). The initial phases of ongoing randomized controlled trials have shown that more aggressive BP reduction is feasible and most likely safe (Anderson et al., 2008; Qureshi et al., 2010).

SUBARACHNOID HEMORRHAGE

In patients with acute aneurysmal SAH, it is often recommended to keep a systolic BP below 160 mm Hg until the ruptured aneurysm is secured in order to prevent re-bleeding. It should be noted that this widespread practice of aggressive BP lowering is not based on solid scientific data. After the aneurysm is secured, BP should not be lowered, since these patients are at risk for delayed ischemia from vasospasm. Hemodynamic augmentation therapy, often including the use of vasopressors, is indicated in patients with symptomatic vasospasm (Rabinstein et al., 2010).

TRAUMATIC HEAD INJURY

Maintenance of an adequate CPP is one of the principal therapeutic goals in the intensive care of severe TBI patients, since secondary ischemic insults are known to have a major detrimental impact on prognosis (Sarrafzadeh et al., 2001). It is advisable to keep the CPP above 60 mm Hg, although it is

unclear whether raising the MAP or lowering the ICP should be the main therapeutic strategy to achieve this goal (Brain Trauma Foundation, 2007). Aggressive fluid resuscitation is the mainstay of hemodynamic treatment in TBI. Vasopressors should be reserved for patients with persistent hypotension after aggressive fluid replacement.

Fluid and Electrolytes

Acute renal failure in acutely ill neurological or neurosurgical patients is most commonly iatrogenic. Mannitol can rapidly cause prerenal azotemia when adequate hydration is not provided to compensate for the fluid lost from osmotic diuresis. This complication can be reliably avoided by adjusting the fluid intake to prevent negative fluid balance, while monitoring serum osmolality. If serum osmolality exceeds 320 mOsm/kg, mannitol infusion is typically withheld to protect renal function. If continuation of osmotherapy is indispensable, mannitol may be continued with relatively low risk of kidney failure, so long as concomitant aggressive hydration is provided. Hypertonic saline may be a valuable alternative in these cases; it is a safer choice than mannitol in patients with chronic renal insufficiency. Radiocontrast-induced nephropathy can be prevented by preemptive hydration, *N*-acetylcysteine, and bicarbonate infusion (Merten et al., 2004; Tepel et al., 2000). Acute interstitial nephritis from drug toxicity (e.g., antibiotics) and (less commonly) pyelonephritis (in patients with chronic indwelling catheters) are also causes of acute renal failure in the NICU.

When renal failure is established, it is essential that the neurointensivist cooperate with the consulting nephrologist to maximize the safety of renal replacement therapy (dialysis). Sudden fluid shifts and changes in BP that would be inconsequential in other patients may have dramatic detrimental effects in patients with cerebral edema or cerebral hypoperfusion. In patients with renal failure, it is also important to closely monitor the free levels of anticonvulsive drugs. These patients not only have heightened risk of developing toxic complications from decreased elimination of the drug, but rapid clearance of the anticonvulsant during dialysis may increase the risk of seizures.

Hyponatremia is the most common electrolyte imbalance encountered in critically ill neurological patients. The two most common mechanisms of hyponatremia in these patients are cerebral salt-wasting syndrome (CSWS) and the syndrome of inappropriate secretion of antidiuretic hormone (SIADH) (Rabinstein and Wijdicks, 2003a). Both mechanisms produce hypotonic hyponatremia with high concentration of urinary sodium (secondary to increased sodium excretion in CSWS and increased water reabsorption in SIADH). In fact, determination of extracellular fluid volume remains the only reliable distinguishing feature between these two conditions: SIADH is a state of volume *expansion*, while CSWS is a state of volume *depletion* (**Table 45.4**). The practical importance of this concept needs to be highlighted because fluid restriction—adequate therapy for SIADH—may be enormously deleterious in patients with CSWS, as is the case in SAH. Symptomatic acute hyponatremia requires tightly controlled infusion of hypertonic saline. Excessively rapid correction of profound chronic hyponatremia may precipitate severe osmotic myelinolysis. The rate of correction should not exceed 10 mmol/L over any 24-hour period to avoid this potentially devastating

Table 45.4 Clinical and Laboratory Features of CSWS and SIADH

Variable	CSWS	SIADH
Extracellular fluid volume	↓	↑
Body weight	↓	↑
Fluid balance	Negative	Positive
Urine volume	↔ or ↑	↔ or ↓
Tachycardia	+	–
Hematocrit	↑	↔
Albumin	↑	↔
Serum bicarbonate	↑	↔ or ↓
Blood urea nitrogen	↑	↔ or ↓
Serum uric acid	↔ or ↓	↓
Urinary sodium	↑	↑
Sodium balance	Negative	Neutral or positive
CVP/PCWP	↓	↔ or slightly ↑

↔, Absent or minor variable change; ↓, decreased; ↑, increased; *CSWS,* Cerebral salt-wasting syndrome; *CVP,* central venous pressure; *PCWP,* pulmonary capillary wedge pressure; *SIADH,* syndrome of inappropriate secretion of antidiuretic hormone.

complication (Laureno and Karp, 1997). **Fig. 45.6** presents an algorithm for the diagnosis and management of hyponatremia in critically ill neurological patients.

Hypernatremia in the NICU is most often produced by therapeutic interventions (e.g., mannitol without sufficient fluid replacement, infusion of hypertonic saline) or diabetes insipidus (DI). Focal brain lesions (most frequently tumors or trauma) or surgery involving the sellar/suprasellar region are the typical causes of DI. Profound DI is also seen at the time of brain death. Diagnosis of DI hinges on the finding of polyuria (characteristically > than 250–300 ML/h for ≥ 2 consecutive hours) with very dilute urine (specific gravity <1.010, urine osmolality <250 mOsm/kg). Treatment demands aggressive fluid replacement. Central DI responds rapidly to administration of vasopressin or desmopressin acetate (DDAVP). Vasopressin is short-acting (2-4 hours), and the recommended dose is 2 to 5 units subcutaneously or intramuscularly every 4 hours. Desmopressin acetate has a longer duration of action and should be administered cautiously in postsurgical patients because, in those cases, DI tends to resolve spontaneously within days or even hours of its presentation. The recommended dose is 0.5 to 4 μg IV or subcutaneously every 12 hours. Serum and urine osmolalities and serum electrolytes should be checked every 2 to 4 hours in every patient with DI.

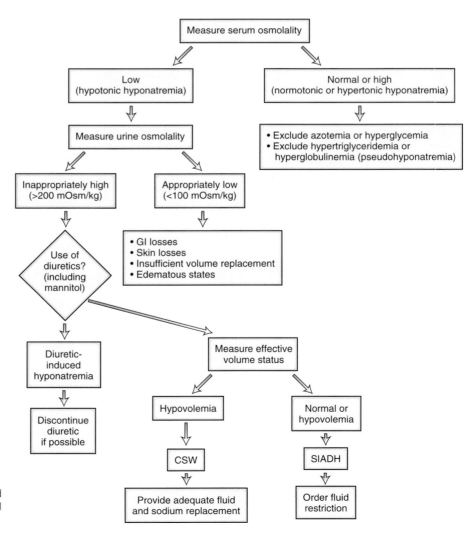

Fig. 45.6 Algorithm for the diagnosis and management of hyponatremia in critically ill neurological patients.

Nutrition and Metabolic Derangements

Adequate nutrition is essential for the recovery of critically ill patients, including those with primary acute neurological conditions. Depressed level of consciousness and abnormal swallowing function are very prevalent in NICU patients, who consequently often require tube feedings. Meanwhile, gastroparesis is also common and may increase the risk of aspiration in patients receiving enteral nutrition. This potential risk demands close monitoring of gastric residuals and positioning of the feeding tube in the distal part of the stomach or first portion of the duodenum. Agents that promote gastric motility (e.g., metoclopramide) may be added in the most severe cases (Booth et al., 2002).

Daily caloric requirement is calculated using the Harris Benedict equation to estimate basal energy expenditure (BEE):

$$\text{For men: BEE} = 66.5 + (13.75 \times W) + (5 \times H) - (6.78 \times A)$$

$$\text{For women: BEE} = 655 + (9.56 \times W) + (1.85 \times H) - (4.68 \times A)$$

For both equations, W is body weight in kilograms, H is height in centimeters, and A is age in years. This is often operationally translated into approximately 25 to 30 kcal/kg/day. Nutritional requirement may be adjusted to the particular disease and nutritional status indicators. For instance, sepsis may require increasing nutritional support by 30%, whereas high-caloric feeding should be avoided in Guillain-Barré syndrome and myasthenia gravis. Adequacy of nutritional support is better assessed using prealbumin (half-life of 2-3 days) rather than albumin (half-life of 20 days). Working closely with a nutritionist specialized in critical care patients is highly advisable to make adequate adjustments.

Enteral feeding is preferred whenever possible to help maintain the integrity of the intestinal mucosal lining. It is recommended to start feeding patients early (ideally within 48 hours of admission); early feeding has been associated with a trend toward better survival and less disability in patients with TBI (Yanagawa et al., 2002). The optimal timing of percutaneous gastrostomy in neurological patients has not been sufficiently studied. There is some evidence that gastrostomy should be performed in patients with dysphagia from stroke persisting after 14 days (Norton et al., 1996).

Hyperglycemia is the most frequent metabolic derangement in critically ill neurological patients. There is solid evidence that hyperglycemia activates neurotoxic oxidative and inflammatory responses after acute ischemia. In patients with acute ischemic stroke, hyperglycemia has been associated with increased risk of hemorrhagic transformation and hyperacute worsening and lower rates of recanalization after thrombolysis (Alvarez-Sabin et al., 2004; Leigh et al., 2004; Ribo et al., 2005). It has also been found to correlate with infarct expansion and worse functional outcome (Baird et al., 2003; Bruno et al., 2002). Similarly, functional recovery is poorer in hyperglycemic patients with ICH and SAH (Frontera et al., 2006a; Passero et al., 2003). Intensive insulin therapy to maintain strict normoglycemia is no longer recommended for critically ill patients, after this practice led to increased mortality in a large randomized trial (Finfer et al., 2009). However, strict blood sugar control could decrease the rate of critical illness polyneuropathy (Van den et al., 2005). In the NICU, intensive insulin therapy carries the risk of inducing neuroglycopenia (with the ensuing risk of energy failure), which may occur in patients with acute brain insults even with serum glucose concentrations within the usual normal range (Godoy et al., 2010; Oddo et al., 2008). Therefore, the treatment of hyperglycemia must be particularly cautious in patients with acute brain disease, and serum glucose concentrations below 100 to 110 mg/dL should be avoided.

Fever and Infections

Fever in a patient with acute brain disease demands prompt diagnostic investigation to determine its cause and symptomatic treatment to avoid the deleterious impact of hyperthermia on the injured brain. Experimental models have consistently shown that even mild hyperthermia worsens cerebral damage after ischemia or trauma (Baena et al., 1997; Dietrich et al., 1996; Kim et al., 1996). Fever has been associated with poor functional outcome in patients with ischemic infarction (Reith et al., 1996; Wang et al., 2000), ICH (Schwarz et al., 2000), SAH (Oliveira-Filho et al., 2001), and TBI (Jiang et al., 2002). Increased metabolic expenditure, exacerbation of excitotoxicity, and elevated ICP may be responsible for the detrimental effects of hyperthermia (Rossi et al., 2001; Thompson et al., 2003).

Fever is very prevalent among NICU patients. Although disturbances in central thermoregulation occur frequently in patients with acute brain disorders (Rabinstein et al., 2007), infections are a common cause of fever in the NICU and should always be excluded (Commichau et al., 2003). Pneumonia, urinary tract infection, and bloodstream infection are the most frequent infectious complications (Dettenkofer et al., 1999). Ventriculitis must always be ruled out in patients with ventriculostomy. The appearance of fever in an NICU patient should be evaluated with cultures of blood, urine, respiratory secretions (ideally collected by bronchoalveolar lavage), and CSF (always in patients with ventriculostomy and when deemed clinically indicated in others). Chest radiograph and urine microscopic analysis are also pertinent. CT scan of the sinuses may be added to the diagnostic evaluation in febrile patients who have been intubated for several days. CT scan of the abdomen and pelvis is sometimes necessary to detect abscesses, pancreatitis, or cholecystitis. The skin should be thoroughly searched for signs of cellulitis or phlebitis. Osteomyelitis and discitis must be included in the differential diagnosis of fever after spine surgery.

When an infection is suspected, empirical antibiotic therapy is reasonable. It should cover for the most likely responsible organisms, depending on the patient's risk factors and the local microbiological resistance patterns of the ICU. Empirical antibiotics may be discontinued after 3 days if no infection is documented. It is always prudent to consider changing indwelling catheters (central venous, arterial, bladder, ventricular) in persistently febrile patients.

Drug reactions, DVT, ethanol withdrawal, pancreatitis, and gout are relatively common causes of noninfectious fever in the NICU. Drug fever is most frequently caused by phenytoin in neurological patients. Signs of anticonvulsant hypersensitivity syndrome (rash, lymphadenopathy, hepatomegaly, eosinophilia, elevation of liver transaminases) must be readily recognized, since failure to discontinue the culprit medication promptly may have the devastating consequence of Stevens-Johnson syndrome (Schlienger and Shear, 1998). Detailed physical examination, venous Doppler, and measurement of liver and pancreatic enzymes should be performed in NICU patients with fever of unclear cause. In chronically immobile patients (especially those with spinal cord injury), heterotopic ossification may be a cause of persistent fever; it may be suspected by marked elevation of the C-reactive protein and sedimentation rate and confirmed by bone scintigraphy.

Central fever remains a diagnosis of exclusion. It occurs most frequently in patients with SAH, and in those patients it is associated with increased risk of vasospasm (Oliveira-Filho et al., 2001; Rabinstein et al., 2007). Patients with central fever often have prolonged hyperthermia with failure to return to normal body temperature, as opposed to the spikes of fever followed by normothermia typically observed with infections. Among patients with TBI, high fevers may be accompanied by other manifestations of *paroxysmal sympathetic hyperactivity* (tachycardia, hypertension, diaphoresis, dystonia) (Rabinstein, 2007).

Multiple measures can be used to normalize body temperature in febrile patients. Antipyretic medications (acetaminophen, ibuprofen) are sufficient in milder cases. However, mechanical cooling methods must be added in patients with more severe or refractory hyperthermia. Ice packs, air- or water-circulating cooling blankets, and effective cooling vests are alternative methods of conductive cooling (Mayer et al., 2004; Seder and Van der Kloot, 2009). Endovascular cooling devices may offer greater control of temperature modulation but require placement of a central venous catheter (De Georgia et al., 2004; Seder and Van der Kloot, 2009). Patients should be monitored for the appearance of shivering, which can be treated with warming gloves, buspirone, meperidine (in patients without high risk for seizures), magnesium infusion, or dexmedetomidine in patients who are awake, but it may necessitate neuromuscular paralysis when severe.

Hematological Complications

The risk of DVT is increased in immobilized patients. The incidence of clinical DVT after acute ischemic stroke ranges between 1% and 5%, and clinical PE occurs in 0.5% to 3.5% of these patients (Kamphuisen et al., 2005). However, the incidence of subclinical DVT is much higher when assessed by ultrasound, venography, or nuclear scans (Kamphuisen et al., 2005). The risk of DVT is also increased after craniotomy (Hamilton et al., 1994), ICH (Lacut et al., 2005), and in patients with severe neuromuscular weakness. The main diagnostic test for DVT is noninvasive bedside vascular ultrasound (venous Doppler). Physical examination is relatively insensitive to detect DVT in acutely ill hospitalized patients. When PE is suspected, spiral CT angiogram of the chest should be performed.

Early mobilization should be promoted in all patients. Options for prevention of thromboembolic complications in immobilized patients include mechanical methods (compressive stockings, intermittent pneumatic compression) and antithrombotics. Current evidence supports the use of subcutaneous anticoagulants for most patients with acute ischemic stroke (Adams, Jr. et al., 2007; Kamphuisen et al., 2005) and after craniotomy (Iorio and Agnelli, 2000). Unfortunately,

similar data are not available to guide the management of thromboprophylaxis in patients with ICH or large ischemic cerebral infarction. Enoxaparin (40 mg daily) was found to be superior to unfractionated heparin (5000 units twice daily) in one randomized controlled trial of patients with acute ischemic stroke (Sherman et al., 2007). In cases of documented DVT and high risk of hemorrhagic complications from anticoagulation, placement of a Greenfield filter in the inferior vena cava is a valuable alternative.

The optimal hematocrit level in critically ill neurological patients has not been adequately studied and probably varies according to the underlying primary disease process. Mild hemodilution may improve the rheological properties of the cerebral circulation, but excessive anemia may compromise oxygen delivery. Transfusions are only indicated for general critically ill patients when the hemoglobin concentration is lower than 7 g/dL. However, the appropriateness of this conservative practice in patients with acute brain damage (who may be particularly sensitive to local or regional hypoxia) remains to be established.

Thrombocytopenia in the NICU is most commonly associated with exposure to heparin or other drugs (e.g., valproic acid, antibiotics). Heparin-induced thrombocytopenia may be diagnosed by the presence of circulating serum antibodies to platelet factor 4. Discontinuation of heparin results in prompt normalization of the platelet count. In patients with heparin-induced thrombocytopenia who still have indication for continuing therapeutic anticoagulation, a direct thrombin inhibitor (recombinant hirudin or argatroban) should be used instead of heparin.

Cerebral Protection after Cardiac Arrest

Therapeutic hypothermia has been shown to improve clinical outcomes after witnessed out-of-hospital ventricular fibrillation arrest (Bernard et al., 2002; the Hypothermia after Cardiac Arrest Study Group, 2002), and induction of hypothermia has become standard of care for the management of this condition. In fact, many centers have adopted the practice of inducing hypothermia after all cardiac arrests, regardless of the initial rhythm. Therapeutic hypothermia serves primarily as a neuroprotective modality, allowing more patients to recover awareness and improving functional outcomes among survivors.

Protocols for induction of hypothermia after cardiac arrest may vary across centers (e.g., methods of induction ranging from cooling blankets and ice packs to more sophisticated surface or intravascular cooling devices), but there is uniformity of criteria on its main principles: (1) cooling should be started as soon as feasible and continued for 24 hours, (2) target temperature should be ideally maintained at 33°C, (3) shivering is treated with paralytic agents, and (4) rewarming should take place over 12 to 18 hours.

The degree of hypothermia used for treatment of cardiac arrest is usually well tolerated. Electrolyte imbalances, especially hypokalemia during induction and hyperkalemia upon rewarming, are the most common side effects. Hypotension may result from increased diuresis due to peripheral vasoconstriction. Bradycardia is frequent but usually asymptomatic. Life-threatening arrhythmias are rare, even in patients with myocardial ischemia. The risk of pneumonia is frankly increased when the duration of hypothermia exceeds 48 hours but not in cardiac arrest patients cooled for 1 day. Hyperglycemia from decreased insulin sensitivity, reduced intestinal motility, and mild coagulopathy (very infrequently leading to clinically significant bleeding) are also side effects of hypothermia.

References

The complete reference list is available online at www.expertconsult.com.

Chapter **46**

Principles of Neurosurgery

Marvin Bergsneider, Garni Barkhoudarian

The basic principles of neurosurgery include but are not limited to:

- Establishing an accurate diagnosis
- Exercising proper patient selection for surgery
- Thoughtful preoperative surgical planning
- Meticulous surgical technique
- Diligent postoperative care

Although these principles have remained constant over the past century, the practice of neurosurgery has evolved tremendously since the days of Cushing, Dandy, and Penfield.* This dramatic change has occurred as a result of a convergence of advancing technology combined with the exponential growth of neuroscience knowledge and discoveries (Apuzzo, 1996; Kaibara et al., 2000).

No one chapter can even begin to cover the gamut of neurosurgical practice in any meaningful way. This chapter is aimed at the practicing clinical neurologist who interacts with neurosurgeon colleagues. Knowing if, when, and which neurosurgical subspecialists to refer patients to can improve outcome as well as avoid unnecessary utilization of healthcare resources. In the best of both worlds, the neurologist can play a key role in the diagnostic and perioperative management plus the long-term follow-up of patients. This paradigm already exists and works well in many brain tumor programs where the neuro-oncologist is an integral member of the surgical decision-making and postoperative management team (Yasargil et al., 2004).

There are countless "principles" of neurosurgery, ranging from broad to highly specific. Here, the basic principles noted earlier will be individually addressed, with an emphasis on highlighting intrinsic differences between the complementary and sometimes overlapping fields of neurology and neurosurgery.

Establishing the Diagnosis

Inherent to surgical intervention, the vast majority of neurosurgical consultations involve diagnostic neuroimaging. In most cases, referral to a neurosurgeon occurs as a consequence of abnormal imaging results, already creating a unique patient-physician relationship. The neurosurgeon is often confronted with the situation of deciding whether the patient's symptoms or signs, if any, correlate with the neuroimaging findings. This is in stark contrast to neurological practice, in which certain diagnoses such as headache and seizures may not receive diagnostic imaging initially or even at all. Although the finding of a neuroimaging abnormality is not a prerequisite for neurosurgical intervention (such as movement disorder surgery), neuroimaging is required nevertheless (Britz et al., 1995; Kent et al., 1994; and Nijeholt et al., 1998).

The reliance upon diagnostic neuroimaging has changed neurosurgical residency training, necessitating that neurosurgeons achieve a high level of diagnostic neuroradiological competence. For the neurosurgeon, the diagnostic process (and surgical planning) typically hinges upon the imaging, and therefore a considerable amount of time is devoted to carefully, personally reviewing the imaging studies. As a result, when referring a patient for neurosurgical evaluation, it is important to emphasize to the patient that the actual imaging study be physically available for review at the time of the neurosurgical consultation.

It is important to understand the difference between standard diagnostic imaging and the high-resolution neuroimaging required for neurosurgical decision making. For example, routine diagnostic magnetic resonance imaging (MRI) studies of the brain are performed with relatively thick 5-mm slices,

---

*Davey (1999), Fahlbusch, Buchfelder, and Schrell (1985), Ljunggren (1982), Penfield (1935), Preul and Feindel (1991), Preul et al. (1993), Sano (1981), and Shrivastava et al. (2003).

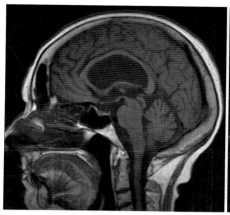 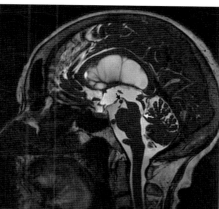

Fig. 46.1 Imaging aqueductal stenosis. *Left,* Midsagittal noncontrast T1-weighted magnetic resonance image (MRI) showing enlarged lateral ventricle, bowing of corpus callosum, and normal-sized fourth ventricle. Cerebral aqueduct appears patent. *Right,* Corresponding constructive interference in steady state (CISS) MRI reveals a distal cerebral aqueduct occlusive membrane *(white arrow).* Premesencephalic cistern has favorable anatomy with a posteriorly placed basilar artery bifurcation *(black arrow)* for endoscopic third ventriculostomy. *(From Bergsneider, M., Miller, C., Vespa, P.M., et al, 2008. Surgical management of adult hydrocephalus. Neurosurgery 62, 643-660.)*

with 2.5-mm skip between slices. Although generally adequate to detect lesions 4 mm in size or larger, partial volume averaging can obscure fine anatomical detail such as the relationship of arteries, veins, and cranial nerves to the lesion. For example, although the diagnosis of hydrocephalus may be obvious on routine diagnostic imaging, establishing the etiology of the ventriculomegaly may require high-resolution constructive interference in steady state (CISS) imaging (**Fig. 46.1**). In this case, a diagnosis of occult aqueductal stenosis would dramatically change the treatment, with endoscopic third ventriculostomy being the preferred treatment rather than a ventriculoperitoneal shunt.

With routine "diagnostic" imaging, the number of different MRI sequences is often limited by the concept of the study being a screening exam rather than one honing in on a certain differential diagnosis. For example, atypical arachnoid cysts can be differentiated from epidermoid cysts if repeat imaging includes a diffusion-weighted imaging (DWI) study (Tsuruda et al., 1990). In this case, an arachnoid cyst may not require referral to a neurosurgeon, whereas the epidermoid cyst should. Consultation with a neuroradiologist, if needed, could lead to proper imaging studies being performed prior to possible neurosurgical consultation.

In other cases, routine diagnostic imaging may be adequate for establishing a diagnosis but inadequate for neurosurgical decision making. In some cases, additional imaging modalities may be required, such as computed tomography (CT) imaging of bony anatomy to supplement abnormal soft-tissue findings on MRI. In other cases, special high-resolution or unique imaging sequences may be required (Barnett et al., 1993; Curtin and Hirsch, 1992). Although beyond the scope of this chapter, suffice it to state that a brief discussion with the neurosurgeon—prior to referral—may in some cases lead to essential imaging studies being obtained prior to the consultation. This may make for a much more productive and useful consultation, obviating the need to have the patient return for an otherwise unnecessary follow-up visit owing to the lack of key imaging studies at the first visit.

Patient Selection for Surgery

Patient selection for surgery is under the purview of the neurosurgeon in most cases, although for many disorders, the neurologist plays an integral and key role. As noted previously, the increasing sophistication and complexity of surgical intervention mandates intimate collaboration between neurologists, neurosurgeons, and other subspecialists. Knowing when to refer to multidisciplinary specialty centers is obviously a function of patient diagnosis and proximity to such centers. In general, community neurosurgeons are well versed in treating a wide range of neurosurgical disorders, although increasingly, many are limiting their practices to mainly treating spinal disorders. Increasing evidence suggests that for specific diagnoses, surgical outcomes are a function of surgical volume load and experience. For example, dedicated brain tumor neurosurgeons performing over 50 brain tumor operations per year generally have better patient outcomes than those only occasionally performing these surgeries (Cowan et al., 2002; and Cowan et al., 2003; D'Agostino et al., 2009; and Shahlaie et al., 2010). Similar findings have been reported for cerebral aneurysm treatment, epilepsy, movement disorders, and pediatric disorders. Most academic centers and some large group private practices have dedicated subspecialty neurosurgeons (as well as the necessary ancillary team) to comprehensively and optimally manage these patients.

Surgeon experience, however, is only part of the equation. Whereas it is highly possible a community neurosurgeon can perform an adequate surgical removal of a brain tumor, neurosurgeons affiliated with a brain tumor center may be able to offer patients clinical studies they might not otherwise be aware of. For some trials, fresh pathological tissue is required, and therefore the operation has to be performed at the site of the trial. Understanding the practice of the neurosurgeons to whom you routinely refer may therefore indirectly improve the care your patients receive.

Patient selection for surgery has become increasingly complex, and new treatment modalities and alternatives have arisen. Just as surgical volume load and experience varies among neurosurgeons, it may be important that the referring physician understand other important factors in patient selection for surgery. An example is vestibular schwannoma (acoustic neuroma) management. As already noted, surgical experience may play a major role with regard to patient outcome. It is important to recognize, however, that fewer patients are choosing surgery for small acoustic neuromas, and instead are undergoing stereotactic radiosurgery or radiotherapy treatment (Andrews et al., 2001; Flickinger et al., 2001; Lunsford et al., 2005; and Meijer et al., 2000). Referring to a neurosurgeon whose practice is located in an area without focal beam radiation capabilities may inadvertently lead to an emphasis on surgical alternatives. A similar situation exists with intracranial aneurysms, in which endovascular coiling has increasingly become the treatment of choice for selected patients. Typically, high-volume neurovascular surgeons are closely affiliated with (or perform themselves) endovascular treatment, and therefore this issue is a moot point (D'Agostino et al., 2009).

Neurosurgery is increasingly subspecialized (as is neurology), and certain diagnoses may require a higher level of expertise. In addition to skull base tumors and neurovascular disorders, others include intractable epilepsy, adult hydrocephalus, movement disorders, and rare conditions such as colloid cysts. A knowledgeable neurologist making the proper initial referral may be a key factor in outcome.

In some cases, the neurologist is the primary determinant of patient selection for surgical intervention. The management of movement disorders is an obvious example. In only a minority of patients is surgical intervention such as deep brain stimulation appropriate Olanow and Koller, 1998). Referral to a movement disorder neurologist first may be appropriate instead of initial referral to a functional neurosurgeon. Other examples include carotid endarterectomy (versus stenting) and cerebrovascular bypass procedures.

To some extent, patient selection for surgery begins prior to neurosurgical evaluation. There are no hard-and-fast guidelines as to what types of neurological diagnoses should be referred for neurosurgical consultation, but in most cases, the decision to refer for neurosurgical consultation is obvious. Symptomatic patients with obvious abnormalities seen on imaging, such as a large cerebral aneurysm, require neurosurgical consultation. There are other cases, however, that may not require neurosurgical consultation and can be managed well and appropriately by the neurologist. Although it may seem obvious and trite, it is important to understand that a neurosurgical practice is a surgical practice. With the increasing use of neuroimaging in our society, so-called incidentalomas are being noted by radiologists (Fainstein et al., 2004; Molitch, 2008; and Molitch, 2009). In some cases, this has led to reflexive referrals to neurosurgeons based solely on the radiology report, without the personal review of the imaging study. Referral of these nonoperative lesions to the neurosurgeon first raises the expectation of the patient that surgical intervention is advised and/or pending, and second takes up a significant amount of the neurosurgeon's clinic time explaining why the lesion does not require surgery. Examples follow.

Arachnoid Cyst

The vast majority of arachnoid cysts are small and asymptomatic and consequently, nonsurgical. A typical location is the anterior middle fossa where the anterior temporal lobe is displaced posteriorly (**Fig. 46.2**). Small arachnoid cysts that do not produce significant mass effect (midline shift, brainstem compression) are rarely a cause of headaches (Pierre-Kahn et al., 1990; Pradilla and Jallo, 2007). If it is equivocal whether the lesion is large enough to warrant surgical intervention, a quick film review by the neurosurgeon is often all that is needed to adequately triage the patient.

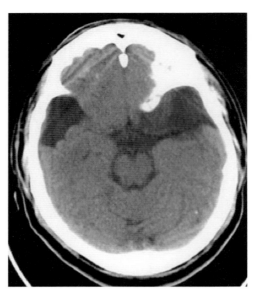

Fig. 46.2 Transaxial computed tomography image demonstrating bilateral middle fossa arachnoid cysts. Although there is displacement of anterior temporal lobes, note the absence of clinically relevant mass effect (i.e., no effacement of basal cisterns). In most cases, reassurance and follow-up imaging is all that is needed.

Tiny Intracranial Aneurysms

With the increasing availability and use of MRI, unruptured intracranial aneurysms less than 7 mm in size are being incidentally discovered during diagnostic imaging. Current international guidelines support repeat imaging of these lesions to ascertain whether they are enlarging or not (Asari and Ohmoto, 1993; Juvela, 2002; Mocco et al., 2004; and Wiebers et al., 2003). Because generally they do not require surgical intervention, referral to a neurosurgeon can be premature. A brief telephone conversation with the neurosurgical colleague may be all that is needed, conserving time and cost for both the patient and surgeon.

Incidental Small Cavernous Malformations

Like small aneurysms, these lesions are rarely surgical and can be followed with neurosurgical consultation (Gross et al., 2009; Robinson et al., 1991). Most neurosurgeons will gladly review imaging studies in order to differentiate which patients should be referred for consultation.

Intervertebral Disk Bulges and Annular Tears

Here, the correlation of neuroimaging findings and neurological symptoms and signs is key (Fujiwara et al., 1999) (**Fig. 46.3**). Clinically insignificant disk bulges are so common in our aging society that a neurosurgical spine specialist could easily be inundated with nonsurgical consultations, stealing time from a practice tailored to helping appropriately referred patients (Stabler et al., 1996; Stabler et al., 1997). Admittedly, inappropriate patient referral to neurosurgeons for asymptomatic disk bulges is infrequent by neurologists, given their training and understanding of neural anatomy.

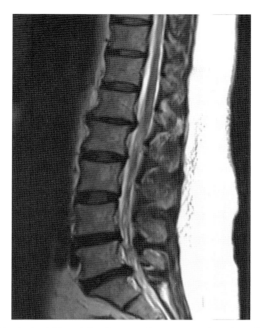

Fig. 46.3 Sagittal T2-weighted magnetic resonance imaging of lumbar spine showing a disk bulge at L5-S1 level. Referral to a neurosurgeon (or other spine specialist) would be indicated if corresponding neurological symptoms existed.

In some cases, certain diagnoses may not require immediate neurosurgical referral. A prototypical example is pseudotumor cerebri (idiopathic intracranial hypertension). It is generally accepted that surgical intervention is one of the last treatment options for this condition (Acheson, 2006; Kelman et al., 1992; Rosenberg et al., 1993). Although many, if not most, neurologists primarily manage this condition, some initiate a referral to neurosurgery for consideration for a cerebrospinal fluid (CSF) shunt procedure. Again, this sometimes raises patient expectations and leads to frustration and delay of (medical) treatment. As diuretics and weight loss are the primary treatment modalities, neurosurgical consultation may never be necessary. However, with rapid visual deterioration, optic nerve fenestration or CSF diversion may be indicated. Also, consideration of intracranial venous occlusive disease should be made for non-obese pseudotumor patients (Mokri et al., 1993; Owler et al., 2003; Owler et al., 2005). A telephone conversation with the neurosurgical colleague could direct the completion of a contrast MR venogram or CT venogram to rule out venous sinus abnormalities.

Equally important to averting unnecessary neurosurgical consultation is avoiding delayed referral. Again, the scope of this chapter does not allow a detailed list of possible diagnoses, but a few examples are given for demonstrable purposes.

Neurosurgical Emergencies

Certain neurological conditions require emergent evaluations. Acute elevation of intracranial pressure, particularly when associated with a Cushing-type response (hypertension, bradycardia, altered respirations) requires emergent evaluation with an immediate head CT. Naturally, mass lesions with herniation syndromes are quite concerning, especially with a rapidly progressing clinical course. Other concerning conditions, including spinal cord compression, cauda equina syndrome, subdural empyema, and spinal epidural abscess, should be urgently evaluated when there is an acute change in the patient's clinical picture.

Long-Standing Overt Ventriculomegaly in Adults

It is common teaching that minimally or asymptomatic patients with overt hydrocephalus simply be monitored, and treatment considered only when the patient becomes significantly symptomatic (Fukuhara and Luciano, 2001; Kelly, 1991). Often these patients have undiagnosed aqueductal stenosis. The basis of this conservative "watch-and-wait" approach presumably arose as a consequence of the historically high complication rate associated with CSF shunt procedures in these patients (Pudenz and Foltz, 1991). This hesitance to consider early neurosurgical intervention is not unique to neurologists and underscores the importance of proper referral considerations. Our understanding and state-of-the-art management of adult hydrocephalus has significantly advanced over the past 2 decades. A neurosurgeon with particular interest in adult hydrocephalus will know that this is not a benign disorder, and that the natural history is inevitable symptomatology, nearly always prior to age 60, and that unfortunately, once a patient becomes symptomatic, it may be too late to effectively intervene. Moreover, the surgical techniques and CSF shunt technology has advanced significantly as well (Dusick et al., 2008; Feng et al., 2004). Many older-generation practicing neurosurgeons were not trained to perform endoscopic third ventriculostomies, which may be the preferred treatment, and therefore default directly to a CSF shunting procedure. Likewise, the use of outdated shunt valve technology may expose the patient to unwarranted risks of postoperative complications. The key point, which will be repeated in this chapter, is that the practice of neurosurgery has become increasingly subspecialized for certain diagnoses. For patients living in rural or even certain urban communities, longer travel to see a subspecialist may offer a better outcome.

Intractable Epilepsy, Trigeminal Neuralgia, and Hemifacial Spasm

These diagnoses have in common the clinical scenario of conditions typically treated primarily pharmacologically, and then consideration given to neurosurgical intervention only with "failure" of medical management (Sidebottom and Maxwell, 1995; Zakrzewska and Thomas, 1993). What constitutes "medically intractable" is clearly the issue at hand, and a detailed description is beyond the scope of this chapter. However, evidence suggests that prolonged (inadequate) medical management may lower the chances of improvement with surgery, and therefore earlier neurosurgical consultation should be considered (Li et al., 2004; Tyler-Kabara et al., 2002). Continued medical education with up-to-date knowledge of current guidelines is recommended.

Preoperative Surgical Planning

The initial patient encounter marks the beginning of surgical planning. As discussed earlier, high-resolution three-dimensional (3D) multimodality neuroimaging is increasingly used on a routine basis. There are several factors the neurosurgeon takes into account for each case. Many are specific to the type of pathology. For intracranial lesions, there is increasing use of 3D reconstructions depicting the relationship between the pathology and surrounding structures.

Vascular lesions are often best characterized by digital subtraction angiography, in some cases augmented by 3D angiography techniques. This modality provides functional and temporal information of the vasculature and is most helpful to characterize arteriovenous malformations (AVMs), complex aneurysms, and various tumors. Magnetic resonance angiography (MRA), however, is rarely helpful to characterize AVMs and aneurysms and therefore is a waste of medical resources if ordered. In some cases, CT angiography (CTA) is adequate for presurgical planning for straightforward intracerebral aneurysms (Papke et al., 2007) (**Fig. 46.4**).

Brain tumor surgical planning can be quite complex. The location of the tumor is often the defining variable. Again, technology has significantly advanced the surgical treatment of brain tumors. Surgical planning for skull base tumors such as meningiomas and vestibular schwannomas may involve consideration of several different surgical corridors, each with inherent advantages and risks. Deep-seated intra-axial tumors that require transcortical approaches ideally should be performed with intraoperative stereotactic neuronavigation that incorporates functional imaging (fMRI), diffusion tensor imaging, white-matter tractography, and sometimes MR spectroscopy (MRS). Fiber tractography (**Fig.**

46.5) can help avoid damage to axonal structures like the optic radiations and arcuate fasciculus, whereas MRS can aid in biopsy site choice (Dowling et al., 2001; Kamada et al., 2005; Kamada et al., 2007). These imaging modalities are not universally available and require experienced technicians and complex postprocessing. For the neurologist, awareness of these considerations and possibilities should play a role in deciding where to refer patients. High-volume neurosurgical subspecialists who routinely use this technology should be sought for appropriate cases.

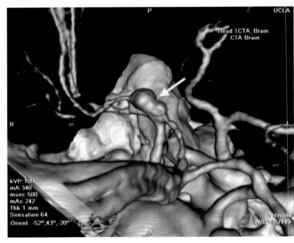

Fig. 46.4 Three-dimensional (3D) reconstruction of a bilobed right internal carotid artery bifurcation aneurysm *(arrow)* visualized using computed tomographic angiography (CTA). The 3D anatomy gives the neurovascular surgeon important insight into aneurysm configuration and orientation.

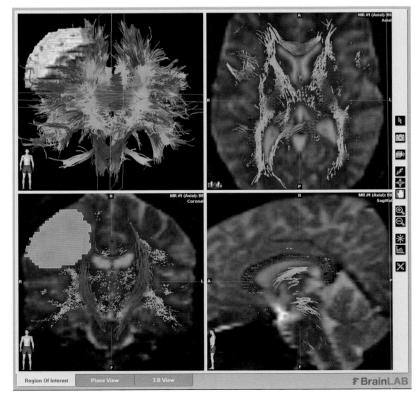

Fig. 46.5 Diffusion tensor magnetic resonance imaging (MRI) can be used to construct white-matter fiber representations (tractography). Combined with anatomical cues and sometimes functional MRI (fMRI) data, the relationship of specific key white-matter bundles can be determined relative to brain tumor location. This data, and often other data such as MR spectroscopy and/or positron emission tomography imaging, can be fused and imported into the surgeon's stereotactic neuronavigation unit. Brain mapping has revolutionized brain tumor surgery, allowing safer, more effective surgery.

Epilepsy surgery requires a different set of diagnostic and surgical decision-making tools. When the location of the epileptogenic focus is not clear or may be attributable to numerous lesions, studies to help determine the culprit lesion are necessary. Cortical surface electrode electroencephalography (EEG), magnetoencephalography (MEG), or depth electrodes may be needed to identify the source of seizures; such modalities are generally only available at dedicated epilepsy centers (Collura et al., 1990; Matsumoto, 1990).

Spinal pathology adds additional diagnostic challenges to differentiating causes of pain and weakness. Dynamic studies such as flexion-extension spinal films can determine instability or ligamentous injury (Elsig and Kaech, 2006). Epidural or facet joint steroid injections can be both diagnostic and therapeutic in the treatment of back pain and radicular pain, directing surgical planning (Cuckler et al., 1985; Koes et al., 1995). Electromyography (EMG) and nerve conduction studies can help pinpoint the source(s) of peripheral nerve pathology (Levin et al., 1996; Tullberg et al., 1993).

The goals of surgery must be clear and direct prior to entering the operative suite. Surgical goals depend on the underlying pathology. These goals include establishing a diagnosis, decompression of neural structures, stabilization, reconstruction, and often cure. The neurosurgeon is ethically mandated to discuss nonsurgical options with the patient or family. The preoperative discussion is essential to emphasize goals and expectations during and after surgery. Expected and unexpected neurological outcomes are discussed, as well as the inpatient and outpatient postoperative course. A common misconception is that surgery will be curative, and patients will be able to return to work immediately. A preoperative discussion can be helpful to provide more realistic expectations.

Similar to medical management of diseases, surgical management may require multiple procedures to achieve the goals of care. Such examples include performing a surgical biopsy prior to surgical resection, approaching a spinal deformity anteriorly prior to a posterior approach, or resecting a lesion prior to placing a ventriculoperitoneal shunt. Advising patients and their families of future events will help prepare them for the treatment process and instill confidence in the surgical team.

"Half of the surgery is done before an incision is made!" This statement is most applicable in the field of neurosurgery. It is not uncommon for the pre-incision activities to take as long as the surgery itself. Attention to specific details such as airway management, intracranial pressure (ICP) management, neuromonitoring, image guidance, brain retraction, and incision planning help ensure safe surgery and plan for untoward events.

As important as a patient's decision to have surgery is the surgeon's decision to offer surgery. The "big picture" must be evaluated for each patient. For example, surgical resection of a small meningioma may be indicated in a healthy young adult but may not be suitable for the vasculopathic, emphysematous, octogenarian smoker. An appropriate preoperative evaluation should also be performed by medical specialists to evaluate for cardiac function, pulmonary capacity, infectious risk, and endocrinopathies. This can help stratify risk for the patient and assist the anesthesia and surgical teams to anticipate intraoperative and postoperative complications.

Surgical Technique

Neurosurgery entails several key considerations. The type of anesthesia is tailored to the patient's pathology and surgical plan. For example, patients with cervical stenosis and myelopathy cannot tolerate direct laryngoscopy and cervical manipulation because of the risk of cervical spinal cord injury. Therefore, awake fiberoptic intubation is performed to avoid cervical hyperextension and allow the patient to control their cervical musculature (Fuchs et al., 1999). Sometimes it is the neurologist, who has the time to comprehensively assess patients preoperatively, who diagnoses conditions such as spinal stenosis, even if it is not the primary condition requiring surgical intervention. Another example is the patient who is dependent on optimal cerebral perfusion pressure, such as in carotid stenosis or compressive cervical myelopathy, and does not tolerate the significant hypotension that is otherwise forgivable with general anesthesia. To combat this, invasive arterial blood pressure monitors are placed prior to induction, and mean arterial pressure (MAP) is kept normotensive throughout the surgery (Epstein, 1988).

Intraoperative neuromonitoring is routinely performed in a variety of neurosurgical operations. Modalities include EEG to monitor for vascular compromise, somatosensory evoked potential (SSEP) and motor evoked potential (MEP) monitoring for cortex through spinal cord viability, brainstem auditory evoked response (BAER) monitoring for acoustic nerve and brainstem injury, and direct nerve stimulation with EMG for cranial nerve and peripheral nerve monitoring. If a change from baseline is encountered in any of these monitoring modalities, surgical or anesthetic adjustments are performed (Minahan, 2002). Examples include repositioning an aneurysm clip if there is a decrease in SSEPs, EEGs that raise concerns of cortical ischemia, tailoring the extent of spinal cord tumor resection if there is a decrease in SSEP and MEP signals, or adjusting spinal pedicle screw trajectories if there is EMG conduction through the neural foramina (Dehdashti et al., 2006). Medical interventions can include increasing MAP for patients exhibiting ischemia, or inducing cortical burst suppression on EEG as a neuroprotective measure (Lavine et al., 1997).

One major advancement of modern neurosurgery is intraoperative stereotactic neuronavigation. The technology entails registering (co-aligning) the patient's head to a preoperative 3D high-resolution image (MRI or CT). The location of the tip of a pointer is then depicted on the imaging monitor (**Fig. 46.6**). This technology has proven helpful in determining the extent of tumor resection, especially if intraoperative CT or MRI is performed (Knauth et al., 1999). Stereotactic biopsy of lesions has become increasingly accurate (Moriarty et al., 2000). On the other hand, neuronavigation can help the surgeon avoid eloquent cortical regions such as the Broca area, Wernicke region, the corona radiata of the primary motor and sensory tracts, and the arcuate fasciculus. Concomitant fMRI and diffusion tensor imaging (DTI) with postprocessing is required to implement this technology (Wu et al., 2007). Lastly, this technology allows smaller incisions and craniotomies compared to those of the past.

Along with utilizing complex technology to avoid neurological complications is the more straightforward concept of passive brain retraction and venous drainage. Much intraoperative morbidity can be prevented by patient positioning. For

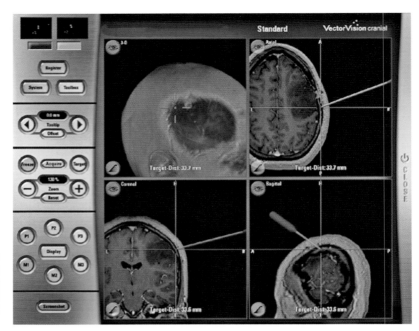

Fig. 46.6 Screen capture taken from an intraoperative neuronavigation system. Virtual pointer displayed on image corresponds to tip of an actual pointer being used by the surgeon. Neuronavigation allows for precise localization of craniotomies and delineation of tumor (lesion) boundaries that are sometimes not apparent by direct vision.

intracranial surgeries, the head position can be adjusted to let gravity retract the brain from the lesion (Rolighed Larsen et al., 2002). The use of the falx cerebri as a natural retractor is helpful for interhemispheric lesions (Stone et al., 1990). Although these technical nuances may not be relevant to a neurologist's daily practice, again it underscores the responsibility of the referring physician to guide patients to specialists who are highly experienced and use modern techniques that minimize operative morbidity.

In some highly specialized neurosurgical procedures, the neurologist plays an integral intraoperative role. One example is awake craniotomies for cortical mapping of eloquent language areas (Costello and Cormack, 2004). Another is epilepsy lesionectomy procedures in which the interpretation of intraoperative corticography is required.

Postoperative Management

The postoperative period can be critical to surgical success. In many larger hospitals, the neurointensive care unit incorporates a neurologist as the neurointensivist. This hospitalist provides minute-to-minute care that cannot be provided by a neurosurgeon while in the operating room. In general, prevention of complications is ideal. Early neurological examination establishes a postoperative neurological baseline. Improvement or decline from preoperative examination should be noted. Early identification of neurological deficits can help diagnose a hematoma, ischemia, or edema that at times can be reversible. Therefore, thorough, frequent, and sometimes continuous neuromonitoring is essential for quick identification and intervention of surgical complications (Bhatia and Gupta, 2007). Many modern intensive care units offer continuous EEG monitoring, again highlighting the natural marriage of neurointensive care with neurology (Guerit, 1999; Guerit et al., 2009).

Postoperative seizure prophylaxis is a controversial topic but is typically initiated intraoperatively and maintained up to 1 week following surgery using established antiepileptic (AED) agents (Horwitz, 1989). Although this has not been proven to decrease the incidence of postoperative seizures or epilepsy, AED use is justified to prevent catastrophic seizures that may lead to increased morbidity and mortality (Glantz et al., 2000). The neurologist can play a key role in postoperative management in this regard, helping determine the best AED agent and duration of treatment.

Another key role neurologists should play is in the long-term management and follow-up of patients with neurosurgical problems. This includes recovery from neurotrauma, intracerebral hemorrhage, hydrocephalus, brain tumor, and epilepsy surgery. Management of chronic neurological conditions is intrinsic to neurological training, and the neurologist is in many ways ideally poised to offer this care. The management of certain neuromodulatory devices such as deep brain stimulators and vagal nerve stimulators is ideally performed by trained neurologists who have a detailed understanding of the patient's neurological status and can titrate stimulator settings much like medications (Okun et al., 2005). Although all neurosurgeons desire to be updated on the long-term sequelae of their intervention, neurosurgical practice is tailored to providing the best perioperative management of patients. It is important to understand that a minor percentage of a neurosurgeon's practice involves outpatient encounters, and therefore this precious clinic time should be largely dedicated to evaluating and treating surgical conditions.

Summary

The neurologist can play a key role in the surgical management of patients. This includes making the diagnosis, ordering appropriate preoperative imaging, referring to the best neurosurgeon for that given patient, educating the patient with regard to treatment options and pitfalls, and actively participating in the long-term management of the patient.

References

The complete reference list is available online at www.expertconsult.com.

II

Chapter 47

Principles of Endovascular Therapy

William Mack, Joshua R. Dusick, Neil Martin, Nestor Gonzalez

Neuroendovascular therapy is an evolving discipline that employs the vessel lumen as an access conduit for the diagnosis and treatment of pathological processes localized in the brain, head, neck, and spine. The femoral artery and vein are the most common routes of entry. However, the carotid, brachial, and radial arteries, the jugular vein, and the intracranial sinus can serve as viable alternate means of access. Initially, endovascular techniques were focused primarily on diagnosis and used for therapeutic purposes only in patients unsuitable for open surgical intervention. Parallel innovations in the fields of neuroimaging and bioengineering have generated rapid advancement in the breadth and capabilities of both diagnostic and therapeutic neuroendovascular procedures. Flat-panel fluoroscopy systems with high-resolution capabilities coupled with three-dimensional software and advanced road-mapping techniques have enabled detailed visualization of the angioarchitecture necessary to treat complex vascular lesions. Concurrent advancement in microcatheter technology has facilitated navigation through previously inaccessible vessels with a high degree of precision and safety, so the incidence of procedural complications has decreased markedly. Material science and device development has allowed for an expanding array of treatment options targeting a host of disease processes previously relegated exclusively to the realm of open surgery.

With a broad range of complex therapeutic capabilities, the performance of thorough diagnostic angiography prior to intervention is critical. In addition to delineating the suspected pathology, this enables visualization of collateral pathways, dangerous anastomoses, and dynamic processes not discernible on noninvasive imaging modalities. Interpretation in multiple angiographic projections affords both a detailed anatomical characterization of the target lesion and an understanding of the regional vascular anatomy. Functional aspects of cerebral blood flow and vascular pathology are provided exclusively by catheter-based angiography.

In a relatively short period of time, neuroendovascular therapy has rapidly evolved into a primary treatment option for a growing number of neurological processes. Among the diseases effectively treated are ischemic stroke, carotid artery disease, intracranial atherosclerosis, brain aneurysms, arteriovenous malformations (AVMs), fistulas, and tumors. Neurointerventional surgery is a less invasive procedure with short hospital stays and, in many cases, superior outcomes compared to traditional surgical methods. The vascular tree is a natural access avenue to any tissue in the human body. As techniques and materials continue to improve, so too will the reaches of our diagnostic and therapeutic capabilities.

Ischemic Stroke

Acute Stroke Treatment

Stroke is the third leading cause of death and the most common reason for disability worldwide (Rosamond et al., 2008). The majority of ischemic strokes result from vessel occlusion secondary to thromboembolic or atheromatous processes (Sussman and Fitch, 1958). To date, timely revascularization and reperfusion of ischemic brain tissue is the most effective therapeutic strategy. Intravenous (IV) thrombolysis has been restricted to a very narrow 3-hour time window based on the NINDS trials (The National Institute of Neurological

828

1A. Level of consciousness (0-3)
1B. Month/age (0-2)
1C. Commands eyes open/closed (0-2)
 2. Best gaze (0-2)
 3. Visual (0-3)
 4. Facial palsy (0-3)
 5. Best motor arm (0-4)
 6. Best motor leg (0-4)
 7. Limb ataxia (0-2)
 8. Sensory (0-2)
 9. Best language (0-3)
10. Dysarthria (0-2)
11. Neglect (0-2)
Normal/near normal examination (0-1)
Minor stroke (1-4)
Moderate stroke (5-15)
Moderate/severe stroke (15-20)
Severe stroke (>20)

Disorders and Stroke rt-PA Stroke Study Group, 1995). Using modified clinical selection criteria, the third European Cooperative Acute Stroke Study recently demonstrated a benefit of IV thrombolysis up to 4.5 hours after symptom onset (Hacke et al., 2008). Nonetheless, the main restrictions on IV recombinant tissue plasminogen activator (rtPA) remain the narrow time window for administration and the nondiscerning systemic mode of delivery. Coupled with an insufficient public awareness, these factors have limited the use of IV thrombolysis to less than 5% of eligible candidates (Barber et al., 2001). Endovascular methods of acute stroke treatment have been developed to help address these shortcomings.

Although inclusion criteria vary for each of the endovascular acute stroke trials, careful patient selection and prudent utilization of recanalization therapies are critical. Treatment algorithms are predicated on clinical and radiographic criteria. Precise assessment of the National Institutes of Health Stroke Scale (NIHSS) (**Box 47.1**) and time of symptom onset determines risk/benefit stratification. Axial imaging (computed tomography [CT], magnetic resonance imaging [MRI]) is used to quantify infarct size and screen for hemorrhage. CT or MR angiography (CTA, MRA) can determine vessel patency, whereas perfusion-weighted MRI helps characterize salvageable tissue in the ischemic penumbra.

Intraarterial Thrombolysis

Compared to IV approaches, intraarterial (IA) administration of thrombolytics via a microcatheter positioned in the cerebral vasculature affords rapid local delivery of greater therapeutic treatment concentrations to the site of vascular occlusion. The selective nature of the delivery system maximizes lysis while limiting systemic conversion and resultant hemorrhage. Intraarterial thrombolysis represents a targeted strategy that lengthens the total therapeutic window for acute stroke intervention. The technique entails performing a catheter-based cerebral angiogram to confirm the point of occlusion. Under fluoroscopic guidance, a microcatheter is advanced though a

larger guide catheter to the base of, into, or distal to the clot. Once positioned, a thrombolytic agent is injected over a 1- to 2-hour time period as intermittent control angiograms are performed (Gandhi et al., 2009). Clinical trials have been performed using streptokinase, urokinase, rtPA, recombinant prourokinase, and reteplase. These agents differ in fibrin selectivity, stability, half-life, and mechanism of action (Gandhi et al., 2009; Schellinger et al., 2001). The Prolyse in Acute Cerebral Thromboembolism II (PROACT II) trial demonstrated the effectiveness of IA prourokinase when given within 6 hours of acute stroke caused by middle cerebral artery occlusion (Furlan et al., 1999). Patients were randomized to IA recombinant prourokinase and IV heparin or heparin alone. The primary clinical outcome, the proportion of patients with minimal or no disability at 90 days (modified Rankin Scale [mRS] score ≤ 2), was achieved in 40% of the treatment group (patients administered heparin and IA prourokinase) and 25% of the controls (patients administered heparin only).

Although IA thrombolysis is an effective treatment, the time delay required for cerebral angiography and microcatheter positioning is an inherent shortcoming. To address this, bridging strategies have employed a combined IV/IA approach. The first such trial was the Emergency Management of Stroke Bridging Trial (Lewandowski et al., 1999). This was a double-blind randomized placebo-controlled phase-I trial of IV rtPA or placebo followed by immediate IA treatment with rtPA. Although recanalization was significantly greater in the IV/IA rtPA group, there was no difference in 3-month functional outcomes, and an increased incidence of death was observed in that treatment group.

The Interventional Management of Stroke (IMS) study investigators compared acute stroke patients treated with a bridging IV rtPA dose (0.6 mg/kg) followed by IA rtPA, with historical controls given only the traditional IV dosing regimen from the NINDS trial. The IMS I study was an open-label single-arm feasibility study using a standard microcatheter to infuse a total dose of up to 22 mg of IA rtPA over 2 hours (IMS Study Investigators, 2004). The objective of the second IMS study (IMS II) was to continue investigating the feasibility of a combined IV/IA approach, permitting the use of the EKOS MicroLysUS (EKOS Corp., Bothell, Washington) micro-infusion catheter, which incorporates sonographic technology to increase permeability and penetration of the intraluminal clot (IMS II Trial Investigators, 2007). The IMS study cohorts demonstrated better functional outcomes and a decreased mortality rate compared to historic controls. The rate of symptomatic intracranial hemorrhage was similar to that of the IV rtPA group in the NINDS trial (IMS Study Investigators, 2004; IMS II Trial Investigators, 2007; National Institute of Neurological Disorders and Stroke rt-PA Stroke Study Group, 1995). These data suggest that bridging protocols combining IV therapy and subsequent endovascular procedures may improve recanalization rates and functional outcome following acute stroke (Mazighi et al., 2009). Definitive evidence to support this combination may not be available, however, until the prospective randomized IMS III trial is completed.

Mechanical Recanalization

Although outcomes following acute stroke have improved with the administration of IV/IA thrombolytics, there are many patients who are not candidates for these treatment

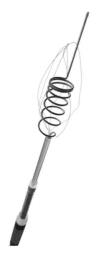

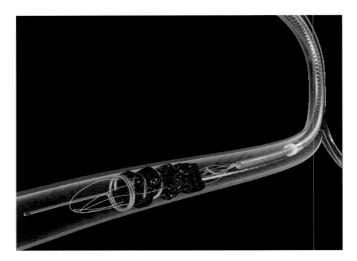

Fig. 47.1 MERCI clot retrieval device *(left)* and diagram demonstrating mechanism of action *(right)*. Spiral loops and suture material are designed to engage the clot and mechanically remove it from the vessel. *(Picture courtesy Concentric Medical Inc.)*

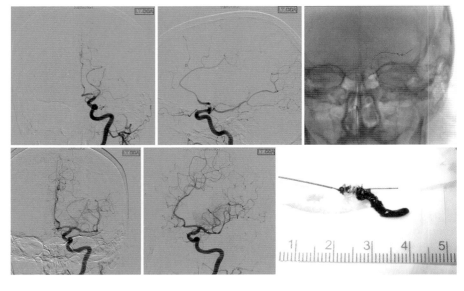

Fig. 47.2 Anteroposterior (AP) *(top left)* and lateral oblique *(top middle)* angiogram demonstrating a left carotid terminus thrombus with no filling of the middle cerebral artery. X-ray image showing the MERCI clot retrieval device deployed in left middle cerebral artery *(top right)*. AP *(bottom left)* and lateral oblique *(bottom middle)* angiograms demonstrating recanalization after mechanical thrombectomy with the MERCI device. Photograph demonstrating an extracted thrombus on the MERCI retrieval device *(bottom right)*.

schemes (Furlan et al., 1999; Williams et al., 2009). Narrow time windows and the risk of hemorrhage associated with thrombolytic agents have prompted the design and application of mechanical thrombectomy devices. Endovascular clot retrieval provides potential for rapid restoration of flow, with a decreased incidence of clot fragmentation and distal embolism (Nogueira et al., 2009). Catheter-based retrieval/aspiration systems are used in acute stroke patients who are either ineligible for or have failed IV rtPA administration; they may be used in conjunction with thrombolytic infusion. Clot-retrieval devices have effectively lengthened the treatment window for acute stroke.

The first device to have received U.S. Food and Drug Administration (FDA) approval for IA stroke treatment is the MERCI clot retriever (Concentric Medical Inc., Mountain View, California). This retrieval system includes the MERCI retrieval device, a compatible microcatheter, and a balloon guide catheter. The retriever is a flexible tapered nitinol wire with radiopaque helical loops at the distal tip (**Fig. 47.1**). Newer-generation retrievers (L series and V series) have cylindrical rather than tapered loops (X series) and a bound suture material that enhances clot capture. An 8F or 9F

balloon guide catheter is advanced into a proximal vessel and inflated to cease anterograde blood flow and thus prevent distal emboli during clot extraction. The microcatheter is advanced coaxially over a microguidewire into the target vessel and through the clot. Once situated in the distal vessel, the microguidewire is exchanged for the clot retriever. The device is unsheathed to position several loops distal to the clot, and the retriever/microcatheter unit is then withdrawn into the balloon guide catheter under constant manual suction (**Fig. 47.2**).

Results from the nonrandomized Mechanical Embolus Removal in Cerebral Ischemia (MERCI) trial demonstrated safety and efficacy of the X-series clot retrieval system in restoring the patency of occluded intracranial vessels within the first 8 hours of acute stroke (Smith et al., 2005). Some 48% of occluded vessels were recanalized, a rate significantly higher than that of the control arm in the PROACT II trial (18%) (Furlan et al., 1999; Nogueira et al., 2009b). After adjuvant therapy (IA rtPA, angioplasty, snare), the rate of recanalization was 60.3%. The overall rates of good outcome (mRS score ≤2) and mortality were 27.7% and 43.5%, respectively, with a clinically significant procedural complication rate of 7.1%.

Revascularization was found to be an independent predictor of decreased mortality and favorable neurological outcome at 90 days.

More recently, the Multi-MERCI Stroke Trial was conducted. This was an international multicenter, prospective, single-arm trial similar to the previous MERCI trial (Smith et al., 2008). However, this study included patients receiving IV rtPA with persistent arterial occlusion and allowed utilization of a newer-generation retrieval device (L5). Treatment with the retriever alone resulted in successful recanalization of 55% of treatable vessels. Recanalization rate was 68% after adjuvant therapy. The overall rates of good outcome (36%) and mortality (34%) were substantially improved when compared to those of the original MERCI trial. Once again, good outcomes were more frequent and mortality was lower with successful recanalization. The authors concluded that mechanical thrombectomy after IV rtPA seems as safe as mechanical thrombectomy alone, and that thrombectomy is efficacious in opening intracranial vessels during acute stroke in patients who are either ineligible for or have failed to recanalize with IV rtPA.

The Penumbra System (Penumbra Inc., Alameda, California) is an aspiration device through which a thromboembolic clot can be retrieved following acute stroke (**Fig. 47.3**). The device removes thrombus via aspiration, mechanical disruption, and extraction. Multiple aspiration catheters of varying luminal diameters are available for use in the cervical and intracranial vasculature, depending on vessel caliber. The aspiration device is advanced coaxially to the level of the thrombus through a guide catheter. Once positioned just proximal to the target lesion, an aspiration pump is connected to the reperfusion catheter. The separator is then advanced through the catheter into the distal clot and repeatedly retracted and advanced, aiding in the debulking process. A multicenter prospective, single-arm, phase I trial of the Penumbra reperfusion catheter was designed to assess safety and efficacy (Bose et al., 2008). The primary endpoint was revascularization, defined by a Thrombolysis in Myocardial Infarction (TIMI) score of 2 or 3. Recanalization was achieved in all vessels in which the device was deployed. A secondary endpoint of mRS score of 2 or less or improvement of NIHSS score by 4 or better was achieved in 45% of patients. The Penumbra device has recently received FDA approval (**Fig. 47.4**).

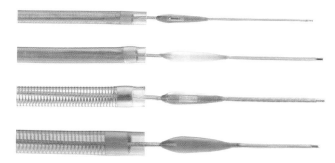

Fig. 47.3 Penumbra reperfusion catheters and separator wires of different sizes. Wire is used to fragment clot as catheter provides suction/aspiration. *(Picture courtesy Penumbra Inc.)*

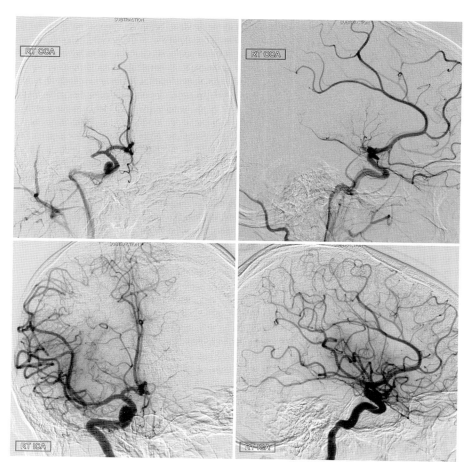

Fig. 47.4 Anteroposterior *(top left)* and lateral *(top right)* angiogram demonstrating right M1 segment middle cerebral artery occlusion. Aspiration with Penumbra catheter resulted in complete recanalization of middle cerebral artery *(bottom left and right).*

No other mechanical embolectomy device is currently approved by the FDA for use in acute stroke. The Phenox Clot Retriever (Phenox GmbH, Bochum, Germany), Neuronet Endovascular Snare (Guidant Corp., Temecula, California), Catch Mechanical Thrombus Retriever (Balt, Montmorency, France), Alligator retriever (Chestnut Medical Technologies Inc., Menlo Park, California), Amplatz GooseNeck Snare (ev3 Inc., Irvine, California), and TriSpan device (Boston Scientific, Natick, Massachusetts) have all been used successfully in a limited number of acute stroke patients, without large-scale demonstration of safety or efficacy (Gandhi et al., 2009; Katz et al., 2006; Nogueira et al., 2009a).

Angioplasty and Stenting

Despite increased experience with IA thrombolytic administration and technical advancements in the development of embolic retrieval or aspiration devices, many intracranial thrombi remain recalcitrant to thrombolysis or embolectomy. Mature fibrinous clots are often difficult to treat pharmacologically, and thrombi adherent to the vascular intima or associated with underlying atheromatous disease pose inherent structural risks to mechanical embolectomy procedures. Percutaneous transluminal angioplasty (PTA) and stenting procedures have been successful in acute coronary revascularization. Recanalization in the absence of clot dissolution or extraction may be sufficient for successful acute stroke treatment (Levy et al., 2009). Several small studies have reported improvement in clinical outcome following angioplasty and thrombolytic administration in the setting of acute stroke (Nogueira et al., 2008; Ringer et al., 2001; Yoneyama et al., 2002). Recently a single-arm prospective trial of primary intracranial stenting for acute stroke demonstrated promising results. The authors reported 100% TIMI 2-3 recanalization in a cohort of 20 patients treated with intracranial stenting. Self-expanding stents (Wingspan [Boston Scientific, Natick, Massachusetts]; Enterprise [Cordis Neurovascular Inc., Miami Lakes, Florida]) designed exclusively for cerebral indications facilitated access and navigation through tortuous craniocervical anatomy. Although adjuvant IA antiplatelet therapy was used in 50% of patients, the authors reported only a 5% rate of symptomatic intracranial hemorrhage. At 1 month, 60% of patients had mRS scores of 3 or below, and 45% had mRS scores of 1 or below. These results are encouraging. Larger studies are needed, however, to adequately assess the safety and efficacy of this treatment modality.

Alternative Reperfusion Strategies

Alternatives to recanalization strategies focus on collateral perfusion as well as flow reversal following acute stroke. One such mechanical approach to flow augmentation is the NeuroFlo catheter (CoAxia Inc., Maple Grove, Minnesota), a dual-balloon catheter designed for partial occlusion of the descending aorta, above and below the renal arteries (**Fig. 47.5**). Temporary partial aortic occlusion is thought to augment cerebral blood flow through mechanical flow diversion. Multicenter clinical trials are currently being conducted to assess the safety and efficacy of this treatment modality (Liebeskind, 2010; Nogueira et al., 2009a; Uflacker et al., 2008). If efficacious, such alternate reperfusion strategies may serve to supplement existing recanalization treatments or represent a novel paradigm for patients ineligible for direct revascularization.

Carotid Artery Disease

Extracranial carotid artery disease and its management has remained a long-standing focus in efforts targeting stroke prevention. Indications and outcomes for carotid endarterectomy (CEA) have been extensively studied in the setting of large-vessel extracranial steno-occlusive disease. Multicenter randomized clinical trials have convincingly demonstrated that compared to medical therapy alone, CEA and aspirin therapy significantly reduce the incidence of stroke and death in both symptomatic and asymptomatic patients with severe carotid stenoses.

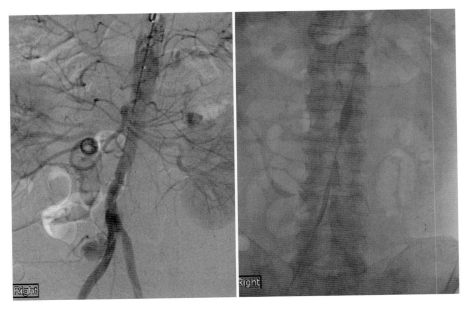

Fig. 47.5 X-ray images of the NeuroFlo device. Balloons are inflated in suprarenal and infrarenal segments of aorta to divert blood flow to collateral cerebral circulation.

The two large landmark randomized controlled trials that enrolled symptomatic carotid stenosis patients were the North American Symptomatic Carotid Endarterectomy Trial (NASCET) and the European Carotid Surgery Trial (ECST) (European Carotid Surgery Trialists' Collaborative Group, 1996; Barnett et al., 1998). The NASCET investigators revealed that carotid endarterectomy reduced the risk of ipsilateral stroke (9%) at 2 years, compared to best medical therapy (26%) in patients harboring carotid stenoses of 70% to 99%. A more modest yet still significant reduction in the 5-year rate of ipsilateral stroke was evident in patients with 50% to 70% stenoses. The overall perioperative stroke and death rate for patients treated with CEA was 5.8%. Using a technically varied measurement criterion for quantifying luminal stenosis, the ECST arrived at a similar result. Data demonstrated that surgically treated patients with stenoses greater than 80% had a lower estimated risk of death or major stroke when compared to those managed medically.

The Asymptomatic Carotid Atherosclerosis Study (ACAS) and the Asymptomatic Carotid Surgery Trial (ACST) addressed indications for CEA in asymptomatic patients (Executive Committee for the Asymptomatic Carotid Atherosclerosis Study, 1995; Halliday et al., 2004). Both studies demonstrated that compared to those treated with best medical therapy, the 5-year incidence of ipsilateral stroke or death was reduced in the carotid endarterectomy group. The degree of benefit for asymptomatic patients was substantially less than previously documented in symptomatic individuals. The 5-year stroke and death rate was 11% for patients in the medical therapy cohort, while the stroke risk was 5.1% for patients treated with CEA. The benefit was evident predominantly in men.

Based on such results, the American Heart Association guidelines recommend CEA for symptomatic patients with 50% to 99% stenosis if the perioperative risk of stroke or death is less than 6%, and for asymptomatic patients with stenoses of 60% to 99% if the perioperative risk of stroke or death is less than 3% (Biller et al., 1998; Sacco et al., 2006).

Carotid Artery Angioplasty and Stenting

Carotid angioplasty and stenting (CAS) has evolved in part because of a need for alternative, less invasive treatment modalities for patients deemed poor operative candidates on the basis of anatomical or clinical parameters. A percutaneous transluminal approach is used to gain endovascular access to the stenotic lesion.

ANGIOPLASTY AND STENTING PROCEDURE

In anticipation of carotid artery angioplasty and stenting, double antiplatelet therapy is initiated prior to the intervention to decrease the risk of thromboembolic complications. Most procedures are performed awake or under monitored anesthesia care, allowing for continuous neurological assessment. Following a diagnostic cerebral angiogram, a guide catheter or shuttle sheath is advanced into the common carotid artery. These delivery systems effectively maintain position and accommodate most stents. If more stability is necessitated, a "buddy" wire can be placed in the external carotid artery. Based upon the diagnostic angiograms, measurements of the stenotic diameter, the length of the lesion, and the diameter of the native common carotid and internal carotid arteries are obtained.

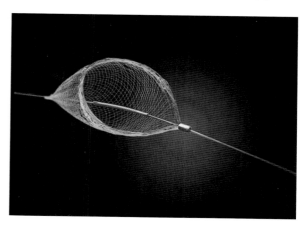

Fig. 47.6 Over-the-wire distal embolic protection device (EPD). Filter is positioned in distal cervical internal carotid artery (beyond stenotic segment) to prevent embolic debris from reaching intracranial circulation.

Next, embolic protection is secured in all attainable cases. Carotid plaques may be extremely friable, and even minor manipulation can result in distal embolization or vessel occlusion. Cerebral protection devices of varying construction are used to prevent embolic complications during CAS procedures. Most commonly, over-the-wire distal filters measured to the diameter of the native cervical internal carotid artery (ICA) are navigated past the stenotic lesion to capture embolic material (**Fig. 47.6**). Such devices allow continuous cerebral perfusion through pores in the filter baskets. Following angioplasty and stenting, the device is collapsed and withdrawn and embolic material retrieved. Alternatively, balloon occlusion devices may be used to completely prevent anterograde flow within the ICA. Any displaced material can be aspirated prior to balloon deflation. However, temporary carotid occlusion may not be well tolerated in all patients, limiting the applicability and utility of this strategy. Guide catheters with distal occlusion balloons may be inflated in the common carotid artery to achieve proximal control and distal flow reversal. Concomitant balloon inflation in the external carotid artery results in more thorough protection. Temporary proximal occlusion is generally performed when distal deployment of an embolic protective device (EPD) is not feasible owing to vessel size, tortuosity, or other anatomical restrictions.

Once embolic protection is achieved, balloon predilatation of tight stenoses can help ensure safe advancement of a self-expanding stent past the target lesion. Balloon inflation is done slowly to lessen the incidence of thromboembolism. Deflation must also be undertaken in a controlled, deliberate fashion. An experienced anesthesiologist and open communication are critical during this portion of the procedure. The endovascular surgeon must inform the anesthesia team of possible bradycardia associated with balloon inflation. This way, changes in the heart rate can be managed in a timely and proper fashion during angioplasty. Stent diameter is calibrated to 100% of the common carotid artery diameter, and length is measured to traverse the entire lesion with a margin of several millimeters both proximally and distally. Tapered stents are available to accommodate the larger diameter of the common carotid artery and the smaller lumen of the ICA. Depending on residual stenosis and distal perfusion, post-stent balloon dilatation may be undertaken.

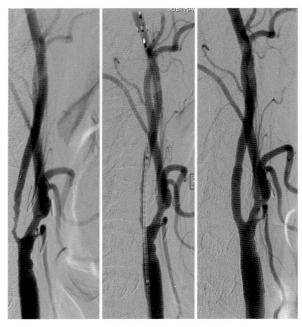

Fig. 47.7 Lateral angiogram demonstrating critical proximal internal carotid artery stenosis *(left)*. Embolic protection device (EPD) is opened in distal cervical internal carotid artery *(top of picture, middle)*. Following balloon dilatation, stent is positioned across stenotic segment *(middle)*. Lateral angiogram showing stent deployed in distal common and proximal internal carotid artery, with minimal residual stenosis *(left)*.

It is critical that balloon angioplasty remain within the confines of the stented arterial segment to prevent dissection of unprotected vascular intima (**Fig. 47.7**).

CLINICAL TRIALS

Since the advent of CAS procedures, there have been multiple clinical trials of relevance. Recent data suggest that carotid stenting procedures can be performed safely. Studies have demonstrated that CAS confers benefit in high-risk surgical patients and represents a rational alternative to CEA in a subset of lower-risk candidates.

When carotid angioplasty procedures were initially introduced more than 25 years ago, they were performed without stenting or distal embolic protection. Despite these limitations, early data suggested the promise of percutaneous intervention (Yadav et al., 1997). The first multicenter randomized trial that compared carotid angioplasty and CEA was the Carotid and Vertebral Artery Transluminal Angioplasty Study (CAVATAS Investigators, 2001). This trial enrolled symptomatic patients with clinically significant (>80%) ICA stenosis. Only 26% of patients (those enrolled later in the study) underwent stenting in addition to transluminal angioplasty. Nonetheless, the 30-day risk of death or stroke was similar between the percutaneous and surgical groups.

The first multicenter randomized CAS study in the United States, the Carotid Wallstent Trial, was conducted using the tracheobronchial Wallstent device (Boston Scientific, Natick, Massachusetts) in symptomatic patients deemed standard risk for carotid endarterectomy. The trial was terminated prematurely, and although the outcomes for stenting and surgery were not statistically different, a strong trend favored surgery (Alberts, 2001). Many believe that relatively limited operator

Box 47.2 Patients at High Risk for Carotid Endarterectomy

Defined as having significant comorbidities and/or anatomical risk and would be poor candidates for carotid endarterectomy (CEA) in the opinion of a surgeon.

Significant comorbid conditions include but are not limited to:
1. Congestive heart failure class III/IV
2. Left ventricular ejection fraction <30%
3. Unstable angina
4. Contralateral carotid occlusion
5. Recent myocardial infarction
6. Previous CEA with recurrent stenosis
7. Prior radiation treatment to the neck; and
8. Other conditions that were used to determine patients at high risk for CEA in the prior carotid angioplasty followed by stenting (CAS) trials

experience and early-generation nondedicated devices profoundly affected the outcome of the stenting cohort in this investigation. The efficacy of a nascent technique was being compared to that of a refined surgical procedure.

Through the 1990s, dedicated improved stent implants and EPDs were developed. Randomized CAS trials and registries targeted patients at high risk for endarterectomy, a cohort of individuals for which previous data were either lacking or revealed suboptimal surgical outcomes, The multicenter randomized Stenting and Angioplasty with Protection in Patients at High Risk for Endarterectomy (SAPPHIRE) trial enrolled high-risk symptomatic and asymptomatic patients (Yadav, 2004). The primary endpoint (death, stroke, and myocardial infarction (MI) at 30 days, plus ipsilateral stroke or neurological death at 1 year) occurred at a rate of 12.2% for stenting and 20.1% for surgery patients ($P = 0.05$). In addition to achieving noninferiority of the primary outcome, the study demonstrated significant decrease in target-vessel revascularization (repeat procedures) and cranial nerve palsies in the CAS cohort ($P <0.05$). On the basis of these data, the FDA recommended approval of the Cordis PRECISE stent and ANGIOGUARD distal filter device (Cordis Corp., Miami Lakes, Florida) for symptomatic patients at high risk for CEA. Three-year follow-up data demonstrated no significant difference in long-term outcomes between CAS and CEA (Gurm et al., 2008). Following the SAPPHIRE trial, a series of multicenter registries was undertaken to gain approval (ongoing or completed) for similar device configurations marketed by various manufacturers. Based on the results from these trials and registries, the Centers for Medicare and Medicaid Services (CMS) approved coverage for CAS with distal embolic protection in high-risk symptomatic patients with stenoses of 70% or greater (**Box 47.2**). Additionally, coverage was provided for high-risk symptomatic patients with between 50% and 70% stenoses and high-risk asymptomatic patients with 80% or greater stenoses in accordance with category B investigational device exemption (IDE) clinical trials regulation and enrollment in CAS postapproval studies.

Supplementing the results generated by the SAPPHIRE trial and subsequent registry studies was the Carotid Revascularization Using Endarterectomy or Stenting Systems (CARESS) trial (CARESS Steering Committee, 2003). This nonrandomized investigation examined all patient subsets (not limited to high risk) and allowed practitioners to determine treatment allocation. In a more realistic clinical paradigm, the study sought to address whether CAS with distal embolic protection was comparable to CEA in patients with symptomatic and asymptomatic carotid stenosis. One-year outcome data demonstrated a trend toward fewer strokes and death in the CAS group, but the difference was not statistically significant (13.6% CEA versus 10% CAS).

Results from two randomized European trials were published simultaneously in 2006. The Stent Protected Angioplasty versus Carotid Endarterectomy (SPACE) trial was a German study that enrolled symptomatic patients with stenoses greater than 50% (by NASCET criteria) and randomly allocated them to CAS or CEA (Ringleb et al., 2006; Stingele et al., 2008). The primary endpoint was ipsilateral stroke or death at 30 days. The steering committee terminated the trial early because of insufficient funding and the large projected number of patients required to demonstrate noninferiority. Nevertheless, primary outcome data appeared to demonstrate near equivalence among the two groups, despite a lack of EPD utilization in the majority of CAS patients.

The French Endarterectomy versus Stenting in Patients with Symptomatic Severe Carotid Stenosis (EVA-3S) trial had inclusion criteria similar to SPACE (symptomatic, >60% stenosis) (Mas et al., 2006). Primary outcome included any stroke or death at 30 days. The investigation was terminated prematurely owing to objective concerns for safety and futility. The primary endpoint was achieved in 9.6% of CAS patients and 3.9% of CEA patients ($P = 0.01$). Detractors claim that the infrequent use of EPDs and deficiencies in the experience of stent operators (as few as five lifetime procedures) may have contributed to poor outcome in the CAS cohort. Nonetheless, the disparate SPACE and EVA-3S results further complicated questions regarding CAS indications in standard-risk symptomatic patients. Furthermore, a secondary analysis of pooled data generated from the SPACE and EVA studies failed to demonstrate that outcome event frequency (stroke or death) was directly related to the use of EPDs, suggesting that not all embolic complications could be avoided with device utilization (Tietke and Jansen, 2009).

The large randomized prospective Carotid Revascularization Endarterectomy versus Stenting Trial (CREST) enrolled a total of 1326 symptomatic patients with greater than 50% stenoses and 1176 asymptomatic patients with greater than 60% stenoses deemed good candidates for either CEA or CAS (Hobson et al., 2004). Primary endpoints included death, stroke, and MI at 30 days or ipsilateral stroke at 1 year. Initial data suggested noninferiority of carotid artery angioplasty and stenting in this broad cohort. Findings indicated that the primary endpoint was not significantly different between the two arms (7.2% versus 6.8%). Additionally, the incidence of death, MI, or stroke at 30 days was similar between the two arms (5.2% versus 4.5%). Periprocedural strokes were significantly higher in the CAS arm (4.1% versus 2.3%), but the incidence of debilitating and major strokes was similar between the two arms (0.9% versus 0.7%). The incidence of MI was significantly lower in the CAS arm, compared with the CEA arm (1.1% versus 2.3%). Cranial nerve palsies were also significantly more common in the CEA arm. Long-term follow-up suggested that the incidence of ipsilateral stroke after the periprocedural period (approximately 4 years of follow-up) was similar between the two arms (2.0% versus 2.4%). Subgroup analyses indicated no difference based on gender, but there seemed to be evidence of effect modification by age such that patients 69 years of age or younger did better with CAS, whereas those aged 70 or older did better with CEA (Brott et al., 2010). These results will likely encourage expansion of indications for CAS procedures.

The International Carotid Stenting Study (ICSS), also known as *CAVATAS II*, is a European trial in symptomatic carotid stenosis patients. It was designed to revisit the questions raised in the original investigation while using stents in all percutaneous procedures (Ederle et al., 2010). Initial results were published at the same time the CREST data were revealed. ICSS enrolled 1713 patients and demonstrated a higher incidence of ischemic stroke and related events after stenting. The incidence of stroke, death, or procedural MI was significantly elevated in the stenting group (8.5%) compared to that the endarterectomy group (5.2%). Risks of any stroke and all-cause deaths were higher in the stenting group than in the endarterectomy group. There was an increased number of cranial nerve palsies in the CEA group.

The conflicting initial results generated by the CREST study, which was performed in the United States, and the largely European ICSS trial raised further questions regarding the indications for these two procedures. It must be noted, however, that the studies were designed (and hence executed) differently. While CREST evaluated both symptomatic and asymptomatic patients, ICSS examined only those with symptoms. Furthermore, the ICSS integrated no "lead-in time" or operator training period, a control measure incorporated into the CREST trial.

Several other trials addressed the indications for CAS in patients who are not high risk for surgery. The ongoing ACT I investigation compared stenting and endarterectomy in standard–surgical risk, asymptomatic patients (Ricotta and Malgor, 2008). The proposed Transatlantic Asymptomatic Carotid Intervention Trial (TACIT) aimed to incorporate an optimal medical management arm comparing the best modern medical treatment regimen to CEA and CAS (Gaines and Randall, 2005; Ricotta and Malgor, 2008). Results generated from investigations such as these will help clarify the future role for CAS procedures. Lessons learned from prior studies will likely translate to rapid development of novel technology and refinement of clinical parameters explored in future CAS trials.

With an extended array of optimal medical therapy, the treatment of marginal asymptomatic carotid stenosis cases by either CEA or CAS is now debatable. Prior to reporting of the CREST and ICSS results, CEA was the preferred treatment for both symptomatic and asymptomatic high-grade carotid artery stenosis—an efficacious procedure with a relatively low complication rate. CAS was reserved for symptomatic high-risk surgical candidates. Results from the CREST investigation will likely increase interest in ongoing and future CAS studies and translate to expanded future indications for CAS procedures.

Intracranial Atherosclerotic Disease

Intracranial arterial stenosis is a common etiology of cerebrovascular disease, responsible for at least 9% of all ischemic strokes (Sacco et al., 1995). The prognosis for individuals afflicted with this pathology remains poor owing to a paucity of therapeutic options and a relative inefficiency of medical treatment. The Warfarin-Aspirin Symptomatic Intracranial Disease (WASID) trial and subset analyses demonstrated that patients who had suffered an ischemic cerebrovascular event and harbored more than 70% stenosis of a referable intracranial artery were at an exceptionally high risk for recurrent stroke (Chimowitz et al., 2005). A reported 23% of enrolled patients experienced a subsequent ipsilateral stroke over the course of the next year despite aggressive medical therapy (Chimowitz et al., 2005). This high event rate was experienced equally regardless of whether or not patients had failed antithrombotic therapy at the time of their qualifying event (Turan et al., 2009).

The development and widespread success of angioplasty and stenting for peripheral and coronary atheromatous disease has promoted adaptation of these techniques to treat lesions in the cerebral vasculature. Modern imaging modalities and rapid technological advancements in catheter and device design have enabled endovascular treatment of intracranial atherosclerotic disease (ICAD).

Intracranial Angioplasty

Balloon angioplasty was the first percutaneous transluminal technique evaluated. In a large retrospective study, Marks et al. (2006) reported on 120 patients with intracranial stenoses treated by primary angioplasty. The authors calculated a combined periprocedural stroke and death rate of 5.8% and a total yearly event rate of 3.2%. This and other investigations have reported posttreatment residual vessel stenoses in the range of 40% (Marks et al., 2006; Terada et al., 1996). High incidences of angiographic vessel dissection have been documented, although they have rarely been noted to manifest as clinical events (Kiyosue et al., 2004; Marks et al., 2006; Mori et al., 1998; Wojak et al., 2006). Durability of primary angioplasty has also been questioned, with documented retreatment rates near 20% (Siddiq et al., 2008). Mori et al. (1998) investigated lesion-specific features that predicted successful angioplasty and low restenosis rates. They determined that short segment, concentric narrowing, and subtotal angiographic occlusion correlated with the lowest incidence of restenosis following percutaneous transluminal angioplasty (PTA). By contrast, features that portended poor outcome or higher rates of restenosis were eccentricity, extreme angularity, length greater than 10 mm, or excessive tortuosity of the proximal vessel segment. Additionally, the success rate was significantly lower for lesions treated greater than 3 months from the time of stroke.

Experience in the coronary literature indicated that the shortcomings of primary angioplasty (plaque dislodgement, acute elastic recoil, vessel dissection, recurrent stenosis) could be overcome by subsequent stent deployment (George et al., 1998; Savage et al., 1998; Serruys et al., 1994). These concepts were translated directly to the intracranial vasculature.

Intracranial Angioplasty and Stenting

Several early case reports described angioplasty and stenting of cerebral vessels using coronary artery techniques (Chow et al., 2005; Feldman et al., 1996; Gomez et al., 2000; Yu et al., 2005). Device rigidity and vascular tortuosity rendered navigation difficult, resulting in periprocedural morbidity and mortality rates greater than that of angioplasty alone (Chow et al., 2005; Gomez et al., 2000; Jiang et al., 2004; Kim et al., 2004; Levy et al., 2001; Yu et al., 2005). The multicenter non-randomized Stenting in Symptomatic Atherosclerotic Lesions of Vertebral and Intracranial Arteries (SSYLVIA) trial reported the safety and efficacy of a balloon-mounted stent (Neurolink, Guidant Corporation, Indianapolis, Indiana) designed specifically for craniocervical application; 43 patients with symptomatic intracranial disease and 18 with extracranial vertebral artery stenoses were evaluated. Successful stent placement was achieved in 95% of patients. The investigators reported a 6.6% periprocedural stroke rate and an additional 7.3% incidence of stroke at 1-year follow-up. However, angiographic restenosis was documented in 35% of patients and was symptomatic in over one-third of these individuals (SSYLVIA Study Investigators, 2004). Based on these data, the FDA granted the stent a humanitarian device exemption (HDE) for the treatment of high-risk patients with significant intracranial and extracranial atherosclerotic disease who had failed medical therapy. More recent studies have investigated modified balloon-mounted stenting systems designed exclusively for the cerebral vasculature. Jiang et al. (2004) documented a 91.7% rate of technical success with the Apollo intracranial stent (MicroPort Medical, Shanghai, China) in patients harboring stenoses greater than 50%. The primary endpoint, ischemic stroke in the target lesion arterial territory or any stroke/death within 30 days, occurred at a rate of 4.3 per 100 patient-years. A restenosis rate of 28% was reported. The Vitesse Intracranial Stent Study for Ischemic Therapy (VISSIT), designed to evaluate the Pharos Vitesse system (Micrus Endovascular, San Jose, California), is currently underway (Kurre et al., 2008b).

The Wingspan stent is the first self-expanding system designed solely for intracranial application (**Fig. 47.8**). A nitinol (nickel and titanium metal alloy with shape memory

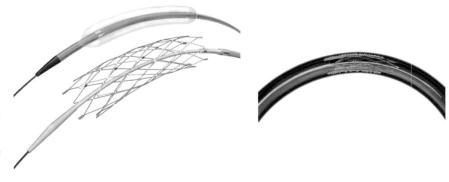

Fig. 47.8 Gateway balloon and Wingspan stent *(diagrammatic rendering on left)*. Stent deployment across an intracranial stenotic lesion with resultant opening of vessel lumen *(right)*. *(Pictures courtesy Boston Scientific.)*

and superelasticity) construct with high radial force allows navigation of small and tortuous intracranial vessels. Recently the FDA granted an HDE approval for the Wingspan Stent System with Gateway PTA balloon catheter (Boston Scientific, Natick, Massachusetts) for symptomatic ICAD referable to an intracranial vessel with greater than 50% stenosis and refractory to medical therapy. Endorsement was predicated on a safety study conducted in Europe and Asia (Bose et al., 2007). In that initial investigation, technical success was achieved in 98% of patients, and the 6-month death or ipsilateral stroke rate was 7%, with an all-cause stoke rate of 9.7%. In the more recent NIH Multicenter Wingspan Intracranial Stent Registry Study, 129 patients with symptomatic 70% to 99% intracranial stenoses were enrolled. The technical success rate was 97%. The frequency of any stroke, intracerebral hemorrhage, and death within 30 days or ipsilateral stroke beyond 30 days was 14% at 6 months (Zaidat et al., 2008). The reported frequency of angiographic restenosis was 25%.

In-stent restenosis has decreased following cardiac angioplasty and stenting procedures with the advent of drug-eluting stents (Regar et al., 2002). While this generation of stents may be useful in reducing myointimal hyperplasia, no platforms have been specifically designed and approved for use in the small and tortuous intracranial vessels.

ANGIOPLASTY/STENTING PROCEDURE

Intracranial angioplasty and stenting with the Gateway/Wingspan system is most often performed under general endotracheal anesthesia. Dual antiplatelet therapy is initiated in anticipation of the procedure. A diagnostic cerebral angiogram is performed to assess degree of stenosis, length of diseased segment, flow restriction, and the presence of leptomeningeal collaterals. A shuttle sheath or guide catheter is used to maintain proximal position and accommodate the angioplasty/stenting platform. Some operators use a distal support catheter in patients with particularly tortuous anatomy. After a microcatheter/microguidewire system is advanced past the lesion, an exchange-length microwire is used to advance, in series, the balloon angioplasty and stent catheters to the level of stenosis. The lesion is initially dilated with a PTA balloon sized to 80% of the native vessel luminal diameter, using the slow inflation technique advocated by Connors and Wojak (Connors and Wojak, 1999). After initial

vessel dilation, the balloon catheter is exchanged for the self-expanding stent system, which is deployed across the stenotic lesion. Post-stenting balloon dilation is discouraged by the manufacturer (**Figs. 47.9 and 47.10**). At the conclusion of the procedure, the average reported residual stenosis (30%) is less than that observed following PTA alone (40%) but more than noted after balloon-mounted stent deployment (10%) (Fiorella and Woo, 2007; Henkes et al., 2005). Follow-up angiograms have demonstrated restenosis rates exceeding 30%, presumably due to elastic recoil, myointimal hyperplasia, and vascular remodeling (Garas et al., 2001). Coating stents with antiproliferative agents such as sirolimus and paclitaxel has been effective in reducing restenosis rates in the cardiology literature (Ong et al., 2006; Stone et al., 2004). Several recent studies have demonstrated encouraging results for the treatment of ICAD patients with drug-eluting stents (Gupta et al., 2006; Qureshi et al., 2006). Difficult vessel navigation with more rigid stenting systems and prolonged postoperative treatment with dual antiplatelet therapies are among the potential limitations to the successful translation of drug-eluting technology to pathologies of the intracranial vasculature.

CLINICAL APPLICATION

There remains controversy as to whether intracranial stent placement is superior to primary angioplasty in the treatment of ICAD. Studies have addressed the angiographic and clinical outcomes associated with each procedure, but relatively few comparative investigations have been reported. A multi-institutional (three tertiary care centers) retrospective study compared the clinical outcomes between primary angioplasty and stent placement for symptomatic intracranial atherosclerosis (Siddiq et al., 2008, 2009). Stroke and combined stroke and/or death were identified as primary clinical endpoints during the periprocedural and follow-up period of 5 years. The authors noted significantly fewer residual stenoses in the stent-treated cohort, but there was no significant reduction in stroke or mortality among the patients who underwent stenting procedures.

In a systematic literature review and meta-analysis, Siddiq et al. (2009) compared primary angioplasty and stent placement in patients with symptomatic intracranial atherosclerosis. They noted technical success rates of 80% in the angioplasty

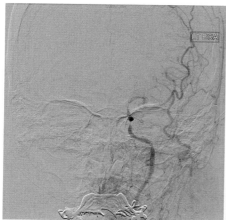
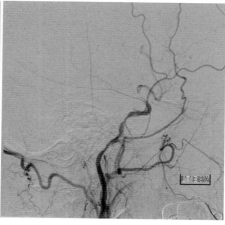

Fig. 47.9 Anteroposterior *(top left)* and lateral *(bottom right)* angiograms demonstrating critical tandem petrocavernous and supraclinoid left internal carotid artery stenoses with no filling of left anterior cerebral artery and diminished flow through right left middle cerebral artery.

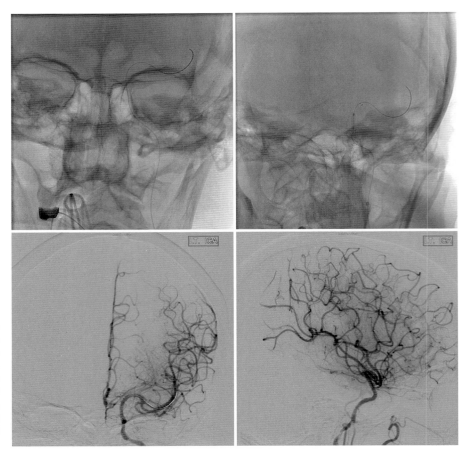

Fig. 47.10 Same patient as in Fig. 47.9. Top x-rays demonstrate balloon positioned across petrocavernous stenosis (black marker is the midpoint of the balloon, *left*) and stents deployed across petrocavernous and supraclinoid lesions *(right)*. Anteroposterior *(left)* and lateral *(right)* post-stenting angiograms on the bottom demonstrate increased flow through stenoses and filling of both anterior and middle cerebral arteries on left.

group and 95% in the stent cohort. There was no difference in the perioperative stroke and death rate between the two treatment groups (9% angioplasty, 8% stent). The pooled incidence of 1-year stroke and death was 20% in patients treated with primary angioplasty and 14% in those treated with stenting, signifying a statistically significant difference in outcome. Also noted was a significantly higher restenosis rate in the primary angioplasty group. Importantly, the authors demonstrated no discernable effect of study publication year on the risk of stroke and death.

Debate remains as to the precise indications and preferred treatment strategies for symptomatic ICAD. The Stenting and Aggressive Medical Management for Preventing Recurrent Stroke in Intracranial Stenosis (SAMMPRIS) study is an ongoing large-scale randomized investigation comparing intracranial angioplasty and stenting (Wingspan stent/ Gateway balloon) and intensive medical management with optimal medical management alone. Patients with 70% to 99% intracranial stenosis who suffered a stroke or transient ischemic attack (TIA) within 30 days of enrollment are randomized and followed for up to 4 years. This marks the first large-scale randomized study comparing the efficacy of endovascular therapy and medical management in patients with ICAD (Rasmussen, 2009). Intracranial angioplasty with or without stenting is an emerging technique that may have a pivotal position in the treatment of symptomatic intracranial atherosclerosis. The results of SAMMPRIS and other ongoing investigations will better address the precise indications.

Hemorrhagic Stroke

Cerebral Aneurysms

Intracranial aneurysms are abnormal focal dilatations of the cerebral arteries, with thinning and weakening of the vessel wall. Aneurysms constitute a common cerebrovascular pathology, with a reported adult prevalence of 0.2% to 9% worldwide (Inagawa and Hirano, 1990). Vessel degeneration and hemodynamic factors contribute to changes in focal sheer stress and flow patterns that ultimately may result in aneurysmal enlargement or rupture.

Most unruptured aneurysms remain undetected, but an increasing number of incidental aneurysms is being discovered during diagnostic imaging studies (Wakhloo, 2008; Wiebers et al., 2003). Although patients harboring intracranial aneurysms may present with symptoms resulting from mass effect or thromboembolism, the most common and perilous clinical manifestation is that of subarachnoid hemorrhage (SAH). It is estimated that 10 of every 100,000 intracranial aneurysms rupture annually. Aneurysmal rupture carries a roughly 50% mortality rate, with 10% to 20% of survivors failing to regain long-term functional independence (Ellegala and Day, 2005; Hop et al., 1997; Schievink, 1997).

Decision Matrix
RUPTURED ANEURYSMS

Following rupture of an intracranial aneurysm, recurrent hemorrhage occurs at a high frequency. Jane et al. (1985)

documented that the incidence of rebleeding among patients with SAH and untreated aneurysms was 50% in the first 6 months and 3% per year thereafter. Because of the high risk of subsequent rupture, these aneurysms are nearly always treated urgently.

The randomized prospective multicenter International Subarachnoid Aneurysm Trial compared the efficacy of endovascular treatment with that of surgery in patients with ruptured intracranial aneurysms suitable for either treatment modality (Molyneux et al., 2002, 2005). A total of 2143 patients were randomized. Recruitment was prematurely terminated after a planned interim analysis demonstrated reduced disability in the endovascular treatment group. In an intention-to-treat analysis, the proportion of patients who were dead or disabled at 1 year was significantly lower in the endovascular therapy group compared to the surgical cohort. Additionally, the risk of perioperative seizures was lower following coiling procedures. However, the requirement for a second procedure was higher with endovascular treatment. The 1-year risk of rebleeding from the ruptured aneurysm was 2 per 1272 patient-years for individuals allocated to embolization and 0 per 1081 in the cohort allocated to open surgery. The investigators noted that the low rates of late rebleeding and potential periprocedural complications associated with retreatment in the endovascular group were unlikely to alter the treatment benefit at 1 year. They concluded that endovascular coil embolization of ruptured intracranial aneurysms when a patient has a good clinical grade (World Federation of Neurosurgical Societies grade I-III) and the aneurysm anatomy is suitable for endovascular treatment is more likely than not to lead to independent survival at 1 year those receiving neurosurgical treatment. Results may be generalized to good-grade patients harboring anterior circulation aneurysms. Statistical comparisons were difficult in poor-grade patients and those with posterior circulation aneurysms, as the vast majority of these individuals were not randomized due to treating physicians' overwhelming preference for endovascular therapy.

To address issues regarding incomplete occlusion and recanalization following endovascular therapy, rerupture rates after treatment for aneurysmal subarachnoid hemorrhage were further investigated in the Cerebral Aneurysm Rupture After Treatment (CARAT) study (Johnston et al., 2008). All ruptured saccular aneurysms treated between 1996 and 1998 in nine institutions were evaluated for rerupture. A total of 1010 patients (711 surgically clipped, 299 treated by coil embolization) were contacted by written questionnaire or telephone. Rerupture of the treated aneurysm after 1 year occurred in one patient who underwent coil embolization (904 person-years of follow-up, 0.11% annual rate) and no patients treated with surgical clipping (2666 person-years). Aneurysm retreatment after 1 year was more frequent in the endovascular cohort. However, major complications were rare during follow-up treatment. The authors concluded that late events are unlikely to overwhelm differences between the procedures at 1-year follow-up.

INCIDENTAL ANEURYSMS

The decision matrix for treatment of incidentally discovered unruptured aneurysms is based on natural history data and the risk/benefit stratification for the applicable treatment modalities.

Rupture rates for intracranial aneurysms vary with size and location, as reported by the International Study of Unruptured Intracranial Aneurysms (International Study of Unruptured Intracranial Aneurysms Investigators, 1998; Wiebers et al., 2003). The prospective observational arm of this large study investigated 2686 unruptured, untreated cerebral aneurysms in 1692 patients. Individuals with no history of SAH who harbor incidental aneurysms located in the anterior circulation (ICA, anterior communicating or anterior cerebral artery, middle cerebral artery) had 5-year cumulative rupture rates of 0%, 2.6%, 14.5%, and 40% for aneurysms of less than 7 mm, 7 to 12 mm, 13 to 24 mm, and 25 mm or greater, respectively. Rupture rates for aneurysms of the same sizes located at the posterior communicating artery or in the posterior circulation were 2.5%, 14.5%, 18.4%, and 50%, respectively. Patients with a prior history of SAH resulting from rupture of an aneurysm distinct from that being studied had a 5-year cumulative rupture rate of 1.5% for aneurysms less than 7 mm in the anterior circulation, compared with 3.4% for aneurysms of the same size located at the posterior communicating artery or in the posterior circulation. Aneurysms greater than 7 mm in this cohort had similar rupture rates to the group with no prior history of SAH (Wiebers et al., 2003).

Therefore, it is generally believed that incidental aneurysms less than 7 mm, located in the anterior circulation, and in patients with no prior history of SAH may be managed expectantly with serial imaging. However, patient-specific desires or the presence of factors such as irregular morphology, documented growth, or a family history of intracranial aneurysms may encourage consideration of surgical or endovascular treatment even in this low-risk cohort (Broderick et al., 2009). Recent studies have focused on quantitative hemodynamic analysis using computer-generated flow models to predict aneurysmal growth and rupture (Chien, 2009). While these methods hold great promise, further development and application to large patient cohorts is required to develop reliable algorithms that accurately predict rupture risk in the clinical setting. According to the ISUIA data, aneurysms of any size located in the posterior circulation and those in patients who have experienced prior SAH carry a significant 5-year cumulative rupture risk and warrant treatment consideration (Wiebers et al., 2003).

There exist no large randomized controlled trials favoring endovascular or surgical management of unruptured intracranial aneurysms. Individualized algorithms must be tailored to specific clinical and anatomical factors when selecting an appropriate treatment paradigm (Raja et al., 2008).

Several large retrospective studies document very low morbidity and mortality rates for surgical clipping in the hands of experienced neurosurgeons (Bederson et al., 2000; Deruty et al., 1996; Dickey et al., 1994; Komotar et al., 2008a; Moroi et al., 2005; Raaymakers et al., 1998). Many authors promote microsurgical treatment in young patients with small anterior circulation aneurysms, suggesting that surgical clipping provides a more durable repair than coil embolization (Komotar et al., 2008a).

Observational studies have advocated surgical clipping for broad-necked aneurysms (Ogilvy et al., 2002; Raftopoulos et al., 2000, 2003; Regli et al., 1999, 2002) and for those with critical vessels emanating from the base (Johnston et al., 2001; Raftopoulos et al., 2000; Regli et al., 1999, 2002).

In 2003, Ogilvy and Carter retrospectively reviewed a series of 604 unruptured aneurysms in an attempt to identify risk factors associated with outcome following surgical treatment. The authors found patient age, aneurysm size, and location within the posterior circulation to be independent predictors of poor outcome (Ogilvy and Carter, 2003).

Emerging data on the endovascular treatment of unruptured intracranial aneurysms suggest low morbidity and mortality rates. Large studies indicate an overall morbidity of 5% to 10%, with mortality rates very close to zero (Johnston et al., 2001; Pouratian et al., 2006; Wiebers et al., 2003). Johnston et al. (2001) compared the safety of endovascular coiling and microsurgical clipping in 2069 patients treated in California between 1990 and 1998. In-hospital mortality and discharge to an alternate facility (rather than home) were significantly less frequent in the endovascular cohort. Mortality was 0.5% in the endovascular group and 3.5% in the open surgical cohort. These results are striking given that the investigation was conducted during the relatively early development of endovascular coiling technology. More recent data from the ISUIA study suggest that endovascular morbidity and mortality may be lower at 1 year than that reported for open surgical treatment in both patients with (7.1% versus 10.1%) and without (9.8% versus 12.6%) prior SAH (Wiebers et al., 2003). Furthermore, outcome following endovascular procedures appeared to be less dependent upon patient age. Direct comparisons were not generated, however, because the endovascular cohort was relatively small. Physician preference led to coil embolization treatment of a greater percentage of older medically ill patients and those with aneurysms located in the posterior circulation.

Endovascular Treatment Modalities
COIL EMBOLIZATION

Diagnostic cerebral angiography is necessary prior to coil embolization of both incidentally discovered and ruptured intracranial aneurysms. Often a focused angiographic examination is sufficient when treating an incidental aneurysm in a patient with thorough noninvasive preoperative cerebrovascular imaging. It is critical, however, to evaluate the entire craniocervical vasculature for potential sources of subarachnoid hemorrhage. While many institutions rely upon high-quality CTA or MRA for this purpose, digital subtraction angiography remains the diagnostic gold standard. In the event no aneurysm or vascular malformation is discovered after a complete intracranial angiogram (bilateral internal carotid/vertebral arteries), it is necessary to assess the ascending cervical and posterior deep cervical branches of the subclavian artery and the bilateral external carotid arteries for the presence of a dural arteriovenous fistula. Delayed repeat angiography is often warranted in cases with a comprehensive negative initial study and a suspicious pattern of subarachnoid blood.

Following diagnostic cerebral angiography, aneurysm morphology and regional vascular anatomy are carefully assessed to determine the safety and feasibility of coil embolization. Certain anatomical configurations render endovascular treatment more difficult. Aneurysms with larger neck-to-dome ratios and those that incorporate the origins of critical vessels are less amenable to primary coil embolization.

Once coil embolization is selected as the treatment modality, a microcatheter is advanced over a microguidewire through a larger diagnostic or guide catheter. Under real-time digital subtraction fluoroscopy, the microsystem is advanced into the aneurysm. From this position, coils may be deployed.

Dr. Guglielmi first introduced electrolytically detachable platinum microcoils in 1990. Initially, only aneurysms judged to be high risk for microsurgical clipping were treated by coil embolization. Since that time, rapid technological advancements have resulted in more efficacious endovascular treatment of complex aneurysms. Improved detachment mechanisms, stretch-resistant coils, three-dimensional complex shapes (Piotin et al., 2003; Wakhloo et al., 2007), varying degrees of softness, and coil lattice incorporating a bioabsorbable polymer (Fiorella et al., 2006; Linfante et al., 2005; Murayama et al., 2003) or hydrogel (Cloft, 2006; Gaba et al., 2006) have been designed to minimize procedural complications and help prevent delayed recanalization.

Coil embolization technique involves the careful placement of a framing coil into the aneurysm dome under real-time digital subtraction fluoroscopy. Once appropriate position is confirmed, the coil is detached. Proper selection and methodical placement of the first coil is of paramount importance, as this often establishes technical ease and safety of the entire procedure. If residual aneurysm filling is noted, additional coils of various shapes and successively diminishing sizes are deployed until complete occlusion is obtained (**Fig. 47.11**).

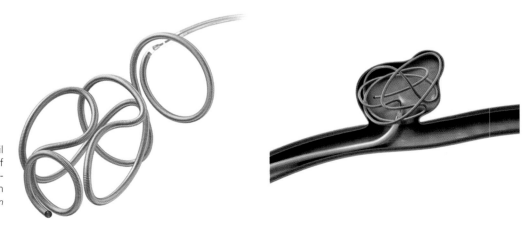

Fig. 47.11 Three-dimensional coil *(left)* and diagrammatic depiction of coil deployment through a microcatheter positioned in an aneurysm *(right)*. *(Pictures courtesy Boston Scientific.)*

BALLOON REMODELING

Initially described by Moret et al. (1997), the balloon remodeling technique affords an ability to effectively treat broad-necked cerebral aneurysms by mechanically protecting the parent vessel from coil prolapse or protrusion. Positioned within the parent artery, a small balloon occlusion microcatheter is intermittently inflated and deflated across the aneurysm neck (**Fig. 47.12**). This provides temporary structural support against which coils are then deployed through a second microcatheter located within the aneurysm dome. Anterograde flow is completely reestablished within the parent artery after successive balloon deflations. This adjunctive technique extends the indication for endovascular aneurysm treatment to cases with less favorable anatomy. It is suggested that remodeling leads to higher packing densities and more effective parent vessel reconstruction (Kurre et al., 2008). In a review of their initial experience, the Moret group documented complete angiographic occlusion in 20 of 21 broad-necked cerebral aneurysms treated via balloon-assisted coil embolization. They reported sustained occlusion without recanalization at angiographic follow-up of at least 4 months. The authors noted complication rates that were no greater than those experienced with primary coil embolization techniques (Moret et al., 1997). These results have been corroborated by several more recent clinical series (Cottier et al., 2001; Lefkowitz et al., 1999; Malek et al., 2000). Balloon assistance has greatly facilitated the endovascular treatment of wide-necked ruptured cerebral aneurysms in the acute phase, allowing for mechanical coil support and vessel remodeling in the absence of prolonged antiplatelet therapy.

STENT-ASSISTED COIL EMBOLIZATION

In more challenging broad-necked cerebral aneurysms, balloon remodeling may not be sufficient to prevent coil protrusion into the parent vessel. In such cases an endoluminal/

endovascular approach uses a permanently deployed intracranial stent as supportive scaffolding. Nitinol self-expanding stents with either open or closed-cell configuration have been designed exclusively for use in the intracranial vasculature (Akpek et al., 2005; Higashida et al., 2005) (**Fig. 47.13**). Many groups deploy a stent across the aneurysm neck and then introduce the coiling microcatheter into the sac through the stent interstices. An alternative method is to first position the coiling microcatheter within the aneurysm dome and then "jail" the distal tip in position through subsequent stent deployment. With either strategy, stent placement precedes positioning and detachment of the coils within the aneurysm (**Figs. 47.14 and 47.15**). Clinical studies have documented favorable results, with initial occlusion rates over 80% (Lylyk et al., 2005). While prospective studies have documented persistent complete or near-complete angiographic occlusion at 20 months, long-term data are necessary to determine sustained viability of stent-assisted coiling techniques (Fiorella et al., 2004). Studies have reported the use of complex stent-assisted techniques such as telescoping/overlapping multiple stents for the treatment of fusiform aneurysms (Crowley et al., 2009) and Y-stent configurations for bifurcation aneurysms (Chow et al., 2004). To date, stent-assisted coil embolization has been largely reserved for the treatment of unruptured aneurysms. Most physicians are reluctant to deploy stents in the setting of SAH, because they require aggressive long-term antithrombotic regimens to protect against thrombosis and embolic events.

Alternative Treatments

Substantial incomplete occlusion and subsequent recanalization rates following coil embolization have raised concerns regarding the durability of endovascular treatment for cerebral aneurysms with unfavorable geometry (Debrun et al., 1998; Fernandez Zubillaga et al., 1994; Guglielmi et al., 1992; Piske et al., 2009; Taha et al., 2006). Experimental models have demonstrated that coils occupy less than 40% of aneurysmal volume. Therefore, residual flow may remain even in tightly packed lesions (Piotin et al., 2000, 2003). This has prompted the development and application of novel techniques such as liquid embolic agents and flow-diverting stents.

Liquid embolic agents may permit more efficient aneurysmal dome and neck filling. Onyx LES (liquid embolic system [ev3 Inc., Irvine, California]) is an embolic system initially developed to treat high-flow lesions such as AVMs and fistulae. It is an ethylene vinyl alcohol dissolved in the organic solvent, dimethyl sulfoxide (DMSO), that precipitates to form a polymer cast when contacted by aqueous solution. The Cerebral Aneurysm Multicenter European Onyx (CAMEO) study assessed the safety and efficacy of Onyx HD-500 in treating aneurysms that presented difficulties for surgical or endovascular alternatives (wide necks/unfavorable geometry). Balloon remodeling was required in all cases. At 12-month follow-up, the authors reported higher occlusion rates, better outcome, and similar complication rates when compared to those reported with traditional embolization methods in comparable study cohorts (Molyneux et al., 2004). Similar results were noted in several other large case series (Cekirge et al., 2006; Piske et al., 2009).

The advent of flow-diversion devices represents a potential paradigm shift in the treatment strategy for broad-necked

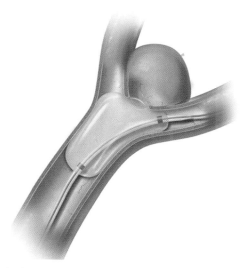

Fig. 47.12 Diagram demonstrating balloon remodeling technique with HyperForm balloon (ev3 Inc., Irvine, California) prior to coil placement. Balloon is positioned across neck of aneurysm to temporarily prevent coil herniation into parent vessel.

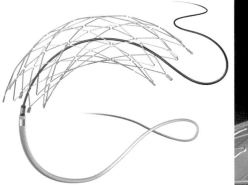

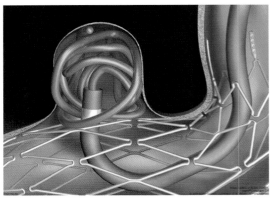

Fig. 47.13 Picture of a Neuroform stent with open-cell design *(left)* and diagrammatic depiction of stent-assisted coil embolization through a microcatheter positioned in an aneurysm *(right)*. Note that stent provides permanent scaffolding for stabilization of coil mass. *(Pictures courtesy Boston Scientific.)*

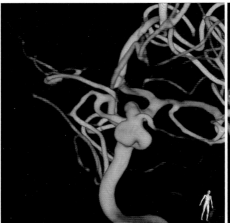

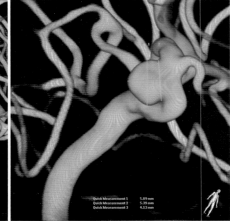

Fig. 47.14 Three-dimensional reconstruction of a left superior hypophyseal region aneurysm *(left)*. Measurements *(right)* demonstrate cranial-caudad (1) and transverse (3) dimensions of aneurysm and size of the neck (2).

intracranial aneurysms. Circumferential endoluminal parent-vessel reconstruction may allow for complete aneurysmal occlusion in the absence of direct endovascular embolization. The Pipeline Embolization Device (PED [ev3 Inc., Irvine, California]) is specifically engineered to reconstruct a segmentally diseased vessel. Lylyk et al. (2009) detailed a large initial experience with the PED; 53 patients with 63 wide-necked aneurysms were treated. The study reported a mean follow-up time of 5.9 months. Complete angiographic occlusion was achieved in 95% of aneurysms, and no major complications were encountered. The investigation found the device to be safe, durable, and curative for selected wide-necked large or giant aneurysms.

Although initial data appear quite promising, further large-scale investigations are needed to determine the clinical efficacy and long-term durability of liquid embolic agents and flow-diversion devices in the treatment of cerebral aneurysms. The rapid emergence of new device technology has vastly increased the number of aneurysms treatable by endovascular methods. However, fusiform aneurysms and those with broad necks or critical branches emanating from the dome are still optimally treated with craniotomy and clip ligation.

Management of Cerebral Vasospasm

Cerebral vasospasm, a delayed reversible narrowing of the intracranial vasculature, is the leading cause of stroke, morbidity, and mortality following neurosurgical and endovascular treatment of aneurysmal subarachnoid hemorrhage (aSAH). Occurring most frequently between 3 and 14 days after aSAH, vasospasm causes a decrease in blood flow and a resultant lowering of cerebral perfusion pressure (Janardhan et al., 2006; Macdonald et al., 2007). Medical treatments including oral nimodipine and induced hypervolemia, hemodilution, and hypertension ("triple-H therapy") have been employed to enhance cerebral oxygenation in the setting of vasoconstriction. Despite maximal medical measures, 15% of patients who initially survive aSAH experience stroke or death secondary to vasospasm (Mayberg, 1998). For vasospasm refractory to medical management or in patients with treatment contraindications, endovascular therapy has emerged as an alternative or supplementary therapeutic modality (Brisman et al., 2006; Newell et al., 1992). Both balloon angioplasty and IA vasodilator infusion have established roles in the management of medically intractable vasospasm. The optimal method and timing of endovascular treatment, however, remain controversial.

Balloon Angioplasty

A technique first applied by Zubkov et al. in 1984, percutaneous transluminal angioplasty commonly results in permanent mechanical reversal of cerebral vasospasm (Zubkov et al., 1984). The precise mode of action remains poorly understood. Proposed mechanisms for smooth-muscle dysfunction include endothelial denudation, collagen fiber stretching, and rupture

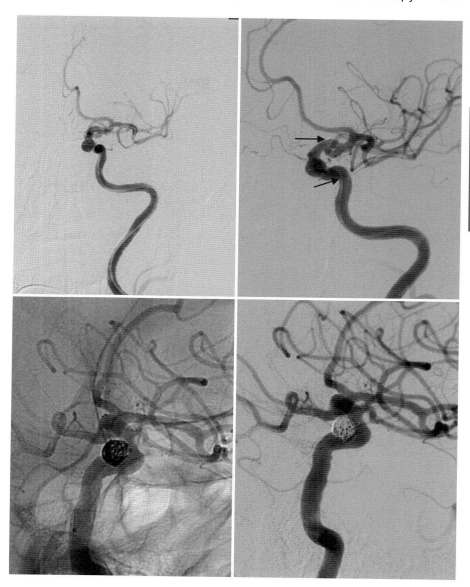

Fig. 47.15 Same aneurysm seen in Fig. 47.12. Large size of aneurysm neck compared to dome led to stent-assisted coiling technique being employed. *Top left,* Working projection oblique angiogram demonstrating stent tines positioned across neck of aneurysm. *Top right,* Arrows point to proximal and distal stent tines. *Bottom left,* Unsubtracted view demonstrating stent position and coil mass. *Bottom right,* Postintervention angiogram in working projection showing no residual aneurismal neck and no filling within coil mass.

of internal elastic lamina (Chan et al., 1995; Honma et al., 1995; Macdonald et al., 1995; Yamamoto et al., 1992).

If severe vasospasm is suspected, percutaneous balloon angioplasty is typically performed under general anesthesia with full muscle paralysis. A noncontrast head CT is obtained immediately prior to angiography to rule out rebleeding, hydrocephalus, or completed infarct. If available, careful examination of a prevasospasm angiogram or vascular study is critical. This allows for assessment of congenitally hypoplastic vascular segments and avoidance of dangerous balloon inflation in unaffected vessels. Vigilant blood pressure control and intracranial pressure monitoring are maintained throughout the treatment. The patient is anticoagulated, and a guide catheter is positioned in the proximal segment of the target vessel. Next, a balloon catheter is advanced over a microguidewire to the level of vessel narrowing. Two differing balloon technologies have been employed. Our preference is the more compliant Hyperglide/Hyperform (ev3 Inc., Irvine, California) or Sentry (Boston Scientific, Natick, Massachu-

setts) balloon catheters. The catheter lumen distal to the balloon tapers and is effectively occluded by a microguidewire, causing injected contrast to expand the balloon. The guidewire is left in place during balloon inflation and a 50:50 mixture of contrast and saline is used to ensure adequate angiographic opacification. Dilatation is performed until vessel conformation is noted in the shape of the balloon. Other groups employ less pliable noncompliant balloon devices such as the Gateway system or Maverick coronary balloon (Boston Scientific, Natick, Massachusetts) (Eddleman et al., 2009). In either case, the balloon is slowly inflated over the length of the accessible spastic segment, attempting to attain dilatation to greater than 50% of the original vessel caliber. Abrupt overdilation is avoided to decrease the risk of rupture and arterial dissection. Balloon angioplasty is generally restricted to larger proximal vessels of the circle of Willis and, less commonly, the smaller immediately more distal branches. Balloon angioplasty can also be effectively used to open proximal vessels and facilitate catheterization of small

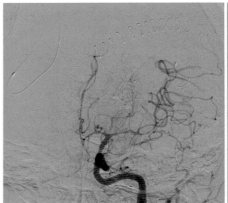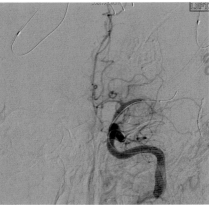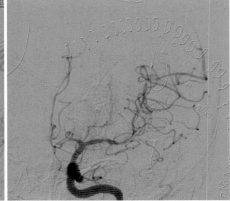

Fig. 47.16 *Top left,* Anteroposterior (AP) angiogram demonstrating severe narrowing of M1 segment of left middle cerebral artery and moderate stenosis of A1 segment of left anterior cerebral artery. *Top right,* Hyperglide balloon positioned across narrowed middle cerebral artery segment. Note two radiopaque markers that confirm position of balloon. *Bottom left,* Post-dilatation AP angiogram demonstrating an increase in caliber of proximal left middle cerebral artery.

distal vessels previously inaccessible to microcatheters. This permits potential for subsequent injection of IA vasodilators in the respective distal vascular territories (**Fig. 47.16**).

An analysis of six retrospective series reporting treatment of cerebral vasospasm by balloon angioplasty demonstrated a mean clinical improvement of 65% (Komotar et al., 2008b). Eskridge et al. (1998) conducted the largest study, examining 50 patients and 170 arterial segments; 61% of patients demonstrated sustained clinical improvement within 72 hours of balloon angioplasty treatment. In a 2005 literature review, Hoh and Ogilvy (2005) found an overall clinical improvement in 62% of patients treated for vasospasm with balloon angioplasty. Rosenwasser et al. (1999) sought to ascertain the time period during which balloon angioplasty was maximally effective. The authors determined that 70% of patients treated within 2 hours of symptom onset demonstrated clinical improvement. By contrast, only 40% of those treated beyond the 2-hour window sustained recovery. Rates of angiographic vasospasm resolution were similar between the two cohorts, indicating that earlier treatment of patients with medically resistant cerebral vasospasm results in superior clinical outcome despite similar radiographic results. Preemptive balloon angioplasty has been advocated for vasospasm prophylaxis in high-risk patients (Muizelaar et al., 1999). A multicenter phase II study published in 2008 that evaluated prophylactic balloon angioplasty in patients with Fisher grade III SAH demonstrated no significant difference in Glasgow Outcome Score when compared to patients treated with standard-of-care therapy. While a statistically significant decrease in the need for therapeutic angioplasty was reported, four procedure-related vessel perforations and three resultant deaths were documented in the prophylaxis cohort (Zwienenberg-Lee et al., 2008).

Intraarterial Vasodilators

Intraarterial vasodilator therapy is often used to treat mild to moderate clinical vasospasm or disease affecting the more distal intracranial vasculature. Administration of IA pharmacological therapy is achieved in a technical fashion similar to that of balloon angioplasty, although often performed under conscious sedation. A guide/diagnostic catheter is advanced

into the proximal portion of the affected vessel. The vasodilatory agent is then injected either directly through the larger catheter or via a microcatheter advanced to a more selective distal position within the target vessel. A slow infusion rate coupled with meticulous monitoring is critical in order to avoid systemic hypotension or undesired increases in ICP. To date, the most robust data regarding efficacy of IA pharmacological therapy for the treatment of cerebral vasospasm has been accumulated with papaverine. An opium alkaloid and nonspecific smooth muscle–cell relaxant, papaverine causes vasodilation through cyclic adenosine and guanosine monophosphate phosphodiesterase inhibition and has a half-life of nearly 2 hours. Investigations have documented incidences of immediate angiographic vasospasm relief ranging between 57% and 90% (Firlik et al., 1997; Kassell et al., 1992; Milburn et al., 1998). Hoh and Ogilvy reported in their systematic review that although papaverine produced clinical improvement in 43% of treated patients, the effect was temporary, and individuals often needed multiple treatment sessions. High rates of relapse in clinical vasospasm have been documented within 48 hours of treatment (Hoh and Ogilvy, 2005; Komotar et al., 2008b).

Concerns regarding the toxicity profile and short effect of papaverine have prompted the off-label use of IA calcium channel antagonists in the treatment of cerebral vasospasm (Smith et al., 2004). Feng et al. (2002) reported a 45% increase in vessel diameter and 33% clinical improvement following verapamil administration. Similarly, neurological improvement was documented in 42% of patients receiving IA nicardipine (Badjatia et al., 2004). Biondi et al. (2004) demonstrated a 43% rate of vessel dilation and a 76% incidence of clinical improvement in the first 24 hours following IA administration of nimodipine. The most significant shortcoming associated with the use of IA vasodilator therapy is the transitory efficacy. Repeat endovascular instillation is often necessary (Brisman et al., 2006; Hoh and Ogilvy, 2005). Furthermore, studies have demonstrated that longer durations of vasoconstriction are less responsive to treatment (Scroop, 2004). Side effects including systemic hypotension and increased ICP have further limited the effectiveness of these therapies, each directly related to rate of infusion (McAuliffe et al., 1995).

Cerebral Arteriovenous Malformations

A brain AVM is an aggregate of arterial and venous communications with no intervening capillary network. Studies suggest that the incidence of brain AVMs is 1.21 per 100,000 person-years (Stapf et al., 2002). Despite their congenital nature, cerebral AVMs may become symptomatic at any time, with a mean presentation age of 31.2 (Hofmeister et al., 2000). Over 50% of AVMs manifest with rupture (Brown et al., 1996; Hofmeister et al., 2000), yielding an annual hemorrhage rate between 2% and 4% (Kondziolka et al., 1995; Ondra et al., 1990). Although the resultant blood pattern is most often intracerebral, subarachnoid or intraventricular hemorrhage may occur. In total, AVM rupture accounts for roughly 2% of all intracranial hemorrhages (Stapf et al., 2001, 2002). The risk of rebleeding in patients who initially present with rupture may approach 6% to 17% during the first year before stabilizing to a baseline level after 3 years (Forster et al., 1972; Graf et al., 1983; Mast et al., 1997). Several demographic and anatomical factors including age, deep brain location, and deep venous drainage have been associated with hemorrhage at presentation in patients harboring brain AVMs (Stapf et al., 2006a; Turjman et al., 1995). As many as 35% of patients present with seizures or ischemic symptoms secondary to regional vascular steal phenomenon (Sekhon et al., 1997).

Because the distinct natural history of unruptured AVMs remains uncertain, A Randomized Trial of Unruptured Brain Arteriovenous Malformations (ARUBA) is currently being conducted. This multicenter trial compares a treatment strategy consisting of endovascular, microneurosurgical, and/or radiosurgical therapy to that of conservative management (Stapf et al., 2006b).

AVM angioarchitecture has been characterized as plexiform or fistulous, depending on the rate and degree of vascular shunting. Hemodynamic changes often produce arterial aneurysms and venous stenoses or varices. Changes in flow dynamics and sheer stress often lead to proximal aneurysms in the circle of Willis. These lesions should be treated independently either by surgical or endovascular techniques. Feeding artery and intranidal aneurysms are directly dependent on the nidal flow pattern of the AVM and represent high-risk features effectively addressed by embolization.

The modern management of cerebral AVMs relies upon the combination of three distinct therapeutic modalities: endovascular embolization, microneurosurgery, and stereotactic radiosurgery. Endovascular management of brain AVMs focuses on eliminating high-risk angiographic features such as aneurysms and high-flow fistulae, in addition to minimizing the lesion size or associated technical challenges prior to definitive radiosurgical or operative procedures. When an AVM harbors a relatively small number of feeding arteries and draining veins, endovascular cure may be achievable.

Embolization Procedure

A detailed superselective diagnostic cerebral angiogram is necessary to determine the angioarchitecture and flow patterns associated with an AVM prior to endovascular treatment. Penetration of the nidus with embolic material, rather than simple occlusion of the feeding vessels, decreases the incidence of recanalization via flow through collateral channels (Vinuela et al., 1986). Procedural staging reduces the likelihood of edema or hemorrhagic complications secondary to normal perfusion breakthrough (Andrews and Wilson, 1987; Spetzler et al., 1987). Superselective Wada testing with sodium Amytal allows for functional assessment in an awake patient. Infusion may reveal vascular supply to eloquent cortical tissue via en passage vessels not apparent on angiographic assessment (Purdy et al., 1991).

Angiography and embolization are usually performed under general anesthesia with muscle paralysis. If superselective Wada testing is desired, however, the patient is maintained awake for the diagnostic portion of the procedure and is then intubated and administered general anesthesia. Following a detailed diagnostic cerebral angiogram, a guide catheter is positioned in the proximal aspect of the target vessel. Under constant real-time roadmap guidance, an over-the-wire or flow-guided microcatheter is advanced to a distal intracranial position. Most often the microcatheter is advanced into the nidus without the use of a wire, limiting the potential for vessel trauma or perforation. If nidal catheterization cannot be achieved, a more proximal position may be accepted. Biplane superselective angiography is obtained and carefully analyzed for en passage vascular segments or cerebral capillary blush (**Fig. 47.17**). Several agents have been used for AVM embolization, discussed next.

Polyvinyl Alcohol

Polyvinyl alcohol (PVA) particles (Boston Scientific, Natick, Massachusetts) were the first material approved by the FDA for intravascular use. Dependent on flow, they are sized to the caliber of the target vessel. Consequently, the microcatheter lumen must be able to accommodate the particle diameter and prevent occlusion secondary to aggregation. Particle embolization occurs in a slower fashion than liquid embolic occlusion. Often, low-flow shunts are disconnected first, leading to increased pressure in the remaining feeding arteries and nidal vessels and rendering the AVM susceptible to rupture. Transient and permanent morbidity rates of 14.3% and 8.6%, respectively, have been reported following particle treatment (Schumacher and Horton, 1991). Nidal recanalization is the most significant failing associated with particle embolization. Following proximal occlusion, development of collateral supply results in persistent shunting through the malformation. In a large series, Sorimachi et al. (1999) reported a 43% rate of enlargement following particle embolization and an 80% nidal recanalization rate in completely occluded lesions. Mathis et al. (1995) demonstrated a 12% recanalization rate in AVMs embolized prior to stereotactic radiosurgery.

n-Butyl Cyanoacrylate

n-Butyl cyanoacrylate (nBCA) (TRUFILL [Cordis Neurovascular Inc., Miami Lakes, Florida]) is an adhesive liquid monomeric agent that polymerizes and solidifies upon coming into contact with an ionic solution such as blood (Debrun et al., 1997). Administration results in marked chronic inflammation, fibrosis, and vessel occlusion (Kish et al., 1983; Klara et al., 1985; Wikholm et al., 2001). The safety of nBCA in AVM embolization was assessed in a prospective randomized

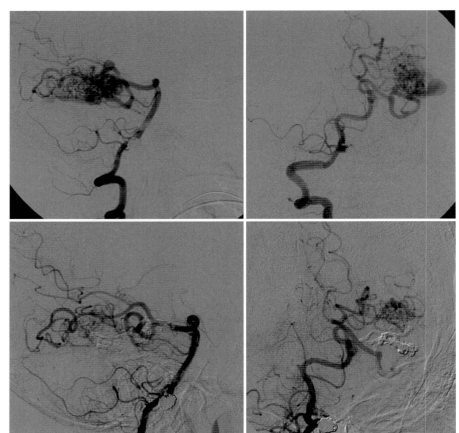

Fig. 47.17 Anteroposterior *(left)* and lateral *(right)* angiograms before *(upper)* and after *(lower)* embolization of a 3-cm arteriovenous malformation (AVM) at the inferior and middle left temporal gyri. AVM was supplied by two inferior temporal branches of the posterior cerebral artery. Following *n*-butyl cyanoacrylate (nBCA) embolization to superior branch and Onyx-34 to inferior branch, there was approximately 25% reduction in total nidal volume, with no opacification of a lateral perinidal aneurysm. This patient received radiotherapy after embolization and in long-term follow-up had complete obliteration of the AVM.

non-inferiority trial demonstrating that nBCA was equivalent to PVA in achieving target embolization volume goal and reduction in feeding vessel number. The rates of permanent occlusion were more favorable in the nBCA group, with very low incidences of recanalization (n-BCA Trial Investigators, 2002). These results led to FDA approval for this indication. More recent investigations confirm that nBCA embolization results in complete, durable vessel occlusion. Yu et al. (2004) reported no recanalization at 17- to 32-month follow-up in a series of AVMs treated with nBCA. Wikholm et al. (2001) demonstrated a lack of recanalization at 5-year follow-up. Achieving nidal penetration requires modification of polymerization and viscosity parameters according to the hemodynamic characteristics of the lesion. Such factors are adjusted by varying the relative concentrations of Thiodol and nBCA in the treatment mixture. Some groups advocate changing the pH of the solution with an organic acid such as glacial acetic acid to lengthen polymerization time (Lieber et al., 2005). Outcomes following nBCA embolization by experienced operators are favorable. In a series of 103 patients, Liu et al. (2000) reported transient and permanent complications of 4.9% and 1.9%, respectively, as well as two deaths. Gobin et al. (1996) documented morbidity and mortality rates of 12.8% and 1.8%, respectively.

Disadvantages of nBCA include short delivery times and the potential for microcatheter retention, which can result in vessel rupture or adverse ischemic sequelae. Additionally, proper administration requires precise understanding of the polymerization kinetics of acrylate. The nBCA in dextrose solution is injected through a microcatheter under constant real-time roadmapping technique until adequate nidal penetration is achieved with minimal reflux. The microsystem is then quickly withdrawn to avoid catheter retention within the glue cast. In lesions with high-flow fistulous components, coils may be deployed prior to nBCA injection to prevent venous egress of liquid adhesive material. The embolization of feeding artery aneurysms is performed by placing the microcatheter tip in or proximal to the aneurysm and allowing glue to infiltrate the AVM nidus while casting the aneurysmal sac.

Ethylene Vinyl Alcohol Copolymer

Ethylene vinyl alcohol copolymer was first proposed for the treatment of AVMs by Taki in 1990 (Taki et al., 1990). Subsequently, many groups have reported on its use as a liquid embolic agent (Jahan et al., 2001; Murayama et al., 1998). As noted earlier, Onyx consists of an ethyl-vinyl copolymer dissolved in DMSO, with tantalum powder added for increased radiopacity. Slow solidification permits prolonged controlled injections, with allowance for continuous assessment and deeper nidal penetration with each catheterization (Katsaridis et al., 2008; Murayama et al., 1998). Onyx was first tested in a phase I investigation conducted by Jahan et al. (2001). The group demonstrated a 63% volume reduction in 23 AVM patients with 129 targeted feeding artery pedicles. They reported a 12% transient and 4% permanent associated morbidity. Van Rooij and colleagues treated 44 patients with Onyx, embolizing 138 pedicles in 52 sessions.

They documented an average volume reduction of 75%, with complete occlusion of 7 lesions (van Rooij et al., 2007). A morbidity rate of 8.5% and a mortality rate of 3.2% were reported. More recently, several large single-center case series have assessed potential for complete AVM occlusion with Onyx embolization. Katsaridis et al. (2008) reported a 53.9% rate of complete occlusion, with an associated morbidity and mortality of 3.7% and 1.4%, respectively, per embolization session. Using a combination of Onyx and nBCA therapy (Onyx as the first-line agent), Mounayer et al. (2007) reported a 49% complete occlusion rate, with similar incidences of complications (8.5% morbidity, 3.2% mortality).

Although it has revolutionized the way many groups treat brain AVMs, Onyx LES carries inherent limitations and disadvantages. It can be used only with DMSO-compatible catheters. This prohibits the use of most flow-guided microsystems that facilitate access to small distal intracranial vessels. Additionally, DMSO can be directly angiotoxic if injected too rapidly into the cerebral vasculature (Jahan et al., 2001). Furthermore, limited opacification may prevent adequate visualization of reflux into small vessels supplying viable cortical tissue (van Rooij et al., 2007). Recent studies have also suggested that Onyx AVM embolization requires increased fluoroscopy and procedure times compared to nBCA (Velat et al., 2008).

Cerebral Arteriovenous Fistulas

Cranial Dural Arteriovenous Fistulas

Cranial dural arteriovenous fistulas (DAVFs) are direct shunts between arteries and venous sinuses or cortical veins with no transitional capillary network. The mean age of presentation is 50 to 60 years, without gender predilection or evidence for familial inheritance (Zipfel et al., 2009). Although most are presumed to be idiopathic, DAVFs may be associated with trauma, craniotomy or venous thrombosis (Berenstein, Lasjaunias, and Ter Brugge, 2001; Chung et al., 2002). These lesions account for 6% of supratentorial and 35% of posterior fossa vascular malformations (Newton and Cronqvist, 1969). DAVFs present with symptoms according to anatomical localization and pattern of venous drainage. Lesions draining into the cavernous sinus often result in proptosis, chemosis, ophthalmoplegia or increased ocular pressure (Ito et al., 1983; Kim et al., 2002; van Dijk et al., 2004). By contrast, those with venous egress into the transverse or sigmoid sinus frequently present with pulsatile tinnitus (Brown et al., 1994). Posterior fossa DAVFs may cause lower cranial nerve deficits or brainstem findings (Borden et al., 1995; Kim et al., 2002). Lesions draining into the superior saggital sinus can manifest with nonspecific cortical symptoms such as hydrocephalus, seizures, or mental status change (Hirono et al., 1993; Hurst et al., 1998; Kim et al., 2002).

The natural history of DAVFs is directly influenced by cortical venous drainage (CVD), which if present, substantially increases the risk of intracranial hemorrhage and nonhemorrhagic neurological deficits (Borden et al., 1995; Cognard et al., 1995; Zipfel et al., 2009). The critical impact of CVD has been reflected in the angiographic classification systems of Borden and Cognard (**Box 47.3**), both of which categorize fistulas with cortical venous reflux as high-grade dangerous lesions (Borden et al., 1995; Cognard et al., 1995). Other associated angiographic features, such as venous ectasias and

---

Box 47.3 Borden and Cognard Classification Systems

Borden Classification System

Type I: dural arteriovenous fistula drainage into a dural venous sinus or meningeal vein with normal anterograde flow. Usually benign clinical behavior.

Type II: anterograde drainage into dural venous sinus and onwards, but retrograde flow is into cortical veins. May present with hemorrhage.

Type III: direct retrograde flow of blood from fistula into cortical veins, causing venous hypertension with a risk of hemorrhage

Cognard Classification System

Type I: normal anterograde flow into a dural venous sinus

Type IIa: drainage into a sinus, with retrograde flow within the sinus

Type IIb: drainage into a sinus, with retrograde flow into cortical vein(s)

Type II a + b: drainage into a sinus, with retrograde flow within the sinus and cortical vein(s)

Type III: direct drainage into a cortical vein, without venous ectasia

Type IV: direct drainage into a cortical vein, with ectasia > 5 mm and 3 times larger than the diameter of the draining vein

Type V: direct drainage into spinal perimedullary veins

From Borden, J.A., Wu, J.K. Shucart, W.A., 1995. A proposed classification for spinal and cranial dural arteriovenous fistulous malformations and implications for treatment. J Neurosurg 82, 166–179; and Cognard, C., Gobin, Y.P., Pierot, L., et al., 1995. Cerebral dural arteriovenous fistulas: clinical and angiographic correlation with a revised classification of venous drainage. Radiology 194, 671–80.

---

varices, have also been correlated with poor outcome. More recent studies report that individuals who present with symptoms of cortical venous hypertension have a substantially higher risk of new neurological events than those who present incidentally or with symptoms consistent with increased dural sinus drainage (Soderman et al., 2008; Strom et al., 2009).

MRI can reveal the presence of a DAVF through flow voids or edema secondary to venous hypertension. Furthermore, dilated vessels may be evident on either CTA or MRA. A catheter angiogram, however, remains the most accurate method of diagnosis and is critical in the assessment of lesional angioarchitecture and venous outflow pattern. Data suggest that lesions with dangerous CVD be addressed urgently (Duffau et al., 1999; van Dijk et al., 2002). Although angiographically benign fistulas may be managed conservatively, those with persistent clinical manifestations often warrant treatment for symptomatic relief.

Treatment options include endovascular occlusion, surgical disconnection, and stereotactic radiosurgery. Embolization, which is the preferred treatment option at most institutions, may be achieved through a transarterial or transvenous access route. Liquid embolic agents such as Onyx or nBCA are typically used alone or in conjunction with thrombogenic coils to attain fistula occlusion. Complete embolization via infiltration of the venous pouch and outflow tract is the ultimate objective. However, partial treatment with selective CVD disconnection is indicated in cases where normal venous drainage through an affected sinus precludes total fistula obliteration. Surgical treatment is typically reserved for lesions not amenable to endovascular therapy or select anterior cranial fossa DAVFs supplied by ethmoidal branches of the ophthalmic artery. Stereotactic radiosurgery is an effective treatment modality used either alone or in conjunction with endovascular therapy (Chandler et al., 1993; Guo et al., 1998; Pollock et al., 1999). However, obliteration occurs over the course of several years, with an inherent interim risk of hemorrhage and neurological events according to the natural history of the specific lesion.

Carotid-Cavernous Fistulas

Carotid-cavernous fistulas (CCFs), abnormal arteriovenous communications in the cavernous sinus, represent a unique subset of cranial arteriovenous fistulas. These lesions may be classified on the basis of etiology (traumatic or spontaneous) or angioarchitecture (direct or indirect). The most commonly used classification system was proposed by Barrow et al. (1985) and segregates lesions according to arterial supply (**Box 47.4**).

The classic presentation of direct CCFs is the sudden onset of exophthalmos, conjunctival injection, and a cephalic bruit. Associated cranial nerve palsies and visual decline are common. Indirect CCFs typically have a more gradual onset and mild presentation but may manifest in a similar clinical

fashion. Proposed etiologies include pregnancy, sinusitis, trauma, and cavernous sinus thrombosis (Kwan et al., 1989).

Axial CT and MRI may reveal proptosis, flow voids, an enlarged cavernous sinus, or a prominent superior ophthalmic vein. Digital subtraction angiography is essential in classifying the CCF and elucidating the precise fistulous site and pattern of venous drainage. Injection of the vertebral artery while manually compressing the ipsilateral common carotid artery (in the presence of a posterior communicating artery) often aids in localization, as the reduced flow facilitates visualization of the fistula.

Direct CCFs can be approached through transarterial or transvenous access. The standard endovascular treatment of direct CCFs had been transarterial disconnection with a detachable balloon. However, technical problems forced removal of this device from the U.S. market. Current strategies employ the use of detachable coils, liquid embolic agents, and covered stents via either a transarterial or transvenous approach. The transvenous route usually involves a posterior approach through the inferior petrosal sinus (IPS). However, if the IPS is occluded or absent, the superior ophthalmic vein (via the angular branch of the facial vein), inferior ophthalmic vein, superior petrosal sinus, pterygoid plexus, or sphenoparietal sinus may be used for access. A temporary balloon can be inflated in the ICA, across the communication, to assist with visualization and protect the integrity of the vessel lumen. Endovascular occlusion with parent-vessel preservation may not be achievable or necessary for direct CCFs caused by extensive injury to the ICA or those associated with significant steal. In such circumstances, occlusion of the parent artery may be the best (or only) viable management option (**Fig. 47.18**).

Indirect fistulas may thrombose without vascular intervention (Higashida et al., 1986). However, persistent indirect CCFs are embolized through arterial or venous access routes (listed earlier) in the manner previously described for cranial DAVFs, in general.

Spinal Vascular Malformations

Spinal vascular malformations are a rare and under-diagnosed entity that, if not treated properly, can result in progressive spinal cord symptoms with considerable

Box 47.4 Grading Scale for Carotid Cavernous Fistulas

Type A (direct): direct communication between the internal carotid artery (ICA) and the cavernous sinus. Usually arises as a result of traumatic laceration or aneurysmal rupture and presents with high flow rate.

Type B (indirect): supplied only by the dural branches of the ICA. Most often arises spontaneously and presents with a lower flow rate.

Type C (indirect): supplied only by dural branches of the external carotid artery (ECA). Most often arises spontaneously and presents with a lower flow rate.

Type D (indirect): supplied by dural branches of the ICA and ECA. Most often arises spontaneously and presents with a lower flow rate.

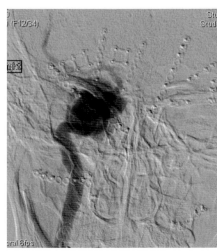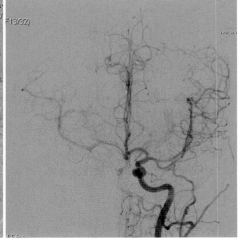

Fig. 47.18 Anteroposterior angiograms before *(left)* and after *(right)* embolization of large posttraumatic carotid-cavernous fistula. Injection of right carotid artery before embolization *(left)* shows filling of cavernous sinus. Cavernous segment of carotid artery was completely embolized with coils and liquid embolic material. Postembolization angiogram *(left)* demonstrates flow to both hemispheres through left carotid artery.

associated morbidity (Krings and Geibprasert, 2009). A majority of the lesions occur in males and are located in the thoracic or lumbar region of the spinal cord. Dural AVFs frequently cause gradual ascending paraparesis or bowel and bladder dysfunction, whereas intramedullary spinal cord malformations typically present with hemorrhage. While MR studies may reveal flow voids or conus medullaris edema, spinal digital subtraction angiography is necessary for diagnosis, characterization of lesional angioarchitecture, and treatment planning. Spinal angiography is most often performed under general endotracheal anesthesia to limit patient movement due to breathing and facilitate visualization of small segmental vessels.

The arterial supply to the spinal cord is derived from a single anterior spinal artery (ASA) and paired posterior spinal arteries (PSAs). The ASA originates from both vertebral arteries, typically just proximal to the vertebrobasilar junction. It courses through the anterior sulcus of the spinal cord and receives tributaries from radiculomedullary branches of the segmental arteries. The most robust anastomotic supply is provided in the cervical lower thoracic and lumbar regions, with a paucity of radicular connections at the upper thoracic levels. One such anastomotic branch, the artery of lumbar enlargement or artery of Adamkiewicz, provides the main arterial supply to the spinal cord from the lower thoracic region to the conus medullaris. It most often originates from a radicular vessel on the left, between the T8 and L4 levels (McCutcheon et al., 1996). The PSAs originate more proximally from the bilateral vertebral arteries. The paired vessels course along the posterolateral aspect of the spinal cord and anastomose with multiple radiculopial branches of the segmental arteries, which enter the dura through the nerve root sheaths. Classification schemes for spinal vascular malformations are based upon this arterial anatomy (Kim and Spetzler, 2006; Spetzler et al., 2002).

Spinal Dural Arteriovenous Fistula (Type I)

These lesions represent the most common type of spinal vascular malformation and may be supplied by one (type 1a) or multiple (type 1b) dorsal radiculomedullary vessels, which form a fistulous connection with the coronal venous plexus upon entering the dura at the root sleeve (Anson and Spetzler, 1992; Kim and Spetzler, 2006; Sivakumar et al., 2009). They occur most frequently in men older than 50 years of age and classically present with progressive myelopathy secondary to chronic venous hypertension. Endovascular treatment consists of embolization of the fistulous origin, including the proximal portion of the draining vein (van Dijk et al., 2002). Open surgical disconnection may be employed to achieve a similar result.

Glomus Arteriovenous Malformation (Type II)

Most similar to intracranial AVMs, these lesions are supplied by perforating braches of the anterior or posterior spinal arteries and drain into the venous plexus surrounding the spinal cord (Kim et al., 2006; Spetzler et al., 2002; Wakhloo, 2008). A high-pressure, high-flow nidus may be diffuse or compact and is often associated with a feeding artery or intranidal aneurysms. These lesions most frequently occur in younger men and women and frequently present with hemorrhage. Embolization is usually employed as an adjunct to surgical resection.

Juvenile/Metameric Arteriovenous Malformation (Type III)

Found predominantly in children and young adults, these lesions are fed by multiple arterial pedicles and affect bone and soft tissue in addition to spinal cord parenchyma (Kim and Spetzler, 2006; Spetzler et al., 2002; Wakhloo, 2008). Involvement of an entire metamere including skin, soft tissue, bone, and spinal cord parenchyma is referred to as *Cobb syndrome*. Multimodality therapy is frequently indicated because of the complex nature of these malformations.

Perimedullary Arteriovenous Malformation (Type IV)

Vascular supply to these intradural extramedullary fistulas is derived from either the anterior (most commonly) or posterior spinal arteries. They occur most frequently between the ages of 30 and 60 and often present with progressive neurological deficits (Anson and Spetzler, 1992; Heros et al., 1986). The treatment paradigm is dependent on the angioarchitecture of the lesion, including the number of feeding pedicles and rate of fistulous flow. Surgical disconnection has been successfully employed for low-flow fistulas supplied by a single feeding artery, while a combination of endovascular and surgical techniques have commonly been used for the management of more complex lesions.

Tumor Embolization

Preoperative embolization of extracranial head and neck or intracranial tumors is a useful adjunct to microsurgical resection. Tumors most commonly treated by this means are meningiomas, glomus tumors, juvenile nasopharyngeal angiofibromas, hemangioblastomas, sarcomas, head and neck squamous cell carcinomas, and choroid plexus tumors (Eskridge et al., 1996; Scholtz et al., 2001). These lesions are often quite vascular, so preoperative embolization can ease complete resection by diminishing surgical time and intraoperative blood loss (Dowd et al., 2003; Gruber et al., 2000; Macpherson, 1991; Manelfe et al., 1986). Many cranial-base tumors are characterized by vascular pedicles that are medially located with respect to the operative approach (Rosen et al., 2002). In such cases, the surgical corridor is often narrow and deep, which amplifies the difficulty of resection. In addition to improving operative safety and visualization, preoperative embolization is believed to reduce transmitted forces to adjacent neural tissues during surgical resection by causing ischemic necrosis and a resultant softening of the tumor mass (Yoon et al., 2008). In selected patients who are not suitable candidates for surgery, embolization can be used for palliation, with a goal of size and tumor growth reduction. Because the primary blood supply is most frequently derived from the external carotid artery, a thorough understanding of the head, neck, and intracranial vascular anatomy is critical.

Embolization Procedure

It is imperative to perform a thorough diagnostic cerebral angiographic evaluation prior to tumor embolization. Interpreted in conjunction with findings evident on noninvasive imaging, this will enable a detailed appraisal of the dural, pial, and extracranial arterial supply to the mass and assessment of the patency and drainage pattern of the venous sinuses. Superselective angiograms afford an opportunity to delineate the nature of dangerous anastomoses involving the internal carotid and vertebral arteries and identify small branches that supply the cranial nerves. Anatomical variants must be noted. Internal carotid artery occlusion testing may be necessary when carotid tumor encasement is present. Rapid technological advances in the development of microcatheters and embolic materials have resulted in greater procedural efficacy and increased safety.

After a diagnostic cerebral angiogram is performed to identify blood supply and assess for feasibility and safety of embolization, a microcatheter is advanced over a microguidewire through the larger diagnostic or guide catheter. Under real-time digital subtraction fluoroscopy, the microsystem is advanced into the vascular pedicle supplying the tumor. Superselective angiography is performed through the microcatheter to confirm proper position, identify any distal branches supplying normal tissue, and assess for the presence of dangerous anastomoses. Provocative testing with IA sodium Amytal or lidocaine may aide in the detection of unsafe collaterals or cranial nerve supply distal to the microcatheter tip (Dowd et al., 2003; Yoon et al., 2008). After proper positioning of the microcatheter, injection of embolic material is performed under constant real-time digital subtraction fluoroscopy. Distal tumoral penetration prevents flow to the mass via collateral vessels and results in devascularization and subsequent tumor necrosis (**Fig. 47.19**). Direct tumor puncture is an alternate means of accessing hypervascular neoplasms of the head and neck (Abud et al., 2004; Chaloupka et al., 1999). This technique may be used alone or in conjunction with transfemoral embolization.

Embolization Materials

A number of agents have been used to embolize tumors, including particles (Bendszus et al., 2000; Wakhloo et al., 1993), nBCA (Capo et al., 1991), Onyx (Shi et al., 2008), platinum coils (Guglielmi, 1998), ethanol (Jungreis, 1991), fibrin glue (Probst et al., 1999), and gelfoam pledgets (Manelfe et al., 1986; Richter and Schachenmayr, 1983). Particulate agents are generally favored over liquid embolic materials owing to their ease of use and relative safety. The precise penetration capacity of particles is dependent on their size, so appropriate selection precludes infiltration into the small arterioles supplying cranial nerves. Since the vasa nervorum are small, the use of particles larger than 150 microns in diameter has been suggested to lessen the risk of ischemic cranial nerve injury (Bendszus et al., 2005; Carli et al., 2010). PVA particles are believed to remain occlusive in vessels for weeks, after which vascular recanalization may occur (Kuroiwa et al., 1996). This property is suitable for preoperative tumor embolization. Because the tumor mass is excised during definitive surgical resection, a long-term durable embolization is not necessary. These agents have been shown by several groups to be safe and effective in decreasing intraoperative blood loss in paraganglioma surgery (Persky et al., 2002; Tikkakoski et al., 1997). After particle embolization is performed, a platinum coil or gelfoam pledget may be placed more proximally in the treated vessel to help prevent recanalization and aid in surgical transection (Dowd et al., 2003). In contrast to particles, liquid embolic materials such as nBCA and Onyx can more easily enter anastomotic channels that supply cranial nerves or cortical vessels not evident on the initial diagnostic angiogram. The operator must be acutely aware of this possibility when using such agents for tumor embolization. Additionally, microcatheter retention can result in vessel rupture or ischemic sequelae. As more aggressive liquid embolic agents are often used for palliative embolization, care must be taken to avoid proximal reflux of any embolic material into eloquent vascular branches.

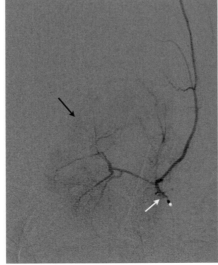
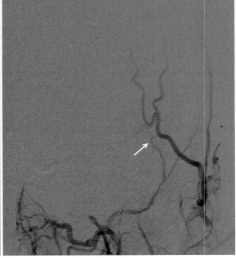

Fig. 47.19 Anteroposterior angiograms before *(left)* and after *(right)* embolization of a left sphenoid wing meningioma. Pre-embolization film shows microcatheter in anterior branch of middle meningeal artery *(white arrow)* and tumoral blush *(black arrow)* after superselective injection. After embolization with polyvinyl alcohol particles, angiogram on right shows an external carotid artery injection with no tumoral blush and a stump at the middle meningeal artery *(white arrow)*.

Vessel Selection

Determining target vessels for endovascular therapy may be difficult. Embolization can effectively obliterate high-flow arteriovenous shunting through the tumor vasculature. Most agree that large external carotid artery branches that directly supply a tumor mass and are distant from dangerous anastomoses may be treated. However, intracranial tumors supplied by both the external and internal carotid artery are reported to exhibit increased pial supply subsequent to embolization of external branches (Manelfe et al., 1986). Augmented blood flow and hypertrophy of the small, deep intracranial vessels may increase the difficulty of the surgical resection, since this vascular supply is often not encountered until the end of the operation. Unless necessary, preoperative embolization of pial blood supply is generally avoided; the benefit of embolization is usually outweighed by the potential risk of ischemia.

Clinical Evidence

Several large case series document angiographic, histological, and surgical benefit following meningioma embolization (Dean et al., 1994; Gruber et al., 2000; Macpherson, 1991; Manelfe et al., 1986; Wakhloo et al., 1993; Yoon et al., 2008). Endovascular treatment of juvenile nasopharyngeal angiofibromas has been shown to reduce both perioperative blood loss and the duration of surgical resection (Davis, 1987; Economou et al., 1988; Roberson et al., 1979). Other reports question the benefit, citing no differences in operative time, blood loss, or clinical outcome (Bendszus et al., 2000). Some groups reserve preoperative embolization for difficult skull-base lesions, referencing complication rates deemed unacceptable for straightforward surgical resections (Rosen et al., 2002). The optimal timing of resection following tumor embolization has been debated. Some operators contend that timing of surgery does not affect outcome, but others have advocated delayed resection to allow for interval tumor necrosis. A comparative retrospective analysis of 50 patients who underwent preoperative embolization for meningioma resection indicated that delaying resection more than 24 hours after embolization can decrease intraoperative blood loss (Chun et al., 2002). Other groups have suggested that the optimal interval between embolization and resection is between 7 and 9 days, as this permits maximal tumor softening (Kai et al., 2002). A significantly long interval between particulate embolization and surgical resection, however, may allow for recanalization of blood vessels supplying the tumor.

Significant neurological deficits have been reported following preoperative tumor embolization. Causes include distal vessel occlusion, reflux of embolic agents, cranial nerve injury, and tumor swelling or hemorrhage following devascularization (Bendszus et al., 2005; Carli et al., 2010; Marangos and Schumacher, 1999). Therefore, potential benefits of embolization must be carefully weighed against the risk of adverse outcome. Patients harboring large hypervascular tumors supplied primarily by external carotid artery branches that are located in anatomical regions difficult to access surgically likely derive the greatest benefit from preoperative embolization.

References

The complete reference list is available online at www.expertconsult.com.

Chapter 48

Principles and Practices of Neurological Rehabilitation

Bruce H. Dobkin

Neurological rehabilitation fosters assessments and practices that extend into every aspect of the care of patients with acute and chronic neurological disabilities. Managing the rehabilitation needs of patients should be a priority for the clinical neurologist who seeks opportunities to lessen impairments and disabilities and to meet the requests of patients to increase their ability to participate in daily home and community activities (Dimyan et al., 2008). To best assist patients, the clinician must determine how a patient's physical and cognitive deficits cause disabilities; consider what tasks patients can and cannot perform independent of assistance and at the speed and accuracy necessary for daily activities; design practice and training paradigms with health-related professionals to lessen disabilities that are important to patients and their caregivers; consider interventions that manipulate the fundamental mechanisms that induce neural adaptations for cerebral reorganization and learning; and anticipate and manage the neuromedical and psychosocial complications of immobility, loss of motor control, cognitive impairment, and functional dependence.

Goals and Structure of Rehabilitation

Rehabilitation training reduces physical and cognitive impairments and their related disabilities in an effort to improve functional independence and health-related quality of life. Training involves an active learning process that requires motivation, guidance, goal setting, progressive practice, and social support.

Aims

Neurological rehabilitation employs multidisciplinary services to improve functional and cognitive skills such as walking and language, reduce disability in personal care and other daily activities, lessen the burden of care provided by family and society for disabled persons, and prevent and manage complications such as dysphagia, contractures, pressure sores, and depression. Although the links between disease pathology, physical and cognitive impairments, disabilities, participation, and handicap are not always clear, physicians and therapists ultimately target the health-related quality of life of patients by maximizing functional independence for home and community pursuits. Patients, caregivers, and families must be fully involved in the rehabilitation process if they are to successfully facilitate self-management, compensatory adaptations, and more independent skills.

The quality of a rehabilitation care plan is only as good as the assessment it is based on. Accurate assessment means getting to the bottom of the mechanisms behind problems that adversely affect patient functioning. Neurorehabilitation assessment includes identifying the most productive focus for interventions and the most appropriate setting in which better outcomes can be achieved within expected time frames. Clinical evaluation initiates a treatment program that is continually revised in light of successive assessments. Over the long run, the clinician monitors for complications and functional changes that present new opportunities to return patients to a higher level of function and participation.

An expert assessment acquires sufficient information to allow a reasonably accurate initial prediction of the potential outcome for the patient after a course of rehabilitation. Both short- and long-term goals take into account the amount of likely neurological recovery and the amount of residual disability. The long-term goal often can be broken down into component steps that move steadily toward the final outcome. Progressive goal setting is a technique to encourage the patient as each short-term objective is achieved, as well as serving to monitor efficacy and identify emerging confounders of gains. Short-term goals must be relevant, motivating, explicit, attainable, measurable, and agreeable to the patient.

To achieve these aims, the rehabilitation process differs from the usual medical model of care by including personnel from multiple disciplines, problem-solving strategies that include methods to engage mechanisms of neuroplasticity, standardized outcome measures, and the organization of home and community services to meet the patient's needs.

Personnel and Strategies

A team approach to inpatient and outpatient care best manages the diverse problems faced by disabled patients and their families (**Fig. 48.1**). In a multidisciplinary model, each member with specialty training treats particular disabilities. In an interdisciplinary model, roles blend. An interdisciplinary approach is oriented toward problem-solving to improve functional outcomes, rather than being bound by individual disciplines. For example, training procedures for motor and cognitive learning or behavioral modification are reinforced by all members of an interdisciplinary group, using agreed-on strategies. These interaction styles are not mutually exclusive. Most teams move between the two models when they formally

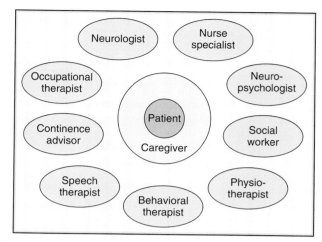

Fig. 48.1 The multidisciplinary rehabilitation team approach centers on the patient and caregiver.

meet to discuss the patient's progress and to adjust goals and treatments.

The care milieu created by the team of therapists, nurses, social workers, neuropsychologists, and physicians, with its emphasis on lessening disability, is one of rehabilitation's most powerful tools. Studies of inpatient stroke rehabilitation, for example, support the team approach as an efficient way to organize services for patients with functional disabilities. With traumatic brain injury (TBI) or spinal cord injury (SCI), the special needs of affected patients suggest that interdisciplinary inpatient and outpatient care will lead to fewer medical and psychosocial complications.

Physicians

An understanding of the underlying disorder, including the mechanisms of disability, potential outcomes, and natural history of the disease being managed, is critical in planning a rehabilitation program for a patient. This expertise may be provided by the growing number of neurologists with expertise in neurorehabilitation who can bring principles from their increasing storehouse of knowledge to bear on recovery, and by rehabilitation physicians or physiatrists, who also have broad experience in musculoskeletal, orthopedic, and cardiopulmonary rehabilitation issues. Orthopedists, urologists, psychiatrists, plastic surgeons, neurosurgeons, and podiatrists often are consulted during rehabilitation and for long-term management of disabled patients.

The clinician superimposes the contributions of neurological, musculoskeletal, cardiopulmonary, and other impairments on a map of the patient's functional abilities and disabilities. For example, does tender musculoligamentous tissue cause pain or limit movement, or does spasticity lead to loss of motor control? Does a medication or metabolic abnormality lessen concentration, the ability to learn, or endurance for exercise? Physicians tend to be the facilitators of the multidisciplinary team, especially during inpatient care. Here, the physician may conduct a weekly team conference that reviews the patient's progress in reaching the functional goals that will permit a discharge to the home. To do this well, the physician must help build the team's infrastructure and understand the practices of its disciplines. Rehabilitation physicians should serve as clinician-scientists as well. The physician can encourage therapists to weigh, formulate, and test strategies. Drawing on current literature and collaborating with basic and clinical researchers, the neurological rehabilitation specialist can optimally assess and develop interventions and creative solutions (Dobkin, 2003).

Physicians should explain to both patient and primary care doctor the indications for medications, measures for secondary prevention of complications, management of risk factors for recurrence or exacerbation of the disease, and the type and duration of rehabilitative interventions. Increasingly, doctors must address the risks and possible benefits of not only medications and usual rehabilitative approaches to care but also potential research interventions such as cellular transplantation (Dobkin et al., 2006b). During outpatient care, physicians must provide informed counseling about exercise and home practice for motor and cognitive retraining. The clinician reviews the details of what the patient is practicing to improve walking, the functional use of an affected upper extremity, language and memory skills, and socialization. Education should be offered about how task-specific practice may alter the brain's representations of these activities and improve the patient's abilities, even years after the initial neurological illness. For patients with chronic diseases that progress, such as multiple sclerosis (MS), practice is perhaps even more important because it may spur gradual neural reorganization to maintain function. Clinicians can encourage patients to increase their strength, speed, and precision of multijoint movements and to build cardiovascular fitness. The physician also should monitor outcomes with serial tests of the activities that are targeted to best determine the optimal dose of a treatment. For example, if the gait pattern is suboptimal, the clinician can test walking speed for 50 feet or the distance walked in 2 minutes to reassess progress in mobility at each visit. By documenting the effects of treatment, the physician can best advocate the continuing goals of rehabilitation to patients and insurers.

The Internet has many sites from which to develop educational materials that physicians and the therapy team can offer patients (e.g., http://www.uclahealth.org/body.cfm?id=1174), as well as lectures and articles about recovery and about experimental interventions.

Rehabilitation Nursing

Traditionally, the nursing role has been one of providing care and support during a phase of illness and doing for others the things they would normally do for themselves. Nurses have particular expertise in bowel and bladder management and have developed the post of continence advisor, particularly for teaching chronic intermittent self-catheterization (CISC) and scheduled voiding programs. They teach skin care and pressure sore management. In an inpatient unit, nurses are in constant contact with the patient undergoing rehabilitation. This extended contact with patients allows nurses to address the issue of carryover of skills from physical and occupational therapy sessions to other areas fundamental for function in the community. Each activity is integrated with others; for instance, continence management through CISC may require improvements in upper limb coordination, trunk control, mobility, lower limb tone, medications to optimize bladder and sphincter control, and strategies to facilitate problem solving. Nurses in community programs also have

become involved in the management of individual chronic diseases including MS, amyotrophic lateral sclerosis (ALS), and Parkinson disease (PD), especially attending to gaps in services needed by patients. A nurse practitioner can be a valuable asset to the physician and team on a busy inpatient service, especially in a university hospital, where patients tend to have complex medical illnesses and needs. The Association of Rehabilitation Nurses has excellent resources for continuing education (www.rehabnurse.org).

Physical Therapists

Physical therapists (PTs), or physiotherapists relate voluntary motor control and patterns of multijoint movements, sensory appreciation, range of motion of joints, strength, balance, and endurance to the training needs for bed and wheelchair mobility, standing up, walking, and functional mobility during activities. PTs bring expertise to the team in wheelchair design, assistive devices, and orthoses. They manage compensatory strategies for carrying out activities of daily living (ADLs) such as the use of a walker and offer interventions to lessen specific impairments. PTs play a primary role in managing musculoskeletal and radicular pain, contractures, spasticity, and deconditioning.

Two broad categories of physical therapy, therapeutic exercise and the so-called neurophysiological and neurodevelopmental techniques, were the bulwark of the approaches used by therapists in the past (**Box 48.1**). Newer concepts related to practice-induced neuroplasticity, motor control, and skills learning have taken greater hold beginning in the past decade.

EXERCISE AND COMPENSATORY FUNCTIONAL TRAINING

Most therapy programs emphasize education about impairments and disabilities, compensatory techniques for ADLs and mobility, and repetitive exercises to build from less complex to more functional multijoint movements. Traditional exercise programs employ repetitive passive and active joint-by-joint exercises and resistance exercises in anatomical planes to optimize strength and range of motion. The approach aims to

---

Box 48.1 Practices in Physical Therapy

Therapeutic exercise and re-education
Resistance exercises
Fitness training
Neurofacilitation techniques:
    Proprioceptive neuromuscular facilitation
    Bobath technique
    Others
Motor control approaches:
    Motor skill learning
Shaping more complex, accurate movements:
    Task-oriented practice
    Forced use
    Massed practice
Biofeedback
Musculoskeletal manipulation techniques
Orthotics (e.g., ankle-foot orthosis), assistive devices (e.g., quad cane)

prevent the complications of immobilization such as contractures, muscle atrophy, and spasticity. In the therapeutic exercise approach to stroke, SCI, and other upper motor neuron (UMN) diseases, residual motor skills in affected and unaffected extremities are used to compensate for impairments. The acquisition of self-care and mobility skills may take precedence over the quality of movement so long as the patient's safety can be ensured. Upper and lower extremity orthotics and assistive devices tend to be used early to promote functional compensation. PTs also use breathing and general conditioning exercises and teach energy conservation techniques, particularly to reduce the energy cost of a pathological gait.

CONDITIONING AND STRENGTHENING

Light resistance exercises for any UMN or lower motor neuron (LMN) disease, from stroke and SCI to ALS, the postpolio syndrome, and the muscular dystrophies, generally are safe and effective in improving strength and sometimes function. Strength can be increased without inducing spasticity in patients with UMN diseases and without muscle tissue injury in those with neuromuscular diseases. Concern about falls, disability, and muscle atrophy in older adults has led to many studies that show that a strengthening program can benefit any sedentary person. Resistance training can lead to an increase in strength without any improvement in muscle bulk, probably by augmenting the amount of supraspinal input that is recruited to the task. Thus, strengthening can be considered a form of motor learning. Isometric resistance exercises probably are the safest approach for weak patients and can be performed without equipment. For example, flexing the elbow of one arm about 60 degrees and pressing down on that forearm with the palm of the other arm to reach an equilibrium of tension in each arm will enhance strength in the shoulder girdle, elbow flexors and extensors, and forearm groups. To build muscle mass requires the subject to perform 1 or 2 sets of 8 to 15 repetitions 3 times a week against 50% or more of the maximum resistance manageable in a single lift. Pool therapy can be used to augment fitness and strengthening exercises. Patients may work against the resistance of the water, for example, by repeatedly flexing, extending, abducting and adducting each leg at the hip while standing on the other or by using swim strokes. Practice walking in a pool allows the patient to make use of the water's buoyancy, but light refraction within the water may make visual cues for foot placement less reliable.

Small trials of medications that act on the neuromuscular junction (e.g., pyridostigmine), those that work on muscle metabolism (e.g., β₂-adrenergic agonists, creatine), potassium channel blockers that act on demyelinated axons (e.g., aminopyridines), and hormones such as androgens and human growth factor, which may lessen disuse atrophy, have revealed modest efficacy when combined with resistance exercise.

Fitness training is valuable in UMN, extrapyramidal, and LMN diseases. Repetitive exercise, at least in animal models of stroke and SCI, also has induced potential reparative biological effects such as neurogenesis and increased expression of neurotrophic factors. This finding may be used to motivate patients. Treadmill walking can be used as an aerobic workout for the older adult with hemiparetic stroke. After a complete SCI, cardiovascular conditioning exercise is limited by the upper body's small muscle mass, by pooling of blood in the leg muscles, which reduces cardiac preloading, and by impaired cardiovascular reflexes. Functional electrical stimulation (FES) of the lower extremities during cycle ergometry can improve both peripheral muscular and central cardiovascular fitness. Clinical trials suggest that FES exercise in sets of 10 to 15 repetitions against an increasing load resistance of 1 to 15 kg over 12 weeks will increase muscle bulk, improve strength, and reduce fatigability for the FES activity. Although psychological and other physiological benefits have been attributed to FES in paraplegic subjects, long-term home programs require much motivation.

NEUROPHYSIOLOGICAL SCHOOLS

Many schools of physical therapy have developed approaches that focus on enhancing the movement of paretic limbs affected by UMN lesions. These approaches may be especially valuable when initiating motor therapies in patients with profound weakness. Techniques include using sensory stimuli and reflexes to facilitate or inhibit muscle tone and single- and whole-limb muscle movements in and out of mass actions called *synergies*. Most approaches try to sequence therapy in a progression reminiscent of the neurodevelopmental evolution in infants from reflexive to more complex movements. The emphasis is on normal postural alignment before any movement. Some techniques permit mass movement patterns early in treatment; others inhibit spastic overflow synergistic movements. For example, mobility activities may proceed in a developmental pattern from rolling onto the side with arm and leg flexion on the same side, followed by extension of the neck and legs while prone, then lying prone while supported by the elbows, and then doing static and weight-shifting movements while crawling on all four extremities. These mat activities are followed by efforts for sitting, standing, and finally walking. This progression is used most often in children with cerebral palsy, but some therapists also apply it to stroke and TBI rehabilitation.

Different schools vary in their attempts to activate or minimize reflexive movements and how they train the functional movements needed for ordinary activities. These schools have not emphasized strengthening exercises. Their use of reflexive movements, vibration to stimulate a muscle contraction, cutaneous stimulation to facilitate a voluntary contraction, and loading a joint to increase extension is reasonable from a physiological point of view, but any carryover of responses into functional or volitional movement is uncertain.

Neurodevelopmental practitioners believe that the optimal facilitation of movement requires normal postural responses, that abnormal motor behaviors are compensatory, and that the quality of motor experiences and the integration of whole-body somatosensory information will train patients for more normalized movements. The *Bobath hands-on approach* is a particularly popular neurodevelopmental technique. It aims to facilitate normal movement and desired automatic reactions and to restore postural control while inhibiting abnormal tone and reflex activity using specific motor patterns. Bobath therapists avoid provoking mass flexor synergies from the shoulder, elbow, and wrist or extensor synergies at the knee and ankle. The coordination of patterns of muscle group activity is viewed as more important than the actions of individual muscles. Most practitioners take a problem-solving and task-oriented approach with patients. A typical exercise routine may work on stance and trunk control with a large ball and careful hand placement by the therapist to evoke movements out of synergy (**Fig. 48.2**). These methods originally were developed for children with cerebral palsy but have

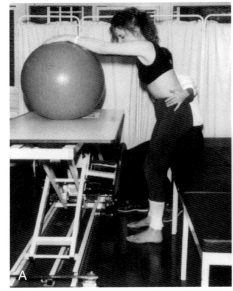
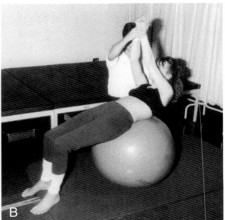

Fig. 48.2 Gymnastic ball used to facilitate standing and postural adjustments for standing up **(A)** and flexion and extension of the trunk and reaching **(B)**.

been adapted for stroke and other neurological disorders. In comparison with other neurophysiological approaches and task-oriented motor learning for gait, upper extremity function, and overall level of functional independence, use of Bobath techniques has led to equivalent outcomes or, in several small trials, modestly inferior outcomes (van Vliet et al., 2005). Given the underlying theory of Bobath, however, outcome measures ought to examine the quality of task-related movements as much as functional gains.

MOTOR LEARNING APPROACHES

Movement science and the bases for learning motor skills have become key concepts for understanding normal movement and analyzing motor dysfunction. The motor control approach may incorporate techniques to eliminate unnecessary muscle activity and provide feedback about performance and practice during task-specific or task-oriented therapies. In rehabilitation settings, little attention has been paid to whether training procedures—not what is taught but how it is taught—optimize gains in cognitive skills, motor functions, self-care, and community activities. The essence of therapy for any disability, as with acquisition of any novel motor or cognitive skill, is practice. Although a practice session can have a powerful effect, such effects are only temporary. Practice that improves performance during a training session may not lead to long-term learning. The goal of practice should be a permanent effect. Research studies of interventions, however, rarely include deliberate reinforcement strategies or dose-response curves to establish how much practice is needed to achieve a retraining goal. For example, practice of functional activities using the hemiparetic arm for reaching and grasping items that includes the contextual interference of intermixing other tasks such as pointing and touching during learning, may lead to better retention over time than blocks of repetitive practice of the same task.

TASK-ORIENTED PRACTICE

Motor learning emphasizes visual, verbal, and other sensory feedback to achieve task-specific movements, in contrast with neurophysiological techniques, which rely on cutaneous, pro-

prioceptive, and other sensory stimuli to elicit facilitation and inhibition of movement patterns. A key aim of the PT is to put the patient in the best position to be able to practice progressively. Constraint-induced therapy (CIT) for the upper extremity, body weight–supported treadmill training (BWSTT) for walking, mental practice, electromyography (EMG) and other forms of biofeedback (BFB) during functional movements, and training in a virtual reality (VR) environment are among many task-oriented approaches to improve motor control for particular tasks.

Studies of the efficacy of particular schools of therapy have not revealed differences between approaches. These studies, primarily in patients with stroke, used outcome measures that emphasize independence in ADLs and not an outcome directly related to the primary focus of the specific technique of physiotherapy, which is motor performance and patterns of movement. Studies of efficacy should concentrate on the best well-defined practice for an important goal such as reaching, grasping items, and walking that may in theory be modulated by the intervention. Another emphasis must be on the optimal intensity and duration of sessions of training. Most therapists take an eclectic experimentalist's approach, not unlike what physicians do in daily practice, but this may not be conducive to an optimal outcome for the patient. Indeed, the best evidence to date is that a mixed approach leads to more functional independence than a placebo or no active therapy, but no one approach to a particular set of upper extremity or mobility functions has been shown to be superior to another (Pollack et al., 2008).

ADAPTIVE EQUIPMENT

Canes and walkers improve stability through a lever arm that can share the body's weight between the leg and device, keep the pelvis level during stance on the weak leg, and generate a joint moment to assist the hip abductors and reduce loading on the knee. Devices must be fitted properly. For example, handgrips should be at a height that allows approximately 20 to 30 degrees of elbow flexion. The cane should swing forward with the involved limb and bear the most weight during stance on that leg.

Box 48.2 Wheelchair Characteristics

Frame:
    Material
    Weight
    Foldable structure
Seat:
    Weight, width, depth, angle
    Sling or cushioned, inserts
    Cushion (foam, air, fluid, gel, gelfoam)
Back:
    Weight, fixed or reclining, headrest
    Flexible, custom-molded; foam or gel inserts
Armrests:
    Weight (fixed or adjustable)
    Fixed, removable, swing-away
    Arm troughs, clear plastic lap board, power controls
Leg and footrest:
    Weight, adjustment from edge of seat, knee flexion angle
    Fixed, removable, swing-away; straps
Rear wheels:
    Materials (alloys, plastic)
    Tires (width, tread; pneumatic or solid)
    Camber for speed and turning radius
Handrims:
    Power-assisted
Front casters
Brakes (locking, backsliding)
Anti-tip bars
Power supply, control system

Wheelchairs are of two main types, companion-operated and patient-operated. The latter can be manual or power-assisted. Lightweight and very lightweight patient- or companion-operated wheelchairs must be fitted with at least a dozen characteristics in mind (**Box 48.2**). Severe spasticity, poor head or trunk control, the amount of upper extremity function, and the type of work and sports engaged in may necessitate additional modifications. Very lightweight wheelchairs tend to be most manageable and durable for the patient with paraplegia. Models with power-assisted wheels have become more affordable and are practical for use by patients with weakness or pain in the upper extremities. Motorized wheelchairs can be maneuvered by joystick switches and chin or sip-and-puff mouth controls. The high cost of custom-designed wheelchairs means that therapists, vendors, patients, and families need to work together to obtain what is most appropriate and cost-effective. Wheelchairs also require maintenance. A wobbly front wheel or poorly aligned main rear wheel adds to the energy cost of mobility and may cause shoulder and wrist injuries. Most rehabilitation centers that manage patients with myelopathies offer a wheelchair clinic and have close links to durable medical equipment suppliers.

Occupational Therapists

Occupational therapists (OTs) facilitate the practical management of disability. The philosophical foundation of OT is that purposeful activity helps prevent and remediate dysfunction and elicits maximum adaptation. Goal-oriented tasks are meant to be culturally meaningful and important to the needs

Box 48.3 Adaptive Aids for Daily Living

Feeding

Utensil: thickened handle, cuff holder
Dish: food guard, suction holder
Cup: no-spill covers, holders

Bathing

Shower seat, transfer bench
Washing: mitt, long-handled scrub brush
Safety: grab bars

Dressing

Hook-and-loop closures for shoes, pants
Button hook, zipper pull
Low clothes rods in closet
Long-handled comb or brush

Toileting

Safety rails, raised seat, commode

Mobility

Prefabricated ramp
Powered stair lift
Wheelchair, standing wheelchair
Transfer devices and ceiling-mounted track lifts
Automobile and van: lifts, hand controls

Communication

Cellular phone, handheld Internet device

Computer Workstation

Environmental controls
Communication: printing, voice synthesis
Interface adaptations: keyboard, microswitch, voice activation

Miscellaneous

One-handed jar opener
Doorknob extension for better grip
Book holder, page turner (electronic or mouth stick)
Holder for one-handed cutting
Long-reach jaw grabbers ("lazy tongs")

of clients and their families. Activities include daily life and work skills, exercise, recreation, and crafts. Occupational therapy also is concerned with improving the patient's interaction with the environment and maximizing the patient's role in society in terms of relationships, occupation, and personal standing. The OT implements a program to enable patients to learn or relearn specific activities, develop new or compensatory skills, adapt their behavior to what is feasible, make adjustments to increase the accessibility of their environment, and perform leisure activities.

A program may include the use of appliances to improve independence, ranging from simple devices (e.g., a thickened grip to better grasp cutlery or a pen) to complex ones (e.g., use of an environmental control unit). Such adaptive aids for daily living are listed in (**Box 48.3**). Hemicuff and Bobath slings are used to reduce shoulder subluxation and prevent pain in patients with upper limb paralytic disorders (**Fig. 48.3**). A balanced forearm orthosis can support the upper arm and allow a modest biceps and triceps contraction to swing

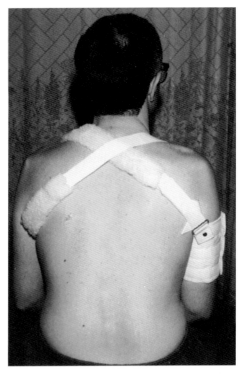

Fig. 48.3 A cuff support to prevent pain and lessen the subluxation of the glenohumeral shoulder joint in a patient with left hemiplegia after stroke.

the arm over a table, which may be especially effective for the patient with a level C5 SCI. For patients with stroke and brain injury, OTs work closely with the neuropsychologist to address visuospatial inattention, memory loss, apraxia, difficulties in problem solving, and the skills needed for return to school or employment. Some OTs manage dysphagia and interpret modified barium swallow (MBS) studies.

Task-oriented and motor learning strategies have gained attention in formal occupational therapy research. Using this approach, the OT presents activities in a way that elicits the retention and transfer of particular skills for use in a functional setting. For example, in one study, limb kinematics improved in normal and hemiparetic subjects when training included purposeful goals with relevant items used daily. Thus, practice in object-related tasks, rather than simple repetition of reaching and grasping of items that have no significance for the client, may provide more concrete sensory information and offer rewards that motivate performance. In many instances, OT strategies evolve from problems that arise in daily living that require a solution. For example, adaptive equipment and an OT educational intervention in stroke patients to remediate the lack of confidence and increase the amount of information patients had available to them reduced the barriers to outdoor mobility and participation in the community (Logan et al., 2004).

Speech and Cognitive Therapists

Speech and language therapists are trained in many aspects of communication and cognition, including phonetics and linguistics, attention and memory, audiology, and developmental psychology, and provide expertise in the investigation and management of dysphagia. These therapists treat primarily

patients with dysarthria, aphasia, and cognitive dysfunction that interferes with daily activities.

Interventions to improve the patient's speech intelligibility, volume, and fluency include exercises of affected oromotor structures. For example, patients may be trained to slow their articulation, use shorter sentences, maximize breath support, extend jaw motion, adjust placement of the tongue, and exaggerate articulatory movements. Communication aids include voice amplification and computer assistive and voice recognition devices. These therapists also provide guidance for persons with swallowing difficulties; assessment may include the MBS study during videofluoroscopy.

Treatment for aphasia generally is based on clinical evaluation of the patient's cognitive and linguistic assets and deficits. The therapy plan is fine-tuned according to standardized language and neuropsychological test results, knowledge of the cortical and subcortical structures damaged, and the ongoing response to specific therapies. Speech therapists attempt to circumvent, deblock, or help the patient compensate for defective language behaviors. Stimulation-facilitation approaches, listed in (**Box 48.4**), are commonly employed. Views on the value of speech therapy for aphasia vary. Most randomized controlled trials demonstrate a significant benefit for aspects of expression and comprehension in moderately impaired subjects. The amount of practice is a key variable for enhancing outcomes for any particular approach.

Recreational Therapists

Recreational therapists involve patients on an inpatient unit in group games, crafts, cooking, playing with pets, and other activities to help them socialize, practice skills, and enjoy the physical and emotional value of recreation despite new disabilities. In addition, the recreational therapist joins with the PT and the OT to teach patients how to reintegrate into the home and community. Outpatient recreational activities carried out in a wheelchair or with one hand also foster socialization and fitness. More than 200 local, national, and international organizations have developed rules and equipment for at least 75 sports and recreational activities that take into account a range of functional abilities.

Psychologists

Neuropsychologists with skills in clinical psychology help define and manage cognitive impairments and mood and behavioral disorders. Detailed psychometric testing is fundamental to establishing a rehabilitation program for a patient with cognitive impairment. These tests of aspects of memory, learning, perception, language, and executive function, however, do not represent the range of cognitive skills needed for real-world activities. The neuropsychologist often takes the lead in the management of mild to severe brain injury resulting from trauma or stroke and plays an important role in counseling patients, caregivers, and staff. When working with amnestic patients after TBI, the neuropsychologist may design operant conditioning paradigms or a token economy to reinforce appropriate social interactions, awareness of deficits, and learning. The neuropsychologist also develops relaxation techniques for anxiety states and behavioral approaches for the management of chronic pain.

Social Workers

Social workers deal with the psychosocial aspects of disability and provide counseling and often brief psychotherapy. Their concerns extend to the ability of the patient and family to cope with disability in and out of the hospital. They play a key role in apprising the rehabilitation team about family issues, supports needed for best management of the disabled patient, and appropriate care services in the community. The close interactions of social workers and patients or caregivers during inpatient rehabilitation often provide valuable insight into the dynamics of family involvement and the adequacy of resources. Social workers serve as liaisons to private and government agencies and to case managers from insurance companies. Smooth discharge planning from an inpatient service requires their assistance.

Orthotists and Bracing

Expertise in the manufacture, selection, and application of orthotic devices is another key component of a rehabilitation service. The PT or the OT works with an orthotist to select external devices that modulate directional forces from the body and joints in a controlled manner. Although many orthotic devices are mass-produced, the expertise of a trained orthotist is invaluable in choosing and constructing orthoses and supervising their fitting and adjustment. Orthoses include ankle and ankle-knee braces, finger-wrist and shoulder splints, spinal braces, collars, and corsets. The material most often used in manufacture of these devices is a malleable type of plastic, but light metals may be used when large biomechanical forces have to be managed. The effects of pressure, shear forces, and heat retention with sweating also must be considered during fitting to protect the skin.

With shortened inpatient rehabilitation stays, especially after stroke, ankle-foot orthoses (AFOs) that fit inside a shoe tend to be used early to more quickly assist foot clearance during ambulation in patients with a central or peripheral

lesion. Observation of gait usually is enough to determine the need for a trial with an AFO in a patient with hemiparesis or footdrop. Indications include inadequate dorsiflexion for initial heel contact or for toe clearance during early and mid-swing, excessive hip-hiking during swing, medial-lateral subtalar instability during stance, tibial instability during stance, and uncontrolled foot placement caused by sensory loss. An orthosis also may be needed after operative heel cord lengthening. If the knee of the hemiplegic buckles during stance, angling the AFO in slight plantar flexion will extend the knee earlier. Dorsiflexing the AFO by 5 degrees can decrease knee hyperextension and help prevent the snapping back that causes instability and pain in midstance. Ankle inversion may necessitate greater rigidity and longer anterior foot trim. The AFO worn in a shoe ought to improve weight-bearing on the affected leg, increase single-limb stance time, and perhaps lessen postural sway. This may improve safety, especially on uneven surfaces, and walking velocity. **Fig. 48.4** shows a thermoplastic AFO that fits in a shoe to limit plantar flexion and rotation and help control the knee. Orthoses may be static, such as a rest splint worn at night, or dynamic, with joints that may be lockable or free moving. **Fig. 48.5** shows a thermoplastic AFO with a hinged joint that allows flexibility on rising to stand and at heel strike to start the stance phase of the gait cycle. Toe clawing can be managed with a metatarsal pad that spreads the toes. Some patients who have footdrop from a neuropathy such as Charcot-Marie-Tooth disease or diabetes may find that a fashionable boot with a flat heel that fits snugly above the ankle can improve gait by lessening its steppage quality, yet allow toe clearance. An orthotist can assess the potential for shoe modifications and inserts to improve

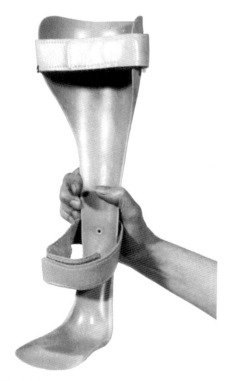

Fig. 48.4 This fabricated ankle-foot orthosis is designed for ankle and knee control of a hemiparetic patient who has minimal hypertonicity. A wider lateral flange and hook-and-loop straps across the front of the ankle would provide greater ankle control.

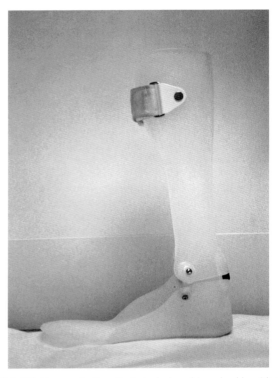

Fig. 48.5 This thermoplastic orthotic includes a hinged ankle with a stop to allow approximately 5 degrees of dorsiflexion when the subject goes from sitting to standing and in portions of the stance phase.

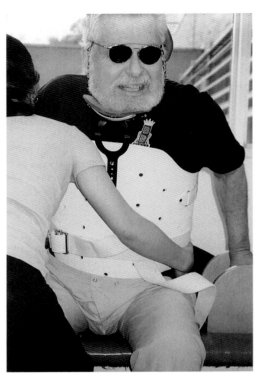

Fig. 48.6 This thoracolumbar support orthotic was molded to the patient's chest to limit upper thoracic vertebral motion after a high spinal cord injury and surgical fusion. The chin brace and stiffness of the jacket limit early progress in mobility tasks for transfers. The riser grips that the patient holds make it easier to practice pushing down into the mat to raise the buttocks.

balance and pressure points. Multiple small trials in patients with hemiplegic stroke show that walking activity increases and impairments in walking and balance decrease with the use of an AFO (Tyson and Kent, 2009). Functional electrical stimulation of the peroneal nerve timed to the gait cycle has equivalent or somewhat better effects on walking speed.

A metal double-upright brace offers greater rigidity for mediolateral foot instability and allows more versatility in adjustments for the amount of plantar and dorsiflexion but can be expensive, heavy, and cosmetically unappealing to the hemiplegic patient. Metal bracing systems are used more often by selected subjects with paraplegia from spinal injuries and in those with polio. Lightweight plastic knee-ankle-foot orthoses (KAFOs) with locking metal knee joints also can assist patients with severe polyneuropathy, muscular dystrophy, meningomyelocele, or SCI. Reciprocal gait orthoses (RGOs) with wire cables that link flexion of one hip to extension of the opposite hip are available for paraplegics. Short-distance ambulation for exercise also can be aided in the patient with SCI by variations on a KAFO or other devices. Bracing in persons with SCI has been combined with functional electrical stimulation to improve stepping and decrease its energy cost.

The thoracolumbar support shown in **Fig. 48.6** was molded to the patient to lessen neck motion after a high thoracic vertebral injury and surgical stabilization. Static orthoses allow no motion of the primary joint. Solid wrist-hand orthoses usually are set between neutral and 30 degrees of extension. Upper limb orthoses, however, have not been shown to improve arm or hand function, increase range of motion or lessen the incidence of pain, based on small trials after stroke. Dynamic orthoses use elastic, wire, or powered levers that

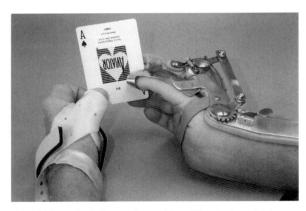

Fig. 48.7 This card-playing patient with a C6 spinal cord injury uses a molded thumb-opposition splint to pinch better with the right hand, and a lightweight metal tenodesis orthotic that pinches the thumb to the next two fingers when he dorsiflexes his wrist.

compensate for weakness or an imbalance in strength and allow some controlled movement. **Fig. 48.7** shows the paretic left hand of a patient with a level C6 SCI holding a playing card with the aid of a thumb opposition splint. The weaker right hand needs wrist extension to mechanically oppose the thumb to the second and third digits. Such custom-made devices can be produced with lightweight metals and plastics. Functional neuromuscular electrical stimulation electrodes can be embedded in a wrist splint to enable grasp and release or over the peroneal nerve to trigger ankle dorsiflexion at appropriate times during the stepping cycle.

Measurement Tools

Outcome measurement is essential to demonstrate the effectiveness of an intervention for an individual and for clinical trials that aim to develop better evidence-based practices. Many of these measurement tools can also be employed within usual clinical care to monitor for declines. The complete discussion of this topic is available in the online version of this book at www.expertconsult.com.

Organization of Services

Service Provision

The way in which services are organized depends to some extent on the disease being managed. The most fundamental differentiation is between acute-onset diseases with different pathophysiological characteristics such as brain and spinal cord trauma and stroke; chronic conditions such as cerebral palsy and polio, in which disability may increase with aging and overuse of muscles and joints; and progressive disorders such as MS, muscular dystrophies, ALS, and PD. Service provision also should be driven by the philosophy underlying rehabilitation: to return the patient home and optimize home and community activities as soon as possible. The speed with which this is done depends as much on the services available in the community and the capacity of the family and caregivers to look after the patient as it does on the severity of the disability. Some tension arises between inpatient services in which all of the necessary ingredients are gathered under one roof, which appeals to patients and families, and community services, which are less centralized but support patients in their own environment. Most important is the smooth interface between these two settings when patients are discharged from an inpatient service.

INPATIENT REHABILITATION UNIT

The most efficient rehabilitation setting is an inpatient unit designed and staffed specifically for this purpose. In the United States, approximately 1200 inpatient sites are covered under Medicare. The benefits of dedicated units for stroke management have been convincingly demonstrated. Patients managed in stroke units are significantly less likely to die than those cared for on ordinary wards. Death, institutionalization, and dependency all are significantly less common in stroke unit patients, in part because of a reduction in secondary complications of stroke and a milieu dedicated to managing disability. Early functionally oriented therapies by an organized team tend to get patients independent enough to return home sooner than sporadic therapy that does not articulate specific attainable goals for mobility, self-care, and family training. These benefits persist for up to 5 years after discharge and improve quality of life. With inpatient stroke rehabilitation in the United States usually starting within 10 days of onset, and with the average length of stay less than 24 days, planning is imperative.

Several studies of TBI suggest the benefit of coordinated care starting during the inpatient stay. Investigators randomly assigned 120 active-duty military personnel who suffered moderate TBI to a standardized inpatient milieu–based cognitive rehabilitation program or to a home program with weekly phone support from a nurse and mental and physical exercises carried out on their own for about 30 minutes a day (Salazar et al., 2000). The inpatient program used both didactic cognitive and functional experiential approaches. Treatment lasted 8 weeks. Outcomes did not differ 1 year later in standard cognitive tests, social adaptation, mood, behavior, or fitness for military duty. More than 90% returned to work. Aggression increased in both groups, suggesting the need for ongoing support.

The role of inpatient rehabilitation units in managing progressive conditions such as MS and PD is much less well defined, although some evidence suggests a benefit in progressive MS. Inpatient care also may return patients home at a higher level of functioning after implantation of a deep brain stimulator for PD or after an exacerbation of walking disability caused by a hip fracture in a patient with a chronic hemiparesis.

COMMUNITY-BASED SERVICES

Although community-based rehabilitation appears to have a number of advantages from the perspective of the disabled patient, few studies have addressed its efficacy (Legg, 2004). This lack may relate at least in part to the methodological difficulties in defining the training team's level of expertise, the patient's level of disability, the amount of caregiver support, and the frequency, duration, and type of therapy. One large randomized stroke trial compared rehabilitation at home after an average 12-day inpatient stay with another week of inpatient care followed by hospital-based outpatient treatment. Patients who lived alone either were independent in transfers when they left the hospital or needed to be assisted by a caregiver. Similar outcomes 12 months after a stroke were achieved at lower cost because of less use of hospital beds by the early discharge group. An intention-to-treat randomized trial with 250 subjects showed that rehabilitation in an inpatient unit after a brief stay in an acute stroke unit or general medical ward produced better outcomes in moderate to severely disabled patients (BI score less than 50) compared with rehabilitation treatment in the community. No differences in quality of life were found, and levels of activity outside the home were not measured. Smaller trials confirm similar positive outcomes at 3 to 6 months for home to those for various forms of outpatient care, with the home group having fewer in-hospital days and greater gains in instrumental ADLs.

A day treatment program for approximately 100 patients who were unable to work for 1 to 2 years after TBI provided a range of interventions during group therapy for a mean of 190 days. The investigators found a significant reduction in physical disability, increased self-awareness and emotional self-regulation, and more effective participation in interpersonal activities. At 1 year after completion, 72% lived independently and 57% were employed.

A brief stint of outpatient therapy for a well-defined goal, such as to improve transfers in a patient who declines from MS or to make walking safe again after an illness that causes deconditioning in a patient with chronic hemiparesis, is an invaluable means for patients to maintain their highest level of independence and avoid placement in a nursing home. A few therapy sessions a week for a few weeks plus a home program may accomplish this when provided for a task-specific goal that relieves caregivers of new burdens. For example, a bout of therapy for aerobic conditioning and muscle strengthening lessened disability in patients with the chronic effects of a prior stroke. A randomized trial assigned 110 patients with mostly chronic TBI to an outreach program in the community or to provision of written material about resources for patients and families (Powell et al., 2002). The outreach group met about twice a week for a mean of 27 weeks. The outreach group made modest but significant gains in scores on the BI and a brain injury outcome measure 2 years after the start of this late intervention.

The most efficient structure for rehabilitation services in many countries includes a two-tiered system of service delivery. Regional specialists can manage complex and profound disabilities, and local community services provide neurological disability teams from local hospitals or the community. Regional neurological rehabilitation centers provide experts familiar with the management of complex and severe disabilities; serve as a focus for education, training, and research; and should be linked to university teaching centers. Such centers can offer care for patients with high-level SCIs and severe TBI, manage specialized orthopedic and plastic surgery procedures, and provide wheelchair and special seating needs, custom orthotics and prosthetics, rehabilitation engineering, functional electrical stimulation devices for walking and upper extremity movement, neuroprostheses, communication aids and environmental controllers for quadriparetic patients, and driving assessments.

Most disability services can be provided locally, which is likely to be both cost-efficient and cost-effective. Services provided by a multidisciplinary neurological disability team based in a local hospital can develop community outreach into clinical centers and homes. Resources often are not adequate for this approach, however. A community-based rehabilitation model developed by the WHO has suggested how communities can develop their own support mechanisms for disabled people, often with locally trained workers supervised by qualified staff. Telerehabilitation services may prove especially useful in supporting patients who live far from available services or are too disabled to leave the home.

Biological Bases for Rehabilitative Interventions

The potential to enhance neurological recovery by manipulating the biological adaptability of the brain, spinal cord, and peripheral nerves has become remarkably relevant to clinical practice (Dobkin, 2003). Basic neuroscience studies suggest that physical and cognitive training, extrinsic stimulation, and pharmacological interventions, along with natural biological reactions to injury, could inhibit or enhance the restoration of motor and cognitive functions. **Box 48.7** lists some of the potential mechanisms that contribute to changes in impairments and disabilities. These are not discrete mechanisms. They overlap, and many depend on each other over periods of variable duration. In addition, biological therapeutic approaches such as use of tissue implants may enhance these mechanisms when applied to human studies of recovery in the near future. These potential mechanisms, drawn mostly from in vitro and in vivo experiments with invertebrates and vertebrates, are the subject of much ongoing investigation (Carmichael, 2008; Blesch and Tuszynski, 2008). Although care must be taken in extrapolating from animal studies of recovery to their implications for human interventions, at

---

Box 48.7 Mechanisms That May Support Recovery of Function

Network Plasticity

Recovery of neuronal excitability:
  Resolve cell and axon ionic dysequilibrium and conduction block
  Resolve edema, resorb blood products
  Reverse diaschisis
Increased activity in neurons adjacent to injured ones and in partially spared pathways
Representational adaptations in neuronal assemblies:
  Expansion of representational maps
  Recruitment of cells not ordinarily involved in an activity
Recruitment of parallel and subcomponent pathways:
  Altered activity in distributed cortical and subcortical networks
  Activation of pattern generators (e.g., for stepping)
  Recruitment of networks not ordinarily involved in an activity
Modulation of excitability by neurotransmitters
Use of alternative behavioral strategies

Neuronal Plasticity

Altered efficacy of synaptic activity:
  Activity-dependent unmasking of previously ineffective synapses
  Learning tied to activity-dependent changes (e.g., long-term potentiation, long-term depression) in synaptic strength in periinjury and remote regions
  Increased neuronal responsiveness from denervation hypersensitivity
  Delayed decline in number of neurons (e.g., from apoptosis)
  Change in number or variety of receptors
  Change in neurotransmitter release and uptake
Regeneration and sprouting from injured and uninjured axons and dendrites:
  Angiogenesis
  Expression of developmental genes for cell viability, growth, and remodeling proteins
  Modulation by neurotrophic factors, neurotransmitters, and signaling molecules
  Dendritic spine remodeling
  Inhibition of growth cone extension (e.g., myelin-associated glycoprotein, Nogo receptor activation)
  Actions of chemoattractants and inhibitors in the milieu for growth cone function and targeting
Remyelination
Neurogenesis and gliogenesis with cell migration

Adapted with permission from Dobkin, B., 2003. The Clinical Science of Neurologic Rehabilitation. Oxford University Press, New York.

---

least a few of these potential mechanisms suggest strategies that the rehabilitation team can use to improve outcomes.

Recovery of Neuronal Excitability

Reversal of toxic-metabolic insults to neurons, axons, and glia plays an early role in recovery of function. Recovery of impairments may be delayed until intracellular and extracellular edema, acidosis, and ion fluxes resolve and until protein synthesis restarts, the mass and toxic effects of blood from a hemorrhage lessen, and other intracellular and membrane functions return to normal. Some of the gains in the first days to few weeks after TBI, SCI, and stroke seem related to these mechanisms. Acute medical interventions to spare the penumbra of hypometabolic tissue on the edge of an infarct have been a mainstay of approaches to neuroprotection in stroke. The extent of the recovery of cortical penumbral and peri-infarct tissue has been modestly correlated with recovery of function in patients after stroke. The surviving penumbra may be a locus for long-term potentiation (LTP), representational plasticity and synaptogenesis, and activity-driven structural reorganization, as well as for the promotion of axonal regeneration and the attraction of new neural cells from the subventricular zone (Cramer, 2008). Infarcts, diffuse axonal injury after TBI, and much of the damage after SCI occur within white matter tracts, so concepts of penumbral sparing may not apply.

Remote effects of an injury, caused by a lack of transsynaptic activity along a neural pathway after one of its links has been damaged or due to the loss of modulation by noradrenergic, serotonergic, dopaminergic, or cholinergic neurotransmission, also could transiently limit recovery. This transsynaptic functional deactivation, called *diaschisis*, has been demonstrated in autoradiography and positron emission tomography (PET) studies as neurovascular uncoupling and aberrant neurotransmission. After a thalamic infarction, for example, hypometabolism of frontoparietal cortex that had received input from thalamic projections often is found. Hypometabolism of the dorsolateral frontal cortex after a stroke in the caudate nucleus and anterior limb of the internal capsule is another example of diminished activity in spared tissue. Although resolution of remote functional deactivation has been suggested as a mechanism of motor recovery in animal studies, human studies with functional imaging have not clearly revealed a relationship between the degree of impairment of recovery and regions of anatomically remote hypometabolism.

Activity in Partially Spared Pathways

Partial sparing of neuronal clusters, as in periinfarct tissue or in tracts such as the posterior limb of the internal capsule, provides a substrate to lessen impairment and disability over days to months after injury. Experimental studies reveal that as little as 20% sparing of one corticospinal tract can provide the minimal residual structure necessary for fair upper or lower extremity motor control. For example, symptoms of PD evolve after approximately 75% of dopamine-containing neurons have died, and locomotor function decompensates when 95% are lost. In a classic human study, Bucy relieved hemiballismus by incising a portion of the cerebral peduncle. Within 24 hours, the patient's flaccid hemiplegia began to improve. By 7 months, the patient plateaued with a very mild hemiparesis, independent gait, and the ability to hop on the contralateral leg. At autopsy, only 17% of the axons in the medullary pyramid persisted. An estimated 90% of precentral giant cells of Betz suffered retrograde degeneration.

Partial wallerian degeneration of the corticospinal tract sometimes can be seen on MRI scans after stroke (**Fig. 48.8**). On computed tomography (CT) images, sparing of more than 60% of the cerebral peduncle, including the medial portion,

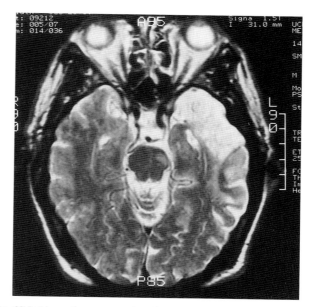

Fig. 48.8 Magnetic resonance imaging 6 months after a left hemisphere stroke reveals atrophy of the ipsilateral cerebral peduncle of approximately 40% relative to the homologous peduncle on the right, and wallerian degeneration of the basis pontis involving a moderate amount of the corticospinal tract. After an initial hemiparesis, the patient was able to oppose his thumb to all fingers, use the hand in activities of daily living, and walk 50 feet in 14 seconds (normal) with minimal gait deviations. The imaging is consistent with enough pathway sparing to have allowed retraining of residual sensorimotor pathways for this functional gain.

predicts the recovery of a precision grip and, to a lesser degree, the force of the grip. Greater sparing of the primary motor cortex (M1) and less extensive wallerian degeneration are associated with better hand function in studies that involved functional neuroimaging. The typical hemiplegic posture of elbow, wrist, and finger flexion followed 60% shrinkage, which corresponds to a loss of roughly 88% of the descending fibers. Better motor and functional outcomes also have been associated with sparing of metabolic activity in the ipsilesional primary motor cortex, the thalamic-and-basal ganglia–frontal network, and with sparing of the basal ganglia ipsilateral to the stroke. Approximately 20% sparing of the ventral or ventrolateral funiculi after SCI permits fair motor function, and 35% sparing of the dorsal funiculus allows appreciation of dorsal column sensory inputs.

The recovery of vision after an occipital stroke may depend on spared parts of the vision-associated areas of the cortex. Patients who recover from a hemianopsia tend to activate bilateral extrastriatal cortex during hemifield stimulation to the affected occipital lobe. Involvement of primary and extrastriatal cortex leaves a persistent field loss.

Residual neurons and axons of an injured tract may need rehabilitation to help drive training-induced, activity-dependent plasticity. When the number of corticospinal fibers that synapse with spinal motor pools is too small to generate adequate excitatory postsynaptic potentials, a descending volley will not excite the spinal neurons. Recovery of an adequate excitatory postsynaptic potential, however, may follow practice that strengthens synaptic efficacy. Other contributors to spared pathway functioning include changes in ion channels along partially demyelinated axons, increased strength of output from undamaged cortical and brainstem neurons that also descend onto spinal neurons such as propriospinal pathways, dendritic sprouting, and up-regulation of the number of motor neuron and interneuron excitatory receptors. In addition, the ipsilateral motor cortex, via the uncrossed ventral corticospinal tract, often has been invoked as a pathway that may provide some of this input, thereby compensating for a contralateral cerebral injury. The fibers of the ventral tract synapse especially with motor neurons for axial and limb girdle muscles. Some projections of the lateral corticospinal tract cross and then recross under the central canal of the cord. Thus, deafferentation of one side of the ventral horn from loss of descending fibers may induce further sprouting of recrossing fibers to enhance motor control of the affected limb (Rosenzweig et al., 2009). Functional neuroimaging studies of the upper extremity, leg, and language suggest that better gains with training are associated with greater cortical activation near the primary representation than when homologous regional activity of the intact hemisphere is most apparent (Baron et al., 2004).

Alternative Behavioral Strategies

Many functional activities can be accomplished by compensatory behavioral adaptations that allow greater independence in ADLs despite persistent impairments. Motor functions can appear to have fully recovered when in fact residual neural activity is supporting behavioral plasticity (Levin et al., 2009). For example, after a unilateral pyramidal lesion in the rodent or monkey, reaching for a pellet of food gradually improves and at first glance may appear to have recovered fully. A closer analysis of the movement reveals better control of the proximal than of the distal portion of the affected limb. The animal reaches with a grasp, brings the pellet to its mouth without the normal supination of the hand and forearm, turns its head to chase after the food, and cannot easily release its grip. The hand-to-mouth movement pattern of the hemiparetic patient is similar to the lesioned animal's strategy. Functional ambulation often improves in part by biomechanical adaptations that are revealed by kinematic deviations in the gait pattern and by use of braces and assistive devices. Behavioral adaptations, of course, also have a neural substrate that includes training-induced cortical representational reorganization and increased efficiency in the incorporation of residual pathways. Cognitive impairments that affect learning and problem solving, however, may limit the use of compensatory strategies. Rehabilitation efforts often train patients to use compensatory behavioral strategies to accomplish a task. Rather than performing tasks using the original neural network, alternative strategies may be emphasized. Substitution by a different neural network, however, may interfere with the activity-dependent reorganization that is needed to achieve further recovery from a specific impairment or disability.

Distributed Networks of Neuronal Circuitry

A distributed system is a collection of processing units (i.e., dynamic neuronal assemblies with similar functional properties and anatomical connections) that are spatially separate and exchange messages. Hierarchical, parallel, and quasi-serial linking operations are made with the afferent and efferent

Box 48.8 Characteristics of Distributed Systems in Neural Circuitry

- Signal flow follows a number of pathways.
- Action may be initiated at any of the nodal loci in a system.
- Local lesions in a system may degrade but not completely eliminate a function.
- Dynamic reorganization may be more important than modification of structural connections.
- In a reentrant system, nodes are open to externally and internally generated signals.

systems of the brain (**Box 48.8**). The nodes in such systems cooperate to manage the diverse information necessary for the rapid and highly flexible control of, for example, cognition and multijoint movements. These circuits lend themselves to an understanding of the neuroplasticity that may contribute to spontaneous and training-induced recovery of function.

The executive motor system has been the subject of recovery-related studies. The primate primary motor cortex (M1) has separate clusters of output neurons that can facilitate the activity of a single spinal motoneuron. Also, a single cortical motor neuron can project to the spinal motoneurons for several muscles, even those that may act across a joint. In addition, neurons in overlapping M1 territories are activated to produce movements of different body parts. This overlapping organization contributes to the control of the complex muscle synergies for voluntary movement of the arm and leg within the ordinary workspace of the body (Graziano et al., 2002). Thus, complex movement representations within cortical and subcortical maps may be reexpressed after injury as usual patterns of movements. It seems likely, then, that retraining ought to engage patients in the practice of complex movements rather than single joint actions or exercise of single muscles.

Multiple representations also have been demonstrated in nonprimary motor regions. They are found in the premotor cortex of Brodmann area (BA) 6, the supplementary motor area, and the region immediately rostral to it, and in BA 23 and BA 24 by the cingulate sulcus. These motor regions have interrelated and some overlapping functions, with direct and indirect anatomical connections. Each area has an independent set of inputs from adjacent and remote regions, and most have parallel but separate outputs to the brainstem and spinal cord. The effective unit of operation in such a distributed system is not a particular neuron and its axon but a group of cells with similar functional properties and anatomical connections.

The capacity of motor-related cortices to redistribute their function is apparent from PET and functional magnetic resonance imaging (fMRI) studies that have looked at subjects with recovered hand function after a stroke. For example, after a striatocapsular infarction in patients who recovered finger tapping and hand squeezing, bilateral rather than just contralateral activation of cortical motor neurons was found, along with greater involvement of motor areas that ordinarily would not be visibly activated for that task. Other regions related to selective attention and intention also show increases in blood flow and metabolism, which suggests that they must play a larger role when the substrates for a movement reorganize. Regions that are activated in normal subjects when greater force is exerted, such as insular, premotor, and anterior opercular cortex, may also be activated during movement of a hemiparetic limb (Baron et al., 2004), in parallel with the increased effort needed to move that some patients describe.

Parallel segregated circuits process different variables for movement throughout their integrated pathways in the striatum, thalamus, cerebellum, brainstem, and spinal cord. The cerebellum receives and modulates locomotor cycle–related signals. The neocerebellum monitors the outcome of every movement and optimizes movements using proprioceptive feedback. In view of the great computational interest the cerebellum has in the details of afferent information from joints and muscles, rehabilitation therapies for walking and upper extremity actions should aim to provide this key motor center with the sensory feedback that the spinal cord and cerebellum recognize as typical of normal walking and reaching-related inputs. The motor functions that the cerebellar inputs and outputs attend to, such as timing and error correction for accuracy as the hand approaches an object, are especially important for patients to practice when a lesion undermines motor control. Thus, individual channels can control separate functional units of motor cortex, and in turn each is independent in its control of subcortical motor nuclei. After an injury, the balance of activities of these networks is reset. Although these systems are not likely to be highly redundant, they may provide a partially reiterative capacity for some sparing or compensation after a sensorimotor network injury. The intact parallel systems from cortical and subcortical areas may partially compensate or substitute for nonfunctional ones when their activity is enhanced by specific cognitive and motor rehabilitative retraining. For example, if the premotor cortex is damaged, compromising visually cued movements, the patient may be taught to use an internally cued strategy mediated especially by the spared supplementary motor area. Patients with a paretic hand, then, can be encouraged to pre-shape the hand before they reach for an object, to lessen the need for automatic visuomotor input from the premotor hand region.

The brainstem and spinal cord also include important subcomponents of distributed motor functions. For example, they contain their own intrinsic networks for aspects of locomotion. Although cortical and peripheral sensory input is essential for normal locomotion under disparate environmental conditions, the timing of synergist and antagonist muscle activity for stepping appears to be primarily the task of a self-oscillating lumbar interneuronal network. Even an isolated section of lumbar spinal cord in mammals can produce cyclical outputs that rhythmically flex and extend a joint. This locomotor circuit is called a *central pattern generator* and especially depends on glutamate and glycine for alternating excitation and inhibition.

Both distributed and hierarchical organization and plasticity are just as evident for higher cortical functions. Cognitive domains appear to be mapped at multiple sites that are highly connected with feedback connections. PET and fMRI studies have begun to reveal changes in the organization of these interactions for particular tasks after a cerebral injury. Cognitive rehabilitation strategies have been developed based on the notion that recovery may be mediated by tapping into the localizable and distributed grids of connectivity that are intact.

Cortical and Subcortical Representational Adaptations

Many lines of animal research suggest that partial restoration after a central or peripheral injury can result from a functional shift to neighboring neurons. In the adult as well as the developing animal, and in humans, the sensory and motor representations of the brain are distributed, dynamic, and capable of much physiological and structural reorganization. As noted earlier, the neurons of the ischemic penumbra of an acute cerebral infarction may play an important role in functional gains. Very early overuse of these neurons was shown to cause greater injury in rat models of stroke and trauma. Such profound overuse shortly after an injury is unlikely in human subjects, however. Indeed, early practice appears important. A primate model of a less than 1-mm injury to the hand area of M1 found that perilesional representations for the digits decreased when the monkey failed to practice using the hand to scoop pellets out of a narrow well. Neighboring representations for the digits, wrist, and forearm increased with practice. Thus, cortical representational changes are especially likely to arise during training paradigms that involve learning and the acquisition of specific skills, although the relationship between the regional cortical change and the behavioral gain may not coincide, because the focal cerebral adaptation may be one of many. This plasticity probably arises from the unmasking of previously silent synapses and increases in synaptic efficacy in thalamocortical and intracortical circuits. Over weeks and months, it might arise from sprouting of dendrites over short distances. In animal studies of recovery of forelimb function, only 12 hours of a specific therapy for the affected limb leads to behavioral gains and cortical representational changes. In human subjects after stroke, representational plasticity for the ankle movers after locomotor training or the wrist and fingers after upper extremity task-related training can be shown after as little as 12 to 18 hours of practice.

The combination of mutable neuronal assemblies that represent movements and sensation and multiple representational maps in a parallel distributed system offers a sound basis for developing rehabilitation interventions. Behaviorally relevant tasks that are shaped by an optimal schedule of practice and feedback to neural networks may potentially increase functional gains. The optimal duration and intensity of training are uncertain for human rehabilitation strategies, but greater intensity of practice seems to enhance subsequent performance (Kwakkel et al., 2004). Unfortunately, most patients get only a few months of formal inpatient and outpatient retraining of modest intensity that is spread across many tasks.

Biological Interventions

The molecular processes that are induced by injury and by activity in neurons, axons, and dendrites are under intense investigation. Morphological changes such as axonal regeneration over short distances, dendritic arborization, and synaptogenesis have been observed after a brain and cord injuries. When inputs from one pathway to the dendritic tree of a neuron are lost, intact axons can sprout and form synapses on denervated receptors. The net effect of this change in the weight of inputs could have a positive or a detrimental effect on neural function. Can such changes be manipulated? Basic neuroscience studies of biological approaches offer some exciting approaches to complement neurorehabilitation strategies.

Sprouting and regeneration of injured axons in the central nervous system has been demonstrated over very short distances, perhaps no more than 1 cm in rodent models. Growth depends in part on production of regeneration-associated genes, receptors on the surface of cells and the axon growth cone, and pro- and antigrowth signaling molecules in the extracellular matrix. Tissue culture and vertebrate models have shown that substances in the extracellular matrix and on the surface of oligodendrocytes inhibit elongation of the axonal growth cone. Antibodies and receptor blockers have been made to these substances, including the inhibitor Nogo-A, the receptor Nogo-66, Rho, and other membrane and intracellular steps that affect cytoskeletal proteins. Blockers lead to some growth of axons in the rat and mouse after a partial spinal or a brain injury, but no one blocker is enough to drive robust regeneration in these complex signaling systems. When they are combined with a growth factor such as neurotrophin-3 or brain-derived neurotrophic factor, axonal growth may increase further, although this is more evident in serotonergic and adrenergic axons than in corticospinal fibers. In nonhuman primates after stroke, focal TBI, and SCI, inosine has led to greater sprouting in the cord and brainstem by driving growth-promoting gene activity, and chondroitinase injected locally has reduced milieu inhibitors to enable sprouting and regeneration within the injection site. Clinical trials have been proposed for these and similar techniques. Neurotrophic factors have been used to protect neurons from apoptosis, as well to signal neuronal machinery to make the intracellular scaffolds necessary for neurite outgrowth.

Cultured Schwann cells, transplanted olfactory ensheathing cells, neural progenitors, embryonic tissue implants, neurotrophic factors delivered by engineered fibroblasts, and peripheral nerve bridge implants, with a combination of other biological manipulations, also have met with some success in permitting several populations of axons to regenerate across or around a rodent SCI. Bone marrow stromal cells have been injected into the blood after experimental stroke and seem to produce a trophic factor or other support for enhancing plasticity. Cortical and subcortical transplants of stem cells, engineered cells, human embryonal cells that take on the characteristics of local neurons, and progenitor cells for neurons and glia also have been introduced into the brain to promote recovery in animal models. Physical activity alone can regulate the expression of neurotrophic factors in the cortex and spinal cord and induce endogenous neurogenesis, especially in the hippocampus and spinal cord.

Published cell transplant experiments in humans include numerous interventions for PD; most have been unsuccessful overall, but recent trials are more promising and aim to eliminate induced movement disorders. Studies in animal models already have led to several safety studies of human interventions for stroke. These include intravenous injection of autologous mesenchymal stem cells about 40 days after a hemispheric stroke and implantation of human neuronal cells (LBS neurons) into the edge of deep infarcts near the basal ganglia. Further studies of bone marrow–derived stem cells are anticipated. Safety studies in SCI have proceeded with injection of human fetal spinal cord tissue into a syrinx, autologous activated macrophage injections into the acute injury,

and injections of porcine oligodendrocyte progenitors into chronic injuries, as well as recent dural or intrathecal infusions of Rho and Nogo inhibitors. No serious complications have been described to date, but reports are often vague. Recent uncontrolled but prospective safety trials from Australia and Portugal point to the safety of autologous olfactory ensheathing glia implanted in the spinal cord. At conferences and on websites, but not in peer-reviewed published reports, clinicians at hospitals in China (www.stemcellschina.com) and at least 100 sites around the world have built stem-cell spas to treat a broad range of neurological and other diseases. They claim to use fetal, olfactory ensheathing glia, bone marrow stromal, and other cell types for injection or implantation in uncontrolled and poorly documented experimental therapies in patients (Dobkin et al., 2006b). The sites offer hope at $20,000 to $50,000 for their services. These unpublished interventions tend to be based on a misinterpretation of preclinical experiments in rodents. Of interest, the patients who go for these interventions and then commit to a lengthy postoperative course of rehabilitation are usually the ones who report very modest changes.

Clinical trials in neural repair will be complex. No single intervention is likely to succeed, a similar situation to trials of neuroprotective agents. Too many biological pathways must be manipulated together and in series over time to get robust regrowth and effective connectivity or to incorporate new cells. To optimize the applicability of animal models to human translational research, clinicians will need to put the results of models into perspective and participate with basic neuroscientists in combining training and transplant technologies. In addition, strict adherence to best scientific practices for the conduct of randomized clinical trials will be needed, as suggested by guidelines from the International Campaign for Cures of Spinal Cord Injury Paralysis. Clinicians should encourage patients to read the educational materials about participating in neural repair experiments, such as the guidelines available at www.icord.org.

Pharmacological Interventions

Drugs that affect neurotransmission, intracellular second messenger signaling, excitation and inhibition, and the cascades associated with long-term potentiation and long-term depression are candidates to enhance learning and the reacquisition of skills after a brain injury or an SCI. At least five neurotransmitter projections have modulating effects on wide regions of the cortex and spinal cord. A lesion may transsynaptically interrupt this neurotransmitter output to cortex and cord, limiting the drive to uninjured regions and producing behavioral deficits. For example, dextroamphetamine augments specific cognitive processes by increasing the signal-to-noise ratio; cholinergic projections serve as a gate for behaviorally relevant sensory information. Cholinergic modulation is essential for motor cortex learning (Conner et al., 2005). Animal studies have provided preliminary evidence that a variety of pharmacological agents may facilitate or inhibit the rate or degree of recovery of sensorimotor function and walking after a cerebral injury. After being given dextroamphetamine, both rats and cats that underwent a unilateral or bilateral ablation of the sensorimotor or frontal cortex exhibited an accelerated rate of recovery, although not necessarily greater gains than in the control subjects, in the ability to walk across a beam. This effect endured well past the single or intermittent dosing schedule of the drug. Amphetamine and other drugs to be discussed have shown promise in small human trials. Thus, specific training paradigms combined with agents may enhance gains. Functional imaging studies with transcranial magnetic stimulation and fMRI may aid in the selection of drugs to combine with rehabilitation (Bute-fisch et al., 2002).

Drugs that may affect neural repair have also been tried, such as fibroblast growth factor, but side effects have exceeded expectations. Erythropoietin, granulocyte stimulating growth factor, an anti-Nogo antibody, and other factors are currently in clinical trials for patients with stroke and spinal cord injury. The designs of these trials suggest uncertainty about the mechanism of action, neuroprotection versus plasticity, in that they are initiated within 1 to 5 days of onset. Some drugs have more clear-cut mechanisms of action. For example, the conduction of action potentials along demyelinated axons may be increased by pharmacological agents such as 4-aminopyridine, which blocks potassium channels. This approach has met with some success in the responders with MS, who improved their ability to walk (Goodman et al., 2009). In some patients with motor neuron disease and Guillain-Barré syndrome, peripheral anticholinesterase-inhibiting medications, acting on neuromuscular junctions with altered structure and function, have reduced fatigability and improved strength in a modest way.

Genetic studies may become of value in identifying patients who have polymorphisms in a single nucleotide that affects memory, learning, cortical morphology, and other critical functions. If patients are predisposed to lower levels of brain catecholamines as a result of enzyme activity (catechol-O-methyltransferase Val versus Met polymorphism) or have higher or lower neurotrophin activity (brain-derived neuro-trophic factor [BDNF] Val versus Met polymorphism), these differences may be amplified after brain injury, potentially affecting outcomes. Medications could be used in a more focused fashion with genetic screening to identify persons most likely to benefit.

Drug studies in humans pose confounding problems. The type, location, extent, and age of the lesion and the specific drug, its dosage, time of initiation, duration of use, and adverse effects and the accompanying physical or cognitive therapy that may add to a drug's effect must be determined. What is clear is that clinicians should select medications with special care in the months after a cerebral injury and must monitor for effects that may impede recovery.

Neuromedical Problems During Rehabilitation

Neurological and systemic complications often interfere with progress during inpatient and outpatient rehabilitation. With shorter acute hospital and inpatient rehabilitation stays, physicians, nurses, and therapists must anticipate, recognize, and treat medical conditions that may impede progress in the rehabilitation process. Some of these problems will arise from new medications, neurological impairments, immobility, transient infections and metabolic abnormalities, and underlying systemic illness. In addition, patients and caregivers must be trained to prevent errors of omission and commission

that arise in using medication, performing daily care, and managing risk factors such as hypertension that lead to late morbidity.

As noted, some but not all studies suggest that specialized stroke, SCI, and TBI hospital programs appear to lead to better early outcomes than with treatment on general medical units. Differences in morbidity, mortality, and length of hospital stay have been associated with more organized services. For example, protocols that use prophylactic subcutaneous heparin, hold oral intake until completion of a screening test for safety of swallowing, avoid indwelling bladder catheters, and assess postvoid residuals by ultrasound examination to avoid unnecessary intermittent catheterizations or overfilling, can reduce medical complications.

Frequency of Complications
Complications in Patients with Stroke

Medical complications often interfere with a patient's ability to participate in therapy (**Table 48.5**). Medical and

Table 48.5   General Frequency of Inpatient Stroke Rehabilitation Neuromedical Complications

Complication	% of Patients
Urinary tract infection	40
Musculoskeletal pain	30
Depression	30
Urine retention	25
Falls	25
Fungal rash	20
Hypertension	20
Hypotension	15
Incipient pressure sores	15
Hypoglycemia or hyperglycemia	15
Azotemia	15
Toxic-metabolic encephalopathy	10
Pneumonia	10
Arrhythmia	10
Congestive heart failure	5
Angina	5
Thrombophlebitis	5
Allergic reaction	5
Gastrointestinal bleeding	5
Pulmonary embolus	<5
Myocardial infarction	<5
Decubitus ulcer	<5
Recurrent stroke	<5
Seizure	<5

Adapted with permission from Dobkin, B., 2003. The Clinical Science of Neurologic Rehabilitation. Oxford University Press, New York.

neurological complications occur at rates of approximately 4 and 0.6 per patient, respectively, during an average course of inpatient rehabilitation. A urinary tract infection, urinary retention, musculoskeletal pain, or depression will develop in approximately one-third of patients. Up to 20% will experience a fall, exhibit a rash, or need continuous management of blood pressure, hydration, nutrition, and glucose levels. In approximately 10%, a transient toxic-metabolic encephalopathy, pneumonia, cardiac arrhythmias, pressure sores, or thrombophlebitis will develop. Up to 5% will have a pulmonary embolus, seizures, gastrointestinal bleeding, heart failure, or other systemic complications. When feasible, prophylactic measures for these potential problems are essential. Because many patients in the United States are transferred from the acute hospital to a rehabilitation unit less than 7 days after a stroke, the rate of neuromedical complications may be higher at some centers. Side effects during the adjustment of new medications are especially prevalent, including orthostatic hypotension from antihypertensives or dialysis, drowsiness from anticonvulsants and analgesics, and a statin-induced myopathy with normal serum creatine kinase. Across rehabilitation centers, 5% to 15% of patients must be transferred back to an acute hospital setting.

Complications in Patients with Spinal Cord Injury

Medical complications of a somewhat different nature are common in the acute and chronic phases after SCI. In this younger group of patients, chronic comorbid systemic medical problems are less common than in patients with stroke. Prior substance abuse and emotional and behavioral disorders, however, are much more likely to complicate therapy. In the first 6 weeks after SCI, reparative operative procedures affect what can be done in rehabilitation. Approximately half of patients undergo spinal fusion and internal fixation. Acute spinal care also entails the use of external stabilization techniques such as a halo vest and Philadelphia collar for cervical injuries and a thermoplastic, custom-molded, thoracolumbar fixation shell (see **Fig. 48.6**). These devices limit head and trunk mobility, which makes self-care tasks that involve balance, management of the lower extremities, and CISC more difficult. Lower extremity fractures, especially of the femur, occur in about 5% of patients with acute SCI, which can further limit mobility and increase the risk of deep vein thrombosis and skin breakdown. **Table 48.6** lists the complications found during a prospective clinical trial of methylprednisolone for acute SCI in 487 patients.

Early morbidity is greater with cervical and upper thoracic injuries and with complete lesions than with lower level or incomplete lesions. Ventilatory dysfunction, aspiration, dysautonomia with upright hypotension or paroxysmal hypertension, a neurogenic bowel with impactions, a neurogenic bladder with retention and infections, a catabolic state, and gastric atony are especially likely to complicate early inpatient rehabilitation. Hypercalciuria or hypercalcemia related to immobilization may also necessitate therapy. Central and musculoskeletal pain and grief reactions warrant immediate attention.

Table 48.6   Medical Complications Within 6 Weeks of Acute Spinal Cord Injury

Complication	% of Patients
Urinary tract infection	46
Pneumonia	28
Decubitus ulcer	18
Paralytic ileus	9
Arrhythmia	6
Sepsis	6
Thrombophlebitis	5
Wound infection	4
Gastrointestinal hemorrhage	3
Pulmonary embolus	3
Congestive failure	1

Complications in Patients with Traumatic Brain Injury

Systemic and neurological complications are common after serious TBI. The older patient carries more systemic comorbidity, whereas the younger patient may have alcohol or drug abuse as a comorbid condition. Unrecognized fractures and heterotopic ossification as a cause of pain, in addition to other bodily injuries may complicate rehabilitation along with any of the complications that may accompany stroke and SCI. Physicians must also monitor for pituitary-hypothalamic dysfunction with endocrinopathies and disorders of homeostasis including cerebral salt wasting and inappropriate secretion of antidiuretic hormone, as well as cerebral hygromas and obstructive hydrocephalus. Ventricular enlargement develops in 30% to 70% of patients with severe TBI. Most have hydrocephalus ex vacuo, which is passive enlargement of the ventricles from the loss of gray and white matter. In the patient with enlarging ventricles who reaches an early plateau or declines in mobility and cognition, a diagnosis of symptomatic normal- or high-pressure hydrocephalus must be considered.

Patients who are in a persistent vegetative state often are evaluated by the rehabilitation team for prognostication and for a trial of stimulation. After TBI, the prognosis is not quite so grim as after hypoxic-ischemic coma unless hypotension accompanied the TBI. **Table 48.7** shows the outcomes during the first year after brain injury determined for a 1994 study by the Multi-Society Task Force on Persistent Vegetative State.

Management of Neuromedical Problems
Dysphagia

Neurogenic dysphagia is the potential cause of a pulmonary infection in any patient with stroke, TBI, motor neuron disease, MS, advanced PD, cervicomedullary disorders such as a syrinx, Guillain-Barré syndrome, myasthenia gravis, and most neuromuscular diseases. Indeed, swallowing disorders affect 10% of acutely hospitalized older adults and 30% of nursing home residents. Even transient dysphagia can lead

Table 48.7   Post–Brain Injury Outcomes for Adults in Persistent Vegetative State Beyond 1 Month

Outcome	% of Cases		
	3 Months	6 Months	12 Months
TRAUMATIC BRAIN INJURY			
Death	15	24	33
PVS	52	30	15
Conscious	33	46	52
Severe disability	—	—	28
Moderate disability	—	—	17
Good recovery	—	—	7
NONTRAUMATIC BRAIN INJURY			
Death	24	40	53
PVS	65	45	32
Conscious	11	15	15
Severe disability	—	—	11
Moderate disability	—	—	3
Good recovery	—	—	1

Data from a 1994 study by the Multi-Society Task Force on Persistent Vegetative State, using the Glasgow Outcome Scale classification for recovery of consciousness and function.

PVS, Persistent vegetative state.

to malnutrition, dehydration, aspiration pneumonia, and airway obstruction with asphyxiation. It increases the patient's risk of death and institutionalization.

The natural history of recovery from dysphagia after stroke and TBI is good. For example, a British study diagnosed dysphagia in 30% of 357 conscious patients within 48 hours of a unilateral hemispheric stroke; the patients were rated as having impaired deglutition if they exhibited delayed and prolonged swallowing or if they coughed on 10 mL of water. Lethargy, gaze paresis, and sensory inattention were present more often than in those who swallowed normally. By 1 week, 16% had dysphagia. At 1 month only 2% and at 6 months only 0.4% of survivors were still impaired. Symptoms and signs that suggest a risk of aspiration include lethargy, coughing or a hoarse and gurgly voice after feeding, slow eating or drinking (<10 mL of water per second drunk from a cup), dysphonia, and poor oropharyngeal movement. The limitations of bedside indicators have led to the use of the MBS with videofluoroscopy as the method of choice to rule out silent aspiration. The relationship between small-volume aspiration as seen on MBS and clinical complications is uncertain, however, and requires clinical judgment. The MBS also visualizes the effects of dietary texture and compensatory techniques. In attentive stroke rehabilitation inpatients, coughing or a wet-hoarse quality of the voice noted within 1 minute of continuously swallowing 90 mL of water from a cup had a sensitivity of 80% and specificity of 54% for aspiration detected by an MBS study. The bedside test had a sensitivity of 88% and specificity of 44% for large-volume aspiration, which may be clinically more significant. Fiberoptic endoscopy also can identify mechanisms of dysphagia and can be performed at the bedside.

Dysphagia management must be addressed through all phases of recovery from stroke and TBI and during the progression of disorders such as PD, ALS, and myasthenia gravis (see Chapter 12B). Lesions in the pathways for swallowing interfere with the oral, oral preparatory, and reflex or pharyngeal phases of deglutition. Common deviations include loss of the ability to form a bolus and inadvertent trapping of liquids in the vallecula, with subsequent trickling over the vocal cords. The initial emphasis for care is placed on protecting the airway and maintaining adequate alimentation and hydration, with use of a nasopharyngeal feeding tube if necessary. A large single-site randomized trial found that a standardized daily therapy for swallowing and dietary modification for up to 1 month after stroke, compared with usual care or with standard care provided only 3 days a week, reduced dysphagia-related medical complications such as pulmonary infection and significantly increased the number of patients who regained swallowing function. As in many other rehabilitation trials, it may be that the intensity of a treatment is as important as the strategy to achieve greatest efficacy.

Swallowing may improve by downsizing a tracheostomy tube or eliminating it as soon as possible. Oral pooling of secretions and drooling, which predispose the patient to aspiration, can be managed with suctioning and sometimes with use of a low titrated dose of an anticholinergic drug such as glycopyrrolate. Good oral hygiene and prevention of tooth caries by oral rinsing with chlorhexidine gluconate and stannous fluoride can lessen the likelihood of carriage of bacterial infection into the lungs by oral secretions. Therapeutic efforts focus on the use of stimulation and compensatory approaches designed to reduce the swallowing impairment or to minimize the functional disability resulting from that impairment (**Table 48.8**). For example, postural adjustments may be made on the basis of the MBS findings. A chin tuck narrows the airway opening, tilting the head to the stronger side of the pharynx directs a bolus away from the weak side, and head rotation toward the weak pharyngeal muscle channels a bolus toward the stronger side. Modification of diet texture includes choosing thickened or gelled liquids, which are less likely to be aspirated than thin liquids. Purees and formable solids such as applesauce or mashed potatoes usually are safer than foods that require chewing and oral manipulation. Pharyngeal stimulation by the therapist may help drive representational plasticity for these muscles on the unaffected side of the brain after stroke to improve swallowing.

The FOOD Trial Collaboration reported that early placement of a nasogastric tube to feed aphagic patients after stroke improved nutrition and reduced deaths and poor outcomes compared with no enteral feeding, but early use of percutaneous gastrostomy caused a 1% absolute increase in complications. Gastrostomy may not lessen the risk of reflux aspiration any more than a nasopharyngeal feeding tube for patients with persisting aphagia. Percutaneous endoscopic gastrostomy can be complicated by gastric perforation, peritonitis, hematoma, fistula formation involving the lung, stomal infection, cellulitis, and bleeding at the insertion site. Jejunostomy may lessen the risk of reflux but increases the risk of the dumping syndrome. Rarely, esophagostomy or pharyngostomy may be better suited for the patient with neurological dysfunction and prior gastrointestinal disease or surgery. Clinical trials related

	Table 48.8 General Therapies for Dysphagia		
Compensation	**Sensorimotor Exercises**	**Direct Interventions**
Postural adjustments:	Oral sensory stimulation (thermal, vibration)	Palatal prosthesis
Head positioning	Resistance and placement exercises of tongue and jaw	Surgery
Chin tuck	Chewing, oral manipulation of bolus	Cricopharyngeal myotomy
Head rotation to weak pharyngeal side	Laryngeal adduction	Epiglottopexy
Dietary modifications: Softer food Thicker liquids Lower intake volume	Biofeedback	
Slower intake pace		
Compensatory maneuvers: Double swallow Supraglottic swallow Laryngeal elevation		

to the efficacy of types of tube feedings and other interventions for dysphagia are monitored by the Cochrane Review. Dysphagia therapies provided by the family under the guidance of a therapist may be as efficacious as hands-on therapy by a professional. With outpatient care, patients and family members assume greater responsibility for integrating and adapting recommended procedures to suit their individual needs and priorities.

Skin Ulcers

Education in skin management during rehabilitation provides an important opportunity for preventing later morbidity and mortality. Ischemia of the skin and underlying tissues occurs particularly in weight-bearing areas adjacent to bony prominences. The American Model Systems data for patients hospitalized within 24 hours of traumatic SCI showed that pressure sores subsequently developed in 4%, and 13% of these were graded as severe. The lesions occurred over the sacrum, heel, scapula, foot, and greater trochanter of the hip. Lower-grade skin lesions developed over the genitals. Sores related to sitting most often are located over the ischial tuberosities, where tissue pressure can exceed 300 mm Hg on an unpadded seat. A 2-inch-thick foam pad decreases the local pressure to 150 mm Hg. Even with the use of cushions designed to distribute pressure evenly over weight-bearing skin surfaces, pressures in the sitting position are far above the pressures of 11 to 33 mm Hg in the capillaries and venules. Raising the head of the bed by only a few inches especially increases shearing forces over the sacrum.

A standard classification for degrees of integument breakdown, prophylactic measures, and wound care is available from the Agency for Health Care Policy and Research in Washington, DC. Rubor, induration, and blistering are signs that precede a break in the skin. Pressure relief by turning and repositioning is the best approach, performed every half hour after a complete SCI and every 2 to 3 hours in patients with intact sensation after stroke or other disabling injuries. Patients must develop a skin care program based on their general health, nutrition, continence, toughness of their skin, most commonly used positions, type of wheelchair seat, presence of old skin scars, and other factors.

Deep Vein Thrombosis and Pulmonary Embolus

In controlled trials of prophylaxis, DVT has been found in 20% to 75% of untreated patients within 2 weeks of stroke; 5% to 20% suffered a pulmonary embolus (PE), which was fatal in approximately 10%. Intermittent calf compression for the paretic leg, intermittent low-dose heparin given as 5000 units every 8 or 12 hours, and low-molecular-weight heparinoid are far more effective than no intervention or the use of antiembolism hose alone. Across several studies, anticoagulants have reduced the incidence of DVT by a factor of two- to sevenfold, and of PE by about two- to fourfold. If a DVT is diagnosed, patients usually can restart activities out of bed after 2 days of intravenous heparin.

For those with SCI or head injury complicated by bone fractures, the incidence of DVT and PE is particularly high. After an SCI without a fracture, the risk of DVT, detected by a radiolabeled fibrinogen scan, impedance plethysmography, or Doppler blood flow study, appears greatest in the first 12 weeks, especially in combination with paraplegia and flaccidity. Symptomatic thrombophlebitis and PE are less common. In one study, thromboembolism was detected in 31% of plegic patients who were randomized to receive 5000 units of subcutaneous heparin twice a day within 72 hours of injury. It was detected in only 7% of patients whose activated partial thromboplastin time was prolonged to 1.5 times control values by dosage adjustment every 12 hours. Over 7 weeks of anticoagulation, the incidence of bleeding complications was greater in the adjusted-dosage group, especially at trauma sites. Most patients with uncomplicated SCI continue anticoagulation until discharge from inpatient rehabilitation.

Contractures

Across studies, approximately 15% of patients with SCI admitted for rehabilitation and 80% admitted after moderate to severe TBI lost more than 15% of the normal range of motion of at least one joint. Hemiparetic patients with stroke fall between these extremes. Contractures are found especially in the lower extremities in neuromuscular diseases, affecting at least 70% of outpatients with Duchenne muscular dystrophy. Contractures limit functional use of a limb and impair hygiene, mobility, and self-care. Serious contractures can cause pressure sores, pain, and, especially in youngsters, emotional distress when odd postures distort the body. After an acute UMN lesion, proper positioning of the arm in abduction and hand in extension and of the leg in hip abduction with knee flexed and ankle in neutral position can protect the affected extremities. Any source of pain will increase tone and predispose to contractures. Serial casting and surgeries occasionally are necessary for contractures that interfere with skin care or functional use of a limb.

Ectopic bone formation—heterotopic ossification (HO)—below the neurological level of injury may cause functional impairment in up to 20% of patients with SCI, usually in the first 4 months after injury. Patients with a complete lesion, pressure sores, spasticity, and age older than 30 years may be at greatest risk. After TBI, HO especially tends to affect the proximal joints of comatose patients. During rehabilitation of less responsive and cognitively impaired or aphasic patients, pain caused by undetected musculoskeletal injury and HO can add greatly to agitation and limit participation. HO develops when multipotential connective tissue cells transform into chondroblasts and osteoblasts, presumably under the influence of locally induced growth factors. The hips, knees, and shoulders are affected most often. Swelling, erythema, and decreasing range of motion are among the first clinical signs. A three-phase technetium 99m–labeled methylene-diphosphonate bone scan reveals focal uptake before radiographic visualization of bone. Early treatment with disodium etidronate suppresses mineralization of the osteoid. Range-of-motion exercises, aspirin, nonsteroidal antiinflammatory drugs, and a wedge resection of mature heterotopic bone can decrease pain and immobility.

Seizures

Seizures occur in 5% to 8% of patients within 24 hours to 2 weeks of an ischemic stroke. The risk of epilepsy after TBI varies with the severity of injury and time after onset of injury. In a population study of more than 2700 patients with mostly nonpenetrating TBI, 2% experienced a seizure in the first 2 weeks after injury. Those with brain contusions, hematomas, or 24 hours of unconsciousness or amnesia had a 7% 1-year and 11.5% 5-year risk of seizures. Within the first 2 weeks in these severe cases, children younger than 15 years of age had a rate of 30%, compared with 10% in adults. After a moderate injury, defined as a skull fracture or 30 minutes to 24 hours of unconsciousness or amnesia, 0.7% of patients at 1 year and 1.6% at 5 years had a seizure. The risk after a mild injury with brief unconsciousness or amnesia was 0.1% to 0.6%, the same as for the general population. With a 25% rate of first seizures regardless of anticonvulsant prophylaxis beyond the first week after serious brain injury, it does not seem productive to continue anticonvulsant therapy beyond the first 2 weeks after a serious TBI, especially because an anticonvulsant medication can increase cognitive impairment.

Dysautonomia

Bedrest, dehydration, cardiac and antihypertensive medications, antidepressants, and autonomic reflex dysfunction from diabetes mellitus contribute to postural hypotension in the patient with stroke and TBI. Supine and standing blood pressures should be checked as mobilization proceeds during rehabilitation. Autonomic reflexes may fail in patients with SCI levels above T6. Symptomatic postural hypotension is common in the first weeks after injury and may persist in quadriplegic patients.

Initial therapies for OH include gradual reconditioning of postural reflexes on a tilt table, sleeping in a reverse Trendelenburg position to prevent overnight diuresis, wearing full compression leg hose, and application of an abdominal binder. In the inpatient setting, fluid loading with saline or albumin may aid the effort to compensate for venous pooling, decreased cardiac output, and impaired vasoconstriction and venoconstriction from interruption of sympathetic outflow. Fludrocortisone increases the intravascular volume and peripheral vascular resistance. The dosage can be pushed gradually to 0.5 mg per day. Salt tablets should be added to the diet. Hypokalemia and edema with pressure sores can complicate use of mineralocorticoids. While the patient is upright, ephedrine, 25 to 100 mg, up to every 3 hours; ergotamine, 2 mg, up to several times daily; or midodrine, up to 10 mg 3 times a day can be tried. Episodic autonomic hyperreflexia related to uninhibited sympathetic outflow may affect 50% to 90% of SCI patients with high-level SCI, usually beginning several months after injury. It is caused by visceral and joint pain, HO, pressure sores, bowel and bladder distention, fecal impaction, urinary infection and cystitis, ingrown toenails, pregnancy and labor, venous thrombosis, and late development of a syrinx. Wearing tight clothing, a particular supine position, or oropharyngeal suctioning also can cause bradyarrhythmias. Often it has no evident precipitating cause. Hypertension, headache, diaphoresis, anxiety, reflexive bradycardia, nasal congestion, flushing above and pallor below the SCI level, extensor spasms, and piloerection can result. The instigating agent must be removed. Acute therapies include upright positioning, search for an unemptied bladder or rectum using lidocaine on a catheter or finger when probing, and treatment of blood pressure that exceeds 180/100 mm Hg. A beta-blocker such as labetalol, a short-acting calcium channel blocker, vasodilators such as hydralazine, and occasionally phenoxybenzamine, prazosin, clonidine, or nitroglycerin usually lower the pressure safely. Some quadriplegic patients have very labile responses to antihypertensive drugs and suddenly become hypotensive with these treatments. For frequent bouts of hypertension, maintenance therapy includes low dosages of any of these oral agents but with dosage adjustments based on the finding of supine hypertension coupled with sitting hypotension. For paroxysmal bradycardia, propantheline or a pacemaker may be needed. Scopolamine and propantheline can prevent bouts of sweating.

Bowel and Bladder Dysfunction

Urinary incontinence occurs in up to 60% of patients in the first week after a stroke, but function tends to improve without a specific medical treatment. This likelihood must be considered in the context of an incidence of urinary dribbling and involuntary emptying of approximately 30% in the population of healthy, noninstitutionalized adults older than 65 years of age. Across studies, about 18% of those who were incontinent at 6 weeks after a stroke are still so at 1 year. By the end of inpatient rehabilitation, the incidence is about 10% in patients with a motor-only stroke and about 30% with large hemispheric strokes. A Cochrane Database systematic review of the prevention and treatment of urinary incontinence after stroke found insufficient evidence for most physical, behavioral, and pharmacological interventions, but specialist management tended to reduce the number of urinary tract infections.

After SCI, the bladder detrusor reflex may not return for 6 weeks to 12 months. In the absence of spontaneous bladder emptying, intermittent catheterization is done on a schedule that prevents the accumulation of more than 400 mL. Patients should measure their output from time to time and develop a voiding schedule that takes into account variations in fluid intake and the use of alcohol and caffeine. Catheters can be washed, stored in a plastic bag, and reused. If sensorimotor impairments persist, nearly all patients with an SCI lesion that spares the S2 to S4 micturition center will develop dyssynergia between the detrusor and the external sphincter. These uncoordinated contractions lead to incontinence and intermittent outlet obstruction. Urodynamic studies and an intravenous pyelogram are indicated as a baseline and to assist in therapy, especially in patients with SCI (see Chapter 50C). Obstruction can cause recurrent infections, urosepsis, vesicourethral reflux, urolithiasis, and hydronephrosis.

Patients should learn the signs of bladder fullness, such as sweating, changes in temperature, increased spasticity, and an increase in heart rate. Some palpate the area of the bladder to determine fullness. Once awareness of fullness develops, the person can aid in initiating or completing micturition by tapping over the bladder, rubbing the skin over the pubis or on the inner thighs, pressing on the abdominal wall (Credé maneuver), and bearing down or coughing. These maneuvers are particularly helpful in those with an LMN bladder with an open sphincter. Most patients with SCI also learn the signs of an early bladder infection, such as a change in clarity or odor, as well as more spasms, and work out a system with their physician to obtain a culture and antibiotics immediately.

Pharmacological treatment can be understood in relation to problems in bladder filling, storage, and bladder emptying with any neurological disease (**Table 48.9**). Urodynamic studies often aid in the choice of drug trial. The goals are continence and regular emptying that is achieved without high intravesicular pressure and with less than 100 mL of residual volume after voiding. Many males after stroke who have an enlarged prostate benefit from an alpha-blocker. If the goal for micturition is not achieved, several alternatives to the use of an indwelling catheter on a long-term basis are available. To prevent inadequate emptying at low pressure at the price of external sphincterotomy and resultant incontinence, long-term CISC can be used in combination with anticholinergic medications or bladder infusion of botulinum toxin to partially paralyze detrusor function. This procedure has become increasingly accepted as an effective alternative in the management of low intravesicular pressure. An external collecting device also can be used to ensure dryness. The patient must be trained to adjust fluid intake and the timing of catheterization to meet the flexible needs of community living. The absence of an effective external collecting device for female patients makes it necessary to continue long-term intermittent catheterization in women with paralysis of detrusor function. A waterproof undergarment may be worn between catheterizations to avoid embarrassment. The difficulties of this regimen cause many women to choose constant indwelling catheter drainage despite its drawbacks. Augmentation enterocystoplasty, reservoirs, conduits, and electrical stimulation techniques are less often needed. The VOCARE Bladder System for patients with UMN SCI allows patients to stimulate sacral nerves that have been implanted with electrodes to empty the bladder and bowel.

The optimal management of spina bifida in children includes self-catheterization. Through cartoons and drawings, children can be taught how to prevent germs from growing in the bladder. Intermittent self-catheterization of the bladder usually can begin by age 5 years or by the time the child starts school.

Bowel evacuation can be brought under control in a majority of cases of SCI or other causes of myelopathy or cauda equina injury. The goals include continence, the prevention of impaction and discomfort caused by inadequate elimination, prevention of rectal bleeding, and a reasonable amount of time for bowel care. Some people with SCI can identify a signal of rectal distention, such as sweating or an increase in spasticity. It is particularly useful to establish a fixed time, usually after a meal, for evacuation. Once a pattern has been established with stimulatory suppositories, patients often get by with dilatation of the anal sphincter, either digitally or by a glycerin suppository. Those who cannot develop enough intraabdominal pressure to defecate may need manual evacuation several times a week.

Fatigue

Although most commonly associated with MS, various forms of fatigue occur in all patients with central and peripheral neurologic diseases. Fatigue may encompass malaise, lack of energy, and depression. Underlying mechanisms may include disease-related autonomic, endocrine, and inflammatory dysregulation, as may occur in MS. Cognitive processing effort that is increased by the presence of cerebral lesions may induce a form of fatigue in carrying out mental and physical activities. One of the least recognized forms of fatigue that will interfere with ADLs occurs with repetitive use of muscles. This fatigability especially affects overused girdle muscles during walking but can be so insidious in the course of a motor activity that patients do not realize why they employ a slow gait with short stride. Clinically, this fatigability can

Table 48.9 **Pharmacological Manipulation of Bladder Dysfunction**		
Medication	**Indication(s)**	**Mechanism of Action**
Bethanechol, 25 mg bid-50 mg qid	Facilitate emptying	Increase detrusor contraction
Prazosin, 1 mg bid-2 mg tid; or tamsulosin, 0.4 mg daily	Decrease outlet obstruction Prostatic hypertrophy	Alpha blockade of external sphincter to decrease tone
Hyoscyamine, 0.125 mg hs-0.25 mg tid; oxybutynin 2.5 mg hs-5 mg qid	Urge incontinence	Relax detrusor, increase internal sphincter tone, decrease detrusor contractions
Tolterodine, 2 mg daily; or imipramine, 25-100 mg hs	Frequency Enuresis	

bid, Twice daily; *hs*, at bedtime; *qid*, four times daily; *tid*, three times daily.

be detected by testing strength immediately before and after 10 leg lifts by a supine or prone subject or after a 30-meter walk. It arises from problems as diverse as the more familiar fatigability found in myasthenia gravis and in lumbar stenosis with intermittent compression of the cauda equina. Impaired drive of motor units from the motor cortex due to less cortical excitability or greater inhibition, loss of corticospinal projections, conduction blocks along the descending projections, spinal mechanisms of reciprocal inhibition, disruption of firing rates of fast and slow motor units, and muscle atrophy can contribute. Medications such as the statins may cause a myopathy that induces weakness and greater fatigability that takes 6 to 12 weeks to resolve. Strengthening and conditioning exercises, as well as use of techniques for energy conservation, may lessen motor fatigability. Medications such as antidepressants, modafinil, and methylphenidate or noradrenergic modulation may reduce symptomatic fatigue.

Central Pain

A major source of disability can be pain from a thalamoparietal stroke or SCI. One of the most common patient complaints a year or more after SCI is burning pain at and below the level of the lesion. Approximately half of these patients gauge their symptoms as moderate or severe. Some patients need only assurance that the pain does not represent a serious complication or a warning signal of another stroke. Others will need the help of the physician in setting goals and identifying interventions to moderate the severity, frequency, and duration of the pain, also taking into consideration the usual time of day for pain onset. Tricyclic and selective serotonin reuptake inhibitor antidepressants, carbamazepine, clonidine, gabapentin, lamotrigine, benzodiazepines, and baclofen are among the drugs that diminish dysesthetic or lancinating pain in some patients. Intrathecal clonidine, baclofen, and morphine can be efficacious when oral approaches fail (see Chapter 44).

Sleep Disorders

During rehabilitation, insomnia, sleep apnea, and excessive daytime sleepiness can interfere with attention and learning. Stimulants, alcohol, medications, pain, anxiety, depression, and chronically poor sleep habits contribute. Central and obstructive sleep apneas have been associated with a higher risk of stroke. Pharyngeal muscle weakness and impaired neural control during sleep of the nasopharyngeal and pharyngolaryngeal muscles caused by a stroke or TBI contribute to the risk of obstructive apnea. Up to one-third of stroke inpatients may have a sleep disorder. Polysomnography is indicated when the rehabilitation team observes a hypersomnolent, confused, and snoring or apneic patient. One study found an average of 52 sleep-disordered breathing events per hour in selected subjects within 1 year of stroke. The number of oxygen desaturation events and the oximetry measures during sleep-disordered breathing correlated with poorer functional recovery scores at 1 and 12 months after stroke. It is especially important to address the possibility of apnea with outpatients with any type of neurological disease, especially stroke, TBI, thoracic SCI, and myasthenia gravis.

Spasticity and Upper Motor Neuron Syndrome

Spasticity is found in less than 20% of hemiplegic patients after stroke. Patients with bilateral weakness from TBI, especially if hypoxic injury occurred, are likely to have signs of spasticity as well. After SCI, spasticity is more prominent with incomplete than with complete motor and sensory impairments, especially with cervical and upper thoracic lesions.

The most important UMN problems that cause disability are the decrement in motor control associated with dyssynergic patterns of muscle activation and the coactivation of agonist and antagonist groups during movements, which are associated with paresis, slow movements, loss of dexterity, and fatigability with repetitive contractions. Spasticity per se does not produce weakness and these other aspects of impaired motor control. Exaggerated cutaneous and autonomic reflexes and involuntary flexor and extensor spasms are the most disabling episodic problems associated with spasticity for patients. During rehabilitation, the most visually striking signs associated with the UMN syndrome tend to be treated, and sometimes overtreated. These include hyperreflexia; flexor synergy of the elbow, wrist, and fingers; plantar flexion of the ankle; and the dystonic postures, rigidity, and contractures that may accompany weakness.

MECHANISMS

Clinical signs of hypertonicity can also be the consequence of interactions between central and peripheral factors. The mechanical velocity-dependent resistance to passive movement at a joint arises from the elastic and viscous properties of muscle, tendon, and connective tissue, as well as from reflexively mediated stiffness. Some investigators have proposed that secondary changes in muscle such as an increase in connective tissue and loss of muscle fibers or change in their properties explain at least some of the increased stiffness in patients. Hyperexcitability of motoneurons probably plays a larger role in this resistance but especially leads to hyperreflexia and clonus. A number of ill-defined mechanisms could alter membrane properties and morphologically and physiologically reorganize spinal circuits, leading to hypertonicity. A variety of neurotransmitters act within these systems, although their net effects are uncertain. Thus, drug interventions produce hard-to-predict changes in muscle tone and the incidence and severity of spasms.

ASSESSMENTS

For routine assessments and for clinical trials of antispasticity interventions, a number of measures of hypertonicity have been used. The Ashworth Scale (**Table 48.10**) has had good interrater reliability in studies of stroke, SCI, and MS. The relationship between this score and disability is not so evident, however. Hypertonicity, clonus, and spasms vary in relation to positioning of the limbs, posture, and activities. A clenched, plegic hand may lead to disability if pain or maceration of the palm develops, but a treatment that lowers the Ashworth score is unlikely to improve motor control. Other measurement techniques require instrumentation.

TREATMENT

Therapists usually can manage pathologically increased tone, spasms, and poor range of motion in patients with hemiplegia

Table 48.10 **Clinical Measures of Spasticity**

Score	Measure
ASHWORTH SCALE	
1	No increase in tone
2	Slight increase, producing a catch when joint is moved in flexion or extension
3	More marked increase in tone but easily flexed
4	Considerable increase, passive movement difficult
5	Affected part rigid in flexion or extension
SPASM SCORING SCALE	
0	No spasms
1	Mild spasms induced by stimulation
2	Spasms less than 1/h
3	Spasms more than 1/h
4	Spasms more than 10/h

by aiming to maintain normal length of the muscle and soft tissue across a joint, eliminating shoulder and other sources of pain, and helping patients to avoid abnormal flexor and extensor patterns at rest and during movement. Splinting to extend the wrist and the long finger flexor muscles is a common practice in the first month after stroke, but in randomized trials, this intervention has not clearly reduced the likelihood of a wrist contracture without employing other modalities. Spasms and dystonic postures should be treated more aggressively when they interfere with nursing care and perineal hygiene or evolve into contractures and pressure sores. Treatment often is needed for patients with myelopathies who endure painful spasms or involuntary flexor or extensor trunk and leg movements during transfers and after minor cutaneous stimulation. Measures to lessen hypertonicity can be useful when hypertonicity appears to restrain voluntary upper or lower limb movements through co-contraction of agonist and antagonist groups. In most cases, however, upper extremity flexor postures during voluntary movement may be best explained by abnormal muscle contraction evoked by action. For example, the typical synergistic response to attempted shoulder abduction causes flexion torques at the elbow, probably because the usual coactivation that stiffens the elbow to stabilize it fails as a result of an imbalance in strength of the opposite extensor action.

Hypertonicity and spasms have potential value. For example, spasms can decrease muscle atrophy and bone demineralization and increase venous return. An extensor thrust can provide the rigidity needed for weight-bearing stance. Learning to induce an extensor spasm can assist bed transfers in patients with a myelopathy. Determining how and when hypertonicity interferes with a patient's activities is the most useful way to determine whether an intervention is needed. Bouts of clonus and flexor and extensor spasms during ambulation, driving, wheelchair push-up pressure releases, transfers, self-care activities, bed mobility, sleep, and sexual activities can be counted over the course of a day or week. Any intervention should aim to greatly lessen recurrences.

Nociception can exacerbate hypertonicity and trigger flexor and extensor spasms and dystonic postures. A painful shoulder can cause the hemiplegic arm to flex at the elbow and wrist. Even an ordinarily innocuous stimulus like tight clothing or sunburn can abruptly increase tone, much as it can cause autonomic dysreflexia in the patient with a cervicothoracic SCI. Treatable pain stimuli include bowel and bladder distention, urinary tract infection, epididymitis, joint pain especially on range of motion, unrecognized fractures, pressure sores, ingrown toenails, and DVT. Resistance exercises, although generally useful during rehabilitation, can increase flexor or extensor tone, especially if the exercise brings out associated movements. Selective serotonin receptor inhibitors used for managing anxiety and depression can exacerbate spasms. The only way to make this diagnosis is to taper off the possibly offending drug and see if improvement follows by 2 weeks after cessation.

An overall approach to the management of pathological hypertonicity and spasms includes reversing any noxious stimulus, using physical interventions before adding drug trials, and reserving more invasive techniques such as nerve blocks and orthopedic or neurosurgical procedures for a few recalcitrant situations.

PHYSICAL MODALITIES

Slow stretching movements and daily passive range-of-motion exercises will reduce motion-sensitive symptoms of spasticity and the risk of contractures. Static stretching with splints probably will not prevent contractures when motor control is absent. Serial casting can reduce stretch reflex activity and contractures as the joint angle gradually increases. Muscle cooling, tendon vibration, pressure exerted over a tight muscle belly, postural adjustments, loading a limb by weight bearing on an extended arm or, for paraplegics, standing in a support frame (**Fig. 48.9**), and electromyographic BFB can complement a stretching program. Electrical stimulation of motor and sensory nerves, muscles, and dermatomes by a variety of paradigms may reduce tone at the ankle and knee and in the forearm and finger flexors. A single session of stimulation usually decreases resistance and clonus for a few hours.

PHARMACOTHERAPY

Controlled trials of antispasticity agents have varied widely in the target symptoms managed and the outcome assessments used. Functional gains related to locomotion and voluntary use of the upper extremity usually are marginal in any UMN disease. A medication that prevents disabling spasms, however, may improve quality of life. **Table 48.11** lists useful first- and second-line drugs.

After an SCI, about 25% of patients are discharged with an antispasticity agent, and half are still using medication by 1 year. Patients with American Spinal Injury Society (ASIA) grades A and D (see Chapter 50C) are less likely to have been treated than those with grades B and C. Baclofen, tizanidine, and clonidine are especially useful in reducing clonus and extensor spasms caused by a myelopathy. The latter two drugs are α_2-agonists that inhibit the excitatory influences of peripheral sensory inputs on motoneurons. Medications with short-lasting effects, such as tizanidine, may be especially useful in limiting spasms during sleep or brief activities like transferring from wheelchair to bed. Baclofen, dantrolene, and the benzodiazepines can cause muscular weakness and difficulty with weight bearing. Children with cerebral palsy and patients with hemiplegic stroke often need their extensor tone to

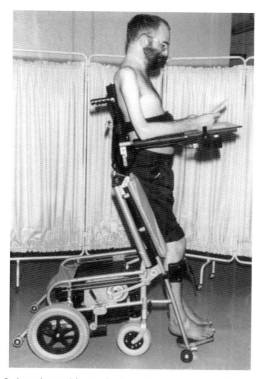

Fig. 48.9 A patient with quadriplegia from a spinal cord injury uses a standing wheelchair to try to reduce ankle and knee contractures and overall muscle tone. Subjects who can use their upper extremities may use a wheelchair like this one to perform tasks while upright, such as washing dishes.

Table 48.11　Dosages of Medications for Symptomatic Spasticity	
Drug	**Dosage**
FIRST-LINE AGENTS	
Diazepam	2 mg bid-15 mg qid
Dantrolene	25 mg bid-100 mg qid
Baclofen	5 mg bid-40 mg qid
Clonidine	0.05 mg daily-0.2 mg tid
Tizanidine	2 mg bid-8 mg qid
Gabapentin	400 mg tid-900 mg qid
OCCASIONALLY USEFUL ADDITIONS	
Intrathecal baclofen	50-150 µg trial dosages; intrathecal infusion with pump
L-Dopa or carbidopa	25 or 100 mg bid, respectively
Phenytoin	Serum concentration 10-20 µg/dL
Phenobarbital	Serum concentration 10-30 µg/dL
Cyproheptadine	4 mg bid-8 mg qid
Chlorpromazine	10 mg daily-50 mg tid
Dronabinol	2.5 mg daily–tid

bid, Twice daily; *qid,* four times daily; *tid,* three times daily.

ambulate on a paretic leg. Dantrolene tends to be most useful in managing hypertonicity of the upper extremity after stroke and TBI. Less than 0.5% of users develop hepatotoxicity after several months of intake. L-Dopa may be of additive value to lessen spasms in selected adults after stroke or SCI. All these drugs can also cause sedation, confusion, or hypotension; may add to bowel and bladder dysfunction; and can produce other central and systemic side effects. Great care must be taken in using them in the patient who has neurogenic dysphagia or a pseudobulbar palsy and is at risk for aspiration. Whenever a drug appears to be useful, it is worth tapering the dosage down from time to time so that the patient can help reassess continued benefits.

For refractory spasms and pain, intrathecal baclofen or clonidine given by an implanted programmable pump infusion generally has replaced a surgical myelotomy, intrathecal morphine, and electrical spinal stimulation. It also has replaced selective dorsal rhizotomy, except in some children with spastic diplegia from cerebral palsy. The functional effects on mobility and self-care are more difficult to discern, but some patients achieve modestly better walking speeds with intrathecal agents.

CHEMICAL BLOCKS

Chemical agents such as phenol have been injected into the lumbar theca, nerve, motor point, or muscle to lessen inappropriate muscle co-contraction, spasms, and dystonic postures. Because motor point blocks can partially spare voluntary

movement and could reduce reciprocal inhibition when given to an antagonist muscle, they could improve some aspects of motor control. Intramuscular infiltrative injections of 50% ethanol or botulinum toxin reduce focal resistance to passive movement for approximately 3 months.

Botulinum injections have seemed most efficacious for the wrist and finger flexors and plantar flexors of the ankle. Interpretation of the results of clinical trials using botulinum toxin requires attention to how well the outcome measure reflects clinical effectiveness for an important problem. Is a change in ease of passive range of motion, as in the Ashworth Scale, as meaningful as an increase in functional use of the limb? A few trials in children with cerebral palsy and spastic diplegia reveal modest 10% increases in walking speed after injections. The great majority of studies report a 1- or 2-point decrease in the Ashworth Scale score and support this finding by offering a global physician score that in reality probably reflects a perception of a decrease in tone around one or more joints. A randomized trial compared injection of type A toxin into forearm muscles with vehicle injection in patients after stroke who scored 3 or more on the Ashworth Scale for the wrist and 2 or more for the fingers (Brashear et al., 2002). A statistically significant decrease in the Ashworth score occurred at 6 and 12 weeks (e.g., a change from 0.1 in controls to 0.8 in the finger flexors of the treated group). Significant changes also were found in the Disability Assessment Scale, which was said to reflect functional disability. This disability is only a subjective measure of change in hand hygiene, pain, positioning, and dressing that does not require use of the hand. It would be easy to misinterpret the data as revealing better functional use of the hand after botulinum toxin injection, but the real meaning is that with the wrist and finger flexors loosened, the hand was easier to keep open passively, and the arm may then be easier to manage when, for example, the patient tries to put it through a shirt sleeve. Trials of botulinum toxin that are sponsored by the pharmaceutical industry have not included a control intervention that uses rehabilitative passive or active range of motion or treatments for pain that may decrease tone. Also, these studies have not tried to maintain the effect of greater passive ranging by adding physical therapy after an injection to try to prolong any benefit.

SURGICAL INTERVENTIONS

A variety of surgical procedures including tendon lengthening, tenotomy, and tendon transfer can correct deformities induced by spasticity and improve function. A gait analysis with EMG helps determine which of these procedures may aid mobility. Physical therapy must follow any surgery. Tenotomy of the hip adductors and iliopsoas and tendon lengthening of the hamstrings, Achilles, and toe or finger and wrist flexors are among the more common interventions. Lower-extremity surgeries are performed most often in children with cerebral palsy, although the data are difficult to interpret in terms of meaningful clinical gains. Achilles tenotomies for Duchenne muscular dystrophy and a variety of foot surgeries, including triple arthrodesis, for Charcot-Marie-Tooth disease may be beneficial.

Posterior rhizotomy has been carried out, especially in children with spastic diplegia. Selective division of posterior nerve rootlets of the second lumbar to the second sacral level is based on intraoperative EMG responses of lower extremity muscles to posterior nerve rootlet stimulation. Youngsters with the most dramatic functional improvements are bright, ambulatory patients with spastic diplegia who have minimal fixed contractures and good strength. Some clinicians argue that such patients would do well with any intensive therapy. Indeed, controlled trials suggest that the intervention is no better than routine physical therapy in terms of functional walking.

Therapies for Impairments and Disabilities

For problems of mobility and use of the upper extremities, therapeutic exercise and neurodevelopmental approaches are merging with strategies related to engaging neural systems for activity-dependent plasticity, motor control, and motor and cognitive learning. Success in motor retraining during rehabilitation requires attention to the movement components of a task; residual sensory and motor control; how performance is reinforced; the patient's mood, motivation, attention, and memory for carryover of what is taught; minimizing environmental distractions and physical barriers; family and community support; and creative problem solving. All can influence how motor and cognitive programs are built, shaped, and refined as the patient acquires a new skill. Overall, trials suggest that repetitive practice of related motor sequences aimed at a defined functional goal will lead to better gains, especially for walking and increased use of a paretic arm and hand (French et al., 2009). A few well-specified approaches to therapy have gained and lost momentum as the results of well-designed clinical trials have been published.

Locomotor Training

Observation of the gait cycle for temporal asymmetries of the legs and for the kinematics at the hip, knee, and ankle during the stance and swing phases reveals deviations that the clinician can identify and target to help train patients. The timing of loading the stance leg and unloading the swing leg after it approaches 10 degrees of hip extension for toe-off (**Fig. 48.10**), for example, provides proprioceptive information that is important for driving reciprocal stepping movements. **Table 48.12** lists components of the gait cycle that are often used in kinematic and kinetic gait analyses. The therapist identifies and tries to modify serious deviations that interfere with the

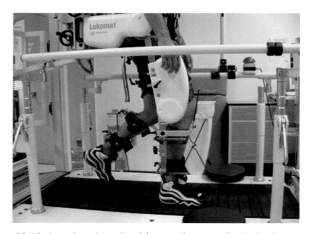

Fig. 48.10 A patient is assisted by an electromechanical robotic exoskeleton (Lokomat by Hocomo Inc.) throughout the gait cycle. The right foot is in mid-stance, and the left hip is extended and the foot is at toe-off, which initiates the swing phase of that leg. This device actively controls hip flexion and knee extension and permits the subject to assist in these phases. The treadmill passively extends the leg at the hip.

Table 48.12 Easily Observed Components of the Gait Cycle	
Gait Phase	**Component**
STANCE	
Pelvis	Lateral and horizontal shift to the stance leg
Hip	Extension to approximately 10 degrees
Knee	Slight flexion upon loading Extension at midstance Flexion at foot pushoff
Ankle	Dorsiflexion to 10 degrees at heel contact Dorsiflexion as the lower leg moves over the foot Plantar flexion to 20 degrees with a propulsive rocker motion of the foot for pushoff
SWING	
Pelvis	Drop at toe-off, then forward rotation
Hip	Flexion to 20 degrees to "shorten" the leg
Knee	Flexion to 65 degrees to "shorten" the leg, then extension just before heel contact
Ankle	Dorsiflexion to 10 degrees for heel strike

safety and energy requirements of ambulation as the patient walks on a flat surface. Temporal features of the gait cycle, such as the symmetry of each leg's stride length, time in stance and swing phases, and overall cadence and walking speed, are other key targets for management. These parameters have been enhanced by stationary bicycling, treadmill walking, and rhythmic auditory stimulation, which may help entrain the timing of more automatic stepping.

The threshold velocity for home ambulation is 40 cm/sec (45 cm/sec = 1 mile per hour [mph]). Therapy ought to aim for faster walking speeds and for more energy-efficient traveling distances to permit unlimited community activities. Community ambulation requires a walking velocity of approximately 80 cm per second, or more than 1.5 mph. Therefore, task-oriented training over ground or on a treadmill ought to try to exceed 1.5 mph as patients progress. In contradistinction to this outcome goal, typical disability measures such as the FIM and the BI assess only the level of independence to walk 15 to 45 meters at any velocity.

The notion of task-oriented training led to many small trials of treadmill training, circuit training around obstacles, bicycling, and related walking activities for patients with hemiplegic stroke, SCI, TBI, MS, and other entities. The specificity of the training aims to improve walking safety and velocity, leg strength, and fitness to reduce the energy cost of walking. The addition of partial body weight support to treadmill training (BWSTT) has shown promise in patients with stroke, SCI, PD, and cerebral palsy. Subjects wear a chest harness that is attached to an overhead lift. The amount of weight borne by the lower extremities is adjusted to optimize the stance and swing phases of gait. One or more therapists may manually assist the lower extremities and pelvis during step training to optimize the step pattern. In theory, BWSTT allows the spinal cord, brainstem, and supraspinal locomotor-related regions to experience sensory inputs that are more like ordinary stepping than the atypical inputs produced by compensatory gait deviations and difficulty with loading a paretic limb. More normal proprioceptive and cutaneous input may improve the timing and increase the activation of residual descending locomotor outputs onto the lumbosacral motor pools. In patients with complete SCI, segmental sensory inputs related to the level of loading and to treadmill speed may modulate the electromyographic output during BWSTT when the legs are fully assisted during the step cycle. Most important, BWSTT allows repetitive practice guided by the verbal and physical cues of the therapist to improve components of the step cycle. This approach, then, offers many elements that may enhance motor relearning. Aims of this task-specific intervention include greater independence in walking, as well as attaining walking speeds that permit home and community ambulation.

Spatiotemporal asymmetries within the stance and swing phases clearly improve on the treadmill during step training. In patients with recent stroke, however, randomized clinical trials started during inpatient rehabilitation to date have not led to more independent ambulation or clinically meaningful increases in velocity compared with conventional therapies that emphasize gait training. When trials tested patients with more chronic stroke who walked poorly, gait speeds often improved by 10% to 30%, but a control intervention for walking usually was included, so the superiority of BWSTT is uncertain (Mehrholz et al., 2008a; Moseley et al., 2005).

Training at treadmill speeds of about 2 mph usually led to faster overground walking speeds than training at slower speeds, regardless of the initial overground walking velocity. Patient selection (e.g., severity of paresis and walking impairment), duration of harness support before full weight bearing is allowed, the use of treadmill speeds that reach for faster overground velocities yet allow subjects to have time during the gait cycle to make adjustments in their kinematics, explicit information about what is meant to be practiced on the treadmill, the intensity and duration of treatment, feedback paradigms, the use of orthotics, explicit strategies to carry over what is trained on the treadmill into overground practice, best outcome measures, and adequate sample sizes need attention for clinical trials. A U.S. trial called the *Locomotor Experience Applied Post Stroke* (LEAPS) Trial (Duncan, et al., 2007) randomized 400 subjects who still walked slowly at 2 and at 6 months after stroke (Duncan et al., 2011). It compared usual care to BWSTT with overground practice and to progressive strengthening and balance exercises in the home for 36 sessions. Improvements were significant for exercise and for BWSTT compared to usual care when started at 2 months, and the two interventions were equal in their effects at 12 months. When the usual care group received the same amount of BWSTT starting at 6 months, no difference was found in walking speed at 12 months compared to early BWSTTT and home exercise. The proportion of subjects with moderate and severe walking disability did not differ in gains. The trial confirmed that progressive, challenging, mobility-related exercise is better than less structured therapies.

BWSTT originally was developed to replicate features of training spinal-transected cats for hind limb stepping on a treadmill belt. Uncontrolled studies and reports that employed historical controls suggested that patients with recent and chronic SCI who walked poorly could improve their ability to take steps. The Spinal Cord Injury Locomotor Trial (SCILT) compared 12 weeks of step training with BWSTT with overground practice to a defined overground mobility intervention for patients with incomplete traumatic SCI within 8 weeks of onset (Dobkin et al., 2006a). This single-blinded randomized trial entered 107 ASIA C and D subjects and 38 ASIA B subjects with lesions between C5 and L3 who were unable to walk on admission for rehabilitation at a mean of 4.5 weeks after onset. The tests for walking speed and distance, among other measures, were performed by blinded observers, and the data were collected at 3, 6, and 12 months later. No significant differences were found in outcomes that included the FIM's scoring system for locomotion (FIM-L), walking speed used over 15 meters, walking distance in 6 minutes, and lower extremity motor score at 3, 6, and 12 months after entry. Very few subjects graded ASIA B recovered the ability to walk, but greater than 90% of the ASIA C subjects walked. Their mean velocity met criteria for unlimited community ambulation. Thus, for early use of BWSTT, the natural history of recovery in ASIA C subjects is too great when given either type of locomotor training to show greater efficacy for either one. Also, BWSTT does not appear to improve the prospects for walking in ASIA B patients who still cannot walk without maximum assistance by 8 weeks after SCI.

BWSTT has been combined with functional neuromuscular stimulation (FNS) with surface or implanted electrodes for patients with hemiplegic stroke and SCI. Peroneal nerve stimulation to dorsiflex and clear the foot during swing is the

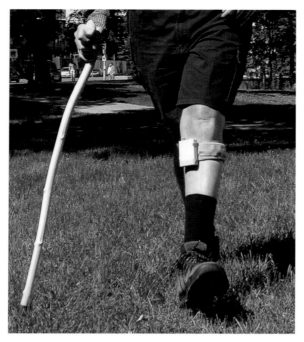

Fig. 48.11 Stimulation of the peroneal nerve under the cuff on the right leg is in response to a signal from an accelerometer, leading to dorsiflexion from toe-off to heel strike to help clear the hemiparetic leg (WalkAide from Innovative Neurotronics, Inc.).

oldest approach to aid overground gait, with a variety of newer and possibly more efficient devices commercially available (**Fig. 48.11**). In patients with paraplegia, peroneal stimulation also aids reflexive hip and knee flexion during swing. The results to date show modest improvements in walking speed and kinematics within subjects, but only small clinical trials with selected patients have been reported. Electromechanical assistive devices for stepping on a treadmill or oscillating footplates have proved to be at least equal to BWSTT in small studies (see later section on robotic-assistive devices). This approach aims to take the physical burden of step training off therapists.

Constraint-Induced Therapy

Constraint-induced therapy (CIT) is a task-oriented strategy that calls for forced use of the affected upper extremity to overcome what is theorized as "learned nonuse" of the paretic limb, along with gradual shaping of a variety of functional movements, to increase the effective daily use of the hemiparetic arm and hand. The theory of learned nonuse was derived from studies of monkeys in which one forelimb had been deafferented by dorsal rhizotomy and then stopped being employed in association with profound sensory loss. Of course, this model of impairment is very different from that in patients with hemiplegia and impaired motor control. The translational intervention uses a variety of techniques to limit the use of the unaffected hand by placing it in a sling or glove and having the patient practice skills and ADLs with the affected arm.

The first rendition of this approach for the upper extremity provided a course of 6 hours of practice with the affected arm on a series of functional tasks combined with restraint of the unaffected one throughout the day for 2 weeks. The key requirement for participation has been the ability to dorsiflex the wrist and extend several fingers of the paretic arm at least 10 degrees. The key treatment focus is as much practice as tolerated of progressively more complex and difficult tasks (shaping) that involve reaching in various planes to grasp or pinch items of different weights and sizes. The most important aspect of this approach is massed practice. Gains in the amount of hand use have been accompanied in some but not all small studies by cortical reorganization of the hand region based on transcranial magnetic stimulation and fMRI. These adaptations were consistent with the effects of practice and skills learning (Sawaki et al., 2008), but the physiological and clinical significance of these brain-behavior correlations is uncertain.

Several randomized inpatient trials for hemiparetic stroke have found modest or no benefit from CIT compared to equal intensity of conventional therapy (Dromerick et al., 2009). A well-powered multicenter randomized trial (Wolf et al., 2006) entered patients who had sustained a first stroke within 3 to 9 months of enrollment. They received 2 weeks of training for 6 hours daily, a home practice program, and wore a mitt on the unaffected hand during formal therapy and at home. Statistically significant and clinically relevant improvements in paretic arm functional skills, measured by the Wolf Functional Motor Test and perceived daily use, were found compared to participants who received no training and restraint. The improvements persisted up to 1 year and were not influenced by age, gender, or initial level of paretic arm function. The design and follow-up of subjects of this trial were outstanding, although the comparison of a very intensive form of treatment against no treatment, a decision that was made for reasons of funding, leaves open the issue of possible value for less intensive interventions.

Other investigators have tested modified CIT strategies by eliminating or reducing the use of the restraining mitt and decreasing the intensity of formal practice with a therapist from 6 hours to 1 to 3 hours a day over 2 to 4 weeks of training. As in many small trials with selected subjects, some show 10% to 20% improvements in an outcome measure, and some reveal no difference compared to an active control intervention. Styles of practice such as the use of shaping, optimal reinforcement schedules, and the most cost-effective intensity of treatment, then, are works in progress. Compared with no formal intervention, CIT does improve functional use of the arm in patients with chronic disabilities who meet the stringent criteria for residual wrist and finger extension, but this gain can be interpreted as an intensity of practice effect, rather than confirmation of the efficacy of restraint. The approach is applicable to no more than 20% of hemiparetic patients but confirms the impact of greater intensity of therapy for specific impairments and disabilities, even when applied beyond the first few months after stroke.

The notion of constraint with therapy has been invoked for interventions for walking and aphasia, because the underlying style of therapy aims for massed practice of specified activities and attempts to optimize responses and limit patient errors. The intensity and focus of the practice paradigm seem more important than concerns about restricting the use of an unaffected arm, leg, or language response, however.

Bimanual Upper Extremity Therapy

Bimanual training is based on the hypothesis that in-phase voluntary movements of the intact arm may facilitate mechanisms of motor synergies for interlimb coordination to improve the paretic arm. The substrate for this bilateral motor control includes the primary, premotor, and supplementary motor cortices and may involve both excitation and disinhibition. Indeed, functional neuroimaging studies show that the motor deficit of patients with a single subcortical lesion is associated with pathological interhemispheric interactions among these motor areas. Several techniques and devices have been developed to aid proximal and distal upper limb training. For example, the Bi-Manu-Track (Reha-Stim, Berlin, Germany) promotes bilateral elbow pronation-supination and wrist flexion-extension, as well as unilateral movements, and can accommodate neuromuscular electrical stimulation to facilitate these movements. Hundreds of repetitive movements can be made in four directions in highly impaired subjects with stroke. Small trials suggest a modest gain in proximal and distal strength and some aspects of motor control in chronic hemiparetic patients with mild to moderate impairment after 20 to 30 hours of bilateral arm training with or without special devices. Trials to date are too heterogeneous and include too few subjects to determine whether the bimanual approach is better than primarily unilateral practice with the affected arm.

Instrumented Biofeedback

Biofeedback includes a variety of instrumented techniques that try to make the subject aware of physiological information that can be used to better perform an activity. Electromyographic BFB to improve upper and lower extremity muscle activity, decrease co-contraction of muscles, and increase functional movements has been tested in groups of 3 to 12 subjects across many UMN and LMN diseases. Its efficacy usually is modest at best. Across controlled trials of ambulation in selected patients after stroke, electromyographic BFB using a visual or auditory cue seems useful as a way to increase ankle dorsiflexion. BFB also can be combined with EMG-triggered neuromuscular stimulation. A minimal voluntary movement such as slight wrist extension of a paretic hand fires low-amplitude motor units. If this reaches the gain that is preset, radial nerve stimulation is triggered for increased motor unit activity of the extensors. This BFB modality may increase cortical and spinal excitation and cognitive-motor resources to gradually increase voluntary EMG and wrist control. The strategy has led to modest functional gains for handgrip in several small studies.

Biofeedback can improve performance during training, but not necessarily when visual or auditory guidance is withdrawn. For example, postural control, which often is considered a prerequisite for walking, has been a focus of visual feedback systems. The Balance Master has been used to provide continuous visual feedback on the position of the center of gravity when patients stand on its force plate. The system detects postural sway and asymmetries of weight distribution on each leg, and patients get feedback when they shift in ways that improve symmetry. Although greater symmetry of weight bearing would be a reasonable goal for a hemiplegic patient, meta-analyses across trials find that improved postural control on the force plate does not carry over to a significant increase in symmetry of stance or improved gait performance over ground. Lack of generalization is not unexpected, in part because hemiplegic patients probably need to center their weight toward the unaffected leg to compensate for weakness and the use of synergies when standing and stepping.

Acupuncture

A variety of acupuncture methods are widely used in China and Korea after stroke. Many of the reports from these countries are uncontrolled and impossible to interpret in terms of efficacy. Several small Asian and Western trials of acupuncture in subjects who had moderate hand paresis after a pure motor stroke showed gains in speed of hand manipulation or ADLs with the intervention. Better-controlled trials and meta-analyses of these trials using sham acupuncture compared with traditional treatment have not shown clear benefit (Wu et al., 2008). As a general intervention during stroke rehabilitation, acupuncture does not appear to improve skills for ADLs or functional use of a hand. Studies focused on particular types of dysfunction and combined with motor learning strategies, however, have yet to be carried out in a well-designed trial with an adequate sample size.

Mechanical and Robotic-Assistive Devices

An *orthosis* typically describes a device that is used to assist a person with limb pathology. Active assist exercise uses external physical assistance to aid participants in accomplishing intended movements. Robotic devices have been developed to provide this assistance for the paretic arm and leg to increase the intensity and reproducibility of practice. Portable exoskeleton devices have both mechanical structures and associated actuators, viscoelastic components, sensors, and control elements that work in concert with the subject's movements. One goal is to decrease mechanical loading on the paretic leg and improve kinematics and energy cost of walking at faster speeds. Myoelectric controlled AFOs and KAFOs may use artificial muscle fibers. These engineered devices are a work in progress, limited by cosmetics, power source, weight, and flexibility, but they are also advancing rapidly. Many experimental models and a few commercial ones have been developed for the leg and arm. Recent devices employ impedance-, counterbalance-, EMG- and adaptive-based controllers that adjust forces and kinematics to assist movements based on the patient's performance.

An increasing number of robotic devices have been developed commercially to aid practice of walking on a treadmill and of reaching and grasping while seated. Devices aim to allow subjects to practice movements repetitively in order to increase motor control and to use the arms or legs in a maximally functional manner, potentially with only intermittent therapist oversight. These approaches are still under development. Researchers must address the best time after onset of injury for each etiological disorder to initiate training, identify the level of arm or walking disability that is most appropriate to target, determine the movements that are best practiced with robotic assistance, define how much the device will assist components of movements or confine them, define the best cognitive and physical cues and feedback to improve specific aspects of practice, perform dose-response studies to estimate the optimal frequency and duration of training, define how robotic training will be used to augment strengthening exercises and fitness training, and ascertain how to transfer robotic exercise to the practice of daily activities and overground walking.

Upper Extremities

A passive device, the Therapy Wilmington Robotic Exoskeleton (T-WREX), was designed to support the paretic arm against gravity, measure arm motion, and trace hand grasp as the user interacts with computer games. After 24 sessions, patients assigned to the device or to an equal intensity of table-top exercises had equally modest gains. Such devices may yet show better outcomes, based on their built-in entertainment value for repetitive practice and feedback about results. The first in its class to reach commercial development, the MIT-MANUS, is a robotic device that manipulates a patient's paretic elbow and shoulder much as a therapist might provide hand-over-hand therapy for reaching in a single plane. Power and control at the shoulder have improved with this robotic training, consistent with the greater intensity of practice using those muscle groups, but it is uncertain that the device offers better outcomes than active therapy for reaching (Volpe et al., 2008). A multicenter trial of a more complex three-part device for the arm in multiple planes, wrist, and hand that incorporates the principles of the MIT-MANUS technology and visual feedback during tasks (Interactive Motion Technologies, Cambridge, MA) showed that the robotic assist was equal in effectiveness to the same amount of intensive conventional therapy in moderately impaired patients (Lo et al., 2008). The more components and degrees of freedom a device incorporates, the more challenging it will be to develop best rehabilitation training procedures.

Walking

Two robotic-assistive devices have been available commercially for years: the Gait Trainer 1 (GT) (Reha-Stim, Berlin, Germany) and the Lokomat (Hokoma AG, Volketswil, Switzerland). Both devices stand the subject in a parachute-type harness attached overhead. The GT powers ellipsoid motion to the legs via footplate attachments. The backward movement of the footplates simulates the stance phase, and the forward motion simulates swing. Posterior leg motion during stance is accomplished as if on a treadmill, with passive hip extension after the mid-stance phase. Settings for swing can be varied between 30% and 50% of the gait cycle. The tip of the plate moves in an arc and the rear lifts, which puts the footplate on an incline during swing. Stride length and phase duration can be adjusted using the fixed "sun and circulating planet gears" in a box behind the subject. The Lokomat (see **Fig. 48.10**) attaches each thigh and lower leg to a motorized exoskeleton while fixing the hips in its frame. Reference trajectories based on the gait of healthy subjects are adjusted by on-line optimization that adapts the parameters of the trajectory of the hip and knee to minimize the measured forces of interaction. Both devices maintain a kinematically repetitive stepping pattern in the sagittal plane.

RCTs revealed that the GT and the Lokomat produce results at least as good as other practice strategies, but so far, no robotic device has been superior to treadmill or overground training for stroke, SCI, and MS (Hidler et al., 2009; Hornby et al., 2008; Lo and Triche, 2008; Mehrholz et al., 2008b; Westlake and Patten, 2009). Indeed, some studies reveal that overground training may be superior. In contradistinction to the strategy of massed practice of kinematically sound stepping, which is an aim of motor-driven devices, the clinical efficacy of a stereotypical assisted-step pattern with relatively unvarying sensory inputs still has to be demonstrated. The reduced degrees of freedom the GT and Lokomat permit during gait may or may not be a limitation for neurologically impaired patients, and certainly not for patients who cannot walk without maximal assistance. Modifications of these devices and of new entries may allow more effective feedback and errors during practice that challenge subjects and increase motor learning.

Functional Neuromuscular Stimulation

Functional neuromuscular stimulation systems activate one or more muscle groups synchronously or sequentially to enable single-joint and multijoint movements. Surface and intramuscular electrical stimulation systems have become more widely available in the past 5 years, but despite extensive study and commercial development, they have not come into sustained use. The discontinued FreeHand provided hand grasp and release in C5 and C6 tetraplegic patients. Electrode wires were implanted in the appropriate muscle of one forearm, and a controller device at the opposite shoulder allowed patients to complete upper-limb grasp, pinch, and release after training. The first commercial surface electrode-driven device for grasping is the Ness System, which has found some use in quadriplegic patients with at least C5 intact and in hemiplegic patients with poor hand function (**Fig. 48.12**). Electrodes attached to a molded forearm orthosis that reaches across the wrist stimulate the wrist and finger flexors and extensors in synchrony. The external control unit operates from a button managed by the patient for the level of output that allows grasp, holding, or release. Small studies suggest that the combination of task-oriented training and assisted grasping in patients who cannot otherwise incorporate the hand may provide better outcomes than either strategy alone.

FNS systems also can aid standing and ambulation. Peroneal nerve stimulation to aid foot dorsiflexion to clear the foot during the swing phase can increase step length and walking speed in hemiparetic persons. A growing number of commercial devices are available that use an accelerometer to switch on the below-the-knee stimulus (**Fig. 48.11**). Used alone or combined with other assistive and bracing devices such as a reciprocal gait orthosis, these systems can allow walking as an exercise and in some instances permit stepping for indoor distances. However, a lengthy strengthening and fitness program must precede the use of these devices by paraplegic patients. The first commercial device to assist stepping, the Parastep System, used six surface electrodes to stimulate the gait cycle as subjects held a rolling walker. Stimulation of the quadriceps muscles and push-off with the arms permitted standing up. Constant stimulation maintained standing. A button on the walker was pressed to stop the quadriceps firing and to stimulate the peroneal nerve to initiate a triple flexion response for swing. The patient released the button after the hip flexed, which fired the quadriceps stimulator for stance. Patients with a complete UMN SCI may exercise with a bicycle ergometer. Bilateral surface electrodes are placed over the

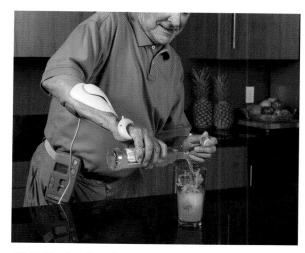

Fig. 48.12 The hemiparetic right arm is assisted by an orthosis with functional neuromuscular stimulation that helps dorsiflex the wrist and produce a palmer grasp or finger pinch (NESS by Bioness, Inc.).

quadriceps, hamstrings, and gluteal muscles to sequentially activate leg forces on the pedals. As muscle strength increases, contractions are made against greater ergometer resistance to increase muscle bulk and aerobic fitness.

It is increasingly conceivable that cosmetically acceptable exoskeletal prostheses will become available and affordable for the arm, hand, and leg. Smaller motors and batteries, more efficient and stronger power sources, lighter materials, and progress in electromechanical prostheses for amputees may enable industry to replace most FNS and robotic-assistive devices in this decade.

Neural Stimulation

Subthreshold cortical electrical stimulation at an optimal frequency and amplitude aims to increase cortical excitability and synaptic efficacy during training. Possible mechanisms include reinforcement by Hebbian plasticity, modulation of neurotransmitters, and remote effects on excitation-inhibition. Transcranial magnetic stimulation over the primary motor cortex as well as ulnar and median peripheral nerve stimulation have led to modest increases in motor control for at least a short time in healthy subjects and in several small controlled trials after stroke (Dimyan and Cohen, 2010). Repetitive transcranial magnetic stimulation also has been used to inhibit a cortical region to improve activation of the homologous contralateral hemisphere. A randomized controlled trial of motor cortex stimulation via an epidural electrode placed over primary motor cortex combined with arm therapy found no overall better functional gains than by the same therapy alone after stroke (Harvery, 2009). Somewhat better function was likely in more mildly paretic subjects.

Spinal cord stimulators have been placed over the dorsal spinal cord in the epidural space to reduce some types of central pain and hypertonicity after SCI. Stimulation of the upper lumbar cord also has produced rhythmic leg movements in subjects with complete SCI and has been used to try to improve the gait pattern of a few patients with spastic quadriparesis. Electrode microarrays are in experimental stages for direct spinal cord stimulation, perhaps of spinal primitive modules and central pattern generators to elicit

oscillating leg movements. Nerve cuffs placed around a portion of a peripheral nerve can provide a permanent electrochemical interface to selectively initiate or record electrical signals or modulate the nerve's responses. Their initial experimental use has been for ankle dorsiflexor stimulation during walking, but may find use for sacral nerve stimulation for bowel and bladder emptying or central excitation.

Virtual Reality Training

Virtual reality training can be used in an immersive and nonimmersive fashion and in both active and passive modes. Practice in a virtual reality environment increase the ecological soundness of the training environs toward real-world settings. Whether in the home or a laboratory, measurements of movement patterns can be integrated with the training and reinforcement paradigms provided as tasks are carried out. For example, walking on a treadmill surrounded by a complex indoor or outdoor environment may restore visual flow and lessen the influence of distracters. VR systems have also been combined with robotic steppers; gains carried over to community walking (Mirelman, 2009). Performing upper-extremity tasks such as putting a letter into a mailbox or pinching moving objects in a virtual field while wearing a Polhemus sensor on the hand allows repetitive practice and useful measures of the trajectory of the hand. Playing games in a VR setting may increase motivation while improving balance and the timing of movements. Small clinical trials also have revealed encouraging results for cognitive rehabilitation assessment and for the treatment of attention and spatial memory deficits and apraxia.

Imagery

Observing another person make a movement activates mirror neurons; imagining a movement evokes activity in cell recordings and by fMRI in some of the same neurons in the primary and nonprimary motor regions and parietal lobe as with performing the movement. The motor cortex may represent the form, speed, and kinematic sense of a movement, whereas the parietal cortex represents conceptual information and kinesthetics. The ability of patients with stroke, PD, and other diseases to use imagery may vary. This form of practice is routinely used by athletes and dancers before a performance to reactivate in working memory the representation of a motor memory. Small randomized trials suggest that motor imagery for particular hand tasks can improve function, at least for a short time after training and perhaps longer. The level of residual motor function necessary, the capacity for imagery in patients with brain lesions, the necessary intensity of practice, and efficacy are uncertain.

Neural Prostheses

Up to 2 million Americans and many others worldwide may be without any voluntary control due to ALS, a locked-in syndrome after stroke or trauma, MS, cerebral palsy, or muscular dystrophy. To aid these highly disabled persons to manage their surroundings and communicate, a variety of brain/computer interfaces have been developed (Daly, 2008). The devices use surface and intracortical neural signals from defined regions of the brain to drive, for example, an FNS system or a computer mouse. Signals are acquired from field potentials over the surface of the scalp, dura, or subdural regions or from the spike potentials of small clusters of neurons picked up by microelectrode arrays from motor cortex or cognitive planning regions. Selected signals such as the amplitude of an evoked potential, a specific rhythm from sensorimotor cortex, or the firing rate of cortical spikes are digitized and processed by algorithms to extract specific features. A translation algorithm converts the particular electrophysiological features chosen to simple commands to a device such as a word processor or keyboard, a website, or an upper-extremity neuroprosthesis. The error rate, often in the range of 10% to 20%, can be frustrating to a patient who tries to make binary changes in the amplitude of a cortical signal to choose a letter or word. Major improvements in signal processing and interfaces should offer greater utility by paralyzed patients and, perhaps, become a tool to increase training-related neural adaptations during routine rehabilitation.

Pharmacological Adjuncts

A stroke or other brain injury that diminishes the availability of a neurotransmitter projection system from the brainstem may degrade synaptic adaptation and learning during rehabilitation. Neurotransmitters and neuromodulators given in pharmacological dosages could be supplied to augment neural activity within a network during a specific motor or cognitive task. It takes much study to find a drug with a dose/response ratio that produces positive effects with no adverse effects. Human clinical trials of drug interventions have had small sample sizes. Investigators often screen 20 subjects for every one who meets entry criteria. Several trials of dextroamphetamine, methylphenidate, L-dopa, piracetam, and L-threodopa have revealed motor gains when the agent is combined with motor therapies, but other studies have not. A promising approach is to use functional imaging or transcranial magnetic stimulation to screen patients for trials of a particular agent, based upon a transient change in regional cortical activity or excitability induced by the drug. Short-term effects, however, may not predict long-term benefits. For inpatient and outpatients, N-of-1 experiments with simple outcome measures for short-term trials that alternate placebo versus active medication can be safe and occasionally beneficial.

Therapies for Cognitive and Behavioral Disabilities

Overview of Cognitive Therapy

Cognitive and behavioral disorders are common with stroke, TBI, MS, PD, and other degenerative diseases. **Box 48.9** lists some of the cognitive impairments dealt with by the rehabilitation team. One mechanism, for example, is interruption of inputs and outputs from the hippocampus after stroke or trauma. These impairments can seriously impede gains in mobility, ADLs, and community reintegration. Prospective studies of patients with an acute stroke reveal that 15% to 35% have greater memory impairments 3 months to 1 year after onset than age-matched controls. Cognitive and behavioral dysfunction, especially from diffuse axonal injury, is especially common after TBI. Greater severity and longer duration of impairments are associated with a lower Glasgow Coma Scale score on acute admission and longer duration of

---

Box 48.9 Cognitive Impairments Managed During Rehabilitation

Language

Aphasia
Affective expression

Attention

Alertness
Speed of mental processing
Awareness of disability and impairment
Focused attention on a single stimulus
Sustained attention to a task
Selective attention during distraction
Divided or alternating attention between tasks

Memory

Retrograde, antegrade
Immediate, delayed, cued, and recognition recall

Learning

Visual, verbal, and procedural or skill

Perception

Visual
Auditory
Visuospatial

Executive

Planning
Initiation
Organization skills
Maintaining goal or intention
Conceptual reasoning
Hypothesis testing and ability to shift responses
Self-appraisal
Self-monitoring

Intelligence

Verbal
Performance
Problem solving
Abstract reasoning

---

posttraumatic amnesia. Up to half of patients with an SCI have cognitive impairments from an associated TBI that may not be obvious early in postinjury care.

The amount and rate of recovery of neuropsychological function vary with the sophistication of the measures used; type and severity of impairment; type, severity, and distribution of lesions; time since onset; and age at onset and follow-up. More subtle factors such as the interactions of diseases, associated sensorimotor and cognitive impairments, and premorbid intellect and education can affect the efficacy of a particular therapeutic approach. Comparisons between interventions often are confounded by the intensity and duration of treatment, lack of specification of the treatment methods, personal interactions between the therapist and patient, and the family's ability to reinforce desired behaviors.

General management approaches include training in particular functional adaptive or compensatory skills, behavioral modification, and remediation of specific cognitive processes. In the adaptive approach, therapy tries to circumvent the effects of cognitive impairments on targeted daily activities. Repetition, cues (both internal and environmental), and cognitive assistive devices are used for training. Learning to do a particular task usually does not generalize to other tasks that are not closely related. Behavioral modification techniques most often are used in acute and transitional living settings for patients with TBI. Rewards are given for accomplishing a task or reducing antisocial actions. In the cognitive remediation approach, the subcomponents or hierarchical organization of a given cognitive skill are addressed. The strategy assumes that at least some of the parallel and hierarchical neural networks for cognitive processes are understood. More often, techniques emphasize interventions meant to boost intact domains to help compensate for more impaired ones.

A modest number of studies of insufficient sample size suggest a benefit with use of a particular approach or combination of approaches for a specified set of cognitive impairments compared with no treatment or a placebo or psychosocial intervention, as well as with conventional training in ADLs (Cicerone et al., 2005). Techniques usually merge as the rehabilitation team experiments with interventions that address the most deleterious problems. Indeed, outpatients with a TBI are the most likely group to need multimodality programs that stress training in task-specific skills by remediative techniques, awareness about impairments and limitations, and an emphasis on the skills needed for independent living and work.

Aphasia

The incidence of language disorders has varied across studies of patients with stroke and TBI. In a British health district of 250,000 people, new cases of stroke-induced aphasia for 1 year numbered 202. By 1 month after stroke, 165 survivors were potential candidates for speech therapy. A prospective, community-based Danish study of acute stroke found that 38% of 881 patients were aphasic on admission, with 20% of the admissions rated as severe on the Scandinavian Stroke Score. Nearly half of the patients with severe aphasia died soon after stroke onset, and half of those with mild aphasia recovered by 1 week. Only 18% of community survivors were still aphasic at the time of their rehabilitation hospital discharge. Up to 28% received early speech therapy as needed. Patients were retested over the subsequent 6 months; 95% with mild aphasia reached their best level of recovery at 2 weeks, those with moderate aphasia peaked at 6 weeks, and patients with severe aphasia reached best language function within 10 weeks. Only 8% of those with severe aphasia fully recovered by 6 months on the scoring system used. The best predictor of recovery was less severe aphasia close to the time of the stroke.

Treatments

Some 20% to 50% of aphasic patients have partial features of the traditional aphasia subtypes (see Chapters 12A and 12B). For rehabilitation therapy, the broadly defined features used to classify patients often do not address in enough detail the underlying disturbances of language, so they may not be optimal for directing treatment. A neurolinguistic assessment of aphasia aims to specify the types of representations or units of language (e.g., simple words, word formation, sentences, discourse) that are abnormally processed during speech, auditory comprehension, reading, and writing. For each unit, the therapist ascertains how the disturbance affects linguistic forms such as phonemes, syntactic structures, and semantic meanings.

Speech therapists most often attempt to find ways for the patient to circumvent, unblock, or help compensate for defective language function by using a great variety of stimulation-facilitation techniques (see **Table 48.4**). These include visual and verbal cueing techniques such as picture matching and sentence completion tasks, along with frequent repetition and positive reinforcement as the patient approaches the desired responses. Phoneme-based treatment, for example, would aim to lessen anomia by increasing phonological production and reduce non-word repetition. Strategies for therapeutic training have also been drawn from hypotheses about activity-dependent adaptations and learning. Since action words and the actions themselves have overlapping neural networks, language tasks perhaps ought to be practiced within relevant physical activities. Massed practice, avoidance of learned nonuse of words due to prior failures, and linking words to actions and daily relevance has been advocated to maximize Hebbian-type plasticity (Pulvermuller and Berthier, 2008). In addition, use-dependent learning suggested constraint-induced language therapy in which intensive training of either nouns or verbs with an emphasis on phonemic cues led to increased use of the taught words, but not of untrained words.

Initial treatments often use tasks that relate to self-care, the immediate environment, and emotionally positive experiences. To prevent withdrawal and isolation, it is especially important to quickly find a way to obtain reliable verbal or gestural "yes-no" responses. Behavioral techniques, particularly for patients with TBI, can be used to improve skills in maintaining eye contact, initiating and staying on a topic, turn-taking during conversation, adapting to listener needs, and using speech to warn, assert, request, acknowledge, or comment. Beyond the stimulation-facilitation approach to therapy, a variety of theoretical models for therapy have been proposed, such as the modality, linguistic, processing, functional communication, and minor hemisphere mediation models.

Specific therapy techniques have been designed for defined aphasia syndromes and neurolinguistic impairments as well. For example, the efficacy of melodic intonation therapy (MIT) has been especially good. In MIT, therapists and patients melodically intone multisyllabic words and commonly use short phrases while the therapist taps the patient's left hand to mark each syllable. Gradually, the continuous voicing and tapping are withdrawn. MIT works best in persons with Broca aphasia who exhibit sparse or stereotypical nonsense speech and good auditory comprehension. If a single sound, word, or phrase overwhelms any other attempted output, the Voluntary Control of Involuntary Utterance Program can help the patient gain control over perseverative intrusions. Some mute or nonfluent aphasics can acquire a limited but useful repertoire of gestures using, for example, American Sign Language. Comprehension in persons with the global and Wernicke forms of aphasia has been managed with the Sentence Level Auditory Comprehension Program. It trains patients to discriminate consonant-vowel-consonant words that are the same or differ by only one phoneme (e.g., "bill, pill, fill"). They then try to associate the word sounds with the written word and later try to identify the target word embedded in a sentence. For persons with global aphasia, nonverbal communication using pantomime has decreased limb apraxia and improved auditory comprehension through a technique called *visual action therapy*. Use of an electronic device that provides delayed auditory feedback by about 200 msec after the aphasic person voices each phoneme can be tried as a means to improve awareness of paraphasic errors and intelligibility. Recent case studies also suggest that focal cortical stimulation using TMS may be able to activate or deactivate a node in the language network to enhance the effectiveness of simultaneous training.

Pharmacological Adjuncts

A few studies suggest that intensive therapy combined with a drug that enhances vigilance or learning may benefit patients who have adequate language comprehension. Piracetam, a derivative of γ-aminobutyric acid (GABA) but with no GABA activity, may facilitate cholinergic and aminergic neurotransmission. A randomized placebo-controlled trial included 50 moderately aphasic patients who had a stroke a mean of 10 months before starting the 6-week intervention of 10 hours of speech therapy weekly. The drug-treated group had a significantly better total score on the Aachen Aphasia Test, although the clinical impact is not clear. In a randomized trial of 24 patients, use of piracetam also was associated with some language subtest gains and higher cerebral blood flow in left hemisphere language regions during a word repetition task. Other cholinergic agents have improved naming in patients with moderately severe Wernicke aphasia or dysnomia, especially by reducing perseveration. Amphetamines, memantine, and dopaminergic agents have improved aspects of language in some small studies but not all. Short-term trials of such agents can be carried out in combination with language therapy and standardized tests in individual patients to look for responsiveness.

Outcomes

A meta-analysis was performed on 55 trials of speech therapy in persons with stroke-induced aphasia. Significant effects were found for patients who received treatment at all stages of recovery, with the greatest improvement found when therapy was started in the acute stage. Treatments of more than 2 hours per week gave greater gains than lesser amounts of therapy. In another meta-analysis, treatments given for approximately 100 hours over 11 weeks were more efficacious than when given for 45 hours over 22 weeks. Persons with severe aphasia showed large gains when their management included treatment by a speech-language pathologist. Treatments for aphasia average 45 to 60 minutes, provided up to three times a week in community practices. The family tries to continue what therapists recommend at home. The Cochrane Library's systematic review of group trials in stroke (http://update-software.com/publications/cochrane) concluded that speech and language therapy for aphasic people after stroke has not been shown to be clearly effective or ineffective due to the design of clinical trials. Still, even a delayed pulse of a specific language therapy often improves a goal-directed aspect of aphasic communication in individual patients. The trials do suggest that therapy for aphasia can

improve aspects of language and social communication, but the components of training, intensity, and augmentation by home-based computer assisted training are still uncertain.

Apraxia

Many forms of apraxia have been defined (see Chapter 10). Approximately 25% of patients will have an ideational or ideomotor apraxia that affects the sequential performance of tasks and knowledge of how to use a limb or deploy objects. This disability interferes with ADLs, but some recovery is likely over several months with both left and right cerebral lesions. Oromotor apraxia often accompanies nonfluent aphasia. Most approaches are compensatory rather than building on an understanding of the cognitive bases for the impairment. Practice of limb gesturing and structured behavioral training, training in specific strategies for necessary ADLs that use relatively errorless learning, and sensory cues lead to moderately positive effects on praxis and may generalize to untrained but related ADLs. Theoretically driven therapies such as strategies that activate the action-observation system of mirror neurons can be explored as well.

Attentional Disorders

Sustained, focused, alternating, and divided attention often are affected by the frontal lobe and diffuse injuries induced by TBI and MS, after stroke that disconnects thalamic–basal ganglia–frontal pathways, from mass effect or vasospasm, and with any toxic-metabolic complication such as a urinary tract infection. Real-time feedback about performance (during visual, verbal, sequential, and environmental tasks), reinforcement paradigms as varied as praise and earned tokens, and compensatory strategies to manage increasingly complex tasks often are part of the rehabilitation of attention. Cognitive processes associated with increasingly difficult attentional demands have been a focus of treatments. These include processing speed, flexibility, interference and distraction thresholds, and use of working memory. Computer programs for attention that emphasize gains in processing speed and reaction times usually have not generalized to improved focused or divided attention, however. The entire rehabilitation team must develop and reinforce attentional strategies across ADL in the hope that the approaches will generalize. Aspects of attention often improve during inpatient rehabilitation rather spontaneously. Severe impairment may continue in patients with TBI or hydrocephalus. Clinical trials of specific approaches for persistent difficulties during outpatient care do not point to greater efficacy of any particular strategy.

Memory Disturbances

Memory disturbances can have a profoundly negative influence on compensation and new learning in the patient undergoing neurorehabilitation. The therapy team depends on teaching that can be encoded and retrieved. Patients with TBI, a remarkably large percentage of those with stroke, and elderly persons with degenerative neurological diseases most frequently are affected by memory problems. Clinical trials of therapies are complicated by variation in the severity of the amnestic syndrome, time since onset, and difficulties in "teasing out" spared and affected components of implicit and explicit memory processes, and in specifying the exact nature of the treatment strategy.

Frequency of Memory Disturbance Across Diseases

The frequency of and risk factors for memory loss and dementia caused by one or more strokes have become increasingly appreciated. The prevalence of memory disturbance in population- and community-based studies is nine times greater in the first year after a stroke than in an age-controlled group and doubles in each subsequent year. Other studies find a risk of memory dysfunction of approximately 20% at 3 months after a stroke. The frequency of dementia rises with increasing age and varies with the definition used. Even a mild aphasia may affect verbal memory and can interfere with verbal learning during rehabilitation.

Memory impairments after TBI have been related to the time between injury and assessment, to the nature of the memory task, and to the severity of the injury. Tasks that require divided attention are especially useful to tease out executive dysfunction caused by a TBI. Natural history studies have reported varying outcomes. For example, in a group of 102 patients with TBI (ages 10 to 60 years) who were hospitalized for any period of unconsciousness, for posttraumatic amnesia lasting for more than 1 hour or for evidence of cerebral trauma, the TBI group performed significantly worse on the Wechsler Memory Scale and the Selective Reminding Test 1 month later than did a control group. Those who could not follow a command for the longest times beyond 24 hours after injury scored below the control subjects on more subtests of the Wechsler Memory Scale. Tests that required storage of new information for later use were superior to tests of orientation and short-term memory in their ability to reveal memory deficits. At 1 year, patients performed better than they had at 1 month after onset. Many patients who were hospitalized for serious TBI are found later on to underestimate their memory and emotional impairments, even as they acknowledge physical and other cognitive problems. Without insight or concern, they deny having the impairment and withdraw or become angry with attempts at rehabilitation. The rehabilitation team must provide the counseling and insight therapy needed to overcome this.

Treatments

Clinical evidence from RCTs neither supports or denies the effectiveness of rehabilitation techniques for memory impairments after stroke or TBI, but many strategies for the diverse types of patients, impairments and disabilities have been tried with some sense of benefit for some patients (Nair and Lincoln, 2007). Most rehabilitative efforts aim to help patients encode new information and recognize and retrieve declarative memories of facts and events. Previous exposure to verbal and especially to nonverbal information, with cues and prompts, can allow many amnestic patients after TBI to recall that information, a phenomenon called *priming*. Priming does not require semantic processing for encoding. It is specific to the properties of the input and relies on perceptual representations stored by modality-specific memory subsystems such as those that process word forms and visual objects. Tests of recognition memory are especially sensitive methods for detecting residual memory in patients with severe amnesia. This implicit memory neocortical mechanism can even support the rapid acquisition of novel verbal and nonverbal material. It is relatively independent of the hippocampal and diencephalic structures that relate to amnesia. Priming seems especially useful during rehabilitation to enhance procedural memory for skill acquisition. The best training paradigm for implicit learning in markedly amnestic patients after TBI appears to be errorless learning rather than trial-and-error learning. The latter tends to produce better consolidation of what has been learned in healthy and mildly affected subjects.

Cognitive remediation of amnestic disorders aims to train patients to use the theoretical subcomponent processes that underlie declarative and nondeclarative memory. Therapists can then take a restorative or compensatory approach to affect particular memory skills for functionally important activities. For example, therapists may address attentional impairments that could interfere with memory training by strategies for improving focused, sustained, selective, alternating, and then divided attention. Impairments in encoding and recall of information are then addressed. This approach uses associative and external cues that are meant to prompt an action after increasingly longer intervals have passed, as well as external aids, rehearsal, and visual imagery.

After a moderate to severe TBI, repetitive paper-and-pencil or electronic drills on names, appointments, orientation, and daily routines may have little impact on daily functional recall and memory outside of the training session. Learning to make associations and "chaining" tasks in a sequence has had better results for daily activities. External aids such as calendars, lists, appointment diaries, and pagers have been shown in clinical trials to be better than no aids. The devices listed in **Box 48.10** may improve daily activities if patients can be reminded to use them. Indeed, prospective memory for upcoming activities is a valuable target for training. The acceptance of particular aids and their value for ADLs varies considerably among patients.

Computers have been used extensively in cognitive remediation and skill training. Although software programs abound for working on reaction times, aspects of attention, language, problem solving, and other cognitive tasks, almost no data demonstrate the efficacy of such programs. Some patients have learned tasks such as data entry, database management, and word processing by taking advantage of preserved cognitive abilities, including the ability to respond to partial cues and acquire procedural information, even in the presence of a marked amnestic syndrome. This knowledge often does not generalize to even modest changes in the tasks, however. Through procedural memory, verbal and visual mnemonic strategies have been used to teach subjects a computer graphics program. Cooking and vocational tasks were taught with an interactive guidance system that cued each subtask to build up to the desired task.

A growing number of animal and human studies suggest that aerobic exercise itself can improve aspects of cognition, including memory, reaction times, and attention. This work has been applied to patients with stroke and Alzheimer disease (AD) with fair evidence of modest gains.

Pharmacological Adjuncts

Studies of single subjects and small groups suggest that the drugs listed in **Box 48.11** may benefit some patients with amnestic and attentional impairments. TBI may lead to

---

Box 48.10 Aids and Strategies for Memory Impairment

External

Reminders by Others
Tape recorder or portable voice organizer
Notes written by hand or entered into PDA

Time Reminders
Alarm clock or phone call
Personal organizer or diary
Calendar or wall planner
Orientation board

Place Reminders
Labels
Codes (colors, symbols)

Person Reminders
Name tags
Clothes that offer a cue

Organizers
Lists
Personal organizer or diary
Numbered series of reminders
Items grouped for use
Radio pager
Calendar and event alarm on cell phone or handheld computer

Internal
Mental retracing of events
Visual imagery
Alphabet searching
Associations to what is already recalled
Rehearsal
First-letter mnemonics
Chunking or grouping of items

PDA, Personal digital assistant, iPhone, Blackberry, etc.

Box 48.11 Possibly Useful Medications for Attentional and Memory

Cholinergic Agonists

Physostigmine
Tacrine
Donepezil, rivastigmine
Metrifonate
Cytidine diphosphocholine
Choline and lecithin precursors

Catecholamine Agonists

Dextroamphetamine
Methylphenidate
L-Dopa
Amantadine
Bromocriptine and other dopamine receptor agonists
Desipramine

Modafinil

Serotonergic Agonists

N-methyl-D-aspartate Receptor Agonists

Ampakines

Nootropics

Pramiracetam
Piracetam

Neuropeptides

Vasopressin and analogs

---

damage in a particular neurotransmitter system such as cholinergic neurons. Presynaptic cholinergic neurotransmission was abnormal in a human postmortem study of TBI. Therefore, rehabilitation trials of cholinergic-enhancing drugs such as donepezil and cytidine diphosphocholine seem warranted. Some patients with stroke improve in some facets of cognition with anticholinesterases, although this could reflect pre-stroke early dementia. Replacement therapies for other neurotransmitters, such as bromocriptine and noradrenergic agents, have a few human case studies to commend them. The diversity of lesions after TBI (e.g., diffuse axonal injury, damage to the dorsolateral prefrontal cortex or hippocampus) and stroke necessitates empirical short-term individualized approaches to pharmacotherapy. Repetitive TMS and direct cortical stimulation are being tested to alter excitation and inhibition of relevant pathways to improve attention and memory. Many other compounds that act on signaling pathways (e.g., cyclic AMP response element–binding [CREB] protein) are likely to become available to induce or increase synaptic adaptations that enhance the acquisition and retention of information (Lee and Silva, 2009).

Outcomes

Although memory-related processes are found to improve over the first 3 months after a stroke, reports on the natural history of ongoing cognitive sequela suggest that both inpatient and outpatient rehabilitation efforts must include ongoing attention to the need for compensatory aids and other strategies for these patients. After mild TBI, memory usually recovers by 3 months. This varies with the test used to measure severity, the time from injury to testing, and the comparison group. The patients who exhibit the greatest impairment at 1 year after a serious TBI initially are unable to follow a command for more than a day and have posttraumatic amnesia for more than 14 days and a Glasgow Coma Scale score of 8 or less. At 1 year after a severe closed head injury, patients followed in the Traumatic Coma Data Bank had greater impairments in verbal and visual memory and in other neurobehaviors, such as naming to confrontation and block construction, compared with normal controls. Selective rather than global cognitive impairments were likely at 1 year. Memory was disproportionately impaired compared with overall intellectual functioning in 15% of the moderately injured and 30% of the severely injured patients. After moderate to severe TBI, children plateau in recovery by 1 year after onset, with little change in the next 2 years, and do not catch up to their peers in terms of memory, problem-solving ability, and academic performance. Late changes do evolve in some. In a long-term outcome study of mostly young adults, Wilson and colleagues reassessed 26 patients who had a TBI resulting in 1 hour to 24 weeks of coma, followed by rehabilitation. At 5 to 10 years later, 58% were unchanged, 31% performed better, and 11% did worse on the Rivermead Behavioral Memory Test and Wechsler Memory Scale. Many needed to rely on memory aids.

Hemineglect

Hemineglect can arise from injury to any node in the cortical-limbic-reticular network, which directs attention and integrates the localization and identification of a stimulus and its importance to the person. Unilateral neglect arises from injuries of the posterior parietal cortex, the prefrontal cortex, which encompasses the frontal eye fields, and the cingulate gyrus. These regions include representations for sensation, for motor activities such as visual scanning and limb exploration, and for motivational relevance, respectively. Subcortical areas such as the thalamus, striatum, and superior colliculus coordinate the distribution of attention. Atrophy of frontal white matter and the diencephalon contributes to persistent anosognosia. The anterior and posterior extent of a lesion also may produce impairments in attentional and intentional processes that contribute to neglect. Therefore, the most severe and subtle hemiattentional disorders can be expected in focal stroke and more diffuse TBI.

Frequency

Community-based studies of stroke survivors detect visual neglect in 10% to 30% of patients. The neglect is modestly associated with poorer ADL scores and slower recovery, although severe neglect is rare beyond 6 months. Visual neglect is greater in right than in left hemisphere strokes. Right-sided inattention, when looked for, has been detected in 15% to 40% of nonaphasic patients with acute left cerebral infarcts, although it is clinically the most prominent after right brain injury. Patients with anosognosia, visual neglect, tactile extinction, motor impersistence, or auditory neglect have the lowest BI scores at 1 year, even after the data are adjusted for initial ADL scores and for poststroke rehabilitation. During rehabilitation, patients with left hemiplegia and neglect tend to improve on the motor portion of the FIM more than those with neglect and anosognosia.

Recovery across reports has been most rapid in the first 2 weeks, regardless of the side of stroke. By 3 months, most patients have little visual neglect. Severe visual neglect and anosognosia in the first week tend to predict some level of persistent impairment at 6 months. Many patients have more subtle and lingering impairments that depend on the test used to detect them. For example, early after a right hemisphere stroke, a group of patients showed a strong and consistent rightward attentional bias, in addition to an inability to reorient their attention leftward. Twelve months later, the attentional bias continued, but now the patients could fully reorient to left hemispace when performing line bisection and cancellation tasks.

Treatments

The initial choice of an intervention may depend on the proposed mechanism of unilateral neglect or hemispatial inattention. For example, the patient can be treated for an underaroused right hemisphere that has difficulty processing sensory inputs. After a right brain injury, a powerful bias of the left hemisphere for attention to contralateral space could lead to an imbalance, necessitating intervention to lessen the bias. A selective inability to disengage from inputs from ipsilateral space may need to be addressed. Other strategies may have to be developed if the mental representation of contralesional space has been degraded or if a unilateral impairment in the activation of motor programs delays or prevents the intention to move to the contralesional side. Repetitive TMS has been used with some success to inhibit or disinhibit one side of the brain after stroke and lessen hemineglect.

If the initial theory-based intervention is not successful, then others should be tried. **Box 48.12** lists some of the traditional and clever ways clinicians have tried for the management of hemineglect. For example, prisms have been used to transform sensorimotor coordinates, and passive prosthetics can be worn during tabletop activities. A 10-degree prism that shifts objects to the right in a patient with left hemi-inattention causes the patient to reach to the left when the glasses are removed. After adaptation to wearing the prism for 5 minutes, the patient's internal visual and proprioceptive map apparently realigns in the direction opposite to the optical deviation. Functional imaging revealed a realignment of visuomotor coordinates processed by the cerebello-cerebral projections. The aftereffects of the prism may include significant improvement in drawing objects and performing cancellation tasks in left hemispace and in ADLs for a few weeks.

Spatial and visual cues, visuomotor feedback, and combined training of visual scanning and reading, copying and describing pictures and figures are more commonly employed strategies. A variety of attempts have been made with some success to help patients recalibrate or realign the work space or frame of reference that is at the center of a task. Noradrenergic and dopaminergic stimulants including guanfacine, methylphenidate, modafinil, and bromocriptine may modulate vigilance for tasks and is worth trying in recalcitrant cases.

Box 48.12 Interventions for Hemineglect

- Multisensory visual and sensory cues, then fading cues
- Verbal elaboration of visual analysis
- Environmental adaptations (bed position, red ribbon at left book margin)
- Computer training
- Video feedback
- Monocular and binocular patches
- Prisms
- Left limb movement in left hemispace
- Head and trunk midline rotation
- Vestibular cold caloric stimulation
- Contralesional cervical nerve stimulation
- Repetitive transcranial magnetic stimulation of unaffected hemisphere
- Reduction of hemianopic defects by a few degrees
- Pharmacotherapy trials

Adapted with permission from Dobkin, B., 2003. The Clinical Science of Neurologic Rehabilitation. Oxford University Press, New York.

Behavioral Disorders

A great variety of behavioral changes can follow any hypoxic-ischemic injury or TBI. Alterations in personality have been reported in up to 75% of patients 1 to 15 years after a TBI and tend not to improve spontaneously beyond 2 years after onset. **Box 48.13** lists some of the more common changes. Agitated motor and verbal behaviors, although not easy to define or treat after TBI, are found in more than 10% and restlessness in 35% of patients during acute inpatient rehabilitation. As cognition improves, agitation declines, but directed and non-directed aggressive, impulsive behavior may evolve. Persistent aggression and emotional dyscontrol suggest premorbid mood and behavioral disorders.

Interventions include a medical assessment for exacerbating problems such as pain and drug-induced confusion, behavioral modification with positive and consistently applied reinforcements, a structured milieu for the most impaired, instruction in formal problem-solving techniques, individual and group psychotherapy, and medication (useful drugs are listed in **Box 48.14**). Interventions to improve self-awareness of deficits in self-regulation and self-monitoring have not been successful in small trials of patients with TBI. Improvements have been reported even years after onset when a focused program of rehabilitation is provided. Some patients who exhibit hypoarousal improve with stimulants such as methylphenidate and amphetamine or with dopamine agonists. Aggressive behavior sometimes is decreased by dopaminergic or noradrenergic receptor blockade. Beta-blockers can decrease irritability. A randomized trial of propranolol with dosage escalation to 420 mg a day showed a reduction in the intensity of agitation, but not the frequency of episodes, compared with placebo. Hypomanic behavior may respond to lithium or anticonvulsant medications that are used in the management of bipolar disorders. Anticonvulsants such as carbamazepine sometimes prevent outbursts related to episodic dyscontrol.

Box 48.13 Potential Changes in Behavior and Personality After Traumatic Brain Injury and Cerebral Hypoxia

Disinhibition
Impulsivity
Aggressiveness
Irritability
Lability
Euphoria
Paranoia
Lack of self-criticism and insight
Irresponsibility and childishness
Egocentricity
Selfishness
Sexual inappropriateness
Self-abuse
Poor personal habits
Apathy, indifference
Indecision
Lack of initiation
Blunted emotional responses
Poor self-worth
Passive dependency

Affective Disorders
Incidence

Depression is very common after stroke and mild TBI. The community-based Framingham Study diagnosed depression in 47% of 6-month stroke survivors, with no difference found in the incidence between those with left- and right-sided lesions, compared with 25% of age- and sex-matched controls. In a population-based cohort of Swedish stroke patients whose mean age was 73 years, the prevalence of major depression was 25% at hospital discharge, 30% at 3 months after stroke, 16% at 1 year, 19% at 2 years, and 29% at 3 years. In this and many other studies, a left anterior infarct, dysphasia, and living alone contributed to the prediction of depression upon discharge. At 3 months, greater dependence in ADLs and relative social isolation were associated with depression. Few social contacts at 1 and 2 years contributed.

Anxiety is another stroke-related affective disorder. Although less often studied, a generalized anxiety disorder was present in 28% of recent stroke victims and was associated with greater social isolation and greater dependence in ADLs. Apathy was found in approximately one-fourth of patients within 10 days of a stroke, associated with greater cognitive impairment, poorer ability to perform ADLs, and some cases of major but not minor depression. Depressed people with an SCI report spending more time in bed and fewer days out of the house. They receive more personal-care assistance than better-adjusted patients with SCI at 2 to 7 years after injury. Suicide rates may be two to four times that in the general population within 5 years of SCI. Anxiety and depression also can arise from a posttraumatic stress disorder associated with the event that led to the SCI. After TBI, 25% to 60% are diagnosed with depression. Late-onset depression has been associated with premorbid psychiatric history and lower psychosocial function. Poor social adjustment can cause long-term depression and anxiety.

Treatment

Clinicians should manage mood disorders aggressively, especially when progress in rehabilitation falls short of expectations. Psychosocial support, individual and group therapy, and support groups appear to help across diseases. In general, patients with depression respond to all classes of antidepressant medications and can be managed with the same judicious care in finding the optimal dose that is necessary for managing

---

Box 48.14 Drug Interventions for Aggressive Behavior, Restlessness, and Episodic Dyscontrol

Anticonvulsants (carbamazepine, valproate, gabapentin)
Beta-blockers (e.g., propranolol)
Lithium
Antidepressants (e.g., amitriptyline, fluoxetine)
Stimulants (e.g., methylphenidate, pemoline)
Neuroleptics (e.g., risperidone)
Benzodiazepines (e.g., clonazepam)
Clonidine
Calcium channel blockers

the elderly. For example, by 6 weeks after initiation of fluoxetine or citalopram therapy, two-thirds of depressed subjects after a stroke recover, compared with 15% given a placebo. The same medications can help alleviate pseudobulbar emotional incontinence with its involuntary weeping, grimacing, and laughing. Close clinical monitoring for adverse reactions to the antidepressants is important during inpatient and outpatient rehabilitation. Such reactions include sedation, insomnia, constipation, inability to void, reduced salivation, orthostatic hypotension, cardiac arrhythmias, anxiety, extrapyramidal symptoms, and a serotonin syndrome.

Functional Outcomes with Rehabilitation

The most important outcomes for the rehabilitation team include the degree of independence in ADLs and community living. Thus, functional measures that reflect the level of care needed and the quality of life achieved by people with neurological disabilities are used in outcome studies more often than measures of change in sensorimotor and cognitive impairments. The scores on the FIM at admission for inpatient rehabilitation and at discharge offer an interesting snapshot of clinical status of a large number of patients with stroke, TBI, and SCI from American institutions that participate in the Uniform Data System for Medical Rehabilitation. Over the past 15 years, data reveal that the time from onset of neurological illness to transfer for rehabilitation has dropped about 30%. The length of stay in rehabilitation has followed a similar decline.

Stroke

A meta-analysis of 36 trials carried out before 1992 showed that the average patient who received a program of focused stroke rehabilitation or a particular procedure performed better than approximately 65% of the patients in the comparison group. Larger treatment effect sizes were associated with earlier timing of the intervention and younger age. This trend has continued over the past 15 years. Interventions for a well-defined disability (e.g., functional use of an affected hand, walking, swallowing, speech intelligibility, community activities), as well as impairments in areas such as muscle strength and fitness, show a moderate benefit from rehabilitation services of optimized intensity and specificity.

Rehabilitation studies of patients with stroke generally show that 50% of 6-month survivors have no motor impairment, 70% to 80% can walk 150 feet alone, and 50% to 70% are independent in ADL based on the BI. These gains in subjects with the best outcomes do not imply that they can walk or function efficiently in the community. Most studies suggest that 50% to 75% of survivors do not return to their pre-stroke level of activities in the community. **Table 48.13** presents a compilation of admission and discharge data for ADLs as measured by the seven-part FIM.

Ambulation

A community-based population study in Copenhagen prospectively followed 800 acute stroke survivors. On admission, 51% were unable to walk, 12% walked with assistance, and

Table 48.13 Summary of Medical Rehabilitation Data for First-Stroke Admissions*

Measure	Admission	Discharge
	Mean Subscore	
Self-care	3.5	5.2
Sphincter	3.7	5.4
Mobility	3.0	5.0
Locomotion	2.1	4.3
Communication	4.2	5.2
Social cognition	3.5	4.6
Total Functional Independence Measure (FIM) score	62	86
Age (years)	70	
Onset (days)	12	
Stay (days)		20
DISCHARGE OUTCOMES (%)		
Community	76	76
Long-term care	15	14
Acute care	7	6

*Data compiled from publications for the year 2000 from the Uniform Data System, Buffalo, New York.

37% were independent. In the same facility, all who needed rehabilitation received services for an average total stay of 35 ± 41 days. At discharge, 22% could not walk, 14% walked with human assistance, and 64% of survivors walked independently by BI criteria. Recovery of ambulation correlated directly with leg strength. About 80% of those who initially were nonwalkers reached their best walking function within 6 weeks, and 95% achieved this within 11 weeks. If patients walked with assistance at stroke onset, 80% reached their best function within 3 weeks and 95% within 5 weeks. With rehabilitation, 34% of the survivors who had been dependent and 60% of those who initially needed assistance achieved independent walking for at least 150 feet.

Life table analysis of patients from different impairment groups reveals a somewhat different pattern of gains. During their rehabilitation, 90% of patients with a pure motor (M) deficit become independent in walking 150 feet by week 14 after stroke onset, but only 35% of those with motor and proprioceptive or sensory (SM) loss by week 24, and 3% of those with motor, sensory, and hemianopic deficits (SMH) by week 30. The probability of walking more than 150 feet with assistance increases to 100% with M impairment by week 14. It increases to 90% in those with SM loss by week 26 and in those with SMH deficits by 28 weeks. At 1 month and 6 months after stroke for all survivors, 50% and 85%, respectively, of M subjects recover walking, 48% and 72% of SM subjects recover, and 16% and 38% of SMH subjects walk without human assistance.

Although many patients become independent in gait, stroke patients who needed rehabilitation most often have self-selected walking speeds that peak in 3 to 6 months at one-third to one-half of normal for age. Speed is a good reflection of the overall gait pattern and, as noted earlier, reflects capabilities for walking in the home and community.

Self-Care Skills

In the Copenhagen Stroke Study, ADL measured by the BI were assessed weekly in the hospital and at 6 months. Some 20% of survivors had a severe disability and 8% a moderate disability after a mean hospital stay of 37 days. Functional recovery peaked by 13 weeks after stroke onset in 95%. The highest BI score was reached within 13 weeks by those with moderate impairments and within 20 weeks in those with severe impairments by the Scandinavian Stroke Scale. A BI score greater than 60 is associated with a home discharge. Using the impairment grouping schema, the cumulative probability of reaching a BI score greater than 60 and greater than 90 at 6 months after stroke is 95% and 70%, respectively, 85% for M subjects, 62% for SM subjects, and 52% and 35% for SMH patients (Patel et al., 2000). Similarly, approximately 65% of inpatients during rehabilitation achieve a BI score greater than 95 by 15 weeks if they have only M deficits and by 26 weeks with SM loss. Only 10% score that high with SMH deficits after 18 to 30 weeks. However, 100% achieve a score greater than 60 by 14 weeks with M loss only, 75% by 23 weeks with SM deficits, and 60% by 29 weeks with SMH loss.

For patients admitted for stroke rehabilitation, the admission BI or FIM score predicts later burden of care. The FIM score on admission positively correlates with discharge FIM and negatively correlates with length of stay, except in patients under age 50. The largest FIM change over time occurs in patients with admission FIM scores of 40 to 80. Patients with admission scores greater than 80 and age younger than 55 years routinely return home. A score of less than 40 and age older than 65 leads to a nursing home discharge for 60%.

Much of self-care depends on making use of the unaffected hand and trying to incorporate the affected one. If no recovery of wrist and finger extension has evolved by 4 weeks after hemiplegic stroke, functional dexterity of the hand rarely develops (Kwakkel et al., 2003). When selective flexion and extension are present, gains in use of the hand may evolve for as long as patients practice specific tasks such as reaching into their workspace to grasp and perform key and pincer pinches. Patients must work on accuracy, precision, speed, and endurance. For example, putting a key into a lock at home, if difficult to perform, should be done 20 to 30 times a day in sets of 10 until this becomes a more functional movement.

Spinal Cord Injury

The Uniform Data System database described the average age of patients with traumatic SCI as 43 years. The mean time from onset to admission for rehabilitation was 22 days, and the mean length of stay was approximately 33 days. The FIM score increased from about 63 to 89. A decrease from ASIA A (sensorimotor complete) and B (sensory present) grades of injury to ASIA C (less than useful motor return) injury occurred in only about 10% of patients during inpatient rehabilitation after a cervical or thoracic SCI. These patients tend to regain some sensorimotor function one level below the initial level of impairment. Gains may be a bit better for these ASIA-level patients with conus and cauda equina injuries.

A clinical trial of GM1 ganglioside found the following changes in 760 patients assessed between 72 hours and 26 weeks after they suffered a traumatic SCI of the cervical or thoracic cord (Geisler et al., 2001). Approximately 80% of patients with a central cord injury became able to walk at least 25 feet. Only 4% of ASIA A patients at onset recovered any ability to walk, whereas 40% of ASIA B subjects regained this function. At least 70% of ASIA C subjects recovered unlimited walking. ASIA A patients almost never recovered normal bowel and bladder function. Approximately 15% of subjects with incomplete injuries recovered these functions. The drug, of note, did not alter outcomes compared with a placebo. More detailed outcomes about walking have helped investigators develop designs for clinical trials after recent SCI (Dobkin et al., 2006a; Fawcett et al., 2007).

Self-care skills depend especially on the level and completeness of an SCI. For ASIA A patients, the absence of recovery of movement two levels below a cervical traumatic SCI injury at 8 weeks predicts little likelihood of gains. Any movement one level below anticipates ongoing gains in strength in the muscles at that level. For ASIA B patients, no motor gains by 16 weeks after SCI markedly diminishes the likelihood that useful motor function will develop. ASIA C patients, however, are highly likely to continue to make gains in motor function. For patients with complete lesions at C4 or above, ventilatory support and assistive devices are needed along with physical help. With C5 intact, self-feeding is achieved with devices such as a balanced forearm orthosis and wrist splints with attachments for utensils. Patients can use a power-assisted wheelchair with a hand control. With C6 intact, wrist extension allows the thumb and fingers to oppose, but a tenodesis orthosis may be needed. Upper-extremity dressing, self-catheterization, manual wheelchair propulsion, and sliding board transfers are feasible. With C7 intact, these activities are performed more efficiently, and use of a suppository for the bowel program is feasible. With C8 intact, long finger flexion permits most ADLs to be accomplished from a wheelchair.

The strength of the lower extremities determines the amount of work that must be performed by the upper extremities for support, which in turn determines the energy cost and feasibility of ambulation. A study using the ASIA Motor Score found that 20 of 23 patients with incomplete tetraplegia who had an ASIA lower extremity motor score of 10 or more (the maximum normal score is 50 for 5 muscle groups of each leg on a 5-point scale of strength) at 1 month after injury became community ambulators with crutches and orthoses by 1 year. They subsequently achieved nearly effortless community ambulation if the lower-extremity motor score improved to at least 30. This finding was confirmed in the Spinal Cord Injury Locomotor Trial (Dobkin et al., 2006a). By comparison, scores of 20 or less were associated with limited ambulation at slower average velocities, higher heart rates, greater energy expenditure, and greater peak axial loads on assistive devices. Paraparetic community ambulators usually need to have pelvic control with at least movement against gravity in the hip flexors and one knee extensor, so that they at most require one KAFO to step with a reciprocal pattern.

Patients need encouragement and resources to be able to return to work or school. Those with education beyond high school are far more likely to return to work and stay employed. Aging with SCI poses problems for many. One-fourth of patients who sustained their injuries 20 or more years ago

Table 48.14   Data Summary for Traumatic Brain Injury Model Systems Project*

Variable	Mean Value	Rehabilitation Discharge	1 Year After Injury
Age at onset, years	36		
% Male	75		
% Vehicle related	52		
% Alcohol related	41		
% Employed	59		24
% Living at home	97		85
% Loss of consciousness	94		
% Posttraumatic amnesia	98		
≥30 days	34		
8-29 days	34		
1-7 days	8		
Lowest GCS score	7		
Duration of coma, days	3.8		
Acute hospital stay, days	22		
Rehabilitation inpatient stay, days		32	
Total FIM score	56	97	115
Disability Rating Scale	12.6	6	2.9

From Traumatic Brain Injury National Data Center (www.tbims.org).
GCS, Glasgow Coma Scale; *FIM,* Functional Independence Measure.
*For the years 1989 to 2000 and a total of 2553 cases.

evolve a greater need for physical assistance over time, especially for help with transfers. They report shoulder pain, fatigue, weakness, weight gain, and a decline in the quality of life more often than patients who do not need more assistance. Clinical surveillance is needed to anticipate when a pulse of therapy for an increasing impairment or disability or a change in assistive devices or wheelchair is needed.

Traumatic Brain Injury

In general, after moderate to severe TBI, self-care and mobility improve from admission for inpatient rehabilitation to discharge, and gains are maintained or continue to increase for approximately 6 months. About 50% return to work at 6 months. Socialization and leisure activities generally do not return to premorbid levels. **Table 48.14** shows some of the characteristics of injury and rehabilitation in a well-defined group of American patients who did not include children.

In a series of 243 consecutive admissions to a rehabilitation unit, a significant inverse relationship was found between the Glasgow Coma Scale score and the duration of coma, along with a strong positive relationship between the duration of coma and posttraumatic amnesia (PTA). Of 119 patients with diffuse axonal injury, no one in a coma for more than 2 weeks or with PTA for more than 12 weeks had a good recovery by the Glasgow Outcome Score at 1 year after injury. Two-thirds of the small subgroup with coma for more than 2 weeks improved to moderate disability when the coma lasted 2 to 4 weeks; only a third achieved this level if in coma for more than 4 weeks. Among patients with PTA for less than 2 weeks, 80% had a good recovery. Half of those with PTA lasting 2 to 8 weeks were moderately disabled at 1 year after admission. At another inpatient facility, patients who had a Glasgow Coma Scale score of 3 to 7 within 24 hours of onset of TBI had lower admission and discharge FIM scores for motor and cognitive function during their rehabilitation. In many communities, approximately 10% of patients return to former jobs, and less than 30% are employed 2 years after severe TBI.

Parkinson Disease

Parkinsonian patients can reduce their symptoms and improve their function with focused physical and occupational rehabilitation therapies to maintain range of motion, flexibility, proximal strength, mobility, freezing, safety, and fitness (Goodwin et al., 2008). Speech therapy improves prosody, breath support for speaking, and intelligibility. Patients have been trained to increase the speed of a skilled movement such as buttoning, although with more practice than normal controls need. Also, twice-a-week practice for 3 months in whole-body movements such as sitting, kneeling, standing up, and throwing, along with problem solving for these activities, improves the speed of movements needed for mobility in moderately disabled parkinsonian patients. A randomized crossover study compared regular activity with 1 hour of repetitive stretching, endurance, balance, gait, and fine motor exercises in moderately disabled patients. Exercises were performed 3 times a week for 4 weeks, with a progressive increase in the number of repetitions. The total United Parkinson Disease Rating Scale score and the ADL and motor subscores, particularly the bradykinesia and rigidity components, significantly improved with exercise. Without an ongoing formal exercise program, these gains were lost 6 months later. Walking to auditory cues and treadmill training have lessened hypokinesia and bouts of freezing.

Multiple Sclerosis

Evaluating the impact of rehabilitation in MS presents difficulties because it is a chronic condition continuing over many decades that is variable, unpredictable, and subject to spontaneous improvement in many patients. A study of patients with the relapsing-remitting form of the disease at onset found that the median times to reach scores of 4, 6, and 7 on the Kurtzke Disability Status Scale were 11, 23, and 33 years, respectively. The scores represent a change from limited walking up to 500 meters (EDSS 4), to walking with unilateral support no more than 100 meters without rest (EDSS 5), to walking no more than 10 meters while holding objects for support (EDSS 6). Scores for patients with progressive disease from onset declined at 0, 7, and 13 years, respectively. In a disease with a clinical course up to 40 years in duration, about 50% of affected persons will use aids for walking, and about 25% will require a wheelchair by 15 years after onset. Thus, plenty of opportunities arise for rehabilitative interventions for specific disabilities, education, and monitoring to prevent unnecessary complications. Rehabilitation for patients with MS is especially challenging because no therapies significantly reduce the movement disorders, ataxia, and visual impairments that often accompany the cognitive and motor-related disabilities that evolve over time.

Randomized controlled trials of both inpatient and outpatient rehabilitation programs in patients with MS suggest that strengthening and aerobic exercise and interventions for mobility can help improve ADLs, and that gains typically are maintained for 3 to 6 months beyond the end of the treatment. For example, a randomized trial compared 3 weeks of inpatient rehabilitation with a home exercise program in 50 patients. No change in impairment was found, but the more intensively treated inpatient group had a decrease in disability on the FIM motor domain for self-care and locomotion (which may include wheelchair use). This gain persisted for 15 weeks. Improvement in perceived quality of life (SF-36) in the mental composite score also was present for 9 weeks. These results emphasize the importance of continuity of care between the rehabilitation environment and the community and social service sectors, if the needs of the person with MS or another chronic neurological disease are to be met effectively over the long term. The effect of an extended outpatient rehabilitation program on symptom frequency, fatigue, and functional status has been modest. Although not yet studied by a scientific design, a day program may include general physical fitness exercises, practice in ADLs, group recreation, gardening, and local travel to help maintain or build self-care and community skills, along with psychosocial supports for clients and caregivers. Treadmill training, with or without weight support or robotic assist, has not revealed greater gains than mobility training of equal intensity.

Other Diseases

Critical illness–related polyneuropathy and myopathy associated with sepsis, organ transplantation, and prolonged disease have become a common cause of diffuse weakness, deconditioning, and disability necessitating inpatient rehabilitation. Exercise management is similar to that for patients with Guillain-Barré syndrome. As soon as feasible, these patients need to enter a milieu that encourages them to assist themselves, stay out of bed, and do light resistance exercises throughout the day. Patients are encouraged to work their arms and legs against the resistance of a stretchable rubber exercise band for 10 to 15 repetitions in various planes every hour, even when resting in bed, or to do isometric exercises with a family member. Nearly all patients with critical illness–induced weakness improve their strength from movement only against gravity at admission to offering resistance in proximal muscles within 3 weeks of the inpatient stay. The average length of stay needed to achieve the ability to stand up and walk 50 feet or more with an assistive device is approximately 18 days.

Resistance, stretching, and conditioning exercises ought to be part of any maintenance program for people with diseases of the motor unit as well, along with instruction from therapists if greater disability evolves. Even patients with moderate AD appear to benefit from exercise and retraining in basic ADLs.

Aging with Neurological Disabilities

Aging is associated with a variety of muscle and central and peripheral nervous system changes that can worsen the impairments and disabilities of people who have had neurological diseases and injuries earlier in life. These degradations in signal processing along with relative inactivity can diminish the neural representations for skills that had been regained through rehabilitation and compensatory training and problem solving. Patients should be encouraged to maintain their fitness with exercise and to practice motor and cognitive skills they wish to maintain.

Future Directions

Well-designed clinical trials for theory-based interventions are leading to more evidence-based practices. These trials will lead to a solid armamentarium of therapies for specific needs. Many interventions for cognitive and motor skills are likely to be applicable across diseases, since they are aimed at the level of impairment and disability in subacute and chronic stages post injury. Traditional therapies are limited to spared neural function, however. To go beyond this barrier, clinicians will have to work with basic scientists to develop and incorporate biological and pharmacological interventions to enable neural repair and enhance learning. These potential therapies also will require more optimal outcome measurement tools and well-defined treatments that foster activity-dependent plasticity during the retraining of skills that are important to patients.

References

The complete reference list is available online at www.expertconsult.com.

Index

Page numbers followed by "f" indicate figures, "t" indicate tables, and "b" indicate boxes.

Entries preceded by ⊙ can be found online. See inside front cover for details.

Volume I • pp 1–892 • Volume II • pp 893–2162

Entries preceded by ⊘ can be found online. See inside front cover for details.

Entries preceded by ☉ can be found online. See inside front cover for details.

Entries preceded by ◎ can be found online. See inside front cover for details.

Entries preceded by ☉ can be found online. See inside front cover for details.

Volume I • pp 1–892 • Volume II • pp 893–2162

Entries preceded by ☁ can be found online. See inside front cover for details.

Volume I • pp 1–892 • Volume II • pp 893–2162

Entries preceded by ⊙ can be found online. See inside front cover for details.

Volume I • pp 1–892 • Volume II • pp 893–2162

Entries preceded by 🌐 can be found online. See inside front cover for details.

Volume I • pp 1–892 • Volume II • pp 893–2162

Entries preceded by ◎ can be found online. See inside front cover for details.

Volume I • pp 1–892 • Volume II • pp 893–2162

Entries preceded by ⊙ can be found online. See inside front cover for details.

Volume I • pp 1–892 • Volume II • pp 893–2162

Entries preceded by ⊙ can be found online. See inside front cover for details.

Volume I • pp 1–892 • Volume II • pp 893–2162

Entries preceded by ○ can be found online. See inside front cover for details.

Entries preceded by ⊕ can be found online. See inside front cover for details.

Entries preceded by ⊙ can be found online. See inside front cover for details.

Volume I • pp 1–892 • Volume II • pp 893–2162

Entries preceded by ◑ can be found online. See inside front cover for details.

Entries preceded by ☉ can be found online. See inside front cover for details.

Entries preceded by ⊛ can be found online. See inside front cover for details.

Volume I • pp 1–892 • Volume II • pp 893–2162

Entries preceded by ⊙ can be found online. See inside front cover for details.

Volume I • pp 1–892 • Volume II • pp 893–2162

Entries preceded by ○ can be found online. See inside front cover for details.

Entries preceded by ⓞ can be found online. See inside front cover for details.

Entries preceded by ⊙ can be found online. See inside front cover for details.

Volume I • pp 1–892 • Volume II • pp 893–2162

Entries preceded by ⊙ can be found online. See inside front cover for details.

Volume I • pp 1–892 • Volume II • pp 893–2162

Entries preceded by ☉ can be found online. See inside front cover for details.

Volume I • pp 1–892 • Volume II • pp 893–2162

Entries preceded by ⊙ can be found online. See inside front cover for details.

Desmoplasia, 1118

Desmoplastic infantile astrocytoma (DIA), 1172

Desmoplastic infantile ganglioglioma (DIG), 1172, 1172f

Desmopressin (desamino-D-arginine-vasopressin, DDAVP)
  for bladder dysfunction in multiple sclerosis, 1304-1305
  for diabetes insipidus, 770
  in neurointensive care, 816
  for neurogenic bladder, 681-682

Desmoteplase, for acute ischemic stroke, 1044-1045

Desmoteplase in Acute Ischemic Stroke (DIAS) study, 1044-1045

Determinant spreading, 747

Detrol (tolterodine), for bladder dysfunction, 872t
  in Lewy body dementia, 1561

Detrunorm (propiverine), for neurogenic bladder, 681t

Detrusitol (tolterodine IR), for neurogenic bladder, 681t

Detrusitol XL (tolterodine ER), for neurogenic bladder, 681t

Detrusor leak-point pressure (DLPP), 975

Detrusor muscle, neurological control of, 668-669, 669f

Detrusor myomectomy, for spinal cord injury, 976

Detrusor–external sphincter dyssynergia (DESD), 975, 975f, 975t

Development
  of axons and dendrites, 1405-1406
    disorders of, 1405-1406
  biosynthesis of neurotransmitters in, 1407
    disorders of, 1407
  Cajal-Retzius neurons of fetal brain in, 1408, 1408f
  concepts of, 65
  electrical polarity of cell membrane in, 1406
    disorders of, 1406
  embryological and fetal, 1396-1398
  of fissures and sulci, 1404-1405, 1405b, 1405f
    disorders of, 1405
  neuroblast migration in, 1401-1402, 1402f
  mitotic proliferation of neuroblasts (neuronogenesis) in, 1399-1400
    disorders of, 1400, 1400f
  molecular, 1396
  myelination in, 1407-1408
    disorders of, 1408
  neuroblast migration in, 1401-1404, 1401f-1402f
    disorders of, 1403-1404, 1404f
      early, 1417-1419
      with inborn errors of metabolism, 1449, 1450t
      late, 1419
    major mechanisms of, 1402-1403, 1402f

Development (Continued)
  neurulation in, 1399
    disorders of, 1399, 1412-1413
  programmed cell death (apoptosis) in, 1400-1401
    disorders of, 1401
  suprasegmental influences on muscle maturation in, 1408-1409, 1409f
  synaptogenesis in, 1406-1407
    disorders of, 1406-1407
  typical and atypical, 65, 66t

Developmental coordination disorders (DCDs), 1436-1438
  and ADHD, 1436
  clinical features of, 1436-1437, 1437t, 1438b
  defined, 1436
  diagnosis of, 1436, 1436b
  evaluation and etiology of, 1436-1437, 1438b
  handedness in, 1436
  motoric difficulties in, 1436, 1436b
  natural history of, 1436-1437, 1437t
  treatment of, 1438
  visuospatial problems in, 1437, 1438b

Developmental delay
  epidemiology of, 65
  global. See Global developmental delay (GDD).
  red flags for, 65

Developmental disability(ies), 1422-1443
  autism spectrum disorders as, 1429-1432
    clinical features of, 1429-1430
      of communication, 1430-1431
      of intelligence and cognition, 1430
      restricted range of behaviors, interests, and activities as, 1431
      of social skills, 1431
    diagnostic criteria for, 1429, 1429b
    etiology of, 1431-1432
      genetic, 1432
      neuropathologic, 1432
      neuropsychological, 1431-1432
    evaluation of, 1431-1432
    management of, 1432, 1433t
    medical disorders associated with, 1429, 1430b
  cerebral palsy as, 1422-1424
    clinical features of, 1422-1423
    diagnosis and etiology of, 1423-1424
    prevention and management of, 1424
  intellectual disability as, 1424-1429
    clinical features of, 1424-1425
    diagnosis and etiology of, 1425-1427, 1425t-1426t
    management of, 1427-1429
    metabolic disorders associated with, 1427, 1428t
    neuroimaging for, 1427

Developmental disability(ies) (Continued)
  learning disabilities as. See Learning disability(ies) (LDs).
  prognosis for, 71

Developmental disorder(s), 1396-1421
  cerebellar, 1419-1421
    Chiari malformation as, 1411t, 1420
    craniosynostosis as, 1421
    Dandy-Walker malformation as, 1404f, 1411t, 1419-1420
    focal cerebellar dysplasia as, 1420, 1420f
    global cerebellar hypoplasia as, 1400, 1411t, 1420, 1420f
    selective cerebellar hemispheric aplasia as, 1419
    selective vermal aplasia as, 1419
  clinical expression of, 1410-1421, 1411t
  etiology of, 1409-1410
  of fissures and sulci, 1405
  genetic loci of known mutations in, 1396-1398, 1397t-1398t
  with inborn errors of metabolism, 1449, 1450t
  due to ischemic encephalopathy in fetus, 1409-1410
  of membrane polarity, 1406
  due to midline malformations of forebrain, 1413-1417
    agenesis of corpus callosum as, 1411t, 1416-1417, 1417f
    colpocephaly as, 1411t, 1417
    holoprosencephaly as, 1411t, 1413-1415, 1414t, 1415f
    isolated arhinencephaly and Kallmann syndrome as, 1415
    rhombomeric deletions and ectopic genetic expression as, 1416
    septo-optic-pituitary dysplasia as, 1411t, 1415-1416
  molecular genetic classification of, 1410
  of myelination, 1408
  neonatal seizures due to, 2113t
  of neurite growth, 1405-1406
  of neuroblast migration, 1403-1404, 1404f
    early, 1417-1419
    with inborn errors of metabolism, 1449, 1450t
    late, 1419
    lissencephaly (agyria, sometimes with pachygyria) as, 1403, 1411t, 1417-1418
      in Miller-Dieker syndrome, 1403, 1411t, 1417-1418, 1418f
      in Walker-Warburg and related syndromes, 1403, 1404f, 1411t, 1418
    X-linked recessive, with abnormal genitalia, 1418
    pachygyria as, 1403, 1411t

Developmental disorder(s) (Continued)
  polymicrogyria as, 1403
  schizencephaly as, 1419
  subcortical laminar heterotopia (band heterotopia) and bilateral periventricular nodular heterotopia as, 1403, 1419
  of neuronogenesis, 1400, 1400f
  of neurotransmitter synthesis, 1407
  of neurulation, 1399, 1412-1413
    anencephaly (aprosencephaly with open cranium) as, 1399, 1412
    cephalocele (encephalocele, exencephaly) as, 1399, 1412, 1412f
    congenital aqueductal stenosis as, 1411t, 1413, 1413b
    meningomyelocele (spinal dysraphism, rachischisis, spina bifida cystica) as, 1399, 1412-1413
  of programmed cell death, 1401
  ☉ structural imaging of, 482
  of symmetry and cellular lineage, 1410-1412
    hemimegalencephaly as, 1410-1412, 1411t
  of synaptogenesis, 1406-1407
  uniqueness of, 1398

Developmental dyscalculia (DD), 1438
  clinical features of, 1438
  evaluation and etiology of, 1438
  management of, 1438

Developmental history, 4, 65-66

Developmental malformation(s). See Developmental disorder(s).

Developmental milestones, 65, 66t

Developmental quotient, 66

☉ Developmental venous anomaly (DVA)

Deviation(s)
  ocular
    dissociated vertical, 589-590, 597
    downward, 47
    inward, 47
    lateral, 47
    periodic alternating gaze, 625-626
    physiological hyper-, 589-590
    primary vs. secondary, 591, 591f
    skew, 47, 621, 630
      alternating, 630
      with combined vertical gaze ophthalmoplegia, 212
      paroxysmal, 630
    standard, 363
      in neuropsychological evaluation, 574f, 574t

Devic disease, 173, 749, 1287, 1302-1303

DeVivo disease, 1472

Dexamethasone
  for brain metastases, 1184
  for cerebral edema, 1139-1140
  for migraine, 1725
  for spinal cord compression, 1191

Volume I • pp 1–892 • Volume II • pp 893–2162

Entries preceded by ⊙ can be found online. See inside front cover for details.

Volume I • pp 1–892 • Volume II • pp 893–2162

Entries preceded by ⊙ can be found online. See inside front cover for details.

Volume I • pp 1-892 • Volume II • pp 893-2162

Entries preceded by ☉ can be found online. See inside front cover for details.

Volume I • pp 1–892 • Volume II • pp 893–2162

Entries preceded by ○ can be found online. See inside front cover for details.

Entries preceded by ☉ can be found online. See inside front cover for details.

Entries preceded by ⊙ can be found online. See inside front cover for details.

Volume I • pp 1–892 • Volume II • pp 893–2162

Entries preceded by ⊙ can be found online. See inside front cover for details.

Volume I • pp 1–892 • Volume II • pp 893–2162

Entries preceded by ⊙ can be found online. See inside front cover for details.

Volume I • pp 1–892 • Volume II • pp 893–2162

Entries preceded by ◐ can be found online. See inside front cover for details.

Volume I • pp 1–892 • Volume II • pp 893–2162

Entries preceded by Ⓢ can be found online. See inside front cover for details.

Volume I • pp 1–892 • Volume II • pp 893–2162

Entries preceded by Ⓢ can be found online. See inside front cover for details.

Entries preceded by ◎ can be found online. See inside front cover for details.

Volume I • pp 1–892 • Volume II • pp 893–2162

Entries preceded by ☯ can be found online. See inside front cover for details.

Entries preceded by 🔵 can be found online. See inside front cover for details.

Entries preceded by ⊙ can be found online. See inside front cover for details.

Entries preceded by 🌐 can be found online. See inside front cover for details.

Entries preceded by ☉ can be found online. See inside front cover for details.

Volume I • pp 1–892 • Volume II • pp 893–2162

Entries preceded by ◎ can be found online. See inside front cover for details.

Inborn errors of metabolism (IEM)
(Continued)
animal models of, 1456
Canavan disease as, 1471
categorization of, 1444-1445
cerebrotendinous xanthomatosis
(cholestanolosis) as,
1464-1465
clinical manifestations of,
1444-1445
congenital defects of glycosylation
as, 1468-1471, 1469t-1470t
of copper metabolism, 1465
Menkes syndrome as, 1465
Wilson disease as, 1465
creatine deficiency syndromes as,
1472
defects in leukotriene synthesis as,
1472
defined, 1444
dementia due to, 1582
diagnosis of, 1445-1448
cardiomyopathy in, 1446
carnitine profile for, 1447, 1450t
clinical findings in, 1447t
commonly requested tests for,
1445, 1446t
course in, 1446
CSF abnormalities in, 1445,
1447t
early, 1445
genetic tests for, 1448
hepatosplenomegaly in,
1445-1446
histological examination for,
1447-1448
imminent death prior to, 1452
mutation analysis in, 1448
special considerations in, 1448
neuroimaging in, 1449-1452
neurologic deterioration in, 1445
ophthalmologic findings in,
1445, 1448t
tandem mass spectroscopy for,
1446-1447, 1449t
dyslipidemias as, 1463-1464
abetalipoproteinemia and
hypobetalipoproteinemia as,
1464
neutral lipid disease (Chanarin-
Dorfman syndrome) as,
1464
sterol synthesis defects as, 1464
Tangier disease as, 1464
epidemiology of, 1444
glucose transporter protein
deficiency (DeVivo disease) as,
1472
inheritance of, 1445
involving complex molecules,
1456-1460, 1457t
lysosomal storage disorders as,
1456-1460
biochemical features of, 1457t
classification of, 1456,
1457t-1458t
clinical features of, 1459
pathophysiology of,
1456-1459
rare variants of, 1459

Inborn errors of metabolism (IEM)
(Continued)
transmission of, 1459
treatment of, 1459-1460,
1459f
mitochondrial disorders as,
1457t
peroxisome disorders as, 1457t,
1460, 1460t
involving small molecules,
1460-1463, 1461t
aminoacidopathies and organic
acidemia as, 1449t,
1461-1462, 1461t
citrin deficiency as, 1462
hyperinsulinism-hyperammo-
nemia syndrome as, 1462
disorders of energy metabolism
as, 1462-1463
carbohydrate (sugar)
intolerance as, 1461t
disorders of gluconeogenesis
as, 1463
disorders of glycolysis as,
1463
disorders of ketogenesis and
ketolysis as, 1463
fatty acid oxidation defects as,
1447t, 1461t, 1463
glycogen storage diseases as,
1462-1463
hyperammonemia as,
1461-1462, 1461t
due to urea cycle defects, 1447t,
1461-1462, 1461t
Lowe oculocerebrorenal syndrome
as, 1465
management of, 1452-1455
during anesthesia and surgery,
1455
bone marrow/hematopoietic
stem cell transplantation for,
1454-1455
diet in, 1452-1453
enhancing excretion or
detoxification of toxic
metabolites in, 1453, 1453f
enzyme replacement therapy for,
1454
genetic counseling in, 1455
individualized approach to,
1452
organ transplantation in, 1455
symptomatic treatment in,
1455
strategies for, 1452
substrate reduction therapy in,
1453-1454, 1453f
substrate replenishment in,
1454, 1454t
molybdenum cofactor and sulfite
oxidase deficiency as, 1465
neurotransmitter and small peptide
defects as, 1471
nondiabetic hyperglycinemia as,
1471-1472
pathogenesis of, 1444
porphyrias as, 1467-1468, 1468t
during pregnancy, 1456
psychiatric symptoms of, 1456

Inborn errors of metabolism (IEM)
(Continued)
of purine and pyrimidine
metabolism, 1465-1467,
1466t-1467t
screening for, 1445
serine deficiency syndromes as,
1472
Inching technique, in nerve
conduction studies, 397,
398f-399f
Incidence proportions (IPs), for
metastatic brain tumors, 691
Incidence rates
defined, 687-688
for epilepsy, 692-693, 692f
for multiple sclerosis, 693-694
for neurological disorders
less common, 701t
most common, 701t
for Parkinson disease, 698
of primary brain tumors, 690-691,
690f
of stroke, 689
for West Nile Virus infection,
699-701
Inclusion body myopathy (IBM)
hereditary, 1469t-1470t,
2071t-2072t, 2086
autosomal recessive, 2086
with early respiratory failure,
2071t-2072t, 2079
muscle weakness in, 309
Inclusion body myositis (IBM),
2106-2107
amyloid deposits in, 2107, 2107f
arm weakness in, 306
CD8+ cytotoxic cells in, 2107
clinical features of, 2106
diagnosis of, 2106-2107
dysphagia in, 156
etiology and pathogenesis of,
752
immune mediation in, 752
immunohistochemistry of, 2107
leg weakness in, 306
muscle biopsy for, 2107, 2107f
rimmed vacuoles in, 2107,
2107f
Incomplete penetrance,
in dystonia, 432
Incontinence
bladder. See Neurogenic bladder
dysfunction.
fecal. See Neurogenic bowel
dysfunction.
Incontinentia pigmenti (IP),
1522-1523
achromians. See Hypomelanosis
of Ito (HI).
cutaneous features of,
1522-1523
genetics of, 1523
neurological features of, 1523
Incremental bicycle ergometry, for
muscle weakness, 303
Indinavir (Crixivan), for HIV infection,
1216t
Indirect excitotoxicity, in Huntington
disease, 1787

Indirect (I) wave
in motor evoked potentials, 390
in transcranial magnetic
stimulation, 421-422
Individualized Education Plan (IEP),
70
Individualized Family Service Plan,
70
Indoles, in mushrooms, 1374t
Indomethacin (Indocin), for chronic
pain, 792t
Inducer T cells. See Helper T cells (T_H
cells).
Inducible nitric oxide synthetase
(iNOS), in brain edema,
1384
Indwelling catheters
for neurogenic bladder, 683
for spinal cord injury, 976
Inertial acceleration models, 932
Infancy
benign sleep myoclonus of,
1685
familial hyperinsulinemic
hypoglycemia of, 1489t
severe myoclonic epilepsy of,
1593, 1600
Infant(s). See also Newborn(s).
brain tumors in. See Children,
brain tumors in.
hypotonic (floppy). See Hypotonic
infant.
Infantile beriberi, 1346
Infantile botulism, 2064
hypotonic infant due to, 327
Infantile facioscapulohumeral
dystrophy, hypotonic infant due
to, 324
Infantile free sialic acid storage
disease, 1457t-1458t
Infantile myotonic dystrophy, 2089,
2089f
Infantile neuroaxonal dystrophy,
hypotonic infant due to, 325
Infantile neuroaxonal dystrophy
(INAD), 1796
Infantile neuronal ceroid-lipofuscino-
sis, 1457t-1458t
Infantile nystagmus syndrome (INS),
600-603
Infantile spasms, 1590
EEG of, 375, 375f
Infantile spinal muscular atrophy
with respiratory distress type 1,
hypotonic infant due to,
326
Infantile-onset olivopontocerebellar
atrophy, 1809
Infarction
cerebral
headache due to, 1710
hyperhidrosis after, 2021t
monoplegia due to, 279
periodic lateralized epileptiform
discharges due to, 375,
377f
myocardial
cardioembolic stroke due to,
1018-1019
and sleep, 1687

Entries preceded by 🌐 can be found online. See inside front cover for details.

Entries preceded by ⊘ can be found online. See inside front cover for details.

Volume I • pp 1-892 • Volume II • pp 893-2162

Entries preceded by ⊕ can be found online. See inside front cover for details.

Volume I • pp 1–892 • Volume II • pp 893–2162

Entries preceded by 🔘 can be found online. See inside front cover for details.

Volume I • pp 1–892 • Volume II • pp 893–2162

Entries preceded by ⊘ can be found online. See inside front cover for details.

Volume I • pp 1–892 • Volume II • pp 893–2162

Entries preceded by 🔄 can be found online. See inside front cover for details.

Volume I • pp 1–892 • Volume II • pp 893–2162

Entries preceded by 🕲 can be found online. See inside front cover for details.

Entries preceded by ⊙ can be found online. See inside front cover for details.

Magnetic resonance imaging (MRI)
(*Continued*)
T1 weighting in, 445-446, 445f-446f, 447t
T2 contrast in, 445-446
T2 (spin-spin) relaxation in, 444, 444f
T2 weighting in, 445-446, 445f-446f, 447t
time to echo in, 444-445
tissue contrast (T1, T2, and proton density weighting) in, 445-446
transverse magnetization in, 443-444
water molecules as basis for, 1381
Magnetic resonance imaging (MRI)-based disease severity scale (MRDSS), for multiple sclerosis, 1299
Magnetic resonance (MR) neurography, of peripheral nerve injury, 992, 993f
Magnetic resonance spectroscopy (MRS)
of brain tumors, 539
prior to epilepsy surgery, 1615-1616
of hepatic encephalopathy, 1324
for inborn errors of metabolism, 1451-1452
of migraine, 1720
for movement disorders, 258
for multiple sclerosis, 1299-1300, 1300f
for stroke in children, 1087
of upper motor neuron disorders, 1857
Magnetic resonance (MR) tractography
prior to epilepsy surgery, 1614-1615
of peripheral nerve injury, 992, 994f
Magnetic search coil technique, 660-661
Magnetic source imaging, prior to epilepsy surgery, 1616
⊗ Magnetization transfer imaging (MTI) for multiple sclerosis, 1300-1301
⊗ Magnetization transfer ratio (MTR) for multiple sclerosis, 1300-1301
Magnetoencephalography (MEG), 382
prior to epilepsy surgery, 1616
Magnocellular layers, in visual pathways, 634-635
Ma-huang, ischemic stroke due to, 1025
"Mainlining", 1365
Maintenance of wakefulness test (MWT), 1694
Maitotoxin, 1374
Major depressive disorder (MDD). *See also* Depression.
electroconvulsive therapy for, 114-115
genetic basis for, 98
repetitive transcranial magnetic stimulation for, 115

Major histocompatibility complex (MHC) antigens
in immune response, 736, 738-739, 739f
in CNS, 745
in multiple sclerosis, 1289
Major histocompatibility complex (MHC) class I restricted T cells, 738-739, 739f
Major histocompatibility complex (MHC) class II restricted T cells, 738-739, 739f
Major histocompatibility complex (MHC) restriction, 738-739, 739f
Mal de débarquement syndrome, 271, 599
Malabsorption syndromes, neuropathy associated with, 1995-1996
Male sexual dysfunction
management of
for ejaculation dysfunction, 685
for erectile dysfunction, 684-685, 685t
due to spinal cord injury, 674, 980-981
Male sexual response, 670
Malignancies. *See* Cancer.
Malignant atrophic papulosis, ischemic stroke due to, 1025-1026
Malignant brain edema, with traumatic brain injury, 953
"Malignant" external otitis, 1981
Malignant hypertension, optic disc swelling due to, 179
Malignant hyperthermia, 761, 1363, 1489t, 1497
ryanodine receptor in, 2089-2090
Malignant inflammatory sensory polyganglionopathy, 1985-1986
Malignant peripheral nerve sheath tumor (MPNST), 1132
management of, 1153-1154
pathology and molecular genetics of, 1132
Malignant plexopathy, 1198-1199
brachial, 1198-1199
lumbosacral, 1199
with spinal cord compression, 1189, 1190f
Malignant spinal cord compression (MSCC), 1188-1189
Malingering, 2148, 2157-2158
Mallampati classification, for obstructive sleep apnea, 1668, 1668f
Mallory body myopathy, 2071t-2072t, 2079
Malnutrition. *See also* Deficiency disease(s).
protein-calorie, 1352
Mammillary body, in memory, 61, 61f
Mammillothalamic tract, in memory, 61f
Management, of neurological disorders, 8
Management of Atherothrombosis with Clopidogrel in High-Risk Patients (MATCH) trial, 1039-1040

Mandibular nerve
anatomy of, 1746f, 1750-1751, 1751f
clinical lesions of, 1752
Manganese, occupational exposure to, 1360
Manganese metabolism, encephalopathy due to disorders of, 1338
Manganese toxicity
dementia due to, 1582
parkinsonism due to, 1782
Mania
neuroanatomy corresponding to, 93t
after stroke, 100
Manifest latent nystagmus (MLN), 602
"Man-in-the-barrel" syndrome, 1316, 1316t
Manipulative automatisms, 1584
Mannitol
for brain edema, 1389
for traumatic brain injury, 949, 950t-951t, 952b
a-Mannosidosis, 1457t-1458t
b-Mannosidosis, 1457t-1458t
Mannosyltransferase I deficiency, 1469t-1470t
Mannosyltransferase II deficiency, 1469t-1470t
Mannosyltransferase VI deficiency, 1469t-1470t
Mannosyltransferase VIII deficiency, 1469t-1470t
Manual automatisms, 1584
MAOIs (monoamine oxidase inhibitors), 112-114, 113t
for migraine prophylaxis, 1725
MAP (mean arterial pressure)
and cerebral perfusion pressure, 804
with spinal cord injury, 969-970
Maple syrup urine disease (MSUD)
clinical findings in, 1447t
disorders of neurotransmitter synthesis in, 1407
incidence of, 1461t
tandem mass spectrometry for, 1449t
MAPT gene, in frontotemporal dementia, 1552-1553, 1553f
MAR (melanoma-associated retinopathy), 1209-1210
Maraviroc (Selzentry), for HIV infection, 1216t
Marburg variant, of multiple sclerosis, 1287
Marburg virus, 1258
March, clonic activity without, 1584
Marche à petits pas, in parkinsonism, 239, 270
Marchiafava-Bignami disease, 1349-1350
Marcus Gunn pupil, 187, 636-637, 637b, 637f
Marfan syndrome, 1827
dural ectasia in, 1827
stroke due to
in children, 1086-1087
ischemic, 1028

Marginal glioneuronal heterotopia, 1404
Marie, Pierre, 1806
Marie ataxia, 1806, 1812
Marijuana use, and seizures, 1602
Marine neurotoxins, 1374-1376, 2065
from ciguatera fish, 1374-1375
from puffer fish, 1375
from shellfish, 1375-1376
Marinesco-Sjögren syndrome, 1811
Markers. *See* Biomarkers.
Markesbery-Griggs distal myopathy, 2071t-2072t, 2079
Maroteaux-Lamy disease, 1457t-1458t
Martin-Gruber anastomosis, nerve conduction studies with, 399
MASS (mitral valve, aorta, skeletal, and skin involvement) syndrome, 1827
Mass lesions, psychiatric manifestations of, 105
Mastitis, in viral CNS disease, 1234t
Mastocytosis, in postural tachycardia syndrome, 2028
MATCH (Management of Atherothrombosis with Clopidogrel in High-Risk Patients) trial, 1039-1040
Maternal brachial plexus neuropathy, 2134
Maternal inheritance, 717-718, 717f
of mtDNA, 1474-1477
Maternal obstetric palsy, 2134
Maternally inherited diabetes and deafness (MIDD), 1484-1485
Maternally inherited Leigh syndrome (MILS), 1476t, 1484
Matrix metalloproteinases (MMPs)
in bacterial meningitis, 1385
in immune response, 741
in vasogenic edema, 1384-1385
Maturation
anatomic and physiological correlated of neurological, 1398
defined, 1396
insults that adversely affect, 1398
Maxalt (rizatriptan), for migraine, 1723t-1724t
in children, 1743-1744
Maxillary nerve
anatomy of, 1746f, 1750-1751, 1751f
clinical lesions of, 1752
Maxillary sinusitis, headache and facial pain due to, 1713-1714
Maximum intensity projection (MIP), in MR angiography, 507-509, 512f
Mayo Asymptomatic Carotid Endarterectomy Trial, 1047
MBP (myelin basic protein), in multiple sclerosis, 1287
MC. *See* Myotonia congenita (MC).
MCA. *See* Middle cerebral artery (MCA).

Entries preceded by ⊙ can be found online. See inside front cover for details.

Volume I • pp 1–892 • Volume II • pp 893–2162

Entries preceded by ☉ can be found online. See inside front cover for details.

Volume I • pp 1–892 • Volume II • pp 893–2162

Entries preceded by ⊙ can be found online. See inside front cover for details.

Volume I • pp 1–892 • Volume II • pp 893–2162

Entries preceded by ○ can be found online. See inside front cover for details.

Volume I • pp 1–892 • Volume II • pp 893–2162

Entries preceded by ⊙ can be found online. See inside front cover for details.

Entries preceded by ◉ can be found online. See inside front cover for details.

Volume I • pp 1–892 • Volume II • pp 893–2162

Entries preceded by 🕓 can be found online. See inside front cover for details.

Entries preceded by ⊙ can be found online. See inside front cover for details.

Entries preceded by ⊙ can be found online. See inside front cover for details.

Entries preceded by ⊛ can be found online. See inside front cover for details.

Entries preceded by ◎ can be found online. See inside front cover for details.

Entries preceded by ☉ can be found online. See inside front cover for details.

Entries preceded by ⊗ can be found online. See inside front cover for details.

Entries preceded by ⊙ can be found online. See inside front cover for details.

Volume I • pp 1–892 • Volume II • pp 893–2162

Entries preceded by 🔫 can be found online. See inside front cover for details.

Entries preceded by ☉ can be found online. See inside front cover for details.

Volume I • pp 1–892 • Volume II • pp 893–2162

Entries preceded by ⊙ can be found online. See inside front cover for details.

Entries preceded by ○ can be found online. See inside front cover for details.

Entries preceded by ❂ can be found online. See inside front cover for details.

Volume I • pp 1–892 • Volume II • pp 893–2162

Entries preceded by ⊙ can be found online. See inside front cover for details.

Pediatric brain tumors (Continued)
central neurocytoma as, 1173-1174, 1173f
desmoplastic infantile astrocytoma or ganglioglioma as, 1172, 1172f
dysembryoplastic neuroepithelial tumor as, 1172-1173
ganglioglioma as, 1171-1172, 1172f-1173f
oligodendroglioma as, 1174
treatment-related complications with, 1180-1181
due to chemotherapy, 1181
due to radiation therapy, 1180-1181
due to surgery, 1180
Pediatric brainstem tumors, 1168t
Pediatric patients. See Children.
Pedigree diagram, 713f
PEDS (Parents' Evaluation of Developmental Status), 65-66
Peduncular hallucinosis, after stroke, 100
Pedunculopontine nucleus (PPN), 1763, 1765-1766
Pedunculopontine tegmental (PPT) nucleus, in REM sleep, 1643-1644
Peek sign, 194
in myasthenia gravis, 2047, 2048f
Peer review process, 366
PEF (parietal eye field), in horizontal eye movements, 616-617
PEG (percutaneous endoscopic gastroscopy), for amyotrophic lateral sclerosis, 1884
Pegvisomant, for acromegaly, 773
Pegylated interferon alfa-2b, for viral infections, 1238t
Pelizaeus-Merzbacher disease, copy number variation in, 727t
Pellagra, 1345, 1993
Pellagra neuropathy, 1993
Pelvic floor electromyography, 679-680
of penilocavernosus reflex, 680
of pudendal nerve terminal motor latency, 680
of pudendal somatosensory evoked potentials, 680
sphincter
for cauda equina lesions, 679
for multiple system atrophy, 679-680, 679f
for urinary retention in young women, 680
Pelvic floor incompetence, due to cauda equina lesion, 686
PEM. See Paraneoplastic encephalomyelitis (PEM).
Pemetrexed, for brain tumors, 1143, 1144t-1145t
Penetrance, 707t, 713-714
incomplete, in dystonia, 432
Penetrating artery disease, ischemic stroke due to, 1017-1018
Penetrating brain injury (PBI) model, 932

D-Penicillamine, neurological complications of, 901
D-Penicillamine–induced myasthenia gravis, 2060
Penile prosthesis, for erectile dysfunction, 685
Penile tumescence, during sleep, 1649t
Penilocavernosus reflex, 680
Penis, dorsal nerve of, 1910f
Pentazocine (Talwin), during pregnancy, 2126t
Pentobarbital, for status epilepticus, 1632, 1632t
Pentobarbital coma, for traumatic brain injury, 952b, 953
Penumbra intracranial aspiration device, 569, 831, 831f
PEO. See Progressive external ophthalmoplegia (PEO).
PEPCK (phosphoenolpyruvate carboxykinase) deficiency, 1463
Pepstatin-insensitive lysosomal peptidase, inborn errors of metabolism of, 1457t-1458t
Peptic ulcers, sleep disturbances with, 1687-1688
Peptides, inborn errors of metabolism of, 1457t-1458t
Percentage in stanine, in neuropsychological evaluation, 574f
Percentiles, in neuropsychological evaluation, 574f, 574t
Perceptual disturbances, in delirium, 27-28
Ⓖ Perched facet
Percocet (oxycodone), for chronic pain, 795t
Percussion concussion, 931-932
Percussion wave, in intracranial pressure monitoring, 804-805
Percutaneous balloon compression, for trigeminal neuralgia, 1742
Percutaneous disc decompression, for pain, 797t, 799
Percutaneous endoscopic gastroscopy (PEG), for amyotrophic lateral sclerosis, 1884
Percutaneous gastrostomy, in neurointensive care, 817
Percutaneous Nucleotome, for disc herniation, 799
Percutaneous radiofrequency thermocoagulation, for trigeminal neuralgia, 1741-1742
Percutaneous transluminal angioplasty (PTA)
for acute ischemic stroke, 832
for intracranial arterial stenosis, 836
Perfusion, maintenance of adequate, for neonatal hypoxic-ischemic brain injury, 2117
Ⓖ Perfusion-weighted imaging (PWI) of ischemic stroke, 462, 463f
Pergolide (Permax)
for Lewy body dementia, 1561
for Parkinson disease, 1773, 1773t

Perhexiline, neuropathy due to, 2001t, 2004
Periaxin gene, in Charcot-Marie-Tooth disease, 1940-1941
Pericarditis, in viral CNS disease, 1234t
Pericytes, in neurovascular unit, 1379, 1380f
Pericytic proliferation, 1118-1119
Perifascicular atrophy, 2070
in dermatomyositis, 2103-2104, 2103f-2104f
Peri-infarct depolarizations, posttraumatic, 937
Perilymph, 645, 646f
Perilymph fistulae, dizziness due to, 648t, 652, 654
Perimedullary arteriovenous malformation, endovascular therapy for, 849
Perimeters, in visual field testing, 639
Perineal nerve, 1910f
Perineurioma, 1936, 1937f
Perineurium, 401, 985
Periodic alternating gaze deviation (PAGD), 625-626
Periodic alternating nystagmus (PAN), 602t, 605t, 606-607, 626
Periodic breathing, neurological complications of, 923-924
Periodic lateralized epileptiform discharges (PLEDs), 375, 377f
Periodic limb movements in sleep (PLMS), 1671
features of, 1672b
polysomnographic recording of, 1673f
treatment of, 1699-1700
Periodic limb movements in sleep (PLMS) index, 1691
Periodic paralysis(es), 1488
in Andersen-Tawil syndrome, 1496
fluctuating weakness in, 307
hyperkalemic, 1494-1495, 2091
clinical features of, 1493t, 1494
diagnosis of, 1494
genetic basis for, 1489t, 1491f
pathophysiology of, 1494
secondary, 2092
treatment of, 1494-1495
hypokalemic, 1492-1494
clinical features of, 1492, 1493t
diagnosis of, 1493, 1493t
familial, 2090
genetic basis for, 1489t
pathophysiology of, 1492-1493
secondary, 2090
fluctuating weakness in, 307
treatment of, 1493-1494, 1494t
type 1, 2090
type 2, 2092
potassium-sensitive, 2091
thyrotoxic, 913, 1493
Periodic pattern, in hypoxia, 380, 381f
Perioperative causes, of delirium, 32t, 33
Peripheral benzodiazepine receptor (PBR), in chemical imaging, 551t, 552

Peripheral innervation, disturbances of, neurogenic bladder dysfunction due to, 675-676
Peripheral motor conduction time, in transcranial magnetic stimulation, 422
Peripheral myelin protein 22 (PMP22) gene
in Charcot-Marie-Tooth disease, 1940-1941
in hereditary neuropathy with liability to pressure palsies, 1944
Peripheral nerve(s)
anatomy of, 333f, 401, 984-985, 1916
axon in, 985, 985f
peripheral nerve trunks in, 985, 985f
palpation of, 1922
pathological processes involving, 1916-1917, 1917f-1919f
Peripheral nerve degeneration, 987-989
distal segment changes in, 987
proximal segment changes in, 988
segmental demyelination in, 987
wallerian degeneration in, 987-988, 987f
Peripheral nerve enlargement, with muscle weakness, 299
Peripheral nerve hyperexcitability (PNH), paraneoplastic, 1207-1208
clinical findings in, 1207
immune responses in, 1207-1208
treatment of, 1208
tumor association of, 1207
Peripheral nerve lesions
classification of, 401
hemiplegia due to, 278
monoplegia due to, 280-284
sensory deficit due to, 331t, 332, 333f-334f
Peripheral nerve metastases, 1199
Peripheral nerve regeneration, 988-989, 988f
Peripheral nerve sheath tumor (PNST)
benign, 1153
malignant, 1132
management of, 1153-1154
pathology and molecular genetics of, 1132
Peripheral nerve syndromes, leg pain due to, 356-358
Peripheral nerve trauma, 984-1002
classification of, 986-987, 986f, 986t
closed, 993-994, 995f
dystonia after, 1796
evaluation of, 990-992
clinical, 990-992
electrodiagnostic, 991-992
history in, 990-991, 991b
imaging studies for, 992
MR neurography in, 992, 993f
MR tractography in, 992, 994f
myelography in, 992, 992f
ultrasonography in, 992

Volume I • pp 1–892 • Volume II • pp 893–2162

Entries preceded by Ⓖ can be found online. See inside front cover for details.

Entries preceded by ⊘ can be found online. See inside front cover for details.

Entries preceded by ⊙ can be found online. See inside front cover for details.

Entries preceded by ☺ can be found online. See inside front cover for details.

Volume I • pp 1–892 • Volume II • pp 893–2162

Entries preceded by ☉ can be found online. See inside front cover for details.

Entries preceded by ◎ can be found online. See inside front cover for details.

Entries preceded by ⓢ can be found online. See inside front cover for details.

Volume I • pp 1–892 • Volume II • pp 893–2162

Entries preceded by ⊙ can be found online. See inside front cover for details.

Volume I • pp 1–892 • Volume II • pp 893–2162

Entries preceded by ☉ can be found online. See inside front cover for details.

Entries preceded by ☉ can be found online. See inside front cover for details.

Volume I • pp 1–892 • Volume II • pp 893–2162

Entries preceded by ⓢ can be found online. See inside front cover for details.

Entries preceded by 🔗 can be found online. See inside front cover for details.

Volume I • pp 1–892 • Volume II • pp 893–2162

Entries preceded by ☉ can be found online. See inside front cover for details.

Entries preceded by ⊙ can be found online. See inside front cover for details.

Volume I • pp 1–892 • Volume II • pp 893–2162

Entries preceded by ⊙ can be found online. See inside front cover for details.

Volume I • pp 1–892 • Volume II • pp 893–2162

Entries preceded by ○ can be found online. See inside front cover for details.

Entries preceded by ◎ can be found online. See inside front cover for details.

Entries preceded by ⊘ can be found online. See inside front cover for details.

Volume I • pp 1–892 • Volume II • pp 893–2162

Entries preceded by ⊙ can be found online. See inside front cover for details.

Entries preceded by ⊙ can be found online. See inside front cover for details.

Entries preceded by ⊙ can be found online. See inside front cover for details.

Volume I • pp 1–892 • Volume II • pp 893–2162

Entries preceded by ⊙ can be found online. See inside front cover for details.

Volume I • pp 1–892 • Volume II • pp 893–2162

Entries preceded by ⊘ can be found online. See inside front cover for details.

Entries preceded by ☉ can be found online. See inside front cover for details.

Entries preceded by ⊙ can be found online. See inside front cover for details.

Entries preceded by ☉ can be found online. See inside front cover for details.

Entries preceded by ☉ can be found online. See inside front cover for details.

Volume I • pp 1–892 • Volume II • pp 893–2162

Entries preceded by ⊙ can be found online. See inside front cover for details.

Entries preceded by ⊙ can be found online. See inside front cover for details.

Volume I • pp 1–892 • Volume II • pp 893–2162

Entries preceded by ⊙ can be found online. See inside front cover for details.